Muir's Textbook of Pathology

Muir's Textbook of Pathology

Twelfth Edition

Edited by J. R. Anderson

CBE, LLD, BSc, MD, FRCP(Glasg), FRCP(Lond), FRCPath, FRS(Edin)
Emeritus Professor of Pathology, University of Glasgow

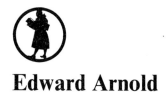

Edward Arnold

© J. R. Anderson, 1985

First published 1924
by Edward Arnold (Publishers) Ltd.
41 Bedford Square, London WC1B 3DQ

Edward Arnold (Australia) Pty Ltd,
80 Waverley Road, Caulfield East,
Victoria 3145, Australia

Edward Arnold, 3 East Read Street, Baltimore,
Maryland 21202, U.S.A.

Reprinted, 1924, 1926, 1927
Second edition, 1929
Reprinted, 1930, 1932
Third edition, 1933
Fourth edition, 1936
Fifth edition, 1941
Reprinted, 1944, 1946
Sixth edition, 1951
Reprinted, 1956
Seventh edition, 1958
Eighth edition, 1964
Reprinted, 1968
Ninth edition, 1971
Reprinted, 1972, 1973, 1975
Tenth edition, 1976
Revised reprint, 1978
Reprinted, 1979
Eleventh edition, 1980
Reprinted, 1981, 1982
Twelfth edition, 1985
Reprinted, 1987

ELBS edition of Eighth edition first published 1964
Reprinted, 1967, 1968, 1969
ELBS edition of Ninth edition, 1971
Reprinted, 1974, 1975
ELBS edition of Tenth edition, 1976
Reprinted, 1979
ELBS edition of Eleventh edition, 1980
Reprinted, 1981, 1982, 1983
ELBS edition of Twelfth edition, 1985
Reprinted, 1987

British Library Cataloguing in Publication Data

Muir, *Sir* Robert
  Muir's textbook of pathology. — 12th ed.
  1. Pathology
  I. Title   II. Anderson, J.R. (John Russell)
  616.07   RB111

  ISBN 0-7131-4458-0

Filmset in 'Monophoto' Times 10 on 11 pt
and printed and bound in Great Britain by
Butler & Tanner Ltd, Frome and London

Contributors

J. H. Adams, MB, ChB, PhD, FRCP(Glasg), FRCPath, Titular Professor of Neuropathology, The University of Glasgow, Scotland

J. R. Anderson, CBE, LLD, BSc, MD, FRCP(Glasg), FRCP(Lond), FRCPath, FRS(Edin), Emeritus Professor of Pathology, The University of Glasgow, Scotland

M. E. Catto, MD, FRCPath, Reader in Orthopaedic Pathology, The University of Glasgow, Scotland

W. J. K. Cumming, BSc, MD, MRCP, Consultant Neurologist, Department of Neurology, Withington Hospital, Didsbury, Manchester

S. Fleming, BSc, MB, ChB, Lecturer in Pathology, The University of Southampton, England

A. K. Foulis, BSc, MB, ChB, MRCPath, Consultant Pathologist, Department of Pathology, Royal Infirmary, Glasgow, Scotland

H. Fox, MD, FRCPath, Professor of Reproductive Pathology, University of Manchester, England

R. B. Goudie, MD, MRCP, FRCP(Glasg), FRSE, Professor of Pathology, The University of Glasgow, Scotland

D. I. Graham, MB, ChB, PhD, MRCP, FRCPath, Titular Professor of Neuropathology, The University of Glasgow, Scotland

D. Heath, DSc, MD, PhD, FRCP, FRCPath, Professor of Pathology, The University of Liverpool, England

J. V. Hurley, PhD, MB, MRACP, FRCPA, FRCPath, Professor of Pathology, The University of Melbourne, Australia

J. M. Kay, MD, FRCPC, FRCPath, Professor of Pathology, McMaster University, Hamilton, Ontario, Canada

F. D. Lee, MD, MRCP(Glasg), FRCPath, Consultant Pathologist, Royal Infirmary, Glasgow, Scotland

W. R. Lee, MD, FRCPath, Titular Professor of Ophthalmic Pathology, The University of Glasgow, Scotland

G. Lindop, BSc, MB, ChB, MRCPath, Senior Lecturer in Pathology, The University of Glasgow, Scotland

S. B. Lucas, MA, BM, BCh, MRCP, MRCPath, Senior Lecturer in Histopathology, University College Hospital and the London School of Hygiene and Tropical Medicine, The University of London, England

D. G. MacDonald, RD, BDS, PhD, MRCPath, Reader in Oral Medicine and Pathology, The University of Glasgow, Scotland

A. McQueen, MB, ChB, FRCPath, Senior Lecturer in Dermatological Pathology, The University of Glasgow, Scotland

R. N. M. MacSween, BSc, MD, FRCP(Glasg, Edin), FRCPath, FRC(Edin), Professor of Pathology, The University of Glasgow, Scotland.

I. A. R. More, BSc, MD, PhD, MRCPath, Senior Lecturer in Pathology, The University of Glasgow, Scotland

J. Stewart Orr, DSc, Professor of Medical Physics, Royal Postgraduate Medical School, The University of London, England

R. M. Rowan, MB, ChB, FRCP(Glasg), Senior Lecturer in Haematology, The University of Glasgow, Scotland

N. P. Smith, MBBS, MRCP, Consultant Dermatologist, Department of Histopathology and Experimental Pathology, The Institute of Dermatology, St. John's Hospital for Diseases of the Skin, London, England

K. Whaley, MD, PhD, MRCPath, FRCP, Titular Professor of Immunopathology, The University of Glasgow, Scotland

Preface

As medical knowledge increases ever more rapidly, teachers in medical schools must necessarily be more selective in the information they impart to students. Such selection will obviously be influenced by the patterns of disease in different countries. For example, parasitic diseases, malnutrition and bacterial infections are of major importance in many developing countries, where coronary artery disease and cancer (the two foremost causes of death in most of the developed countries) are *relatively* unimportant. This book attempts to allow for such regional differences by providing an account suitable for students in most parts of the world. The result is a text which provides too much systematic pathology for most medical students to assimilate during the undergraduate course in pathology, and guidance by their teachers on which topics deserve their special attention is necessary. I hope that the book will continue to be of use throughout the 'clinical' years of the curriculum, and also during the vocational postgraduate training which is now an essential prelude to independent medical practice.

A brief introductory chapter defines pathology, explains its importance in the medical curriculum, in the care of patients, and in the advancement of medical knowledge. The remainder of the book consists of twelve chapters on 'general pathology', thirteen chapters on 'systematic pathology', and a new chapter on diseases caused by parasites.

The twelve chapters on general pathology describe pathological processes of fundamental importance, starting with a new chapter on genetic causes of disease and continuing with the nature of cell injury, the inflammatory response to various types of injury, the processes of healing and regeneration. The rapid advances in immunology are reflected in two chapters, one on the physiological functioning of the immunity system and the other on disease resulting from disorders of immunity. A very brief account of host-parasite relationships is followed by a description of various types of microbial infection. A chapter is devoted to the causes and effects of general and local impairment of blood flow and disturbances of body fluids, and there is a short chapter on deposition of some normal and abnormal metabolites. Finally, the general section contains two chapters on tumours: the first describes the general features of tumours and gives illustrative examples: descriptions of individual tumours are included in the systematic chapters. The second chapter on tumours is devoted entirely to their causes, including the exciting developments on the role of oncogenes.

The basic pathological processes mostly apply to mammalian species in general, and while they are illustrated mainly by human diseases, full account is taken of the experimental work which has contributed so greatly to these topics. The length of the general chapters has been determined largely by the importance of each subject in the understanding of disease processes known to be of importance in the practice of medicine. Material mainly of abstract scientific interest has been kept to a minimum on the basis that medical students already have an extremely demanding course. For example, the complex subject of the mediation of the acute inflammatory reaction has been studied extensively, but very few potential mediators have been shown to play an important role, and a detailed account seems unnecessary. By contrast, disturbances of immunity play an important part in many types of disease and immunology and immunopathology therefore require to be considered in some detail. Similarly, molecular biology has become increasingly important in the understanding of disease processes in general and particularly genetic disorders, mechanisms of cell injury, immunology, and the aetiology of cancer. In spite of these and various other advances, the length of the general section has not been increased significantly. Although written mainly for medical, dental and veterinary students, I hope it may also prove of interest to students of the biological sciences in general.

The systematic section consists of fourteen chapters, each of which describes the more important diseases of a particular organ or system—the blood vessels and heart, respiratory, haemopoietic and nervous systems, alimentary tract, etc. Emphasis has been placed on the aetiology of those diseases and their effects on structure and function, together with brief clinicopathological correlations. The whole text has been revised and most of the systematic chapters have been extensively re-written. The accounts of the aetiology of atheroma, diseases of the heart valves, the leukaemias and lymphomas, the neuromuscular disorders and soft-tissue tumours have been extended in accordance with recent advances or increasing importance. The number of illustrations remains at about 1200, but some photographs have been replaced and new diagrams have been included. Overall, the systematic section has inevitably increased in length, but greater use has been made of small print to indicate sections of more importance to postgraduate students.

Bibliography at the end of each chapter consists mainly of longer texts and recent reviews. It includes some references to classical work and to original papers representing major advances, but we have not appended long lists of references to recent, often unconfirmed reports. Advances in many aspects of pathology are now so rapid that reading lists must change continuously and it is the duty of the teacher to guide students in their search for further information.

Acknowledgements

I am grateful to all my fellow authors, not only for their contributions but also for granting me wide editorial licence to achieve uniformity of style and nomenclature, to avoid unnecessary repetition, and hopefully to provide a balanced account. I accept responsibility for errors of fact and judgement.

In addition to named contributors, I have received helpful advice or short contributions on particular topics from Drs J. Douglas Briggs (renal diseases), J. W. Kerr (atopy), Sebastian Lucas (leprosy and fungal infections) and Professors David Hamblen (locomotor system), M. R. S. Hutt (Kaposi's sarcoma, Burkitt's lymphoma and cardiomyopathies) and M. C. Timbury (viral infections).

My thanks are due also to colleagues who have contributed to previous editions, parts of whose contributions are still embodied in the text. They include Professors A. J. Cochran, M. J. Davies, B. Lennox and N. Woolf and Drs J. F. Boyd, C. D. Forbes, E. L. Murray, the late Dr A. T. Sandison, Dr J. M. Vetters and members of the MRC Hypertension Research Unit (Drs J. J. Brown, A. F. Lever and J. I. S. Robertson). In particular, I must acknowledge the contribution of the late Professor D. F. Cappell, author of the 6-8th editions of this book. Many of his illustrations are still included in the present edition.

All my colleagues in this Department have been most helpful in making useful suggestions, providing illustrations and participating in the correction of proofs. Illustrations provided by colleagues outwith the Department are acknowledged in the legends.

I wish to thank Mr David McSeveney, FIMLT and his colleagues for their willing co-operation and skill in providing histological preparations and electron micrographs of the highest quality. Mr Peter Kerrigan, assisted by Mr David McComb, has once again contributed an enormous amount of skilful and painstaking work in the preparation of photographs and diagrams.

I am particularly grateful to Mrs Maureen Ralston and Miss Helen Scott who have dealt successfully with a considerable amount of typing, often from scarcely legible manuscripts. Mrs Jean Lyall has been most helpful in chasing up references and ensuring the availability of excellent library facilities.

It is a pleasure once more to thank Messrs Edward Arnold, and particularly Miss Barbara Koster and Miss Ailsa Andrew for their enthusiastic co-operation and determination to overcome delays in publication.

Many readers have sent me useful comments on the previous edition. I hope it will continue.

Finally, I wish to thank my wife. Not only has she advised me on bacteriological topics and helped with proof reading, but she and our family have been unfailing in their support in spite of my pre-occupation and irritability during the preparation of this edition.

J. R. ANDERSON

Glasgow, November 1984

Contents

1

Introduction

What is pathology?

Pathology is the study of disease by scientific methods. Disease may, in turn, be defined as an abnormal variation in the structure or function of any part of the body. There must be an explanation of such variations from the normal—in other words, diseases have causes, and pathology includes not only observation of the structural and functional changes throughout the course of a disease, but also elucidation of the factors which cause it. It is only by establishing the cause (*aetiology*) of a disease that logical methods can be sought and developed for its prevention or cure. **Pathology may thus be described as the scientific study of the causes and effects of disease.**

Methods used in clinical pathology

Clinical pathology originated in 'siderooms' adjacent to hospital wards, in which simple diagnostic tests were carried out by doctors, nurses and students. As the number and complexity of diagnostic tests grew, a centralised laboratory was set up, and one of the hospital clinicians usually assumed responsibility for the laboratory investigations. Inevitably, the work of the hospital laboratory continued to expand, and soon required the full-time attention of a doctor—the pathologist—and non-medical assistants. The story has been one of rapid expansion in the scope of laboratory work, and nowadays the pathology laboratories of large hospitals comprise a number of departments, each with its own specialist pathologist(s) and non-medical scientific staff. The pathology specialties include the following:

(*a*) **histology** and **cytology**, in which the structural changes in diseased tissues are examined by naked-eye inspection, or by light and electron microscopy of tissue sections or smears; (*b*) **biochemistry** (chemical pathology), in which the metabolic disturbances of disease are investigated by assay of various normal and abnormal compounds in the blood, urine, etc.; (*c*) **microbiology**, in which body fluids, mucosal surfaces, excised tissues, etc., are examined by microscopical, cultural and serological techniques to detect and identify the micro-organisms responsible for many diseases. (*d*) **haematology**—investigation of abnormalities of the cells of the blood and their precursors in haemopoietic tissue and of the haemostatic, including the clotting mechanisms; (*e*) **immunology**, the detection of abnormalities in the immunity system responsible for specific immune responses and other defence mechanisms against infection. Further specialisation includes the division of microbiology into bacteriology and virology, and the development of highly specialised pathology departments associated with clinical departments of dermatology, neurosurgery, gastro-enterology, etc.

The use of immunological techniques illustrates the increasing range and sophistication of methods in all branches of pathology. Large numbers of polyclonal and monoclonal antibodies to various constituents of human cells and their products are now available: they are used extensively by the biochemist in immunoassay, by the microbiologist to identify micro-organisms, and by the haematologist and histopathologist to identify various types of normal and abnormal cells.

Another specialty, which is advancing rapidly, is **medical genetics**. An increasing number of genetic defects which cause severe disability can now be detected early enough in pregnancy to induce abortion where this is considered desirable, while in other instances the chances of pregnancy resulting in a disabled child can be predicted with accuracy and the prospective parents can be given appropriate advice. Accordingly, departments of medical genetics have been set up in major centres and make use of various techniques, including those of the molecular biologist. The degree of specialisation in pathology varies greatly in different countries. Even in those with highly developed medical services it is inevitable that pathologists in the smaller hospitals in sparsely populated areas have to provide services in more than one pathological specialty. The relative importance of the several branches of pathology varies for different types of disease. In some instances, for example in diabetes mellitus, biochemical investigations provide the best means of diagnosis and are of the greatest value in the control of therapy. By contrast, recognition of the nature of many diseases, for example tumours, and so the choice of the most appropriate therapy, still depend very largely on examination of the gross and microscopic features. For most diseases, diagnosis is based on a combination of pathological investigations. To give an example, biochemical tests may indicate that a patient is suffering from impairment of renal function, but the nature of the renal disease responsible for this commonly requires removal of a piece of renal tissue for histological and immunological examination (*renal biopsy*). Another example is provided by anaemia, which may have many causes. The changes in the cells of the blood and the bone marrow may suggest deficiency of a factor essential for erythropoiesis, and biochemical and physiological tests are then indicated to confirm the deficiency, e.g. of vitamin B_{12} or folic acid. Alternatively, anaemia may result from blood loss and this may be due to a parasitic infection, ulceration or cancer of the gastro-intestinal tract or the effects of disordered endocrine function on the endometrium, diagnosis of which may require histological examination.

The hospital pathologist is becoming much more clinically orientated. He must co-operate closely with clinicians, not only in diagnosis, but also by applying his skills to assessment of the effects of treatment, e.g. by examination of multiple biopsies of cancers and other lesions, removed serially during the course of treatment. He must also make use of laboratory techniques to monitor patients for unwanted effects

of treatment, e.g. the harmful effects of some drugs on the cells of the liver, kidney, immunity system or haemopoietic tissue.

Finally, it is important to emphasise the continuing value of the clinical autopsy. In the past, when diagnostic procedures were relatively limited and primitive, a high proportion of diagnoses were made in the post-mortem room. In many cases, the more sophisticated diagnostic procedures now available have not diminished the value of the autopsy, even in hospitals providing a very high standard of patient care (Cameron and McGoogan, 1981). The important role of post-mortem examination in elucidating the natural history of disease processes is well illustrated by the extensive studies of Willis (1973) on the spread of tumours within the body. This role of the autopsy is still important, for it is revealing the changes in the patterns of many diseases, and also new and unwanted effects, resulting from use of the ever-increasing number and variety of powerful drugs and therapeutic procedures available to the clinician.

Why learn pathology?

Most medical students are not going to become pathologists. It is nevertheless essential that the medical school curriculum should include a course of pathology which provides a clear account of the causes, where these are known, and of the pathological changes, of the more important diseases. Most disease processes bring about structural and functional changes and these usually provide a logical explanation for the symptoms and signs and commonly also for the biochemical changes. A clinician without an understanding of the structural and functional effects of various disease processes must base his or her diagnoses on memorisation of lists of symptoms and signs of individual diseases, an exercise which seems more suited to a computer than to the human brain. This applies not only to the clinical diagnostician but also to the surgeon, who must also recognise the nature of the structural changes exposed at operation and act accordingly, and to the radiologist who must be familiar with the structural changes of diseases in order to interpret the changes observed in images provided by x-radiology, ultrasonography and nuclear magnetic resonance. To the research worker, histopathology and electron microscopy are superb techniques; both can be adapted to enzymic and other chemical investigations (**histochemistry**), including immunohistological techniques which make use of the exquisite specificity of antigen–antibody reactions to detect tissue and cell constituents and abnormal substances (see Fig. 22.21, p. 22.22 and Fig 26.1, p. 26.2).

Accordingly, pathology is of central importance to the medical student, regardless of the branch of medicine he intends to pursue.

How to learn pathology

Pathology is no exception to the general rule that learning is dependent mainly on the student's own effort. Most medical schools provide lectures and/or small-group tutorials, demonstrations and practical classes in pathology, but self-education by reading, preferably supplemented by audio-visual aids, is essential. The student should also take full advantage of opportunities to compare the clinical features of patients' illnesses with the underlying pathology. Clinicopathological conferences on selected cases, held for teaching purposes, are helpful, but one of the best places to see pathology and to compare the clinical features of disease with the pathological changes is the post-mortem room. A well-conducted autopsy, presented jointly by a clinician who cared for the patient and the pathologist performing the autopsy, is still unsurpassed as a teaching method. Students should also gain experience by following the progress of the patients they examine, noting the results of laboratory investigations and examining the lesions removed surgically or revealed at autopsy.

Pathology in the medical curriculum

There is a logical sequence in the traditional pattern of teaching of most medical schools. After courses in the basic sciences—chemistry, physics, biology—often provided before starting at medical school, the student is introduced to normal human structure (anatomy and histology) and function (physiology and biochemistry), followed by courses in pathology (the causes, features and effects of diseases) and pharmacology, and finally concentrates on the clinical subjects, i.e. the diagnosis and treatment of patients. Classically, the subjects are dealt with on a broad front. For example, the courses in anatomy and physiology deal with the whole of the body. In many medical schools, this policy has been replaced by what is variously termed 'integrated', 'topic' or 'systems' teaching, in which each of the body's major systems (cardiovascular, alimentary, respiratory, etc.) is the subject of a teaching course provided by a multidisciplinary team. Thus the course on, say, the alimentary system may include its anatomy, physiology, biochemistry, pathology, pharmacology, diagnosis and treatment. Each method has its advantages, but it has become abundantly clear that the second method requires considerable organisation and good co-operation between departments in the preparation and delivery of the course on each system. At present, there is a tendency to revert to the classical type of curriculum, or to compromise between the two.

A block course in pathology, spanning the gap between the preclinical and clinical subjects, has the great advantage of providing the student, in the early part of his hospital experience, with a basic knowledge of the diseases he is likely to encounter most often in the wards and clinics. By contrast, the 'integrated' course must either be brief and intensive or must extend over much of the curriculum, with the result that some systems come very late, leaving little time for their personal clinical study by the student.

Pathological processes

It was first pointed out by Virchow that all disturbances of function and structure in disease are due to cellular abnormalities and that the phenomena of a particular disease are brought about by a series of cellular changes. Pathological processes are of a dual nature, consisting firstly of **the changes of the injury** induced by the causal agent, and secondly of

reactive changes which are often closely similar to physiological processes. If death is rapid, as for example in cyanide poisoning, there may be little or no structural changes of either type. Cyanide inhibits the cytochrome-oxidase systems and thus halts cellular respiration before histological changes can become prominent. Similarly, blockage of a coronary artery cuts off the blood supply to part of the myocardium and death may result immediately from cardiac arrest or ventricular fibrillation. When this happens, no structural changes are observed. If, however, the patient survives for some hours or more, the affected myocardium shows changes which occur subsequent to cell death and the lesion becomes readily visible both macroscopically (Fig. 15.10, p. 15.11) and microscopically (Fig. 3.32, p. 3.32). Reactive changes may be exemplified by enlargement of the myocardium in the patient with high blood pressure i.e. systemic hypertension (Fig. 5.31, p. 5.25). In this condition, there is an increase in the resistance to blood flow through the arterioles and consequently the normal rate of circulation can be maintained only by a rise in blood pressure. Reflex stimulation of the heart results in more forcible contractions of the left ventricle, and in accordance with the general principle that increased functional demand stimulates enlargement (**hypertrophy**) and/or proliferation (**hyperplasia**) of the cells concerned, the left ventricular myocardium increases in size. Although part of a disease state, this reactive hypertrophy of the myocardium is closely similar to the physiological hypertrophy of the skeletal muscles in the trained athlete. To give another example, the invasion of the body by micro-organisms, in addition to causing cell and tissue injury, stimulates reactive changes in the lymphoid tissues, with the development of immunity. The distinction between the changes due to injury and those due to reaction are not usually so well defined as in the above examples. In many instances where cell injury persists without killing the cells, the cytological changes are complex and those due to injury often cannot be distinguished from those due to reaction. Some examples of the various types of cell injury and reaction are provided in Chapter 3.

In order to facilitate the understanding of pathological processes, it is helpful to group together those which have common causal factors and as a consequence exhibit similarities in their structural changes. For example, bacterial infections have certain features in common, and may with advantage be further sub-divided into acute and chronic infections. The features and behaviour of neoplasms (tumours) are sufficiently similar to classify most tumours into two categories, benign and malignant, and to provide a general account of each group. The changes resulting from a deficient blood supply are similar for all tissues. Accordingly, the next twelve chapters of this book are of a general nature and deal with the causes and structural and functional features of the major categories of disease. They assume that the reader has a basic knowledge of molecular and cellular biology (e.g. see Albers *et al.*, 1983). The remaining chapters are systematic and describe the special features of disease processes as they affect the various organs and systems.

The causes of disease

Causal factors in disease may be genetic or acquired. *Genetically-determined disease* is due to some abnormality of base sequence in the DNA of the fertilised ovum and the cells derived from it, or to reduplication, loss or misplacement of a whole or part of a chromosome. Such abnormalities are often inherited from one or both parents. *Acquired disease* is due to effects of some environmental factor, e.g. malnutrition or micro-organisms. Most diseases are acquired, but very often there is more than one causal factor and there may be many. Genetic variations may influence the susceptibility of an individual to environmental factors. Even in the case of infections, there is considerable individual variation in the severity of the disease. Of the many individuals who become infected with poliovirus, most develop immunity without becoming ill; some have a mild illness and a few become paralysed from involvement of the central nervous system (Fig. 21.41, p. 21.35). This illustrates the importance of **host factors** as well as causal agents. Spread of tuberculosis is favoured by poor personal and domestic hygiene, by overcrowding, malnutrition, and by various other diseases. Accordingly, disease results not only from exposure to the major causal agent but also from the existence of **predisposing** or **contributory factors.**

Congenital disease

Diseases may also be classified into those which develop during fetal life (congenital) and those which arise at any time thereafter during post-natal life. Genetically-determined diseases are commonly congenital, although some present many years after birth, a good example being adenomatosis (polyposis) coli, which is due to an abnormal gene and consists of multiple tumours of the colonic mucosa, appearing in adolescence or adult life (Fig. 19.72, p. 19.64). Congenital diseases may also be acquired, an important example being provided by transmission of the virus of rubella (German measles) from mother to fetus during the first trimester of pregnancy. Depending on the stage of fetal development at which infection occurs, it may result in fetal death, or involvement of various tissues leading to mental deficiency, blindness, deafness or structural abnormalities of the heart. The mother may also transmit to the fetus various other infections, including syphilis and toxoplasmosis, with consequent congenital disease. Ingestion of various chemicals by the mother, as in the thalidomide disaster, may induce severe disorders of fetal development and growth. Another cause of acquired congenital disease is maternal–fetal incompatibility. Fetal red cells exhibiting surface antigens inherited from the father may enter the maternal circulation and stimulate antibody production: the maternal antibody may pass through the placenta and react with the fetal red cells, causing a haemolytic anaemia.

Genetically-determined disease is discussed in the next chapter.

Acquired disease

The major causal factors may be classified as follows:

(1) Deficiency diseases. Inadequate diet still accounts for poor health in many parts of the world. It may take the form of deficiency either of major classes of food, usually high-grade protein, or of vitamins or elements essential for specific metabolic processes, e.g. iron for haemoglobin production. Often the deficiencies are multiple and complex. Disturbances of nutrition are by no means restricted to deficiencies, for in the more affluent countries obesity, due to overeating, has become increasingly common, with its attendant dangers of high blood pressure and heart disease.

(2) Physical agents. These include mechanical injury, heat, cold, electricity, irradiation and rapid changes in environmental pressure. In all instances, injury is caused by a high rate of transmission of particular forms of energy (kinetic, radiant, etc.) to or from the body. Important examples in this country are mechanical injury, particularly in road accidents, and burns. Exposure to ionising radiations cannot be regarded as entirely safe in any dosage. While radiation is used with benefit in various diagnostic and therapeutic procedures, any pollution of the environment with radio-active material is potentially harmful to those exposed to it and probably to subsequent generations.

(3) Chemicals. With the use of an ever increasing number of chemical agents as drugs, in industrial processes, in agriculture and in the home, chemically-induced injury has become very common. The effects vary. At one extreme are those substances which have a general effect on cells, such as cyanide (see above) which causes death almost instantaneously, with little or no structural changes. Many other chemicals, such as strong acids and alkalis, cause local injury accompanied by an inflammatory reaction in the tissues exposed to them. A third large group of substances produces a more or less selective injury to a particular organ or cell type. Hepatocytes play a major role in absorbing and metabolising many toxic chemicals. They are therefore liable to injury by various chemicals, including paracetamol and alcohol in high dosage. Many toxic chemicals or their metabolites are excreted by the kidneys, and because of their concentrating function the renal tubular epithelial cells are exposed to high levels of such substances. Accordingly, toxic hepatic and renal tubular cell death are common. Fortunately both types of cell have a high regenerative capacity. Specific effects of chemicals are illustrated also by injury of neurons by overdosage of barbiturates and lung injury by drinking a solution of paraquat (Fig. 16.37, p. 16.54).

(4) Infective micro-organisms. These include bacteria, protozoa, small metazoa, lower fungi and viruses. In spite of the advances in immunisation procedures and the extensive use now made of antibiotics, many important diseases still result from infection by micro-organisms, and the danger of widespread epidemics, e.g. of influenza and cholera, has been enhanced by air travel. The disease-producing capacity of micro-organisms depends on their ability to invade and multiply within the host, and on the possibility of their transmission to other hosts. The features of the disease produced by infection depend on the specific properties of the causal organism. Bacteria bring about harmful effects mainly by the production of chemical compounds termed **toxins**, and the biological effects of these, together with the response of the host, determine the features of the disease. Viruses multiply in host cells, usually with a direct cytopathic effect: features of virus disease depend largely on which cells are invaded and on the response of the host. Some viruses also become integrated, i.e. viral genes are inserted into the genome of the host cell, and this is probably a contributory cause of some forms of cancer. Of the protozoa, the malaria parasite is of enormous importance as a cause of chronic ill health in whole populations.

(5) **Metazoan parasites** are also an important cause of disease in many parts of the world. Hookworm infection of the intestine and schistosomiasis are causes of ill health prevalent in many tropical countries.

(6) **Immunological factors.** The development of immunity is essential for protection against micro-organisms and parasites. Harmful effects, both local and more widespread, can, however, result from the reaction of antibodies and lymphocytes with parasites, microbes and their toxic products. Also, the immunity system does not distinguish between harmful and harmless foreign antigenic materials, and injury may result from immune reactions to either. Such **hypersensitivity reactions** are numerous and complex. Local examples include hay fever, asthma and some forms of dermatitis, while hypersensitivity to many foreign materials,

including penicillin and other drugs, can cause generalised, sometimes fatal, reactions. Hypersensitivity reactions may also result from the development of **auto-immunity** in which antibodies and lymphocytes develop which react with and injure normal cells and tissues: examples include chronic thyroiditis, commonly progressing to hypothyroidism, and the excessive destruction of red cells in auto-immune haemolytic anaemia.

In another group of disorders, the immunity system is deficient, and the patient lacks defence against micro-organisms: this may result from abnormalities of fetal development, as an effect of various acquired diseases, or it may be induced by immunosuppressive therapy.

(7) **Psychogenic factors.** The mental stresses imposed by conditions of life, particularly in technologically advanced communities, are probably largely responsible for three important and overlapping groups of diseases. First, acquired mental diseases such as schizophrenia and depression, for which no specific structural or biochemical basis has yet been found. Second, diseases of addiction, particularly to alcohol, various drugs and tobacco: these result in their own complications, for example alcohol predisposes to liver damage (Fig. 20.27, p. 20.24) and causes various neural and mental disturbances, while cigarette smoking is the major cause of lung cancer (Fig. 16.47, p. 16.67) and chronic bronchitis, and is concerned also in peptic ulceration and coronary artery disease. The third group of diseases is heterogeneous, and includes peptic ulcer (Fig. 19.30, p. 19.23), high blood pressure and coronary artery disease (Fig. 15.2, p. 15.7). In these three important conditions, anxiety, overwork and frustration (all of which are experienced by editors of textbooks) appear to be causal factors, although their modes of action are obscure.

References

Albert, B., Bray, D., Lewis, J., Raff, M., Roberts, K. and Watson, J. D. (1983). *Molecular biology of the cell*, pp. 1146. Garland Publishing, Inc, New York and London.

Cameron, H. M. and McGoogan (1981). A prospective study of 1152 hospital autopsies. *Journal of Pathology*, **133**, 273–300.

Willis, R. A. (1973). *The spread of tumours in the human body*, 3rd edn., pp. 400. Butterworths, Sevenoaks and London.

2

Genetics and Disease

A knowledge of genetics is essential for the understanding of four groups of diseases. These are attributable to (a) chromosome imbalance in the fertilised ovum and thus in all the individual's cells; (b) inheritance of mutant genes from one or both parents; (c) an interplay between environmental factors and the genetic constitution of the sufferer, and (d) genetic defects (chromosomal imbalance or gene mutation) which are not inherited from the parents but arise in somatic cells during the life of the individual.

(a) *Major chromosome imbalance* is found in approximately 0·5% of live-born children. A well known example is Down's syndrome, in which characteristic physical abnormalities and mental retardation are usually due to inheritance of an extra chromosome.

(b) *Inheritance of abnormal genes*, e.g. in haemophilia and certain muscular dystrophies, occurs in about 0·25% of children born in this country. The variety of inherited disorders is enormous and most of them are uncommon or rare. However, in Africa and around the Mediterranean up to 5% of individuals have hereditary forms of anaemia due to abnormal haemoglobins. The widespread occurrence of these disorders almost certainly has a Darwinian explanation, namely that carriers of the abnormal gene have increased resistance to malaria and therefore a survival advantage. Many inherited diseases can now be largely prevented either by genetic counselling of members of affected families, by population screening for carriers of metabolic defects, and by identifying and aborting affected offspring at an early stage of gestation. Some metabolic defects can also be treated effectively if they are detected at birth before there has been irreversible cellular damage. These disorders are also of considerable scientific interest as 'experiments of nature' which provide unique physiological and pathological information about functions which cannot readily be investigated otherwise.

(c) The third category, diseases which depend not only on the particular *genetic constitution* of the individual (**genotype**) but also on the effect of *environmental factors* (i.e. both nature and nurture), is much more common, accounting for about 10% of chronic adult disease. There are, for example, many disorders in which foodstuffs, drugs, organic dusts, radiation and infection have unduly severe effects on some individuals because of their genetic background. A classical example is acute intermittent porphyria in which an inherited partial deficiency of the enzyme uroporphyrinogen-1-synthetase remains latent until the metabolic pathway is stressed with barbituates, which leads to the excretion of porphyrins in the urine accompanied by an attack of abdominal pain and other symptoms. It should be emphasised that in some instances the relevant genetic traits are regarded as normal, e.g. the inheritance of a fair skin which makes the individual unduly prone to those skin disorders which are provoked by exposure to sunlight. Another striking example is the predisposition of individuals with particular cell-surface glycoproteins (termed HLA antigens) to develop certain types of disease. The HLA antigens are determined by genes at the major histocompatibility complex. They are of considerable genetic interest and of importance in transplantation of tissue, and are considered on p. 2.12. The scientific study of a disease in which a particular environmental agent has variable effects on different individuals because of their genetic make-up poses special problems because experimental studies on other individuals or species may be partially or totally irrelevant.

(d) The fourth category, *genetic disorders*

occurring *in the somatic cells* of a hitherto normal individual, has only recently come into prominence with the development of new techniques in cellular and molecular biology. It now seems clear that many tumours arise from a single somatic cell as a result of mutation or other genetic change which allows it to divide more rapidly or survive longer than its normal counterparts. Logically, somatic cell genetics is an important aspect of the pathology of virus infection (which introduces new genes into the cell) but at present little is known of the details of the genetic interactions involved except in the case of some tumour viruses.

Interestingly, there is some overlap between all the above categories. Thus, an individual who inherits an abnormal gene for sickle cell haemoglobin from one parent may remain healthy until sickling of the red cells is provoked environmentally by hypoxia (as may occur while flying at high altitude or during general anaesthesia for a surgical operation). Another example is the rare disease xeroderma pigmentosum in which a genetically-determined enzyme defect leads to increased susceptibility of epidermal cells to the damaging effect of the ultraviolet radiations in sunlight, with the consequent development of multiple skin tumours.

This chapter assumes some previous familiarity with genetic principles at the molecular and cellular levels. It is not intended to be exhaustive and the topics and examples of disorders have been chosen to give a simplified account of the principles which must now be grasped in order to understand how disease results from genetic disturbances. As knowledge increases these principles will undoubtedly be modified and will contribute further to our understanding of the nature of human disease.

Organisation of genetic material in mammalian cells

Genes and the genetic code. DNA is the material in which genetic information is stored. This information is coded in 3 letter words (codons) made from an alphabet composed of 4 letters. The letters are organic bases, namely the purines adenine (A) and guanine (G) and the pyrimidines thymine (T) and cytosine (C). Each DNA word codes for an amino acid, e.g. TTC for lysine, GCA for arginine and CCT for glycine. There are two or more different codons for some amino acids (e.g. TTC or TTT for lysine).

The DNA molecule is long and threadlike, consisting of a backbone of alternating deoxyribose and phosphate groups which serves like a paper tape on which the letters are written in meaningful order in a single line. For example (3') TTC—GCA—CCT (5') codes for the amino acids lysine—arginine—glycine in that order in a polypeptide molecule (Fig. 2.1). 3' and 5' refer to the deoxyribose-phosphate linkages which define the direction in which the DNA is copied and read (see below).

As words are used to form sentences, so codons are grouped to form genes, each gene carrying the instructions for the entire amino-acid sequence of a single protein or poly-

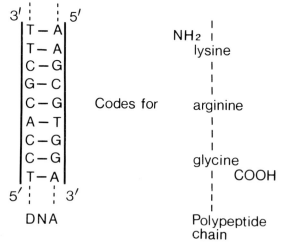

Fig. 2.1 Part of a double stranded DNA molecule and the corresponding part of the polypeptide chain for which the gene (on the left DNA strand) codes. The vertical lines on each side of the DNA molecule represent the deoxyribose-phosphate backbones which hold the bases in order. Note that the right strand of DNA is complementary to the left and in this instance does not code for polypeptide.

peptide chain. Except in bacteria, genes also contain sequences of codons which do not

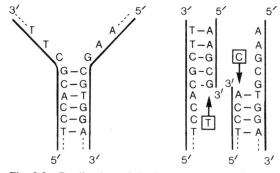

Fig. 2.2 Replication of double stranded DNA molecule shown in Fig. 2.1. The strands first separate and each serves as a template for the other by complementary base pairing. The new strands grow at their 3′ ends (*arrows*).

serve as instructions for the amino-acid sequence of its polypeptide product. These non-contributory sequences, known as **introns**, divide the instructional DNA of the gene into a series of **exons**.

DNA replication. Although the genetic information in DNA is coded as described above, the DNA molecule does not consist of a single threadlike strand: it forms a double helix with a second strand which also consists of a deoxyribose-phosphate backbone and the bases A,G,T and C, which pair selectively with those on the first strand (Fig. 2.1). A on one strand always pairs with T on the other and G on one with C on the other. Hence if bases on one strand were TTC GCA CCT the opposite ones on the second strand would be AAG CGT GGA. This arrangement is of major importance in DNA replication preceding mitosis, in which each strand acts as a template for the other (Fig. 2.2).

How genes are switched on and off. While the DNA encodes the order in which the various amino acids are arranged in the polypeptide chain, the process is an indirect one involving **messenger RNA (mRNA)**; this closely resembles single stranded DNA with ribose replacing deoxyribose in the backbone, and uracil replacing thymine among the bases. Before a polypeptide is synthesised, an mRNA copy must be **transcribed** from the DNA of the gene (Fig. 2.3). The transcription of genes is controlled by *promoters*, stretches of DNA which act as switches and lie some distance 'upstream' (in the 3′ direction) on the strand containing the gene to be transcribed. The function of the promoter can be increased by other stretches of DNA in its neighbourhood—*enhancers*—and can be activated or repressed by regulatory polypeptides produced by other genes. Some of these regulatory genes are themselves controlled by the binding to them of metabolites or hormones.

Following transcription, mRNA is modified in various ways, including a process called *splicing* which removes superfluous information transcribed from the extra sequences (introns) present in the DNA of the genes. The mRNA corresponding to the exons of the gene is then ready to thread through the ribosomes and direct the order in which the various **transport (t)RNAs** present their specific amino acids for the synthesis of the polypeptide chain—a process called **translation**. Both mRNA splicing and translation are also subject to regulation and so influence gene expression.

A very important aspect of control of gene expression in somatic cells involves post-translational modification of polypeptides—phosphorylation, methylation etc.—by enzymes which are the products of other genes. Much of the switching of genes on and off produces short-term reversible effects which serve the immediate metabolic requirements of the cell.

Demonstration of genes. Originally genes were recognised as hereditary factors producing conspicuous effects which are handed down from generation to generation in statistically predict-

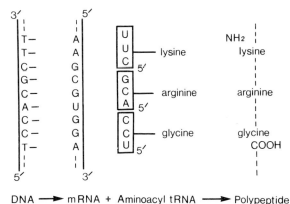

DNA ⟶ mRNA + Aminoacyl tRNA ⟶ Polypeptide

Fig. 2.3 Transcription of DNA to mRNA and translation of mRNA to polypeptide with the help of tRNA depend on complementary base pairing. Transcription occurs when a promoter is active upstream (3′) on the same strand of the double stranded DNA as the gene. For simplicity, the complementary strand of DNA is not shown.

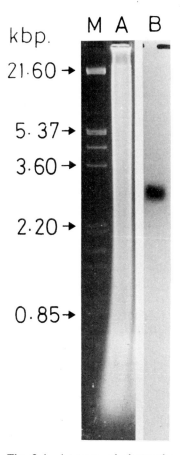

kbp.

21·60 →

5·37 →

3·60 →

2·20 →

0·85 →

M   A   B

Fig. 2.4 Agarose gel electrophoresis of restriction fragments of DNA. Track A: human DNA stained with ethidium bromide; the bands formed by different fragments are too numerous to resolve with this stain. Track B: autoradiograph of Southern blot of track A, hybridised with ^{32}P-labelled DNA copy of the human gene c-myc; the electrophoretic mobility of the restriction fragment containing c-myc is easily seen. Track M: fragments of DNA of standard bacteriophage stained with ethidium bromide; each band represents a fragment of known molecular weight. The rate of migration of DNA fragments depends on the number of bases they contain. Migration rates for various sized fragments expressed as kilobase pairs (kbp) are shown on the left. (Ms. Sheila Graham, Beatson Institute for Cancer Research.)

able ways, the appearances or disease produced in the individual being referred to as that individual's **phenotype**. Phenotype can also be described in terms of the actual proteins produced by many genes e.g. by measurement of their enzyme activity, or analysis of their amino-acid sequences. Now the DNA structure of genes

can be studied by a variety of biochemical and biological methods. The most important of these involves treating the DNA with enzymes called **restriction endonucleases** which cut it at specific sites to form a set of fragments ('**restriction fragments**') which can be separated from each other and are easier to investigate. The fragment containing the relevant gene can be identified by hybridisation with a highly radioactive DNA copy of the gene, the process involving bonding of two molecules which have complimentary base sequences. The molecular weight of restriction fragments can be assessed by their electrophoretic mobility on agarose gel, which acts as a molecular sieve (Fig. 2.4). If small enough fragments can be isolated, their base sequences can be determined chemically and compared with the amino acid sequence of the gene product. A functional test for activity of an isolated gene can sometimes be performed by introducing a restriction fragment containing it into a culture of cells ('*transfection*') and observing a change in their properties.

Chromosomes. The total DNA in a single mammalian cell is about a metre long and it would be quite unwieldy were it not divided into shorter pieces and stored in a compact form, just as a particularly long tape would for convenience be divided up and stored in spools of manageable size. Each of these shorter pieces forms a *chromosome*—a complex structure composed of a series of compact bead-like coils of DNA known as *nucleosomes*—held together by a protein scaffold.

Human gametes are *haploid*, i.e. they have one complete set of genes packaged in 23 chromosomes—22 autosomes and an X or Y sex chromosome in sperm, or 22 autosomes and an X in ova. Fertilisation of the ovum by a sperm leads to an embryo which is *diploid* i.e. its cells contain two complete sets of chromosomes, one set from each parent. Most somatic cells are diploid.

The chromosomes are particularly compact during cell division and at this time can be distinguished fom one another microscopically by their size, the position of the centromere and characteristic banded appearances which can be seen with special histological stains (Fig. 2.5). The gene coding for each particular polypeptide normally occurs on one particular chromosome, e.g. that for the enzyme glucose-6-phosphate dehydrogenase is on the long arm

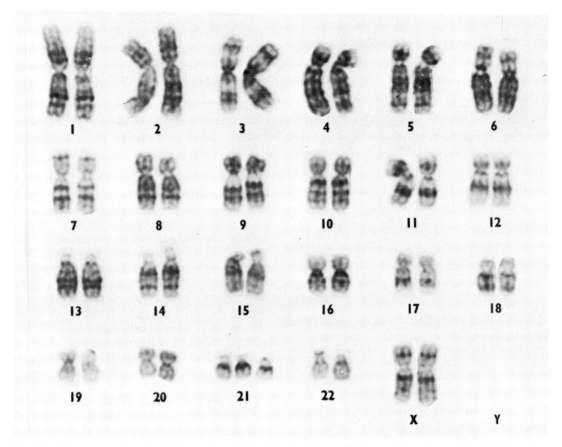

Fig. 2.5 Karyotype (trypsin-Leishman banded) of female infant with Down's syndrome. The chromosomes, obtained from a cell during mitosis, have been arranged as homologous pairs, each of which is numbered according to size, position of centromere (constriction) and pattern of transverse banding. The child has trisomy 21 (three 21 chromosomes instead of two). (Professor M.A. Ferguson-Smith.)

of the X chromosome at a fixed position (*locus*) relative to neighbouring genes (e.g. that determining haemophilia) with which it is said to be *linked*. Each pair of *homologous chromosomes* (the equivalent members of the set inherited from each parent) thus has a duplicate set of genes. The base sequence in the two genes at a particular locus may differ in detail, in which case the alternative forms are called **alleles**, the character (e.g. protein product) is referred to as **polymorphic**, and the individual as being **heterozygous** at that locus.

Cell division

Mitosis. As a rule, division by mitosis produces two separate daughter cells, each genetically identical to the cell which has just divided. Mitosis is characterised by the splitting of each chromosome longitudinally into two chromatids which then migrate to opposite poles of the cell and become the chromosomes of the two new cells which arise when the cytoplasm divides. As a result of mitosis one diploid cell divides into two diploid cells. At the molecular level, mitosis involves duplication of the DNA in each chromosome. This is achieved by separation of the two strands of the double helix and synthesis of a complementary strand on each of the two separated strands. An identical copy of each chromosome is thus provided (see Fig. 2.2). If errors occur in the base sequence during the copying process these are usually identified by nuclease enzymes which recognise an irregularity in the double helix, excise the defective portion and allow the gap to be filled correctly.

Meiosis. As already mentioned, gametes are haploid i.e. they contain one set of 23 chromo-

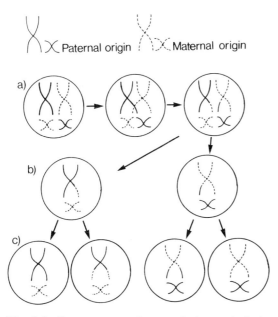

Fig. 2.6 Reassortment of genes during meiosis in hypothetical diploid cell with 4 chromosomes (*a*) Homologous recombination by crossing over; (*b*) products of first meiotic division, each with two chromosomes; (*c*) products of second meiotic division showing further segregation of parental genes.

somes. They arise from diploid precursor cells during the course of two special meiotic divisions. In the first, the 46 chromosomes line up as 23 homologous *pairs* and the members of each pair migrate to opposite poles of the cell which then divides to form two haploid cells, each with 23 chromosomes (reduction division). During the second meiotic division each duplication of DNA is followed by longitudinal splitting of each chromosome as in mitosis, giving rise to two haploid daughter cells.

Meiosis is not only important in producing haploidy in gametes; it allows reassortment of genes. Before the first meiotic division, stretches of DNA may be exchanged between corresponding loci on homologous chromosomes (*homologous recombination by crossing over*) and during the division the pairs of chromosomes (one inherited from each parent) segregate randomly and independently to the two poles of the cell so that all post-meiotic germ cells contain an assortment of parental chromosomes (Fig. 2.6).

Genetic variation within the species

Most of the processes described above are concerned with the conservation of genetic information which has accumulated in the DNA of the species over millions of years. When conservation is effective, no new genes emerge though almost infinite variation and evolution is still achieved by reassortment of existing alleles during meiosis and following fertilisation of the ovum by the sperm.

A second and potentially much more radical form of variation is qualitative and quantitative change in the DNA itself—from alteration of a single base in a gene (**point mutation**), through rearrangement, duplication or loss of parts of one or more chromosomes, to **aneuploidy** due to acquisition or loss of whole chromosomes. If these changes have any phenotypic effect at all, they are usually disadvantageous, resulting in a non-viable embryo or abnormal offspring. Rarely, mutations prove to be advantageous and sometimes they are a mixed blessing (e.g.

the sickle-cell haemoglobin mutation which causes anaemia and other problems but affords partial protection from malaria).

Point mutations may not be clinically apparent if they cause an amino-acid substitution at a functionally unimportant part of the protein molecule. Even if an important site is affected and the product of the mutant gene is nonfunctional, the protein coded by the normal allele at the corresponding locus on the homologous chromosome may be adequate for good health and the ill effects of the mutant gene then only become apparent in an unfortunate member of a later generation who inherits the defective gene from both parents. Characters expressed only in such **homozygous** individuals are said to show **recessive inheritance**. Many so-called inborn errors of metabolism, the result of production of functionally impaired enzyme molecules, are in this category, e.g. albinism—an inherited absence of pigment in the skin and eye due to failure of one step in the conversion of tyrosine to melanin. Less often, a mutant gene exercises a positive effect even in a heterozygous individual (i.e. even in the presence of a normal allele), in which case the character is said to be **dominant**. The A and B blood group antigens are inherited in this way. The best examples of clinical disorders showing dominant inheritance are due to mutations in genes which regulate the activities of other genes (e.g. in brachydactyly, where the normal developmental program for fingers and toes is disturbed). Ultimate proof of a point mutation depends on amino-acid sequencing of the poly-peptide gene product or on base sequence analysis of the relevant gene or the mRNA transcribed from it.

Frequency and causes of mutation. *Most changes in DNA appear to occur spontaneously.* The frequency of mutation varies at different loci but is of the order of 1 in 10^5 per locus per generation. One of the main known causes of mutation is *ionising radiation*. The amount of genetic damage increases with duration and intensity of exposure (short of that producing cell death) and is to a large extent cumulative. Agents which cause mutations are termed **mutagens**; *heat* is a potent one as are *various chemical agents* which alter base pairing and DNA repair, e.g. alkylating agents such as cyclophosphamide, epoxides, etc. Mutation rate also appears to rise with *increasing age*.

Karyotypic abnormalities

The changes just described affect one or a small number of contiguous bases in the DNA molecule and produce no alteration in the app-earance of the chromosome. Grosser changes result in an abnormal karyotype i.e. a change in the number or morphology of the chromo-somes. They can be observed on microscopic examination of the chromosomes during mitosis and may be classified as follows.

Chromosomal nondisjunction. This occurs at the first meiotic division in gamete formation. Instead of two particular homologous chromo-somes separating and moving to opposite poles of the dividing cell, both move to the same pole so that one germ cell receives both and the other neither. For example, instead of a 46,XY diploid cell producing one 23,X and one 23,Y haploid cell nondisjunction may result in a 24,XY and a 22,O haploid cell. Germ cells de-ficient in one or more chromosomes never pro-duce viable offspring except when a 22,O cell combines with a normal 23,X cell. This leads to a 45,XO individual with *Turner's syndrome* which is characterised by a female phenotype with rudimentary gonads (*gonadal dysgenesis*), small stature and other physical abnormalities.

Fertilisation with a gamete containing extra chromosomes is sometimes compatible with life. For example, fusion of a 24,XX gamete with a 23,Y produces a 47,XXY individual with *Klinefelter's syndrome*, in which a male pheno-type is associated with testicular atrophy, the presence of a sex chromatin body in the nuclei (p. 2.11), and sometimes excessive breast de-velopment and mental retardation. In a second example, combination of a normal gamete and one containing two copies of chromosome 21 leads to the karyotypic abnormality of trisomy 21 (Fig. 2.5): this is the usual cause of *Down's syndrome*—mental subnormality, a character-istic facial appearance, tendency to congenital heart disease, etc.

Translocation means exchange of fragments between non-homologous chromosomes e.g. between 14 and 21—t(14;21). This particular translocation (Fig. 2.7) leads to Down's syndrome in those members of the family whose cells also contain two normal copies of chromosome 21.

Deletion. A striking example of deletion (loss of part of the DNA from a chromosome) occurs in certain familial cases of retinoblas-toma—a malignant and frequently bilateral tumour of the eye which develops in childhood. All of those affected in such a family have an abnormal chromosome 13 with a micro-scopically visible deletion. The presence of such a chromosome is almost always associated with development of the tumour (i.e. dominant inheritance). It should be noted that many de-letions are too small to produce a karyotypic abnormality visible with the microscope and can be demonstrated only by molecular techniques.

A feature of all the syndromes described above due to karyotype abnormalities is that the affected individuals have an abnormal dose of many genes though it is unknown precisely which genes are responsible for the abnormal-ities observed, nor how they bring them about.

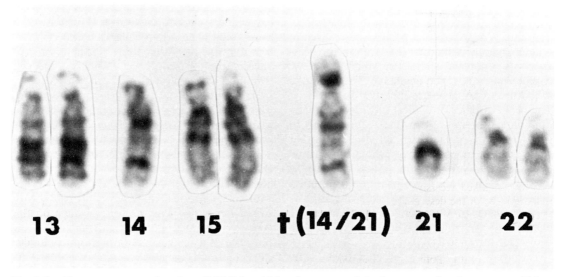

13   **14**   **15**   **†(14/21)**   **21**   **22**

Fig. 2.7 Chromosome translocation t(14/21) in which a large part of the long arm of a chromosome 21 has exchanged with part of the short arm of chromosome 14. Inheritance of such a chromosome, together with two normal copies of chromosomes 21 (instead of only one, as in this case), is the cause of some cases of Down's syndrome. (Professor M.A. Ferguson-Smith.)

Modes of inheritance

Examples of **monogenic inheritance** have already been given in which an allele at a single locus causes a profound effect on the individual. In affected families, expression of monogenic characters follows laws which were first described by Mendel (1866) and can readily be understood from the way chromosomes segregate during meiotic division to form gametes. Thus a true dominant character is expressed in at least one parent and is expected in half the offspring (Fig. 2.8) while a recessive character (expressed only in homozygotes) is evident in a quarter of the siblings born to parents who both happen to be heterozygous and therefore do not themselves express the character.

A distinctive family history is seen with disease caused by an X-linked recessive trait: the female carriers of the abnormal gene on one X chromosome are unaffected due to the presence of the normal allele on the other X chromosome, while half of the male offspring inherit the abnormal gene and suffer from the disease because the relevant gene does not occur on the Y chromosome (Fig. 17.46, p. 17.66). Fig. 2.9

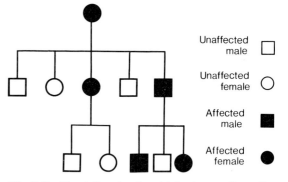

Unaffected male □

Unaffected female ○

Affected male ■

Affected female ●

Fig. 2.8 Mendelian dominant inheritance. Part of a pedigree of human brachydactyly.

shows part of the family tree of Alice of Hesse who inherited haemophilia, an X-linked recessive, from Queen Victoria. About 70% of unaffected female carriers of haemophilia can now be recognised by demonstrating the presence of a biologically inactive (mutant) form of anti-haemophilic globulin in their blood.

Certain characters show **dominance with incomplete penetrance**—i.e. they may or may not

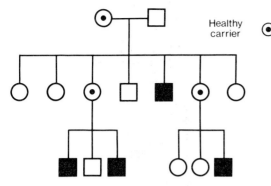

Fig. 2.9   X-linked recessive inheritance of haemophilia in some of the descendants of Alice of Hesse, a daughter of Queen Victoria.

be expressed in heterozygotes, even in the same family. Presumably some factor in addition to the gene itself is needed. In some examples, alleles at other loci are involved, and the inheritance is then said to be **polygenic**. Alternatively, or in addition, the abnormality in question may depend on interaction between the gene and some environmental factor (**multifactorial inheritance**).

Obviously the molecular mechanisms involved in polygenic inheritance are much more difficult to work out than those in which a single gene is concerned, and the difficulty in distinguishing hereditary from environmental effects is correspondingly greater. This problem can be approached by a study of the differences (*discordance*) between individuals of the same genotype (i.e. monozytotic twins) and by the rates of occurrence of a particular character in different classes of relative.

Precision in diagnosis and knowledge of the mode of inheritance of genetic defects and of the probability of a couple having diseased children, is obviously of great importance in genetic counselling. Tables 2.1–2.4 list some examples of genetic defects, most of which are discussed elsewhere in this book.

Table 2.1   Some diseases with autosomal recessive inheritance

---

Adrenal virilism
Albinism
Alkaptonuria
Alpha-1-antitrypsin deficiency
Cystic fibrosis
Gaucher's disease
Glycogen storage disease
Hepatolenticular degeneration
Hurler's syndrome
Metachromatic leukodystrophy
Phenylketonuria
Sickle cell disease
Tay-Sachs disease
Xeroderma pigmentosum

Table 2.2   Some diseases with X-linked recessive inheritance

---

Agammaglobulinaemia (Bruton)
Androgen insensitivity (testicular feminisation) syndrome
Christmas disease
Chronic granulomatous disease of childhood
Colour blindness
Duchenne muscular dystrophy
Glucose-6-phosphate dehydrogenase deficiency
Haemophilia
Lesch-Nyhan syndrome

Table 2.3   Some diseases with dominant inheritance

Achondroplasia
Adult polycystic kidney
Brachydactyly
Haemorrhagic telangiectasia
Hereditary angio-oedema
Hereditary spherocytosis
Huntington's chorea
Hyperbetalipoproteinaemia
Hypertrophic cardiomyopathy
Neurofibromatosis
Osteogenesis imperfecta
Otosclerosis
Polyposis coli
Retinoblastoma
Tuberous sclerosis

Table 2.4   Some diseases partially due to heredity

Allergic asthma
Ankylosing spondylitis
Haemochromatosis
Insulin dependent diabetes
Pernicious anaemia
Psoriasis
Rheumatoid arthritis

Somatic cell genetics

As already explained the DNA is the coded information by which our heritage from millions of years of evolution is handed down from generation to generation. The amount of information is immense—of the order of 50 000 structural genes coding for different polypeptides—and there is 30 times as much DNA again whose precise function is not yet known. From a study of different mature tissues of the body it is estimated that each cell produces roughly 15 000 different polypeptides: of these, approximately 12 000 are common to most cells and are involved in functions essential for the life of the cell, such as ATPase, glycolytic enzymes etc. The remaining 3 000 are concerned with specialised functions associated with the differentiated state. Some of the ways in which individual structural genes are switched on and off have already been mentioned. (p. 2.3). The central problems of somatic cell genetics are how the control of these switches is organised to permit the harmonious operation of the various intracellular functions from moment to moment and the long term co-ordinated development of the specialised cells which make up the tissues of a multicellular organism. Especially relevant to this chapter are the pathological effects which result when these mechanisms break down.

We must now consider the overall series of events which is responsible for orderly growth, development and function of the human body, an organisational problem of great complexity about which much remains to be discovered.

Clones

One very important principle is that in the very early embryo all the cells have the same potential for the expression of genes i.e. the cells can be interchanged without harmful effect. As development proceeds, the potential of each somatic cell becomes restricted by a series of self-perpetuating steps which, in effect, make less and less of the genome available to it and its descendents. Since these steps are not the same in all cells, there arise a number of distinct families or '*clones*' of cells, the word 'clone' meaning 'the mitotic progeny of one cell in which a specific constellation of gene loci first

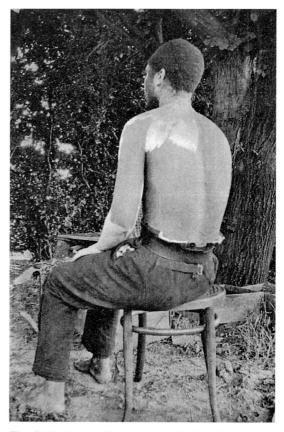

Fig. 2.10 Patch of cutaneous albinism in a negro, probably due to somatic mutation in early embryonic life. There were fifteen complete albinos in the family.

becomes active or derepressed and has remained active as a cell heredity' (Mintz, 1971). This principle of heritable differentiation is fundamental to the allocation of cells to particular lines of development during embryogenesis. For example, certain ectodermal cells which happen to be at the edge of the neural plate at a particular stage of development become committed to form clones of neural crest cells; subsequently they migrate from the neural crest and become even more narrowly committed when they, in turn, form clones of melanocytes, autonomic neurones or chromaffin cells, depending on the anatomical destination they reach. *Thus the differentiated form of a somatic cell and the particular structure it goes to form (e.g. arm or leg) depends on the cell lineage* (*clone*) *to which it belongs and the regulative effect of its microenvironment.* Conversely, a single specific micro-environment may have quite different effects on different clones.

It should be noted that the cells of some clones tend to adhere to each other preferentially, forming relatively large discrete cellular masses which may be readily apparent (Fig. 2.10). In contrast the cells of some other clones become intimately mixed with those of neighbouring clones and do not form circumscribed masses which are easily recognised. A further point of great importance is that most specialised cells of most tissues, e.g. the hepatocytes, do not consist of a single clone derived from one founder cell but are formed from several similar clones derived from a corresponding number of founder cells (in the liver about 3) the balanced development of which is controlled by intercellular regulation.

Finally, it must be emphasised that the adult body contains numerous relatively undifferentiated stem cells. When a stem cell divides it produces two daughter cells which are different from each other; one remains a stem cell and the other gives rise to a new clone of more highly differentiated cells. For example, adult bone marrow contains pluripotent stem cells called colony forming units. These can proliferate to form monoclonal colonies, each of which has the potential to follow any one of several lines of differentiation e.g. to form clones irreversibly committed to produce progeny which are entirely erythrocytes or granulocytes etc. The proliferation of erythrocyte clones is controlled by the glycoprotein hormone erythropoietin.

Genetics of clone formation. What changes in the DNA make one clone differ from another? One well recognised mechanism in mammalian cells is the conversion of the loosely-packed DNA of *euchromatin*, which is readily transcribed to mRNA, to densely-packed *heterochromatin* whose DNA is inaccessible for transcription. This is why the chromatin in the nuclei of mature differentiated cells is much denser than in embryonic cells. A well known example of clone formation by this mechanism occurs in the somatic cells of normal females and is called *lyonisation of the X chromosome* after its discoverer, Mary Lyon. At an early stage of development one of the two X chromosomes in each cell becomes heterochromatic,

forming a dense *sex chromatin body* on the inner aspect of the nuclear membrane, (Fig. 25.18, p. 25.20); this chromosome is thereafter inactive in that cell and its clonal descendants. The choice of which X chromosome is inactivated in each cell is random and therefore the human female is a mosaic composed of a roughly equal number of clones expressing either the paternal or maternal X chromosome.

Another method of clonal development and restriction of genetic potential is seen in cells allocated to form B lymphocytes. These cells are destined to synthesise antibody and at an early stage random deletions occur in parts of the genes coding for the polypeptide chains from which antibody molecules are formed (p. 6.15). The extent of the deletions in one particular cell determines the final structure of the antibody genes in that particular cell and hence the specificity of the antibody which that cell and its clonal descendants will make. There is also evidence that the diversity of antibody-forming clones is further increased by point mutations occurring during somatic development in the part of the gene coding for specificity.

Experiments involving nuclear transplantation between specialised cells of different types show that irreversible genetic changes of the type seen in mature B lymphocytes are probably exceptional. More often, other self-perpetuating but potentially reversible mechanisms seem to be involved in differentiation. These may include chemical modification of DNA (e.g. heritable methylation of cytosine which inactivates genes), chromosomal re-arrangements whereby stretches of DNA are inserted into or excised from the neighbourhood of an active promoter, or regulation of promoter activity by specific protein activators or repressors of gene activity.

Recognition of somatic cell clones. At present individual cell clones can be recognised with confidence in human tissue only in the following special circumstances. (1) As a result of lyonisation of the X chromosome in females of appropriate genotype. If the female is heterozygous for an X-linked gene with two or more variants (e.g. glucose-6-phosphate dehydrogenase) the tissue forms a mosaic of clonal patches distinguished by which variant they express. (2) In B lymphocytes by virtue of the various genetic changes (see above) associated with antibody specificity. (3) When the founder cell has developed a conspicuous genetic abnormality e.g. a karyotype different from the rest of the cells in the body, as often occurs in tumours. **Abnormal clones.** From what has been said above, the clone is clearly a key unit in the genetics of normal somatic development. Its relevance in pathology is that abnormal clones may develop when genetic abnormalities such as mutations and chromosomal rearrangements arise in somatic cells. Such a change is of little significance if expression of the abnormal mutant gene is recessive, or if it is lethal and other cells can take over, or if it occurs so late in development that the abnormal clone never attains a significant size. Somatic mutations or genetic rearrangements early in embryonic life may produce striking developmental abnormalities as illustrated in Fig. 2.10, but by far the most important abnormal clones are those which form tumours, a subject discussed in Chapter 13.

The major histocompatibility complex (MHC)

This complex of genes is of particular genetic importance because of its unusual degree of polymorphism, the role of the gene products in cell-cell interactions and their associations with certain diseases.

When living cells, tissues or organs (skin, kidney, etc.) are transferred between individuals of the same species, the recipient usually develops an immune response to antigenic components of the donor's cells and in consequence the graft is destroyed (graft rejection). This has brought to light the presence of antigenic glycoproteins on the surface of all human cells except erythrocytes and perhaps trophoblast. These antigens are encoded by a closely-linked group of genes which in man are termed the HLA (human leucocyte antigen) genes. They occupy four loci or regions, A, B, C and D, on chromosome 6, and the allelic genes at each locus exhibit marked variation, so that their products, the HLA antigens, are unusually polymorphic. Two HLA genes (one from each parent) are expressed at each locus, so that each individual has eight antigens. Because they are closely linked, the genes are inherited as haplotypic sets: there are thus four possible genotypes in the children of any particular family: 25% of the children will have the same two haplotypes and their HLA antigens will be identical; 50% will have one haplotype in common, and 25% will differ in both haplotypes (Fig. 2.11). Because of the number of allelic genes for each locus, the chance of two unrelated individuals having the same HLA antigens is small. These considerations are important in clinical transplantation, for the greater the HLA antigenic

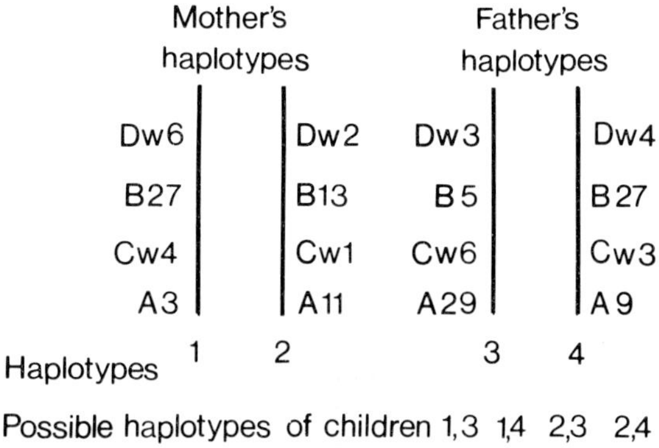

Mother's haplotypes		Father's haplotypes	
Dw6	Dw2	Dw3	Dw4
B27	B13	B5	B27
Cw4	Cw1	Cw6	Cw3
A3	A11	A29	A9
Haplotypes 1	2	3	4

Possible haplotypes of children 1,3 1,4 2,3 2,4

Fig. 2.11 The inheritance of HLA genes. Two hypothetical haplotypes are shown for each parent. The particular allelic genes at each locus, D, B, C and A (the order in which they lie on chromosome 6) are detected by the antigens they express at the cell surface. Being closely linked, the genes are inherited in haplotype combinations and each child will thus receive *either* haplotype from each parent, giving the possible combinations shown. The determination of haplotypes requires family studies. (The letter w in some of the genes refers to the numbers allocated to them at international workshops).

disparity between recipient and donor, the more likely is graft rejection.

Because genetic recombinations occur during the meiotic divisions to form germ cells and following fertilisation of the ovum, the combinations of genes in HLA haplotypes would be expected to be random, depending solely on the incidence of each gene in the population. Some genes are, however, observed to occur in association more often than expected, e.g. HLA-A1 is commonly associated with B8 and

DR3, and A2 with B7 and DR2. This is termed **linkage disequilibrium** and is presumably the result of some advantage for survival conferred by particular combinations of genes during evolution. This advantage is likely to have been resistance to infections, for the histocompatibility antigens play a role in intercellular collaboration necessary for immune responses (p. 6.16) and also in the destruction of infected cells once immunity has developed (p. 7.20). It is thought that viral infection of cells modifies their surface HLA antigens and that they are, in consequence, treated as abnormal by cells of the immunity system. Transplanted cells possessing different HLA antigens from those of the recipient are similarly regarded as abnormal and stimulate a remarkably strong immune response. The development of **HLA antibodies** is thus stimulated by transplantation of incompatible tissue and by the leucocytes and platelets in blood transfusion. Antibodies are also found in about 30% of parous women as a result of stimulation during pregnancy by fetal HLA antigens inherited from the father. Antibodies from the above sources are used for detection of HLA antigens (p. 7.31). HLA–D antigens, however, are detected by the reaction of lymphocytes rather than antibodies, although the closely related (and possibly identical) DR (D-related) antigens are detected by antisera.

The HLA system and disease

If the products of allelic genes can be detected by a simple technique, it is possible to determine whether the presence or absence of a particular gene is associated with any particular disease. The detection of such a correlation indicates that genetic factors play a causal role in that particular disease. The highly polymorphic HLA antigens provide an especially good opportunity for such investigations, and a high incidence of one or more HLA antigens has indeed been observed in various diseases. The strongest association is seen in ankylosing spondylitis (AS) in which rigidity of the spine results from ossification of ligaments and joints. In this disease, which affects males predominantly, 90% of patients possess the HLA–B27 gene (c.f. 9% in the general population). This association is world-wide and about 1 in 10 B27 + ve males develop some degree of AS, i.e. about 100 times greater than the risk in B27–ve

males. The aetiology of AS is unknown and the nature of the association with B27 is obscure. B27 is less closely associated with several other diseases, including a rare form of fibrosis of the thyroid gland (de Quervain's thyroiditis— p. 26.21). Infections with certain bacteria are sometimes complicated by inflammatory lesions of joints (reactive arthritis—p. 23.47) and this complication occurs much more frequently in B27 + ve than in B27 − ve patients.

In some diseases characterised by auto-immunity to cellular constituents of the affected tissues (the *auto-immune diseases*—p. 7.24), there is a raised incidence of HLA–B8, while in one of these diseases, *type 1 diabetes mellitus*, the incidence of BW15 is also raised. The chronic disabling disease, *multiple sclerosis*, is associated with a raised incidence of B7 and Dw2. These associations are unexplained. One possibility is that particular HLA genes are in linkage disequilibrium with nearby genes which play a causal role. The HLA genes form part of a stretch of DNA on chromosome 6 termed the **major histocompatibility complex (MHC)**: it includes the allelic Ir (immune response) genes which control the strength of the immune responses to individual antigens, and also allelic genes for three components (C4, C2 and B) of the complement system (p. 7.2). It is of interest that some of the diseases associated with HLA genes are characterised by infections (reactive arthritis) or disturbances of the immunity system (the autoimmune diseases), and linkage disequilibrium with Ir genes is a plausible explanation of the associations, while there is also some evidence of disturbances of the complement system in *systemic lupus erythematosus*, (p. 23.60) in which the incidence of several HLA genes is increased. The incidence of the various HLA genes varies in different communities and racial groups, and the genes associated with some diseases, e.g. type 1 diabetes, differ in the different racial groups. This supports the possibility that linkage disequilibrium with adjacent genes is involved. Another possibility is that microbial antigens might be closely similar to one or other HLA antigen, '(*molecular mimicry*') and this might result in either a poor immune response to infection with that organism, or an immune response which attacked not only the microbe but also the host cells.

The nature of MHC antigens. The products of the HLA–A, –B and –C genes are of similar structure and are termed *Class I MHC antigens*: they consist of a larger glycopeptide chain linked to a smaller peptide chain (β_2 microglobulin) which is the product of a gene on chromosome 15. The sequences of amino acids in both chains resemble those in parts of the two chains of immunoglobulin (antibody) molecules. The diversity of these HLA antigens lies in the large chain, the β_2 microglobulin being homogeneous for any particular species.

The products of the D, DR and Ir genes (*Class II MHC antigens*) consist of two glycopeptide chains, both of which are products of MHC allelic genes. These chains also show some homology with immunoglobulins. Little is known about human Ir genes and their relationship to D and DR genes.

Class I antigens are expressed in nearly all types of nucleated cells, but Class II antigens are normally restricted to subsets of lymphocytes and to cells of the mononuclear phagocyte system.

Much of what is known about the MHC and its function has been discovered from study in inbred mice of a system of H–2 antigens which are closely homologous to the human HLA antigens. Indeed, all mammals so far investigated have been found to possess a similar MHC of species-specific allelic genes.

References and Further Reading

Alberts, B., Bray, D., Lewis, J., Raff, M., Roberts, K. and Watson, J.D. (1983). *Molecular Biology of the Cell*, pp. 1146. Garland, New York.

Connor, J.M. and Ferguson-Smith, M.A. (1984). *Essential Medical Genetics*, pp. 280. Blackwell Scientific, Oxford.

Goodenough, U. (1984). *Genetics* 3rd edn. pp. 912. Holt-Saunders, Philadelphia.

Mintz, B. (1971). Clonal basis of mammalian differentiation. In' Davis, D.D., Balls, M. eds. *Control mechanisms of growth and differentiation* XXV p. 345–370. Cambridge University Press, Cambridge.

3

Molecular and Cellular Pathology of Tissue Damage

Most forms of tissue damage start with, or rapidly give rise to, molecular abnormalities in cells, and the resulting effects on cell structure and function are a central theme in pathology, important not only for a fundamental understanding of disease but also for rational prevention and treatment.

Cells are complex machines which are themselves composed of smaller machines—subcellular organelles and macromolecules such as enzymes. There are many causes for breakdown in cellular machinery. These include faults in the plans, that is in the DNA, causing inherited defects, and environmental factors such as lack of fuel and building materials, radiation and other forms of physical damage and a host of toxic chemical substances. A great many kinds of cellular abnormality at the molecular level can result from these causes—in theory at least one for each gene, of which there are at least 50 000!

As a result of great advances in chemistry and biology, enough is now known of normal cell structure and function to discuss tissue damage in general terms of a few vital processes; the maintenance of appropriate intracellular environments for specific metabolic functions, the production of energy in a form which can be used for the needs of the cell, the maintenance of an intracellular pool of small molecules for cellular fuel and building materials, the synthesis of macromolecules, digestion and degradation of macromolecules, cell form and movement, communication between cells, cell growth and replication, and differentiation. This chapter is largely devoted to these processes and to the causes and effects of their breakdown. However, because of their special importance, sections have been added on the effects of ionising radiation and on cell death, the end-point of many forms of tissue damage.

In practice, the production of energy and the control of intracellular environment are of most immediate importance for the survival of each individual cell. Interestingly, damage to one of these two processes rapidly upsets the other, leading to similar effects, and disorders of both play a very important part in many common human diseases. Cellular lesions due to lack of fuel or building materials are frequent in malnourished populations in many parts of the world, while in prosperous societies, dietary excess is a more important cause of cell damage. Apart from disorders of cell replication and differentiation which result in developmental abnormalities or in tumour formation, primary damage to each of the other vital processes is relatively uncommon, although knowledge of them is of theoretical interest in viewing tissue damage as a whole and of great practical value in individual patients, particularly in counselling of families with rare inherited defects, genetic aspects of which were considered in Chapter 2.

1. Maintenance of special intracellular environments

The interior of the cell is separated from the extracellular fluid by the plasma membrane which consists of various kinds of protein molecules floating in a lipid bilayer. The latter is composed mainly of lecithin and other phospholipids with some cholesterol and glycolipid.

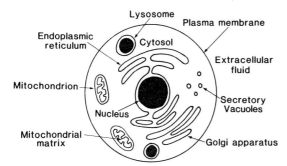

Fig. 3.1 Simple diagram of cell membranes which sequester ions and molecules and produce special intracellular environments for the chemical activities of the cell.

It is relatively impermeable, allowing the passage only of water and some small nonpolar organic molecules such as glycerol. Many of the membrane proteins traverse the lipid bilayer and project from each side of it: some act as receptors of information from the environment, others as channels through which specific inorganic ions, amino acids or sugars diffuse passively across the membrane, while still others function as pumps, actively driven by energy derived from ATP, and transport ions across the membrane against a concentration gradient.

The interior of the cell is further divided up by specialised lipid membranes enclosing intracellular organelles which have special internal environments suited to their own particular metabolic functions (Fig. 3.1). Thus the inner mitochondrial membrane encloses a matrix relatively rich in Ca^{++} and poor in H^{+}, a milieu required by the proteins responsible for ATP

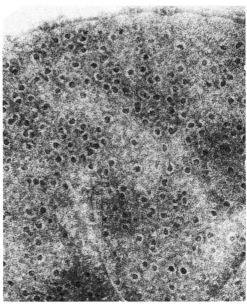

Fig. 3.3 Electron micrograph of part of the cell membrane of *Esch. coli* treated with antibody and complement followed by treatment with trypsin. Activation of complement at the sites of antigen-antibody reaction has resulted in lesions—apparently holes—in the cell membrane, and these are accentuated by trypsin. Cytotoxic antibody and complement produce similar lesions in human cells. × 140 000. (Dr. R. Dourmashkin.)

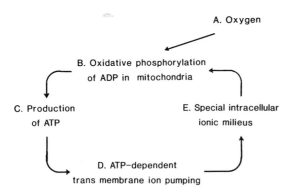

Fig. 3.2 Interdependence of ATP production and transmembrane ion pumping.

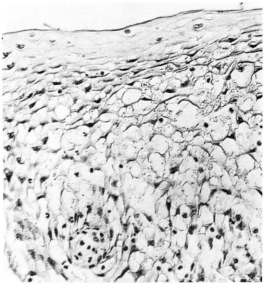

Fig. 3.4 Osmotic swelling leading to ballooned appearance of epithelial cells due to bacterial toxic injury in acute laryngitis. × 250.

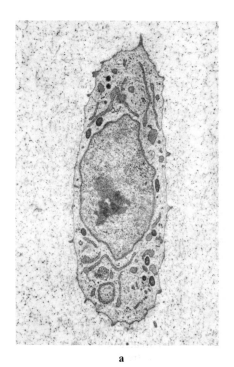

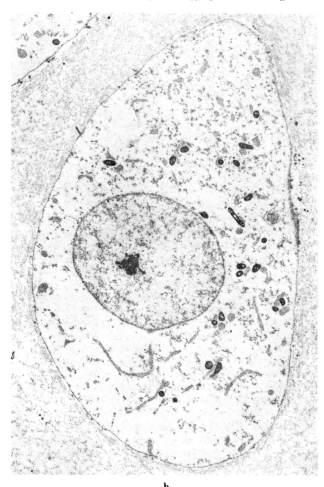

Fig. 3.5 Electron micrographs of chicken cartilage cells (**a**) before and (**b**) after injury by glutamylaminoacetonitrile. The damaged cell is swollen and the organelles separated due to accumulation of water in the cytosol. × 6 000. (Dr Morag McCallum.)

synthesis by aerobic respiration. In contrast, the membranes of lysosomes maintain a high H^+ concentration necessary for the activity of the special digestive enzymes (acid hydrolases) they contain. Cellular organelles thus form specialised compartments which allow the cell to perform various incompatible chemical reactions simultaneously.

Causes of membrane damage. From what has just been said, it follows that the special intracellular environments can be upset in several ways.

(1) One of the most important in medical practice is failure of the active pumping of ions due to lack of ATP. This often occurs because of inadequate supply of oxygen for the formation of ATP by oxidative phosphorylation in the mitochondria (Fig. 3.2 **a**, **b**, **c**).

(2) Alternatively, membrane permeability can be affected by the action of substances which specifically poison the ion pumps of the cell membranes. One such is the glycoside ouabain, used in small doses to treat cardiac failure because of its effect on Na^+ and K^+ transfer across myocardial cell membranes. It acts by competing with K^+ for a special site on Na^+ K^+ dependent ATPase.

(3) A third way in which the intracellular environment can be upset is by damage to and increased permeability of the cell membrane by the digestive action of complement, an enzyme system activated by combination of antibody with antigen on the cell membrane (Fig. 3.3). Certain bacterial enzymes such as the alpha toxin (lecithinase) of *Cl. welchii* are also causes of primary cell-membrane injury.

(4) Rupture of the plasma membrane due to mechanical causes. This may not be lethal to the cell if the lesion is small (e.g. in experimental nuclear transplantation by

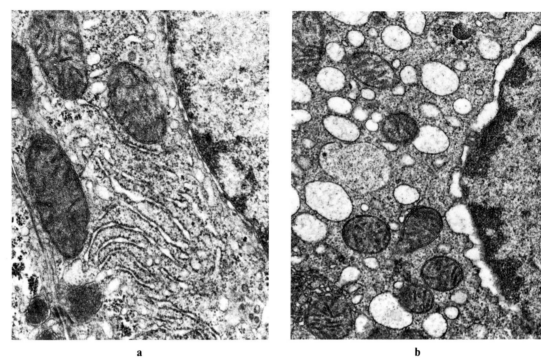

a   b

Fig. 3.6 Osmotic swelling of cisternae of rough endoplasmic reticulum. (**a**) Part of a normal mouse liver cell. Note the regular parallel plates of rough endoplasmic reticulum and discrete clusters of ribosomes. (**b**) Part of a mouse liver cell 4 hours after oral administration of carbon tetrachloride. The cisternae of the rough endoplasmic reticulum are dilated and appear as oval vesicles. Note that many of the ribosomes have been detached as a result of membrane damage. × 23 000.

microsurgery) in which case the defect closes spontaneously.

Effects. Each of the widely different mechanisms described above alters the permeability of cell membranes and the selective partitioning of inorganic ions and small molecules in the various compartments. These changes in turn can lead to osmotic swelling of the cell (Fig. 3.4, 3.5) and its organelles (Fig. 3.6). In addition, the altered internal environment of the cell (probably particularly the raised level of Ca^{++} in the cytosol) further inhibits mitochondrial ATP production and intensifies the disorder of membrane permeability due to lack of energy to drive the ion pumps (Fig. 32 **d**, **e**, **b**). Other energy-requiring functions of the cell fail and the moribund cell finally ruptures (lysis).

Membrane damage can be studied conveniently in cell suspensions in culture by observing changes of permeability to dyes such as trypan blue which are normally excluded from the nucleus and cytoplasm (Fig. 3.7). Alternatively, membranous components of the living cells

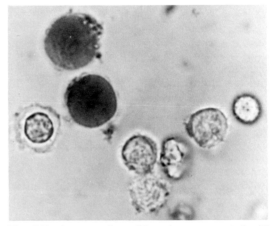

Fig. 3.7 A suspension of lymphocytes treated with cytotoxic iso-antibody and complement. Some of the cells have been killed, and have become stained by trypan blue dye present in the suspending fluid: other cells have survived and are unstained. × 1250.

may be labelled with radioactive isotopes such as ^{51}Cr or ^{32}P: subsequent severe injury to the cell, probably lethal, is recognised by release of radioactivity from the cells into the culture medium.

The above examples illustrate two important general aspects of cell damage. (1) A set of functionally related structures such as those controlling selective membrane permeability can have their action impaired by a variety of causes which act in different ways to produce a similar effect. (2) Damage to one process eventually leads to impairment of others.

2. Production of cellular energy

Most of the energy used by the cell for such vital processes as ion pumping, chemical synthesis and cell movement is obtained by the breakdown of a high energy phosphate bond in the conversion of ATP to ADP, ATP being analogous to a battery which provides energy for electric motors in the various subcellular machines. The reconversion of ADP to ATP requires fuel in the form of food, particularly carbohydrates and fats, which release energy when they are broken down to smaller molecules. In anaerobic conditions, breakdown of one molecule of glucose to pyruvic acid provides energy for the formation of two molecules of ATP, whereas oxidative catabolism of one molecule of glucose to CO_2 and H_2O provides energy for the formation of about 36 ATP molecules. The latter reaction involves the citric acid cycle whose enzymes are dissolved in the matrix within the inner compartment of the mitochondria, and a chain of respiratory proteins which are embedded in the inner mitochondrial membrane and function best when there is a high concentration of Ca^{++} in the inner compartment. The synthesis of ATP itself depends on energy given up by protons as they pass through a channel of yet another protein complex of the inner membrane, ATP synthetase. Very little energy released in these reactions is wasted as heat.

Causes of diminished ATP production. The two most important causes have already been mentioned. (1) Lack of oxygen in the tissues. This can occur locally e.g. in a piece of tissue supplied by an artery which becomes blocked by thrombus; or it may affect all the cells in the body as a result of severe anaemia or of cardiac or respiratory arrest. (2) Damage to cell membranes which alters the intracellular ionic environment and inhibits mitochondrial function. (3) Poisoning with fluoroacetate: this inhibits the citric acid cycle by blocking the enzyme aconitase which converts citrate to isocitrate (Fig. 3.8). (4) Inhibition of the respiratory chain by poisoning with cyanide, azide or carbon monoxide, all of which bind to and inhibit the enzyme cytochrome oxidase. (5) The small nonpolar molecule dinitrophenol, which has the property of crossing lipid membranes and of binding to protons. In appropriate concentrations, dinitrophenol can destroy the proton gradient across the inner mitochondrial

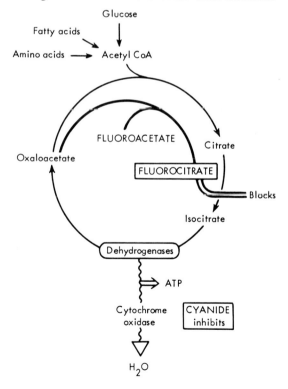

Fig. 3.8 The effects of fluoroacetate and of cyanide on cellular metabolism. Note that fluoroacetate is converted to fluorocitrate which inhibits conversion of citrate to isocitrate by aconitase.

membrane, bypassing ATP synthetase, and releasing the stored electro-osmotic energy as heat instead of ATP. This process is described as uncoupling of oxidative phosphorylation. (6) Lack of substrate for the citric acid cycle which occurs in neurons during severe hypoglycaemia.

Effects. When the production of ATP is severely impaired for one minute, the ATP:ADP ratio may fall to one tenth of its normal value. The cell is thus deprived of its energy (except that provided by anaerobic glycolysis or stored in transmembrane electro-chemical gradients) and all cellular processes requiring energy slow down or stop. Probably the most critical of these processes is ion pumping, and for this reason the sequence of events is due mainly to an altered intracellular environment.

The early stage of damage due to anoxia is reversible for some time, a return of aerobic conditions causing resumption of ATP synthesis by the mitochondria, ion pumping, and restoration of the normal intracellular environment. If, however, the period of anoxia continues, the cell comes to a 'point of no return' at which its death is inevitable. What happens at this point is unknown; electron microscopy of anoxic cells in tissue culture shows that it is marked by profound swelling of the inner mitochondrial compartment, perhaps due to activation of a Ca^{++}-dependent phospholipase or some such mechanism. The synthesis of RNA and protein are also inhibited at this stage but this probably does not influence the outcome (cells from which the nucleus has been removed can survive for long periods). The later stages following the point of no return show the changes of necrosis which are described in detail on p. 3.30 and include rupture and distortion of the membranes of the cell and enzymatic degradation of its macromolecular constituents.

It should be noted that the interval before irreversible damage is produced varies greatly with cell type. Thus neurons of the cerebral cortex have a high energy requirement which depends entirely on aerobic glycolysis, and they die after three minutes of oxygen deprivation, whereas other cells with less stringent metabolic requirements can survive in the absence of oxygen for many hours, forming ATP by anaerobic glycolysis until their supply of glycogen is used up. These facts are of considerable importance in the resuscitation of patients with cardiac or respiratory arrest and in obtaining cadaveric organs for transplantation surgery.

Four important principles emerge from the above discussion. (1) Some forms of cell injury are reversible if the cause is removed. (2) The effects of a single cause of injury may be influenced by the severity and duration of its action. (3) Different kinds of cells vary in their susceptibility to a single kind of injury. (4) Since the morphological changes which follow cell death may take several hours to develop after a cell reaches the point of no return, there is at present no reliable method of recognising recent cell death.

3. Maintenance of the intracellular pool of small organic molecules

The enormously complicated processes of cell metabolism depend on the maintenance of intracellular pools of small organic molecules which are required as fuel and as starting materials for the many synthetic activities of the cell. These include amino acids, fatty acids, monosaccharides, purines, pyrimidines, vitamins etc., and intermediaries such as pyruvate and acetate. The exact composition of the pool in a particular cell to some extent reflects the type of differentiation it has undergone and its functional activity at the time, and these in turn determine the various active enzymes present and the control they exert by positive or negative feedback on their substrates or products. Intracellular pools are also greatly influenced by the state of the whole body pool which depends on many factors including (1) the extent of dietary provision of foodstuffs; (2) effective absorption by the alimentary tract; (3) storage of reserves (mainly in the form of glycogen and triglyceride fat) and their release when required, functions largely controlled by the endocrine and autonomic nervous systems; (4) the recycling of fragments of macromolecules from cells or organelles; (5) the appropriate behaviour of organs of excretion such as the kidneys and liver; (6) the presence of carriers between specialised cell types (e.g. proteins forming water-soluble complexes with insoluble lipids—see Table 3.3); (7) the effective function of specific transport across the plasma membrane to the interior of the cell and (8) biochemical transformations by intracellular enzymes.

Disturbances of any of the factors mentioned above may lead to significant alterations in the intracellular pool of small molecules. By far the most important in practice are dietary causes, both deficiency and excess, and these will be further considered below. Disorders of the alimentary system, including intestinal malabsorption syndromes, predispose to undernutrition and will be described in Chapter 19. Other causes include endocrine disorders (Chapter 26) and impaired functions of individual enzymes due to genetic defects or to poisoning.

Effects

Unlike the forms of damage considered in the two previous sections, which have rather similar consequences in all cells, disturbances of the intercellular pool of small molecules are more heterogeneous and distinctive in their effects.

Deficiency of dietary protein or essential amino-acids leads to decrease in cellular synthesis of protein, with diminution in the appropriate cytoplasmic machinery, ribosomes and rough endoplasmic reticulum, shrinkage in cell size and impairment of cell growth and replication. Tissues which are particularly active in protein synthesis such as the liver and pancreas, are most obviously affected. Reduced albumin synthesis by the liver causes hypoalbuminaemia and contributes to 'famine oedema' (p. 10.34) while globules of triglyceride fat accumulate in the cytoplasm of hepatocytes (fatty change—Fig. 3.9), partly due to diminished hepatic synthesis of the proteins which transport fat from the liver i.e. the apoproteins of the very low density lipoproteins. Severe impairment of production of digestive enzymes by the pancreas leads to intestinal malabsorption and further nutritional difficulties.

During *total starvation*, cellular energy can be provided for about 24 hours from stored glycogen (glycogenolysis), then by formation of carbohydrate from protein breakdown (glyco-

neogenesis). Free fatty acids released from adipocyte stores remain available as a source of energy for a relatively long period and their breakdown is accelerated with increased production of 2-carbon-atom fragments derived from them. Most of these fragments enter the citric acid cycle which, in the absence of carbohydrate, functions less effectively and this leads to the accumulation of ketone bodies (acetone and aceto-acetic acid), and of β hydroxybutyric acid, the latter two tending to cause metabolic acidosis. In the hepatocytes, the increased production of 2-carbon-atom fragments also leads to increased synthesis of triglyceride and this, together with the reduction in apolipoprotein production already mentioned, leads to *fatty change* in the liver, which is a characteristic feature of starvation. Interestingly, the accumulation of large amounts of fat in liver cells, as in Fig. 3.9, seems not to impair their other functional activities.

Vitamin deficiency. Some aspects of various vitamin deficiencies are summarised in Table 3.1. In some examples the reason for selective involvement of certain cell types is understood. For example, in folic acid deficiency the occur-

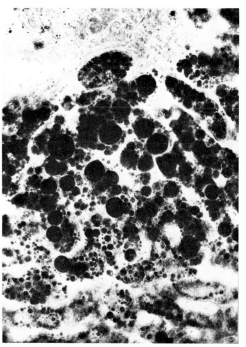

Fig. 3.9 Fatty change of liver. The cells are filled with large globules of fat. (Stained with Sudan IV.) × 190.

Table 3.1   Diverse effects of vitamin deficiencies

Name	Biochemical function impaired	Cell type notably affected	Clinical deficiency
Retinol (A)	Formation of light-sensitive rhodopsin	Retinal rod cells Epithelia	Night blindness Squamous metaplasia
Cholecalciferol (D)	Control of genes influencing calcium metabolism	Enterocyte Macrophage ? Osteocyte	Impaired calcification of cartilage Rickets and osteomalacia
Thiamine (B_1)	Conversion of pyruvate to acetate for use in citric acid cycle	Neurons Cardiac muscle	Beri beri: peripheral neuritis, cardiac failure: Wernicke's encephalopathy: ? neural tube defects in developing fetus
Pyridoxine (B_6)	Formation of NAD and NADP for oxidation-reduction in intermediary metabolism	Presumably many	Pellagra: dermatitis, diarrhoea and dementia
Folic acid	Synthesis of thymine for DNA etc.	Erythrocyte precursor in marrow	Megaloblastic anaemia
Cyanocobolamin (B_{12})	Conversion of tetrahydrofolate for synthesis of thymine	Erythrocyte precursor Epithelial cell Oligodendrocyte and Schwann cell	Pernicious anaemia Demyelination
Ascorbic Acid (C)	Hydroxylation of proline in nascent collagen	Fibroblast	Scurvy (capillary haemorrhage: poor wound healing)

rence of abnormal chromatin in rapidly proliferating red cell precursors in the bone marrow can be explained by the role of folic acid in the synthesis of thymine for the production of DNA. In others, such as Wernicke's encephalopathy, which is due to thiamine deficiency, the curious selective vascular damage in the neighbourhood of the third ventricle of the brain (p. 21.43) is quite unexplained. Despite these problems, it should be remembered that the study of vitamins possibly represents the greatest contribution of medical science to human welfare.

Dietary Excess. Intake of too much food, especially carbohydrate and fat leads to obesity with excessive storage of triglyceride fat, particularly in adipocytes but also in the liver. This is synthesised in the endoplasmic reticulum from 2-carbon-atom fragments derived from surplus glucose and fatty acids and from deaminated amino acids not required for protein production. The triglyceride is stored in the cytoplasm, usually as a single large globule surrounded and kept in suspension by a single layer of phospholipid molecules with their hydrophilic poles towards the aqueous cytosol. Metabolism of excessive dietary alcohol also causes storage of triglyceride fat, especially in the liver. Not only does alcohol provide 2-carbon-atom acetaldehyde molecules for synthesis of fatty acids but the protons released from alcohol by the enzyme alcohol dehydrogenase increase cellular NADPH and this impairs energy production by inhibiting aerobic respiration.

An important form of cell damage, not yet fully understood, is the accumulation of cholesterol and its esters in the myofibroblasts of the arterial intima (Fig. 3.10). This appears to result in part from excessive amounts of dietary animal fat which is composed mainly of triglyceride esters of long chain saturated fatty acids. Population surveys suggest that a relative deficiency of unsaturated fatty acids enhances the effect. In Western societies, the resulting swelling and damage to the arterial wall (atheroma) is a major cause of death and morbidity from ischaemic heart disease and stroke.

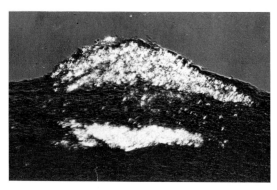

Fig. 3.10   Doubly refractile intimal cholesterol and cholesterol esters in early atheroma of the aorta photographed by polarised light.

In general, ingestion of excessive amounts of vitamins is harmless, though ill effects occur in hypervitaminosis D (p. 23.16) and A.

It should be noted that deficiencies due to inadequate diet or impaired intestinal absorption are frequently multiple. For example, malabsorption of fat is often accompanied by failure to absorb fat soluble vitamins A, D and K. Deficiency diseases are particularly evident during pregnancy and in childhood because of the special requirements for growth. If not fatal, many of the abnormalities of the intracellular pool of small molecules can persist for long periods and their correction by appropriate measures will return the affected cells to normal. However, even if this happens, there may be irreversible tissue damage, e.g. persisting bone deformities in individuals with healed rickets.

4. Synthesis of macromolecules

Synthesis of macromolecules by cells requires small organic molecules as building blocks, energy from ATP, synthesising machines (themselves composed of macromolecules such as nucleic acids and enzymatic proteins), control systems which turn the machines on and off to meet the needs of the body, and mechanisms which direct the delivery of the newly-synthesised molecules to the appropriate part of the cell where they exercise their function. Different macromolecules are synthesised at different sites within the cell. Nucleic acids are mainly produced within the nucleus. The endoplasmic reticulum is concerned with several functions, including synthesis of complex lipids associated with cell membranes, the oligosaccharide component of glyco-proteins and, where ribosomes are attached (the rough endoplasmic reticulum), membrane proteins and proteins for export from the cell as secretory products. Following initial synthesis in the endoplasmic reticulum, further enzymatic modification of the carbohydrate component of glycoproteins takes place in the Golgi apparatus, which also forms membrane-packaged vacuoles whose function is to distribute newly synthesis macromolecules to the appropriate part of the cell (secretions to the cell surface,

acid hydrolases to the lysosomes, etc.). In the cytosol, free ribosomes, often linked to form polyribosomes by thread-like molecules of mRNA, synthesise the enzymes involved in the intermediary metabolism of small molecules, which mainly takes place in that compartment of the cell.

The structure of macromolecules is determined not only by the small molecules of which they are composed, but by the order in which they are arranged. Two distinct mechanisms are involved: (1) those using a template already present in the cell (as in the arrangement of nucleotides in DNA and RNA and amino acids in polypeptides) and (2) those involving enzymatic recognition of each particular intermediate product and the addition of the next specific building block required in the sequence, a feature of the synthesis of all but the simplest carbohydrate and lipid molecules. These two categories are considered separately below.

Disorders of nucleic acid and protein synthesis

The roles of DNA, mRNA, tRNA and ribosomes in protein synthesis have already been outlined in Chapter 2, together with some examples of diseases due to abnormal proteins

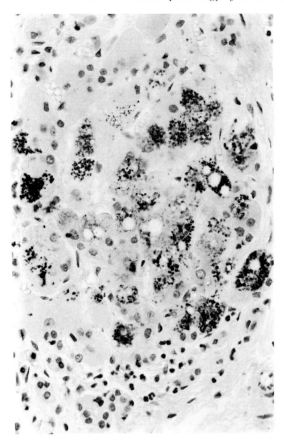

Fig. 3.11 The liver in α_1-antitrypsin deficiency. The hepatocytes have synthesised an abnormal form of protein which they cannot secrete. It is seen as numerous dark cytoplasmic globules which have been specifically stained with peroxidase-labelled antibody. $\times 570$.

whose synthesis is directed by mutant genes. In many of these disorders, such as the muscular dystrophies, the affected genes and their products have still to be identified, while in some it is known which enzyme is abnormal though the molecular basis remains obscure. In an increasing number of genetic disorders, a clear picture of the structural and functional abnormality is emerging at molecular and cellular level. Thus in sickle-cell disease, replacement of glutamic acid by valine in position 6 from the N terminal end of the β polypeptide chain alters the shape of haemoglobin in such a way that in hypoxic conditions the α and β chains of neighbouring molecules can combine to form large polymeric aggregates. As a result, the red cells acquire a characteristic sickle shape and abnormal rigid-ity which makes them unduly prone to mechanical injury and subsequent phagocytosis in the spleen. This explains the haemolytic crises which occur in this condition. Somewhat different effects of a single amino-acid substitution due to point mutation are seen in individuals who are homozygous for the gene which leads to a severe form of α_1-antitrypsin deficiency. Following synthesis, the abnormal protein (which has normal antitrypsin activity) is not released into the blood stream from the hepatocyte. Instead, it accumulates in the endoplasmic reticulum to form characteristic globules which can readily be seen by light microscopy (Fig. 3.11). A common finding in such patients is destruction of alveolar septa due to unopposed action of extracellular proteolytic enzymes in the lung.

A second important group of disorders of protein synthesis, already discussed, results from an inadequate supply of amino-acids and other essential precursor molecules. It has been shown in cultured cells that amino-acid deficiency leads to inactivation of a factor which initiates the assembly of ribosomes from their RNA subunits, thereby slowing the formation of new polypeptide chains in starvation.

There are also various poisons which directly affect the machinery for protein synthesis. Notable among these is the bacterial toxin produced by *Corynebacterium diphtheriae* whose biochemical effects are now well understood. In man and other species with appropriate cell surface receptors, diphtheria toxin enters the cell and catalyses the formation of ADP ribose, an abnormal product which blocks the ribosomal transpeptidase necessary for the formation of peptide bonds during protein synthesis. Even a single molecule of diphtheria toxin can lead to death of a cell.

Table 3.2 lists some other inhibitors of protein synthesis which have been widely used in biological research. In contrast to these, there are some poisons which induce the synthesis of proteins. A well known example is phenobarbitone, which by an unknown mechanism induces hepatocytes to synthesise unusually large amounts of cytochrome P450 and other enzymes responsible for the detoxification and excretion of certain organic compounds from the body. There is a corresponding increase in smooth endoplasmic reticulum, with which these enzymes are associated. While dim-

Table 3.2 Inhibitors of protein synthesis

Inhibitor	Mode of action
Actinomycin D	Binds to DNA Inhibits RNA polymerase
Alpha amanitin	Binds to RNA polymerase
Cycloheximide	Blocks ribosomal transpeptidase
Puromycin	Releases incomplete polypeptide from ribosome

inishing the toxicity of some substances, these changes may actually intensify liver damage due to others (e.g. carbon tetrachloride) by increasing the production of toxic metabolites, effects of considerable importance in clinical pharmacology.

Viral genes commonly lead to serious upsets in protein synthesis in infected cells. The viral proteins synthesised intracellularly can influence the metabolism of the affected cells in various ways, including interference with the production of host proteins and nucleic acids. Proteins of some viruses are incorporated in the membrane of infected cells and they may be treated as foreign antigens. The resulting immune response involves cytotoxic T lymphocytes (p. 7.20) which help to eliminate the infection by destroying cells harbouring the virus. Another mechanism of cell damage when synthesis of viral nucleic acid and protein is complete involves non-immunological rupture of the cell with release of infective virus particles (cytopathic effect).

Disorders of synthesis of other macromolecules

To date, remarkably few disorders of synthesis of lipid or carbohydrate macromolecules have been fully characterised. Two examples of secondary effects of enzyme abnormalities will now be considered, one affecting the normal polymerisation of glucose to form glycogen and the second, the synthesis of the glycocorticoid, cortisol.

Type IV glycogen storage disease. Glycogen is normally stored in cells for short term energy requirements. It consists of a linear 1,4 glycoside polymer of glucose with branches every twelfth unit or so. An extremely rare genetic deficiency of the brancher enzyme 1,4–1,6 transglucosylase leads to an abnormal

molecular form of glycogen which is resistant to digestion with diastase. The disorder, also known as *amylopectinosis* or *Andersen's disease*, leads to death in early childhood from hepatic cirrhosis or cardiac failure.

Congenital adrenal hyperplasia. A number of enzyme deficiencies are known to affect steroid hormone synthesis in the smooth endoplasmic reticulum of the adrenocortical cells. As might be expected, affected children are deficient in cortisol and this leads to hyperplasia of the adrenal cortex due to increased secretion of adrenocorticotropic hormone (ACTH) by the pituitary. Fig. 3.12 shows a female child with congenital adrenal hyperplasia whose external genitalia are masculinised (adrenogenital syndrome) as a result of deficiency of the enzyme 21-α hydroxylase which normally converts the androgenic steroid 17-α hydroxyprogesterone to a nonandrogenic precursor of cortisol.

Defective lipoprotein synthesis

Two rare but theoretically important autosomal recessive defects are recognised in the synthesis of lipoproteins—abetalipoproteinaemia and familial α-lipoprotein deficiency. In order to understand the nature and effects of these disorders, it is first necessary to consider the normal structure and functions of the lipoproteins. Lipoproteins are macromolecular complexes

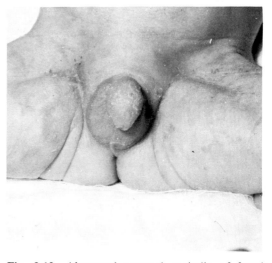

Fig. 3.12 Abnormal external genitalia of female child due to the action of androgen in a case of adrenogenital syndrome with 21-hydroxylase deficiency. (Professor M.A. Ferguson-Smith.)

Table 3.3 Properties of lipoproteins

Class	Density	Electrophoretic mobility	Apoprotein	Main core lipid	Site of formation
Chylomicrons	Extremely low	Alpha-2	C, B, A	Triglyceride	Intestinal epithelium
VLDL	Very low	Prebeta	C, B	Triglyceride	Hepatocyte
LDL	Low	Beta	B	Cholesterol ester	Plasma
HDL	High	Alpha-1	A, C	Cholesterol ester	Hepatocyte

with a water-insoluble lipid core consisting mainly of triglyceride fat or cholesterol esters, coated and held in solution by a film composed of hydrophilic apoprotein, polar phospholipid and cholesterol molecules. There are four classes (Table 3.3). Chylomicrons are synthesised by the epithelium of the small intestine for the onward transport of absorbed dietary triglyceride. The liver synthesises very low density lipoproteins (VLDL) for secretion of triglyceride formed there from fatty acids ori-

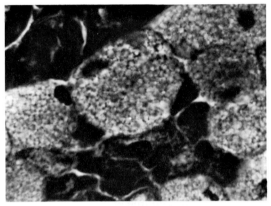

Fig. 3.14 Foamy cells—macrophages distended with multiple fine droplets of doubly-refractile lipid. Photographed through crossed polarising prisms. × 500.

ginating in adipose tissue stores or released from chylomicrons, or synthesised by the hepatocytes themselves when there is superfluous dietary carbohydrate or protein. High density lipoproteins (HDL) are also produced in the liver for the transport of cholesterol esters. The apoproteins of chylomicrons, VLDL and HDL are synthesised in the rough endoplasmic reticulum, while the long chain fatty acids are esterified with glycerol or cholesterol in the membranes of the smooth endoplasmic reticulum, the lipoprotein complexes being assembled in the cisternae prior to leaving the cell in secretory vacuoles. In contrast, low density lipoproteins (LDL) are formed in the circulation by transfer of cholesterol esters from HDL to VLDL 'remnants'—the apoprotein left over after the triglyceride core has been released from VLDL by lipase for use by peripheral tissues.

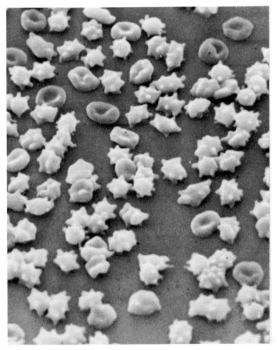

Fig. 3.13 Scanning electron micrograph of the red cells in a patient with abetalipoproteinaemia. Most of the red cells show the deformity of acanthocytes; a few show the appearance of normal biconcave discs. (Professor K.E. Carr.)

Abetalipoproteinaemia. This is characterised by total absence of apoprotein B, which prevents production of chylomicrons, VLDL and LDL. Following ingestion of triglyceride, the epithelial cells of the intestinal mucosa may become packed with fat droplets, the plasma triglyceride level fails to rise and the patient develops fatty diarrhoea. A characteristic feature is the presence of acanthocytes—erythrocytes with prickle-like surface projections (Fig. 3.13) due to the abnormal composition of their surface membranes, which reflects the lipid content of abetalipoproteinaemic serum. Later in life, neurological disorders and retinitis pigmentosa develop and death commonly results from cardiomyopathy.

Familial α-lipoprotein deficiency (Tangier disease) leads in homozygotes to absence of HDL. In this condition, large amounts of cholesterol esters are taken up by cells of the mononuclear phagocyte system and these become distended with lipid to form 'foam cells' (Fig. 3.14). There is enlargement of the spleen, lymph nodes and tonsils, the latter having a bright yellow colour which is pathognomonic of the condition.

Several of the disorders of synthesis of macromolecules described above illustrate the principle that a defect primarily expressed in one tissue may lead to secondary abnormalities in others.

5. Digestion and degradation of macromolecules

The enzymatic hydrolysis of macromolecules to form smaller fragments has several important physiological functions. (1) For transport across membranes, as in the digestion of food in the alimentary tract prior to its absorption by the intestinal epithelium. (2) To meet immediate specific requirements of the metabolic pool, for example the breakdown of muscle glycogen during exercise. (3) To degrade and remove components no longer required by the body. Thus certain rate-limiting enzymes may be destroyed when their products are present in abundance or, at the cellular level, effete erythrocytes are broken down after about a hundred days in the circulation. The small molecules so produced are generally recycled through the metabolic pool. (4) Activation of specific biological functions of a macromolecule by its hydrolysis at a single site, a mechanism used in the conversion of polypeptide prohormones to hormones, of proenzymes to enzymes, and of soluble precursors to insoluble fibrous polymers. Errors of degradation may thus lead to shortage of fuel or of essential building blocks, accumulation within the body of surplus macromolecules which cannot be re-used or excreted, or the impairment of function of specific proteins or polypeptides. The lysosomes are the principal site of intracellular digestion but some molecules are hydrolysed mainly elsewhere in the cell. Glycogen, for example, is converted to glucose mainly in the cytosol. Extracellular digestion takes place not only in the alimentary tract but also in the blood stream and in the interstitial tissues.

Lysosomes and their disorders

Lysosomes are cytoplasmic organelles limited by a single membrane. They contain various hydrolases which digest proteins, nucleic acids, fats, carbohydrates, etc. Under the electron microscope they present very varied appearances and can be recognised with certainty only by histochemical demonstration of their acid hydrolase activity. The enzymes have a low pH optimum and become active when the membrane of the primary lysosome is altered, e.g. by fusion with a phagocytic vacuole to form a secondary lysosome (phagolysosome).

Phagolysosomes which contain cytoplasmic membranes (e.g. derived from damaged mitochondria) are commonly encountered in cells with focal cytoplasmic damage such as follows irradiation. The damaged parts of the cell are taken into an autophagic vacuole which coalesces with lysosomes to form a phagolysosome, and the activated hydrolases digest the contents of the vacuole. Phagolysosomes containing both cytoplasmic and nuclear fragments are seen in cells whose neighbours have been eliminated by **apoptosis** (Fig. 3.15), a special form of cell death which occurs in various physiological and pathological circumstances and is described on p. 3.29. Material resistant to digestion sometimes remains within a

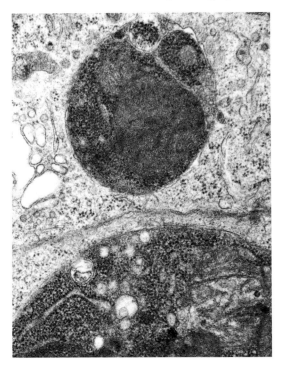

Fig. 3.15 Electron micrograph showing two phagolysosomes in adjacent cells of the intestinal mucosa of a mouse, following radiation injury. Mitochondria and glycogen granules can be identified in the large electron-dense vacuoles. × 57 000.

phagolysosome and forms one variety of residual body seen on electron microscopy. *Lipofuscin* pigment seems to originate from undigested lipid-rich material in this way.

Marked accumulation of metabolites in lysosomes with normal enzymes also occurs as a result of excessive production of substrate e.g. α chains of haemoglobin in red cell precursors in β thalassaemia (p. 17.28). Storage of heavy metals e.g. copper, or iron in the form of ferritin and haemosiderin, occurs in lysosomes when cells are overloaded with these substances.

Lysosomal permeability and cell damage. Lysosomal hydrolases seriously impair the biochemical function and structure of subcellular particles *in vitro* and there has been much speculation on the importance of lysosomal damage in cell injury *in vivo*. Damage to the lysosomal membrane leading to release of lysosomal enzymes into the cytosol of living cells results in various degrees of cell damage up to cell death. This happens in certain bacterial infections, e.g. by streptococci, and appears to

result from the action of bacterial toxins. It is also encountered in hypervitaminosis A where it is attributed to the surfactant effect of the vitamin on the lysosomal membranes. Another example is the necrosis of macrophages which have ingested silica particles; some of the silica of the particles within phagolysosomes is converted to silicic acid and this forms hydrogen bonds with the phospholipids of lysosomal membrane which then ruptures and releases the enzymes into the cytoplasm. Phagocytosis of monosodium urate crystals by neutrophil polymorphs in patients with gout is said to increase lysosomal permeability with resultant cell injury. Some photosensitivity reactions are due to lysosomal membrane damage when certain pigments, e.g. porphyrin, taken up by lysosomes, release energy on exposure to light of appropriate wavelength. Cortisol and chloroquine, drugs known to stabilise lysosomal membranes, diminish cell damage in vitamin A poisoning and in some photosensitivity reactions. In many forms of cellular injury, however, the 'suicidal' release of lysosomal enzymes into the cytosol does not seem to be an important factor. For example, autolysis by lysosomal enzymes in cells injured by hypoxia, carbon tetrachloride and many other poisons, occurs only after the cells have died.

Inherited deficiency of lysosomal enzymes. In individuals lacking an enzyme necessary for the catabolism of membrane-derived lipids, cells may accumulate lipids derived from the normal turnover of the plasma membranes and organelles. The accumulation of lipid is often especially prominent in macrophages because of their phagocytic function. A good example is **Gaucher's disease** in which there is a genetic deficiency of a lysosomal β-glucosidase. Normally, old worn-out red cells are phagocytosed and digested by macrophages, mainly in the spleen. In Gaucher's disease, the glucocerebrosides of the red cell membrane accumulate in phagolysosomes in the macrophages, which consequently become greatly enlarged, develop a characteristic appearance (Fig. 18.3) and are termed Gaucher cells. As a result, there is gross splenomegaly, hepatomegaly, and anaemia due to replacement of the haemopoietic tissue by Gaucher cells. Another form of Gaucher's disease affects the cerebral neurons.

In marked contrast to Gaucher's disease, the lesions of **Krabbe's disease** are confined to the

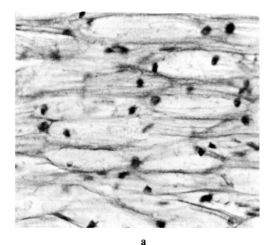

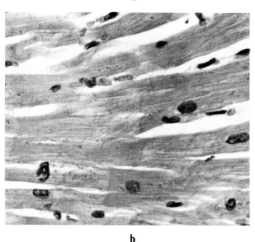

Fig. 3.16 Myocardium in Pompe's disease (**a**), compared with normal myocardium (**b**). The affected muscles fibres are distended with glycogen which does not stain with eosin but gives them a vacuolated appearance. × 460.

and Krabbe's diseases illustrate the great differences between lesions due to inherited deficiency of enzymes responsible for intracellular breakdown of lipids and they demonstrate some of the reasons for these differences.

In **Pompe's disease** there is excessive storage of glycogen in lysosomes due to the inherited deficiency of the lysosomal enzyme, α-glucosidase, which is normally present in all tissues and presumably hydrolyses the small amount of glycogen finding its way into phagolysosomes as a result of autophagy. Much of the stored glycogen is therefore found within greatly enlarged phagolysosomes and it seems likely that the various disorders of cellular function encountered are the result of phagolysosomal rupture and spilling of harmful hydrolases into the cytosol. This explains most of the features of Pompe's disease, namely, generalised glycogen storage, e.g. in the myocardium (Fig. 3.16), skeletal muscles, nervous and lymphoid tissues, and peripheral blood leucocytes. The results include enlargement of organs, cardiac failure, mental deficiency and general muscle weakness.

Failure of receptor-mediated endocytosis. In order to function normally, lysosomes require not only the appropriate digestive enzymes but also mechanisms such as the formation of phagolysosomes to give the enzymes access to their macromolecular substrates. Failure of one of these mechanisms, receptor-mediated endocytosis, is responsible for many cases of hyperbetalipoproteinaemia, a biochemical abnormality of great importance in the development of atheroma. Normally LDL (low density or β lipoproteins) are removed from the bloodstream and degraded by cells when they require cholesterol for the synthesis of new membranes, bile acids, steroid hormones etc. On their surface, such cells have specific LDL receptors and these mediate the uptake of LDL by endocytosis into vesicles which subsequently fuse with lysosomes. Following digestion of the contents, free cholesterol is released into the cytosol. Once the cell has an adequate supply of cholesterol, transcription of the LDL-receptor gene is switched off and uptake of LDL stops. Several different mutations affecting the production or effective function of LDL receptors are responsible for the condition known as **familial hypercholesterolaemia** (one form of hyperbetalipoproteinaemia). Heterozygotes have only half the number

central and peripheral nervous system because galactocerebroside, the substrate of the deficient enzyme, galactocerebroside β-galactosidase, is a major component only of myelin. In infancy, this recessive lysosomal enzyme defect leads to severe central and peripheral nervous dysfunction due to unexplained demyelination of axons. Krabbe's disease is also known as 'globoid leukodystrophy' since the white matter of the brain is particularly affected and the lesions contain macrophages: these are globoid in shape because they are distended with galactocerebroside which has characteristic electron microscopic appearances. Gaucher's

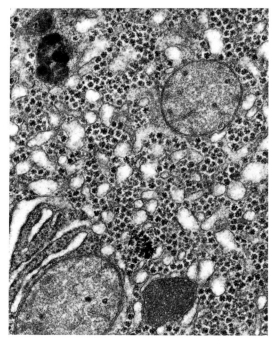

Fig. 3.17 Electron micrograph of normal liver showing the characteristic small, dense, round particles of glycogen. The large dense organelle at the top of the field is a residual body. × 30 000.

cholesterol-laden macrophages which are described as xanthomas when present in skin or tendons and as xanthelasmas in the eyelids. Homozygotes have no LDL receptors at all and develop hyperbetalipoproteinaemia of such severity that they frequently die from atheroma during childhood. It is clear that LDL have evolved not as a transport mechanism to dispose of unnecessary cholesterol, but as a store to conserve available supplies of cholesterol until required. This fact, together with modern dietary habits and the inability of the body either to break down or to excrete cholesterol in significant amounts, largely accounts for the present epidemic of ischaemic heart disease and stroke, both consequences of atheroma, in the Western world.

Non-lysosomal glycogenolysis

In the resting state, many kinds of cell contain free cytoplasmic particles of glycogen, a branching polymer of glucose (Fig. 3.17). Attached to the particles are the enzymes responsible for the main glycogenolytic pathway, failure of which thus leads to the accumulation of excessive amounts of glycogen in the cytosol.

Phosphorylase deficiency. The unbranched parts of the glycogen molecule are broken down by the sequential release of glucose 1-phosphate molecules by phosphorylase enzymes which are tissue-specific. Thus inherited deficiency of liver phosphorylase causes glycogen storage in the liver but not in skeletal muscle, while in **McArdle's syndrome** deficiency of muscle phosphorylase has the opposite effect. In contrast

of normal receptors. This leads to diminished uptake of LDL and high levels of LDL in the plasma, but deficiency of intracellular cholesterol is made good by the cells themselves synthesising new cholesterol molecules. The result is a further increase in the total body pool of cholesterol, further rise in plasma LDL, accelerated development of atheroma, arcus corneae and the formation of yellow masses of

Table 3.4   Components of the cytoskeleton

Component	Diameter (nm)	Chemical composition	Stable form	Unstable form
Microtubule	25	Tubulin	Cilia, flagella	Mitotic spindle
Intermediate filament (IF)	10	Keratin	Epithelial tonofilament	—
		Desmin	Muscle IF	—
		Neurofilament	Neuronal IF	—
		Glial acidic protein	Glial IF	—
		Vimentin	Fibroblasts, Muscle, Glial IF	—
Microfilament	7	Actin	Myofibril	Contractile fibres of non-muscle cells

Note. IF = intermediate filaments

to both of these conditions, deficiency of debrancher enzyme affects both liver and muscle.

To meet the intrinsic metabolic needs of the cell, glucose 1-phosphate is converted to glucose 6-phosphate and this requires to be hydrolysed by glucose 6-phosphatase to provide glucose for release from the liver (and kidney) to maintain the blood sugar level during fasting and exercise. **von Gierke's disease**, which is due to glucose 6-phosphatase deficiency, is thus characterised by hypoglycaemia and glycogen storage in the liver and kidney. Through its inhibitory effect on insulin synthesis, hypoglycaemia also leads to hypertriglyceridaemia, fatty change in the liver cells and xanthomatosis.

6. Cell form and movement

The cytoskeleton consists of arrays of microtubules, intermediate filaments and microfilaments, and is largely responsible for the shapes that cells adopt, for the arrangement of organelles within them, and for cellular movement. Microtubules are composed of polymerised tubulin and microfilaments of polymerised actin, while the intermediate filaments vary in chemical composition in different kinds of cells (Table 3.4). Each structure can be recognised by the use of labelled antibodies and their ultrastructural appearances (including size) are also distinctive. Microtubules and microfibrils can assemble and disintegrate very rapidly, properties which allow them to form transient structures, such as the mitotic spindle, to meet temporary needs of the cell. In contrast, intermediate filaments are stable and long-lasting as are the structural specialisation for movement in muscle cells—myofibrils composed of actin and myosin—and the microtubular cores of the flagella of spermatozoa and the cilia of respiratory and other epithelia. It is not yet known how the structure and functions of the various components of the cytoskeleton are co-ordinated, but the centrioles and the microtubules arising from them probably have an important role.

Abnormalities of microtubules. The movement of cilia and flagella is brought about by the parallel microtubules which lie in their cores and which slide over each other due to changes in the configuration of the protein dynein, an ATPase which links adjacent microtubules.

In **Kartagener's syndrome**, inherited deficiency of dynein (or, in some families of certain other microtubule-associated proteins) results in immotility of cilia and flagella and leads to recurrent respiratory infections and male infertility. In addition, there is a remarkable error in early development in 50% of cases—*situs inversus* (dextrocardia, left sided liver, etc.)—suggesting that cilia or flagella are concerned in the morphogenetic movements which determine laterality in early embryogenesis.

Unstable arrays of microtubules are readily affected by drugs which bind to tubulin. In this way, colchicine leads to disappearance of the mitotic spindle, an effect which is reversed by removal of the drug. The anticancer agents vincristine and vinblastine also inhibit the formation of microtubules and block cells in mitosis.

Microfilament disorders. Poisons such as the cytochalasins, which bind to actin, and so prevent elongation of microfilaments by further polymerisation, interfere with phagocytosis and (except in muscle cells) with contractile movements involved in cell locomotion. Phalloidin, a toxin derived from the toadstool *Amanita phalloides*, also paralyses cell movements but it does so by preventing depolymerisation of microfilaments.

Intermediate filaments. Little is known of the physiological function of intermediate filaments or of their role in disease. Certain long-recognised cytoplasmic abnormalities are due to aggregation of intermediate filaments. For example, the well known effect of high circulating levels of adrenal glucocorticoids on the ACTH-producing cells of the anterior pituitary—Crooke's hyaline change—is seen ultrastructurally to consist of a mass of intermediate filaments in the perinuclear region. Electron microscopy of hepatocytes also shows that Mallory's alcoholic hyalin (p. 20.24) is composed of intermediate filaments.

7. Communication between cells

Intercellular communication is essential for the co-ordination of development and of function in multicellular animals. In general, information can be exchanged between cells by at least three distinct mechanisms.

1. Gap junctions between adjacent cells establish cytoplasmic continuity and allow exchange of ions and small molecules. Gap junctions are undoubtedly of major physiological importance (e.g. in the electrical coupling of myocardial cells) and they are probably equally important in disease, though precise roles have not yet been established.

2. By membrane-associated signalling molecules, such as those of the major histocompatibility complex (p. 2.12), which allow cells in contact to recognise one another. Thus as a rule immunisation normally occurs only if antigen is presented to T (thymic-dependent) lymphocytes by special cells such as macrophages which express HLA-DR markers on their surface. It now seems possible that inappropriate expression of HLA DR by other cells such as thyroid epithelium or insulin-producing B cells of the pancreatic islets may signal T cells to mount abnormal immune responses, thus leading to auto-immune disease.

3. By the release of soluble chemical signals, such as hormones, neurotransmitters or other chemical mediators which modify the behaviour of other cells bearing receptors of appropriate specificity. Steroid hormones, being lipid soluble, pass through cell membranes freely, but once in the cytoplasm they form complexes with specific hormone receptor proteins. These complexes have high affinity for certain parts of the nuclear DNA and selectively alter gene expression in the target cell. In contrast to steroid hormones, most other diffusible signalling molecules, such as polypeptide hormones and the classical neurotransmitters, combine with specific receptors which project from the outer surface of the plasma membrane, the effects within the cell being mediated by 'second messengers' such as cyclic AMP or Ca^{++} (p. 7.4–5). Internalisation of ligands by receptor-mediated endocytosis also occurs but this is probably of importance mainly in 'down regulation' of the number of cell surface receptors.

Most known examples of abnormalities of communication between cells affect soluble chemical signals or their receptors. Sometimes the fault lies in the cell producing the molecular signal (ligand) but often the target-cell receptor is abnormal due to the binding of drugs, poisons or antibodies, or because of a genetic defect.

Abnormal soluble chemical signals. The classical example, the production of androgen instead of cortisol by the adrenal cortex, due to inherited deficiency of the enzyme 21-hydroxylase, has already been described (p. 3.11). It is important to note that different tissues, though containing the same testosterone receptors, respond differently to excess hormone, the Mullerian duct becoming atrophied while the clitoris enlarges.

Failure to destroy local chemical mediators which are normally broken down rapidly leads to abnormal signalling such as is seen in muscle tissue following the administration of anticholinestrase drugs. Furthermore, if cells are presented with unusual substrates, they may synthesise abnormal messengers which have non-physiological effects. For example, an increased supply of the substrate tyramine (in place of tyrosine, to which tyramine is normally converted in the liver) leads to the synthesis by adrenergic neurons of the false neurotransmitter octopamine and this may be a cause of the tremor and coma encountered in severe liver disease ('*hepatic encephalopathy*').

There is interesting preliminary evidence that inappropriate or excessive production of chemical signals by certain cerebral neurons may be involved in the pathogenesis of schizophrenia and depressive illnesses.

Inherited defects of testosterone receptors. Other than the gonads themselves, the embryonic development of most of the genital system in the two sexes is determined mainly by the presence or absence of testosterone produced by the fetal testes at an appropriate stage of development. If no testosterone is produced, female genitalia are formed. This also happens in male embryos with normally functional testes if the cells of the body are unable to respond to testosterone due to inherited deficiency of testosterone receptors—a condition known as the **testicular feminisation syndrome**.

Induced changes in cell surface receptors.
Intercellular signalling may be disturbed due to
the binding of drugs, poisons or antibodies to
cell surface receptors. Thus the arrow poison
curare, now used therapeutically as a muscle
relaxant, blocks access of acetylcholine to its
receptor at the motor end plate in skeletal
muscle. In myasthenia gravis, in which antibody is formed against the same receptor,
curare-like effects are also produced.

It is of interest that two drugs, carbachol and
atropine, which combine with the muscarinic
receptor on smooth muscle cells, have quite
opposite effects. Carbachol mimics the action
of the normal neurotransmitter, acetylcholine,
while this is blocked by atropine. By analogy,
in patients with auto-immune thyroid disease,
there are antibodies against the TSH (thyrotrophin) receptors of thyroid epithelium which
have opposing effects. As its name implies,
thyroid stimulating antibody leads to hyperthyroidism, while certain blocking antibodies
inhibit the normal response of thyroid epithelial cells to TSH and depress thyroid activity.

8. Cell growth and replication

Cell growth and replication are necessary not
only for normal development of the body but
also for its continued maintenance. Growth involves cellular enlargement by the incorporation of additional macromolecules (excluding
those destined for secretion) and is a prelude to
cell replication.

Depending on their origin, most normal cell
types enlarge in tissue culture and undergo a
limited number of mitotic divisions (about
twenty) provided the conditions are right. An
adequate supply of nutrients must be present in
the medium together with certain hormones
and/or other growth factors. For example,
thyrotrophin must be added to obtain growth
of thyroid epithelium, while interleukin 2, a
growth factor produced by helper T lymphocytes, permits *in vitro* proliferation of other T
lymphocytes bearing the appropriate cell surface receptor. Mitosis does not readily take
place in cells which are close together, because
protein synthesis, an essential preliminary to
the synthesis of DNA, is inhibited by overcrowding. This phenomenon, previously attributed to 'contact inhibition' is now known to be
due to closely packed cells assuming a rounded
form rather than the flattened configuration
which favours protein synthesis.

Mechanisms of the above sort also operate *in
vivo*, though clearly they must be regulated by
delicately balanced feedback controls which involve signalling not only between similar cells,
but also between cells of different kinds (e.g.
between ACTH-producing corticotrophs of the
anterior pituitary and cortisol-secreting cells of
the adrenal cortex). In intact organs, the position of a cell in relation to others is an additional factor of major importance in the control
of cell division, mitotic figures in the epidermis,
for example, normally being confined to the
basal layers.

Circumstances in which cells proliferate

In the body, cell proliferation takes place in five
sets of circumstances.

1. As part of normal embryonic, fetal and
postnatal development. At an early stage, the
regulation of growth is remarkably flexible
and even when an embryo splits to form monozygotic twins, each rapidly grows to become
normal in size.

2. In the maintenance of the status quo following cell loss by normal wear and tear. Thus
there is normally an exact balance between
exfoliation of keratinocytes from the surface
of the skin and the production of new cells in
the basal layers of the epidermis.

3. As an adaptive response to loss of tissue
following injury. The processes involved include
replication of specialised cells to replace those
which have been lost—*regeneration* (p. 5.1) or,
if this does not happen, the proliferation of
fibroblasts to fill the space with a collagenous
scar—*repair* (p. 5.4).

4. As an adaptive response to special functional demands. For example, thyroid epithelium undergoes hyperplasia (excessive but
reversible proliferation p. 5.24) in response to
increased pituitary TSH when thyroid hormone

secretion is impaired due to iodine deficiency. Similarly, there is hyperplasia of erythrocyte precursor cells in the bone marrow mediated by the hormone erythropoietin which is produced in response to chronic oxygen lack. Cell division by B lymphocytes following contact with antigen (p. 6.18) is a striking example of a proliferative response to a special environmental stimulus. It is of particular interest because it usually requires a second signal from an activated helper T lymphocyte. It should be noted that certain specialised cells, such as cardiac and skeletal muscle, are unable to divide in the adult and they respond to increased workload by an increase in size rather than number (*hypertrophy* p. 5.24).

5. As part of the abnormal process of tumour formation unrelated to the needs of the body. In general, the excessive proliferation of tumour cells appears to be due to the inappropriate and irreversible expression of one or more genes which take part in the regulation of normal growth. For example, growth of normal epidermal cells is stimulated physiologically by a polypeptide epidermal growth factor which activates an intracellular tyrosine phosphokinase enzyme through a specific cell-surface receptor. It now seems likely that irreversible switching on of the genes coding either for epidermal growth factor or its receptor, or for tyrosine phosphokinase, may each contribute to cell proliferation in different tumours (see pp. 13.9–12 for further discussion).

Hypoplasia and atrophy

These terms are used to indicate a decrease in size and/or numbers of specialised cells as a result of which the relevant tissue never attains its normal size during development (*hypoplasia*) or, having reached a normal size, subsequently becomes smaller (*atrophy*). In addition to being shrunken, atrophic organs are sometimes brown in colour ('brown atrophy') due to the accumulation in the cell cytoplasm of residual bodies containing lipofuscin, a pigment derived from lipids which are resistant to digestion by lysosomal enzymes (p. 11.19). In general, these states are due either to diminished growth or to failure to compensate for increased loss of cells which have been eliminated by apoptosis (p. 3.29). Some of the mechanisms involved are now described.

Hypoplasia may be genetically determined as in achondroplasia, in which growth of the cartilaginous skeleton is impaired, or it may result from endocrine insufficiency as in pituitary dwarfism due to inadequate production of growth hormone. Other mechanisms include cell loss from infection or poisoning. German measles during early pregnancy may damage the fetal heart and lead to incomplete development of the cardiac septa and other congenital cardiac defects, while the anti-emetic drug thalidomide has a specific toxic effect on certain cells of the developing limb buds.

Physiological atrophy. Atrophy is a normal aspect of ageing of many tissues, for example, the loss of thymocytes and shrinkage of the thymus after puberty, the reduction in endometrial cellularity after the menopause and of osteocytes in the ageing skeleton. The biological clock(s) initiating these changes are not understood, but they are probably not a consequence of the limited number of times a normal cell can divide.

Nutritional atrophy. This may be produced locally by arterial disease interfering with the blood supply to a part when the reduction is not sufficiently severe to cause extensive necrosis. Atrophy of the functioning parenchymatous tissue (e.g. renal tubular epithelium or myocardial muscle fibres) is sometimes accompanied by overgrowth of fibrous tissue.

General atrophy occurs in starvation. Emaciation depends chiefly on utilisation of the fat of the adipose tissues, but there is also a general wasting of the tissues, the liver and muscles being particularly affected. (The term **cachexia** is often applied to the combination of wasting, anaemia and weakness, and is mainly seen in severely ill patients in whom loss of appetite and other gastro-intestinal disturbances lead to diminished food intake. In most cases, there usually are additional contributary factors such as the increased catabolism of fever and other, less well-defined effects).

Disuse atrophy. In general, diminished functional activity is associated with reduced catabolism which in turn has a negative feedback effect on anabolism and leads to decrease in size of cells. For example, when the pancreatic duct is obstructed, secretion of digestive enzymes ceases and apoptosis of the exocrine cells leads to shrinkage of the organ. Similarly, the muscles responsible for operating a joint which

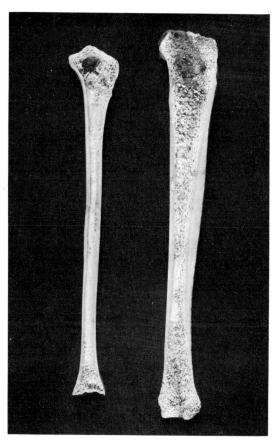

Fig. 3.18 Tibia from a longstanding case of polio-myelitis, showing marked atrophy (*left*). Normal tibia for comparison (*right*). × 0·3.

has been immobile for some weeks become wasted, and in paralysed limbs the bones become atrophic (Fig. 3.18). Unless such atrophy has become extreme, it is reversible and full functional activity may be restored.

Neuropathic atrophy. This happens when there is any destruction of lower motor neurons or their axons. After nerve section, the denervated muscles may lose half their mass. For at least a few weeks anabolic processes continue at a normal rate but catabolism, due to increased lysosome numbers and activity, is greatly accelerated. The affected muscles give pecular electromyographic 'reactions of degeneration' which indicate that the phenomenon is different from disuse atrophy and that complete return to normal is no longer possible.

Endocrine atrophy. Atrophy of thyroid, adrenals and gonads are seen when damage to the pituitary results in diminished secretion of the appropriate trophic hormones. In hypothyroidism, there is marked atrophy of the target organs of thyroid hormones, notably the skin, hair follicles and sebaceous glands, but their structure and function may be restored by oral administration of thyroxine. In contrast, congenital hypothyroidism leads to irreversible neuronal damage within a few weeks.

Atrophy due to increased catabolism. This may occur in fever or following severe trauma. The amount of dietary nitrogen is less than that excreted (negative nitrogen balance) and this is mainly due to increased catabolism and reduced synthesis of protein in skeletal muscle (p. 10.44).

Pressure atrophy. Atrophy of an organ may be brought about by pressure from benign tumours or cysts which interfere with the blood supply or function of the tissue. Interestingly, when bone is subject to pressure it is actively absorbed by osteoclasts.

Post-irradiation atrophy. In contrast to the various forms of atrophy described above, post-irradiation atrophy is not due to altered control of cell division but to chromosomal damage which interferes with the process of mitosis itself. Details are given on pp. 3.24-29.

9. Differentiation

Differentiation is the process of structural and functional specialisation of cells which occurs in multicellular organisms. Differentiated cells such as hepatocytes and lymphocytes are easily distinguished by qualitative and quantitative differences in the macromolecules they contain (enzymes, receptors, secretions, etc.), in their morphological features and in their functional relationship with other cells. These differences depend on the selection of genes which each cell type expresses and this in turn depends on the developmental history of the cell and of its precursors (p. 2.10) and on the signals it is receiving from its environment. Differentiation not

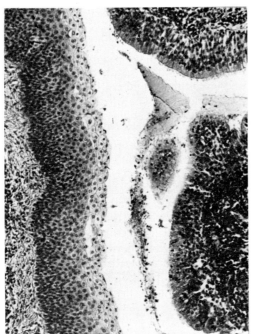

Fig. 3.19 Metaplasia of bronchial epithelium to stratified squamous type is seen on the left side, persistence of columnar ciliated epithelium on the right. × 200.

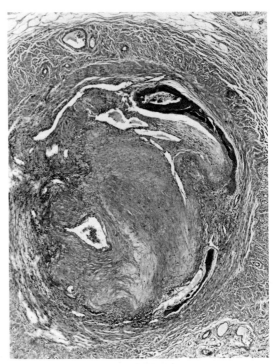

Fig. 3.20 Metaplastic bone formation in the wall of a largely obliterated artery. × 50.

only allows a cell to perform certain specialised functions more effectively, it also restricts its potential to carry out others. Thus, as they mature many differentiated cells irreversibly lose their capacity for mitotic division and the last stage of differentiation often leads to death of the cell, as in the surface layer of the epidermis. Indeed, genetically-controlled programmes leading to the death of certain cells by apoptosis (p. 3.29) is an essential feature of normal development.

Three kinds of abnormal differentiation are conventionally described.

Heterotopia. This arises during embryonic development and is characterised by groups of cells differentiating in a manner which is inappropriate to their anatomical position in the body. An example is the presence of small clusters of pancreatic acini (sometimes with islets) in the wall of the stomach. The pathogenesis is unknown but presumably the lesion results from focal errors in intercellular communication in the developing fetus.

Metaplasia. Metaplasia means the transformation of one type of differentiated tissue into another. An example is provided by the surface epithelium of the bronchi which commonly changes from the normal ciliated pseudostratified columnar type to stratified squamous (Fig. 3.19). In this example it appears that chronic injury or irritation, often due to cigarette smoke, results in adaptive changes in the surface epithelium to a type likely to be more resistant to the cause of the irritation. Similarly, stratified squamous epithelium may form as a result of chronic irritation in the mucous membrane of the nose, salivary ducts, gallbladder, renal pelvis and urinary bladder. In some cases the injurious stimulus is apparent, e.g. when there is a stone in the gallbladder or renal pelvis or in cases of extroversion of the urinary bladder, while in others the cause is obscure. In vitamin A deficiency, in addition to xerophthalmia, stratified squamous epithelium may replace the transitional and columnar epithelia of the nose, bronchi and urinary tract, and the specialised secretory epithelia of the lacrimal and salivary glands. In auto-immune chronic gastritis, in which there is an immunological attack on the mucosa of the fundus of the patient's own stomach, the specialised surface-lining cells and chief and parietal cells of the gastric glands are often replaced by tall columnar cells with striated borders, goblet cells and Paneth cells, i.e. metaplasia to an intestinal type of mucosa.

In the connective tissues, metaplasia occurs between fibrous tissue, myxoid tissue, bone and cartilage. Bone formation occasionally follows the deposition of calcium in such tissues as arterial walls (Fig. 3.20), bronchial cartilage and the uveal tract of the eye. In healing fractures, cartilaginous metaplasia may occur especially when there is undue mobility. The flattened serosal mesothelium of the rabbit pleural cavity becomes cubical, columnar, transitional or even stratified squamous following injection of the dye Sudan III with sodium cholate in olive oil, and the lining of adjacent alveoli also becomes cubical or columnar. Similar changes, which are rapidly reversible, follow the injection of strontium chloride.

The examples of metaplasia described above persumably are due to gene activation and/or repression due to environmental signals.

Metaplastic cells may give rise to tumours which exhibit the same type of metaplasia. Metaplasia may also arise in tumour cells *de novo*, striking examples being seen in the inappropriate synthesis of hormones by tumour cells. Thus certain tumours derived from the pancreatic islets produce the polypeptide hormone gastrin, a phenomenon known as ectopic hormone synthesis since gastrin is not a normal product of islet cells. In such cases it is probable that the switch of biochemical function is not simply a response to environmental signals but the result of a genetic change, such as somatic mutation, in the neoplastic clone. Metaplasia is to be distinguished from encroachment of one tissue upon another. Thus the fatty marrow of the long bones is replaced in certain types of anaemia by red haemopoietic marrow: in this case the haemopoietic tissue has spread by proliferation of haemopoietic stem cells and not by metaplasia of the adipose tissue cells originally present.

Dedifferentiation. Cells frequently lose some of their specialised characters when they become atrophic. A much more important phenomenon, often wrongly attributed to dedifferentiation, is seen in tumours, in which excessive cellular proliferation may be due in part to *failure to differentiate* to a stage of maturation at which mitosis can no longer take place.

Cell damage due to ionising radiation

Because of the widespread use of radiation and radioactive materials in industry and medicine the study of their effects on living matter is now of great importance. Of all the branches of radiation biology—molecular, sub-cellular, cellular, organ and whole animal—cellular radiation biology is the most instructive in the present state of knowledge. This is firstly because the measurement of its effects on proliferation or neoplastic transformation of cells in culture makes quantitation fairly easy. Secondly, it appears that effects on whole organs or whole animals can often, to a first approximation at least, be described or explained on the basis of cellular injury, although it must be emphasised that the effects of radiation on the individual cannot easily be explained fully by its effects on his component cells. The importance of molecular or sub-cellular processes in the development or repair of radiation damage is therefore judged by the roles they play in determining the future of the cell.

Radiation causes its effects by transferring energy to the substance through which it passes. This energy can produce two changes, excitation or ionisation. Excitation is a change in the energy state of some electrons or charged parts of molecules. Radiations which, like ultra-violet light, produce excitations only, are of very low penetrating power and are not discussed in this section. Other radiations produce mixtures of ionisations and excitations.

Measurement of radiation

No widely useful and accurate biological method of measuring radiation dose has so far been developed. The standard methods of measuring radiation dose are purely physical. Three methods are in common use. The first is based on the application of a voltage to an air-filled chamber through which the ionising radiation passes. This voltage has the effect of separating the positive and negative electric charges produced by the ionisations and produces a small electric current.

The second uses x-ray film exposed to radiation through selected filters and processed in a standard way. The third uses thermoluminescent materials (TLD) which emit light when heated after being irradiated.

These methods are calibrated against an absolute method of measuring radiation dose based on the measurement of the total energy absorbed from a beam of radiation by a solid material. The material must be one in which no radiation-produced chemical energy can be stored, all of it being transformed into heat which can be measured by sensitive calorimetry. The unit of absorbed dose is the *gray* (Gy), called after the British scientist who did fundamental work on the oxygen effect described below. Absorbed dose used to be expressed in units called *rads*. The new unit, Gy, equals 100 rads.

Much research has been done on the effects of radiation on aqueous solutions; these are mediated primarily through the decomposition products of the water, and probably reflect the initial damage produced in living biological material. However, this initial damage has never been directly observed in cells. The effects which are observed are the result of an interaction, between the disruptive effects on the normal biochemical processes and the response of the cell or organism in trying to overcome the disruption. From an analysis of these effects much has been learned about the nature of the disruption and repair, but very much more still remains unknown.

Types of ionising radiation

Ionising radiations fall into three categories; electromagnetic radiations (x-rays and γ-rays), charged particles (electrons, protons and heavier nuclei), and uncharged particles (neutrons).

All of these radiations can be administered to animals and human beings externally or internally. External sources include x-ray machines, electron accelerators, γ-ray sources, nuclear reactors and atomic bombs. Internal irradiation arises from the ingestion of any of the hundreds of known radionuclides (radioactive isotopes) many of which are used for medical diagnostic or therapeutic purposes; they are produced in nuclear reactors. The dosage has, in the past, been expressed as *curies* (Ci), but the modern unit is the *becquerel* (Bq) after the French scientist who discovered radioactivity. One Ci equals 3.7×10^{10} Bq. The best known severe radiation damage from accidental ingestion of radioactive material is that produced by radium which was once used extensively in luminising paints. Some sufferers from radium poisoning have been under medical supervision for fifty years and the effects are well documented. Today, in spite of strict regulations and control, occasional accidents occur in nuclear reactors, industry and hospitals, which result in significant radiation of personnel. Ionising radiation for diagnosis and therapy, however, has a secure and important place in modern medicine and has been essential for many research purposes.

Everyone is exposed throughout life to what is called **background radiation**. This includes fall-out from bomb tests, medical radiation and natural background. The last comes from natural radioactivity in our bodies, from the ground and from walls of buildings, from cosmic rays and from the air in houses. The air in poorly ventilated houses can give significant lung radiation.

Cellular radiation effects

Measurement of cellular radiation effects is often based on the survival curve, i.e. on the ability of cells to multiply in appropriate environmental conditions. One of the most marked effects of radiation is the destruction of this ability. The number of cells in which the ability survives can be readily measured by counting the number of clones in cultures of the irradiated cells.

The percentage 'survival', that is, the percentage of cells which still retain the ability to produce clones after irradiation, is plotted on a logarithmic scale and the radiation dose is plotted on a linear scale (Fig. 3.21). Since log per-

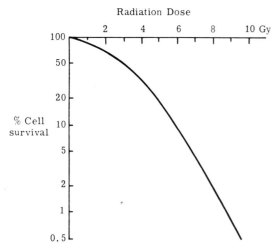

Fig. 3.21 Radiation injury, showing the relationship between percentage cell survival and dose of ionising radiation.

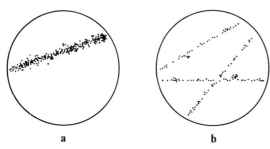

Fig. 3.22 The distribution of ionisations for high LET radiation (**a**) and low LET radiation (**b**).

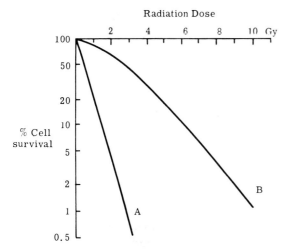

Fig. 3.23 The comparative cytotoxic effects of α-particles (A) and electrons (B).

centage decreases continuously with increasing dosage, the origin is placed in the top left corner of the figure. The resultant curve usually approximates to a straight line after an initial shoulder. This shoulder shows that the cells can repair some of the damage at low doses, but not at higher doses, which are more efficient at killing cells. If, however, heavily irradiated cells are allowed to recover for some hours, it is found that the shoulder reappears, showing that the ability to repair some of the damage has been recovered.

The slope of the portion of the survival curve, which is almost straight on the log-linear plot of Fig. 3.21—the exponential part—represents the rate at which additional lethal damage is produced as additional dose is administered. The fact that this portion of the curve is almost straight means that, irrespective of the damage already created, a given amount of irradiation always reduces the survival by the same fraction.

The available evidence suggests that, within each category of radiation, no great differences exist in the slopes of survival curves for various types of mammalian cells, unless they are hypoxic when irradiated. The magnitude of the shoulder, however, is dependent on the history, the environment, and the biochemical condition of the cells.

Linear energy transfer effect. Survival curves referring to different types of radiation have different shapes. The reason for this is that although, for equal doses of different radiations, the total number of ionisations are equal, the geometrical distribution of these ionisations in the cell can vary greatly. These large variations in distribution have a considerable effect on the mean number of ionisations necessary to produce the kind of biological damage which, after complex development, results in a cell losing its ability to continue to divide.

Heavy charged particles moving relatively slowly produce dense columns of ionisations, while electrons produce sparse lines of ionisations with occasional small clumps (Fig. 3.22). The average amount of energy deposited per micron of track of a particle or photon is called the linear energy transfer (LET) and can be used to characterise the quality of the radiation. A number of ionisations grouped closely together are more likely to initiate a lethal chain of biological events than the same number of

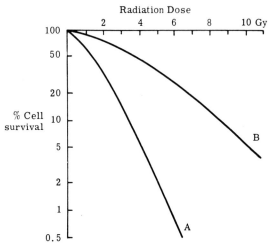

Fig. 3.24 The effect of oxygen on the cytotoxic effect of x-irradiation. A, high oxygen tension; B, low oxygen tension.

ionisations widely separated, perhaps by preventing repair mechanisms from acting effectively. Thus the survival curves for high LET radiation such as α-particles show no shoulder, and have a steeper slope than those for low LET radiation such as x-rays or electrons (Fig. 3.23). For both these reasons a dose of high

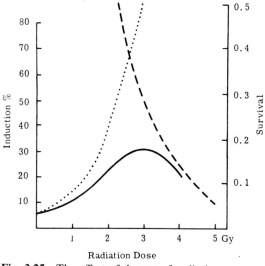

Fig. 3.25 The effect of dosage of radiation on mutation rate in mice. As the dose is increased, the mutation rate rises (dotted line), but the survival rate diminishes (interrupted line). The incidence of mutation-dependent abnormality, in this case leukaemia, is dependent on mutation and survival rates, and is shown by the continuous line.

LET radiation produces far more biological damage than an equal dose of low LET radiation.

Effect of oxygen. Another factor which has a striking effect on survival curves is the presence or absence of oxygen. Oxygen has the ability to combine with freshly severed ends of molecular structures thus preventing them from rejoining, which they commonly do if the opportunity presents itself. Oxygen thus interferes with a natural recovery process—a different one from that which produces the shoulder—and causes a given dose of radiation to be much more damaging than it would be in hypoxic or anoxic conditions. The ratio of the doses required to reduce the survival to the same level in anoxic and normal conditions is called the **oxygen enhancement ratio** (OER) (Fig. 3.24).

There are many other radio-sensitisers and radio-protectors which affect different levels of recovery and repair processes. Estimation of the biological damage produced by a given dose of radiation must therefore take into account both the type of radiation, the environment in which it is administered and the time allowed for repair and recovery.

Mutations and neoplastic transformation. Radiation damage that changes cells without killing them is also important. Errors are produced in the DNA base sequence, the number of errors—mutations—being related to the radiation dose, as illustrated in Fig. 3.25. A given dose of radiation may give rise to the same total number of mutations irrespective of the number of individuals among whom it is distributed. There is therefore no 'safe' level of radiation.

If the mutations are in the germ cells, children of irradiated parents can be affected. If the mutations are in somatic cells (p. 2.10), malignant tumours can be induced by the radiation (p. 13.25). The commonest radiation-induced tumours are leukaemia and tumours of thyroid, breast, bone and lung.

Tissue radiation effects

The effect of radiation in destroying the ability of cells to continue dividing has been discussed above in relation to individual cells. It is important because it plays a major part in causing tissue effects. Cell function which is not related to mitosis and division is relatively insensitive to radiation. Much higher doses of radiation are required to produce gross changes in such function than are required to inhibit cell division. When cell death follows large doses of radiation it has the features of apoptosis (p. 3.29) rather than of necrosis. The typical radiation effect on tissues arises from an inhibition of division.

Tissues whose cells are undergoing continuous controlled division, and whose integrity requires a continual flow of new cells, are therefore the first tissues to show the effects of radiation. The most obvious are the skin, the intestinal tract, the bone marrow and the immunity system. Similar considerations apply to the therapeutic use of radiation for malignant tumours, in which there is excessive division of cells. The initial effect upon a tissue is a reduction in cell numbers as the supply of new cells falls below the normal rate. The drop in cell numbers leads via homeostatic feedback mechanisms to a build up of the population of viable stem-cells from which new cells are produced, and to an increase in the rate of cell division. If this compensation is successful, then in due course enhanced production of cells not only restores the depleted population but commonly results in a temporary hyperplasia or overshoot before the cell numbers return to normal (Fig. 3.26). The inflammatory response to trauma follows injury by irradiation and commonly results in permanent structural changes, e.g. fibrosis.

The fall, rise, overshoot and return to normal of the cell populations exhibiting such behaviour after irradiation can be understood and explained in cellular terms if the appropriate homeostatic feedback mechanisms are known. The normal cell turnover controls the rate at which the cell population falls following irradiation. The extent of the fall depends on the percentage of surviving cells and the rate at which they can divide.

If the cell population of a tissue falls below a critical value the tissue can lose its functional effectiveness. In the cases of the intestinal tract and the bone marrow the result is death of the individual. A rapidly administered x-ray dose of about 8 Gy to the bone marrow and 12 Gy to the intestinal tract reduces the number of surviving cells to such low levels that the delay before an adequate production of cells can be re-established is long enough to allow the cell population to fall below the critical value.

The cells whose reproductive ability has been destroyed by the irradiation often remain in the tissue for some time. Their abortive attempts to divide or prepare to divide can produce gross abnormalities in cytological appearance (Fig. 3.27). Toxic products of cell disintegration can increase the damage. However, the damaged cells are no longer directly relevant to the course of events leading to permanent damage or repair. This course is determined by the number of surviving cells still capable of division and by the kinetics of proliferation in the

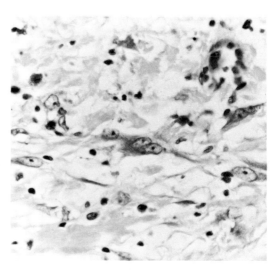

Fig. 3.27 Changes in the sub-epithelial connective tissue of the tongue following irradiation therapy for an epithelial tumour six years ago. Note the abnormally large connective tissue cells, one of which is binucleate. × 340.

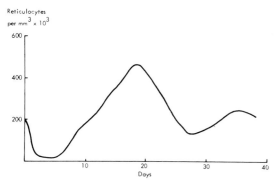

Reticulocytes per mm^3 × 10^3

Fig. 3.26 Changes in the numbers of reticulocytes in the blood following 2 Gy whole-body irradiation.

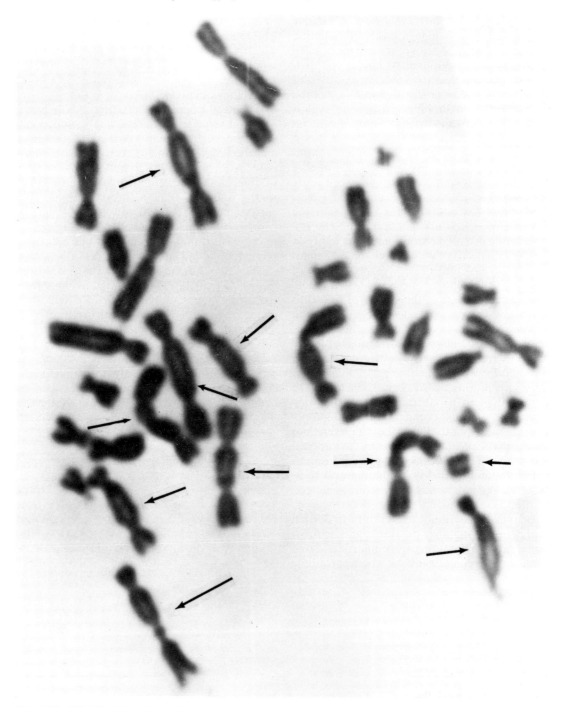

Fig. 3.28 Dividing lymphocyte in peripheral blood culture from a patient with bronchial carcinoma and spinal metastases, treated by five Gy of ^{60}Co radiation to the lumbar spine. This cell shows the result of extensive chromosome breakage due to radiation followed by random fusion of broken ends. There are nine dicentric chromosomes, one possible tricentric, one acricentric fragment and at least three other abnormal chromosomes. 44 centromeres can be counted, indicating elimination of two chromosomes. (Aceto-orcein stain). ×2000. (Professor M.A. Ferguson Smith.)

tissue. Ultimately, however, if a large enough dose is given (about 18 Gy in a single exposure) a tissue condition described as the **limit of tolerance** is reached. Although the nature of this is not understood, it is the determing factor for radiotherapy, and represents an accumulation of permanent, irreparable damage.

Tissues whose cells are long-lived and therefore are not normally dividing show very little effect after doses of several grays. Damage has been done, however, and becomes apparent if the cells are stimulated to divide, even after long intervals of time. Examples of such tissue are the adult liver, adult thyroid and long-lived lymphocytes (Fig. 3.28). Indeed, chromosomal abnormalities can be used as a rough measure of largish radiation doses. Again, the major effect is that many of the cells are unable to divide successfully when called upon to do so.

Radiation damage to the gonads may lead to infertility due to impairment of germ cell division.

Following a substantial dose of radiation, there is a latent interval of hours or days before histological evidence of tissue injury is seen. As already explained, the damage depends on the dose and type of radiation, on the interval following exposure and on the tissue exposed. Early changes in the skin include dilatation of blood vessels and other signs of acute inflammation and these reflect acute tissue injury. With a single dose of 15 Gy mitotic activity of the basal cells is arrested, with subsequent loss of the epidermis and epilation. The walls of the dermal vessels are infiltrated with fibrin; later a characteristic concentric proliferation of intimal fibrous tissue is seen (endarteritis obliterans), followed by replacement with dense homogeneous (hyaline) collagen (Fig. 3.29). Large bizarre fibrocytic nuclei are present in the der-

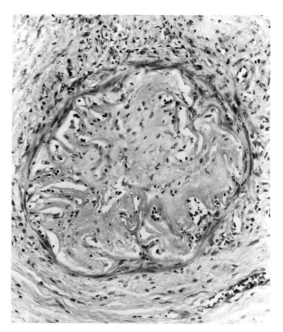

Fig. 3.29 A small artery occluded by hyaline fibrous tissue following radiotherapy. (Same case as in Fig. 3.27.) × 126.

mal connective tissue (Fig. 3.27). With repeated exposure to radiation the dermal collagen becomes very dense and there is a tendency for the dermal fibrous tissue to become necrotic even years after exposure; persistent melanin pigmentation and vascular dilatation are also noted. Comparable changes found in other tissues following irradiation are described later in the appropriate chapters; the detailed findings depend, of course, upon the radiosensitivity of the various types of tissue present, their turnover of cells and potential for cell multiplication, and the architectural features of the tissue.

Cell Death

It is now recognised that cell death can take place in two distinct ways. *Apoptosis* is mainly the result of a physiological process by which cells are eliminated when they are no longer required by the body. *Necrosis*, on the other hand, is invariably a pathological consequence of cell damage.

Apoptosis

Apoptosis (literally 'falling off' as of leaves in autumn) is characterised by shrinkage and compaction of the dying cell. It rapidly breaks up to form 'apoptotic bodies' which are phagocytosed by neighbouring cells. Cells tend to be affected singly rather than in contiguous groups and appear as inconspicuous round or oval eosinophilic structures with dense chromatin inclusions. Electron microscopy shows that apoptotic bodies are bounded by intact plasma membrane and crowded with organelles (Fig. 3.15). There is no inflammatory reaction. It has been shown that, unlike necrosis, apoptosis requires continuing synthesis of RNA and protein and a supply of ATP, features suggesting that the process is one of active self destruction.

Occurrence. Apoptosis is an essential component of normal cell turnover and it corresponds exactly to the rate of cell division in maintaining many organs at a constant size. It is also responsible for programmed destruction of cells (e.g. in the interdigital clefts) during embryonic development, and for endocrine-dependent involution of tissues (e.g. during the menstrual cycle).

In pathological states it occurs as a consequence of special forms of cell injury notably that due to damage by UV or ionising radiation or following attack by cytotoxic T-cells. Thus the shrunken eosinophilic Councilman bodies seen in the liver in viral hepatitis are apoptotic hepatocytes injured by the reaction of cytotoxic T lymphocytes to cell surface antigens modified by intracellular virus.

Apoptosis is also the usual mechanism by which cell numbers are reduced in various forms of pathological atrophy.

Necrosis

In contrast to apoptosis, necrosis usually affects groups of contiguous cells. Unless the cells are killed very rapidly, their death is preceded by osmotic swelling and depletion of ATP, and characterised by rupture of internal and plasma membranes and eventual disappearance of chromatin. There is frequently an associated inflammatory reaction.

Causes of necrosis

(a) Marked impairment of blood supply, usually due to obstruction of an end-artery (that is, one without adequate collaterals) is a common and important cause of necrosis, the necrotic area being known as an **infarct** (p. 10.23).

(b) Toxins derived from bacteria, plants, and animals such as snakes and scorpions, produce toxic organic compounds which even in very small quantities can cause cell damage amounting to necrosis. Some toxins have identifiable enzyme activity; for example, the causal organism of gas gangrene, *Clostridium welchii*, forms a lecithinase which digests the lipid of cell membranes. Diptheria toxin inhibits protein synthesis indirectly through production of ADP ribose, which blocks ribosomal transpeptidase (p. 3.10). Certain bacterial toxins, including those mentioned above, exert their effects not only locally, but are distributed via the bloodstream and other routes and so injure the cells of organs remote from the infection. The necrosis accompanying bacterial infection may be partly due to interference with the circulation brought about by toxic injury to the vascular endothelium with inflammation and sometimes thrombosis.

(c) Immunological injury can result from the reaction of antibody and complement, or of T lymphocytes, with antigenic constituents of cell surfaces. The reaction of antibody and complement with non-cellular antigen can also cause injury to adjacent tissues. These effects are classed as *hypersensitivity reactions* and are described in Chapter 7.

(d) Infection of cells notably by viruses, which are obligate intracellular parasites. This is the cause of necrosis *in vivo* of the anterior horn cells of the spinal cord in poliomyelitis.

(e) Chemical poisons. Many chemicals in high concentration cause necrosis by non-selective denaturation of the cellular proteins (e.g. strong acids, strong alkalis, carbolic acid, mercuric chloride). Others, such as cyanide and fluoroacetate, have much more specific effects and in low concentrations quickly cause cell death by interfering with oxidative production of energy (p. 3.5). The action of some poisons is indirect and less specific. Thus carbon tetrachloride is toxic to liver cells because it is metabolised by the microsomal enzyme P450 to produce free radicals which lead to peroxidation of mRNA and of unsaturated fatty acids in cell membranes.

(f) Physical agents. Cells are very sensitive to heat and, depending on the type of cell, they die after variable periods of exposure to a temperature of 45°C. Cold is much less injurious and, provided certain precautions are taken, cell suspensions and even small animals can be frozen without being killed. Necrosis after frostbite is due to damage to capillaries, resulting in thrombosis which may even extend to the arteries. Mechanical trauma such as crushing may cause direct disruption of cells. Certain disorders of the nervous system are sometimes accompanied by necrotic lesions in the limbs; these 'trophic' lesions were previously attributed to an ill-defined effect of denervation on tissue nutrition but are now thought to result from mechanical trauma which occurs unnoticed because of sensory loss.

The recognition of necrosis

As explained on p. 3.6 it is not possible to determine exactly when a particular cell becomes necrotic—i.e. when the disintegration of its vital functions has reached an irreversible stage. Many of the changes by which necrosis is recognised occur *after* cell death and are due to the secondary release of lytic enzymes normally sequestrated within the cell, e.g. in the lysosomes; this process of **autolysis** is described below.

In organised tissues such as liver or kidney, necrosis is usually recognised by secondary changes seen on histological examination. In preparations stained with haematoxylin and eosin, the nuclei may gradually lose their characteristic staining with haematoxylin so that the whole cell stains uniformly with eosin (Fig. 3.30), although the nuclear outline may persist; this change, the result of hydrolysis of chromatin within the cell after its death, is called **karyolysis**. Sometimes the chromatin of necrotic cells, especially those with already dense chromatin such as polymorphonuclear leucocytes, forms dense haematoxylinophilic masses **(pyknosis)** and these may break up **(karyorrhexis)** to form granules inside the nuclear membrane or throughout the cytoplasm (Fig. 3.31). In many necrotic lesions the outlines of swollen necrotic cells can be recognised but the cytoplasm is abnormally homogeneous or granular and frequently takes up more eosin than normal. In other tissues, e.g. the central nervous system, necrotic cells absorb water and then disintegrate, leaving no indication of the architecture of the original tissue; the lipids derived from myelin etc. persist in the debris of the necrotic tissue. The activities of certain enzymes, e.g. succinic acid dehydrogenase, diminish rapidly after cell death and appropriate tests provide useful indicators of recent tissue necrosis.

Electron microscopy of cells which have undergone necrosis shows severe disorganisation of structure. Gaps are seen in the various membranes and abnormal polymorphic inclusions, presumably derived from membranes, lie

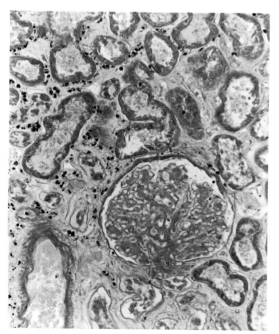

Fig. 3.30 Part of an infarct of kidney, showing coagulative necrosis. A glomerulus and tubules are seen, but the nuclei have disappeared and the structural details are lost. × 172.

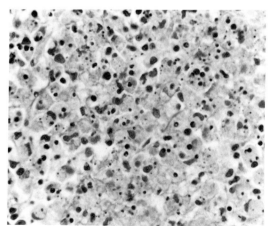

Fig. 3.31 Spreading necrosis with karyorrhexis in lymph node in typhoid fever. Note destruction of nuclei and numerous deeply-stained granules of chromatin. × 312.

in the ground substance. Fragmentation and vacuolation of endoplasmic reticulum and mitochondrial membranes precede the disappearance of these structures. Curious lamellar structures with concentric whorling form from the cell membrane, especially where there have been microvilli. Ribosomes and Golgi apparatus are unrecognisable from an early stage. There is loss of density of the nucleoplasm and large chromatin granules accumulate just inside the nuclear membrane before it disappears.

Necrosis can often be recognised macroscopically when large groups of cells die. The necrotic area may become swollen, firm, dull and lustreless, and is yellowish unless it contains much blood. This appearace is often found in kidney, spleen and myocardium. Histologically the outlines of the dead cells are usually visible (Figs. 3.30 and 3.32) and the firmness of the tissue may be due to the action of tissue thromboplastins on fibrinogen which together with other plasma proteins has been shown to diffuse through the damaged membranes of necrotic cells. This type of necrosis is appropriately described as **coagulative necrosis**. By contrast, necrotic brain tissue, which has a large fluid component, becomes 'softened' and ultimately turns into a turbid fluid (**colliquative necrosis**) with profound loss of the previous histological architecture.

Certain necrotic lesions develop a firm cheese-like appearance to the naked eye and microscopy shows amorphous granular eosin-ophilic material lacking in cell outlines; a varying amount of finely divided fat is present and there may be minute granules of chromatin. Because of its gross appearance this lesion is described as **'caseation'**. It is very common in tuberculosis but essentially similar changes are occasionally seen in infarcts, necrotic tumours and in inspissated collections of pus.

Necrotic lesions affecting skin or mucosal surfaces are frequently infected by organisms which cause putrefaction, i.e. the production of foul-smelling gas and brown, green or black discolouration of the tissue due to alteration of haemoglobin. Necrosis with putrefaction is called **gangrene** (Fig. 3.33). It may be primarily due to vascular occlusion, e.g. in the limbs or bowel where the necrotic tissue is exposed to putrefactive bacteria, but it may also result from infection with certain bacteria, namely the clostridia which cause gas gangrene (p. 9.11) or fusiform bacilli which result in **noma** (p. 9.13).

The special features of **fat necrosis** are described on pages 20.57 and 24.32.

Autolysis

The structural disintegration of cells as a result of digestion by their own enzymes is largely responsible for the softening of necrotic tissues and the associated loss of histological structure. In the intact cell, the enzymes concerned are restricted to specific organelles, such as the lysosomes, and do not have general access to the cytoplasm. After cell death, the lysosomal acid hydrolases are activated by the low pH which prevails in necrotic cells due to acid production from anaerobic glycolysis and the action of phosphatases and proteolytic enzymes. The small molecules produced by hydrolysis of macromolecules lead to osmotic swelling of the necrotic cells and their organelles provided that the membranes are sufficiently intact.

It should be noted that when many polymorphonuclear leucocytes are present in necrotic tissue the enzymes from their abundant lysosomes may contribute to the hydrolysis of other cells. This is an important factor in the liquefaction of pus and in the softening seen in infected organs at autopsy.

If tissue is killed by heating, e.g. to 55°C, or by immersion in fixative such as formalin, the enzymes and other proteins are denatured and the histological features of necrosis attributable

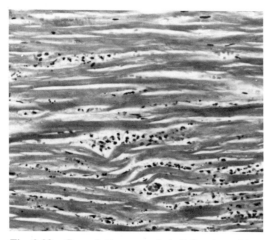

Fig. 3.32 Coagulative necrosis in infarction of heart muscle. The dead fibres are hyaline and structureless; remains of leucocytes, which have migrated from the venules, are present between them. × 125.

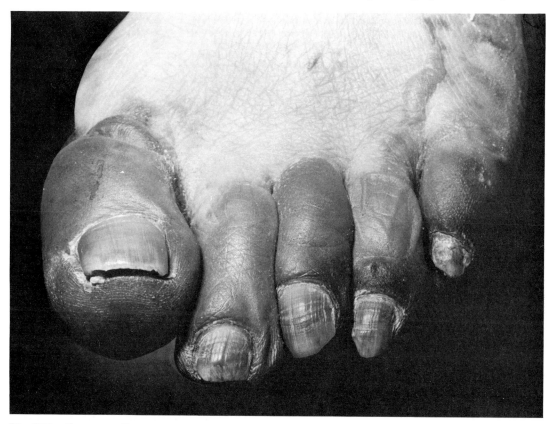

Fig. 3.33 Gangrene of toes.

to autolysis do not develop. By contrast, if a piece of tissue is deprived of its blood supply by removal from the living body and kept at 37°C, the development of autolysis can be observed, with marked osmotic swelling of membrane-bounded structures.

Two points of practical importance in the recognition of necrosis deserve emphasis. First, morphological signs of necrosis are not apparent until autolysis has developed in the necrotic tissue, and this takes 12–24 hours. Second, following death of the individual (somatic death), all cells of the body will in time die due to lack of blood supply and post-mortem autolysis will gradually take place. This is particularly marked in the parenchymal cells of the liver and kidney tubules and when seen at autopsy it may be mistaken for true necrosis, i.e. cell death occurring while the individual was still alive. This problem is of great importance in electron microscopy which shows fine structural evidence of necrosis and of post-mortem autolysis within a very short time.

Somatic death

Though not strictly related to cell necrosis, the interesting subject of somatic death (death of the individual) deserves some consideration. For many years, somatic death was defined as complete and persistent cessation of respiration and circulation. For legal purposes the persistence of the state was arbitrarily taken as five or more minutes, by which time irreversible anoxic damage would have developed in the neurons of the vital centres. However, it is now possible to restore the circulatory and respiratory functions of heart and lungs in many cases of somatic death as defined above, and integrated function both of cells and of organs (excluding those of the central nervous system) can then continue for prolonged periods with the aid of special equipment. This fact is of great importance in obtaining organs for transplantation from cadaveric donors and a legal redefinition of somatic death in terms of extensive and irreversible brain damage is now necessary.

Effects of necrosis

By definition, necrotic cells are functionless. The effect of cell necrosis on the general well-being of the body accordingly depends on the functional importance of the tissue involved, the extent of the necrosis, the functional reserve of the tissue, and on the capacity of surviving cells to proliferate and replace those which have become necrotic. For example, splenectomy is compatible with good health in man (although it increases the risk of certain infections) and extensive splenic necrosis is apparently of little importance. By contrast, extensive necrosis of renal tubular epithelium results in the serious clinical condition of renal failure which is likely to be fatal unless the patient is kept alive (e.g. by haemodialysis) until there is regeneration of tubules by proliferation of surviving cells. Necrosis of a relatively small number of motor nerve cells may produce severe paralysis which persists because nerve cells cannot proliferate to replace those lost. Since myocardial cells have not only a contractile but also a conducting function, quite small necrotic lesions may result in striking alterations in the electrical activity of the heart.

The breakdown of necrotic cells results in escape of their contents. Enzymes such as aminotransferases released into the plasma from necrotic liver or myocardial cells form the basis of clinical tests for necrosis in these tissues. It should be emphasised, however, that abnormal enzyme release occurs from cells with damage short of necrosis (e.g. in muscular dystrophy). In poisoning by alloxan, which kills the β cells of the pancreatic islets, discharge of stored insulin from the necrotic cells results in hypoglycaemia which may be fatal: those animals which survive develop diabetes from lack of insulin.

Reactions to necrosis

Neutrophil polymorphs frequently accumulate in small numbers around necrotic cells (Fig. 3.32). Occasionally infarcts and caseous lesions are invaded by large numbers of these cells and this leads to softening as already described. Such softening is a notable feature in a small proportion of myocardial infarcts (which usually show coagulative necrosis) and may lead to rupture of the heart; it is also common in tuberculosis of the lumbar vertebrae where the caseous material liquifies and tracks down beneath the psoas fascia to form a 'cold abscess' in the groin.

Individual cells killed by toxins rapidly undergo autolysis and are absorbed, especially when the circulation is maintained. They may be quickly replaced by proliferation of adjacent surviving cells. When a large mass of tissue undergoes necrosis, e.g. in an infarct, the necrotic material may be gradually replaced by ingrowth of capillaries and fibroblasts from the surrounding viable tissue so that a fibrous scar results. If this process is incomplete the necrotic mass becomes enclosed in a fibrous capsule, may persist for a long time, and may become calcified. Areas of necrotic softening in the brain are usually invaded by macrophages and eventually become cyst-like spaces containing clear liquid and surrounded by proliferated astroglia.

Old caseous lesions and necrotic fat have a marked affinity for calcium and frequently become heavily calcified.

Further Reading

Alberts, B., Bray, D., Lewis, J., Raff, M., Roberts, K. and Watson, J.D. (1983). *Molecular biology of the cell*, pp. 1146. Garland Publishing, New York and London.

Bondy, P.K. and Rosenberg, L.E. (1980). *Metabolic Control and Disease*, 8th edn., pp. 1870. Saunders, Philadelphia.

Bowen, I.D. and Lockshin, R.A. (Eds.) (1981). *Cell Death in Biology and Pathology*. Chapman and Hall, London.

Cori, G.T. (1952–3). Glycogen Structure and Enzyme Deficiency Glycogen Storage Disease. *Harvey Lecture Series*, Vol. 48, p. 145.

Dingle, J.T. and Fell, Dame Honor (1973 and 1975). *Lysosomes in Biology and Pathology*, 4 vols. North Holland Publishing Co., Amsterdam.

Dixon, K.C. (1982). *Cellular Defects in Disease*, pp. 503. Blackwell Scientific, Oxford.

4

Inflammation

Definition and nature of inflammation

When living tissues are injured, a series of changes, which may last for hours, days or weeks, occurs in and around the area of injury. This response to injury is known as inflammation, the term being derived from the Latin *inflammare* meaning to burn.

The injury is abnormal but the body's reaction, inflammation, is a normal, if complex, physiological reaction—the only one possible in the circumstances of that particular injury. This reactive nature of inflammation was first recognised by John Hunter (1794), who, after his studies of war wounds, concluded: 'Inflammation is itself not to be considered as a disease, but as a salutary operation consequent either to some violence or some disease'.

Many different types of injury may evoke inflammation. They may be classified as follows:

(1) Physical agents, such as excessive heating or cooling, ultra-violet or ionising radiation or mechanical trauma.

(2) Chemical substances, including toxins from various bacteria.

(3) Hypersensitivity reactions. The reaction of antibody or of sensitised lymphocytes with bacterial or other antigens may, by any of the mechanisms of hypersensitivity described in Chapter 7, release substances which cause an inflammatory response.

(4) Microbial infections are a very important cause of inflammation. Micro-organisms may injure tissue in several ways—by release of exo- or endo- toxins, by hypersensitivity mechanisms or by intracellular multiplication followed by cell death as seen in many viral infections.

(5) Necrosis of tissue from almost any cause leads to release of substances which induce inflammation in adjacent living tissues.

The reaction in the first few hours after injury is stereotyped and widely different kinds of injury cause a similar initial response—**the acute inflammatory reaction**. The inflammatory nature of a lesion is usually indicated by the suffix—**itis**. Thus inflammation of the appendix is appendicitis, of the liver hepatitis and so on. There are occasional historical exceptions. Inflammation of the lung is traditionally pneumonia, not pneumonitis, and of the pleura pleurisy not pleuritis. The terms *acute* and *chronic* refer to the duration of the response. Acute inflammation lasts for days or a few weeks; chronic inflammation persists for weeks, months or even years.

The inflammatory response is usually beneficial, indeed it is essential in combating most infections and in limiting the harmful effects of many toxic agents. However it is not always of benefit. There are many situations when destruction of tissue or other untoward effects are due not to the damaging agent but to one or other aspect of the body's response to injury. For example in acute inflammation of the larynx there may be sufficient inflammatory swelling to obstruct the airway and cause death from asphyxia. In both the Arthus reaction (p. 7.13) and the local response to the bites of certain ticks, necrosis of tissue is caused by substances liberated from polymorphonuclear leucocytes which accumulate at the site of injury as part of the inflammatory response: such necrosis does not occur in animals deprived of blood leucocytes by prior treatment with bone marrow poisons such as nitrogen mustard. Inflammation is best considered not as a single process but as a collection of distinct processes, each of which may have evolved for defence against injury, but each of which has also potentially deleterious effects.

This chapter begins with a description of the structural and functional features of the processes which together comprise the initial phase of the inflammatory response and an account of the factors which may be involved in the initiation and control of these processes. This is followed by a description of the appearances of acutely inflamed tissues and an explanation of why these appearances vary considerably in different organs and tissues. Next, the several sequelae of the initial response are described and consideration is given to the factors which determine which course will be followed after any particular injury. Finally, the origin, function and life history of the different types of cell involved in inflammation are described.

The Acute Inflammatory Reaction

Inflammation was known to the ancients by the appearances it produces in the skin and external parts of the body. Its manifestations were summarised by Celsus (30 BC–38 AD) as *rubor* (*redness*), *tumor* (*swelling*), *calor* (*heat*) and *dolor* (*pain*). About 120 years ago, Virchow added a fifth manifestation (*loss of function*), and these five features are known as the cardinal signs of inflammation.

It was not until late in the 19th century that Addison, Waller, Cohnheim and others studied the changes seen after injury to the transparent tongue or foot web of the living frog, that the basis of the cardinal signs became clear. Cohnheim's (1889) vivid and exciting account has never been surpassed and should be read by all students. Others have since shown that similar changes occur after injury to warm-blooded animals, including man, and Cohnheim's account is the basic frame of reference against which information obtained about inflammation by other techniques must be evaluated.

The normal microcirculation

Structure. There is a basic anatomical pattern of small blood vessels throughout the body. Blood enters the microcirculation through a vessel with a thick muscular wall, the arteriole, and leaves by way of a larger, thin-walled venule. Arterioles and venules are joined by metarterioles and capillaries. No smooth muscle fibres are present in the capillary wall, but muscle fibres surround metarterioles to form a pre-capillary sphincter. Some capillaries are large and form preferential channels; others are small, the true capillaries.

Function. Flow through capillaries is intermittent because of irregular contraction and relaxation of arterioles and pre-capillary sphincters. The small diameter requires that erythrocytes pass along capillaries in a single file, but within larger vessels, both arterioles and venules, blood flow is divided into two zones—a peripheral zone of almost cell-free plasma and a central mass of closely packed red and white cells. This distribution, known as **axial flow,** is a hydrodynamic consequence of the streamline or laminar nature of flow in all blood vessels larger than capillaries.

Increased tissue activity—whether it be muscular exercise, glandular secretion or intestinal absorption—is accompanied by increased blood flow through the active area. Intrinsic myogenic activity of the vascular wall and nervous and humoral stimuli are major control factors in arterioles and venules, but extrinsic factors are of minor importance in the terminal vascular bed, where flow appears to be modulated largely by the effects of locally-produced metabolites of tissue activity on the sphincters surrounding metarterioles.

The changes seen after injury

Immediately after injury there may be a transient constriction of arterioles. This does not always occur and is of little importance. The next stage is a widespread dilatation of arterioles and venules and the opening up of many small vessels which had previously been carrying little or no blood (**active hyperaemia**). Blood flow through the injured area may increase as much as tenfold. Initially, flow through the dilated vessels is very rapid and, as a consequence, axial flow is accentuated. After mild stimuli, rapid flow lasts only 10-15 minutes and then returns gradually to normal. After more severe injury, increased flow may last for hours and be followed by a gradual decrease in the rate of flow through still dilated vessels. As flow slows, the axial column of packed cells widens and the outer, plasmatic zone shrinks progressively until flow may cease entirely in some vessels, which are now distended by immobile columns of tightly packed cells. Stasis may persist and end in death and distintegration of the affected vessels, but in many instances flow begins again and gradually returns to normal.

Soon after flow slows, and long before stasis is apparent, leucocytes begin to appear in the marginal stream of the venules and to impinge from time to time on the venular wall. At first they stick momentarily to the wall and then fall back into the flowing blood, but, when injury is sufficiently severe, progressively more leucocytes hit, and become adherent to, the venular wall. The luminal aspect of venules in the injured area becomes coated with a layer of living adherent leucocytes, an appearance which Cohnheim described as **pavementing of leucocytes**.

Many of the adherent cells subsequently pass out through the venular wall into extravascular tissue spaces. This phenomenon is known as **leucocytic emigration** and will be discussed more fully later. In injuries of moderate severity, pavementing and emigration may last for several hours. They then gradually cease and the affected vessels resume an entirely normal appearance.

At about the same time as leucocytes are behaving in this way, protein-rich fluid escapes from the blood vessels into extravascular tissues, producing **inflammatory oedema**. It is not possible to see how this fluid escapes by study of living tissue preparations, and as extravascular fluid accumulates it becomes increasingly difficult to see what is happening in and around the still-dilated vessels. The escape of fluid is termed **exudation** and the fluid is called an **inflammatory exudate**.

Summary of early stages of inflammation

The reactive changes in the first few hours after injury involve three processes:
1. changes in vascular calibre and flow;
2. increased vascular permeability and the formation of inflammatory exudate;
3. escape of leucocytes from blood into extravascular tissue spaces.

These processes result in the accumulation of protein-rich oedema fluid, fibrin and leucocytes in the extravascular spaces of the injured tissues. Recognition of this accumulation is the basis of the histological diagnosis of acute inflammation (Figs. 4.1, 4.2).

Basis of the cardinal signs

1. Redness is due to gross and persistent dilatation of all small blood vessels within the area of injury.

2. Heat. An area of inflammation is hot only when it occurs in or near the skin, which is at a lower temperature than the central part of the body and the circulating blood. The rise in local

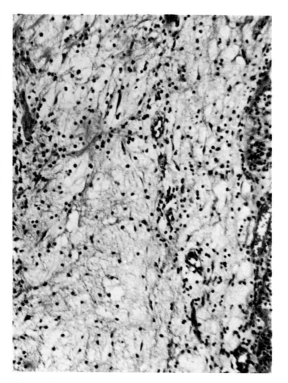

Fig. 4.1 Meso-appendix in acute appendicitis, showing inflammatory oedema with early leucocytic emmigration. × 100.

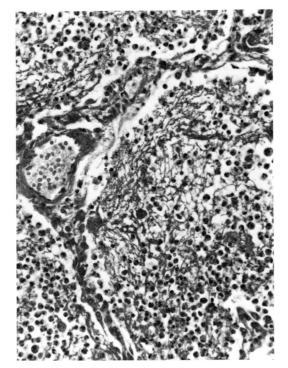

Fig. 4.2 Acute inflammation of the lung in pneumonia. The exudate, which fills the alveoli, is rich in plasma proteins, and this is illustrated by the fine network of fibrin (stained black) which has resulted from clotting of fibrinogen in the inflammatory exudate. (Weigert's fibrin stain). × 150.

temperature in inflammation of surface areas is a direct result of increased local blood flow. Inflammation of internal organs causes no increase in their temperature except as a part of the general rise in body temperature, or fever, which is a feature of many types of acute inflammation.

3. Swelling. The main factor responsible for swelling in an inflamed area is local oedema caused by accumulation of fluid exudate in the extravascular spaces. Extravascular accumulation of leucocytes also contributes, but except in certain types of chronic inflammation its contribution is much smaller than that of local oedema.

4. Pain is the least understood of the cardinal signs. Substances such as bradykinin, serotonin and certain prostaglandins, known to be present in inflamed tissues, cause pain when applied to wounds or exposed connective tissues. A more important factor in producing pain is a rise in tissue tension within the inflamed area. Inflammation in areas which become tense after accumulation of small amounts of oedema—for example the skin covering the ala nasae—is much more painful than a similar degree of inflammation in the peri-orbital and other loose tissues. Pus under tension in an abscess causes extreme pain and its evacuation is followed by an immediate and marked decrease in both pain and tenderness.

5. Loss of function is due in part to reflex inhibition of muscular movement as a result of pain, aided by limitation of movement because of swelling of the inflamed area. There is no evidence of impairment of the function of undamaged cells in areas of inflammation.

Changes in vascular calibre and flow

Arteriolar constriction, when present, appears to be due to a direct response of the vascular smooth muscle to the injurious stimulus.

The subsequent vasodilatation is an active hyperaemia caused by widespread arteriolar dilatation. Both nervous and humoral factors are involved. The role of cutaneous nerves was shown by Lewis (1927) in the classic paper in which he described the so-called *triple response to injury*. However, this type of response appears to be limited to skin, tongue and conjunctiva, and it is known that acute inflammation occurring in denervated tissues presents all the usual features. Clearly, neural factors are not essential in inflammation, and it is likely that Lewis's postulated axon reflex is of little practical importance.

Many endogenous substances which can increase vascular permeability are found in injured tissues and most of them are also vasodilators. However, little is known of their relative importance in different types of inflammation.

Vasodilation increases the escape of fluid but does not itself cause increased leakage of protein. A good example of the separate nature of these two phenomena is seen in muscular exercise when there is great increase in local blood flow and in the volume of lymph draining from the exercising muscle, but no change in the total protein content of lymph. The time course of vasodilatation and increased vascular permeability may differ markedly in many types of inflammation. For example in sunburn, exudation may occur during only a short part of the prolonged period of hyperaemia characteristic of this type of injury. It has, however, been shown recently that for any given level of increased permeability, the amount of protein lost into the injured area varies directly with the rate of blood flow through the leaking vessels. Thus prostaglandin E_1 causes gross hyperaemia but no change in vascular permeability, while bradykinin produces little vasodilatation but induces an immediate increase in permeability. If the two substances are injected simultaneously into the same area, total protein leakage is al-most 100 times greater than when bradykinin is injected alone. Conversely, severe injury may lead to complete vascular stasis and no protein at all may then escape from the widely dilated vessels despite the presence of large gaps in their endothelial lining (see below). The situation is analogous to holes in a garden hose—the rate of loss of water depends directly on how hard the tap is turned on.

The main factor causing **slowing of flow** and eventual **stasis** is increased permeability, which allows escape of plasma but retains erythrocytes within the vessels. The consequent rise in haematocrit leads to an increase in blood viscosity and slowing of flow follows. The rise in tissue pressure caused by rapid escape of fluid into extravascular tissues and also the diminution of the lumen of the small vessels by pavemented leucocytes may also contribute to slowing of the blood flow.

Increased vascular permeability—formation of local oedema

To understand how oedema develops in injured tissues, knowledge is required both of the nature of the fluid which accumulates in the extravascular spaces and of the structure and behaviour of the walls of normal and injured small blood vessels.

Inflammatory exudate

The fluid which accumulates is known as inflammatory exudate and has the following characteristics.

1. A relatively high protein content—35-50 g/l, the proteins being all those present in blood plasma, including fibrinogen. On coming into contact with extravascular tissues, the fibrinogen in the exudate is converted to insoluble fibrin, and local accumulation of fibrin within injured tissues or on an inflamed surface is a prominent feature of the inflammatory response.

2. Exudate is not a static puddle but a high-turnover pool. The best measure of the rate of passage of plasma proteins through a tissue is the quantity of protein in lymph draining from the area: This may increase five to ten-fold in an area of acute inflammation and its protein concentration also rises considerably, indicating a massive passage of protein from blood to lymph.

3. Some degree of sieving, according to molecular size, persists between plasma and lymph during exudate formation.

4. The texture and compliance of tissues influence the volume of exudate. Inflammatory exudate forms too rapidly to allow adaptive remodelling of tissue, and in dense tissues, or in organs with a fibrous capsule, escape of small amounts of fluid leads to a rapid and progressive rise in tissue pressure which limits further exudation. In loose tissues or inflammation of the lining of a body cavity, large volumes of exudate can accumulate rapidly without appreciable rise in tissue pressure.

Structure of normal small blood vessels

In all tissues, small blood vessels are lined by a single layer of endothelial cells, whose cyto-

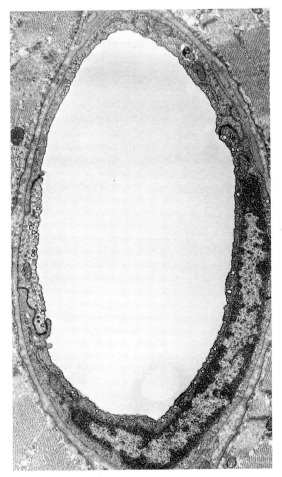

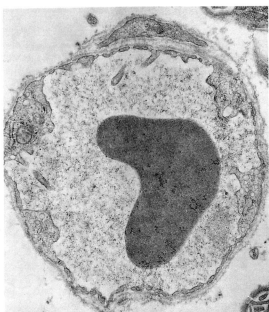

Fig. 4.4 Electron micrograph of small blood vessel of fenestrated type in the mucosa of the small intestine. Fenestrae are occluded by a thin membrane and particles of injected ferritin are visible in large numbers in the vascular lumen. $\times 14\,000$.

Fig. 4.3 Electron micrograph of small blood vessel in skeletal muscle. Note numerous pinocytotic vesicles in endothelial cell cytoplasm and the presence of three closed intercellular injections. $\times 10\,000$) from Miles and Hurley, *Microvascular Research* 1983, **26**, 273).

plasm contains the usual organelles and an extensive system of pinocytotic vesicles. In many tissues, including skin and muscle, endothelial cell cytoplasm forms a complete layer of uniform thickness all round the vessel (Fig. 4.3). In other tissues, including endocrine and exocrine glands, the kidney and intestinal mucosa, the endothelium of capillaries and small venules shows areas of extreme thinning (*fenestrae*) (Fig. 4.4), and vascular sinusoids of the liver, spleen and bone marrow have large endothelial defects (Fig. 4.5). A complete basement membrane is present in all small vessels except sinusoids, where it is incomplete or absent.

Nearly all experimental studies in inflamma-tion have been on tissues whose small vessels have continuous endothelium, and findings from them are not necessarily valid for tissues whose small vessels have fenestrae or defects.

Exchanges across the wall of normal small blood vessels

The wall of small blood vessels acts as a passive microfilter and passage of water and solutes across it does not involve any expenditure of energy by endothelial cells. Two distinct mechanisms are involved in passage of materials across the vascular wall. First, molecules move by diffusion, which will cause net transfer of a substance only when there is a difference in its concentration on the two sides of the vascular wall. Diffusion is the major process by which oxygen and nutrients pass from blood to extra-vascular tissues and by which CO_2 and waste products are removed by the blood. For small molecules, diffusion is very rapid, but for large molecules like plasma proteins it is an extremely slow process. Secondly, bulk transfer of fluid and small solutes occurs by ultra-filtration. First described by Starling in 1896, this type of fluid transport is governed by the dynamic

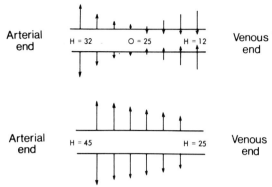

Fig. 4.6. Exchange of fluid by ultrafiltration across the wall of small blood vessels. H and O represent the difference between the hydrostatic and colloid osmotic pressures (mm Hg) of plasma and extravascular space. The arrows indicate the net movement of fluid in and out of vessels along their length.
Upper figure, normal tissue: fluid movement across vessel wall approximates to equilibrium.
Lower figure, acute inflammation: much more fluid leaves vessels than is returned to them. The values of H and O are approximations. In inflammation, H may be less than indicated because of rise of pressure in the extravascular space, and O will also be reduced due to escape of plasma protein (via endothelial gaps) into the extravascular space.

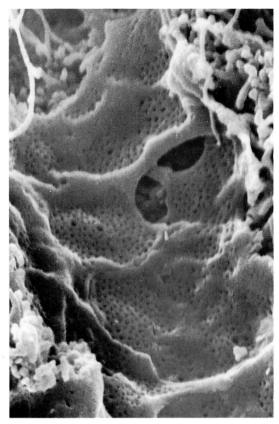

Fig. 4.5 Scanning electron micrograph of sinusoid in rat liver. Note sieve plates of small openings and also scattered larger openings. The very large openings are terminations of smaller branch sinusoids. (Dr P.S. Bhathal.) × 5000.

balance between hydrostatic and colloid osmotic pressures on either side of the vascular wall (Fig. 4.6). Under normal circumstances, fluid is lost at the high-pressure arteriolar end of capillaries and reabsorbed at the low-pressure venular end of the vessel. Despite minor modifications to allow for the much greater area available for ultra-filtration at the venular end of the microcirculation, and continuing doubt as to the precise values of hydrostatic and osmotic pressures in the extravascular space, experiments by Landis and others have fully substantiated Starling's hypothesis. It is generally agreed that both diffusion and ultra-filtration occur via the junctions between endothelial cells (and in fenestrated vessels via fenestrae as well) and not by passage of water and solutes across the cytoplasm of endothelial cells.

Some protein leaks from small blood vessels in all tissues. Any protein which escapes is returned to the blood via the lymphatic system, and hence the total protein content of lymph draining from a tissue is an indication of the degree of leakage of protein from blood vessels in that tissue. Vessels lined by continuous endothelium normally leak little protein, fenestrated vessels lose considerably more, and sinusoids are freely permeable to all plasma proteins. Both continuous and fenestrated endothelium exert a sieving effect on large molecules, and provide a barrier to macromolecules which increases with their molecular weight.

The route by which protein escapes from normal small blood vessels is not clear. Physiologists have postulated the existence of a system of 'large pores' to explain protein leakage, but there is no general agreement amongst electron microscopists about the morphological equivalent of these pores. In sinusoids, the many large openings in endothelium are adequate to explain the massive protein leakage from this type of vessel and in fenestrated vessels there is evidence that protein may escape via the fenestrae.

In continuous endothelium, Palade and his associates ascribe a major transport function to pinocytotic vesicles, but most authorities do not agree with this hypothesis. Many believe that some junctions between endothelial cells are permeable to protein and that protein may seep down apparently unaltered junctions. Another possibility is that large pores are not a fixed anatomical entity, and that transient gaps of the type which occur in the endothelium of small vessels in areas of acute inflammation (see below) may form from time to time in uninjured vessels.

The basis of increased vascular permeability in acute inflammation

After injury, inflammatory exudate accumulates rapidly within the injured area. The accumulation cannot be due to decreased lymphatic drainage as the lymph draining from the injured area increases markedly in both volume and protein concentration. Hence exudate formation must be due to increase in the rate of escape of water and protein from small blood vessels i.e. to increased vascular permeability. Cohnheim appreciated this over 100 years ago and wrote of a 'molecular change' in the wall of inflamed blood vessels, but the nature of this change remained entirely obscure until, roughly 30 years ago, it became possible to examine biological specimens by electron microscopy.

In recent years, detailed knowledge has accumulated of the degree and time course of leakage of fluid and protein in many types of inflammation, and the structural basis of the increased permeability that follows injury is now well understood.

The response to histamine-type permeability factors—vascular labelling. Local injection of histamine-type permeability factors provides the simplest model of increased vascular permeability. Injection of histamine or bradykinin in appropriate dosage into skin and muscle causes leakage of plasma protein which begins immediately, rises rapidly to a maximum and ceases abruptly 10-15 minutes later. In 1961, Majno and Palade showed that the structural basis of this type of leakage is the appearance of transient openings of $0.1-0.4\,\mu m$ diam. between the endothelial cells of small vessels (Fig. 4.7). There is no evidence of concurrent damage to endothelial cell cytoplasm, and when the gaps close, leakage ceases, and the endothelial lining reverts to normal (Fig. 4.8). Majno and Palade located the site of leakage by injecting large marker particles of colloidal carbon or mercuric sulphide intravenously before applying the permeability factor. When gaps form in endothelium, plasma and circulating marker particles are forced out through the gaps by intravascular hydrostatic pressure. Plasma passes through the basement membrane but carbon and mercuric sulphide particles are too large to do likewise and accumulate on the luminal aspect of the basement membrane. Marker particles in circulating blood are removed within 30-60 minutes by phagocytic cells in the liver and spleen but particles trapped between endothelium and its basement membrane remain in that position after the gap in the overlying endothelium has closed. If colloidal carbon is used as the marker, such labelled vessels can be detected easily by light- or electron-microscopy of sections or in cleared specimens of the injured area. This is the basis of the vascular labelling technique which allows the detection of leakage from individual vessels within an area of injury.

The formation of endothelial gaps has been shown to depend upon the activation of a contractile protein within the cytoplasm of vascular endothelial cells. To date, this protein has not been visualised by electron microscopy, presumably because of the known lability of actin filaments and of aggregation of contractile proteins within cells.

Vascular labelling studies indicate that *the leakage induced by histamine and all other known permeability factors is restricted to venules and small veins and does not involve capillaries (Fig. 4.9)*. The reason for this localisation is not clear. It is not due to selective venular localisation of the contractile protein as immunofluorescence studies show this to be present in the endothelium of vessels of all sizes from the aorta to capillaries.

Leakage in other types of inflammation. In naturally-occurring or experimentally-induced acute inflammation, increased vascular permeability commonly lasts for hours—much longer than the brief leakage seen after application of histamine-type permeability factors.

The time course and magnitude of leakage vary with the type and severity of the injury, but can always be accommodated by the com-

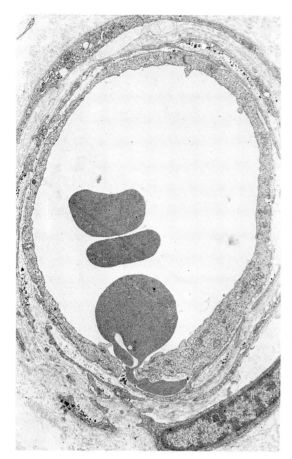

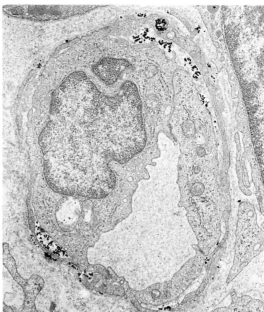

Fig. 4.8 Electron micrograph of venule in muscle of rat injected intravenously with carbon at the time of local application of histamine and killed 30 min. later. Intercellular junctions are now closed, but carbon trapped in vascular wall beneath them indicate that gaps were present in the period immediately after injection of histamine. × 9000.

bination, in varying degrees, of the following three basic patterns of response (Fig. 4.10).

1. *The immediate transient response.* This is seen after application of histamine and other endogenous permeability factors and its characteristics are described above. It may occur as an isolated event in very mild injuries, or may precede another type of leakage, as for example the initial phase of the response to mild thermal injury.

2. *The immediate sustained reaction.* This is seen after severe injuries such as thermal burns, crushing injuries or application of chemical or bacterial toxins in high concentration. Leakage begins immediately, may be sustained at a high level for many hours and is associated with obvious damage to both the endothelium of the leaking vessels and surrounding tissues.

3. *Delayed prolonged leakage.* This is a very common pattern of response, seen after mild degrees of physical injuries such as thermal or ultraviolet burns or injury induced by x-ray, application of chemical or bacterial toxins, or delayed (type 4) hypersensitivity reactions.

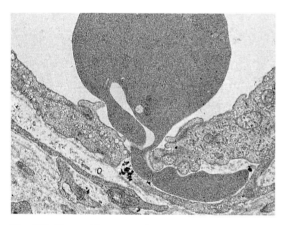

Fig. 4.7 *Upper.* Electron micrograph of small venule in muscle 2 min. after application of histamine solution. A large gap is present in endothelium of normal appearance. Carbon particles and portion of an erythrocyte lie within the gap. × 4500.
Lower. Higher magnification of the region of the gap. × 10 000.

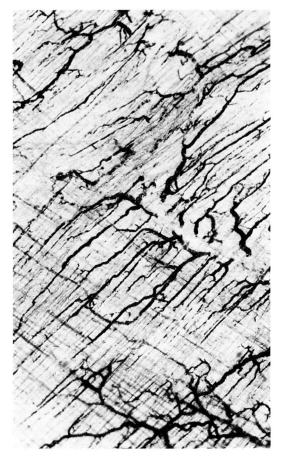

Fig. 4.9 Portion of a cleared specimen of the cremaster of a rat injected locally with histamine and intravenously with colloidal carbon and killed 60 min. later. Carbon deposition in the walls of small venules has produced a candelabra-like pattern of vascular labelling. Unlabelled capillaries can be seen as a series of indistinct parallel lines. × 15.

In delayed prolonged leakage, there is a latent interval of varying duration between injury and the start of leakage, which once begun may last for many hours. Leakage of this type is often preceded by immediate transient leakage of histamine-type, giving the whole response a biphasic pattern. Lesions which evoke a delayed prolonged response do not usually cause obvious tissue necrosis.

Endothelial changes

The morphological basis of increased permeability in all types of inflammation is the presence of defects in vascular endothelium. The

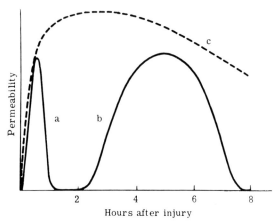

Fig. 4.10 The time course of the 3 basic patterns of increased vascular permeability. (**a**) = immediate transient—histamine type; (**b**) = delayed prolonged; (**c**) = immediate sustained—severe direct vascular injury. The time course illustrated is for mild thermal injury. Other types of injury produce delayed-prolonged leakage with a different time course.

defects may vary in size from small gaps induced transiently by histamine to total destruction of parts or the whole of endothelial cells. There may or may not be ultrastructural evidence of damage to the endothelium of the leaking vessels.

Prolonged leakage over several hours may occur from individual vessels, both those that are injured severely and those whose endothelium appears little damaged.

The topography of vascular leakage

Not all types of injury cause the venular pattern of labelling (see above) found after application of endogenous permeability factors. Labelling patterns vary with both the type and stage of injury examined and with the tissue that has been injured. Labelling may be purely venular, purely capillary, or involve vessels of all sizes within the area of injury.

Unless there are endogenous mediators, as yet unidentified, capable of causing leakage from capillaries, some other mechanism must contribute to the formation of inflammatory exudate. This mechanism is direct injury to vascular endothelium.

It has been known for many years that severe injuries—chemical, physical or bacterial—cause leakage by direct vascular injury. The major

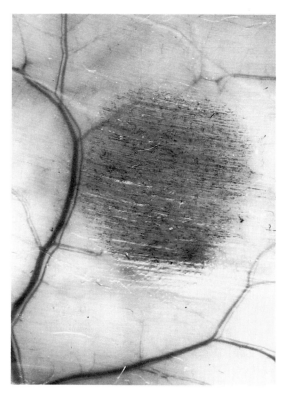

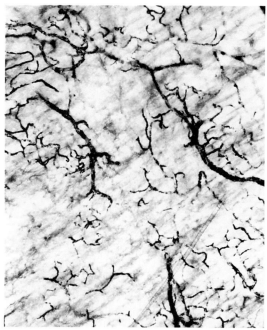

Fig. 4.11a Peritoneal surface of the abdominal wall of a rat after heat injury at 53°C for 20 secs. Carbon injected 30 min. before killing. A sharply defined zone of blackening is visible which corresponds precisely with the area in contact with the hot iron. No carbon is visible outside this area. × 4.

Fig. 4.11b Higher magnification of portion of burn shown in Fig. 4.11a. Carbon deposits are visible in large and small venules, and also in capillaries which form a mesh on the surface of the muscle. Capillaries situated more deeply are also blackened but not visible at this plane of focus. × 28.

part of fluid and protein loss in injuries which provoke an immediate sustained type of increased permeability, including clinically significant burns, occurs in this way.

Lesser degrees of injury by many chemical or physical agents cause a delayed prolonged or biphasic pattern of leakage. Detailed study of thermal injury to skin and to muscle shows that delayed prolonged leakage is confined strictly to the injured area. It is not the size of vessels but their proximity to the source of heat which determines which vessels will leak. In the skin, where all sub-epidermal vessels are capillaries, leakage occurs only from capillaries: in muscle, where vessels of all sizes lie on the surface, arterioles, capillaries and venules all contribute to exudate formation (Fig. 4.11). In both skin and muscle, there is electron-microscopic evidence of damage to the endothelium of the leaking vessels (Fig. 4.12). *Delayed prolonged leakage in thermal burns is clearly not a mediated response but a consequence of direct vascular injury (Fig. 4.13)*. The delayed prolonged response to many other injuries—ultraviolet or x-ray injury, and chemical and bacterial toxins—has similar characteristics. Leakage caused by direct vascular injury can be identified by the following criteria: leakage and labelling should be confined strictly to the injured area; the pattern of labelling should reflect the intensity of injury to which vessels are exposed and not vascular calibre; there should be electron-microscopic evidence of damage to endothelial cells.

Little is known of the intimate nature of leakage due to direct vascular injury. It does not, however, appear to depend upon the contractile mechanism responsible for mediated leakage.

The roles of mediators and of direct endothelial injury

The relative importance of liberation of mediators and of direct endothelial damage after different types of injury is not fully established. In

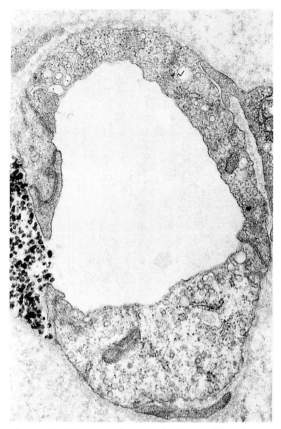

Fig. 4.12   Electron micrograph of a capillary in rat muscle 3 hr. after mild thermal injury. An intramural deposit of carbon lies under a large gap in the endothelium which shows gross swelling and mild but definite evidence of injury. × 15 000.

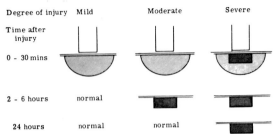

Fig. 4.13   The phases of increased vascular permeability following varying degrees of heat injury to the skin by a hot tube. Two effects are observed. Firstly, an immediate transient increase in the permeability of venules (lightly shaded), due to release of histamine. This occurs with all degrees of injury short of necrosis and extends well beyond the area of injury. Secondly, more persistent leakage (heavily shaded) which results from direct heat injury to the endothelium of both capillaries and venules. This leakage is confined to the zone of injury. Its onset is delayed after moderate injury, but leakage begins immediately after severe injury.

severe injuries, which evoke an immediate prolonged response, the major part of loss of fluid and protein is certainly due to direct damage to small blood vessels.

In most examples of less severe injuries, evoking a biphasic response, the brief immediate phase, in which relatively little fluid and protein is lost, is mediated by the release of histamine, and the delayed prolonged phase, during which most fluid and protein loss occurs, is due to direct vascular injury. However, in a few experimental systems leakage in both immediate and delayed phases is of mediated type.

Blood vessels of similar size and structure in different tissues vary in their response to permeability factors. Venules in skin, subcutaneous tissues, muscle, serous membranes, conjunctiva and the mucosa of the trachea and main bron-

chi are sensitive to histamine and similar agents. Vessels in solid organs, including the central nervous system, and in the small bowel mucosa and the walls of pulmonary alveoli, are insensitive to permeability factors. The basis of this difference is unknown but it does not reflect variations in the actomyosin content of endothelial cells in different organs. It seems likely that all leakage in organs whose vessels are unresponsive to the known permeability factors is due to direct vascular injury.

No evidence is available about the basis of leakage in clinically important infective inflammation like pneumonia and peritonitis.

Recognition of the major role of direct vascular injury in exudate formation is important because it follows that attempts to inhibit excessive and prolonged loss of plasma protein, as for example in extensive burns, should aim at diminishing the effects of endothelial injury rather than the suppression of endogenous chemical mediators.

Summary

The invariable basis of exudation of protein-rich fluid in acute inflammation is the presence of gaps in the endothelium of small blood vessels. Gaps may be formed by active contraction of endothelial cells induced by histamine or other permeability factors, or they may result from direct damage to vascular endothelium. Mediators are responsible for the brief initial phase of leakage after most mild injuries and may also play a role in the later phases after some types of injury. However, direct damage to endothelium appears to be the basis of leakage of protein after severe injuries and also during the delayed phase of many types of less severe injury.

Composition of inflammatory exudate

Although always high, the protein content of inflammatory exudate varies considerably in different types of acute inflammation. This is because two processes contribute in varying degree to exudate formation. The formation of gaps in vascular endothelium allows free escape of plasma from injured vessels: the raised intravascular pressure resulting from inflammatory vasodilatation increases transudation of protein-free plasma ultrafiltrate into the injured tissues, but it only increases the leakage of protein when gaps are present (p. 4.5). There is no close correlation between the duration and magnitude of gap formation and of vasodilatation and this accounts for the variable composition of inflammatory exudates.

Emigration of leucocytes

Accumulation of leucocytes within an area of injured tissue is the histological hallmark of acute inflammation. Initially the cells which escape are almost all neutrophil polymorphs, but later, depending on the nature of the injury, monocytes, eosinophils and lymphocytes may also escape in varying numbers into the inflamed area.

Study of living tissues reveals three distinct stages in the escape of leucocytes. First, they adhere to the inner aspect of venular endothelium within the area of injury, a process graphically described by Cohnheim as **margination** or **pavementing* of leucocytes** (Fig. 4.14). Many of the adherent cells subsequently pass through the vascular wall into extravascular spaces—a process known as **leucocytic emigration.** Having escaped from the vessels, the cells may wander at random, or move in an apparently directed manner towards a focus of dead tissues or a clump of bacteria. This directed movement is attributed to **chemotaxis**, in which the direction of cell movement is determined by concentration gradients of dissolved substances known as **chemotaxins**.

Pavementing of leucocytes

This can be studied only in living tissues and is one of the least understood aspects of acute inflammation. Pavementing occurs only in

* For North American readers, the British call sidewalks pavements.

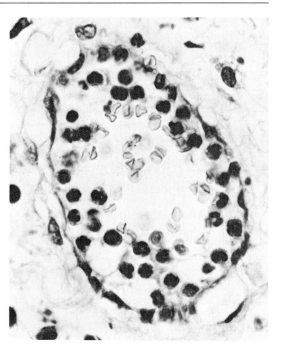

Fig. 4.14 Section of venule in acute inflammation. Showing pavementing of polymorphonuclear leucocytes. × 1000.

venules, and depends upon some change in the vascular wall rather than in the cells which stick to it. Leucocytes impinge from time to time on venular endothelium in normal tissues, but pavementing is seen only after injury. If localised injury is inflicted on the endothelium of one side of a venule, cells stick only to the

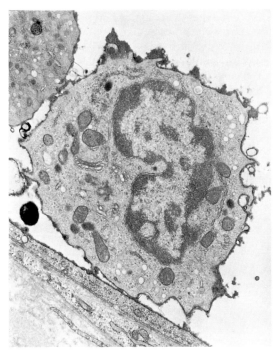

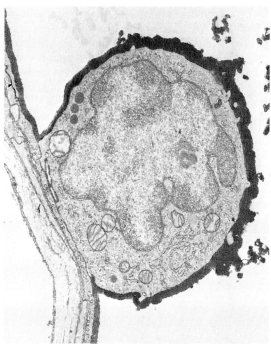

Fig. 4.15 Electron micrograph of a venule in inflamed muscle. A leucocyte lies partly in contact with vascular endothelium. Both leucocyte and endothelial cell are covered with a uniform layer of densely stained material (lanthanum-alcian blue stain). × 9000.

Fig. 4.16 Electron micrograph of a venule in inflamed muscle. A leucocyte is intimately apposed to vascular endothelium. A layer of densely stained material covers both endothelium and leucocyte but is absent in the area of contact between the two cells. (lanthanum-alcian blue stain.) × 9000.

damaged side. This experiment was performed on tissue which had grown into an ear-chamber (a shallow transparent chamber with open sides) inserted into a rabbit's ear. Pavementing is not a consequence of slowing of blood flow. It begins within a few minutes of injury in dilated vessels while flow is still extremely rapid, and is usually well established before the onset of the slowing of flow characteristic of the later stages of the inflammatory reaction. Pavementing can develop without any apparent change in the ultrastructure of endothelium or of the mucopolysaccharide layer which covers its inner surface (Figs. 4.15, 4.16). Adherent leucocytes can be released by local application of the chelating agent, EDTA, or of prostacyclin, but the significance of these findings is not clear.

The changes responsible for the adherence of circulating leucocytes to vascular endothelium must be highly specific. The cells which stick to inflamed venules are neutrophil polymorphs and occasional monocytes and eosinophils. By contrast, in the specialised high-endothelial venules of normal (non-inflamed) lymphoid tissue, lymphocytes adhere but other types of leucocyte do not, while in the early stages of thrombosis, platelets stick to the damaged vascular wall which fails to attract any type of leucocyte.

Leucocytic emigration

Leucocytes escape from venules and small veins, and only very occasionally from capillaries. Leucocytes emigrate by active amoeboid movement, polymorphs taking 2–9 minutes to pass through the vascular wall and thereafter moving through extravascular tissues at up to 20 μm per minute. Leucocytes have been observed to migrate from vessels in which flow has stopped completely, so intravascular hydrostatic pressure is not a prerequisite for leucocytic emigration.

In addition, some red cells escape, but this is entirely passive, the red cells being pushed by intravascular hydrostatic pressure through tiny

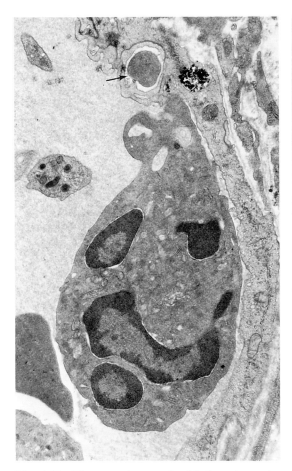

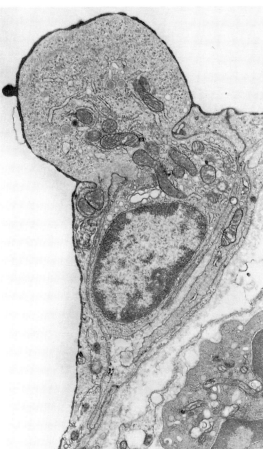

Fig. 4.17 Electron micrograph of inflamed muscle, showing part of a venule. A polymorph has inserted a pseudopod (→) into an intercellular junction in the endothelium of the venule. Endothelial-cell cytoplasm appears normal. × 9700.

Fig. 4.18 Electron micrograph of inflamed muscle. A leucocyte passing through venular endothelium. Densely stained material covers both endothelium and the escaping cell except that part of the leucocyte which lies beneath the surface of the endothelium (lanthanum-alcian blue stain). × 9000.

breaches in the vascular wall. Commonly a number of red cells escape in rapid succession through the same defect before it closes and prevents further escape of cells. This process is called *diapedesis* of red cells, a term used by Cohnheim to denote escape of cells in the absence of a permanent tear in the vascular wall. The more severe the vascular injury, the greater the escape of red cells, and a haemorrhagic exudate indicates severe damage to vascular endothelium.

Electron-microscopic study of serial sections shows that neutrophil polymorphs, monocytes and eosinophils escape from inflamed venules by dissecting their way down the junctions between vascular endothelial cells (Figs. 4.17,

4.18). This does not damage the endothelium, normal junctions re-forming behind the escaping cell. It is of interest that as early as 1875 Arnold claimed that leucocytes left vessels via areas stained by silver nitrate, i.e. intercellular junctions, and gave clear drawings of his observations (Fig. 4.19). It is now established that lymphocytes cross the endothelium of venules in lymphoid tissue by passing between cells in the same manner as other types of leucocyte.

The emerging leucocytes penetrate the basement membrane by producing gaps which close soon after the cell has passed through. The basement membrane does, however, seem more resistant to emigrating leucocytes than the apparently more substantial endothelium, and

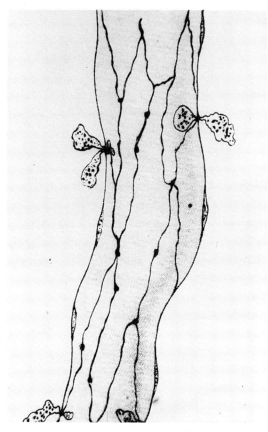

Fig. 4.19 A small inflamed venule from the tongue of a frog. The intercellular borders have been stained with silver. Leucocytes are passing through the wall at points on intercellular junctions (from Arnold, *Virchows Arch. Path. Anat.* **62**, 487, 1875).

escaping cells are seen more often between endothelium and basement membrane than in the act of passing between endothelial cells. The mechanisms of disruption and repair of endothelial cell junctions and basement membrane are not understood.

Chemotaxis

Since the earliest studies of experimental inflammation, it has been believed that leucocytes in extravascular tissues are attracted towards higher concentrations of specific chemical substances in solution by a process known as *chemotaxis*.

Two methods have been used to detect chemotactic agents. In the 1950s, Harris incubated a suspension of leucocytes in a slide-coverslip

preparation in which he could follow the movement of individual cells by time-lapse photography. He was able to demonstrate chemotactic activity towards bacteria but not towards dead or damaged tissues. In 1962, Boyden devised a novel assay for chemotactic substances in solution. A suspension of leucocytes is separated by a Millipore membrane from the test solution: if this is chemotactic, leucocytes crawl towards it through the pores of the membrane (Fig. 4.20), and measurement of their rate of advance provides a quantitative assay of chemotaxis. Appropriate control tests must be used to exclude the effects of so-called *chemokinetic agents*, which enhance random motility of leucocytes without influencing their directional motility.

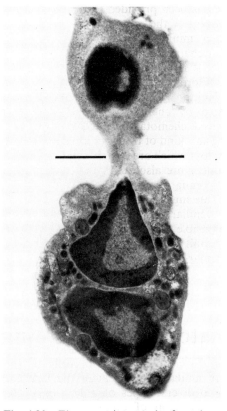

Fig. 4.20 Electron micrograph of a polymorph migrating through a Millipore membrane in response to a chemotaxin. Most of the organelles have passed into the cytoplasm which, together with two lobes of the nucleus, has moved downwards through a pore, the site of which is indicated by the heavy line. $\times 14\,300$ (by courtesy of Professor P.C. Wilkinson and Churchill-Livingstone).

By the use of the Boyden chamber, chemotactic and chemokinetic factors with influences on one or more types of leucocyte have been described to account for all the types of cellular infiltration seen in different kinds and stages of inflammation. These factors include products liberated from the complement cascade, certain lymphokines, factors liberated from polymorphs which can attract more cells of the same type, and two small peptides, ECF-A, liberated from mast cells which are specifically attractive to eosinophils. Features of the more important of these factors are described later.

Despite conclusive evidence that chemical concentration gradients can influence both the rate and direction of movement of leucocytes *in vitro*, direct evidence that chemotaxis occurs *in vivo* is very slender. Virtually the only direct evidence has been provided by time-lapse cinephotography of the movement of polymorphs towards a minimal area of tissue injury in rabbit ear chambers (p. 4.14). Local accumulation of cells is not necessarily due to chemotaxis. As Florey pointed out, cells may arrive at a site of injury by random movement, perhaps accelerated by chemokinesis and, once they have arrived, chemotaxins may keep them there by acting as a kind of trapping mechanism.

All factors which are chemotactic in the Boyden chamber are also active in inducing rapid leucocytic emigration after local injection into tissues. This suggests that, once leucocytes have stuck to venular endothelium, the same factors are responsible for their passage through the vascular wall as for the later movements in extravascular tissue spaces.

Increased vascular permeability and leucocytic emigration as separable phenomena

If carbon labelling (p. 4.8) is used as the indicator of increased permeability, study of histological sections shows that massive leucocytic emigration can occur without any increased permeability of the same venule. In histological sections of areas of experimental inflammation, some vessels are blackened with no visible emigrating leucocytes, others show active leucocytic emigration but no carbon in the vascular wall, and yet others show both leucocytic emigration and carbon labelling. Even at the greater resolution of electron microscopy, leucocytes may pass through the vascular wall without any accompanying escape of either carbon or ferritin. It appears that an effective 'protein-tight' seal can be maintained between endothelial cells and an emigrating leucocyte at all stages of its escape.

However it has been shown recently that leucocytic emigration and increased permeability are not always unrelated and that certain types of prolonged vascular leakage in rabbits can occur only in the presence of concurrent leucocytic emigration. The basis of this leucocyte-dependent leakage is not known. The escaping leucocytes may release a permeability factor, or suitably activated emigrating leucocytes (p. 4.26) may cause leakage by damaging vascular endothelium. The time course of the increased permeability favours the latter explanation.

Mediators of the acute inflammatory reaction

The close similarity of the acute inflammatory reaction to diverse types of injury, the highly ordered succession of events extending over many hours which follow an injury lasting only a brief period, and the spread of the inflammatory reaction to adjacent uninjured tissues all suggest that chemical substances, liberated within injured tissues (**endogenous chemical mediators**), play a role in the genesis of the acute inflammatory reaction.

Endogenous mediators appear to be responsible for both vasodilatation and leucocytic emigration (including chemotaxis), and also to cause those forms of increased vascular permeability which are not a result of direct injury to endothelial cells (p. 4.11). A large and increasing number of endogenous substances which can reproduce one or more features of acute inflammation have been identified in injured tissues and in inflammatory exudates, but little is known for certain about which of these potential mediators are of importance in particular types of inflammation.

Proof of the participation of a specific mediator requires the detection of its presence in active form and effective concentration during the relevant period, and inhibition of the response by prior administration of specific antagonistic drugs. These criteria have not been satisfied for any mediator except **histamine** which has been shown to be responsible for the brief, and relatively unimportant, initial phase of leakage after many types of injury. It is therefore not appropriate to give a detailed account of the possible chemical mediators of inflammation, and the notes which follow on their production and actions are intentionally brief.

Possible endogenous mediators

These may be divided into those formed in plasma and those arising from tissue cells.

Plasma factors

These include products of activation and interaction of four major cascade systems—the kinin, complement, coagulation and fibrinolytic systems.

1. **The kinin system.** On a molar basis the most potent known vascular permeability factor is **bradykinin**, a nonapeptide formed by digestion of a plasma glycoprotein, *kininogen*, by a proteolytic enzyme, *kallikrein*, found in normal plasma as its inactive precursor, *prekallikrein*. Contact of plasma with damaged tissues or with a foreign surface activates *Hageman factor* (factor XII of the coagulation cascade) which converts prekallikrein to kallikrein. Enzymes with kallikrein activity are present in many tissues, in urine and in glandular secretions. Several peptides closely related to bradykinin can be released by similar enzyme systems and are also powerful permeability factors (i.e. increase vascular permeability). Kinins are destroyed rapidly by kininases in plasma and in tissues, both of which also contain kallikrein antagonists.

Before the kinin system was characterised, a part of it was described by Miles and Wilhelm under the name of PF/dil, which is probably a

combination of several elements of the kinin system and not a specific substance.

2. **The complement system.** This is described on pp. 7.2–4. Its activation by the 'classical pathway' is a cascade reaction in which nine major components, some of which are pro-enzymes, react sequentially, resulting in a cytolytic complex which disrupts the integrity of cell membranes. A second sequence of activation, the alternative pathway, involves additional components and by-passes the first three stages of the classical complement cascade.

At various stages along the complement cascade, biologically active by-products are released by enzymic cleavage of complement components. Some are permeability factors and others have chemotactic or chemokinetic effects on blood leucocytes. These active by-products can be generated also by the direct action of various proteolytic enzymes, present in damaged tissues, on complement components, especially C3 and C5.

Complement by-products include the following.

(a) C5a, a cleavage product of the fifth component of complement (C5), which has both chemotactic and permeability-increasing properties. The latter effect is partly a direct one on venular endothelium and partly mediated by triggering release of histamine from mast cells. C3a, a product of C3, has similar but weaker properties, and C3a and C5a are widely but inappropriately known as anaphylatoxins (see p. 7.4).

(b) A high molecular weight complex of C5, 6 and 7, which has been claimed to have chemotactic activity.

Formation of a kinin-like substance by cleavage of C2 has long been suspected but it now seems likely that this is really a kinin, production of which is inhibited by C1-INH which also inhibits activation of complement.

In the complex environment of acute inflammation, the complement system can be activated in various ways, notably as follows.

(*i*) *In infections*, union of antibodies with micro-organisms or their antigenic products can activate complement. The endotoxins of Gram-ve bacteria can activate complement at the C3 stage and enzymes secreted by some bacteria are capable of activating C3 and C5.

(*ii*) *In tissue injury*, e.g. ischaemic necrosis of

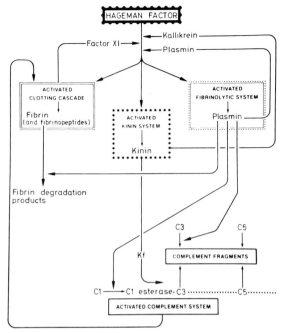

Fig. 4.21 Schematic representation of possible interactions of mediator systems in plasma. (Ryan and Majno, 1977. *Amer. J. Path.* **86**, 183–276.)

heart muscle, enzymes capable of activating C3 and C5 are released from the dying cells.

(*iii*) Activation products of the *kinin, clotting* and *fibrinolytic systems* (see below), are capable of activating complement.

3. **The coagulation and fibrinolytic systems.** These are described in Chapter 10. The coagulation or clotting system brings about the conversion of soluble fibrinogen to insoluble fibrin. Biologically active peptides are released during this conversion and in the subsequent lysis of fibrin by **plasmin**, an enzyme present in inactive form, plasminogen, in normal plasma. These peptides can affect both vascular permeability and the movement of leucocytes.

The different cascade systems outlined above are related in a variety of ways, and each can enhance the activity of the others. An outline of these interactions is shown in Fig. 4.21. **Hageman factor** plays a key role. It is activated by contact with extravascular tissue elements, including basement membrane, by bacterial enzymes and by certain proteolytic enzymes. Once inflammation has begun, Hageman factor leaking through gaps in the endothelium of small blood vessels can activate all three media-

tor systems. Elements in each system can, in turn, activate more Hageman factor.

Despite these complex interactions, it seems likely that the major inflammatory end products of the three plasma cascades are bradykinin and complement activation products C3a and C5a.

Factors released from tissue cells

Histamine is present in inactive form in mast cells, eosinophil and basophil leucocytes and platelets. It can be released from these depots by inflammatory stimuli, by complement activation products C3a and C5a (see above) and by a lysosomal protein secreted by polymorphs. Its release in certain types of immunological reaction is described in Chapter 7. Histamine can also be synthesised by the enzyme histidine decarboxylase present in other types of cell.

Histamine causes active hyperaemia and increased vascular permeability lasting 10–15 minutes. It is responsible for the immediate transient phase of increased permeability seen after many types of mild injury (p. 4.8).

Serotonin (5-hydroxytryptamine) is found in large amounts in mast cells and in platelets and in lesser amounts in many other types of cell. In rats and mice, serotonin increases vascular permeability in a similar way to histamine. In man it is a potent vasoconstrictor but does not increase vascular permeability.

As well as histamine and serotonin, stimulated mast cells can release other active products including SRS-A (see below) and an eosinophil chemotactic factor of anaphylaxis, ECF-A, which is strongly chemotactic for eosinophils (p. 7.8).

Prostaglandins (PG) and leukotrienes. *Prostaglandins* are long-chain hydroxy-fatty acids which can be synthesised and released by most types of cell, but are not stored within cells. Individual prostaglandins differ in their effects. Some, including E_1 and E_2, are powerful vasodilators and potentiate greatly the increased permeability induced by other agents. Despite earlier claims, they do not themselves increase vascular permeability. Other prostaglandins can inhibit certain of the processes of inflammation. Prostaglandin I_2 (prostacyclin), secreted by vascular endothelium, has a powerful inhibitory effect on platelet aggregation and appears to inhibit also the adherence of leucocytes to vascular endothelium. Thromboxane A2, liberated from blood platelets, has the opposite effect, being a most powerful platelet-aggregating agent. Firm evidence of the role of prostaglandins in inflammation is scanty, but the anti-inflammatory effect of aspirin and related drugs has been shown to be due to inhibition of prostaglandin synthetase (cyclo-oxygenase), an enzyme concerned in the synthesis of prostaglandins (p. 10.8).

Leukotrienes. More recently, compounds termed leukotrienes (LTs) have been proposed as mediators of acute inflammation. They are produced by the action of lipoxygenase on arachidonic acid. LTB4 is secreted by neutrophil polymorphs in inflammatory lesions: it is chemotactic for neutrophil and eosinophil polymorphs and monocytes. Once a few neutrophil polymorphs have migrated into inflamed tissues, release of LTB4 presumably promotes the accumulation of more polymorphs. LTC4 and LTD4 are secreted by activated mast cells: they are capable of inducing vascular dilatation and increased venular permeability. **SRS-A** (*slow-reacting substance of anaphylaxis*) is a mixture of LTC4 and LTD4, and has been shown to be involved in the bronchospasm of asthma (p. 7.8).

Lysosomal components. Potential mediators may be released from lysosomes, especially from neutrophil polymorphs, but also from other cells including macrophages and platelets. The most important lysosomal products in inflammation appear to be *cationic proteins* and *neutral proteases*. Cationic proteins can increase permeability, either directly or via mast cells, and are chemotactic to monocytes. The neutral proteases are involved in tissue damage after many types of injury, and can generate chemotactic factors by cleaving C5 and probably also C3.

Lymphokines are proteins released when sensitised T lymphocytes are exposed *in vitro* to the sensitising antigen. None has been characterised chemically. Some lymphokines increase vascular permeability, others are chemotactic factors or mitogenic agents. They are important mediators of delayed hypersensitivity reactions (p. 7.21) but some of them are also involved in immune responses (p. 6.25).

Conclusions

The available evidence suggests the following roles of endogenous mediators in contributing to those features of acute inflammation which are not attributable to direct endothelial injury.

1. Vascular dilatation. Histamine, prostaglandins (notably PGE_2) and complement components C3a and C5a have all been shown to be capable of causing vasodilatation and are present in the inflammatory exudate.

2. Increased vascular permeability. The immediate transient phase is caused by histamine: kinins and leukotrienes may be of importance in the prolonged phase and prostaglandins enhance the effects of these permeability factors.

3. Emigration of leucocytes. C5a and leukotriene LTB4 are potent chemotactic agents for neutrophil polymorphs and monocytes and the cationic proteins of neutrophil polymorphs are chemotactic for monocytes. All three agents induce emigration of leucocytes *in vivo*. Prostaglandins appear to be chemotactic for leucocytes in some species, but apparently not in man.

It is no accident that vertebrate animals have evolved such complicated systems to mediate their responses to injurious stimuli. Mechanisms such as the kinin and complement systems enhance both the range and control of the body's response, and allow physical agents and insoluble irritants to evoke, by indirect means, responses which they are unable to produce by direct action on small blood vessels and inflammatory cells. Inflammation is a vital defence mechanism and the existence of multiple mediator systems ensures that if one mechanism of producing inflammation is impaired, others are available to take its place.

The macroscopic appearances of uncomplicated acute inflammation

Although the basic phenomena of the early stages of acute inflammation are always the same, there is considerable variation in the macroscopic appearances of acutely inflamed tissues. The variation depends in part on the relative magnitudes of the fluid and cellular responses to any particular type of injury, but more importantly upon the nature and texture of the organ which is inflamed and upon the degree of tissue damage produced by the injury which caused the inflammation.

The appearances of mild acute inflammation in the *skin* form the basis of the cardinal signs and have been described already. More severe injury to the skin may cause local accumulation of exudate in the form of blisters, or to loss of a patch of epidermis with the formation of an acute inflammatory ulcer.

The macroscopic characteristics of acute inflammation in *serous membranes* are very different from those in the skin. Normal serous membranes—pleura, pericardium and peritoneum—are thin, shining and transparent. The first recognisable change in acute inflammation of a serous membrane is an enormous increase in the number of visible small blood vessels within the inflamed area. This reflects the vasodilatation characteristic of the early stages of inflammation and is termed *injection* by surgeons. Next, the inflamed membrane loses its normal sheen and becomes dull and slightly opaque due to deposition of small amounts of fibrin on the serosal surface. At the same time, clear or **serous exudate** begins to accumulate in the adjacent pleural or peritoneal cavity. This stage is called **serous inflammation**. As the inflammation continues, more and more fibrin is deposited and within a few hours the inflamed surface becomes covered with an opaque creamy layer of fibrin which obscures the

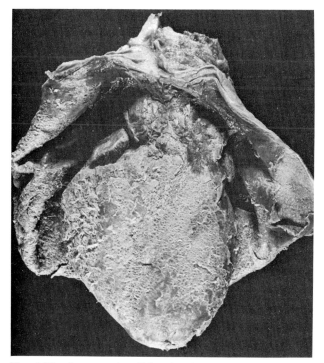 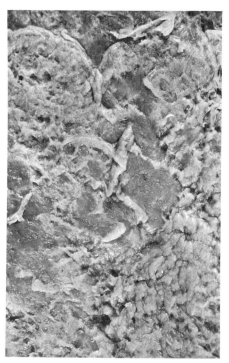

Fig. 4.22 Acute pericarditis; showing a thick, irregular deposit of fibrin on the pericardial surface. The appearance has been likened to that when a butter sandwich is pulled apart ('bread and butter' pericarditis) **Left**, × 0.7. **Right**, × 3.

underlying tissues, including the still-dilated small blood vessels. This stage is termed **fibrinous inflammation**. Exudate increases in volume and becomes **seropurulent**, i.e. progressively more opaque due to accumulation within it of flakes of fibrin and polymorphs. If visceral and parietal layers of the inflamed serous membrane are kept apart by exudate, the fibrin coating the inflamed area has a smooth appearance, but if little exudate forms, or if what does form is removed rapidly via lymphatics, the parietal and visceral serous layers become stuck together by fibrin. Separation of the adjacent layers imparts a characteristic rough irregular— so-called 'bread and butter'—appearance to the inflamed serous membrane (Fig. 4.22). In some acute bacterial infections, massive emigration of polymorphs results in a **purulent** exudate, also called **pus**. It is a creamy fluid, yellow or bloodstained, and often viscid (p. 4.29).

Mild inflammation of a *mucous membrane*, commonly termed **catarrhal inflammation**, is typified by a common cold (coryza). The virus causing the cold multiplies in the epithelial cells of the nasal mucosa and excites an acute inflammatory reaction. This leads to reddening (vasodilatation) and swelling (local accumulation of exudate) of the nasal mucosa, and to the nasal obstruction seen in the early stages of a cold. Some epithelial cells are killed by the virus and desquamate into the nasal cavity. Mucosal glandular cells are stimulated to secrete a thin mucous fluid, and this, mixed with exudate leaking from areas of epithelial desquamation, forms the thin, irritant nasal discharge seen in the early stages of a cold. Various bacteria normally resident in the nose colonise and multiply within the bare areas of mucosa and aggravate the inflammation. The nasal discharge becomes increasingly **purulent** due to emigration of large numbers of polymorphs, until it consists of a mixture of mucous secretion and pus. The inflammation, originally catarrhal, has thus become **mucopurulent**. When the infection is finally overcome, the inflammatory reaction ceases, swelling and vasodilatation subside, the denuded areas of epithelium are restored by proliferation and migration of surviving epithelial cells and discharge from the nose ceases. Other examples of catarrhal inflammation are bacillary dysentery of moderate severity, the acute enteritis of mild infective 'food poisoning', and the inflammation which

follows inhalation of formalin or other irritant vapours.

More severe injury to mucous membranes may result in different appearances. If the injury is severe enough to cause epithelial necrosis, the dead cells separate and large shallow ulcers are formed. A good example of this type of inflammation is acute ulcerative colitis, where injury to surface epithelium is severe and widespread but there is very often surprisingly little involvement of the deeper layers of the bowel wall. The most severe and dramatic type of inflammation of mucous membranes is **pseudomembranous inflammation**: diphtheric infection of the pharynx or larynx used to be the commonest example, but nowadays this type of reaction is seen most often in the small or large bowel. Hyperacute ulcerative colitis, infections with *Cl. difficule* or with enterotoxin-producing strains of *Staphylococcus aureus*, can all produce this type of change. The basic elements of pseudomembranous inflammation are extensive confluent necrosis of surface epithelium and severe acute inflammation of underlying tissues. The fibrinogen in the inflammatory exudate coagulates within the necrotic epithelium and, together with polymorphs, red cells, bacteria and the debris of dead cells, constitutes the false (pseudo) membrane, which forms a white or cream-coloured layer over the surface of the inflamed mucosa (Fig. 9.2, p. 9.5). If the patient survives, the digestive activity of polymorph-derived enzymes loosens and detaches the pseudomembrane, the epithelium regenerates from surviving cells in the base of gland crypts and the lesions heal, often with some fibrosis (scarring).

Uncomplicated acute inflammation makes little difference to the macroscopic appearance of *solid organs* such as liver, kidney or spleen. These organs normally contain so much blood that vasodilatation is impossible to detect, and their dense texture and firm fibrous capsule ensure that very little exudate can accumulate without causing sufficient rise in tissue pressure to limit further leakage of fluid from small blood vessels. Only when acute inflammation is accompanied by large areas of tissue necrosis (as in hyperacute viral hepatitis), or has progressed to the formation of pus, can it be recognised macroscopically with confidence in these vascular solid organs.

The situation in the *lung* is precisely the opposite. The lung is a collection of intercommunicating airfilled spaces, and large amounts of inflammatory exudate can form and pass from alveolus to alveolus via airways and inter-alveolar pores without causing any rise in tissue pressure. Acute inflammation in the lung is therefore usually associated with the formation of large volumes of exudate. The extreme example is lobar pneumonia, which is best regarded as a spreading inflammatory oedema whose extension is limited only by the visceral pleura. A lobe or lobes can fill rapidly with exudate, whose fluid portion is resorbed by lymphatics to leave a pale solid area of lung with a dry, somewhat granular surface. Histologically, the alveoli are filled with fibrin and polymorphs. This is termed grey hepatisation and is the most characteristic stage of lobar pneumonia (p. 16.37).

The role of lymphatics in acute inflammation

The lymphatics are responsible for removing most of the fluid and all of the protein in the inflammatory exudate. To understand how this occurs it is necessary to review briefly the structure and function of lymphatics.

Structure of lymphatics. Terminal lymphatics are blind-ended thin-walled tubes present in almost all tissues in numbers comparable to blood capillaries. They are inconspicuous in histological sections and it is only by perfusion studies that their true frequency can be appreciated. Terminal lymphatics drain into collecting lymphatics, which pass to ever larger collecting channels, finally draining into the veins in the neck via the thoracic duct or the right lymph duct. Valves are present in all collecting lymphatics, so arranged that fluid can flow only proximally. During its passage from terminal lymphatics to the thoracic duct, lymph passes through one or more lymph nodes which act as filters along the lymphatic system.

Electron-microscopic studies show that lymphatic endothelium is thinner and more irregular than that of blood capillaries and its basement membrane is tenuous and incomplete. Junctions between endothelial cells are simpler in form and gaps are normally present between endothelial cells in some terminal lymphatics (Fig. 4.23). Fine fibrils join the outer surface of the endothelial cells of terminal lyphatics to collagen fibres and other connective tissue structures (Fig. 4.24). Collecting lymphatics have a more regular endothelium and smooth muscle cells are present in their walls.

Function of lymphatics. The main function of plasma proteins is to maintain intravascular volume at a reasonably constant level. They achieve this by exerting an osmotic pressure which balances the hydrostatic pressure within small blood vessels. However, many plasma proteins have other functions as well, and to carry out these functions they need to escape from small blood vessels and come into contact with tissue cells. The extent of physiological leakage of protein into different tissues varies a great deal. It is highest in an organ with a sinusoidal blood supply like the liver, less from the fenestrated vessels of the intestinal mucosa, and lowest in tissues whose vessels are lined by continuous type endothelium.

Once protein has escaped from small blood vessels into extravascular tissues, it cannot return to the blood directly against the gradient of protein concentration that exists between plasma and tissue fluid. Instead, the system of lymphatic vessels has developed with a structure specifically adapted to take up the escaped proteins and return them to the blood. Electron-microscopic study shows that large marker particles, and so presumably plasma-proteins, enter terminal lymphatics via intercellular junctions. If not normally present, gaps appear in the endothelium of terminal lymphatics after trivial or physiological stimuli. The wall of collecting lymphatics is much less permeable, and dyes injected into these vessels do not escape into surrounding tissues.

Flow of lymph along lymphatic vessels is in part a passive process, and is due to the combined effects of the valved structure of lymphatics and pressure from adjacent tissues, especially skeletal muscle. This passive flow is assisted by rhythmical contraction of smooth muscle cells in the wall of collecting lymphatics.

Lymphatics in acute inflammation. When tissues swell due to accumulation of inflamma-

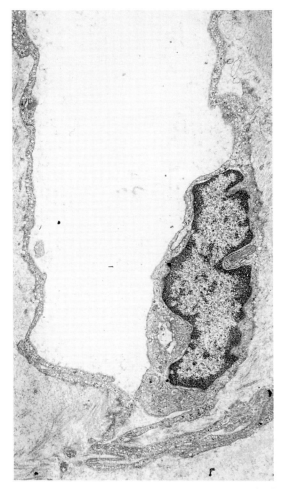

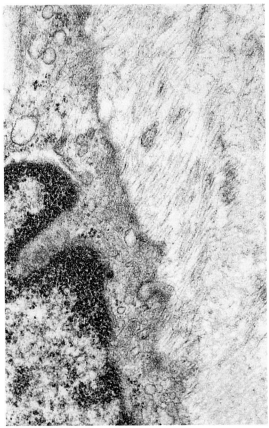

Fig. 4.24 Higher magnification of a portion of the lymphatic shown in Fig. 4.23. Numerous fine fibrils radiate out into the adjacent tissues from the outer aspect of a lymphatic endothelial cell. × 40 000.

Fig. 4.23 Electron micrograph of terminal lymphatic in muscle of rat. The endothelium is thinner and more irregular than that of a blood vessel of similar calibre. × 6000.

tory exudate, the fine anchoring filaments which join the outer aspect of the endothelium of terminal lymphatics to adjacent elements of connective tissue exert an outward pull on the lymphatic wall, rather like the guy ropes of a tent, and terminal lymphatics in areas of acute inflammation become widely dilated. More gaps are present in the endothelium of the distended vessels, possibly as a consequence of the outward pull of the anchoring filaments or due to the action of endogenous permeability factors with an action on lymphatic endothelium. The exudate that escapes from inflamed blood vessels enters the distended terminal lymphatics via these gaps and is carried away by collecting lymphatics.

Lymph draining from an area of acute inflammation is greatly increased in both volume and protein content and, because of its high content of fibrinogen, it usually clots spontaneously on removal from the body. Lymphatics remove fluid and protein from the injured area by processes which are merely an accelerated form of normal lymphatic function. Inflammation will only cause local oedema if the rate of formation of exudate from small blood vessels exceeds the capacity of lymphatics to remove it. The greatly increased flow of lymph from inflamed tissues shows that deposition of fibrin in inflamed tissues does not form an effective barrier to drainage of the exudate. The lymphatic channels only become occluded when they lie within areas of coagulative necrosis caused by severe tissue injury.

As the movement of adjacent muscle plays a

major role in the propulsion of lymph, resting an inflamed area will decrease lymph drainage and diminish the danger of spread of bacteria and toxic substances, both locally and to the lymph nodes and the bloodstream. This is the basis of the long-established clinical doctrine that immobilisation of the inflamed part is of therapeutic value.

Effects of the acute inflammatory reaction

There is no doubt that inflammation is, in general, beneficial. It helps to eliminate invasive micro-organisms, limits the injurious effects of irritating chemicals and bacterial toxins, and participates in the removal of necrotic cells and tissue debris.

Like most beneficial biological processes, acute inflammation is not without its disadvantages: in some instances it appears to confer no obvious benefit, and in others it seems positively harmful.

The **systemic effects** of acute inflammation, leucocytosis and fever, are discussed on pp. 8.15–23.

Beneficial effects

These are conferred partly by the flow of exudate through the inflamed tissues and partly by the phagocytic and microbicidal effects of emigrated leucocytes.

The fluid exudate

This is protective in the following ways.

1. Dilution of toxins. When inflammation is caused by toxic chemicals, including bacterial toxins, the exudate diminishes local tissue injury by diluting the toxins and carrying them away by the lymphatics.

2. Protective antibodies. The proteins in the exudate include antibodies which have developed as a result of infection or immunisation and which are present in the individual's plasma. In acute inflammation due to infection, the exudate may thus contain antibodies which react with, and promote destruction of, the micro-organisms, or which neutralise their toxins. Antibodies promote killing of micro-organisms by rendering them susceptible to lysis by complement and destruction by phagocytes. This is described more fully in Chapter 8.

3. Fibrin formation. Fibrinogen in the exudate is converted to solid fibrin by the action of tissue thromboplastin. A network of deposited fibrin is commonly seen in inflamed tissues, and may form a mechanical barrier to the movement and spread of bacteria. It may also aid in their phagocytosis by leucocytes.

4. Promotion of immunity. Micro-organisms and toxins in the inflammatory lesions are carried by the exudate, either free or in phagocytes, to the local lymph nodes where they may stimulate an immune response. This provides antibodies and cellular mechanisms of defence which appear within a few days and may be maintained for years.

5. Cell nutrition. The flow of inflammatory exudate brings with it glucose, oxygen, etc., and thus helps to nourish the greatly increased numbers of cells: it also carries away their waste products.

The role of leucocytes

Phagocytosis. This is a process in which phagocytic cells ingest solid particles such as bacteria, dead cells, fragments of cells and tissues, fibrin and foreign material. Neutrophil polymorphs are actively phagocytic and become increasingly active when they emigrate into inflamed tissues. Monocytes are only weakly phagocytic but when they emigrate in the late stages of an acute inflammatory lesion they transform into **macrophages**: this involves increase in size, in metabolic activity, motility and phagocytic capacity (p. 4.35).

The first stage in phagocytosis is the attachment of the particle to be ingested to the surface of the phagocytic cell. Adhesion between particle and cell surface depends upon the surface characteristics of the particle and especially on coating of the particle by plasma factors known as **opsonins**: they include antibodies and components of the complement system. This aspect of phagocytosis and also the mechanisms of destruction of ingested micro-organisms by phagocytes are considered with immunological aspects of phagocytosis on pp. 8.9–11.

The next stage is ingestion of the attached particle. The phagocyte extends pseudopodia around the particle and these meet and fuse, enclosing the particle in a **phagocytic vacuole** or **phagosome** which is bounded by plasma membrane and is drawn into the cell. The cytoplasmic granules (lysosomes) come into contact with the phagosome, their membranes fuse, and break down at the site of fusion so that the lysosomes are incorporated into the phagosome to form a **phagolysosome** into which the lysosomal enzymes are released. These consist of about 40 enzymes including proteases, nucleases, lipases, glycosidases, phosphatases, phospholipases, etc. In fact, enzymes capable of digesting most cellular and microbial constituents. Most of them function optimally at a pH of about 5, and this is maintained within the phagolysosome by an H^+ pump mechanism in the membrane. In most acute bacterial infections, bacteria are ingested by neutrophil polymorphs and are killed by mechanisms described on p. 8.10 and digested. Their toxins may, however, kill the polymorph and they are then re-phagocytosed by fresh polymorphs.

Macrophages play only a minor role in phagocytosis and killing of bacteria in most acute inflammatory lesions caused by bacterial infections. They appear late and their main function is removal of dead bacteria, dead cells, damaged red cells, tissue fragments and fibrin—in other words the debris of tissue injury and acute inflammation. Macrophages do, however, play the major phagocytic role in many types of chronic inflammation and in scavenging indigestible material.

Phagocytosis by polymorphs is an important protective mechanism against invasion of tissues by many types of micro-organism causing acute infections. Individuals in whom polymorphs are entirely absent (*agranulocytosis*), greatly reduced in number, or functionally defective, are liable to frequent severe infections, often caused by micro-organisms which are of low virulence and are destroyed rapidly by normal individuals. Such *opportunistic infections* (p. 8.1) have become much more common since the widespread use of cytotoxic drugs for the treatment of disseminated malignant disease, especially lymphomas.

Tissue breakdown by phagocytes. In acute inflammatory lesions, neutrophil polymorphs and subsequently macrophages are not only phagocytic but during phagocytic activity they also secrete lysosomal and other enzymes into the exudate. In this process, lysosomes fuse with the plasma membrane of the cell instead of with phagocytic vacuoles, and discharge their contents at the surface (**exocytosis**). These various enzymes, and particularly cationic proteins and neutral proteases, may contribute to digestion of the inflammatory debris, but released lysosomal enzymes are active only if the pH is low. Being short-lived, most of the neutrophil polymorphs which accumulate in acute inflammatory lesions die locally, and any remaining lysosomal and other enzymes are then added to the exudate.

Active secretion of enzymes by phagocytes may also increase the tissue and cell injury in acute inflammation, and is the major cause of vascular damage in certain Arthus-type reactions in which antigen-antibody complexes are formed or deposited in vessel walls (p. 7.13), e.g. some forms of glomerulonephritis and acute arteritis. Much of the injury to articular cartilage in rheumatoid arthritis appears to arise in this way. Polymorphs can also release agents which increase vascular permeability and induce the migration of more leucocytes into the injured area.

In the absence of infection, removal of dead tissue (debridement) and subsequent repair can proceed in the absence of polymorphs, but if macrophages are also depleted both debridement and repair are seriously delayed. It appears that the macrophage, not the polymorph, is the most important cell in the early stages of wound repair.

Harmful effects

Swelling of acutely inflamed tissues may have serious mechanical effects. For example, in acute laryngitis the lumen of the larynx may be so reduced as to interfere with breathing.

Acute inflammation of tissues which are confined within a restricted space, and so cannot expand, results in a rise of tissue pressure which may impair function directly or may interfere with blood flow and so cause ischaemic injury.

Examples include inflammation of the brain (encephalitis) and meningitis, both of which cause increased intracranial pressure sometimes leading to coma and death. Similarly acute bacterial infection of the bone marrow (osteomyelitis) raises the pressure in the medullary cavity and extensive ischaemic necrosis may occur. A third, painful example is acute inflammation of the testis, usually caused by mumps virus; the tough tunica albuginea prevents much expansion, and ischaemia results, sometimes with permanent residual injury. Fortunately, both testes are seldom severely affected.

Some examples of inflammation are inappropriate and harmful. For example, most people encounter grass pollen in the air without ill effect, but others become sensitised to pollens and react by the acute conjunctivitis and rhinitis of hay fever. There is also a rare condition, angio-oedema, in which acute inflammatory lesions develop spontaneously in various tissues, including the gastro-intestinal tract. It is due to deficiency of a plasma factor which controls activation of the complement and kinin systems.

Subsequent course of the inflammatory reaction

After the initial stages of acute inflammation have developed, subsequent changes within the area of injury may follow any one of four possible courses. (1) resolution (2) healing by fibrosis (*scarring*) with or without regeneration of lost parenchymal cells, (3) suppuration, or (4) chronic inflammation.

The course of any particular injury depends upon the nature and duration of the injurious stimulus, the type of tissue injured, and the degree of destruction caused by the damaging agent.

1. Resolution

This means complete restoration of the injured area to normal. It can occur only if the damaging agent does not cause areas of dead tissue above a certain critical size. In many tissues, single cells or a small group of cells can be killed, their remains removed and the defect filled by division of adjacent cells of the same kind. However, foci of necrosis of more than a few cells in size are replaced by newly formed scar tissue and complete resolution is then no longer possible.

Resolution is the usual sequel to mild chemical or physical injuries of brief duration and to many types of infection in which the causal organism does not induce large areas of tissue destruction. Cellulitis (inflammation of connective tissue), many viral infections and some types of pneumonia, most strikingly lobar pneumonia, fall into this category.

Resolution involves not only subsidence of vascular changes, such as vasodilatation and increased permeability, but also the removal of all abnormal material from the extravascular spaces. The material to be removed includes exudate, polymorphs, fibrin and dead tissue cells and their breakdown products.

When vasodilatation subsides, the balance of hydrostatic and osmotic forces across the wall of small blood vessels returns to its normal resting state. As a result, some of the fluid of the **inflammatory exudate** is resorbed into the venular end of capillaries. However, the bulk of fluid and all the protein in the exudate are removed via lymphatics. The mechanisms by which this occurs and the structure and functions of lymphatics are described on pp. 4.23–5.

Most of the accumulated polymorphs die locally, but some leave via the lymphatics. As noted above, they release various enzymes during phagocytosis and after their death, and these contribute to their own digestion. Dead tissue cells undergo partial digestion by their own lysosomal enzymes and those released by polymorphs and macrophages.

As polymorphs disappear, macrophages come to form an increasing proportion of the extravascular cells in the inflamed tissues, until finally they replace the polymorphs completely. They are actively phagocytic and, as described above, take up and digest much of the debris of cells and tissues destroyed in the inflammatory lesion. When the inflammation subsides, some of the macrophages pass to the draining lymph nodes, while others may remain locally as tissue histiocytes.

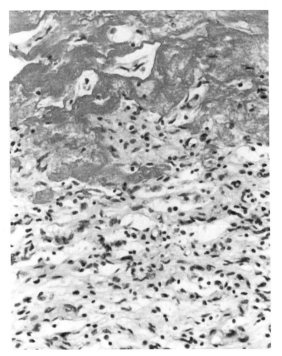

Fig. 4.25 A dense layer of fibrin on the pleural surface, showing organisation, i.e. replacement by vascular granulation tissue, extending from the underlying pleura. × 250.

The replacement of polymorphs by macrophages in resolving inflammation is due to a combination of later emigration of monocytes and the short lifespan of polymorphs in extravascular tissues. Polymorphs and monocytes migrate independently and successively from small blood vessels, and no correlation exists between the numbers of each type of cell escaping after different kinds of injury.

Most of the fibrin deposited in the extravascular spaces is broken down by fibrinolytic enzymes in the exudate and the soluble products are removed via the lymphatics. A relatively small amount of fibrin is engulfed by macrophages.

Enzymes derived from at least three sources remove the fibrin. The most important is plasmin (p. 10.11). The inactive form of this enzyme, plasminogen, is present in plasma and may be activated by material released from damaged tissues. Fibrinolysins are among the enzymes released by polymorphs and macrophages within the area of inflammation (see above), and in addition certain bacteria produce powerful fibrinolysins.

2. Healing by fibrosis

Fibrosis, or scar formation, may result from inflammation in three circumstances:

(*a*) *If heavy deposits of fibrin are formed* in the early stages of acute inflammation, they may not be removed completely within a few days by the fibrinolytic enzymes from the plasma and those released by polymorphs. Fibrin not so removed is gradually replaced by granulation tissue by a process termed **organisation** (Fig. 4.25): macrophages migrate into the fibrin, digesting it as they go, and are closely followed by new capillaries and fibroblasts. The granulation tissue thus formed (like all granulation tissue) gradually changes to dense fibrous tissue. Organisation of fibrin is a common sequel to acute inflammation of serous membranes or of the synovial lining of joints. Adjacent surfaces initially glued together by fibrin become united by granulation tissue and eventually by firm, almost avascular fibrous tissue.

(*b*) If the injury causes *death of a substantial volume of tissue*, the mechanism of removal of the dead tissue depends on its nature. Some highly cellular tissue, e.g. liver, is rapidly digested by lysosomal enzymes as described above, leaving a space containing exudate, polymorphs, etc. This is gradually replaced by granulation tissue growing in from the margin. Other dead tissue, e.g. fibrous tissue, is not readily or rapidly digested, and, like dense deposits of fibrin, is gradually replaced by organisation. In both cases, the result is a fibrous scar which becomes increasingly dense and avascular as it matures.

(*c*) *Progression of acute to chronic inflammation*, described below, is always accompanied by fibrosis.

3. Suppuration

Suppuration, or formation of pus, is a common sequel to acute inflammation. Suppurative lesions are characterised by an exudate containing very large numbers of neutrophil polymorphs, which, sometimes together with dead tissue cells, break down to form a thick creamy, yellow or bloodstained fluid called pus (p. 4.22). Pus may form diffusely in loose tissues or body cavities or be localised in discrete foci which are known as abscesses.

For acute inflammation to proceed to suppuration, the causative stimulus must persist and must be of a type which evokes massive emigration of polymorphs. Suppuration is virtually always caused by infection, usually by certain so-called pyogenic (pus-forming) bacteria, the most important of which are *Staphylococcus aureus*, *Streptococcus pyogenes*, *Streptococcus pneumoniae*, gonococci, meningococci, *Escherichia coli* and related Gram -ve bacilli. Injection of some chemicals, e.g. croton oil or turpentine, may also cause abscess formation.

Pus consists of living polymorphs, polymorphs in all stages of disintegration, living and dead micro-organisms and the debris of dead tissue cells and leucocytes all suspended in inflammatory exudate. The high concentration of nucleic acids derived from cell breakdown is responsible for the sticky, slimy nature of pus.

No matter how long suppurative inflammation continues, all the leucocytes within pus are polymorphs; macrophages are only seen in the exudate when the inflammation is subsiding, after the infection has been overcome, although they may be numerous in the inflamed tissue around chronic abscesses and also in many types of non-suppurating chronic inflammation.

Abscess formation. The mode of development of an abscess can be appreciated by describing the events which follow injection of pyogenic bacteria, for example *Staphylococcus aureus*, into living tissues. The microbes start to multiply rapidly soon after their introduction and liberate increasing quantities of toxins which damage tissue cells. The toxins, and products released from the damaged cells, induce a severe inflammatory reaction. When the concentration of toxin becomes high enough, tissue in the centre of the inflamed area dies.

Eight to ten hours after inoculation, polymorphs have emigrated in large numbers into the oedematous tissues. Many of them are killed, liberating enzymes which produce rapid liquefaction of the dead tissue, and by 48 hours a ragged cavity filled with pus is present in the centre of an area of acutely inflamed tissue (Fig. 4.26).

Later changes in the abscess are a result of two simultaneous processes. Proliferation of

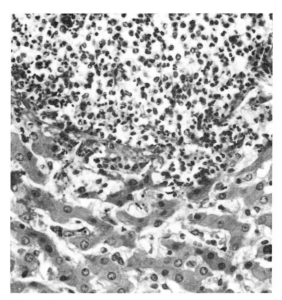

Fig. 4.26 Margin of an abscess cavity in the liver at an early stage in its formation. In the upper part of the field the liver tissue has been destroyed and digested, leaving a space filled with purulent exudate. ×250.

staphylococci continues, more polymorphs accumulate, more polymorphs and tissue cells are killed, and as a result the size of the abscess cavity and the volume of pus in it increase progressively. At the same time, repair processes commence in the surrounding tissue and a layer of granulation tissue begins to form around the abscess, separating it from the adjacent, still inflamed tissue. If this repair process is successful in limiting further extension of infection, then by ten to fourteen days the abscess becomes lined by a well-defined layer of granulation tissue with a thin band of collagen on its outer side (Fig. 4.27). If the abscess does not rupture or is not drained surgically, the collagen layer thickens progressively. Inflammation in surrounding tissues subsides as the wall of granulation tissue develops, but leucocytes can still be seen escaping in large numbers from the newly formed vessels in the granulation tissue and add to the pus in the abscess cavity.

Abscesses may also form in another way. If pyogenic bacteria infect a body cavity, as for example in acute appendicitis extending to the peritoneal surface, the inflamed part of the peritoneal cavity may become walled off from the rest by fibrinous adhesions. Fibrin may glue adjacent serous surfaces together and, aided by

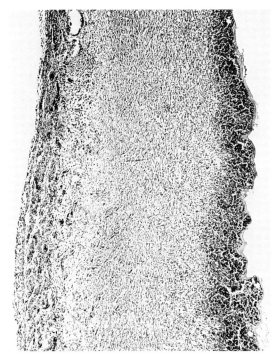

Fig. 4.27 Wall of a ten-day-old experimental abscess in a rat. Pus in the cavity of the abscess (left) is surrounded by a thick wall composed of granulation tissue and developing scar tissue. × 100.

the omentum, form an isolated pocket containing the appendix, bacteria, inflammatory exudate and polymorphs. If the inflammation continues, pus will form progressively within

the walled off zone and the fibrinous adhesions will be invaded by fibroblasts and new blood vessels and converted into fibrous adhesions. In this type of abscess, tissue need not die to form the cavity of the abscess, which is simply a walled off portion of an existing body cavity.

Commonly, an abscess terminates by rupture onto the skin surface or into a hollow viscus, or by surgical incision. Rupture allows escape of most of the viable bacteria and much of the pus. The pressure of the surrounding tissues collapses the abscess cavity and its walls adhere to one another first by fibrin and later by granulation tissue. The residual bacteria are disposed of by polymorphs, discharge ceases and only a scar remains to mark the site of the abscess. By allowing drainage, surgical incision of an abscess has the same beneficial effect. Conversely, if an abscess is allowed to become chronic, considerable scarring results (see below).

4. Progression to chronic inflammation

Long continued tissue injury, for example by persistence of micro-organisms in a focus of infection, results in progression of acute inflammation to a chronic stage. This is discussed below.

Chronic Inflammation

Some types of inflammatory reaction are of much longer duration than those so far described, persisting for weeks or months after the initial injury. Any prolonged inflammation is termed *chronic*, the term referring solely to the duration of the inflammatory process.

There are two main types of chronic inflammation: chronic supervening on acute and chronic *ab initio*, i.e. developing slowly with no initial acute phase.

Chronic inflammation supervening on acute

This is almost always suppurative in type, and presents as a persistent discharge of pus from

an abscess which has ruptured or been drained surgically. There are two common causes of persistent suppuration. The first is delay in evacuation of an abscess. If an abscess remains undrained, its fibrous wall becomes progressively thicker and more rigid. When such a thick-walled abscess is opened, pressure of adjacent tissues cannot collapse the cavity, and it can only be obliterated by ingrowth of granulation tissue from its walls. If, due to inadequate drainage, pus stagnates within the abscess cavity, residual bacteria may multiply and cause re-activation of the inflammatory process. Chronic abscesses may be seen after delayed or inadequate drainage of an empyema thoracis (suppurating pleurisy) or whenever an abscess forms in bone.

The second cause of persistent suppurating infection is the presence of foreign material within the inflamed area. This may be dirt, cloth or wood, etc. driven in from outside, or a metal or plastic prosthesis introduced by the surgeon. Indigestible dead tissue may also have an effect like a foreign body. In a boil or carbuncle, substantial portions of dermal collagen may be killed by bacterial toxins: dead collagen is broken down very slowly by lysosomal enzymes and may persist in the abscess for a considerable time. A piece of dead bone (*sequestrum*) in osteomyelitis (infection of a bone) is another example of a persistent endogenous 'foreign body'. Why a foreign body within an area of suppuration causes the infection to persist is not always clear, but it is a well-established clinical observation that suppuration will continue until the foreign material is removed.

Chronic inflammation *ab initio:*

This type of response occurs after many types of injury. The injury may be physical, chemical, such as the response to talc or asbestos, or may result from poor local circulation, as in the ulceration of the leg often seen in association with varicose veins. Certain micro-organisms, including those that cause tuberculosis, syphilis and leprosy, characteristically induce chronic inflammation. In still other types of chronic inflammation, including rheumatoid arthritis, ulcerative colitis and Crohn's disease, the cause is not known but disturbances of immune mechanisms are believed to play an important aetiological role.

The histological appearances of chronic inflammation vary widely with different causative factors, but all types share the following morphological characteristics.

1. The reaction is usually more productive than exudative, i.e. formation of new fibrous tissue is more prominent than exudation of fluid. Tuberculosis of joints, bones and serous cavities is sometimes an exception to this generalisation.

2. Destruction of tissue and resulting inflammation proceed at the same time as attempted healing.

3. The cellular reaction is pleomorphic,

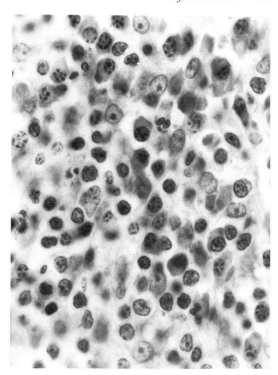

Fig. 4.28 Chronic inflammation showing the confusing variety of cells. In this instance, they include plasma cells, lymphocytes and occasional polymorphs, while the larger nuclei probably belong to macrophages and fibroblasts. × 820.

various cell types being present in the inflamed tissues (Fig. 4.28).

4. There may be suppuration and/or necrosis.

5. The microscopic appearances in most cases are non specific, in the sense that they give no indication of the cause of the condition.

Attempted healing occurs concurrently with tissue destruction and inflammation in all types of chronic inflammation, but the topographical relationships of inflammation and repair vary. In a chronic abscess and in many tuberculous lesions, the two processes are sharply separated. However, healing and inflammation may intermingle to form a mass composed of inflammatory cells, areas of granulation and fibrous tissue, and sometimes foci of necrosis or abscesses. Such a chronic inflammatory mass is traditionally called a *granuloma* (see below).

The many different cell types which may be present in areas of chronic inflammation include neutrophil and eosinophil polymorphs, macrophages and their derivatives (epithelioid cells and giant cells), plasma cells, lymphocytes and fibroblasts. *The presence of a mixture of cell types is the most characteristic histological feature of chronic inflammation.*

In many cases of tuberculosis, the diagnosis can be suspected strongly from the histological appearances alone, but there are dangerous pitfalls as several other conditions may give rise to changes readily mistaken for tuberculosis. Moreover, in this regard tuberculosis is a most atypical chronic inflammation. In most instances of acute or chronic inflammation it is not possible to determine the precise cause from the histological appearances alone. It is true that suppurating inflammation is virtually always caused by bacterial infection, but the particular bacteria responsible cannot be deduced from the histological appearances. *A firm diagnosis of the cause of inflammatory lesions depends upon the recognition of a specific causative agent, or on some other procedure such as serological tests for a specific infection.*

Macroscopic features of chronic inflammation

These are extremely variable. Common forms, which may be seen alone or in combination, are (1) a chronic abscess; (2) a mixture of caseous necrosis (structureless debris of necrotic tissue which may liquefy and discharge, leaving a cavity), granulation tissue and fibrosis, as seen in tuberculosis; (3) a chronic ulcer, such as a peptic (Fig. 19.30 p. 19.23) or varicose ulcer; (4) diffuse thickening of the wall of a hollow organ, as seen in chronic cholecystitis (Fig. 20.56, p. 20.50), or more localised thickening to form an inflammatory stricture, or (5) a chronic inflammatory mass or granuloma as described above.

Fibrosis of an organ without evidence of continuing inflammation is not chronic inflammation. The scarred appendix seen as the end result of severe acute appendicitis is a fibrosed appendix, not chronic appendicitis.

Granuloma and granulomatous inflammation. These terms are widely used with three different meanings. Traditionally they are used to describe a chronic inflammatory lesion in the form of a mass which grossly resembles a tumour, hence the suffix *-oma*, which is usually reserved for neoplasms.

Recently, especially in North America, granuloma has been restricted to lesions composed largely of macrophages, or restricted still further to mean a collection of altered macrophages (epithelioid cells and giant cells) as seen in tuberculosis. To avoid confusion it is wise to indicate this usage by terms such as *macrophage granuloma, epithelioid-cell granuloma* or *tuberculoid granuloma.*

Finally, a number of heterogeneous entities are called granulomas—*malignant granuloma of nose* or *midline granuloma* (a lesion with histological features of chronic inflammation which resembles a tumour in its infiltration and destruction of tissue), *Wegener's granuloma* (due to a polyarteritis) and *eosinophil granuloma of bone* (a mass composed largely of Langerhans cells and eosinophil leucocytes). These terms are distinctive enough to avoid confusion.

Mediators of chronic inflammation

Largely because of the great difference in time scale between chronic inflammation and the experimental systems used to study the inflammatory reaction, little is known of the mediators of chronic inflammation. Persistence of chronic inflammation requires the continued presence of the irritant stimulus. The chemotactic factors which may be involved have been discussed above. Apart from lymphokines (p. 7.21), almost nothing is known of the role of endogenous permeability factors in non-suppurative chronic inflammation.

Types of Cell in Inflammatory Lesions

Polymorphonuclear leucocytes

Neutrophil polymorphs are the predominant cells in most acute inflammatory lesions. Their mode of escape into inflamed tissues, their phagocytic activities and the control of their emigration, have been described earlier in this chapter.

Neutrophil polymorphs are the first cells to arrive in large numbers at the scene of acute tissue injury: they already have their full complement of enzymes, a store of glycogen to provide energy in hypoxic conditions, and are actively motile, responsive to chemotactic stimuli, strongly phagocytic and capable of killing many types of micro-organisms (p. 8.10). They are thus well adapted to counter invasive micro-organisms. As noted earlier, they are short-lived cells, but can be produced in the haemopoietic marrow in huge numbers (p. 8.16 *et seq*).

Eosinophil polymorphs have a similar origin and lifespan to neutrophils and are sluggishly amoeboid and phagocytic. Their granules contain similar enzymes to neutrophils and also a peroxidase and large amounts of basic protein. They react chemotactically *in vitro* to substances which attract neutrophils, to specific eosinophil chemotactic factors released by mast cells, particularly in allergic reactions, and to products of lymphocytes in some immune reactions.

Many eosinophils are present in normal intestinal mucosa and in the uterus after oestrus. They are the predominant cell in immediate type hypersensitivity reactions like asthma and hay fever, and in the reaction around parasitic worms.

The function of eosinophils is not known with certainty. It is believed that, by releasing enzymes like histaminase and aryl sulphatase, they limit and control immediate hypersensitivity reactions (p. 7.7). In parasitic infections, eosinophils are attracted by chemotaxins released by lymphocytes. They may mediate antibody-dependent killing of the parasites, and they are believed to play a major role in resistance to parasites (pp. 28.24 and 43).

Lymphoid cells

Lymphocytes are present in large numbers in many non-suppurative types of chronic inflammation. They are not phagocytic, do not adhere to foreign surfaces, and respond to different chemotaxins to those which attract polymorphs and mononuclear phagocytes.

Lymphocytes are the specific responder cells of the immunity system (see Chapter 6) and are subdivided into T and B types which are indistinguishable by light microscopy. They are not concerned directly in destruction of micro-organisms or disposal of dead tissue. When sensitised T lymphocytes come into contact with the sensitising antigen, they liberate soluble substances, **lymphokines**, which may play an important role in increasing vascular permeability and attracting leucocytes into the site of the reaction. Some T lymphocytes are also capable of effecting the destruction of foreign cells introduced into the body, and, in experimental studies, cancer cells.

Plasma cells. After immunological stimulation, some B lymphocytes are transformed into plasma cells, which are the main source of humoral antibody. Plasma cells may be present in large numbers in areas of subacute or chronic inflammation. They do not usually appear until about a week after the onset of inflammation and are seen in greatest numbers in persistent lesions caused by various micro-organisms.

Macrophages—the mononuclear phagocyte system

The term *macrophage* was first applied in 1905 by Metchnikoff to distinguish large phagocytic cells from the smaller phagocytes, the polymorphs, which he called microphages. Macrophages are amoeboid cells, respond to chemotactic stimuli, are powerful phagocytes of some types of micro-organisms and cell debris, and participate in immune responses and in the immunological destruction of foreign or infected cells, and possibly also tumour cells.

Macrophages in inflamed tissues are derived mainly from emigrated, transformed blood monocytes. This has been established by labelling circulating monocytes with either tritiated thymidine or colloidal carbon, and use of these techniques has shown that all the mononuclear phagocytic cells in the body are members of one system of cells—**the mononuclear phagocyte system**. This system includes many, but not all, of the cells in the *reticulo-endothelial (R-E) sys-*

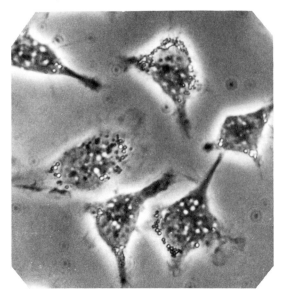

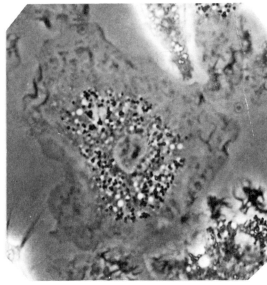

Fig. 4.29   Mouse peritoneal macrophages in culture, viewed by phase-contrast microscopy. Inflammatory exudate has been added to the culture shown on the right. Note the increase in size, content of (phase dense) lysosomes and (phase-lucent) vesicles and extensive cytoplasmic 'ruffling' of the stimulated cell. × 960. (The late Professor W.G. Spector and Mrs Katherine M. Wynne.)

tem as defined in 1924 by Aschoff on the basis of intravital staining with non-toxic protein-bound dyes. As well as phagocytes, Aschoff's R-E system included certain non-phagocytic cells—the reticulum cells of the framework of lymph nodes which may be related to macrophages, and also vascular endothelial cells which are quite distinct in their origin and function. The term 'reticulo-endothelial system' is

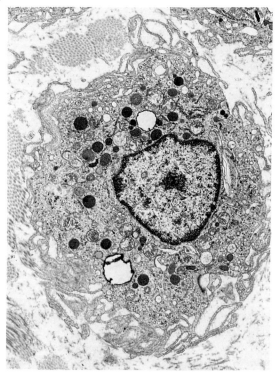

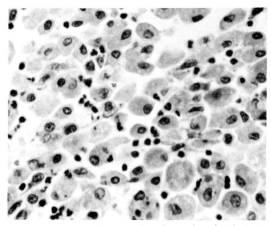

Fig. 4.30   Macrophages of various sizes in the wall of a chronically inflamed gall bladder. Note the ovoid or indented nucleus and abundant cytoplasm. × 405.

Fig. 4.31   Electron micrograph of a macrophage in loose connective tissue. Note the numerous irregular filipodia on the cell surface. The dense bodies in the cytoplasm are phagolysosomes formed by the fusion of lysosomes with phagocytic vacuoles. × 7000.

no longer appropriate to describe mononuclear phagocytes and should not be so used.

It is now known that all cells in the mononuclear phagocyte system are derived from a bone marrow precursor, the **promonocyte**, which is in turn derived from the *haemopoietic stem cell* (p. 17.2). The promonocyte matures to a **monocyte**, which enters the blood stream and circulates for 20–30 hours. Monocytes normally leave the blood and may enter any one of a variety of tissues to become '**free tissue histiocytes**', which may be regarded as macrophages in a resting state. They are found in loose connective tissues, the peritoneum, brain (microglia), lymphoid tissues and lung alveoli, etc. Other monocytes become '**fixed tissue histiocytes**' which lie between endothelial cells lining the vascular sinusoids of the liver (Kupffer cells), spleen, bone marrow, etc., and the lymphatic sinuses of lymph nodes. The **osteoclasts** of bone are also derived from monocytes and the reticulum cells of lymphoid tissues and spleen may be. The turnover of macrophages in most tissues is normally slow, individual cells surviving for several months. In the resting state, histiocytes are small, inconspicuous cells with a condensed nucleus and scanty cytoplasm. When stimulated by tissue injury, etc., they become activated (see below).

Macrophages in inflamed tissues. When monocytes migrate from the venules in inflammatory lesions, they develop into *inflammatory* or *activated macrophages*: this involves increase in euchromatin, protein synthesis, increase in size, in the number, size and enzyme content of lysosomes, and enhancement of motility, phagocytic activity and capacity to kill ingested micro-organisms. In the living state, they exhibit continuously-moving cytoplasmic veils or ruffles which project from the cell surface (Fig. 4.29). In histological sections, inflammatory macrophages range up to 30 μm in diameter, with an ovoid vesicular nucleus and abundant agranular cytoplasm. Phagocytosed debris of various kinds is often present in their cytoplasm (Fig. 4.30) and electron-micrography may show heterogeneous dense bodies which consist of indigestible material within phagolysosomes (Fig. 4.31).

Resting macrophages in the tissues (histiocytes) may become activated, but, as noted above, the macrophages in various experimentally-induced inflammatory lesions, both acute and chronic, are provided mainly by emigration of monocytes.

Macrophages are activated by factors present in the inflammatory exudate, notably a component of complement (see above) and probably other chemotactic factors. In inflammation induced by T lymphocytes, these cells also release lymphokines, one of which activates macrophages, while another arrests them within the inflammatory lesion (p. 7.21).

Cell kinetics. Spector and his colleagues have provided much information about the kinetics of inflammatory macrophages. Monocytes, after emigration and transformation to macrophages, are not end cells but retain a capacity for both limited mitosis and change into other morphological forms. The lifespan of inflammatory macrophages varies with the causal agent. In chronic inflammations caused by agents toxic to cells, macrophages survive for only a few days, the population being replenished constantly by further emigration of monocytes. With more bland stimuli, however, individual cells may survive for weeks or months within the inflamed area, and mitosis of macrophages within the lesion may be almost sufficient to maintain the population.

Functions of macrophages. The phagocytic activity of macrophages in acute inflammatory reactions has already been described (p. 4.25); they can engulf a wider range of foreign material than polymorphs and are much more efficient scavengers of inflammatory debris. When polymorphs ingest micro-organisms, they either kill them or die in the attempt. This is not so with macrophages, which, because of their longevity, may harbour micro-organisms or other foreign material for long periods. Macrophages are more involved in phagocytosis of micro-organisms which are less acutely destructive and cause chronic infections; important examples of micro-organisms which can survive for long periods within them are the tubercle and leprosy bacilli and *Histoplasma capsulatum*. Destruction of such intracellular organisms is dependent on a cell-mediated immune response in which T lymphocytes secrete lymphokines which increase the microbicidal capacity of macrophages. Unfortunately the immune reaction may also result in the death of the infected macrophages, with consequent foci of necrosis (p. 7.20).

Activated macrophages secrete a large num-

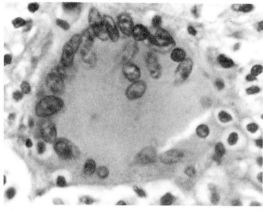

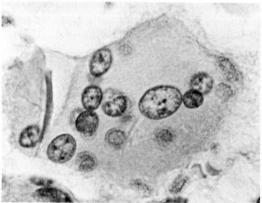

Fig. 4.32 Multinucleated giant cells formed by fusion of macrophages. The upper cell is a Langhans' giant cell in a tuberculous lesion: note the peripheral arrangement of nuclei and abundant cytoplasm. The lower cell is a foreign-body giant cell: the nuclei vary in size and are irregularly distributed, and the cell has engulfed a fragment of suture material. × 750.

ber of biologically active factors, notably lysosomal enzymes, vascular-permeability and chemotactic factors, including some complement components. They also secrete a factor (endogenous pyrogen) which causes fever, and factors which modulate the activity of fibroblasts, lymphocytes and perhaps endothelial cells, and produce antibiotic agents such as lysozyme and interferon. They may thus help to control some bacterial and viral infections.

Macrophages co-operate with lymphocytes in both humoral and cell-mediated immune responses and, as noted above, also act as effector cells in the immune destruction of antigenic material and foreign (transplanted) cells. These

functions are described in Chapter 7. They may also be responsible for killing tumour cells (p. 13.33).

Cells of the mononuclear phagocyte series may be identified by immunocytological staining with monoclonal antibodies to specific cell markers, and by cytochemical methods, e.g. granular staining with sudan black and strong positivity for non-specific esterase (the NASDA reaction) which is inhibited by pre-treatment of the cells with sodium fluoride (p. 17.49).

Modulated forms of inflammatory macrophages

Within areas of chronic inflammation, macrophages may be transformed into two other types of cell—epithelioid and giant cells.

Epithelioid cells, named from their resemblance to cells of epithelial type, have vesicular nuclei and abundant acidophil cytoplasm. They are commonly arranged in groups as in the classic tubercule and the lesions of sarcoidosis, but they also occur in other types of chronic inflammation, and it seems likely that they are induced by delayed hypersensitivity reactions. Epithelioid cells have little phagocytic capacity and appear to have a secretory function. What they secrete is not known.

Giant cells are very large cells with cytoplasm similar to epithelioid cells and contain multiple nuclei—up to 100 or even more in one cell. They are found whenever there is material which macrophages find difficult to ingest. They are especially numerous around insoluble material such as a splinter of wood, urate crystals in gouty deposits or a non-absorbable suture, and are also a characteristic feature of the lesions of both tuberculosis and sarcoidosis. Giant cells are often classified into *foreign body giant cells*, which have irregularly scattered nuclei, and *Langhans' giant cells*, in which the nuclei are arranged peripherally (Fig. 4.32). It has been claimed that Langhans' giant cells are characteristic of tuberculosis, but the distinction is not valid.

Giant cells arise by fusion of macrophages, and it has been suggested that fusion results from a simultaneous attempt by two or more cells to engulf a single particle. However, they commonly come to resemble multinucleated epithelioid cells and have then little phagocytic capacity and no known specific function. They may be a form of biological 'accident' rather than a specific adaptation of macrophages.

Langerhans cells of the skin and **dendritic** and **interdigitating reticulum cells** in lymphoid tissues are now thought to be derived from the mononuclear phagocyte system, but the evidence is inconclusive. These cells are, at most, poorly phagocytic and have special roles in the immune response. Their cytoplasm contains small discoid bodies (*Birbeck granules*), which appear in electron micrographs as straight or curved rods, sometimes with terminal expansions: their nature is unknown.

References and Further Reading

Boyden, S. (1962). The chemotactic effect of mixtures of antibody and antigen on polymorphonuclear leucocytes. *Journal of Experimental Medicine* **115**, 453–66.

Buckley, I.K. (1963). Delayed secondary damage and leucocyte chemotaxis following focal aseptic heat injury *in vivo*. *Experimental and Molecular Pathology* **2**, 402–17.

Chambers, T.J. (1978). Multinucleate giant cells. *Journal of Pathology* **126**, 125–48.

†Cohnheim, J. (1889). Lectures in General Pathology, Vol. 1., pp. 242 to at least 270. (English translation). New Sydenham Society, London. (The classic account of the acute inflammatory reaction observed *in vivo*.)

Dale, M.M. and Foreman, J.C. (Ed.). (1984). *Textbook of Immunopharmacology*. pp. 407. Blackwell Scientific Publications, Oxford, etc. (Includes up-to-date accounts of endogenous mediators.)

van Furth, R. *et al.* (1975). Mononuclear phagocytes in human pathology—proposal for an approach to improved classification. pp. 1–15. In *Mononuclear Phagocytes in Immunity, Infection and Pathology*. pp. 1062. Ed. by R. van Furth. Blackwell Scientific Publications, Oxford. (A comprehensive multi-author text.)

Harris, H. (1953). Chemotaxis of granulocytes. *Journal of Pathology and Bacteriology* **66**, 135–46.

Hurley, J.V. (1983). *Acute Inflammation*. 2nd ed. pp. 157. Churchill Livingstone, Edinburgh. (A detailed account suitable for the general reader.)

Hurley, J.V., Ham, K.N. and Ryan, G.B. (1967). The mechanism of the delayed prolonged phase of increased vascular permeability in mild thermal injury in the rat. *Journal of Pathology and Bacteriology* **94**, 1–12. (The recognition of leakage due to direct vascular injury.)

†Landis, E.M. (1927). Micro-injection studies of capillary permeability. I. Factors in the production of capillary stasis. *American Journal of Physiology* **81**, 124–42. (Work done while a medical student.)

†Lewis, T. (1927). *The blood vessels in the human skin and their responses*. pp. 322. Shaw and Sons, London.

Majno, G. and Palade, G.E. (1961). Studies in Inflammation. I. The effect of histamine and serotonin on vascular permeability: an electron microscopic study. *Journal of Biophysical and Biochemical Cytology*, **11**, 571–605.

Majno, G., Palade, G.E. and Schoefl, G. (1961). Studies in Inflammation. II. The site of action of histamine and serotonin along the vascular tree: a topographic study. *Journal of Biophysical and Biochemical Cytology* **11**, 607–26.

†Metchnikoff, E. (1905). *Immunity in Infective Diseases*. (English translation.) Cambridge University Press, London.

Miles, A.A. (1958). Mediators of the vascular phenomena of inflammation. *Lectures on the Scientific Basis of Medicine* **8**, 198–225. (Criteria for the identification of mediators.)

Ryan, G.B. and Majno, G. (1977a). Acute inflammation. *American Journal of Pathology* **86**, 185–276. (A detailed review with an extensive bibliography.)

Ryan, G.B. and Majno, G. (1977b). *Inflammation*, pp. 80. Upjohn Company, Kalamazoo. (A beautifully illustrated, clear account, of convenient length for the general reader.)

Ryan, G.B. and Spector, W.G. (1970). Macrophage turnover in inflamed connective tissue. *Proceedings of the Royal Society of London* (Series B) **175**, 269–92.

†Starling, E.H. (1986). On the absorption of fluids from the connective tissue spaces. *Journal of Physiology* **19**, 312–26.

Vane, J.R. and Ferreira, S.H. (Ed.). (1978). *Inflammation*. pp. 784. Handbuch der experimentellen pharmacologie, New Series vol. 50/1. (Detailed accounts of many aspects of inflammation by leading workers.)

Wilkinson, P.C. (1982). *Chemotaxis and Inflammation*. 2nd edn. pp. 249. Churchill Livingstone,

† Mainly of historical interest.

Edinburgh. (An authoritative account of chemotaxis including original observations by the author.)

Williams, T.J. (1976). Simultaneous measurement of local plasma exudation and blood flow changes induced by intradermal injection of vasoactive substances, using ^{131}I albumin and ^{133}Xe. *Journal of Physiology* (London) **254**, 4p–5p.

Zweifach, B.W. (Ed.). (1973–4). *The Inflammatory Process*, 3 vols. Academic Press, New York and London. (Accounts on most aspects of inflammation by leading workers.)

Acknowledgement The following illustrations in Chapter 4 appeared in Acute Inflammation, 2nd edn. (1983) by J.V. Hurley. (Churchill Livingstone, Edinburgh). They are reproduced by kind permission of Professor Hurley and Messrs Churchill Livingstone. Figs 4.4, 4.5, 4.7, 4.8, 4.11, 4.12, 4.15–19, 4.23 and 4.32.

5

Healing (Repair) and Hypertrophy

Healing

Reaction of tissues to injury varies greatly in different species of animals and in different tissues. **Regeneration**, i.e. the replacement of a single type of parenchymatous cell by production of more cells of the same kind may be seen in man but different tissues vary in their regenerative capacity. A helpful guide to the expected reaction to damage of any tissue is given by the division of somatic cells into three types.

(a) **Labile cells** are those which under normal conditions continue to multiply throughout life replacing cells that are lost. They include cells of the epidermis, the lining mucosa of the alimentary, respiratory and urinary tract, the endometrium and the haemopoietic bone marrow and lymphoid cells.

(b) **Stable cells** normally cease multiplication when growth ceases but retain mitotic ability during adult life so that some regeneration of damaged tissues may occur. This group includes liver, pancreas, renal tubular epithelium, thyroid and adrenal cortex and many types of mesenchymal cells.

(c) **Permanent cells** lose their mitotic ability in infancy and the classic example of this group is the neuron.

In many instances healing of an organ or tissue occurs by regeneration, the cells lost being replaced by proliferative activity of those remaining. The original structure is more nearly replaced when the supporting stroma is preserved. However, when the injury involves a cell type inherently incapable of regeneration or when other factors, e.g. interruption of blood supply, prevents restoration, healing occurs by the **formation of a fibrous scar** the development of which is best illustrated by the healing of a wound of the skin and subcutaneous tissue.

Healing (repair) of skin wounds

Healing by first intention (primary union)

Primary union occurs when uninfected surgical incisions and other clean wounds without loss of tissue are closed promptly, e.g. by sutures. (Fig. 5.1A) It is characterised by the formation of only minimal amounts of granulation tissue. It is a rapid process and contrasts with healing by **secondary intention** which occurs in an open wound, the edges of which are not brought together by sutures (Fig. 5.1B). Wound infection also prevents healing by first intention. The sequence of events in healing by first intention is as follows: blood clots between the wound edges and on the surface where it dries to form a protective scab. While removal of clot and dead tissue is occurring, firstly by the action of polymorphs and later of macrophages, there is a rapid spread of epithelium beneath the scab to bridge the wound surface within the first two days. Within 3 to 5 days capillaries and fibroblasts grow in beneath the epithelium, and collagen formed by the fibroblasts begins to bind the wound edges together by the end of the first week, reaching a maximum in two to four

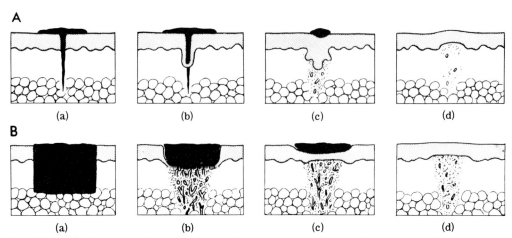

Fig. 5.1A   Healing by first intention (sutured surgical incision). Immediately after injury (**a**) the wound fills with blood clot and a scab forms on the surface. Epithelium which has grown from each side of the wound joins together within about two days (**b**) and later forms a spur of epithelium. A little granulation tissue grows into the wound (**c**). The collagen formed by the fibroblasts in the granulation tissue unites the wound edges. The epithelial spur resorbs and the epithelium does not re-form rete ridges. The narrow fibrous scar gradually becomes less vascular (**d**).

Fig. 5.1B   Healing by second intention (open excised wound). After injury the wound fills with clot (**a**). Epithelium begins to extend under the clot and abundant granulation tissue grows into the base of the wound (**b**). Contraction of the wound occurs and the epithelium finally completely covers the base of the wound (**c**). The vascularity of this more bulky fibrous scar gradually diminishes (**d**).

weeks. Thereafter wound strength slowly increases over many months.

The wound clot and its removal

When an incision is made in the skin and subcutaneous tissue, blood escaping from cut vessels clots on the wound surface and fills the gap between the wound edges which, in sutured wounds, is narrow. The fibrin in the blood clot acts temporarily as a glue which holds the cut surfaces together, while the dehydrated blood clot on the surface forms a scab which effectively seals the wound. Excess of blood clot deeper in the wound delays healing, for it greatly increases the risk of infection and if not evacuated, will only slowly be converted to fibrous tissue (see organisation, p. 5.23). During the first 24 hours, there is a mild inflammatory reaction at the wound edges with exudation of fluid, deposition of further fibrin and migration of polymorphs, monocytes and lymphocytes. Blood clot is digested by enzymes from disintegrated polymorphs and this is aided from about the third day by macrophages, derived mainly from blood monocytes, which ingest and digest the remaining fibrin, red cells and

cellular debris, converting macromolecules into useful amino acids and sugar. Fibronectin, a glycoprotein present in soluble form in the plasma is thought to enhance the phagocytic action of macrophages, which are the dominant cells by 72 hours after wounding. These changes represent the acute inflammatory (exudative) phase of response to injury and are usually mild unless infection supervenes.

Epithelial regeneration

The first tissue to bridge the incisional gap is the squamous epithelium of the epidermis. Within 24 hours and extending from 3–4 mm around the wound edge there is enlargement of the basal cells with some loss of their normally close adherence to the underlying tissue and with flattening of rete ridges. Two processes then contribute to the closure of the gap. Close to the cut edge, cells from the deeper part of the epithelium begin to slide over each other; they *migrate* out over the wound surface and become flattened to form a continuous advancing sheet. The stem cells in the basal layer of the epidermis and adjacent pilo-sebaceous follicles also *proliferate*. Mitosis is rarely seen in

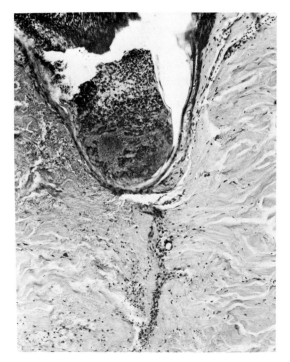

Fig. 5.2 Aseptic abdominal wound showing the stage of healing at five days. The incision is represented merely by a vertical cellular line. The round body on the surface is a small scab beneath which the epithelium has extended down to cover the dermis. × 105.

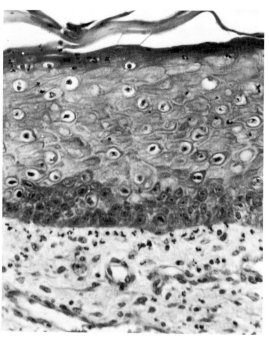

Fig. 5.3 Newly formed epithelium on healed ulcer. The epithelium is several cells thick, but there is little differentiation, and there is no formation of rete ridges. A similar appearance is seen in a healed surgical incision. × 400.

the migrating cells but occurs later in the new epithelium. While the advancing edge of the sheet of new epidermis consists of a single layer of flat cells, the older part at the periphery of the wound becomes stratified so that there is a gradient of thickness. The cells will only migrate over viable tissue. They burrow beneath the superficial part of the blood clot and wound debris, down the cut edges of the dermis; by secreting proteolytic enzymes, they cleave a path between dead and living collagen fibres (Figs. 5.1A and 5.2). Within 48 hours the wound may be bridged by epithelium which rapidly becomes stratified but does not form rete ridges (Figs. 5.3, 5.8). Any epithelium which has grown down into the dermis is later resorbed (Fig. 5.1A).

Suture tracks. Each suture track is a wound, with haemorrhage, death of cells and injury to skin appendages, and in consequence there is a slight inflammatory reaction and fibroblast proliferation (Fig. 5.4). Because the suture prevents closure of the surface epithelium the track is

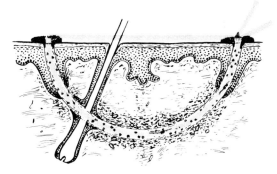

Fig. 5.4 Diagram of suture track a few days after wounding and before removal of sutures. In the centre of the picture the healed epithelium still forms a small projection into the dermis and beneath it the more cellular vertical line of the healing wound is seen.

The surface epithelium and that from a damaged hair follicle have grown along the suture track which is open to the skin surface and is lined by a layer of fibrin containing polymorphs. There is more vascular and fibroblastic proliferation around the suture track than around the original wound.

prone to infection and 'stitch abscesses' are commoner than sepsis of surgical incisions.

Epithelium also tends to grow down suture tracks from both ends (Fig. 5.4). Often much of the epithelium is avulsed when stitches are removed but some may remain and occasionally gives rise either to a small implantation cyst or to a marked inflammatory reaction to keratin, which may simulate infection.

Repair of the dermis and subcutaneous tissue

These tissues heal by proliferation of new blood vessels and fibroblasts to form 'granulation tissue'. Macrophages probably play an important part along with platelets in attracting fibroblasts into the wound and in stimulating their proliferation. They may also promote the formation of new blood vessels (p. 5.11). The migration of cells is aided by a local increase in hyaluronic acid which attracts water and increases the extracellular matrix. The insoluble form of fibronectin present in connective tissue matrices is plentiful in granulation tissue, disappearing as collagen matures. It is thought to have a general influence on cell adhesion and migration, to attract fibroblasts and may form, along with fibrin, a temporary scaffold to which migrating cells can adhere.

From about the third day, **vascular proliferation** is seen as capillary sprouts, which grow from blood vessels at the wound margins (Fig. 5.5), and advance, along the line of least resistance into the wound: the capillary sprouts are produced partly by re-arrangement and migration of pre-existing endothelial cells and partly by their proliferation just behind the advancing tip. The sprouts are often solid at first, but they unite with one another or join a capillary already carrying blood and develop a lumen. These newly formed capillaries are very delicate (Fig. 5.12), lacking a basement membrane and behave as if acutely inflamed: they leak protein-rich fluid with escape of some red cells, and polymorphs emigrate from them. It has been observed in rabbits that if blood flow is not soon established through a new vessel then the lumen disappears, the vessel reverting to a solid cord which then breaks and the ends retract by sliding back of endothelial cells to the nearest vessel carrying blood. Within a few days of the establishment of circulation, some of the new vessels differentiate into arterioles and ven-

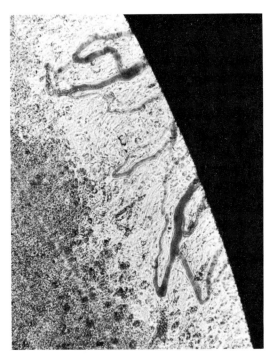

Fig. 5.5 Capillary loops growing into a blood clot in a transparent chamber embedded in a rabbit's ear, photographed *in vivo*. Similar but less marked vascular proliferation is seen in the healing of a simple surgical incision. The rounded dark objects are macrophages which are digesting the blood clot in advance of growing vessels. (The late Professor Lord Florey.)

ules by the acquisition of muscle cells either by migration from pre-existing larger blood channels or by differentiation from mesenchymal cells.

Lymphatic channels are re-established in the same manner as blood vessels.

Fibrous tissue production. After the removal of blood, fibrin and dead cells from the wound, and simultaneously with the development of new blood vessels, long, spindle-shaped fibroblasts (Fig. 5.6a and b) stream from the perivascular connective tissue and begin to proliferate and to move into the wound. Within a few days fibroblasts thus come to lie in the wound: they produce both type I and type III collagen (see below), synthesis being greatest at about 7 days. The collagen fibres come to lie across the incision line and help to unite the cut edges from about the end of the first week after injury. Proteoglycan ground substance, also secreted by the fibroblast, may play an import-

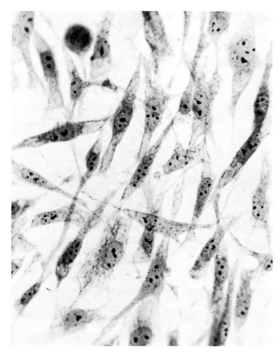

Fig. 5.6a Fibroblasts in tissue culture. (The late Dr Janet S.F. Niven.)

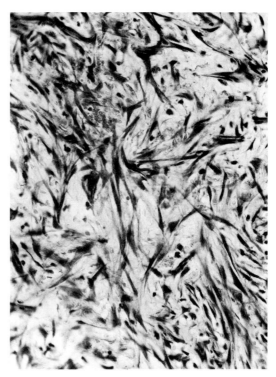

Fig. 5.6b Fibroblasts in a healing wound, showing the characteristic shape and early formation of collagen fibrils. × 350.

ant role in determining fibre size and direction and also later in enhancing crosslinks between collagen molecules (see below). By the third week the total amount of collagen in the wound has almost reached a maximum. In contrast, at this stage the tensile strength of the wound is still low, but it increases over many months by replacement of some of the type III by type I collagen, by further intermolecular bonding between collagen fibrils, and by remodelling of the anatomical configuration of the collagen in response to mechanical stress. Such remodelling involves collagen turnover, i.e. synthesis and lysis, which occurs also in normal (unwounded) tissues (see below).

While healing of a wound by fibrous tissue is clearly beneficial, in some tissues it may also have harmful results, for example narrowing of the oesophagus, stenosis of the mitral valve, or stricture of the urethra. Attempts to modify the fibrotic process by inhibiting collagen formation, promoting its destruction or altering its metabolism by drugs so far have not been very effective.

Collagen synthesis. Collagen is synthesised and secreted by fibroblasts in soluble form, and deposited extracellularly. As with secretory proteins in general, the polypeptide chains of collagen (**pro-α-chains**) are formed on the ribosomes with N and C terminal extension peptides. A distinctive feature of collagen synthesis is the conversion of proline and lysine residues on the growing polypeptide chains to hydroxyproline and hydroxylysine residues. This enzymic hydroxylation requires Fe^{++}, O_2, ascorbic acid and α-ketoglutarate. Glycosylation of some of the hydroxylysine residues then occurs. In the cisternae of the endoplasmic reticulum pro-α-chains are converted to **pro-collagen** by the formation of disulphide bonds and they begin to assume a tri-helical structure. The pro-collagen molecules, of which there are several types, are stabilised by hydroxyproline and are secreted via the Golgi apparatus. Outside the cell the N and C extension peptides, which do not assume the helical form, are removed in some types of collagen by pro-collagen peptidase. This drastically alters the properties of the molecule which precipitates as **tropocollagen**. The tropocollagen molecules, which are rigid rods of $290 \times 1·4$ nm, align side by side, prob-

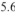

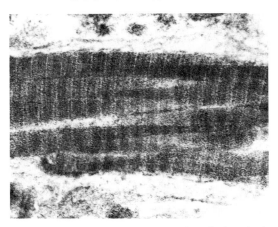

Fig. 5.7 Collagen fibres are seen here in longitudinal section. The characteristic, regular cross banding is evident. × 65 000.

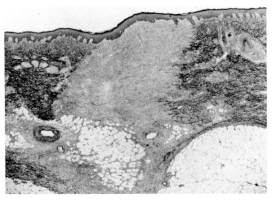

Fig. 5.8 Healed surgical wound of skin of 14 days' duration. The elastic fibres are stained black, and the healed wound is seen in the centre: it is composed of connective tissue in which elastic fibres have not yet formed. × 5.

ably in fives, staggered at a quarter of their length to produce a fibril with a 64 nm periodicity on electron microscopy (Fig. 5.7). The acquisition of tensile strength of the fibrils is dependent on the formation of co-valent links, mainly of aldemine and keto type. Increase in strength results from further alterations in the extent and nature of intermolecular cross-linkage.

Types of collagen. There are at least five different types of collagen derived from different structural genes (see Table 5.1). All have the triple helical configuration and types I, II and III have an identical appearance, banded at 64 nm, on electron microscopy. (Fig. 5.7).

The time needed for their synthesis and secretion varies as does their susceptibility to the various collagenases bringing about collagen lysis. While many tissues contain more than one type of collagen (e.g. adult dermis contains type I and about 10–15% of

type III), mixed fibres are not found. Initially in a healing scar there are more type III (**reticulin**) fibres than in adjacent skin but later these are replaced by type I fibres.

Collagen lysis. Collagenases are formed, at the site where they are required, e.g. in healing wounds, by macrophages, polymorphs and regenerating epidermal epithelium. The collagenase is secreted directly onto the fibre by a closely apposed cell and this splits the fibre so that fragments may be ingested by macrophages. Splitting is more likely to occur in fibres with few or unstable cross links. Within the phagosomes, the fragments are broken down to amino acids or small peptides. In the healing wound, lysis occurs in the early stage of cleaning up the damaged collagen at the wound face and for a depth of about 7 mm into the surrounding tissue. There is also breakdown and replacement of much of the collagen first formed: wound remodelling continues for six months to a year. If the balance between synthesis

Table 5.1 Types of collagen

Type	Molecular form	Tissue
I	Two identical chains $\alpha1(I)_2$ and one $\alpha2(I)$	Dermis, tendon, bone, dentine, cornea; 90% of collagen in body (stains red with Van Gieson, green with Masson and blue with Mallory stains for collagen).
II	Three identical chains—$\alpha1(II)_3$	Cartilage, intervertebral disc, vitreous body.
III	Three identical chains—$\alpha1(III)_3$	Embryonic dermis (and about 10–15% of adult)—early scar tissue, granulomas, cardiovascular tissue, synovial membrane (stains with silver nitrate as reticulin).
IV	Three identical chains—$\alpha1(IV)_3$ but perhaps a heterogeneous group	Basement membrane (non-fibrillar—does not show the typical banded structure on electron-microscopy).
V	Two identical chains $\alpha1(V)_2$ and one $\alpha2(V)$	Interstitial tissue, widespread in small amounts, non-fibrillar.

and lysis is upset by starvation, sepsis, or deficiency of specific protein or of oxygen, then the wound collagen may be extensively digested.

Events following primary wound healing

Once the wound has healed the young scar is commonly raised above the surface due to the underlying proliferative processes and is red as a result of increased vascularity. The blood vessels gradually decrease in number, probably in the manner already described, and the amount of collagen may also diminish. *Elastic fibres* are formed much later than collagen (Fig. 5.8). They form a crosslinked, random-coil structure of fibres or sheets which, unlike the rigid collagen, allows stretch and recoil and gives the skin its elasticity. *Sensory nerves* may grow into the scar in about three weeks but specialised nerve endings such as Pacinian corpuscles do not re-form. The end result of healing by first intention should be a pale linear scar, level with the adjacent skin surface, but sometimes a **hypertrophic scar** or **keloid** forms (p. 23.64).

Healing by second intention (secondary union)

Healing of an open gaping wound with loss of tissue or of an infected closed wound occurs by the formation of granulation tissue which grows from the base of the wound to fill the defect. The vascular and fibroblastic proliferation which together make up the granulation tissue are much more abundant and healing takes much longer than when it occurs by first intention (Fig. 5.1B). Skin grafts are increasingly used to speed the healing of open wounds.

Clean open wounds. As in the closed wound there is haemorrhage and exudation of fibrin from the cut surfaces. This is soon followed by a much greater emigration of polymorphs and subsequently of macrophages, from vessels in the wound: by enzymic action and phagocytosis these cells soften and remove the fibrin and other debris. As in the incised wound, epithelial cells at the margins enlarge and begin to migrate down the walls of the wound in the first day or two after injury. Migration and proliferation together produce a sheet of cells which advances in a series of tongue-like projections beneath any remaining blood clot or exudate

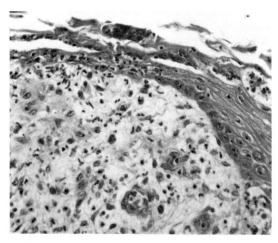

Fig. 5.9 Granulating wound with early growth of epithelium over the surface. The epithelium is growing from the right-hand side and tapers off as a thin layer. × 400.

on the wound surface. As the single layer of cells moves inwards towards the wound centre, there is stratification of the cells near to the wound margin (Fig. 5.9). Since the denuded area is large, the advancing epithelial sheet does not completely cover the wound until the granulation tissue from the base (see below) has started to fill the wound space. Care should always be taken, in removing adherent dressings from an open wound, because the delicate epithelium is easily ripped off. As soon as the wound surface is covered, epithelial cell migration ceases and proliferation, stratification and keratinisation are rapidly completed, though rete ridges are not re-formed.

When the full thickness of the skin is destroyed by a burn re-epithelialisation is slow for the cells, with the help of their collagenases, have to burrow beneath the thick layer of dead coagulated collagen. In contrast, in a burn which destroys only part of the skin thickness, in a superficial wound or the donor site of a 'split thickness' skin graft, re-epithelialisation is relatively rapid as proliferation of epithelium occurs not only from the wound edge but also from the cut mouth of each pilosebaceous follicle. In man, slower and less perfect epithelial regeneration occurs from sweat gland ducts. If skin appendages are destroyed they are not re-formed.

Although epithelium shows the first evidence of reparative activity, within a few days the

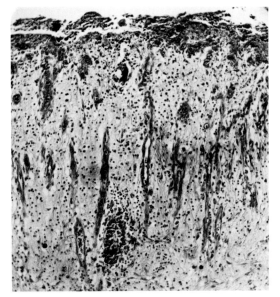

Fig. 5.10 Granulating wound showing the vertical lines of newly formed blood vessels. × 150.

pre-existing vessels in the wound bed produce vascular sprouts which grow upwards, forming loops and coils near the wound surface (Fig. 5.10), giving it a red, granular appearance—hence the term '*granulation tissue*' (Fig. 5.11.) From these new, more permeable vessels (Fig. 5.12), small haemorrhages occur and polymorphs migrate, reinforcing those already present in the exudate on the wound surface and helping to keep down bacterial growth. At the same time as the new capillaries form, fibroblasts, some of which are in mitosis, are seen in the base and walls of the wound, often running parallel to the new capillary walls (i.e. towards the wound surface). This fibrovascular granulation tissue continues to proliferate and to fill the wound space only until epithelium grows over its surface, when the exudative inflammatory changes and the migration of polymorphs also subside. Later the fibroblasts may become orientated parallel to the wound surface (Fig. 5.13) and about the end of the first week collagen is produced and rapidly increases in amount. If epithelialisation is delayed, e.g. by further trauma or infection, granulations may pout from the wound surface. Following healing, there is gradual retraction and disappearance of some of the new vascular channels and further crosslinking and remodelling of collagen (see above) which, over a period of months, becomes progressively less cellular.

Healing of an open, excised wound is aided by **contraction of the surface area** in sites where the skin is mobile and loosely attached to underlying tissue. All edges of the wound do not move together to the same extent, the degree of contraction being related to skin tension. This movement of the edges towards the centre of the wound is brought about by contraction of the fibroblasts which are now accordingly termed **myofibroblasts**. These cells

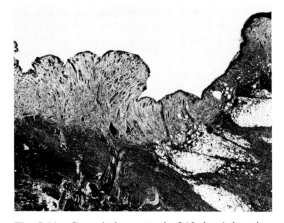

Fig. 5.11 Granulating wound of 12 days' duration. The advancing epithelial margin is seen as the dark surface layer on the right. Granulation tissue projects from the floor of the wound, and can be seen to contain many small blood vessels. × 10.

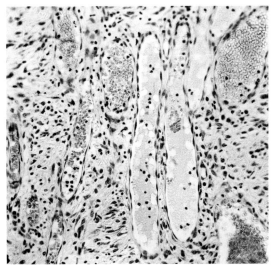

Fig. 5.12 Newly formed thin-walled blood vessels in a granulating wound, the surface of which is to the top. × 150.

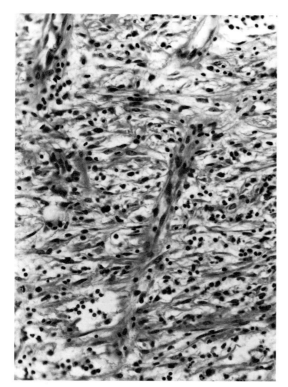

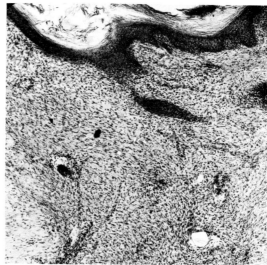

Fig. 5.14 Healing abdominal wound in which infection has delayed the process of healing. Note that the line of cellular tissue is much broader than in Fig. 5.2. × 75.

Fig. 5.13 Deeper part of granulating wound. *Below*, the collagen fibrils are being formed parallel to the surface; *above*, the vessels are seen running in a vertical direction. × 240.

develop temporarily a well-organised system of contractile cytoplasmic microfilaments resembling that of smooth muscle cells and responding to many pharmacological agents which contract smooth muscle. The bundles of parallel contractile microfilaments run longitudinally within the cells and are attached to the cell surface at sites where it is firmly adherent to other cells or to underlying tissue. Sliding of microfilament bundles in a meshwork of myofibroblasts in an open wound may thus pull together the wound edges, in which position they are stabilised by the deposition of collagen fibres. When desirable, as sometimes in flexor surfaces over joints, wound contraction may be inhibited by early skin grafting. The term **contracture** is applied when healing produces distortion or limitation of movement of the tissues. It may result either from contraction of the wound or from scarring of the underlying muscle and soft tissue.

Infected wounds. The repair of infected wounds is accomplished by the same processes already described for clean, open wounds; that is, by the production of granulation tissue, but with a more pronounced acute inflammatory reaction, and also by formation of larger and more numerous blood vessels.

Open wounds, apart from those produced under aseptic surgical conditions, are almost always contaminated by bacteria, and for this reason a careful surgical toilet should include removal of dead tissue, which promotes invasive bacterial growth; this *débridement* is an important part of treatment. Granulation tissue provides a good defence against bacteria because, being rich in small blood vessels, it can mount an effective inflammatory response. These local defensive factors may be aided by antibacterial therapy, which may permit early suture or skin grafting. If infection continues, however, more leucocytes pour into the surface exudate, which then becomes purulent. The result of acute infection on the healing processes is to inhibit both epithelial regeneration and proliferation of fibroblasts, so that healing is delayed. This delay and the greater tissue destruction result eventually in increased fibrous tissue and a larger and denser scar (Fig. 5.14).

Skin grafting. When a skin graft is placed on the recipient site it adheres to this new bed by fibrin and is nourished by diffusion of plasma from the raw surface. Within about three days capillary buds growing from the recipient area begin to unite with those on the undersurface of the graft, while ingrowing fibroblasts produce collagen which anchors the graft more securely. Good vascularity of the bed without haematoma formation, control of pathogenic infection and close, undisturbed contact with the graft, promote a rapid 'take'.

Grafts from the same individual (autografts) persist indefinitely. Grafts from another individual (homografts) are accepted initially but are destroyed within a month or so by an immune reaction by the recipient; they are nevertheless useful to provide temporary cover of extensive raw surfaces, for example large burns, and help to prevent excessive contraction of the area.

Control mechanisms in healing

While the morphological changes of wound healing are well known, the factors controlling the various observed processes are controversial or unknown.

There is evidence from tissue culture that virtually all cells have the ability to move along a surface to which they can adhere. If two cultures of fibroblasts are made on a plane surface the cells grow out as a monolayer from each explant until they collide, when movement virtually ceases because the cells will almost never pile up on one another. This is known as **contact inhibition** and it appears to be tissue specific in some degree.

If the monolayer is scraped to leave a space the cells at the edge of the wound flatten, spread out into the empty space and divide. Experiments with cell culture on surfaces with different degrees of adhesiveness suggest that cell division may be stimulated not so much by loss of contact as by the ability of the cell to *flatten* and spread on its substrate. Certainly the more flattened the cell the faster the rate of protein synthesis and the shorter the cell cycle. These findings suggest that *in vivo* a wound may stimulate cell division by allowing adjacent cells to spread into the wound space and that the relationship between the proliferating cell and its underlying tissue or basement membrane is important.

Inhibitory factors—chalones. It has been suggested that cell growth is controlled by negative feedback in which freely diffusible chemical inhibitors or chalones are produced by functional cells of a tissue and act directly on stem cells of that tissue to prevent their division. In the epidermis, for instance, the Malpighian cells are thought to produce a chalone which inhibits the basal cells. When the number of Malpighian cells are reduced by wounding or stripping of the surface epithelium, the amount of chalone falls and the basal cells are permitted to divide until the loss is made good, when the amount of inhibitory factor increases and reduces the rate of cell replacement to normal physiological levels. While this neatly explains both the induction and cessation of proliferation the chalone hypothesis has not been widely accepted because chalones have not been isolated or identified and the evidence for their existence is indirect and inconclusive.

Growth factors. There is an increasing interest in the possible function in wound healing of various polypeptides which promote cell growth in tissue culture. Though many have been isolated and their amino acid sequences determined, their physiological function *in vivo* remains speculative. Only some of those which might be applicable to wound healing are mentioned here. Somatomedins (the insulin-like growth factors) are mentioned on p. 26.4 and the production of growth factors by tumours on p. 13.12.

1. Platelet derived growth factor (PDGF). Growth of most cells in a monolayer culture requires whole blood serum in the medium but cell-free plasma becomes growth promoting if it is enriched with a platelet extract. The growth-stimulating factor, PDGF, is released from the α granules of platelets and in culture it binds to specific cell surface receptors of vascular smooth muscle cells, fibroblasts and glial cells, stimulating DNA synthesis and cell multiplication as well as being chemotactic to these cells.

It is postulated that *in vivo* PDGF, perhaps synthesised by megakaryocytes, and normally present within the α granules of circulating platelets, is released from the granules when the platelets come in contact with subendothelial collagen exposed after vascular injury as in a wound (p. 10.9). The released PDGF binds with high affinity to receptors on connective tissue cells, such as fibroblasts, promoting their proliferation and so connective tissue formation. Excess PDGF which has not bound to the cells in the wound is thought to be rapidly inactivated and cleared from the circulation. The chemotactic and mitogenic properties of PDGF to vascular smooth muscle cells is discussed in relation to atheroma (p. 14.13) and the similarity of its peptide structure to that of the transforming protein of an oncogene on p. 13.12. It must be emphasised that the response of cells to PDGF *in vivo* is hypothetical.

2. *Epidermal growth factor (EGF).* This substance has been purified from the submaxillary glands of mice and from human urine (urogastrone) and is also present in human Brunner's glands. EGF is known to be active *in vivo* as well as in culture. Its activity as a promoter of epidermal proliferation and keratinisation was first recognized when its injection into newborn mice resulted in premature opening of the eyelids and eruption of the teeth. Its mitogenic activity *in vitro* is not confined to skin and squamous mucosa but extends to fibroblasts, glial and kidney cells. EGF may have an important role in fetal development since many types of ectodermal and mesodermal cells carry its specific receptors and respond to its mitogenic activity.

3. *Macrophage derived growth factor (MDGF).* It seems likely that, in addition to their phagocytic function in wound healing, activated macrophages which gather at the site of tissue damage produce a factor which stimulates fibroblast proliferation and induces endothelial cells to form new capillaries. Neutrophils and lymphocytes are thought to have similar angiogenic activity. MDGF may also, like PDGF, increase vascular smooth muscle in atheroma.

4. *Fibroblast growth factor* has been obtained from bovine brain and pituitary. It promotes synthesis of protein and RNA and stimulates proliferation and migration of many types of mesodermal cell in culture but its *in vivo* activity is unknown.

5. *Nerve growth factor (NGF)* has been isolated from mouse submaxillary glands and is probably necessary both for the development and the survival of sensory and sympathetic neurons and to regulate their neurotransmitter activity. Like the fibroblast, axonal and dendritic growth are promoted in culture by chemotactic factors and by the adhesive property of the underlying substrate.

Most somatic cells in adults are in the G_0 phase, i.e. they are dropouts from the cell cycle

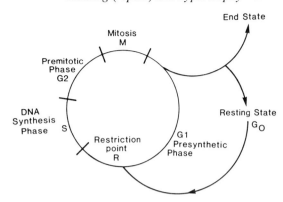

Fig. 5.15 The mitotic or cell cycle, showing the relative duration of each phase. The whole cycle normally takes from about 24 hours to several days, depending largely on the duration of G_1, the phase preceding the synthesis of DNA (S phase). The S phase if followed by a brief (G_2) phase before the cell undergoes mitosis (M). After mitosis the cell may leave the cell cycle permanently or may enter a resting phase G_0 from which it can be recruited to re-enter the cycle in the G_1 phase and proliferate. Towards the end of G_1 there is a restriction point and cells which pass beyond this point are committed to divide.

(Fig. 5.15) and are neither growing nor committed to future mitosis. The action of growth factors is to return the cells to the cycle so that they progress into the S phase of synthesis of DNA. To do this there may be a synergistic interaction with other factors and with local chemical mediators such as prostaglandins. The first steps in this process of returning a resting cell to the cycle is known for example in relation to EGF. Binding of EGF to receptors on the plasma membrane, induces the selective phosphorylation of membrane proteins by the activation of protein kinase. It is not known how this stimulates RNA and DNA synthesis. The cAMP system (p. 7.4) does not appear to be involved.

Much remains speculative or unknown about the regulation of cell migration and proliferation in wound healing but it seems likely that this involves the complex interaction of different processes, including the availability of space and the secretion of inhibitory and stimulatory factors by adjacent cells. So far the evidence of participation of growth factors is much stronger than for chalones.

Factors which impair healing

Healing may be influenced by local factors. Infection delays healing (p. 5.9) as does a poor local blood supply; wounds of the relatively avascular shin tend to unite more slowly than those of the highly vascular scalp or face. This may be due at least partly to the greater risk of infection in hypoxic tissue. Killing of phagocytosed bacteria by polymorphs and macrophages is associated with a burst of oxygen uptake. Defects in collagen formation may result from generalised deficiency of vitamin C or of sulphur-containing amino acids and also from an excess of glucocorticosteroids.

Deficiency of vitamin C (ascorbic acid) and sulphur-containing amino acids. Man, monkey and guinea-pig are unable to synthesise vitamin C, and in the guinea-pig impaired synthesis of wound collagen occurs after even a few days on a diet lacking the vitamin. In man, however, a much longer dietary deficiency is necessary before collagen formation is depressed, although this may occur before scurvy is clinically apparent (p. 23.16). Patients with multiple injuries or extensive burns readily become deficient in vitamin C unless intake is increased. Deficiency of the vitamin disturbs the synthesis of collagen at the stage of intracellular hydroxylation of amino acids so that most of the underhydroxylated collagen remains within the cell and the small amount that escapes is more readily degraded than normal collagen. As a result, although wound contraction is not impaired, the wound is weak and tends to break down after re-epithelialisation and apparent healing: this was a well-known complication of naval surgery on scorbutic sailors. In addition to the reduced amount and abnormality of the collagen formed in the wound, the new capillaries may be unduly fragile because of failure of formation of basement membrane (type IV

collagen). Deficient galactosamine may alter the properties of the ground substance. Similar alteration in collagen production with loss of wound strength may be seen in starving animals deficient in the sulphur-containing amino acids such as methionine, which are essential for collagen synthesis. Even when starvation continues, some of the methionine required for wound healing may be obtained from endogenous tissue proteins but wound strength is increased by providing a diet adequate in protein. In well nourished individuals, protein and vitamin supplements will not speed healing or improve wound strength.

Excess of adrenal glucocorticoid hormones. Large doses of glucocorticoids, especially if given within the first few days after wounding, may suppress repair in experimental animals. In man the usual therapeutic doses seem to have little effect on healing of sutured incisions but may delay closure of open wounds with their higher energy requirements. Polymorphs and macrophages tend to be scanty, fibroblast proliferation and migration and the formation of new blood vessels are all diminished, while epithelialisation and contraction are also deficient. In the steroid-treated patient there is a higher risk of infection in wounds exposed to serious contamination and this is more likely to be undetected clinically. While the administration of vitamin A systemically or topically may counteract some steroid effects, it does not restore wound contraction.

Zinc deficiency. Zinc is necessary for the synthesis of collagen. Oral supplements of zinc may promote wound healing in patients with zinc deficiency, but it is difficult to identify these patients since serum zinc levels may not reflect accurately the overall bodily status of zinc metabolism. Patients with severe burns and intestinal fistulae are most likely to be deficient.

Healing of fractures

Healing in bones bears many resemblances to healing in soft tissues. Primary union of a fracture is however exceptional (p. 5.17), healing by the proliferation of callus (similar to wound healing by secondary intention) being the rule.

There is initial haemorrhage and mild acute inflammation, followed by a proliferative or productive stage in which osteogenic cells play a vital part. Continuity between the bone fragments is first established by a mass of new bony

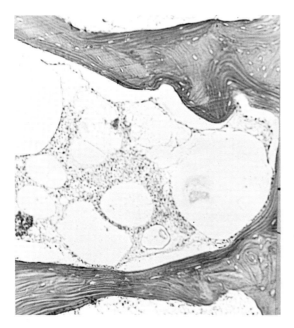

Fig. 5.16 The bone is necrotic and osteocytes have disappeared, leaving empty lacunae. Cell ghosts can be seen in the necrotic haemopoietic marrow. × 100.

trabeculae and sometimes cartilaginous tissue (**provisional callus**). This undergoes slow remodelling, with resorption and replacement so that, under favourable conditions, firm bony union is achieved. Sometimes restoration is so good that the fracture site is later hardly identifiable.

Early stages

A good deal of force is normally required to break a bone, the fragments are usually displaced, and in addition to a relatively small amount of haemorrhage between the bone ends much blood may seep into the tissues from ruptured vessels of the torn periosteum and adjacent soft tissues. In addition to haemorrhage, local inflammatory changes take place with hyperaemia and exudation of protein-rich fluid from which fibrin may be deposited. Polymorphs are scanty unless there is infection, and this is common only in **compound fractures**, i.e. when a bone fragment has torn the overlying skin or mucous membrane. Macrophages also invade and phagocytose clot and tissue debris. Red blood cells are often removed rapidly from the fracture site, leaving a homogeneous mass of fibrin between the bone ends. A large amount of clot and debris between the bone fragments delays healing.

Bone necrosis occurs chiefly as a result of tearing of blood vessels in the medullary cavity, cortex and periosteum: the first recognisable histological evidence is observed within a day or two, the haemopoietic marrow cells showing loss of nuclear staining (Fig. 5.16). Fat released from dead marrow may be taken up by macrophages, and fat 'cysts' form, surrounded by foreign-body giant cells. Damage to the marrow may have serious results when globules of fat enter torn local venules and produce **fat emboli** in the pulmonary bed, brain and kidneys (p. 10.20). Because of its vascular arrangements the cortical bone usually suffers more extensive necrosis than the spongy medullary bone. The amount of bone necrosis depends especially on the local peculiarities of the blood supply; the talus, carpal scaphoid, and the femoral head following intracapsular fracture, are particularly liable to undergo extensive ischaemic necrosis. When there is splintering of bone (**comminuted fracture**) some of the fragments may lose their blood supply; they become necrotic and, if small, are eventually resorbed by osteoclasts. Bone death is recognisable histologically by loss of osteocytes from the bone lacunae (Fig. 5.16) but some cells may remain visible long after their death.

Provisional callus formation

(a) **Periosteal reaction.** The cells of the inner layer of the periosteum proliferate in a fairly wide zone overlying the cortex of each fractured bone end. (Fig. 5.17). A cuff of bone trabeculae is formed around each bone end at right angles to the cortex and anchored to it ((b) in Fig. 5.18)

Further woven bone trabeculae (p. 23.1), less well orientated, form an irregular meshwork whose pattern at this stage is uninfluenced by stress. This formation of new bone is dependent on the blood supply, which derives partly from surviving periosteal vessels but largely from muscle and other surrounding soft tissues. Mixed with this cuff of new bone there are often nodules of hyaline cartilage which usually do not appear until bone formation is well under way (Fig. 5.18). The amount of cartilage which is formed in provisional callus varies greatly from one species to another. Small mammals such as

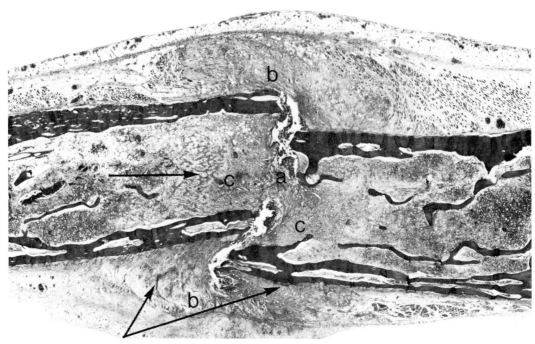

Fig. 5.17 Rib 7 days after fracture. The fracture gap (a) contains fibrin and extends into the adjacent soft tissue. A spindle of highly cellular tissue (b) has formed in the muscle around the fracture site but only a little new subperiosteal bone (arrows) and cartilage have formed as yet. Bone and marrow at the fracture site are dead (c) but there is some early revascularisation of the marrow and a little bony callus is beginning to form in the medullary cavity (arrow). × 10.

mice, rats and rabbits tend to form chiefly cartilaginous callus while in man the amount, though variable, is less. Cartilage formation is thought to be promoted by a poor blood supply and by shearing strains and stresses so that it is particularly abundant in poorly immobilised fractures: bone gradually replaces the cartilage by endochondral ossification.

The two enlarging cuffs of callus advance towards each other and finally unite to bridge the fracture line leaving a gap between the bone ends (Fig. 5.18). This 'bandage' of **external callus** helps to immobilise the fragments in an unstable or poorly fixed fracture. If the two cuffs fail to meet the external callus resorbs.

The amount of bridging periosteal callus varies greatly in different sites and under different circumstances. In intracapsular fractures (i.e. within a joint capsule), such as subcapital fracture of the femoral neck, the periosteum is lacking and union is almost wholly dependent on **internal callus** formed by osteoblasts lying in the medullary cavity (see below). By contrast, fractures of the shaft of large tubular bones, such as the femur and humerus, tend to form much external callus, internal callus in the relatively small medullary cavity not being striking. The formation of bulky external callus probably depends on

plenty of surrounding undamaged muscle as a source of blood supply, for one of the causes of the difficulty in healing of fractures of the tibia is that they are partially covered by relatively avascular subcutaneous tissue and tend to form little callus. Poorly aligned fractures and those with much movement at the fracture site (e.g. the ribs and clavicle) are liable to produce abundant external callus, whereas fractures which are well immobilised by external or internal surgical fixation may unite with relatively little callus formation.

(b) Medullary reaction. The first evidence of healing is the advance of capillaries from the viable into the necrotic marrow (Fig. 5.19) closely followed by macrophages, fibroblasts and osteoblasts. The macrophages phagocytose and remove dead material, while osteoclasts begin to resorb dead spongy bone (Fig. 5.20) and the endosteal surface of the necrotic cortex. The osteoblasts produce new woven bone in the marrow spaces: the new bone is deposited partly on the surface of dead trabeculae which, when surrounded by new bone, may remain unresorbed for months or even years (Fig. 5.21).

In contrast to external callus, cartilage is rare in the medullary cavity, perhaps because it is a rela-

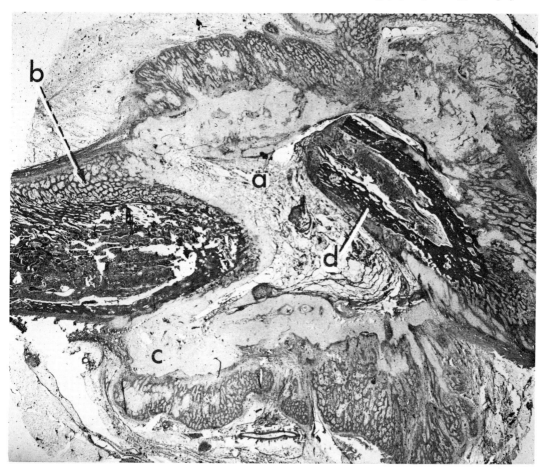

Fig. 5.18 Healing of displaced birth-fracture in the femur of a premature infant. The bone ends are cut obliquely. Bridging periosteal callus has formed but around the bone ends there is still a gap (a) which contains a meshwork of fibrin. The subperiosteal cuff of new bone is well seen at (b). The bridging callus consists partly of woven bone and partly of pale hyaline cartilage (c). The Haversian canals of the living cortex (d) are slightly enlarged by osteoclasis. × 5.

tively vascular site and is protected from mechanical stress. It may form, however, when callus formation reaches the fracture gap (see below).

(c) Cortical reaction. The most striking re-action in the living cortex adjacent to the frac-ture is an increase in osteoclastic resorption with widening of the Haversian canals, presum-ably partly due to disuse atrophy (Fig. 5.22 and p. 3.20). This may be followed later by some osteoblastic activity. Similar changes are seen in the dead cortex of the bone ends once there has been revascularisation of the Haversian canals from adjacent vessels in viable bone or from periosteal and medullary vessels. The re-sorption of necrotic bone may widen the frac-ture gap.

The fracture gap

The periosteal (external) callus unites the frag-ments externally but not directly across the bone ends. As already stated, immediately after fracture, blood clot, exuded fibrin and bony de-bris fill the gap and these are attacked by mac-rophages and by osteoclasts. The fibrin clot, which usually persists between the bone ends (Figs. 5.17 and 5.18), is finally invaded by blood vessels and cellular tissue containing varying amounts of osteogenic cells and fibroblasts, so that bony union may occur in either of two ways.

(a) Direct ossification is brought about by osteogenic cells spreading from medullary and

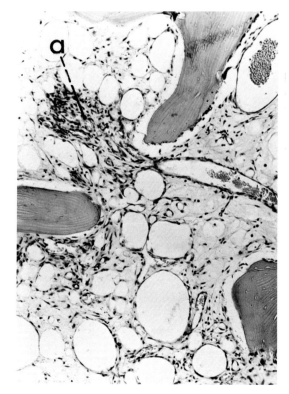

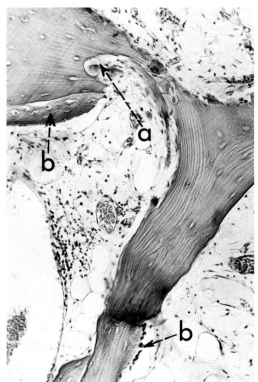

Fig. 5.19 Dead fatty marrow in the medullary cavity is being revascularised. A knot of proliferating capillaries is seen at (a). × 100.

Fig. 5.20 A dead medullary bone trabecula is being removed by osteoclasts at (a) and new bone is being laid down on the surface of dead bone at (b). × 120.

periosteal callus. Cartilage may also be formed and is converted into bone. This process is relatively rapid and effective.

(b) Fibrous union may occur initially. Fibrous tissue grows in from medulla or periosteum or both, becomes densely collagenised, and only then much more slowly becomes ossified (Fig. 5.22). This slower type of union occurs especially when there is instability, separation by excessive traction or marked resorption of the bone ends, massive necrosis, a poor blood supply, extensive periosteal damage, comminution or infection. Sometimes conversion to bone following fibrous union is very slow (**delayed union**) and occasionally it fails to occur (**non-union**). Electrical phenomena appear to be associated with bone healing and when union is delayed osteogenesis may be promoted by electrical stimulation. In non-union the fibrous tissue may become very dense, hyaline and finally fibrocartilaginous. The appearance of an area of eosinophilic fibrinoid necrosis is followed by a linear split which may enlarge

and eventually develop a lining similar to synovium, thus forming a false joint (**pseudarthrosis**) (Fig. 5.23). The bone ends buried in the dense fibrous tissue tend to become very sclerotic.

Later stages: final remodelling

Once bony union has occurred and function has been regained, the bone begins to be remodelled in response to mechanical stresses. If the fracture has united at an angle new bone is incorporated on the concave side while resorption occurs on the convex, so that the bone becomes straighter. In any event excessive callus is resorbed, slowly formed lamellar bone begins to replace the hastily laid down woven bone, and any remaining necrotic bone is removed and replaced (Fig. 5.24). The cortex is re-formed across the fracture gap and gradually medullary callus is removed and the marrow

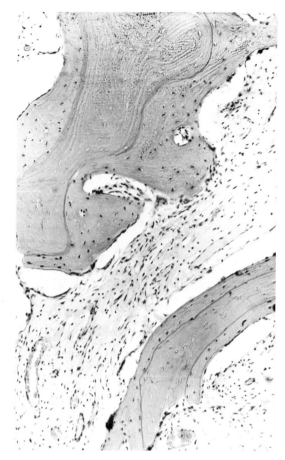

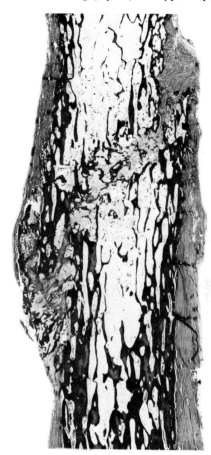

Fig. 5.21 Months after fracture dead bone trabeculae are still recognisable, covered by new living bone. × 70.

Fig. 5.22 This 12-week-old fracture of the distal fibula in an old man has formed a good deal of external callus medially (on the left). The fracture gap itself is filled with fibrous tissue in which a few trabeculae of metaplastic bone are forming. As a result of immobilisation and disuse the fibula is porotic with enlargement of Haversian canals. × 3.

cavity is restored. the whole process may take about a year and is more rapid and complete in children.

General factors and bone healing

Some of the local factors affecting bone healing have already been mentioned but, as in wound healing, general factors are also important. Lack of vitamin C results in depression of both fibroblastic and osteogenic activity so that collagen and bone production are both deficient. Glucocorticosteroids administered to animals with fractures also delay healing but it seems that they have little effect when given to patients in the usual therapeutic doses. In vitamin D deficiency abundant callus may form, but it fails to calcify, remaining soft until the deficiency is made good.

Primary union of fractures

Although primary union of soft tissues is the rule in clean sutured surgical incisions, primary union in bone is a curiosity. It entails bony union with the formation of only minimal amounts of callus and was first described in compression arthrodesis (i.e. excision of the joint) of the knee, the cancellous surfaces of femur and tibia being held together by compression clamps. Bony union occurs in about 4 weeks and biopsy shows only a thin line of new bone at the contact points of opposing trabeculae. While moderate compression

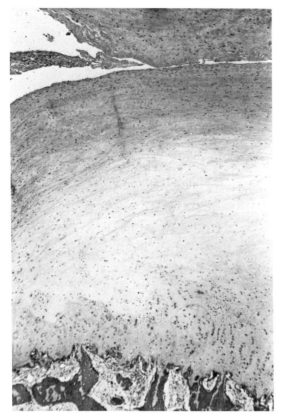

forces may assist union of a fracture, rigid fixation and close apposition of surfaces are probably the major factors. Cortical fractures in dogs, produced by a very fine saw with minimal necrosis, and fixed by a compression plate, have united without periosteal callus. The necrotic ends of the cortical bone were not resorbed but blood vessels entered the Haversian canals and subsequently the bone ends in contact were joined by new osteones (Haversian systems) which involved both bone fragments. At the opposite cortex from the compression device a small amount of new bone, formed from the endosteal cells of the Haversian canals, filled the narrow gap between the fragments and was later replaced by osteones. The healing process is similar to normal bone remodelling. Although a patient with a rigidly fixed fracture can be mobilised early, the more extensive bone necrosis results in slow healing since it depends on the formation of medullary callus and the direct replacement of cortical osteones.

Fig. 5.23 Pseudarthrosis following fracture of the clavicle. The bone ends have become covered by cartilage. At the top of the picture a split in the cartilage has occurred giving a false joint. There is endochondral ossification of the proliferated cartilage in the lower part of the picture. × 40.

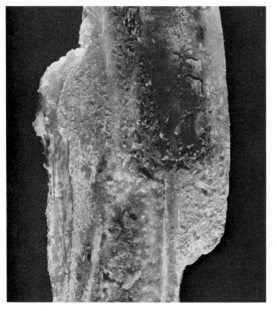

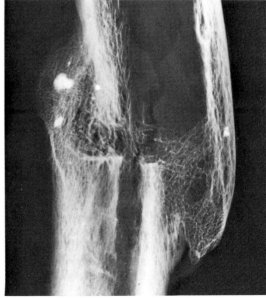

Fig. 5.24 This fracture through the midshaft of the femur united with anterior shift of the proximal fragment. Eighteen months after fracture there is firm bony union. The slab radiograph shows how the provisional callus has become remodelled along lines of stress with buttressing of the posterior and slightly concave part of the fracture line and some retubulation in the medullary canal at the fracture site.

Repair of some other tissues

Repair of articular cartilage

There is evidence that articular cartilage remains metabolically active throughout life, with continuous turnover of the proteoglycans and collagens of the matrix. Following injury, chondrocytes may proliferate to form cell clusters and there is an increase in proteoglycan turnover. The capacity to form new collagen is however limited and it is exceptional for these intrinsic reactions to produce any significant filling in of cartilage defects.

Extrinsic repair may occur by the growth of fibrous tissue over the articular surface from the joint margin. When there is loss of the full depth of the cartilage, fibrous tissue growing from the underlying marrow, through cracks in the exposed subchondral bone plate, may cover the bone end. This collagenous tissue may then acquire a more chondroid matrix, to become fibrocartilage, and is sometimes able to function reasonably well. However, the amount of new tissue formed by extrinsic repair is usually insufficient and of poor quality, especially when the defect is large, so that joint function is only partly restored and tends to deteriorate.

Repair of tendon

A good functional result following healing of a severed tendon requires a strong fibrous union between the ends without loss of a full range of gliding motion. In patients with sutured tendons, repair occurs by ingrowth of fibroblasts and blood vessels from surrounding connective tissue into the fibrin meshwork between the sutured ends. The cells, at first randomly arranged, later become orientated along the line of the tendon and produce collagen fibres. The amount of collagen synthesised is increased for some weeks after injury and, as in a healing wound, there is subsequent remodelling of the fibrous scar. The extrinsic source of vessels and cells during the healing process makes the formation of adhesions inevitable, but a good range of movement is retained when the adhesions are long and consist of loosely arranged areolar tissue. Restricted movement is associated with short adhesions containing large bundles of collagen fibres. Rough operative handling is thought to promote the formation of such adhesions, but little is known of other factors concerned.

Recent experimental evidence suggests that fibrocytes of tendon are not necessarily inert, but have some intrinsic potential for carrying out repair and remodelling. It may be that it is the surgical suture of the severed ends which, by disturbing the local blood supply, impairs this response and makes healing dependent on extrinsic sources. However suture is essential to hold the severed ends together and allow union to occur.

Repair of muscle

(a) Skeletal muscle. Regeneration of muscle is described on p. 21.70.

In **Zenker's hyaline degeneration** the endomysial tube remains intact and regeneration may be complete. This condition may accompany severe toxic infections, especially typhoid fever, and tends to involve most severely the muscles of the abdominal wall, diaphragm and intercostals. When the connective and supporting tissue in muscle is also torn or destroyed, as in more severe injuries, regeneration is less well orientated and a scar composed of fibrovascular tissue and irregularly orientated muscle fibres is formed. This is seen, for example, in **Volkmann's ischaemic contracture** in which ischaemic necrosis of the flexor muscles of the forearm may follow injuries around the elbow: replacement of dead muscle by fibrous tissue results in a characteristic deformity with clawing and restriction of movement of the fingers.

(b) Visceral muscle (smooth muscle). The healing of visceral muscle, e.g. in surgical incisions in the bowel or uterus, occurs by fibrous repair. Smooth muscle cells appear in newly-formed arterioles, but their origin is uncertain and they may arise from other mesenchymal cells. In atheromatous plaques (p. 14.6) they are derived from migration of medial smooth muscle cells. Proliferation with mitotic activity is said to occur in the early months of the physiological uterine enlargement of pregnancy.

(c) Cardiac muscle. Destruction of cardiac muscle by infarction is repaired by fibrous tissue (Fig. 15.12). Effective regeneration occurs in young patients with Coxsackie virus infections or diphtheria, where there is damage to individual fibres with preservation of the endomysium, a situation similar to that of Zenker's degeneration in skeletal muscle.

Repair of neural tissue and nerves

Central nervous system. Once mature nerve cells of the brain, cord or ganglia are destroyed, they are not replaced by the proliferation of other nerve cells. There is also no *useful* regeneration of the axons in the central nervous system: indeed when an axon is severed at any point, the entire axon and the nerve cell body degenerate. Of the neuroglial cells, proliferation in response to tissue damage is restricted to astrocytes and microglia (see also p. 21.5).

Regeneration of peripheral nerves. In contrast to the nerve cells and fibres in the central nervous system, peripheral nerves have considerable regenerative capacity.

When a nerve is transected, the axis cylinders distal to the cut undergo Wallerian degeneration, i.e. the axon and its myelin sheath break down and the debris is absorbed by macrophages (p. 21.5). At the same time the Schwann cells proliferate within the neurilemmal sheath to form pathways along which the axons may regrow. Above the level of transection, myelin degeneration extends upwards only to the first or second node of Ranvier and the nerve cell body characteristically shows reversible changes (central chromatolysis p. 21.3). Axonal sprouts soon emerge from the proximal ends of the interrupted axis cylinders and, if the cut ends of the nerve are in close apposition, they grow into the distal part of the nerve and along the spaces formerly occupied by axis cylinders and now filled with proliferated Schwann cells. The axons grow at a rate of about 3 mm per day. These new axons, which at first are very thin, develop a new myelin sheath and then increase in diameter. They do, however, remain smaller than normal nerves unless they establish satisfactory end-organ connections and functional relationships. This takes some time, and restoration of function is accordingly slow and often imperfect.

A feature of regenerated nerves is that the internodal segments are shorter than in normal nerves.

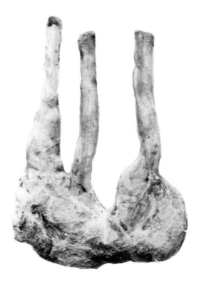

Fig. 5.25 Traumatic neuroma at severed proximal ends of nerves of an amputated arm.

The degree of functional recovery in a damaged peripheral nerve depends principally on the severity of the injury. If nerve fibres only are disrupted and the other components of the nerve trunk remain intact, as in a crush injury and sometimes in a stretching injury, regenerating axons can grow along their original endoneurial tubes, continuity of which is preserved and these fibres can re-establish their original end-organ relationships. If there is considerable disorganisation of the internal structure of individual nerve bundles within the nerve trunk, the continuity of endoneurial tubes is less likely to be preserved: fibrosis then occurs within the damaged segment and interferes with the growth of axons from the proximal segment of the damaged nerve. Some axons never traverse the fibrous barrier, while those that do almost never grow along their original endoneurial tubes. Thus many axons fail to reach their original end-organ and abnormal and incomplete innervation results. When there is subtotal or complete loss of continuity of the nerve trunk, the proliferation of axonal sprouts, fibroblasts and Schwann cells from the proximal end of the nerve results in the formation of a so-called **traumatic** or **stump neuroma** (Fig. 5.25).

In severely damaged nerves, surgical repair after excision of the involved segment or the traumatic neuroma is often the only hope of

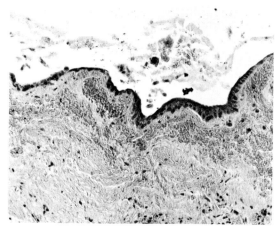

Fig. 5.26 Repair of lining of gallbladder after acute inflammatory desquamation. The epithelial cells extend as a thin flattened layer to reline the viscus. × 150.

achieving any functional recovery, but some residual disability almost invariably persists.

Repair of mucosal surfaces

Cells which line mucosal surfaces, are being lost and replaced continuously throughout life and, like all surface epithelia, have a good potential for regeneration (Fig. 5.26). In general, the raw surface is first covered and only later is there differentiation into more specialised cells.

(a) Gastro-intestinal tract mucosa. Physiological replacement of lost surface cells in the small bowel takes place by proliferation of the cells of the crypt base. Experimental excision of an area of mucosa, e.g. in the stomach, is rapidly followed by re-epithelialisation: epithelial cells of the mucous neck type migrate over the exposed connective tissue, forming first a layer of thin, flattened epithelium, which later becomes cuboidal or columnar. The epithelium of glands and surface cells adjacent to the wound undergo mitosis, and this proliferation increases the supply of migrating cells until the surface is covered. Gland crypts re-form by mucous cells growing down into the underlying granulation tissue and, some weeks later, specialised cells, e.g. parietal cells, differentiate from the mucous cells in the crypts. Failure of re-epithelialisation of chronic peptic ulcers (p. 19.26) is not fully understood. Surgical anastomoses of the mucous membranes heal readily, and the line between the two different types of mucosa remains sharp.

Rectal lesions heal slowly with formation of much granulation tissue, but the small and, to a lesser extent, the large bowel mucosae have a good capacity for repair (Fig. 19.50d, p. 19.37). Repeated ulceration and repair of the colon, as for instance in ulcerative colitis and bilharzial infestation, may lead to overgrowth of the reparative mucosa, producing polypoid projections (Fig. 28.37, p. 28.27).

(b) Respiratory tract mucosa. The basal cells of the tracheal and bronchial lining epithelium proliferate throughout life and replace loss of the surface ciliated epithelium. Many microbial infections result in loss of only part of the thickness of the pseudo-stratified columnar epithelium, and this is readily replaced by cell proliferation. Destruction of the whole thickness of the mucosa is followed by the usual migration and proliferation of cells which at first appear transitional and later become low columnar: eventually the superficial cells develop cilia. Destruction of subepithelial tissue or repeated damage, e.g. in chronic bronchitis, may result in less perfect regeneration, the ciliated cells being replaced by columnar non-ciliated mucus-secreting cells, and under very unfavourable circumstances, as in heavy cigarette smoking, metaplasia of the regenerating epithelium to squamous type may be seen (p. 16.10).

(c) Urinary tract mucosa. The urinary tract mucosa, like the epidermis, responds to injury by migration and proliferation of cells. The transitional-cell epithelium of the bladder has particularly good powers of rapid regeneration, in which all layers of the mucosa participate.

Repair of the kidney

The glomerulus is a highly specialised unit and little effective regeneration follows severe damage. Lost renal substance is replaced by fibrous tissue. If the basement membrane of the tubules remains intact, loss of tubal cells may be followed by proliferation (Fig. 5.27) and slow migration of surviving cells to restore continuity. If however the lost cells are highly specialised, as in the proximal convoluted tubule, it is doubtful whether the regenerated cells develop the same degree of functional efficiency.

Repair of the liver

The hepatic parenchymal cells form a fairly stable population, and few mitotic figures are seen in the normal liver. Replacement of normal 'wear-and-tear' cell loss is by division of neighbouring cells. Some replacement is effected by division of the nucleus and enlargement of the cell, which explains the occurrence of binucleate and multinucleate liver cells, particularly in elderly individuals.

Wounds of the liver are repaired by formation of connective tissue, with minimal replace-

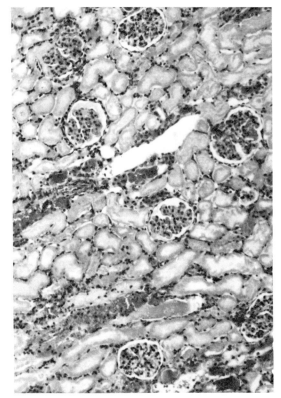

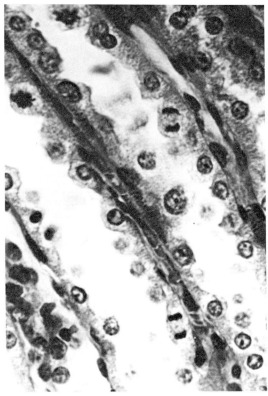

Fig. 5.27a Acute tubular necrosis in the rat. Note the anatomical normality of the glomeruli and the absence of nuclei in the dead tubular epithelial cells. × 150.

Fig. 5.27b Regeneration of renal tubular epithelium following acute tubular necrosis in the rat. Four mitotic figures are present. The adjacent regenerated cells are still of subnormal size. × 450.

ment of parenchymal cells around the margin of the wound.

The outcome of liver cell necrosis depends on the distribution of the cells affected and also upon the presence or absence of an intact vascular system. Occlusion of hepatic arterial branches may be followed by infarction of liver tissue: as in most other tissues, coagulative necrosis occurs and the dead tissue is digested by macrophages and replaced by organisation (see below), eventually leaving a fibrous scar. Necrosis and lysis of individual liver cells scattered throughout the parenchyma, as in the typical attack of virus hepatitis, is followed by replacement by proliferation of surviving cells with restoration to normal. Even when there is widespread destruction of all the hepatocytes in the central and mid-zones of lobules* the periportal cells proliferate and extend into the surviving

*The newer terminology, in which the unit of hepatic parenchyma is the acinus is described on p. 20.1.

vascular framework so that normality is once again achieved. If, however, there is loss of most or all of the hepatocytes of whole lobules and groups of lobules, proliferation of the surviving hepatocytes leads only to irregular nodules of regeneration, the lobular pattern being lost. The reticulin framework in the areas depleted of parenchymal cells becomes collapsed and scarred (Fig. 5.28).

The very high regenerative capacity of liver cells has been demonstrated by subjecting animals to excision of various amounts of liver tissue. After excision of two-thirds of the rat's liver, hyperplasia and hypertrophy of the remaining third result in restoration of a normal liver mass in 15–20 days. The capacity of the liver to regenerate in this way is maintained even when partial hepatectomy is performed monthly for up to one year.

The factors which regulate the extent of liver regeneration are not understood. When partial

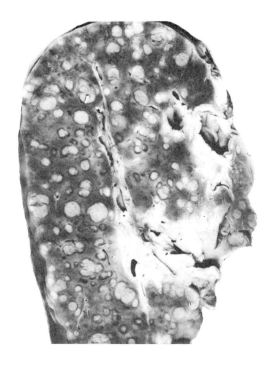

hepatectomy is performed on one member of a pair of parabiotic rats, liver cell proliferation occurs in both animals. This and similar experiments suggest that a humoral mediating factor is responsible for hepatic regeneration. More recent studies in dogs suggest that a humoral growth-stimulating factor is responsible for hepatic regeneration and is released by regenerating liver. If the portal vein is divided and anastomosed to the inferior vena cava before partial hepatectomy, regeneration of parenchyma is impaired, and it thus seems that portal venous flow through the liver affects the degree of restoration. There is evidence that insulin plays a major role in maintaining normal functioning of liver cells and in promoting hepatocellular proliferation. This makes good sense of the drainage of pancreatic venous blood to the liver and not to the systemic venous system.

Fig. 5.28 Following extensive liver necrosis, there has been proliferation of surviving liver cells. These form the pale rounded nodules lying in a background of scar tissue from which dead liver cells have now disappeared.

Organisation

This means the replacement, by fibrous tissue, of solid, non-living material such as fibrin, clotted blood, intravascular thrombus and dead tissue. The process involves the gradual digestion of the material by macrophages. Since these phagocytic cells can only operate within a short distance of capillaries, removal of more than a small amount of dead material requires the ingrowth of capillaries and fibroblasts. This formation of granulation tissue is similar to that in healing, but the term organisation is used only when inanimate material is replaced by it.

An example already familiar is the removal of **fibrin deposited in acute inflammation** (p. 4.28). Thin strands of fibrin are rapidly phagocytosed and digested, but larger deposits, for example the thick layer which forms on the pleural surface in some cases of pleurisy, are removed more slowly by organisation. After the acute inflammation has subsided monocytes continue to emigrate from the vessels in the pleura underlying the adherent fibrin and assume the features of macrophages: they begin to digest the fibrin by a combination of phago-

cytosis and release of lysosomal enzymes. Capillary sprouts develop from the superficial pleural vessels and grow into the spaces created by the macrophages (Fig. 5.29): they anastomose to form a network of capillaries, some of which enlarge and develop into arterioles and venules. The capillaries are accompanied by proliferating fibroblasts which produce collagen and ground substance. A thin layer of granulation tissue thus takes the place of the deepest part of the fibrin and gradually the process extends until all the fibrin has been replaced. Meanwhile, the granulation tissue slowly changes to less vascular, firm fibrous tissue. If the layer of fibrin has glued together the visceral and parietal pleura, organisation proceeds from both surfaces and meets in the middle: in consequence, the lung becomes firmly bound to the chest wall by fibrous tissue.

A second example of organisation is seen when haemorrhage occurs into the tissues and the escaped blood clots to form a solid mass, i.e. a **haematoma**. This is removed by organisation from the surrounding tissues (Fig. 5.30) and progresses to the centre of the clot, eventu-

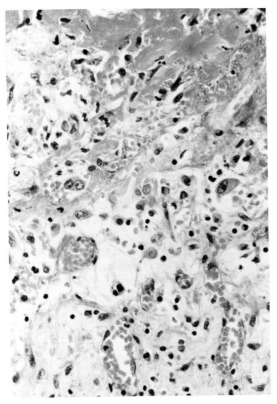

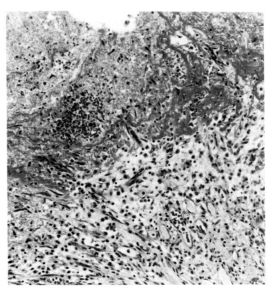

Fig. 5.30 Organisation of a haematoma after 7 days. Capillary sprouts are beginning to grow into the clot and there are also large numbers of macrophages at its margin. × 80.

Fig. 5.29 Dilated capillaries and fibroblasts have grown into and are replacing the dense fibrin on the surface of the lung. × 400.

ally leaving a fibrous scar. A patch of **necrotic tissue** (most commonly seen in the heart, brain, kidneys, etc. as the result of arterial blockage by thrombus, i.e. an infarct) is similarly removed by organisation with consequent scar formation.

When an artery or vein is blocked by **thrombus**, this is removed partly by organisation, but other processes are involved and the fate of thrombi is described on pp. 10.18–19.

Hypertrophy

Stimulation of the parenchymal cells of an organ, usually by increased functional demand or by hormones, result in an increase in the total mass of the parenchymal cells. This may be brought about by enlargement of the cells— **hypertrophy** or by an increase in their number— **hyperplasia**. The relative importance of the two processes varies in different organs. In some, e.g. the skeletal muscles, enlargement is purely by hypertrophy, but in most organs hypertrophy and hyperplasia both contribute.

(a) The response to increased functional demand

This is illustrated by the hypertrophied **muscles** of manual labourers and athletes; the individual fibres increase in thickness but not in number. Similarly, when extra work is demanded of the **heart** as a result of valvular disease or high blood pressure (Fig. 5.31), there may be much thickening of the muscular walls of those chambers which bear the brunt of the extra work. Narrowing of the mitral valve, for example, produces chiefly left atrial and right ventricular hypertrophy, whereas systemic hypertension gives rise predominantly to left ventricular hypertrophy (Fig. 15.5). The heart may increase to twice the normal weight, the degree of hypertrophy being limited by the diffusion of oxygen and nutrients between the capillaries and the thickened fibres. **Smooth muscle** may

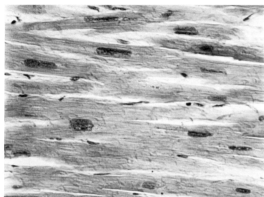

Fig. 5.31a Hypertrophied muscle fibres of heart in a case of arteriosclerosis with high blood pressure. × 250.

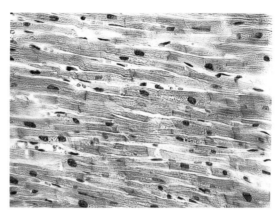

Fig. 5.31b Slightly atrophied heart muscle; to compare with Fig. 5.31a. × 250.

also undergo hypertrophy, for example in the wall of the stomach in a patient with pyloric stenosis, in large bowel proximal to an obstructing tumour (Fig. 19.75. p. 19.66), or in the bladder obstructed by an enlarged prostate (Fig. 25.3, p. 25.8). The muscle in arterial walls also hypertrophies in response to long continued high blood pressure (Fig. 14.14, p. 14.16). Striking hypertrophy is seen in the pregnant uterus, where a combination of increased functional demand and hormonal stimuli results in enlargement of fibres to more than a hundred times their original volume. In early pregnancy, there may be both hypertrophy and hyperplasia of muscle fibres. After parturition, the muscle fibres return to a normal size and this is seen also in hypertrophied heart muscle when the increased work stimulus is removed.

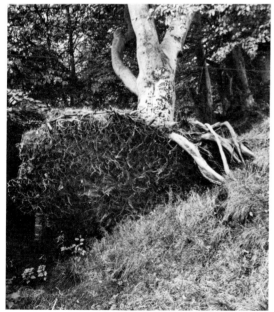

Fig. 5.32 This beech tree was largely uprooted by a gale six years before, and has since leant against its neighbour. It continues to survive because a few roots (on the right) have retained contact with the soil and have become greatly hypertrophied.

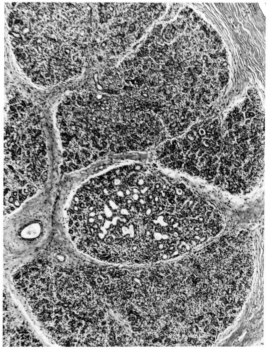

Fig. 5.33 Breast lobule in pregnancy showing marked hyperplasia. × 50.

In some instances, the response to an increased demand is by a pure hyperplasia; for instance, blood loss is not followed by enlargement of red cells and leucocytes but by an increase in their production in the haemopoietic marrow (Fig. 17.13b, p. 17.18).

Compensatory hypertrophy may occur in the survivor of a pair of organs when one is removed. Following nephrectomy, the remaining kidney enlarges and, particularly in young patients, may double its weight. This is brought about by increase in the size of the nephron as a result of both hypertrophy and hyperplasia of the component cells of the glomeruli and tubules. Removal of one adrenal leads to hypertrophy of the opposite cortex, the medulla remaining unchanged. Following removal of a lung, the remaining lung enlarges but this is caused mainly by over-distension, which produces a lasting enlargement of the alveoli; only when it occurs in early life is there any formation of new alveoli. Compensatory hypertrophy is a widespread natural phenomenon, as illustrated in Fig. 5.32.

The testes are exceptional in that, in both man and animals, removal of one in adult life is not followed by enlargement of the other, the number of spermatozoa produced being reduced.

(b) Hypertrophy due to hormonal changes

A balanced activity of certain of the endocrine glands is essential for the normal growth and metabolism of the tissues and many of the examples of hypertrophy and hyperplasia already mentioned require the continued physiological action of the growth hormone of the anterior pituitary as well as an adequate blood supply. Excessive secretion of growth hormone (usually due to a tumour of the somatotrophic cells of the anterior pituitary) results, in adults, in acromegaly (p. 26.6) with bone enlargement and generalised organ and tissue hypertrophy. In childhood or adolescence, the result is even more striking, for excess of hormone in adolescence, before the skeleton matures results in gigantism (p. 26.7). An example of physiological hyperplasia is the enlargement of the breasts in pregnancy, when the formation of mammary gland acini is stimulated chiefly by hormones from the corpus luteum or placenta (Fig. 5.33).

Further Reading

D'Ardenne, A.J. and McGee, J.O'D. (1984). Fibronectin in disease. *Journal of Pathology*, **142**, 235–51.

Peacock, E.E. Jr. (1984). *Wound Repair* 3rd ed. pp. 526. Saunders, Philadelphia.

Tissue Growth Factors. (1984). *Clinics in Endocrinology and Metabolism 13* No. 1, pp. 191–225. Guest editor, Wm. D. Daughaday.

D. Gospodarowicz. 1983. Growth factors and their action *in vivo* and *in vitro. Journal of Pathology*, **141,** 201–33.

S. Sevitt. (1981). *Bone Repair and Fracture Healing in Man.* pp. 316 Churchill Livingstone, Edinburgh.

6

Immunophysiology: The Immune Response

The invasion of the body by living organisms, including viruses, bacteria, and protozoan and metazoan parasites, presents a major threat to the stability of the internal milieu upon which Claude Bernard placed such importance. To counter this threat, certain general defence mechanisms have evolved—a relatively impermeable epidermis, methods of ridding the body of noxious material, such as vomiting, diarrhoea and coughing, the dilution of irritants by increased flow of interstitial fluid in inflammatory oedema, and the destruction of particulate matter by phagocytic cells. In addition, there exists in vertebrates a special defence mechanism of immense potential which is mobilised when the body is invaded by foreign organisms and which is expressly and specifically adapted to overcome the effects of any particular invader. The special mechanism is called **acquired specific immunity** and its study— the science of **immunology**—is of great importance in the understanding and prevention of disease.

The phenomenon of acquired specific immunity has been recognised for centuries in that individuals who had survived an attack of certain clearly recognisable infectious diseases such as smallpox were known to be much less susceptible to the disease during a later epidemic. Such individuals could be said to show **immunity** (i.e. protection) against the disease, **acquired** inasmuch as it did not apparently exist before the first infection, and **specific** inasmuch as an attack of smallpox protected the individual against a further attack of smallpox but had no bearing on his susceptibility to later attacks of measles, diphtheria, etc.

This knowledge has been applied with great success to the prevention of infectious disease by **prophylactic immunisation**, a procedure in which a relatively harmless variant, or modified toxin, of a pathogenic organism is purposely introduced into the body: this results in the development of specific immunity such as would be encountered following recovery from the natural disease. The principle is well illustrated by Edward Jenner's use of fluid from the lesions of cowpox (vaccinia) to vaccinate against smallpox; it was known to Jenner that milkmaids, who had had natural cowpox infection, had developed not only markedly altered reactivity to re-infection with cowpox but also resistance to a first infection by smallpox, a closely related but much more serious disease. In this case the two viruses are so similar that immunity to one is effective also against the other.

When an individual has become immune following natural infection or prophylactic exposure to a pathogenic organism or its toxin, he is said to be **actively immunised** against that organism. Specific resistance to infection can in many instances be conferred upon a non-immune individual by an alternative method, namely the injection of *serum* or *lymphoid cells* from an actively immune individual. The state of **passive immunity** so conferred is not due to transfer of the infecting organism or its toxin but to the transfer of the products of immunisation developed by the actively immunised donor of the serum or lymphoid cells. The *passive transfer* of immunity provides a way of analysing the factors which contribute to the immune state, and by transfer experiments it has been shown that, in some instances, specific immunity results from the presence in the serum of special globulins known as **antibodies**, while in other cases the immune state seems to be mediated directly by **specifically primed (sensitised) lymphocytes** without the participation of serum antibody. Serum containing one or more

6.1

antibodies produced by active immunisation is termed **antiserum** or **immune serum**.

The development of acquired specific immunity is the result of an **immune response**, which may thus take two forms.

1. Antibody production, i.e. the appearance of globulin molecules which have the property of combining specifically with and remaining attached to **antigen** (see below) of the same kind as that which has led to their formation.

2. Cell-mediated immunity, i.e. the production of specifically primed lymphocytes whose presence can be demonstrated *in vivo* by the development of a local imflammatory reaction appearing about 24 hours after intradermal injection of the antigen—a **delayed hypersensitivity reaction**.

Most antigenic stimuli evoke both cell-mediated immunity and antibody production. These responses take place in the lymphoid tissues, and their products, specifically primed lymphocytes and antibody, both capable of reacting with the antigen, are released into the bloodstream.

Under certain conditions, an antigenic stimulus may induce a state of **specific immunological tolerance**, i.e. non-responsiveness to subsequent challenge with the same antigen.

The term '*immunological reaction*' should not be confused with '*immune response*' as described above. An **immunological reaction** is the effect observed when the products of the immune response—antibody or primed lymphocytes—encounter and combine with the appropriate antigen *in vitro* or *in vivo*.

The amount of antibody produced in an immune response following antigenic stimulation can be determined roughly by measuring the level in the serum. A second exposure to the same antigen induces a much more rapid, greater, and more prolonged production of antibody. This is the **secondary immune response** and is dependent on **immunological memory**. Similarly, the cell-mediated immune response to subsequent antigenic stimulation is greater than that following the first encounter with the antigen.

Factors affecting the immune response

The form taken by the immune response depends upon several factors, including the nature of the antigen, the genetic constitution of the individual exposed to the antigen, the route by which the antigen enters the body and the dose administered. These factors are discussed below.

Antigens

An antigen is a substance which is **immunogenic** i.e. capable of evoking an immune response. It is difficult to define precisely the properties which make a substance antigenic, but in general terms antigens are large molecules, usually of molecular weight exceeding 3000, fairly rigid in structure, and either protein or carbohydrate, with or without other constituents, such as lipid. Antigen–antibody reactions appear to be the result largely of stereo-chemical interactions of molecules of complementary configurations, analogous to the interaction of lock and key. For this reason, floppy molecules such as gelatin are poor antigens. Evidence will be presented later that immune responses follow the binding of antigen molecules to specific receptors on the surface of lymphocytes. It seems likely that, to trigger off an immune response, antigen must form a link between these surface receptors: this explains why most antigens are large molecules.

Although some small molecules, such as para-aminobenzoic acid, are not by themselves antigenic, they may become so if they are attached to larger molecules. Injection of *p*-aminobenzoic acid attached by diazotisation to serum albumin may result in formation of some antibody molecules which combine specifically with the *p*-aminobenzoic acid moiety and not with the albumin carrier protein. In these circumstances, *p*-aminobenzoic acid is said to be a **hapten**, i.e. a substance which is antigenic inasmuch as it can take part in an immunological reaction (in this case antigen–antibody combination) but which is not itself immunogenic, i.e. cannot by itself evoke an immune response (in this example, the formation of specific antibody) unless it is conjugated with macromolecular material. The existence of such simple haptens suggests that the antigenic specificity of large molecules may be determined by the three-dimensional configuration of small parts of these molecules (**antigenic determinant sites** or **epitopes**). Study of synthetic polypeptide and polysaccharide antigens has confirmed that specific antigenic determinant sites do consist of a few amino acids or monosaccharides, and it has been shown that most naturally-occurring macromolecules such as plasma albumin contain several antigenic determinant sites of differing specificity. Larger, complex antigenic particles, such as bacteria, contain a correspondingly greater number and variety of epitopes. Both antibody production and cell-mediated immunity evoked by antigenic material are correspondingly complex, each particular kind of epitope being potentially capable of inducing both types of response.

Genetic constitution of the individual. The repertoire of specific immune responses which an individual can mount depends on the selection of genes inherited from two distinct sets—the V genes which code for the various antigen binding sites found on different antibody molecules (pp. 6.15–16) and the Ir (immune reactivity) genes which are not linked with (i.e. on the same chromosome as) the genes coding for antibodies, but lie in the 'I' region of the major histocompatibility complex (p. 2.12). The genetic nature of the responsiveness is clearly shown by crossing inbred strains of mice which exhibit marked differences in their responses to immunisation with simple antigens containing only one type of epitope, such as simple synthetic oligo-peptides. Inheritance of specific responsiveness to most natural antigens is difficult to demonstrate because of the multiplicity and variety of epitopes on natural macromolecules, but the magnitude of response to these antigens is also controlled non-specifically by a number of genes, some affecting such properties as rate of antigen degradation by macrophages (pp. 6.26–27).

Genetic factors also play a large part in determining the antigenicity of tissues, and this field has become particularly important in the practice of blood transfusion and of tissue transplantation. The molecular composition of tissues, including potential antigenic sites, is, of course, genetically determined. In general, when cells or tissues from one individual are injected or transplanted into another, the more genetically dissimilar or foreign the two individuals

are to each other, the easier it is to induce antibody formation and cell-mediated immunity. For example, human red cells injected into rabbits evoke a wide variety of antibodies reacting with a corresponding variety of antigenic determinants on the human red cell; when, as in this case, the antigen is derived from a species other than that of the immunised animal (and this includes bacterial antigens), it is called a **hetero-antigen** and the antibodies are **hetero-antibodies**. Injection or transplantation of one human with the red cells or tissue cells of another may result in the formation of antibodies to antigenic groups not shared by both individuals; e.g. human red cells containing the rhesus antigen D (rhesus positive cells) into a person whose cells do not contain this antigen (rhesus negative) may result in the development of antibodies specific for D antigen; antigens which differ within a species are called **iso-antigens** and the corresponding antibodies **iso-antibodies**. In general, iso-antigens are much less numerous and less likely to evoke an immune response than hetero-antigens. Finally it should be noted that injection of an individual with his own cells (**auto-antigen**) results in **auto-antibody** formation or cell-mediated immunity only in exceptional cases; the subject of **auto-immunity** is considered further on p. 7.24. Unfortunately, the prefixes traditionally used to indicate the relationship between individuals providing antigen and forming antibody are different from those used in the more recent field of tissue transplantation, in which graft rejection is effected mainly by delayed hypersensitivity reactions. Table 6.1 summarises this confusing and irrational situation.

As stated above, the cells and tissues of an individual are antigenic when injected or grafted into an animal of another species or even into a different individual of the same species, yet with certain exceptions the individual does not respond to the antigens of his own cells by the development of auto-antibody or delayed auto-hypersensitivity. Unresponsiveness to auto-antigen is a general physiological principle described by Ehrlich as 'horror autotoxicus'. It may reflect absence of lymphoid cells with the genetic coding necessary for the synthetic processes associated with formation of antibody or cell-mediated immunity against most 'self' components, analogous to the inherited non-responsiveness of certain strains of

Table 6.1   Terminology of antigens, antibodies and tissue grafts

Relationship between donor and recipient	Genetic terminology	Antibody, antigen	Transplantation terminology
Same animal	—	Auto-antibody Auto-antigen	Autograft
Identical twins and inbred strain	Syngeneic (Isogeneic)	—	Isograft
Same outbred species or different inbred strains	Allogeneic	Iso-antibody Iso-antigen	Allograft (Homograft)
Different species	Heterogeneic Xenogeneic	Hetero-antibody Hetero-antigen	Xenograft (Heterograft)

animals to synthetic polypeptide antigens. An attractive alternative explanation, suggested by Burnet and Fenner (1949), proposes that the various potential antigens in an individual's tissues do act on the cells responsible for immune responses but that, instead of causing antibody formation or cell-mediated immunity, they lead during fetal life to **specific immunological tolerance**. The subject is, however, a complex one; it is considered more fully on p. 6.28.

Route of administration of antigen. In most cases, antigens elicit an immunological response only when they are introduced parenterally (i.e. not through the alimentary canal) so that their macromolecular state and the configuration of their antigenic determinants are not destroyed by digestion in the gut. Traces of certain proteins, such as those in heterologous milk, may, in fact, be absorbed from the gut and bring about specific immunisation, especially in infants. In general, however, antigens introduced into the portal circulation are less immunogenic than when administered by other routes.

The relative contributions of cell-mediated immunity and antibody formation to an immune response can be influenced by the route of administration of antigens. For example, many antigens administered intradermally evoke a strong cell-mediated immune response but given intravenously result predominantly in antibody formation.

Dose of antigen administered. The immune response is highly sensitive to the dose of antigen administered. There is not a simple dose-response relationship since many antigens may be immunogenic at certain doses and induce tolerance at others (p. 6.29).

The cellular basis of the immune response

The cytology of immunological phenomena is complex but is worth studying in some detail, not only because of the vital importance of specific immunity, but also because it illustrates the complexity of the systems by which eukaryotic cells communicate with one another and co-ordinate their activities. Most of the advances have been based on the manipulation of cells and tissues of experimental animals, but the features of immune responses and of naturally occurring immunodeficiency states in man, the effects of therapeutic immunosuppression, and investigation of human lymphocytes *in vitro* all indicate that the same basic rules apply.

The main features of the cellular basis of antibody production and cell-mediated immunity may be summarised as follows.

1. Cell-mediated immunity and antibody production are both attributable to lymphocytes capable of recognising and responding specifically to the stimulus provided by an antigen, i.e. **specifically responsive lymphocytes**.

2. At some stage in their development, lymphocytes become 'committed', i.e. capable of responding only to a particular antigenic determinant group, or to closely similar determinant groups. Lymphocyte populations thus consist of individual cells which differ in the antigens to which they can respond. In consequence, no one antigen can stimulate a response in more than a small proportion of them.

3. The specifically responsive lymphocytes which bring about cell-mediated immunity are **thymus-dependent** or **T lymphocytes**. They develop from stem cells in the thymus under the

influence of thymic hormones and other differentiation signals and many of them leave the thymus and reach the various other lymphoid tissues.

4. On encountering an antigen to which it is specifically responsive, the T lymphocyte proliferates in the lymphoid tissues to produce a clone of lymphocytes, all of which are capable of reacting with that antigen—**specifically-primed T lymphocytes**. These include the cells responsible for delayed hypersentitivity reactions.

5. The specifically-responsive lymphocytes which bring about antibody production are **thymus-independent** and are termed **B lymphocytes**. In mammals, they develop from stem cells in the haemopoietic tissue from which many of them migrate and pass to the various other lymphoid tissues.

6. On encountering an antigen to which it is specifically responsive, the B lymphocyte, like the T lymphocyte, proliferates in the lymphoid tissues to form a clone of cells capable of reacting with that antigen. Some cells of the clone differentiate into **plasma cells** and secret **antibody** which also is capable of reacting with the antigen. The plasma cells are thus derived from B lymphocytes.

7. Some of the lymphocytes produced by antigen-induced proliferation of T and B lymphocytes persist as **memory cells**. In other words, antigenic stimulation increases the number of T and B lymphocytes capable of reacting with that antigen, and some of these lymphocytes are long-lived and are responsible for a secondary response on subsequent stimulation by the antigen.

8. Although T lymphocytes do not give rise to antibody-producing plasma cells, they co-operate with B cells in antibody responses. There is a subpopulation of T cells called **helper cells,** whose co-operation with B cells enhances the production of antibody to specific antigens, and whose help is essential for some antibody responses. A different subpopulation of T lymphocytes exists, whose co-operation with B cells is essentially regulatory and suppresses the production of antibody. These latter cells are termed **suppressor T cells**.

9. In some circumstances, antigenic stimulation results in neither antibody production nor cell-mediated immunity, but renders the individual specifically unresponsive to subsequent challenge by that antigen. This unresponsive state is termed **acquired immunological tolerance**. It provides an explanation of why we do not usually respond strongly to antigens in our own cells and tissues, and it plays an important role in successful transplantation of foreign cells and tissues.

These basic features of immune responses are considered more fully below.

The specifically responsive lymphocyte

For the development of specific immunity, it is necessary that cells should recognise specific determinant sites (epitopes) on antigenic molecules, and should respond to them in ways that lead to the production of antibodies and primed lymphocytes, both of which are capable of reacting specifically with the antigen. Much of the credit for demonstrating that these cells—the keystones of the immune response—are lymphocytes, is due to Gowans and others (see Gowans, 1966). They used techniques in which lymphocytes were removed from rats by thoracic duct drainage. By drainage for several days, the cell-free fluid being returned to the rat, depletion of a population of small lymphocytes was achieved and the depleted rats were found to be defective in their responses to antigenic stimulation. For example, when challenged by injection of sheep erythrocytes or tetanus toxoid, they made poor antibody responses, and when grafted with skin from an allogeneic rat they did not reject the graft, indicating failure of the normal cell-mediated response to the graft antigens. These immunological deficiencies were corrected by injection of small lymphocytes from the thoracic duct of a normal rat, and when the donor had been previously immunised, e.g. by a skin allograft or an injection of sheep erythrocytes, the recipient showed the rapid and intense response to antigenic challenge which is characteristic of the secondary response. These observations suggested that small lymphocytes in thoracic duct lymph are essential for primary immune responses, and showed more conclusively that they include specifically responsive cells resulting from a previous immune response, i.e. immunological memory cells (thus explaining the rapidity of the secondary response). Gowans' findings have since been confirmed by many other workers and have been shown to apply to several mammalian and avian species. Animals depleted of lymphocytes by various other methods (p. 6.34) have also been shown to be immunologically deficient and the deficiency is corrected by lymphocytes from histocompatible normal animals. Moreover, in such experiments it has been shown by cell labelling techniques that the donated lymphocytes proliferate and provide the plasma cells which produce antibody and also the lymphocytes responsible for cell-mediated immunity.

By such experiments, it has been firmly established that, *in both primary and secondary immune responses, the cells capable of recognising the antigen, and of responding specifically to it by production of antibody or cell-mediated immunity, are lymphocytes.*

Humoral Immunity

Antibodies

Antibody molecules have the special property of combining specifically with antigen or hapten. In so doing, they may cover up harmful areas on molecules of toxin, in which case they are said to be **antitoxins**, or their combination with cells such as bacteria may lead (with the help of complement—p. 7.2) to death and lysis of the bacteria (**bacteriolytic effect**) or to phagocytosis by polymorphs and macrophages (**opsonic effect**). Chemically, antibodies belong to the **immunoglobulin (Ig)** proteins of the plasma (formerly called γ-globulins because of their predominant electrophoretic mobility). There are five classes: IgG, IgM, IgA, IgD and IgE. All immunoglobulins are composed of one or more similar units, each unit consisting of two pairs of identical polypeptide chains (Fig. 6.1); one pair, termed the **heavy chains**, are about twice the size (molecular weight) of the other pair, which are termed the **light chains**. Digestion of an Ig molecule by papain breaks it into three fragments, of which two are identical and are termed **Fab** (antigen-binding fragments) because each contains a combining site for antigen. The third fragment consists of the C-terminal ends of the heavy chains, and is termed **Fc** fragment; it is readily obtained in crystalline (hence Fc) form. As shown in Fig. 6.1, digestion of IgG by pepsin frees two pFc' fragments but leaves the two Fab fragments united by part of the Fc fragment as a single fragment—F(ab')$_2$. Heavy chains differ structurally for each class of Ig, and the letters γ, μ, α, δ, ε, are used to indicate the heavy chains of IgG, IgM, IgA, etc. respectively. By contrast, there are only two types of light chain, κ and λ,

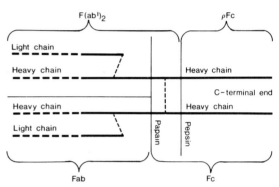

Fig. 6.1   Structure of a monomeric immunoglobulin molecule. In any particular molecule, the two light chains have an identical amino-acid sequence and so do the two heavy chains. Each immunoglobulin class has a distinctive Fc piece (C-terminal end of the heavy chains). The amino-acid sequences of the interrupted portions of the light and heavy chains (the N-terminal ends) vary greatly among immunoglobulin molecules, even of the same class and constitute the specific antigen-binding (Fab) sites, of which there are two on each molecule, each consisting of the N-terminal ends of a light and a heavy chain. The antigen-binding region of the molecule is also known as the idiotype. The light interrupted lines represent disulphide bonds and the light continuous lines the sites of action of papain and pepsin, which divide the molecule respectively into two Fab and one Fc fragment, and one F(ab')$_2$ and two pFc' fragments.

in all Ig classes, and each Ig molecule has *either* κ or λ light chains.

The combination of antibody with antigen is believed to be achieved by hydrogen bonding, electrostatic, hydrophobic and van der Waal's forces; these are effective over a very short range and hold separate molecules together only when they fit snugly. The specificity of antigen–antibody union therefore depends on the antibody combining site having a complementary shape to the antigenic determinant, which permits the necessary close fit. The shape of the combining site is determined by the amino-acid sequence of the N-terminal ends of the heavy and, to a lesser extent, of the light chains. In view of what is now known of protein synthesis, this is of great interest and of fundamental importance in elucidating how antigenic stimulation gives rise to specific antibody formation. In contrast to most other proteins, each one of which in a given individual is of uniform amino-acid sequence, the immunoglobulins in a serum show marked heterogeneity of their N-terminal regions (the **variable regions**), the number of variations amounting to millions. Analysis of the amino-acid sequences of the N-terminal regions of different immunoglobulin molecules has shown that there are three or four areas in the polypeptide chain where most of this sequence variation occurs—**the hypervariable regions**. In the tertiary structure of the immunoglobulins, these hypervariable regions are brought into close proximity with each other at an exposed part of the molecule and constitute the antigen-combining sites of the antibody. This variety is responsible for the great range of antibodies which can develop in response to stimulation by an enormous number of different antigens.

Some idea of the specificity of antibody–antigen union can be gained from study of antibody against chemically defined haptens. Landsteiner, for example, showed that antibody raised against para-aminobenzene sulphonic acid does not combine with the ortho- form but gives a weak reaction with meta-aminobenzene sulphonic acid (Fig. 6.2). The latter is called a **cross reaction** and it implies immunological reactivity with an antigen different from that which has led to the production of antibody. It results from the production of some antibody

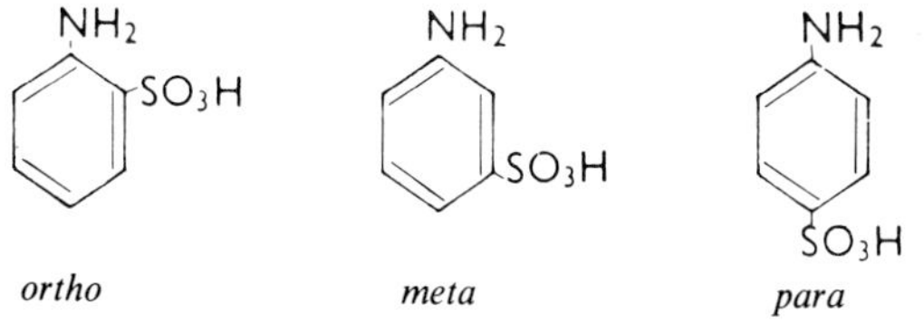

molecules which fit the cross-reacting antigen sufficiently well to permit intermolecular attraction by short-range forces (see above). The closeness of fit between the antigen-binding sites of antibody and an antigen of given configuration can thus vary and this affects the firmness of combination; we therefore speak of high or low **affinity** of antibody for a given epitope. Cross reactions are generally of low affinity.

When an antiserum contains a variety of antibodies reacting with multiple and often heterogeneous epitopes on a macromolecular antigen, the strength of the binding together of antigenic molecules by antibodies is referred to as the **avidity** of the antiserum; this is influenced not only by the affinities of each of the various antibodies reacting with individual epitopes, but also by the number of antigen–antibody linkages formed: although individual antibody-epitope linkages dissociate, those which fit snugly dissociate less readily than poorly-fitting linkages, and large numbers of firm linkages will result in the maintenance of avid binding.

Quite apart from their specific reactivity with antigens, antibodies of different classes possess properties which depend on the Fc part of the heavy (μ, γ, α, etc.) chains.

Properties of the immunoglobulin classes

The various immunoglobulin classes have different functions (beyond that of specific combination with antigen, which is common to all) and this is determined by the structure of the part of the heavy chains included in the Fc fragment.

Table 6.2 compares some of the features of the five known immunoglobulin classes. **IgG** is monomeric (Figs 6.1 and 6.3). It is the most abundant immunoglobulin in the plasma and extravascular fluid. IgG antitoxins are of importance because they combine with and neutralise toxins, thus protecting the individual from their harmful effects. There are receptors for the Fc part of IgG antibodies on polymorphs and macrophages which facilitate adherence and phagocytosis of the corresponding antigens. The reaction of IgG antibody with the corresponding antigen can usually be demonstrated *in vitro* (see below): IgG can cross the human placenta and in this way passive immunity is transferred from mother to child.

Fig. 6.2 Isomeric forms of aminobenzene sulphonic acid.

Table 6.2 Size and plasma (or serum) concentrations of immunoglobulins

Class	Molecular weight (daltons)	Degree of polymerisation	Concentration (normal serum) G/litre
IgG	150 000	Monomer	8–16
IgM	900 000	Pentamer	0.5–2
IgA	mainly 150 000	Mono- and dimer	1·4–4
IgD	185 000	Monomer	0–0·4
IgE	200 000	Monomer	2–45×10^{-7}

There are four sub-classes of IgG (1–4), which differ somewhat in their properties, e.g. capacity to activate complement (see below). These differences are referred to later in relation to topics in which they are of importance. **IgM** is a macroglobulin consisting of pentamers of the basic four-chain units or monomers (each of which has two antigen-combining sites) and one additional polypeptide J chain, which is probably responsible for formation of the pentamer (Fig. 6.3). It is the first Ig class of antibody to be produced following the initial introduction of an antigen (i.e. in the primary immune response). Having 10 combining sites, it is usually of high avidity: it is most effective in activating complement (see below), and its reaction with antigen is readily demonstrated *in vitro*. Except in inflammatory lesions, it is largely confined to the plasma, where it has an important function in destroying micro-organisms. The presence of IgM antibody to a virus indicates recent or continuing infection by the virus. **IgA** is secreted locally by plasma cells in the intestinal mucosa, the lacrimal glands, respiratory passages and salivary glands. It is secreted by the plasma cells in the form of a dimer, the two molecules being linked by a J chain (Fig. 6.3). Such locally produced IgA is taken up by the glandular and lining epithelial cells of these tissues and coupled with a carbohydrate 'transport piece' which renders it more resistant to digestive enzymes. In this form it is secreted in the tears, alimentary and salivary mucus, etc. and forms a lining, sometimes referred to as 'antiseptic paint', over the alimentary and respiratory mucous membranes and conjunctiva. IgA activates complement by the alternative pathway and may enhance the bacteriolytic activity of lysozyme (p. 8.2). It is also present in the

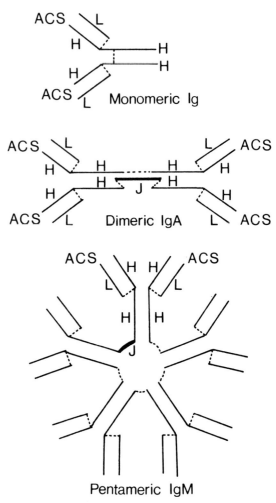

Fig. 6.3 The structure of immunoglobulins. The monomeric Ig molecule consists of two heavy and two light chains (*upper and Fig. 6.1*). IgA (*middle*) is secreted as a dimer, consisting of two monomeric units joined by a J chain (heavy line). Secretory IgA also contains a secretory piece (not shown). *Lower*, the pentameric IgM molecule, consisting of an oligomer of five monomers (one of which is labelled) and one additional (J) chain which may initiate oligomerisation. All the other inter-chain links (interrupted lines) consists of disulphide bonds. Note that each unit has two antigen-combining sites (ACS), so that IgA dimer has four and IgM ten. (The heavy chains of Ig are angulated at the so-called hinge region, so that the unit molecule is Y-shaped: this is not shown in Fig. 6.1.)

plasma in the form of monomers and dimers. **IgE** has the special property of attaching to mast cells and basophil leucocytes, by means of its Fc fragment, leaving the specific combining sites (on the Fab fragments) available for union with antigen. If such union takes place, pharmacologically active substances such as histamine are released by the sensitised cell, with the production of an anaphylactic hypersensitivity reaction within a few minutes (p. 7.6). The biological properties of **IgD** are unknown, but it acts as a lymphocyte surface antigen-receptor (pp. 6.15, 6.18).

Demonstration of antigen–antibody reactions

This section and the following one on demonstration of cell-mediated immunity are largely of a technical nature and are intentionally brief. To some extent, they interrupt the account of the immune response, which continues on p. 6.13. They do, however, illustrate the practical aspects of what might otherwise seem to be largely an academic subject. Accordingly, the reader is advised not to skip them.

The demonstration of antigen–antibody reactions is applicable equally to the detection and assay of antigen by means of a known antibody and of antibody by means of a known antigen.

Antigen–antibody reactions *in vivo*

These may be demonstrated in three ways.

(1) A potentially harmful antigenic substance may be rendered harmless by union with antibody and not have the expected effect. For example, in the Schick test, intradermal injection of a small amount of diphtheria toxin into the skin of a non-immune individual results in an area of inflammation. The diphtheria antitoxin present in an immunised individual neutralises the toxin and so suppresses the inflammation. Similarly, antibodies to pathogenic micro-organisms may be demonstrated by their capacity to protect experimental animals against a lethal dose of the micro-organism.

(2) A normally harmless stimulus may result in tissue injury, i.e. a hypersensitivity reaction. For example, inhalation of grass pollen may induce an attack of hay fever or asthma, mediated by its reaction with antibody specific for grass pollen. In this instance, the antibody is usually of IgE class, but hypersensitivity

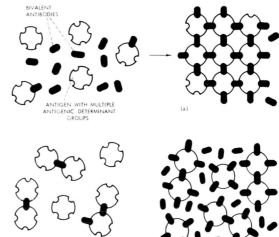

Fig. 6.4 The reaction of antigen and bivalent (e.g. IgG) antibody; (a) in optimal proportions to form large aggregates; (b) in antigen excess; (c) in antibody excess. In (b) and (c) small complexes are formed. In the case of soluble antigens, large aggregates form as in (a), and produce a precipitate, whereas with particulate antigens e.g. bacteria, formation of aggregates is termed agglutination.

reactions may result from the union *in vivo* of other classes of antibody with antigen: they are of considerable importance in disease processes and are described in Chapter 7.

(3) In the special instance of antibodies which

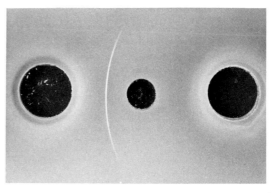

Fig. 6.5 Elek-Ouchterlony technique. The central well contains a solution of antigen. The well on the left contains the corresponding antiserum, and that on the right a negative control serum. A white line of precipitate, composed of antigen–antibody complex, has formed between the antigen and antibody wells. In this instance the antigen is thyroglobulin and the test detects auto-antibody to thyroglobulin in the serum of a patient with chronic thyroiditis.

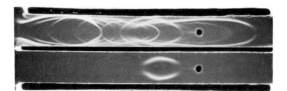

Fig. 6.6 An illustration of the use of immunoelectrophoresis to detect antigens. A mixture of antigens (in this case human serum in the upper well) is subjected to electrophoresis in agar. Antiserum (rabbit antiserum to whole human serum) is then placed in the trough and diffusion allowed to proceed. Each antigen reacts with the corresponding antibody to form an arc of precipitation, the position of which depends on the electrophoretic mobility of the antigen. Use of a single purified antigen (in this case the C3 component of human complement in the lower well) helps to determine whether that antigen is present in the mixture. The upper and middle troughs contain antiserum to whole human serum and the lower trough antiserum to human C3.

react with antigenic constituents of the host cells, death of the target cell may result, e.g. destruction of lymphocytes by anti-lymphocyte serum. There are also rare examples of antibodies which alter the physiological activity of target cells, e.g. increased secretion of thyroxin as a result of the reaction of auto-antibody specific for the TSH-receptor of thyroid epithelium. By binding to the receptor, the antibody has the same effect as TSH.

Antigen–antibody reactions *in vitro*

These may be demonstrated in various ways, depending on the nature of the antigen and the type and amount of antibody present.

1. Visible aggregation of antigen. Since each antibody molecule has at least two combining sites it can bind with two or more antigen molecules. If the antigen molecules contain several antigenic determinants, and if they are in solution, antibody can form cross-linkages between antigen molecules, uniting them in the form of a lattice (Fig. 6.4): if antigen and antibody molecules are present in optimal combining proportions, the aggregates will be large (Fig. 6.4a) and visible as an insoluble precipitate (**precipitin reaction**). Lattice formation and therefore precipitation can be inhibited when an excessive amount of antigen saturates the combining sites on all the antibody molecules, and smaller complexes may then be formed

(Fig. 6.4b). Conversely when gross excess of antibody is present (Fig. 6.4c), each antigen combining site may fix a separate antibody molecule, and, once again, the complexes may be too small to form a visible precipitate (**prozone effect**). Optimum antigen–antibody proportions for lattice formation can readily be achieved by allowing antibody and antigen to diffuse towards each other through agar (Elek-Ouchterlony technique, Fig. 6.5). The interpretation of agar diffusion tests involving antiserum raised against a complex mixture of antigens (as when human serum is injected into rabbits) is facilitated by partial separation of the constituent antigens by electrophoresis prior to the precipitin reaction; this method, called **immunoelectrophoresis**, is illustrated in Fig. 6.6.

When the antigen molecules are associated with a large particle, e.g. the antigenic determinants of the surface of a red cell or bacterium, or are absorbed artificially onto red cells or latex particles, antibody causes aggregation of the particles (**agglutination reaction**). The visible aggregation of large particles such as bacteria can be effected by minute amounts of antibody to their surface antigens.

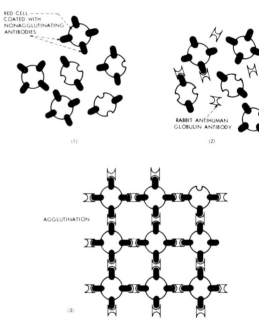

Fig. 6.7 Antigenic particles sensitised with a non-agglutinating antibody are agglutinated by antibody to immunoglobulin (antiglobulin reagent).

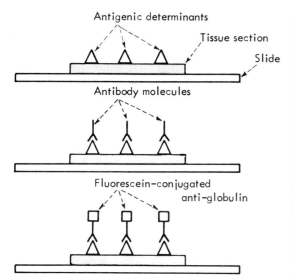

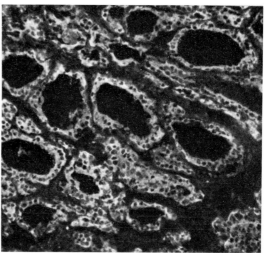

Fig. 6.8 The indirect immunofluorescence technique performed on a tissue section. *Top,* tissue section on slide. *Middle,* section treated with antibody (⅄) to a tissue constituent and washed: antibody molecules adhere to the tissue antigen (△). *Bottom,* section treated with fluorescein-conjugated antibody to immunoglobulin (☐). Sites of antigen–antibody reaction fluoresce in ultraviolet light.

Fig. 6.9 A positive indirect immunofluorescence test for antibody to thyroid epithelium. A frozen section of thyroid tissue has been treated with the serum undergoing test (from a patient with chronic thyroiditis), followed by treatment with fluorescein conjugated anti-human-IgG. Note fluorescence of the thyroid epithelial cytoplasm. (UV microscopy).

2. Methods using anti-immunoglobulin. In certain circumstances, antibody combines with antigen without causing aggregation. This may occur if the spatial arrangement of the antigen (e.g. the rhesus antigen on the surface of red cells) prevents the divalent IgG antibody molecule from combining simultaneously with antigenic determinant groups on two different red cells. In these circumstances, exposure of the rhesus-positive red cells to anti-rhesus antibody merely results in their being coated with IgG. However, the coated cells can be agglutinated by antibody against IgG (**antiglobulin** or **Coombs' reaction**) (Fig. 6.7).

A similar principle is used in the **indirect immunofluorescence (indirect fluorescent antibody) technique** to detect insoluble antigen (e.g. bacterial capsular polysaccharide) in a histological section or smear. When this is exposed to antiserum, the antibody combines with antigen without visible effect. The slide is washed to remove the antiserum, leaving only the specific antibody (which is, of course, an immunoglobulin) attached to the antigen present in the section. Antibody to immunoglobulin, conjugated with a fluorescent dye such as fluorescein iso-thiocynate, is then applied to the section or smear and the site of antigen–antibody combination is visualised by the presence of the fluorescent antiglobulin when the section is examined microscopically with ultra-violet light (Figs. 6.8, 6.9). In the **direct immunofluorescence technique** the tissue or cells are washed to remove free immunoglobulins and treated directly with fluorescein-conjugated antiglobulin reagent. This demonstrates the binding of antibody (or the deposition of antigen-antibody complexes) *in vivo.* Analogous techniques, in which antiglobulin is labelled with an enzyme, e.g. peroxidase or alkaline phosphatase instead of a fluorescent dye, are now used widely in histopathology. The enzyme can be localised by the formation of a coloured deposit after appropriate histochemical treatment, and this is seen within the tissues using ordinary light microscopy (Fig. 26.1, p. 26.2).

3. Methods using radioactive antigen. Radioimmunoassay (RIA), is used to measure the concentration of a solution of antigen: a known amount of the same antigen labelled with a radioactive isotope is added to the solution and a limited amount of the appropriate antibody is then added. The antibody will combine equally with the unlabelled and labelled antigen and the amount of radiolabelled antigen bound is inversely proportional to the concentration

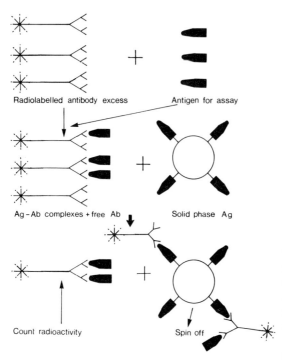

Fig. 6.10 Diagram of the two incubations involved in IRMA. In the first, labelled antibody and soluble antigen combine. In the second, the free antibody remaining after the first incubation becomes bound to antigen present on the solid phase and can thus be separated.

of (unlabelled) antigen originally present in the solution. Free and bound radiolabelled antigen can be separated by various techniques, usually involving precipitation of the antibody. The concentration of antigen in the original solution can then be estimated by measuring the radioactivity of the precipitate.

In the **Farr technique**, which is valuable in measuring antibody to soluble antigen, excess of radiolabelled antigen is added to the test antiserum; the immunoglobulin (including antigen–antibody complexes) is then precipitated by 50% saturation with ammonium sulphate. Provided that the free antigen (uncombined with antibody) is not salted out by this procedure, the amount of radioactivity precipitated is proportional to the amount of antibody in the serum.

In the **antiglobulin co-precipitation technique**, the amount of antibody reacting with a given radioactive antigen can similarly be measured by precipitation with class-specific anti-Ig antibody instead of by a salting out procedure.

4. Methods using radioactive antibody. In **immunoradiometric assay (IRMA),** the concentration of an antigen in solution is measured by addition of excess of the appropriate radiolabelled antibody. Some of the antibody combines with the antigen, while the excess of antibody remains free. Excess of the antigen covalently linked to insoluble material (solid phase antigen) is then added and free antibody binds to it. The solid phase antigen is then removed and the amount of radiolabelled antibody remaining in solution (i.e. bound to the antigen originally present in the solution) is measured, and is proportional to the original antigen concentration (Fig. 6.10).

5. Methods using enzymes. Antigen concentration may be measured by the technique used in radioimmunoassay (see above) but using an enzyme instead of a radioisotope to label the antigen. Calculation of the result depends on measurement of enzymic activity by conversion of a suitable substrate to a coloured product.

In the **enzyme-linked immunosorbent assay (ELISA),** the solution of antigen to be assayed is added to a plastic tube containing antibody bound to its inner surface. A known quantity of enzyme-labelled antigen is then added. The tube is washed out to remove unbound labelled antigen and the amount of bound labelled antigen is determined by adding a suitable substrate for the enzyme. The enzyme activity in the tube is inversely proportional to the concentration of antigen in the test solution.

6. Methods involving damage to cells. Antibody combined with antigen on the surface of intact cells, such as bacteria or erythrocytes, can damage the cell membrane and cause lysis (partial dissolution) of the cells which is readily demonstrable. The lysis is mediated by a complex group of at least twenty factors present in fresh normal serum and known collectively as **complement** (p. 7.2). These factors are activated by the Fc portions of IgM and IgG antibodies which have combined with antigen, and once activated they give rise to a chain of enzyme reactions culminating in digestion of the cell membrane where the antibody is attached. In the course of the reaction, complement is used up or 'fixed'.

7. Complement fixation. Complement is activated or 'fixed' in many antigen–antibody reactions in addition to those involving cell-surface antigens. Invisible antigen–antibody

Mix antigen and antibody	Add complement (C)	Add sensitised RBC
Positive test $Ag^x + Ab^x \longrightarrow Ag^x\!-\!Ab^x$ (union)	$+ C \longrightarrow \begin{matrix} Ag^x\!-\!Ab^x \\ \mid \\ C \end{matrix}$ (complement used up)	No lysis
Negative test $Ag^x + Ab^y \longrightarrow Ag^x + Ab^y$ (no union)	$+ C \longrightarrow Ag^x + Ab^y + C$ (complement not used)	Lysis

Fig. 6.11   The complement fixation reaction depends on the 'fixation' of complement by an antigen–antibody complex (upper line). The fixation of complement is demonstrated by non-lysis of subsequently added red cells coated with a haemolytic antibody. If there is no antigen–antibody reaction (lower line), complement is not used up and lyses the sensitised red cells.

reactions can often be demonstrated indirectly by allowing them to occur in the presence of a measured amount of complement and subsequently adding an indicator system, namely red cells coated with a 'haemolytic' antibody which causes red cell lysis only in the presence of complement. Fixation of complement by the invisible antigen–antibody reaction prevents haemolysis in the indicator system (Fig. 6.11). A more detailed account of complement is given on p. 7.2.

Blocking antibody. In certain circumstances (usually poorly defined), antibody can combine invisibly with antigen which thereby becomes unavailable for participation in a subsequent visible immunological reaction such as agglutination or cytotoxic damage. The presence of blocking antibody in a serum can thus be demonstrated by a two-stage test.

The production of antibody

Injection of an antigen to which an individual has not previously been exposed results in a **primary antibody response**, i.e. the transient appearance in the blood of a small amount of specific antibody, mainly of IgM class, about seven days after the injection. Re-injection of the same antigen at a later date leads to a **secondary** or **anamnestic** (remembering) **response** in which large amounts of specific antibody, most of which is usually of IgG class, appear in the blood rapidly (in four days or so) and continue to be produced, although in gradually diminishing amounts, for weeks, months or even years. The greatly enhanced antibody production of the secondary response

is the reason for the repeated injections of microbial antigens (vaccines) widely used in prophylactic immunisation.

Most of the antibody found in serum is produced by plasma cells in lymph nodes, spleen and bone marrow, but some may also be formed by plasma cells in the lymphoid tissue of the gut and in the inflammatory lesion which forms around injected antigenic material. **Plasma cells** are ovoid, somewhat larger than small lymphocytes, and have a small round nucleus in which granules of chromatin are regularly spaced around the periphery giving a 'cart-wheel' or 'clock-face' appearance. Their

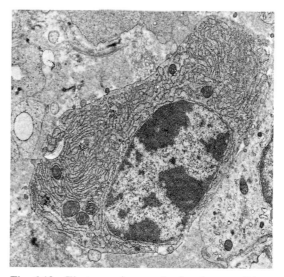

Fig. 6.12   Electron micrograph of a plasma cell in a lymph node, showing the eccentrically placed nucleus with the peripheral chromatin condensation and abundant rough endoplasmic reticulum in which immunoglobulin is being synthesised. × 1300.

cytoplasm contains a large amount of rough endoplasmic reticulum, a characteristic of cells which synthesise and secrete protein (Fig. 6.12). The ribonucleic acid associated with this endoplasmic reticulum gives the cells their characteristic basophilic and pyroninophilic staining reactions (Fig. 4.28, p. 4.31). It has been shown by immunofluorescence that each plasma cell at any given time produces light chains together with heavy chains of only one immunoglobulin class (e.g. IgG or IgM). Furthermore, *following stimulation with two distinct antigens (e.g. diphtheria and tetanus toxins) individual plasma cells will produce antibody to one or the other but not to both of these antigens.*

An additional polypeptide, **the J chain**, is synthesised by plasma cells producing IgM and IgA. It links together the basic 4-chain units of IgM and IgA to form polymers (p. 6.8).

Plasma cells are end-stage cells and are derived from antigen-stimulated differentiation of a subpopulation of lymphocytes concerned with humoral immunity. As noted earlier, these are the lymphocytes of the bursa-dependent lineage (B lymphocytes).

The origin of B lymphocytes

In birds, the *bursa of Fabricius*, like the thymus, develops as an epithelial organ and is invaded in embryonic life by haemopoietic stem cells which proliferate and differentiate into lymphocytes: these, in turn, enter the blood and help to populate the lymph nodes, spleen, etc. They constitute a major population of lymphocytes, termed **B lymphocytes** (B for bursa-dependent), and bursectomy of the embryo results in failure to develop B lymphocytes. Such birds develop T cells normally, and can make cell-mediated immune responses, but they lack plasma cells and cannot make antibodies; accordingly, the plasma is devoid of immunoglobulins ('agammaglobulinaemia').

The haemopoietic marrow of mammals contains large numbers of lymphocytes which are rapidly labelled by ^{3}H-thymidine, i.e. they are an actively dividing population, and the labelled immature cells mature into B lymphocytes, some of which can subsequently be detected in the lymph nodes, spleen, etc. *Haemopoietic tissue is thus a site of production of B*

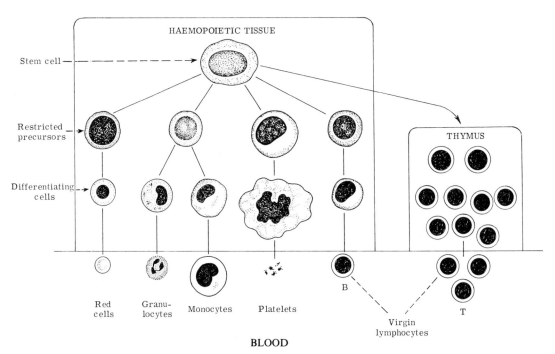

Fig. 6.13 In addition to differentiating into restricted precursors of red cells, granulocytes, monocytes and platelets, the haemopoietic stem cell differentiates into pre-B cells which undergo B-lymphopoiesis (in mammals within the haemopoietic tissue) and provide virgin B lymphocytes. Some stem cells pass into the blood and settle in the thymus, where they rise to virgin T lymphocytes.

lymphocytes from stem cells (Fig. 6.13), *but it is not known whether it is the only site.*

Stem cells entering the haemopoetic tissues are probably committed at least to haemopoietic differentiation (see Fig. 6.13). However those cells destined to become B lymphocytes quickly show evidence of B cell differentiation. This can be demonstrated by the appearance in the cytoplasm of μ heavy chains ($C\mu^+$ cells). Light chains are absent, so that complete antibodies are not formed at this stage and immunoglobulins cannot be detected on the cell surface (SIg^-). These are termed **pre-B cells.** Light chain synthesis and the formation of whole antibody in the cytoplasm occurs later, followed by the expression of immunoglobulin on the cell surface. The immunoglobulin initially expressed is monomeric IgM although this is followed by the synthesis and surface expression of both monomeric IgM and IgD. These $SIgM^+$ $SIgD^+$ B lymphocytes are the **virgin B cells** and are capable of responding to antigenic stimulation.

How B lymphocytes develop specific responsiveness and diversity

Much of the ontogeny of the B lymphocyte is now understood at the genetic level. During differentiation, these lymphocytes become committed to the B cell lineage, synthesise only one type of light chain (*either* κ or λ), and acquire their antigen-specific responsiveness. Since the specificity of antibody depends on the sequence of amino acids in the variable regions of the polypeptide chains, it is a reflection of the sequences of the bases in the DNA of the genes coding for immunoglobulin synthesis. Commitment of the lymphocyte thus implies that it becomes restricted to coding for only one particular sequence for the variable regions of the heavy chain and one sequence for the variable regions of the light chain. Since all the B cells of a proliferating clone are committed to produce the same antibody, commitment must be heritable and irreversible through many cell generations. But individual lymphocytes become specifically committed to produce *different* antibodies, thus providing the great diversity of the antibody response.

We must therefore conclude that either (a) the genome of the individual contains large numbers of alternative genes for the variable

parts of the Ig chains (**V genes**), and that commitment involves the restriction to coding for one light and on heavy chain V gene, (the **germ line theory**) or (b) the genome of the individual contains relatively few V genes, and different sequences of bases develop by **somatic mutation** during early lymphopoiesis (Jerne, 1971). It has not been established with certainty which of these two theories of diversity is the correct one, but present evidence suggests that both mechanisms contribute to antibody diversity: there are a large number of V genes in the genome, but this number is further amplified by somatic mutation.

It is known that each Ig chain is synthesised as a single unit, by translation of messenger RNA carrying the code for the constant and variable regions of the whole chain. It is now believed that the gene selection responsible for lymphocytic commitment and diversity is brought about by the mechanism illustrated for heavy chain synthesis in Fig. 6.14. During sequence analysis experiments on the heavy chain region of the genome, it was found that the V_H genes stopped short of coding for the entire variable region. **Joining (J) segments** (also present in light chain genes) were identified near the genes coding for the constant region of immunoglobulins. Each of four separate J genes codes for a short segment of the polypeptide adjacent to the constant region of Ig heavy chains. The entire amino-acid sequence of the variable regions is still not coded by the V_H and J genes. A missing segment of the polypeptide sequence was found to be encoded by a further group of genes, each of which can combine at random with one V_H gene thus increasing the diversity of the immunoglobulin repertoire. These genes, present on the genome between the V_H and J genes, were therefore designated the **diversity (D) genes.**

In the embryonic germ-line form, heavy chain genes exist as discontinuous segments coding for variable (V_H), diversity (D) and joining (J) regions and for the constant region (C_H) of different classes of Ig, i.e. $C\mu$, $C\gamma$, $C\alpha$, etc. Between these genes there are long stretches of DNA which do not code for any known proteins. Differentiation involves rearrangement of this germ-line form. Probably by the formation and excision of loops of DNA, a single V_H gene is brought into continuity with

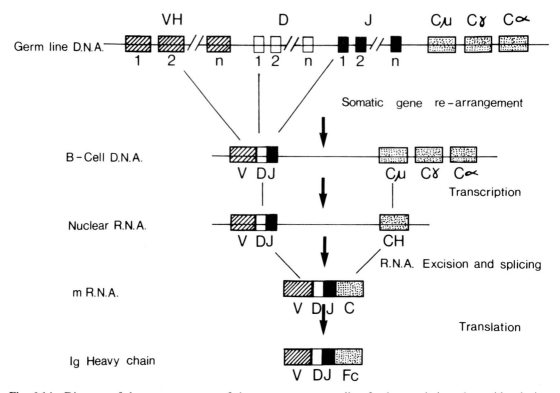

Fig. 6.14 Diagram of the rearrangement of the gene segments coding for heavy chain polypeptides during B cell maturation. Variable (V), diversity (D), and joining (J) segments recombine at the DNA level during differentiation. VDJ_H-C_H recombination occurs by processing of the original transcription form of mRNA.

one D gene and one J gene to form the continuous VDJ_H DNA configuration found in the differentiated B cell. A similar mechanism of somatic gene re-arrangement brings a single V_L gene in apposition to a J_L gene to complete the VJ_L DNA configuration of the light chain variable region genes found in B cells. *Following these events, the individual B cell has a heritable commitment to the production of antibody of a specificity defined by its selected V, D and J genes.* In the mouse κ chains there are approximately 1000 V_L gene segments and 10 'J' segments, giving a repertoire of 10^4 amino-acid sequences. The specificity of antibody depends on the variable regions of light and heavy chains, and if we assume a similar variability (10^4) for the mouse heavy chain, this gives a total repertoire of 10^8 different antibodies, which agrees fairly closely with most estimates based on analysis of the antibodies which develop in response to one particular antigenic determinant. (see Williamson, 1979).

This somatic re-arrangement of genes not only results in the committment of individual B lymphocytes to the production of a specific antibody but also generates the antibody diversity of the repertoire of the B-cell population.

The synthesis of the heavy chain of immunoglobulins incorporating these re-arranged V sequences (VDJ_H) and the appropriate constant region ($C\mu$, etc.) results from translation of one continuous strand of mRNA. Similarly the variable sequences (VJ_L) and constant regions of the light chains are transcribed into a single mRNA strand. In the B-cell genome, however, a long stretch of DNA (termed an *intron*) separates the variable and constant genes and the corresponding sequence in mRNA is excised, leaving the sequences which are translated into the polypeptide chains (Fig. 6.14).

It is now widely accepted that commitment of B lymphocytes occurs spontaneously, probably during lymphopoiesis in the sheltered environment of the haemopoietic tissue, and is not dependent on encounter with an antigen.

The response of B lymphocytes to antigenic stimulation

Both virgin and memory B lymphocytes respond to antigenic stimulation. The primary response does not produce very much antibody, presumably because it depends entirely on virgin lymphocytes, relatively few of which are capable of responding to any particular antigen. The primary response does, however, provide memory cells, and these account for the much greater amount of antibody produced in the secondary response.

The antigen stimulates all those B lymphocytes whose specific surface receptors can bind it sufficiently firmly and each of these cells gives rise to a clone of plasma cells producing its own distinctive antibody molecules. The result is a mixture of diverse antibodies, some of which can bind the antigen more firmly than others, but the total effect of which is exquisite specificity. If the antigen is administered repeatedly in small doses, it is taken up mainly by those lymphocytes which can bind it most firmly and as these proliferate the result predicted would be a progressive increase in the avidity (p. 6.7) of the antibody, which is indeed what happens.

The use of anti-idiotypic antibodies (see p. 6.28) has shown that the expanded clone retains the idiotype of the initial responding cells and, since idiotype is determined by the amino-acid sequence of the variable regions of immunoglobulin, the genetic re-arrangement of the variable region genes for heavy (VDJ_H) and light (VJ_L) chains must be inherited by the daughter cells of the clone. The somatic gene re-arrangement of the immunoglobulin genes must therefore be inherited during clonal expansion.

Heavy chain switching. During the immune response to many antigens, a change occurs in the heavy chain isotype of the secreted antibody. Early in the immune response, IgM predominates: later, however, IgG and IgA antibodies appear. The plasma cells secreting these later antibodies are probably derived from clones which originally had surface IgM as antigen receptor. This heavy chain 'switch' in immunoglobulin synthesis is achieved by the formation and excision of a loop of DNA (similar to that observed in V gene re-arrangements) bringing VDJ_H gene complex in proximity to $C\gamma$ or $C\alpha$ etc. with the loss of the intervening C_H genes. The synthesis of this immunoglobulin polypeptide still requires splicing of mRNA because of intervening sequences of non-translated DNA.

Monoclonal antibodies

Because the specificity of antibody is retained during clonal proliferation, the antibody produced by a clone is homogeneous or 'monoclonal'. It is now possible, by means of cell-fusion techniques, to maintain continuously proliferating ('immortal') clones of antibody-producing 'hybridoma' cells (Kohler and Milstein, 1975). A laboratory animal (usually a mouse or rat of an inbred strain) is immunised with the antigen to which antibody is required. After allowing time for the development of an antibody response, a cell suspension is prepared from the spleen and these 'immune' cells are mixed with cultured cells of a plasma-cell tumour (myeloma) from an animal of the same species. An agent which promotes cell fusion (e.g. polyethylene glycol) is added and hybrid cells, formed by fusion of a spleen cell with a myeloma cell, are cultured individually. The cultures are tested for antibody and those suitable are grown continuously in culture or injected into the peritoneal cavity of mice (or rats), the peritoneal fluid being harvested for antibody. The technique depends on the hybrid cell inheriting the capacity of the spleen cell to produce antibody of the specificity desired and the proliferative capacity of the myeloma cell.

Monoclonal antibody reacts specifically with one particular epitope on the antigen. It does not form precipitates with the antigen unless the latter contains numerous copies of the epitope, and it reacts, often unexpectedly, with other antigens containing a similar epitope. Monoclonal antibodies are nevertheless proving to be extremely useful reagents in immunoassays and identification of particular types of normal and abnormal cells in histological sections and cell suspensions. Their preparation also has the advantage that the original antigen need not be purified.

Cellular response to antigen stimulation

Antigenic stimulation induces proliferation and further differentiation of virgin and memory B lymphocytes. The responding cells enlarge to become 'blast' cells (Fig. 6.15) with an increase

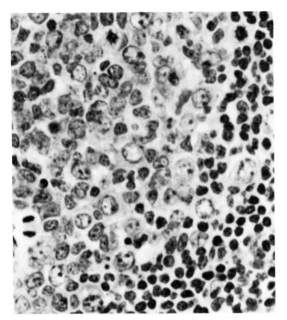

Fig. 6.15 Segment of a germinal centre showing proliferating B 'blast' cells with large pale nuclei and abundant cytoplasm. The centre is surrounded by tightly packed small lymphocytes. × 850.

in both DNA and RNA, the latter giving the cytoplasm its basophilic staining properties. Successive divisions produce large numbers of daughter cells which can differentiate in two ways. Some differentiate into plasmablasts, acquiring rough endoplasmic reticulum and eventually a Golgi apparatus to become the mature plasma cells synthesising and secreting large amounts of a single antibody. Other cells differentiate into B memory cells and join the recirculating pool of lymphocytes: upon subsequent encounter with the appropriate antigen this expanded population provides the more vigorous secondary immune response. The factors which determine the pathway of differentiation of individual lymphocytes are obscure but may depend on the density of antigenic and helper signals or upon other factors in the micro-environment in which the response occurs, for the two cell types—plasma cell and memory cell—seem to differentiate in anatomically different lymphoid sites (see p. 6.35).

How B lymphocytes recognise antigens

To respond to an antigen, a lymphocyte must have surface receptors capable of recognising antigen to which the cell can respond, and union of antigen with surface receptors must stimulate the response. In fact, when lymphocytes from a normal individual are incubated with an antigen which has been labelled, for example with ^{131}I or fluorescein, the labelled antigen can be demonstrated to bind to the surface of very small proportions of both T and B lymphocytes. If the donor has previously encountered that antigen, the number of antigen-binding lymphocytes is increased, but is still only a very small proportion of the total.

The B lymphocyte has surface molecules of immunoglobulin (SIg), which float in the lipid of the cell membrane with the Fab end of the molecules projecting from it. These act as the specific antigen receptors on B cells. Some of the evidence for this is summarised below.

Firstly, treatment of B lymphocytes with an anti-immunoglobulin (anti-Ig) inhibits antigen binding.

Secondly, evidence has been provided by the 'capping' phenomenon. When B lymphocytes are treated with a labelled antigen, the SIg molecules of those

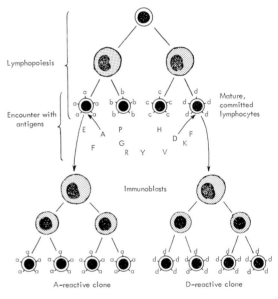

Fig. 6.16 The clonal selection theory of immune response. During lymphopoiesis, each developing T or B cell becomes committed to respond to a narrow range of antigenic determinants: this is reflected by the specificity of the antigen receptors (a, b, c, etc.) on its surface. For example, lymphocytes with hypothetical 'a' receptors can bind an antigen 'A', but not 'D' or 'E', etc. Binding of an antigen stimulates a lymphocyte to proliferate, producing a clone of lymphocytes with identical commitment.

cells which bind the antigen become aggregated into clumps and finally in a single mass or 'cap' at one part of the surface: the effect is the same as that induced by treating B cells with anti-immunoglobulin (Fig. 6.26, p. 6.33). When capping is induced by antigen, the cap can be shown to contain *all* the antigen bound to the cell surface and *all* the SIg molecules, thus demonstrating that all the SIg molecules react with the antigen.

The significance of antigen binding by the surface Ig of B cells. *Those B cells which can bind a particular antigen are responsible for the antibody response to that antigen.* This has been demonstrated by passing lymphocytes through a column of inert material coated with antigen. The cells which bind the antigen are retained and are thus separated from non-binding lymphocytes. The separated cells may be tested for antibody response either *in vitro* or by administering them to an animal whose own lymphocytes have been destroyed (e.g. by x-irradiation) and then

challenging the animal with the same and other antigens. Such experiments have shown that the antigen-binding cells can mount an antibody response to the same antigen. The non-antigen-binding population does not respond to the same antigen, but responds normally to other antigens. These findings suggest that the SIg molecules of B lymphocytes represent a sample of the specific antibody which that cell and its descendants can synthesise and secrete.

Thus antigen has, by binding to surface antibody, 'selected' that population of B cells capable of responding to it and initiated the expansion of the appropriate lymphoid-cell clones. This is the molecular basis of the clonal selection theory (Fig. 6.16) of Jerne (1955) and Burnet (1959). The theory was first proposed in 1908 by Paul Ehrlich who suggested that toxins combine with antitoxin side chains on the cell surface, that the complexes were neutralised, and that the production of additional similar side chains was thus stimulated.

Cell Mediated Immunity

The origin of T lymphocytes: The Thymus

Development. The thymus develops from bilateral epithelial ingrowths of the endoderm of the 3rd and 4th branchial arches accompanied by mesenchyme which is probably of ectodermal origin. In most mammals, these ingrowths fuse to form a single organ. Meanwhile some of the stem cells which develop in the haemopoietic tissue migrate into the blood and settle in the thymus, where they proliferate rapidly and differentiate into lymphocytes. The thymus now appears as a lobulated organ (Fig. 6.17) in which the outer or cortical layer is crowded with proliferating lymphocytes lying in a network of epithelial cells. In the inner or medullary layer, lymphopoiesis is less active and there are aggregates of epithelial cells (Hassall's corpuscles).

Function. Until quite recently the thymus was an organ of mystery. Unlike the other lymphoid tissues (lymph nodes, spleen, tonsils, etc.) it is not a site of significant immune responses following exposure to antigen, and the proliferation of lymphocytes in the thymic cortex, which is maximal around the time of birth but continues throughout life, is quite independent of antigenic challenge. This suggested that the thymus supplies lymphocytes, but many lympho-

cytes produced in the cortex die *in situ*, their nuclear debris being conspicuous in macrophages, and export of thymic lymphocytes remained no more than a likely possibility. Nor did early studies of thymectomy elucidate thymic function, for no important immunological effects were observed.

The important clue to thymic function came from the observation by Good and his co-workers (1964) and others that congenital immunological deficiency states in man were sometimes associated with thymic abnormalities. Miller (1964) then demonstrated that mice thymectomised *at birth* failed to thrive and commonly died of a wasting disease since shown to be due mainly to infections. The thymectomised mice were shown to be defective in cell-mediated immune responses and in their antibody responses to some antigens. They were also deficient in lymphocytes in the blood, thoracic duct lymph, and parts of the lymph nodes, spleen tonsils, etc. These deficiencies were soon shown to be prevented, or completely and permanently corrected, by a syngeneic thymus graft, while lymph node or spleen cells from normal mice were partially restorative. Similar deficiencies occur spontaneously in an inbred strain (*nu nu*) of mice with thymic aplasia.

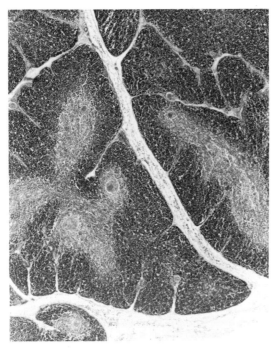

Fig. 6.17   Thymus in childhood, showing lobulation and division into cortex (darker areas) and medulla. × 30.

It thus appears that, in mice, the presence of the thymus is necessary for the development of a major population of lymphocytes which are responsible for cell-mediated immune responses and which also influence antibody production. By preparation and use of suitable antisera, mouse thymocytes have been shown to exhibit various surface antigens, some of which (e.g. θ or Thy-1 antigens) are shared by many of the lymphocytes in the blood, lymph and other lymphoid tissues. It is these lymphocytes with 'thymic markers' which fail to develop following neonatal thymectomy and in *nu nu* mice; accordingly they are termed the **thymus dependent** or **T Lymphocytes**, and mice lacking them are sometimes termed '*B*' mice.

The same immunological and T-cell deficiencies as occur in mice have been shown to follow neonatal thymectomy in several other species, and can be prevented or corrected by thymus grafts. In man, the T lymphocyte population develops long before birth, but congenital failure of thymic development (p. 7.34) is associated with the same features as neonatal thymectomy in mice.

It has also been demonstrated in a number of species that, in conditions much closer to the physio-logical state than in the experiments described above, the thymus supplies lymphocytes to the other lymphoid tissues. This was done by injecting ³H-thymidine into the thymus, so that it became incorporated in the nuclei of dividing thymocytes: labelled lymphocytes were subsequently detected by auto-radiography in the other lymphoid tissues.

Thymus function in the adult. As the thymus slowly involutes following puberty, its lymphopoietic activity diminishes but does not cease entirely, even in old age. The diminishing importance of the thymus is illustrated by performing thymectomy in mice after the neonatal period: the longer it is delayed, the less its effect. This is clearly because the thymus provides much of the T-lymphocyte population shortly after birth. Even in adult mice, however, thymectomy has some effect, for a year or more later the mice show deficient cell-mediated immunity as illustrated by reduced capacity to reject a skin allograft. Similarly in man, thymectomy in young adults (performed therapeutically in patients with myasthenia gravis) has no immediate immunological effect, but defective cell-mediated immunity and a diminution in T lymphocytes in the blood has been reported in patients examined 15 or more years later.

In spite of its involuted state in the adult, the thymus remains capable of replacing the whole T-lymphocyte pool. This is demonstrated by subjecting mice to a dose of x-irradiation which destroys virtually all the body's lymphocytes and haemopoietic stem cells, and administering bone marrow cells to restore the haemopoietic tissue. Regeneration of the T lymphocytes (from haemopoietic stem cells) is dependent on the presence of the thymus and is prevented by concomitant thymectomy.

The thymus thus produces and exports T lymphocytes (Fig. 6.18). This occurs maximally during fetal life or shortly after birth (depending on species). Thymectomy before production of the T-lymphocyte population results in a virtual absence of T cells and consequent severe immunological deficiencies. The thymus continues to supply T lymphocytes after birth but this function becomes progressively less important with age, the T-lymphocyte population, which includes much of the individual's immunological experience stored in memory cells, becoming increasingly self-sufficient.

Thymic lymphopoietic hormone. There is evidence that the thymus produces hormones which stimulate differentiation and proliferation of T lymphocytes. This was first suspected when implantation of thymic tissue enclosed in cell-proof diffusion chambers was found to restore partially the T-lymphocyte population of neonatally thymectomised mice. Subsequently, extracts of thymic tissue have been shown to have a similar effect, and similar activity has been detected in normal human and mouse plasma, but is absent following thymectomy. According to Bach, *et al.* (1975), the plasma activity in man decreases with age, an observation which accords well with the normal process of thymic involution. It thus seems likely that production of T lymphocytes in the thymus is stimulated by the local effect of thymic hormone.

Although administration of thymus extract has some influence on differentiation of T lymphocytes in the thymectomised animal, there is no strong evidence that production of mature T lymphocytes from stem cells can occur without the thymus.

From electron-microscopic and other observations, the thymic epithelium seems the most likely source of these hormones.

The development of monoclonal antibodies and their use as cell markers by binding to surface antigen on lymphocytes has offered the opportunity to analyse T cell ontogeny in more detail. The most fully studied series of markers are the T1, T2 etc. markers described by Reinherz *et al.* (1979). The pathways of T lymphocyte differentiation within this system are shown in Fig. 6.18. Thus markers such as T9 identify primitive T lymphocytes which lose these antigens during differentiation and acquire mature cell markers such as T3. It is also possible to identify, by these antigens, subpopulations of T lymphocytes which are functionally distinct, e.g. T4+ cells which have 'helper' activity and T8+ cells which have

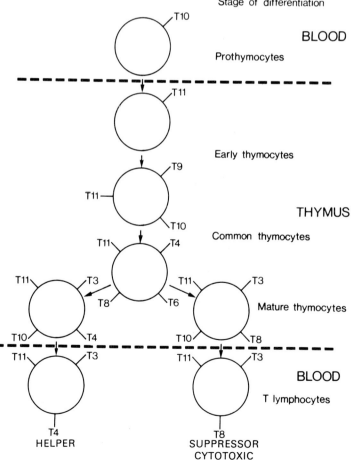

Stage of differentiation

BLOOD

Prothymocytes

Early thymocytes

THYMUS

Common thymocytes

Mature thymocytes

BLOOD

T lymphocytes

T4
HELPER

T8
SUPPRESSOR
CYTOTOXIC

Fig. 6.18 A model of T-cell development defined by monoclonal antibodies. T lymphocytes at different stages of development can be shown to express, on their cell surface, a series of antigens detected by monoclonal antibodies. A pre-thymic, three intrathymic and a post-thymic stage of T cell differentiation can be defined by the monoclonal antibodies. The mature T cells include helper cells (T4 +ve) and suppressor and cytotoxic T cells (both T8 +ve). (Modified from Reinherz *et al.*, 1979.)

suppressor or cytotoxic functions (p. 7.20). It is also apparent that these two separate sub-populations develop at a late stage of differentiation in the thymic medulla.

It is now known that some of these marker antigens are of functional importance in cell recognition during the induction of the T-lymphocyte immune response (see below).

The lymphocytes which leave the thymus have been shown to be mature, functional T cells which are capable of responding appropriately to antigen.

The response of T cells to antigenic stimulation

Antigenic stimulation induces proliferation of responsive T lymphocytes: the proliferating cells (like responding B cells) become enlarged and acquire abundant basophilic (RNA-rich) cytoplasm (Fig. 6.19): they are termed **T 'blast' cells** or **T immunoblasts**. They pass through a succession of divisions during which they differentiate into small T lymphocytes capable of binding the antigen which has induced their production.

Like B lymphocytes, T lymphocytes become committed to respond to a narrow range of antigenic stimuli, and this occurs without antigenic stimulation, probably during lymphocytic maturation in the thymus. Another similarity is that the T lymphocyte recognises antigens by means of surface receptors, but the nature of these is uncertain. In addition, T lymphocytes are capable of responding in large numbers to the 'histocompatibility' alloantigens (in man the HLA antigens—p. 2.12) present on the surface of most cells. This occurs when cells or tissues are transferred from one individual to another and is the major obstacle to transplantation of many types of tissue.

Recent work has shown that T lymphocytes only recognise antigen when it is presented to them in association with self-histocompatibility antigens, e.g. on the surface of viral-infected cells. In an elegant series of experiments, Zinkernagel and Doherty (1979) reconstituted the T lymphocyte population of irradiated mice with cells which were not identical at the major histocompatibility complex and showed that

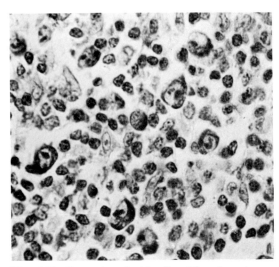

Fig. 6.19 Large lymphoid cells with enlarged nucleus and pyroninophilic cytoplasm (*immunoblasts*) in a human lymph node removed 6 days after a skin allograft. Methyl green pyronin stain. ×480. (Professor D.M.V. Parrot and Dr. M.A.B. de Sousa.)

the recognition of viral antigens by cytotoxic effector T cells (p. 6.23) of donor origin only occurs when both the donor cell population and the viral-infected host cells share common class 1 antigens of the major histocompatibility system. Similar experiments have shown that helper T cells probably recognise antigen only when present on cells with identical Ia antigens (DR antigens in man).

Clearly, the T lymphocytes must in some way recognise both the specific antigen to which they are responding and also the major histocompatibility antigens. This need for dual specificity has obscured further the difficult field of investigation of the nature of the T-cell antigen receptor.

T-cell antigen receptor. The extent and nature of the antigenic repertoire of T cells seems to be similar to those of B cells, but T cells have not been shown to contain measurable cytoplasmic or surface immunoglobulin nor to synthesise these molecules (although they can bind serum IgG or monomeric IgM to their surface by means of receptors specific for the Fc portions of these molecules). The possibility that the T cell antigen receptor may be related to immunoglobulins is, however, supported by the following observations.

By administering to inbred mice or rats a simple antigen which, in these animals, stimulates only a few T and B lymphocytes to clonal proliferation, it has been possible to isolate antibody of a particular idiotype (p. 6.28) and to prepare an anti-idiotype antibody. In such experiments, it has been shown that the anti-idiotype antibody reacts with the receptors of both T- and B-cell clones, which suggests strongly that they are identical, and since the B-cell receptors are known to be the variable ends of Ig molecules, it seems likely that the T-cell receptors are also of this nature. Recently, the human T-cell antigen receptor has been shown to be composed of two different polypeptide chains associated with the T3 surface antigen (see p. 6.21). Analysis of the primary structure of these proteins and of the mRNA sequences coding for them has shown extensive similarities with the variable, joining and constant regions of mouse and human Ig λ chains. The mouse T-cell antigen receptor also shows similarities with mouse κ and λ light chains and parts of human heavy chains. There is extensive polymorphism of these antigen-receptor genes in different T cell clones, at points corresponding to the positions which show variability in the immunoglobulin V genes variable regions—pp. 6.15–16).

It seems very likely that the T-lymphocyte antigen-receptor genes are coded for by a family of genes closely related to the immunoglobulin V genes and that the nature and function of the receptor on the cell membrane are similar to those of B-cell surface Ig receptors.

The nature of the T cell immune response

The T lymphocytes are responsible for the types of responses referred to as cell-mediated immunity (CMI). When antigen-responsive T lymphocytes encounter the appropriate antigen, they enlarge, undergo mitosis and stimulate mitosis in other lymphocytes. They also release biologically active compounds termed **lymphokines** (p. 7.21), one of which causes an acute inflammatory reaction, another immobilises macrophages, others induce the production of certain proteolytic enzymes by macrophages and some regulate lymphocyte proliferation. The exact number of lymphokines is unknown and several different biological effects may be mediated by one substance.

Tests for CMI are based on, and illustrate, these T cell responses. It is demonstrated most readily **in vivo** by intradermal injection of the antigen, which leads to an indurated erythematous lesion in the dermis, maximal in 24–72 hours—the **delayed hypersensitivity reaction.** During the development of the lesion, there is early but transient emigration of polymorphs,

followed by an increasing accumulation of lymphocytes and some macrophages around venules, hair follicles and sweat glands: this is accompanied by inflammatory hyperaemia and oedema (Fig. 7.8, p. 7.19).

A classical example of CMI is that which develops to tuberculoprotein in most individuals who are (or have been) infected with *Mycobacterium tuberculosis* or following inoculation with BCG (an attenuated strain of *Mycobacterium bovis*). The Mantoux test (p. 7.18), in which more or less purified tuberculoprotein is injected intradermally, is a classical delayed hypersensitivity reaction.

Skin tests with appropriate antigens may be used similarly to test for CMI to various other micro-organisms, including viruses and fungi. They are also useful to elicit CMI to certain simple chemicals which, when applied to the skin, act as haptens and, by combining with skin proteins, become immunogenic: examples include *p*-phenylene diamine (in some hair dyes) and nickel salts (derived from nickel clasps on underwear, etc.): once CMI has developed, application of the chemical to the skin results in an inflammatory lesion known as *contact dermatitis*, which is simply a delayed hypersensitivity reaction (p. 7.23).

CMI is also important, and can be demonstrated, during the rejection of tissue allografts: indeed graft rejection has been widely used in experimental animals as a model for CMI.

The cell-mediated killing of viral-infected cells (and transplanted cells expressing foreign antigens) is dependent on an intact T-lymphocyte system. **Cytotoxic T lymphocytes** specific for viral antigens develop after stimulation by viral infection, and are capable of destroying host cells which have become infected by the virus. T-cell killing of target cells depends on the recognition of foreign antigen and of autologous HLA antigens (p. 2.12) on the target cell membranes, on close cell-cell interactions and on a cytotoxic property as yet poorly understood. Having destroyed one target cell, the cytotoxic T cell is then free to move on and attack others.

It should be noted that the demonstration of CMI *in vivo* is by eliciting a delayed hypersensitivity reaction which is a destructive inflammatory lesion and may, if severe, progress to necrosis. Delayed hypersensitivity reactions occur naturally, e.g. in various infections and in contact dermatitis, and are responsible for most of the tissue injury in tuberculosis. CMI does, however, afford protection against various micro-organisms, notably viruses, fungi and many of the bacteria which cause chronic infections. This is well illustrated by children with congenital agammaglobulinaemia who cannot produce antibodies and yet can overcome some viral infections normally unless they are also deficient in CMI.

Recent knowledge has shown that T lymphocyte responses are much more complex. With the discovery of helper and suppressor populations of T lymphocytes and the elucidation of the role of T lymphocytes in most antibody responses, it has become apparent that T lymphocytes are involved in extensive cell-cell co-operations during the development and regulation of the immune response (see below).

In-vitro tests for CMI involve the addition of the antigen to a mixed culture of lymphocytes and monocytes from the test subject. The cells may be examined for morphological evidence of **transformation** to blast cells (p. 6.22) or ³H-thymidine may be added and its incorporation into newly-synthesised DNA assayed. An alternative method is the **macrophage migration inhibition test** in which an open-ended capillary tube containing leucocytes from the test subject is placed horizontally in a culture chamber and the migration of the leucocytes onto the floor of the chamber observed. In a positive test, addition of the antigen to the culture medium inhibits the migration of the leucocytes from the tube, a result of the secretion of macrophage immobilising factor (see above).

Transfer factor

Since 1948, Lawrence has reported investigations which suggest that cell-free extracts of human leucocytes can transfer cell-mediated immunity to non-immunised recipients, and that the responsible agent, transfer factor, has a molecular weight of about 3000 (see Lawrence, 1969). Attempts to demonstrate transfer factor in experimental animals have mostly been disappointing, but it must be appreciated that, in general, man and other primates show much stronger cell-mediated immune responses and delayed hypersensitivity reactions than do lower animals.

A number of reports have appeared on the therapeutic use of transfer factor in the treatment of patients with resistant infections due to immunodeficiencies, and with various diseases of obscure causation (e.g. sarcoidosis, connective tissue diseases and tumours). The degree of success achieved has varied greatly, and it is difficult to draw conclusions. The existence of human transfer factor which enhances immune responses is no longer in doubt, although its mode of action is obscure and its antigen-specificity has not been widely accepted.

Cell co-operation in the immune response

Although we have so far discussed the B and T lymphocyte systems separately, it is now known that there is extensive co-operation between them during the immune response.

T-dependent and T-independent antibody responses. Animals deficient in T cells (e.g. 'B' mice, p. 6.20) are unable to mount antibody responses to many antigens, including foreign proteins. B cells require the co-operation of T cells to produce antibodies to such antigens, which accordingly are called **thymus-dependent antigens**. Some antigens, however, do stimulate 'B' mice to antibody production: these so-called **thymus-independent antigens** are usually of very high molecular weight, with large numbers of one or more particular antigenic determinants (epitopes) e.g. bacterial lipopolysaccharide, pneumococcal capsular polysaccharide or artificially prepared polymers. It appears that, by binding to, and so linking up, large numbers of the surface Ig receptors on a B cell, such antigens can provide the necessary stimulus for clonal proliferation and antibody production (Fig. 6.20). By contrast, smaller molecules, or globular proteins which display a variety of epitopes without a high concentration of any one epitope, would be expected to bind less strongly to B cells and to occupy fewer surface receptor sites: this may be why they cannot stimulate an antibody response without the help of T cells.

The helper function of T cells in antibody responses has been elucidated by complexing a hapten (e.g. dinitrophenyl) to a foreign carrier protein. Using this system, Mitchison (1971) and others showed that an antibody response to the hapten is dependent on the development of cell-mediated immunity to the carrier protein. It seems likely that the binding of molecules of the protein to primed T lympho-

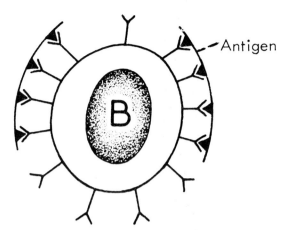

Fig. 6.20 T-independent antibody response induced by an antigen with large numbers of a particular type of antigenic determinant (epitope) which effectively link the surface Ig antigen receptors of an appropriate B cell and stimulates it to respond.

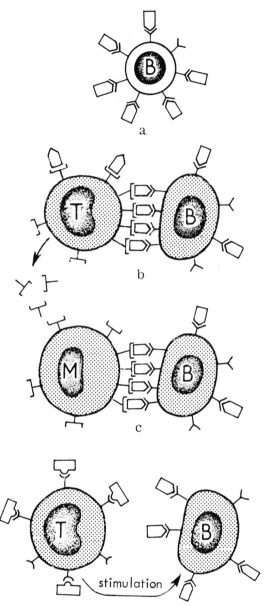

cytes renders the hapten-protein complex immunogenic to B cells, perhaps by presenting the hapten to B cells in such a way that it effectively links together the B cell receptors (Fig. 6.21b). Alternatively, it could be that the T cell binding the protein carrier transmits an additional stimulatory signal to the B cell binding the hapten. Some evidence for this 'second signal' hypothesis is provided by the demonstration that T cells binding and responding to a quite separate antigen (or to mitogens—p. 6.32) can be of some help to the B cell in its response

---

Fig. 6.21 Possible mechanisms of co-operation of T cells in antibody production by B cells. In (**a**), a B lymphocyte has bound an antigen by a particular type of determinant, but is not stimulated by it because it has not cross-linked the specific antigen receptors. If a T cell also binds the same antigen by a different determinant, as in (**b**), it may effectively cross-link the B-lymphocyte receptors and thus stimulate it (indicated here by 'blast' transformation of the B cell). Alternately the T-cell antigen receptors may be transferred to macrophages (**c**) which then become capable of co-operating in B-cell stimulation. Lastly, a T cell which has bound an independent antigen, as in (**d**), can also provide a stimulus to the B lymphocyte. In all these forms of co-operation, the stimulating T cell has itself been stimulated to 'blast' transformation, and indeed the last form of co-operation can be provided by a T cell which has been stimulated non-specifically, e.g. by phytohaemagglutinin.

(Fig. 6.21d). It is also possible that the T cell responding to the protein carrier transfers receptor sites to macrophages, and thus confers on them specific helper capacity (Fig. 6.21c).

Whatever the mechanism of T-cell co-operation in antibody production, it has been shown to be a property of memory T cells and, as indicated above, can be antigen-specific or non-specific. Specific T-cell co-operation is essential for optimal primary and secondary antibody responses to most protein antigens, and even those immune responses which can occur without T-cell help are usually limited mainly to production of antibodies of IgM class. The co-operation of T cells appears to be necessary for the production of large amounts of IgG antibody, as in the secondary response. Indeed, there is evidence that the formation of B memory lymphocytes is less dependent on T-cell help than is the production of antibody-producing plasma cells. The degree of helper T-cell activity in the response of inbred strains of mice to highly artificial T-dependent antigens has been shown to depend on the Ir (immune response) genes which lie within the major his-tocompatibility gene complex (p. 2.13) and code for class II (Ia) antigens.

Although we refer above to antigen-specific T-cell co-operation in antibody production, investigation of the phenomenon with antigen consisting of a carrier-hapten complex (p. 6.2) has shown that the co-operation requires carrier-specific helper T cells and hapten-specific B cells. This is illustrated in Fig. 6.21. It appears to be a general feature of T-cell help that the helper T and B cells recognise different epitopes on the same antigenic molecules.

T helper cells also enhance the clonal prolif-eration of effector T cells in cell-mediated immune responses.

Macrophages and the immune response

In addition to the evidence outlined above for the interaction between T and B lymphocytes and between sub-populations of T lymphocytes, it is known that macrophages also participate in the immune response.

When antigenic foreign macromolecular or finely particulate material penetrates into the body, much of it is engulfed by macrophages. Most of the ingested antigen is digested within phagolysosomes and destroyed, but some anti-genic material becomes bound to the plasma membrane and a small proportion persists within the macrophage where it is protected in some unknown way from digestion and is slowly secreted. Both forms of antigenic material—surface and secretory—persist for at least 2 weeks in immunogenic form (see below).

Macrophages can bind and engulf antigen without the assistance of antibody, but if IgG antibody is present (from previous immunisa-tion) and combines with the antigen to form immune complexes, binding is greatly enhanced because macrophages, like polymorphs and some lymphocytes, have surface receptors for the Fc of the IgG in the complexes. Macro-phages do not have receptors for IgM, but when IgM antibody reacts with antigen, com-plement is activated and the binding of the anti-gen–antibody complexes is then enhanced by surface receptors for the C3b component of complement (p. 7.4). Some sub-classes of IgG antibody are cytophilic for macrophages, i.e.

they bind to the macrophage surface in the absence of antigen, and will enhance the bind-ing of antigen subsequently encountered. These mechanisms of antigen binding are summarised in Fig. 8.2, p. 8.10.

The immunogenicity of macrophage-associated antigen. When living macrophages are incu-bated with an antigen *in vivo* and washed to remove free antigen, they induce an immune response when injected into a syngeneic animal. if the antigen is weak, i.e. induces a poor im-mune response when injected alone, prior pro-cessing by macrophages considerably enhances its immunogenicity. Similar experiments sug-gest that macrophage-associated antigen enhances both primary and secondary antibody and cell-mediated immune responses: it is par-ticularly effective in stimulating the production of B memory cells and so primes the individual for a secondary respose. Both the number of B lymphocytes responding to a weak antigen and the number of cells resulting from the clonal proliferation of each stimulated B cell are in-creased by macrophage participation. Macro-phage activity does not, however, overcome the need for helper T cells in thymus-dependent antibody responses, nor does it induce immune responses in animals which have acquired immunological tolerance to the antigen.

It seems likely that a special sub-population of macrophages present the antigen in im-munogenic form. Antigen is presented to helper

T cells in association with the products of the Ir genes (Ia antigens) of the major histocompatibility complex. The antigen-presenting cells are a small proportion of macrophages which express large amounts of Ia antigen on their surface membrane.

Recent work has suggested that the **Langerhans cells** (p. 6.36) and the closely related **interdigitating reticulum cells** (so-called because of the long cytoplasmic processes these cells possess) may also fulfil this role. These cells, present in the skin and lymphoid tissues respectively, express large amounts of Ia antigen on their surface and are known to be important in the development of T-cell responses to antigens absorbed through the skin (leading to contact dermatitis), and probably also in other cell-mediated immune responses (p. 6.22).

Another type of dendritic cell involved in the immune response is the dendritic cell of the germinal centre (p. 6.36) which holds antigen, in the form of antigen-antibody complexes, on its cell surface; these cells are anatomically related to the rapidly dividing B cells of the germinal centre, and appear to present the antigen in strongly immunogenic form for a long period, thus inducing the production of large numbers of B memory cells.

Interleukins and the immune response

In addition to the presentation of antigen in immunogenic form, macrophages produce one of a family of glycoproteins, **the interleukins,** which may be important in cell co-operation.

Interleukin-1 (IL-1) is synthesised by activated macrophages in inflammatory lesions and probably after ingestion of antigenic material. IL-1 has several biological effects, including endogenous pyrogen activity (p. 8.20), but in the context of cell co-operation it has been shown to amplify the antigen-induced production of helper T cells. Helper T cells recognising antigen presented in association with Ia antigens on antigen-presenting macrophages can, in turn, regulate the proliferation of cytotoxic T cells in response to the antigen. Helper T cells also synthesise a second interleukin (interleukin-2; IL-2). These helper cell activities are enhanced by IL-1.

Interleukin-2 (also known as T-cell growth factor—TCGF) is chemically related to growth hormone. It has been shown to regulate the antigen-induced clonal expansion of cytotoxic T lymphocytes.

Similar mechanisms, possibly involving a third interleukin, may operate in T-B cell co-operation.

Regulation of the immune response

So far we have dealt with the role of lymphocytes, etc. in the production of an immune response but clearly some regulation of the immune response must exist.

Antibodies. The immune response to an antigen can be partially or even completely inhibited by injection of the corresponding antibody either shortly before or shortly after administration of the antigen. Part of the inhibitory effect is due to rapid phagocytosis and destruction of much of the antigen following its union with the injected antibody. There is, however, evidence that antibody can exert an additional inhibitory effect, which is not due to destruction of antigen, and may involve receptors on suppressor T cells (see below) for the Fc of IgG. The inhibitory effects of antibodies are of practical importance in prophylactic immunisation of infants, for maternal IgG antibodies cross the human placenta and may interfere with the response to vaccines during the first few months of infancy. The inhibitory effects of antibody are now used extensively to prevent immunisation of the rhesus-negative mother by a rhesus-positive fetus (p. 7.12).

Suppressor T cells. In addition to T cells which co-operate in the antibody response, it is now known that subsets of T cells have a suppressive effect on B cells. This explains why the antibody response to thymus-independent antigens is often greater in T-deficient animals. In lepromatous leprosy and some other chronic infections, very high titres of antibodies to the causal agent are commonly observed and may be due to relative lack of suppressor T-cell control, for failure of cell-mediated immunity (and

to the micro-organism is a constant feature of lepromatous leprosy.

The complexity is increased by recent evidence that helper T cells (and probably suppressor T cells) exert some control over T cell, as well as B cell, immune responses. The helper and suppressor activities of T cells are complex, but the use of monoclonal antibodies has shown that the cells responsible are of different pathways of intrathymic development, and have different HLA recognition restrictions (p. 6.22).

Anti-idiotypic antibodies. The specificity of an antibody is conferred by the sequences of amino acids in the variable regions of its light and heavy chains (p. 6.7), which compose the antigen-combining sites. These sequences, which are unique for any particular antibody, also confer on the antibody a specific antigenicity. Thus when monoclonal antibody (or a myeloma immunoglobulin—p. 17.60) is injected into an animal, it will develop antibodies which react specifically with the antigen-combining site. As defined by its antigenicity, the antigen-combining site of an antibody is termed an **idiotype** and antibody to it is anti-idiotypic antibody. It has become apparent that anti-idiotypic antibodies develop normally and spontaneously and react with the idiotypes of the individual's own antibodies. This may be of considerable importance in the regulation of antibody responses. Such control does not stop at this level, for anti-idiotype antibodies also act as antigens and may stimulate the development of further anti-idiotype antibodies (anti-anti-idiotypes), and so on. The immune system therefore seems to be an extended network of interacting idiotypes and anti-idiotypic antibodies, with control of the responses resulting from the overall balance of suppressor and helper signals (Jerne, 1975).

Acquired Immunological Tolerance

In some circumstances, exposure to antigen does not result in an immune response, but in the development of unresponsiveness (tolerance) of the individual to that particular antigen, although responses to other antigens remain normal. In addition to true or 'classical' tolerance, suppressor T cells and antibody are both capable of inhibiting specific immune responses (see above), and thus may bring about a state resembling true tolerance.

Classical immunological tolerance. When living cells or tissues are exchanged between genetically dissimilar individuals, the host develops an immune response which results in destruction of the transplanted cells. Yet in 1945 Owen, an American veterinary surgeon, detected red cells of two distinct groups in some bovines, and noted that such animals were always derived from a twin pregnancy. Apparently there is sometimes placental vascular anastomosis between dizygotic twin cattle, with consequent admixture of their blood during early fetal life. Circulating haemopoietic stem cells from each fetus settle in the other and remain functional so that each twin subsequently produces red cells, etc. from its own and from its twin's stem cells.

This observation—that allogeneic cells introduced into the embryo were not rejected by the host—led Burnet and Fenner (1949) to postulate that antigenic challenge during fetal life could result in specific unresponsiveness rather than an immune response. Burnet failed to substantiate this because of an unlucky choice of antigen/host combination. It was, however, subsequently confirmed by Medawar and his co-workers, who showed that injection of living cells from a mouse of one inbred strain (say Y) into a *neonatal* mouse of another inbred strain (X) induced immune unresponsiveness to cells of the donor strain. Thus when the treated mouse matured, it failed to reject a skin graft from a Y mouse, although capable of rejecting normally skin from a mouse of an unrelated strain (Z) (Fig. 6.22). The likely explanation of this form of '**classical' tolerance** is that, on encountering an antigen to which it can respond, the immature lymphoid cell is either destroyed or rendered irreversibly unresponsive. This is supported by the additional finding that when the tolerant X mouse bearing a Y skin graft is injected with lymphocytes from a normal adult X mouse, the Y graft is rejected, i.e. tolerance is abolished.

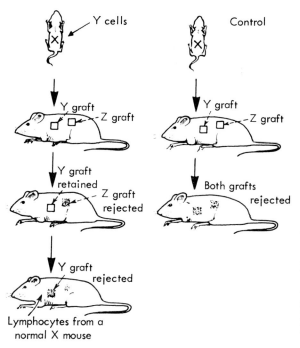

Lymphocytes from a
normal X mouse

Fig. 6.22 Immunological tolerance to allogeneic cells. A neonatal 'X' strain mouse (top left) injected with strain 'Y' cells becomes tolerant to 'Y' 'transplant' antigens, as shown by retention of a subsequent 'Y' skin graft. It rejects an unrelated ('Z' strain) graft normally. Injection of lymphocytes from a normal 'X' mouse results in rejection of the 'Y' graft. (In practice, injection of lymphocytes or haemopoietic cells is commonly used to induce tolerance in such experiments: this raises the complication of the graft versus host reaction (p. 7.30) which, for the sake of simplicity, has been ignored in this illustration.)

Tolerance may be induced also to foreign proteins by injecting them into the fetal or neonatal animal, but to maintain such tolerance it is necessary to administer repeated injections of the antigen. Thus classical tolerance is maintained only so long as the antigen persists in the host. As an explanation, it is suggested that, when lymphocytes become committed to recognise a particular antigen, they pass through an immature stage during which encounter with the antigen promotes their death or non-responsiveness: if antigen is continuously present, it will 'catch' potentially responsive lymphocytes at this stage and tolerance will persist. Mature lymphocytes are more likely to mount an immune response on encountering the antigen. It follows that widely spaced pulses of

antigen should favour an immune response, as indeed they do.

Although tolerance is most readily induced in immature animals, adults may also be rendered tolerant and Mitchison (1967) showed that this could be achieved by administering repeated injections of either very low or very high doses of antigen to adult mice. Intermediate doses induced an immune response. The explanation is that tolerance is readily induced in T lymphocytes by very small or very large doses of antigen, while B-lymphocyte tolerance is induced only by very large doses of antigen (Fig. 6.23). It follows that high dosage suppresses both the T-cell response (cell-mediated immunity) and the B-cell response (antibody production). If the antigen is T-dependent (p. 6.24), as in Mitchison's experiment, then low dosage, by inducing T-cell tolerance, will inhibit also the antibody response. For T-independent antigens, however, low dosage will induce suppression of cell-mediated immunity but there will still be antibody production: this

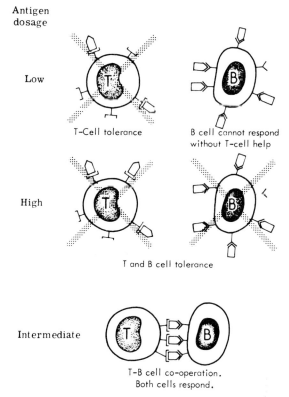

Fig. 6.23 The induction of immunological tolerance to a 'thymic-dependent' antigen by administration of very small or very large amounts of the antigen.

is sometimes termed **split tolerance** or **immune deviation**.

In fact, the situation is more complex than stated above, for any particular antigenic determinant will be bound by many lymphocytes with different specific receptors (p. 6.17). Some of these cells will have receptors which make a 'good fit' with the antigen and bind it firmly; others will bind it less well because it fits their receptors poorly. These factors will influence not only the amount of antibody produced, but also its avidity. A high concentration of antigen which induces non-responsiveness of strongly-binding cells may stimulate an immune response in those binding the antigen less firmly, with consequent production of a relatively small amount of antibody of poor avidity. The same considerations apply to T lymphocytes, and accordingly tolerance is not an all-or-nothing phenomenon. Any antigenic stimulus is likely, in fact, to induce tolerance in some potentially responsive lymphocytes and an immune response in others.

Well-established tolerance to an antigen can sometimes be overcome by administering a closely related, cross-reacting antigen, or by injecting the antigen as an emulsion in Freund's adjuvant (a suspension of killed *Mycobacteria* in mineral oil). The mode of action of Freund's adjuvant is uncertain, but abolition of tolerance by a closely related antigen is probably explained by Mitchison's work with hapten bound to a protein carrier. As already noted (p. 6.24), he showed that antibody production to the hapten is dependent on a T-cell response to antigenic determinants of the carrier protein. If T-cell tolerance to the carrier is induced by low dosage of the hapten-carrier complex, then, as explained above, the antibody response will also be suppressed. If the same hapten coupled to another protein is then injected into the animal, T cells will respond to the new carrier protein and in doing so will provide the co-operation needed by B cells to respond to the hapten. Native proteins each possess various antigenic determinants and, by regarding any particular type of determinant as equivalent to the hapten in Mitchison's experiments, we can explain the breakdown of B-cell tolerance by administration of a closely related, cross-reacting antigen.

Conditions resembling classical tolerance. So far in this account, tolerance has been explained on the basis of a direct and permanent suppression of T cells, and sometimes of B cells also, by a particular antigenic stimulus. However, it was shown by Gershon and Kondo (1971) that the thoracic duct lymphocytes of a mouse rendered tolerant to a particular antigen could confer tolerance on a normal animal of the same strain. This is now regarded as due to the development of suppressor T cells capable of inhibiting T- and B-cell responses to the particular antigen. A form of unresponsiveness to an antigen can also be induced by administration of the corresponding antibody shortly before or after antigenic stimulation (p. 6.27).

The significance of immunological tolerance. The capacity of the immunity system to develop immune responses to countless antigens carries with it the danger of responding similarly to one's own normal body constituents, i.e. auto-immunisation. The ease with which classical tolerance can be induced to specific antigens during fetal and neonatal life is believed to be the major safeguard against auto-immunisation, but it is not always effective and some diseases are attributable to auto-immunity (p. 7.24). Also B cells with surface Ig capable of binding self-constituents, e.g. thyroglobulin or DNA, have been detected in the blood of some normal individuals, indicating a capacity for auto-antibody formation; this is apparently held in check in most individuals either by lack of helper T cells, or by a dominating influence of suppressor T cells, and there is evidence that deficiency of the latter is a feature of auto-immune diseases.

As described above, tolerance may also develop towards the antigens of *foreign* cells or proteins introduced into the animal during fetal or neonatal life, and this can apply also to micro-organisms, with consequent persistence of infection, e.g. in lymphocytic choriomeningitis of mice (p. 8.13).

The fact that tolerance to foreign antigens can be induced throughout life offers a promising approach to the therapeutic transplantation of foreign tissues, for the induction of specific tolerance to antigens of the donor tissue would obviously be preferable to the use of drugs which bring about a general depression of the host's immunity system to all antigens, including those of pathogenic micro-organisms. In fact, administration of such drugs (e.g. azathioprine, glucocorticoids, etc.) together with an antigen, facilitates the induction of tolerance in the adult, and this is probably of importance in clinical renal transplantation, in which the dosage of immunosuppressive drugs can be gradually reduced without rejection of the kidney. Some form of tolerance develops to the allo-antigens of the transplant: this may either be 'classical' tolerance, as described above, or it may be due to production of specific suppressor

T cells or of 'blocking' or 'enhancing' antibody, which suppresses further immune responses, including cell-mediated immunity, to the transplant antigens (p. 7.31).

Histological Features of the Immune Response

The cellular events of immune responses take place mainly in the secondary lymphoid organs, i.e. the lymph nodes, Malpighian bodies of the spleen, tonsils and gut-associated lymphoid tissues. Study of the morphological changes of immune responses is not easy, for the large numbers of micro-organisms in the alimentary and upper respiratory tracts, and on the other exposed mucous membranes, provide continual antigenic stimuli which ensure that the immunity system is never completely inactive. The maintenance of animals in a germ-free environment from birth onwards is helpful, but technically exacting, and does not ensure complete freedom from antigenic stimulation: thus 'germ-free' mice are likely to be infected with mouse leukaemia virus, and do, in fact, show evidence of immune responses in their lymphoid tissues. There is also great regional variation in lymph node responses: when the antigenic stimulus is localised, e.g. in vaccination, the draining lymph nodes usually show the greatest response, but there may be marked differences, even between adjacent nodes.

Study of the lymphoid tissues in animals rendered deficient of T cells (e.g. by neonatal thymectomy, anti-lymphocyte serum or thoracic duct drainage), in fowls rendered B-cell deficient by bursectomy, and in patients with major congenital immunodeficiencies, has helped to distinguish between the histological features of the T-cell-mediated immune response and those of the B cell antibody response.

Lymph nodes

Normal structure. The lymph node consists of cortex, medulla and lymph sinuses (Fig. 6.24). The cortex occupies the superficial part of the node except at the hilar region: the medulla lies centrally, but extends to the hilum. The framework of the node consists of a network of fine

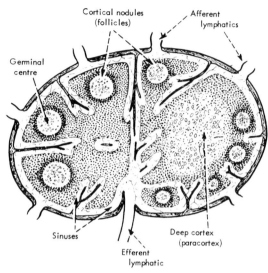

Fig. 6.24 Diagram of a lymph node, portraying the superficial cortex with nodules and germinal centres, and on the right an ill-defined area of deep cortex.

reticulin fibrils which are covered by the cytoplasm of elongated, flat reticulum cells with branching cytoplasmic processes. Many different names have been suggested for these cells, but their origin, nature and function are unknown. The sinuses are simply channels in the reticular framework, and they also are lined and traversed by reticulum cells. Macrophages are present in varying concentrations in all parts of the lymph nodes, including the lumen and walls of the sinuses.

Most of the free cells in the node are lymphocytes, and small lymphocytes usually predominate. In the cortex, the lymphocytes are closely arranged, and *the superficial part of the cortex* consists of foci, termed *primary nodules*, in which lymphocytes are more closely packed. In a stimulated node, as described below, a focus of lymphopoiesis, termed a *germinal centre*, may develop within the primary nodules. The *deeper cortex*, sometimes termed the *paracortex*, consists of ill-defined uniform areas of cortical tissue lying between the superficial

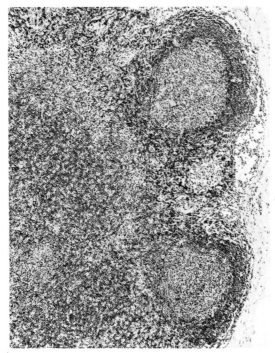

Fig. 6.25 Part of the cortex of a lymph node, showing two large cortical nodules (follicles) with germinal centres. The ill-defined area to the left of these consists of deep cortex. × 40.

cortex and medulla (Fig. 6.25): in the stimulated node, there may be intense proliferation of lymphoid cells here, and this may result in one or more large cellular zones which compress the medulla of the node.

Lymph arriving at the node by the afferent lymphatics enters the peripheral sinus which surrounds the lymphoid tissue of the node and communicates at the hilum with the efferent lymphatic. From the peripheral sinus, cortical sinuses pass radially inwards to the medulla, running between the superficial cortical nodules and traversing the deep cortex. In the medulla the lymph sinuses are numerous and the lymphoid tissue lies between them as the *medullary cords*: the medullary sinuses unite to form the efferent lymphatic.

The lymph nodes have two major functions. One of these is the interception and removal of abnormal or foreign material in the lymph stream passing through them, and is described on p. 18.8: the other is the production of immune responses.

The secondary lymphoid tissues (lymph nodes, spleen, tonsils, Peyer's patches, etc.) contain a complex mixture of T and B cells, and the situation is further complicated by the continuous re-distribution of lymphocytes via the blood and lymphatics. Considerable progress has, however, been made in defining and identifying the major lymphocyte sub-populations in the secondary lymphoid tissues and the blood, and in elucidating their lifespan, function and migratory behaviour. The main features are described briefly in the following sections, but first it is necessary to note some of the methods of recognising T and B lymphocytes.

Identification of T and B lymphocytes

Although morphologically similar, T and B lymphocytes differ in a number of ways. It is, however, important to appreciate that the features of both types of cell change during their life cycle. The situation is further complicated by the existence of subsets of lymphocytes with features not characteristic of either T or B cells, the nature of which is uncertain. Some of the features used for identification are summarised below.

Surface antigens. Depending on their degree of maturity, the lymphocytes of various species, including man, may be identified by hetero-antisera specific for T and B cells. Such antisera may be used to identify individual cells by immunofluorescence or, together with complement, to destroy either T or B cells *in vivo* or *in vitro*. Great advances in the study of lymphocyte differentiation have been made by the use of monoclonal antibodies identifying various cell markers appearing at various stages of differentiation (p. 6.21).

Intracellular esterase activity is readily demonstrable in T, but not in B, lymphocytes.

Response to mitogens. A number of substances induce mitosis preferentially in T or B cells. For example, phytohaemagglutinin and concanavalin A induce mitosis mainly in T cells while bacterial lipopolysaccharides induce B cell mitosis. Using these and other reagents, *in vitro* mitotic activity may be assessed by incorporation of ^{3}H-thymidine, but these tests are used mainly as indirect indications of T or B cell functional activity and are unsuited to identifying individual lymphocytes.

Surface immunoglobulin. As they mature in the haemopoietic marrow, B lymphocytes develop surface immunoglobulin; this is detectable in both virgin and memory B cells, and also up to a late stage of differentiation of B cells into plasma cells. Surface

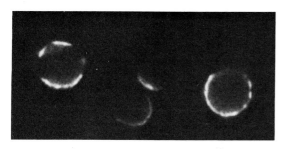

Fig. 6.26 The demonstration of surface Ig in human B lymphocytes by immunofluorescence, using labelled anti-Ig. Surface Ig is seen in four cells: it is forming aggregates on the cell surface, and in the upper central cell exhibits 'capping' (p. 6.19).

Ig may be detected by use of anti-Ig antisera (Fig. 6.26).

Receptors for Fc. B cells and K cells (see below) have surface receptors for the Fc part of IgG which has been aggregated by heat or complexed to an antigen. Fc receptors may be demonstrated by the binding of antibody-sensitised red cells to form rosettes (Fig. 6.27), or fluorescein-labelled antigen–antibody complexes. Some T cells also develop receptors for the Fc of IgG, and these are also a feature of monocytes, macrophages and polymorphonuclear leucocytes. Monocytes and polymorphs and some B cells also bind complement component C3b. On incubation *in vitro*, some T cells develop receptors for the Fc part of IgM.

Receptors for red cells. Human thymocytes and T lymphocytes are capable of binding sheep red cells *in vitro* to form rosettes (Fig. 6.27). This is a chance finding, the significance of which is obscure.

In our experience, approximately 70 per cent of human blood lymphocytes form rosettes with sheep red cells; about 28% form Fc rosettes with antibody-sensitised red cells, and of these rather less than half are B cells (positive for surface Ig) and the remainder ('null' cells) include the K-cell population (p. 7.13).

Electron microscopy reveals differences between T

and B cells, but some cells have features intermediate between the two.

Lymphocyte recirculation

In their experiments on rats, Gowans and others (p. 6.5) showed that when thoracic duct drainage was continued for several days, the number of small lymphocytes in thoracic duct lymph fell rapidly and the lymph nodes and spleen became partially depleted of small lymphocytes. They also showed that lymphocyte depletion was prevented by re-injecting the lymphocytes *intravenously*, and that when the cells were radio-labelled before return to the animal, most of the labelled cells reappeared *in the thoracic duct lymph* within the next few days. It was thus demonstrated that large numbers of small lymphocytes recirculate continuously between the blood, secondary lymphoid tissues and major lymphatics. This has since been shown to apply also to the mouse, sheep, bovines and man. Curiously, recirculation of lymphocytes is much less apparent in the pig.

Normally, about 80% of the thoracic duct small lymphocytes are T cells and the rest are B cells. In thoracic duct drainage, the number of T cells removed falls rapidly, while the fall in numbers of B cells is much slower. Correspondingly, the lymph nodes, spleen and blood are depleted of T cells rap-

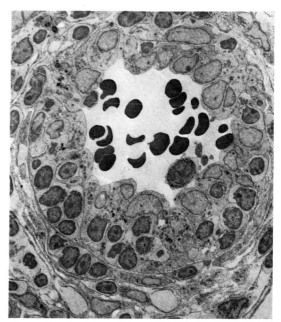

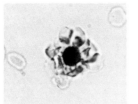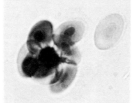

Fig. 6.27 Use of rosette formation to detect lymphocyte surface markers. **a**, a T lymphocyte binding sheep red cells. **b**, a lymphocyte binding (chicken) red cells sensitised with IgG antibody, indicating that the lymphocyte has surface receptors for the Fc of IgG.

Fig. 6.28 Electron micrograph of a post-capillary venule in a Peyer's patch from a rat, showing a lymphocyte on the luminal surface, several lying between endothelial cells, and other in the surrounding sheath. × 1200. (Dr. Gutta I. Schoefl.)

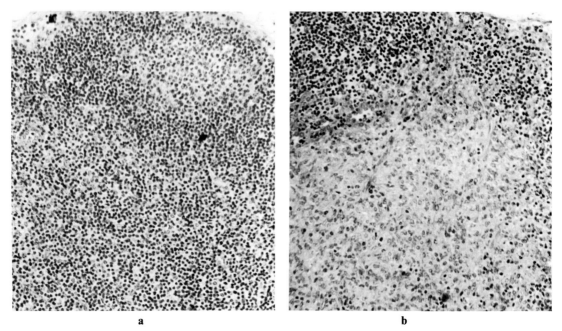

a   b

Fig. 6.29   Mouse lymph nodes, showing the influence of the thymus on the histological appearances. **a**, normal lymph node, showing a cortical follicle (top right), and the deep cortex which occupies the lower two thirds of the field. **b**, lymph node from an athymic mouse: the superficial cortex shows little abnormality, but the deep cortex is almost devoid of lymphoid cells and consists largely of 'reticulum cells'. × 150. (Professor D.M.V. Parrott and Dr. M.A.B. de Sousa.)

idly and of B cells slowly. In the mouse, this difference in depletion rate has been shown to be due partly to the greater rapidity of T-lymphocyte recirculation, and partly to the longer lifespan of T cells. By contrast, B lymphocytes recirculate more slowly and have a shorter lifespan.

The pathway and lifespan of recirculating T lymphocytes. The recirculating pathway of T lymphocytes has been elucidated by Parrott and de Sousa (1971) and other workers, usually by injecting intravenously lymphocytes radio-labelled with ³H-thymidine or ³H-uridine (which is incorporated into RNA) and following their distribution in the body by autoradiography of tissue sections or smears. Such experiments have shown that T lymphocytes in the blood gain entrance to the lymph nodes by migrating through the walls of post-capillary venules in the **paracortex** (also termed **deep cortex**) of the nodes. These venules have unusually tall endothelial cells, and the migrating lymphocytes pass between them (Fig. 6.28) to enter the paracortex, which contains mainly T lymphocytes and has been termed the **T-dependent zone** of lymph nodes. In neonatally thymectomised or athymic (*nu nu*) mice, these zones lack lymphocytes (Fig. 6.29) and similar depletion is produced by thoracic duct drainage or by destroying T lymphocytes by a heterologous anti-lymphocyte serum. Similar depletion of the T-dependent zones is

observed in children with congenital thymic aplasia (p. 7.34). From the paracortex, the lymphocytes migrate to the medullary sinuses, and thus to the efferent lymphatic. They then pass via the lymphatics to the blood, thus completing the cycle (Fig. 6.30). T lymphocytes pursue a similar course through T-dependent zones of the tonsils, Peyer's patches and Malpighian bodies (white pulp) of the spleen. In the mouse, they pass through the Malpighian bodies of the spleen in about 6 hours and through the lymph nodes in about 18 hours.

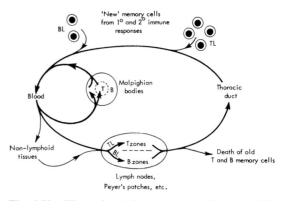

Fig. 6.30   The recirculation pathway of long-lived T lymphocytes (TL) and B lymphocytes (BL).

T lymphocytes also leave the blood, although in smaller numbers, in the various non-lymphoid tissues of the body and return to the draining lymph nodes via the afferent lymphatics.

As explained on p. 6.5, the recirculating small T lymphocytes include memory cells derived from a previous antigenic stimulus. Recent work suggests that virgin lymphocytes supplied by the thymus do not join the pool directly.

In the mouse, the number of virgin T lymphocytes leaving the thymus is much greater than the number entering the recirculating T-lymphocyte pool. When the nuclei of thymic cortical lymphocytes are radio-labelled by injecting ^{3}H-thymidine directly into the thymus, labelled cells can be detected subsequently in the Malpighian bodies of the spleen, but only a few appear in the lymph nodes or thoracic duct lymph. Such cells do not, however, accumulate progressively in the spleen, and most of them apparently die within a few days of leaving the thymus. It has been suggested that, to avoid this fate, the virgin T lymphocyte must encounter an antigen to which it can respond; it then undergoes proliferation and provides effector cells and memory cells. This is supported by the fact that gnotobiotic animals (reared from birth in a germ-free state) fail to develop the recirculating T-lymphocyte pool, although lympho-poiesis in the thymus proceeds normally and some short-lived T lymphocytes (presumably virgin cells) can be detected in the spleen. They may circulate between the blood and lymph nodes, spleen, etc. during their short lifespan, but this has not been established with certainty.

It thus appears likely that the recirculating T-lymphocyte pool consists mainly of memory cells. This being so, they would be expected to be long-lived: this has been confirmed by administering injections of ^{3}H-thymidine over periods of several weeks and observing the rate of labelling of T lymphocytes in the recirculat-ing pool (usually by autoradiography of cells in the thoracic duct or blood), and the duration of their persistence after stopping the injections. In mice it has been estimated that their lifespan is approximately 6 months: in rats it appears to exceed 1 year. The lifespan of human T lym-phocytes is not known, but it is thought to be many years. This is based on the finding of lymphocytes with chromosomal abnormalities incompatible with successful mitosis in the blood of patients treated by radiotherapy (Fig. 3.28, p. 3.28), sometimes many years before.

Analysis of small lymphocytes in the blood, lymph nodes and thoracic duct has shown that 70–80% of them are cells of the recirculating T-lymphocyte pool, and the degree of depletion effected by prolonged thoracic duct drainage agrees with this estimate.

A small percentage of T cells in the blood and thoracic duct are not small lymphocytes but larger 'blast' cells. These have arisen in the proliferative responses to various antigenic stimuli: experimental studies suggest that many of them settle and die in the secondary lymphoid tissues, notably those lining the gut, while a few differentiate into small lymphocytes and join the recirculating pool.

The pathway and lifespan of recirculating B lymphocytes. Most, if not all, of the small B lymphocytes in the blood, thoracic duct and secondary lymphoid tissues are recirculating cells. This has been established by experiments similar to those described above for T cells. They appear to leave the blood by the same route as T lymphocytes, i.e. via the post-capil-lary venules in lymph nodes, tonsils, Peyer's patches, etc., but they then come to occupy **B-dependent zones** of these secondary lymphoid tissues: in the lymph nodes they pass into and through the superficial cortex (cortical nod-ules—Fig. 6.24, p. 6.31) and medulla, and leave by the efferent lymphatic to return to the blood (Fig. 6.30). In the spleen they pass into the peripheral zone of the Malpighian bodies and presumably leave by the venous sinuses of the red pulp. These B-cell zones are depleted by thoracic duct drainage, but this takes longer than T-cell depletion because the small B lymphocytes recirculate less actively, and their lifespan (in mice approximately 6 weeks) is distinctly shorter than that of recirculating T lymphocytes.

There are occasional large B 'blast' cells in the thoracic duct and blood: these cells have arisen in the proliferative response to various antigenic stimuli: many of them differentiate into plasma cells, some in the lamina propria of the gut where they produce IgA antibodies, others in the lymph nodes, etc. where they mostly produce antibodies of other classes.

As with the T cells, it is unlikely that virgin B lymphocytes leaving the primary lymphoid organ (in mammals the haemopoietic marrow) enter directly into the recirculating lymphocyte pool. The number of B lymphocytes leaving the marrow appears to ex-ceed greatly the number of lymphocytes entering the recirculating pool. Like virgin T cells, many apparently die quickly, probably in the spleen, and it may be that the recirculating B lymphocytes are mainly memory cells resulting from proliferation of those virgin cells which meet an antigen to which they can respond by proliferation.

Accordingly, the recirculating T and B lymphocytes, which make up the great majority of small lymphocytes in the secondary lymphoid organs, blood and lymphatics, are likely to consist mainly of relatively long-lived memory cells.

Once antigen has been encountered, the primary immune response will have resulted in addition of specifically responsive T and B memory cells to the recirculating lymphocyte pool. On subsequent encounter with the same antigen, it is these memory cells which are responsible for the rapid and enhanced secondary antibody response and strong cell-mediated immunity.

Antigen-presenting cells

The **Langerhans cells** of the skin have been shown to carry antigen adsorbed on their surface to the regional lymph nodes, where they settle in the paracortex and are believed to present the antigen to T lymphocytes. **Interdigitating reticulum cells** in the paracortex are almost identical with Langerhans cells, from which at least some of them are derived: these cells also are believed to present antigen to T lymphocytes. The specialised **dendritic cells of the germinal centre** have receptors for the Fc of immunoglobulin and for the C3b product of complement activation. Following an antibody response, they bind complexes of antigen, antibody and complement: the antigen persists for several weeks on the cell surface and B lymphocytes capable of responding specifically to it are believed to be arrested and proliferate in the germinal centres. These three specialised cells—Langerhans, interdigitating and dendritic reticulum cells—are highly specialised cells of the mononuclear phagocyte system: they are not actively phagocytic and do not degrade antigen, but retain it on their surface. They also have stable HLA-DR (Ia) molecules on their surface and thus are capable of stimulating autologous T and B lymphocytes. They are, moreover, strategically placed to intercept the T and B lymphocytes as they circulate through the lymphoid tissues: they can thus present antigen to very large numbers of lymphocytes and stimulate those capable of responding to the particular antigen(s) they present.

As noted earlier (p. 6.26), 'ordinary' macrophages degrade much of the antigen they ingest, and yet present a part of it on their surface in highly immunogenic form. They appear to play a particularly important role in T-cell-dependent antibody responses. Following injection, antigen reaching the lymph nodes can first be detected within the macrophages lining the lymph-node sinuses, while in the spleen it is to be found in the marginal zone and red pulp. Much of this antigen disappears rapidly, presumably being degraded in phagolysosomes. It is not clear how some of the antigen reaches the specialised dendritic and interdigitated reticulum cells described above.

Non-specific effects of antigenic stimulation

Antigen also has non-specific effects on the recirculation of lymphocytes. In experiments in sheep, it was found that lymph nodes draining an area of skin into which an antigen has been injected show a large increase in the blood flow through the node, an increased rate of entry of lymphocytes into the node, and a fall in the number of lymphocytes in the efferent lymph. This causes a rapid increase in the size of, and the number of lymphocytes in, lymph nodes draining a site of antigen injection. The exact mechanism of these effects is unknown but recent studies suggest that they may be mediated partly by prostaglandins.

Antigen has also been shown to induce the trapping of specific lymphocytes recirculating through nodes draining sites of local injection of antigen. Thus Ford (1975) and others have shown that the recirculating population becomes depleted of appropriate specific lymphocytes following antigenic localisation in lymph nodes or spleen and that, three or four days later, corresponding blast cells are found in the efferent lymph from such lymph nodes.

Immune responses in lymph nodes

(a) **Cell-mediated immune responses.** In lymph nodes draining the site of an antigenic stimulus of a kind which induces this type of response, e.g. an allogeneic skin graft or application to the skin of the hapten dinitrochlorobenzene, the most conspicuous early change is the appearance of large basophilic (and pyroninophilic) **T 'blast' cells** or **immunoblasts** in the deep cortex of the node. These cells appear 2 days or so after antigenic stimulation; they multiply rapidly and are maximal at about 5 days. Small lymphocytes also increase in number in the deep cortex, which becomes enlarged and conspicuous, causing appreciable increase in size of the node. If the antigenic stimulation is not prolonged, the immunoblasts disappear after a further few days, the main feature then being an increased number of small lymphocytes in the deep cortex.

As explained on p. 6.34, the deep cortex is in the pathway of the recirculating T lymphocytes, which are responsible for cell-mediated immune responses, and the appearance of immunoblasts and subsequently small lymphocytes in the deep cortex represents the clonal proliferation of specifically responsive T cells following antigenic stimulation. The responsive cells may have encountered antigen in the tissues and passed to the lymph nodes, or antigenic material, either free or carried by macrophages, may have reached the draining nodes and there stimulated appropriately responsive cells among the recirculating lymphocytes passing through the deep cortex. The use of tritiated-thymidine labelling has shown that the T immunoblasts in the deep cortex proliferate to produce small T lymphocytes, and that these appear in the recirculating lymphocyte pool at about the time of development of cell-mediated immunity: recirculation will allow such 'primed' cells to encounter, and react with, the corresponding antigen almost anywhere in the body, a factor of obvious importance in combating infections.

(b) Antibody production involves the proliferation of B lymphocytes to provide B memory cells and the plasma cells which synthesise and secrete antibody. As with T cells, the recirculation of B lymphocytes provides opportunity for their encounter with antigens in most of the tissues of the body. The main site of cell proliferation observed during antibody responses is in the superficial cortical nodules, which develop large spherical or ovoid **germinal centres** (Fig. 6.25), consisting of actively dividing, large basophilic B immunoblasts. **Plasma cells** appear in increasing numbers deep to the germinal centres and in the medullary cords, which are the main site of antibody production. Although the function of germinal centres is uncertain, evidence suggests that they may be the site of the clonal expansion of B memory cells

developing in response to a high concentration of antigen on the dendritic cells (p. 6.36).

During antibody responses, which are often most pronounced in the lymph nodes draining the site containing antigen, the proliferating B cells differentiate into both plasma cells and memory B cells. Some of the B immunoblasts leave the nodes via the efferent lymphatic, and are distributed by the blood to other lymph nodes, etc., to the haemopoietic marrow, the lamina propria of the gut, and to the inflammatory reaction which may develop if antigen persists at the site of its introduction in the tissues (see below). Presumably these migrant cells also rive rise to both plasma cells and B memory cells.

Although the histological features of cell-mediated immune responses and antibody production are described above separately, it must be emphasised that many antigenic stimuli induce both responses, and indeed the control of antibody responses by helper (p. 6.24) and suppressor T cells (p. 6.27) requires the combined form of response, although the sites of T–B cell interaction in the lymphoid tissues is not known with certainty.

Immune responses in other lymphoid tissues

Spleen. The structure of the spleen is described briefly on p. 18.2. Immune responses take place in the Malpighian bodies in which the area immediately adjacent to the central arteriole is occupied by T lymphocytes of the recirculating pool, and corresponds to the deep cortex of lymph nodes. The more peripheral lymphoid tissue is occupied by recirculating B lymphocytes: it corresponds to the superficial cortex of lymph nodes and is the site of formation of germinal centres during antibody production. Antibody-producing plasma cells appear at the periphery of the Malpighian bodies and pass into the adjacent red pulp.

Immune responses in the spleen occur particularly when antigenic material gains entrance to the bloodstream, and present morphological appearances similar to those which have been described for the lymph nodes.

Gut-associated lymphoid tissues. The solitary lymphoid follicles and Peyer's patches of the gut and the lymphoid tissue of the appendix all have T- and B-cell areas, and are in the pathway of long-lived T and B lymphocytes (probably mostly or all memory cells—p. 6.36). The gut lymphoid tissue has no afferent lymphatics but lies immediately beneath the surface epithelium which in these sites is cuboidal and includes specialised 'M' cells which have a complex folded surface. Antigen in the gut lumen, including whole bacteria, can penetrate the overlying epithelium and stimulate an immune response in both T and B cells, with the usual histological changes, including germinal centre formation. The B cells of these lymphoid tissues do not specialise in the production of IgA antibodies, this being the function of plasma cells lying in the lamina propria of the gut mucosa and derived from other lymphoid tissues by way of the major lymphatics and blood (p. 6.35).

The thymus. As already indicated, the thymus is a site of T-cell lymphopoiesis. It is not an important site of immune responses, but occasional germinal centres and plasma cells are demonstrable in the medulla of the thymus in a significant percentage of people dying suddenly or after a short illness: this suggests that B lymphocytes, presumably entering the thymus from the blood, are capable of mounting an antibody response. Thymic germinal centres are rarely seen in patients dying after a chronic illness, perhaps because there has been increased secretion of adrenal glucocorticoids, which results in thymic and lymphoid atrophy. Thymic germinal centres are, however, numerous in many cases of myasthenia gravis (p. 21.76), and occur also in the connective tissue diseases.

Immune responses in non-lymphoid tissues

In intensive and prolonged antibody responses, plasma cells may be widespread in various tissues, including the haemopoietic marrow, which can be an important site of antibody production. When antigen gains entrance to non-lymphoid tissues, some of it is carried, either free or by macrophages, to the local lymph nodes where an immune response occurs. If, however, the antigen persists in its original site, as in chronic infections, skin allografts and locally-injected antigen of low solubility, then specifically primed T and B cells derived from the immune response in the lymph nodes may enter the tissue and respond specifically to the antigen: thus after 2 weeks or so there may be

numerous plasma cells and also proliferating T lymphoblasts. Macrophages also accumulate and may play a role in the local immune response by processing the antigen (p. 6.26). If the antigen persists locally for some weeks, lymphoid tissue with germinal centres and T-cell areas may develop, i.e. ectopic secondary lymphoid tissue. This is seen also in the thyroid, etc. in the organ-specific autoimmune diseases (p. 26.19), and in the synovial membrane of joints in rheumatoid arthritis (Fig. 23.51, p. 23.45).

In conclusion

During their maturation in the sheltered environment of the primary lymphoid organs, individual lymphocytes differentiate in such a way that each one becomes capable of responding to only a narrow range of antigenic determinants or epitopes. The result is a continuous supply of virgin lymphocytes of such considerable diversity that no matter what or how many natural or artificially-prepared foreign antigens are introduced into the body, there are likely to be some lymphocytes capable of mounting a specific immune response against each sort of determinant on each antigenic molecule. The restricted responsiveness and diversity of lymphocytes also ensures that only a very small proportion of the available lymphocytes can respond to any one antigen, so that immune responses to many different antigens can proceed simultaneously. The development of this restricted responsiveness of individual lymphocytes comes about by changes in the cell's DNA: it occurs in the genes coding for antigen-specific receptors of both B and T lymphocytes and is heritable and irreversible, so that when a mature virgin lymphocyte meets an antigen to which it can respond, it does so by proliferating and all the cells of the resulting clone have the same restricted specificity of response (Fig. 6.16). Encounter with an antigen thus leads to an increase in the number of lymphocytes which can respond to it. Some of the cells so produced are long-lived memory lymphocytes, which, on subsequently encountering the same or a closely similar antigen, also undergo proliferation. The result is that large numbers of responsive lymphocytes are available for those antigens which are encountered frequently. The development of complex lymphoid organs and recirculation of lymphocytes ensures adequate contact between the recognition and effector arms of the immunity system. Thus the highly complex immunity system has evolved as an exquisitely balanced and controlled mechanism which protects the host against potentially harmful micro-organisms.

References

Bach, J.-F., Dardenne, M., Pleau, J.-M. and Bach, A.A. (1975). Isolation, biochemical characteristics and biological activity of a circulating thymic hormone in the mouse and in the human. *Annals of the New York Academy of Science* **149**, 186–210.

Burnett, F.M. (1959). *The Clonal Selection Theory of Acquired Immunity*. Cambridge University Press.

Burnet, F.M. and Fenner, F. (1949). p. 76. In: *The Production of Antibodies*, 2nd edn. pp. 142. Macmillan and Co. Ltd., London.

Ford, W.L. (1975). Lymphocyte migration and immune responses. *Progress in Allergy*, **19**, 1–59.

Gershon, R.K. and Kondo, K. (1971). Infectious immunological tolerance. *Immunology* **21**, 903–14.

Good, R.A., Martinez, C. and Gabrielsen, Ann E. (1964), Clinical considerations of the thymus in immunobiology. In: *The Thymus in Immunobiology*, pp. 3–47. Ed. by R.A. Good and Ann E. Gabrielsen. Harper and Row, New York.

Gowans, J.L. (1966). Life-span, recirculation and transformation of lymphocytes. *International Review of Experimental Pathology* **5**, 1–78.

Jerne, N.K. (1955). The natural-selection theory of antibody production. *Proceedings of the National Academy of Science (N.Y.)* **42**, 849–57.

Jerne, N.K. (1971). The somatic generation of immune recognition. *European Journal of Immunology* **1**, 1–9.

Jerne, N.K. (1975). The immune system: a web of V domains. *Harvey Lecture Series*, **70**, 93–110.

Kohler, G. and Milstein, C. (1975). Continuous cultures of fused cells secreting antibody of predefined specificity. *Nature*, **256**, 495–7.

Lawrence, H.S. (1969). Transfer factor. *Advances in Immunology* **11**, 196–266.

Miller, J.F.A.P. (1964). Effect of thymic ablation and replacement. pp. 436–60 in *The Thymus in Immunobiology* in. Ed. by R.A. Good and Ann E, Gabrielsen. Harper and Row, New York.

Mitchison, N.A. (1967). Immunological paralysis as a dosage phenomenon. pp. 54–63 in *Regulation of the Antibody Response*, Ed. B. Cinader, pp. 400. C.C. Thomas, Springfield.

Mitchison, N.A. (1971). The carrier effect in the secondary response to hapten-protein conjugates. *European Journal of Immunology* **1**, 10–27.

Owen, R.D. (1945). Immunogenetic consequences of vascular anastomoses between bovine twins. *Science* **102**, 400–1.

Parrott, D.M.V. and de Sousa, M.A.B. (1971). Thymus-dependent and thymus-independent populations: origin, migratory patterns and life-span. *Clinical and Experimental Immunology* **8**, 663–84.

Reinherz, E.L., Kung, P.C., Goldstein, G. and Schlossman, S.F. (1979). Separation of functional subsets of human T cells by a monoclonal antibody. *Proceedings of the National Academy of Sciences (N.Y.)*. **76**, 4061–5.

Williamson, A.R. (1979) Control of antibody formation: certain uncertainties. *Journal of Clinical Pathology*. Supplement (Royal College of Pathologists), **13**, 76–84.

Zinkernagel, R.M. and Doherty, P.C. (1979). MHC-restricted cytotoxic T cells: studies on the biological role of polymorphic major transplantation antigens determining T-cell responsiveness. *Advances in Immunology*, **27**, 51–177.

Further Reading

Advances in Immunology. (1961–85). Academic Press, New York. (A continuing series of comprehensive articles on major immunological topics by leading authorities).

Albert, B., Bray, D., Lewis, J., Raff, M., Roberts, K. and Watson, J.D. (1983). The Immune System. pp. 952–1012 in *Molecular Biology of the Cell*. Garland Publishing Inc., New York and London.

Bowry, T.R. (1984). *Immunology Simplified*, 2nd edn., pp. 220. Oxford University Press. (A clear and brief account of basic and clinical immunology).

Herbert, W.J., Wilkinson, P.C. and Stott, D.I. (Eds.) (1985). *A Dictionary of Immunology*, 3rd edn., in press. Blackwell Scientific, Oxford. (A most helpful compilation of brief descriptions of terms used in immunology).

Immunology Today. Elsevier Medical Press, Amsterdam. (A monthly publication devoted to various immunological topics of current interest).

Janossy, G. (1982). The lymphocytes. *Clinics in Haematology*, **11**. (A series of reviews on topics relating to normal and pathological biology of lymphocytes).

Roitt, I.M. (1984). *Essential Immunology*, 5th edn., pp. 369. Blackwell Scientific, Oxford. (A clearly written and beautifully illustrated account of basic and clinical immunology).

Turk, John (Ed.) *Current Topics in Immunology Series*. Edward Arnold, London. (A series of monographs on basic and clinical aspects of important immunological topics).

See also bibliography for Chapter 7 (pp. 7.37–38).

7

Immunopathology

This chapter is devoted entirely to disease processes which have, or appear to have, an immunological basis. It falls naturally into two parts. First, the **hypersensitivity reactions** which are of an immunological nature. It should be noted that this use of the term hypersensitivity is somewhat restricted. It does not include those conditions in which the subject responds abnormally to a drug as a result of genetically-determined deficiency of an enzyme system necessary for metabolising the drug or because of failure to excrete the drug or its metabolites, e.g. in diseases of the liver or kidneys: this type of undue responsiveness is termed *idiosyncrasy* and is not dealt with here.

The second main section of the chapter describes the **immunological deficiencies** i.e. congenital or acquired conditions in which the subject is incapable of the normal range of immune responses and as a result is unduly susceptible to infection.

Hypersensitivity Reactions

In most instances, hypersensitivity may be defined as a state in which the introduction of an antigen into the body elicits an unduly severe reaction. It follows exposure to the antigen and is due to the presence of antibodies or sensitised T lymphocytes reactive with the antigen. *It is this reaction between the antigen and products of the immune response which produces the lesions of the hypersensitivity disease processes.*

Hypersensitivity reactions may be localised to the site of entry of the antigen, or generalised: the local reactions are mainly of an inflammatory nature, but may also include spasm of smooth muscle. The generalised effects include fever, shock, gastrointestinal and pulmonary disturbances, and sometimes fatal circulatory collapse. One of the earliest examples of hypersensitivity was provided by Richet and Partier (1902) who observed that intravenous injection of small amounts of extracts of sea anemone into dogs was harmless, but a second injection some weeks later was quickly followed by a violent and sometimes fatal reaction with dyspnoea, vomiting, defaecation, micturition and collapse. Since this early report, which illustrates the acute and severe nature of some hypersensitivity reactions, a great deal has been learned, and hypersensitivity reactions may now be classified into four major types (see below).

The definition of hypersensitivity given above refers solely to **foreign antigens** entering the body from outside. However, the term includes also the conditions commonly known as the **auto-immune diseases**, in which antibodies and sensitised lymphocytes appear which are capable of reacting with a normal cell or tissue constituent *in vivo*, with consequent pathological changes. Hypersensitivity reactions may result also from passive immunisation, for example when antibody is produced in the mother by active immunisation by fetal red cells, and crosses the placenta in a subsequent pregnancy to gain entrance to the fetal circulation. Another special example of hypersensitivity of increasing importance is **the rejection process in**

allogeneic or heterogeneic tissue transplants. The increasing diversity and use of drugs has also provided an important group of **drug hypersensitivities** and the same applies to the expanding number of chemicals used domestically and in industry.

The four major types of hypersensitivity reactions are described briefly below and then each is dealt with in more detail. They have been elucidated very largely by animal experiments. Hypersensitivity reactions in man, whether they occur naturally, as a result of transplantation, or from administration of a drug, tend to be complex and often involve more than one of the four types.

Atopic, anaphylactic or type 1 reactions occur in individuals who are predisposed to develop increased amounts of IgE class antibodies in response to antigenic stimuli. IgE antibody binds to mast cells, and subsequent union of the corresponding antigen triggers off release of histamine, etc., from the sensitized mast cells, giving rise to a local inflammatory reaction and smooth muscle spasm, or to a more generalised reaction. Examples include hay fever and asthma.

Cytotoxic antibody or type 2 reactions occur when antibody develops which is capable of reacting with surface antigens of cells. As a result, the cells are injured by subsequent complement activation, phagocytosis, etc. Examples include destruction of red cells and platelets by auto-antibodies to their surface components.

Immune-complex, Arthus-type or type 3 reactions are caused by the reaction of antibody, usually of IgG class, with the corresponding soluble antigen. This can occur locally (Arthus reaction) or in the blood. In either case, immune complexes are deposited in the walls of blood vessels, where they activate complement and induce vascular injury.

Delayed hypersensitivity or type 4 reactions occur when primed T lymphocytes, which develop during the cell-mediated immune response, encounter the corresponding antigen. The specifically reactive T lymphocytes transform to blast cells and secrete a number of factors (lymphokines) which mediate an acute inflammatory reaction, aggregation of more lymphocytes and monocytes, and sometimes necrosis. The tuberculin skin reaction is a good example.

It should be noted that type 1 and 2 reactions occur in subjects predisposed to unusual immune responses, while types 3 and 4 are the result of immune responses of which all normal individuals are capable.

Before considering the types of hypersensitivity in detail, this is a convenient place to describe (1) **the complement system**, which is important in acute inflammation and some types of hypersensitivity reaction, and (2) the systems of 'intracellular messengers' by which the effects of the binding of hormones and other extracellular messengers to surface receptors of their target cells are transmitted within the cell. The most important intracellular messengers are **cyclic adenosine monophosphate (cAMP)** and **calcium ions.**

The complement system

This consists of at least 18 proteins which make up about 10% of the total protein of the plasma. Most, if not all, of the components are synthesised in the liver by hepatocytes, and some are synthesised also by macrophages. Increased macrophage activity, as in inflammation, is accompanied by enhanced production of complement components.

Eleven of the complement components are termed C1–C9 (C1 is a complex of three factors, C1q, C1r and C1s), and when complement is activated by an antigen–antibody reaction these components react in sequential or cascade fashion in the order 1 to 9 except for C4 which is now known to react sequentially between C1 and C2. Such activation is termed the **classical pathway**. A second method of activation, termed the **alternative pathway**, is also initiated by antigen–antibody complexes and by certain bacteria without the necessity for an antigen–antibody reaction: it involves at least four additional factors—factors B, D, P (properdin) and C3b—and triggers off the sequential reaction at the C3 stage, so that C1, 4 and 2 are not involved. Various proteolytic enzymes present in inflammatory exudates, or participating in the clotting and kinin systems, can also activate the complement reaction at the C1 or C3 stages (p. 4.18). Complement activation is modulated by spontaneous decay of some of the activated components and by a number of inhibitory fac-

The Classical Pathway

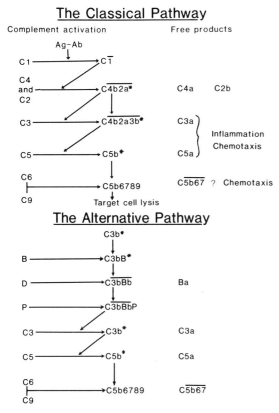

The Alternative Pathway

*Those activated components and complexes which bind to cell surfaces are marked with an asterisk. Activation products with enzymic activity are overlined.

Fig. 7.1 Activation of complement. **The classical pathway** is initiated when C1, which is a pro-enzyme, is activated by binding to the Fe of IgG or IgM antibody complexed with antigen (Ag–Ab). The active enzyme C1 cleaves both C4 and C2 into small fragments (C4a and C2b) and large fragments (C4b and C2a). The large fragments unite to form a second enzyme C4b2a which cleaves C3 into C3a and C3b. The larger fragment, C3b, binds to C4b2a to form a third enzyme, C4b2a3b, which cleaves C5 into C5a and C5b. C6 and C7 then bind to C5b, forming a stable complex, C5b67. C8 binds to this complex which in turn binds C9 to form the C5b-9 lytic complex. **The alternative pathway** requires C3b for its initiation: this is provided by continuous spontaneous low-grade activity of the classical pathway, by splitting of C3 by plasmin, the kinin or clotting systems, or by various proteolytic enzymes released by polymorphs, injured tissue cells, etc. C3b is inactivated by factors H and I, but is protected by the binding of B (and probably also by endotoxin). D splits B in this complex, releasing Ba, leaving C3bBb which binds P (properdin) to form a complex which splits C3, producing more C3b; this amplifies the alternative pathway activation and also contributes to an enzyme complex which splits C5 to provide C5b. The reaction then proceeds as in the later stages of the classical pathway.

tors, the best known of which are C1–INH which inhibits C1 (activated enzymic products of the complement system are indicated by overlining; thus C1 is activated C1) and factor I (C3bINA) which, in the presence of a co-factor, C4b-binding protein, degrades C4b and in the presence of factor H (β1H) degrades C3b.

The classical pathway (Fig. 7.1) is initiated when IgG or IgM antibody reacts with antigen in the presence of complement. As shown in Fig. 7.1, three early stages of the pathway involve enzyme reactions, and since one molecule of enzyme can cleave many molecules of substrate, the sequential reaction is amplified as it progresses. Such amplification is, however, opposed by the rapid spontaneous decay of some of the activated components and by various inhibitory factors.

The alternative pathway. It is probable that small amounts of C3 are continuously converted to a C3b-like form by low-grade hydrolysis.

This C3b-like C3 will bind B in the fluid-phase to form a low efficiency C3 convertase to generate C3b, which is an essential constituent of the alternative pathway (Fig. 7.1). Normally, the alternative pathway is held in check by factors H and I, both of which are necessary to prevent uncontrolled cleavage of C3 by this pathway, and agents which trigger off the alternative pathway do so by interfering with the inhibitory function of either or both of these inhibitory factors. The lipopolysaccharide cell wall material (including endotoxin) of various bacteria is the most important activator of the alternative pathway; it probably acts by binding C3b and rendering it resistant to the action of factors H and I. The alternative pathway is also activated by IgA antibody-antigen complexes, and since C3b is the limiting factor in the alternative pathway, its production in the classical pathway also promotes alternative pathway activity.

Biologically active products of complement.

When complement is activated by either pathway, some of the activation products are released into the surrounding fluid. Of these, C3a and C5a influence the behaviour of various cells. They stimulate mast cells and basophils to release histamine and other vasoactive amines and thus induce vascular exudative changes as in acute inflammation. In these effects, C5a is far more potent than C3a. C5a is also chemotactic for neutrophil polymorphs and monocytes and so promotes emigration and accumulation of these cells. C3a and C5a are commonly, though inappropriately, termed *anaphylatoxins* (p. 4.18). When complement is activated by particulate material, e.g. micro-organisms or host cells sensitised with antibody, or certain bacteria alone, some of the activation products, indicated in Fig. 7.1 by an asterisk, bind to the surface of the target cell and promote its destruction by two methods. Firstly, polymorphs and macrophages have surface receptors for C3b, adherence of which to the target cell (*immune adherence*) thus promotes the binding of polymorphs and macrophages and favours phagocytosis and destruction of the target cell. Secondly, completion of the complement cascade results in the insertion of the C5b–9 complex into the bacterial or target cell membrane which is consequently injured, sometimes causing their death. The mode of injury is not fully understood, but in electron micrographs C8 and C9 appear to form channels in the cell membrane (Fig. 3.3, p. 3.2); the cell absorbs water and electrolytes, swells up and ruptures.

When complement is activated by either pathway, C5b is released and may adhere to adjacent cells not involved in the initial activation. The C5b-9 complex may then build up on these 'innocent' cells, causing their death. This is known as **bystander cell lysis** or **reactive lysis**.

The pathological importance of complement. As explained earlier (p. 4.18), complement is a source of *mediators of the acute inflammatory reaction* and appears to be of importance in the inflammation induced by immunological and various non-immunological stimuli. The role of complement in types 2 and 3 hypersensitivity reactions is discussed later in this chapter.

Probably the most important role of complement is in killing micro-organisms and rendering them susceptible to ingestion and killing by phagocytes (pp. 8.9–8.11).

Complement deficiency. Genetically-determined deficiency of one or other of the complement components is rare. Deficiency of components of the classical pathway predisposes to infection. In addition, deficiencies of some early components, notably C4, C2 and B, have a high incidence in patients with immune-complex diseases (p. 23.62). This emphasises the importance of the complement system in the handling of antigen–antibody complexes.

The best known genetic abnormality of complement is deficiency of C1̄-INH which results in uncontrolled activation of complement and the inflammatory lesions of hereditary angio-oedema (p. 10.31).

Detection of complement components. The measurement of total haemolytic complement activity present in serum is performed traditionally by determining the concentration of serum required to cause 50% lysis of (i.e. escape of 50% of the haemoglobin from) a suspension of red cells sensitised with antibody (p. 6.12). Techniques are, however, available to measure individual complement components, and also their activation products: such tests are now in routine use to detect evidence of activation of complement *in vivo* in various diseases, and to distinguish between activation by the classical and alternative pathways.

Intracellular messenger systems

Cyclic adenosine monophosphate (cAMP). This is synthesised from ATP under the catalytic influence of adenylate cyclase, which is located on the inner side of the plasma membrane. When various extracellular messengers bind to surface receptors, the inner part of the receptor is changed in such a way that it induces a second protein (**G protein**) to bind guanosine triphosphate (GTP). In this form, G protein activates adenylate cyclase, with consequent rapid increase in the cytosol concentration of cAMP (Fig. 7.2).

In order to respond quickly to the body's changing requirements, the level of cAMP must be capable of rapid change. Production of cAMP continues only so long as messenger-receptor complexes persist at the cell surface, and such complexes are rapidly removed by endocytosis, a process similar to the capping

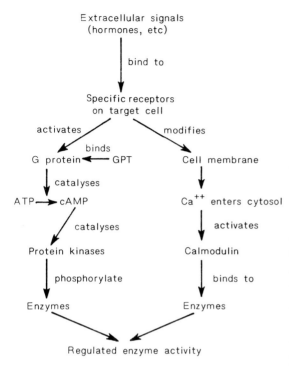

Extracellular signals
(hormones, etc)

bind to

Specific receptors
on target cell

activates ← binds → modifies

G protein ← GPT   Cell membrane

catalyses

ATP → cAMP   Ca^{++} enters cytosol

catalyses   activates

Protein kinases   Calmodulin

phosphorylate   binds to

Enzymes   Enzymes

Regulated enzyme activity

Fig. 7.2 Mechanisms involved in the two major systems of intracellular messengers, the cAMP and Ca^{++} systems.

and endocytosis of the antigen receptors of B lymphocytes (p. 6.19). Also, activated G protein quickly renders itself inactive by hydrolysing its bound GTP, and cAMP in the cytosol is rapidly destroyed by phosphodiesterases. Accordingly, brief signals induce rapid and short-lived changes in cAMP levels.

An outstanding example of disturbance of the cAMP system is provided by cholera, in which the bacterial toxin renders the G protein in intestinal epithelium incapable of hydrolysing its bound GTP: in consequence, the activity of adenylate cyclase is greatly prolonged and a persistent increase in the level of cAMP is responsible for the excessive transfer of water and electrolytes into the lumen of the gut, thus accounting for the severe diarrhoea and dehydration of cholera.

Most stimuli which influence the behaviour of cells by the cAMP system do so by stimulating adenylate cyclase activity and increasing cAMP, but some exert their effect by inhibiting adenylate cyclase activity and thus lowering the level of cAMP. Most cellular activities are in-

fluenced by cAMP levels, although mutant cells incapable of cAMP synthesis can survive and multiply in culture.

The effect of cAMP is to activate phosphorylating enzymes (protein kinases) and dephosphorylating enzymes within the cell: phosphorylation of various enzymes is thus controlled, and this, in turn, regulates their activity.

Cellular activities are also influenced by the **cyclic guanosine monophosphate (cGMP) system,** but its regulating effects appear to be much less important than those of the cAMP system.

As noted below, the cAMP system is closely integrated with another important 'second messenger' system, in which Ca^{++} plays a major role.

Calcium as a second messenger. The overall concentration of intracellular calcium is approximately the same as in extracellular fluid, but most of the intracellular calcium is sequestrated in various organelles or incorporated into calcium phosphate, calcium-binding proteins, etc., and so is not in ionic form. There is thus a steep concentration gradient of Ca^{++} across the plasma membrane and this is maintained by using energy derived from hydrolysis of ATP to pump Ca^{++}, against the gradient, both out of the cell and into its organelles.

The binding of some extracellular messengers to their cell surface receptors produces a local effect on the plasma membrane and the membrane of cell organelles, the result of which is to allow Ca^{++} to enter the cytosol (Fig. 7.2). An important example of the use of Ca^{++} as a second messenger is provided by skeletal muscle: binding of acetylcholine to its specific receptors results in a rise of sarcoplasmic Ca^{++}, which induces contraction. The effect of hormones on secretory target cells is also usually mediated by a rise of cytosol Ca^{++}.

Like cAMP, the level of cytosol Ca^{++} can change rapidly. Entrance of relatively small numbers of calcium ions can increase the concentration to several times the low baseline level, and the level can be reduced rapidly by Ca^{++} pumps.

A rise of Ca^{++} in the cytosol results in increased binding of Ca^{++} to calcium-binding proteins, notably *calmodulin*, an important cell protein which, depending on the number of calcium ions bound, can attach selectively to various enzymes and thus regulate their activity. Some of the enzymes involved in the cAMP system are themselves influenced by calmodulin, and there is thus close integration between the two major regulating systems.

Atopy (anaphylactic, 'immediate' or type 1) hypersensitivity

Approximately 10% of the population suffers from this type of hypersensitivity, although in most of these the symptoms are mild and occasional. The commonest manifestations of atopy are **hay fever** and **extrinsic asthma**, which tend to run in families and are sometimes preceded by **atopic eczema** in infancy and childhood. The sufferer from hay fever develops acute inflammation of the nasal and conjunctival mucous membranes with sneezing and nasal and lacrimal hypersecretion within minutes of exposure to an atmosphere containing the causal agent (**allergen**) — usually grass pollens. Similarly, an attack of asthma, with difficult wheezing respiration due to narrowing of the airways by bronchospasm and mucous secretion, develops rapidly when the asthmatic inhales the agent to which he is hypersensitive, e.g. house dust or animal dander. Atopic individuals, particularly in childhood, may also suffer from '**food allergies**' in which absorption of antigenic constituents of certain foods, e.g. milk or eggs, promotes an acute reaction in the gut with colicky pain, vomiting and diarrhoea.

Urticaria, consisting of acute inflammatory lesions of the skin with wealing due to dermal oedema, is common in atopic subjects and also occurs alone as an acute or chronic condition.

In addition to local disturbances, atopic patients sometimes develop **acute systemic anaphylaxis** (anaphylactic shock) with dyspnoea, urticaria, convulsions, and sometimes death. Generalised reactions occur when the responsible agent is absorbed in amounts which produce a significant level in the blood. Fortunately, severe anaphylactic shock is rare, but it sometimes occurs in hypersensitivity to drugs, notably penicillin, and to the venoms of stinging insects.

Skin tests and provocation tests. Diagnosis of

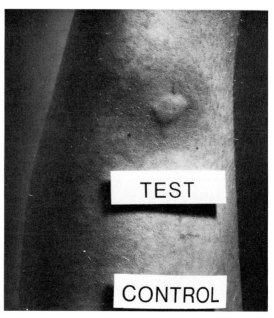

Fig. 7.3 Skin test showing immediate (type I) hypersensitivity reaction. The patient was an asthmatic and the test was performed by intradermal injection of an extract of house dust. Note the oedema and wide zone of reddening. Photograph taken 10 minutes after injection. (Dr Ian McKay.)

atopy depends on an accurate clinical history, which sometimes suggests that acute attacks result from exposure to a particular environmental antigen (allergen). To confirm the state of hypersensitivity, dilute solutions of the suspected antigens (which are commercially available) may be placed on the skin and pricked in with a needle. A positive result is indicated by a local weal and flare reaction, developing within a few minutes (Fig. 7.3) and lasting for an hour or so. Hence the term 'immediate type' hypersensitivity. Although of diagnostic help, skin tests are not infallible. The atopic individual tends to give positive reactions not only to the environmental antigen(s) responsible for attacks of atopy, but also to various others. Also, in a proportion of cases the skin test is negative although the history is very suggestive of atopy to that antigen. A more reliable indication of the causal role of a particular antigen is provided by provocation tests, for example bronchial challenge by controlled inhalation of the suspected antigen by the asthmatic, and nasal application for the hay fever patient: an acute attack implicates the test antigen. In all such tests, careful precautions must be taken to avoid provoking a severe reaction.

The mechanism of atopic hypersensitivity

Passive transfer of immediate type hypersensitivity was demonstrated beautifully 60 years ago by the classical investigation of the two German doctors, Prausnitz and Küstner. Küstner himself regularly developed hypersensitivity reactions immediately after eating fish, and intradermal injection of an extract of cooked fish induced an immediate-type reaction. Injection of a small amount of Küstner's serum intradermally into Prausnitz induced a local state of hypersensitivity, for when cooked fish muscle extract was injected intradermally 24 hours later at the same site an immediate-type reaction occurred, whereas other skin sites were negative.

Passive transfer has been confirmed repeatedly with serum from atopic subjects: it has been shown to be antigen-specific, and the interval between the two injections can be prolonged to 3–4 weeks, demonstrating that the serum factor (reagin—see below) binds to some tissue element in the skin.

Temporary atopic hypersensitivity has also been observed in recipients of blood from atopic donors: the recipient exhibits positive skin tests and may develop clinical atopy if exposed to the relevant antigen(s). Evidence that reagin sticks to various tissues and not just to skin has been provided by the demonstration that fresh bronchial tissue removed from an atopic subject undergoes contraction of the smooth muscle when exposed to the appropriate antigen, and it has been shown that normal tissues of various types can be sensitised passively by the serum of atopic individuals.

Reaginic antibody: IgE. Being antigen-specific, the serum factor responsible for passive transfer of atopy has long been regarded as an antibody, and known as **reagin** or **reaginic antibody**. It has proved difficult to characterise, for it is present in serum in only trace amounts, and is **homocytotropic**, i.e. binds to the tissues of man or related primates, but not to tissues of other genera: this restricts its detection by passive transfer to experiments on man and some monkeys. However, it was eventually shown by Ishizaka *et al.* (1966) to be due to an immunoglobulin of a distinct 'new' class, since termed IgE. Patients with IgE-producing myelomas (plasma-cell tumours) have provided a rich source of IgE. Using this material, it was shown that when a solution of IgE or of its Fc component was injected into the skin, it was found to block the tissue sites of attachment of reaginic antibody, and so inhibited the Prausnitz–Küstner reaction at the same site. This is strong confirmation that reaginic antibody is of IgE class, and shows that fixation to mast cells (see below) is a property of its Fc component. Antibody induced by myeloma IgE is now used to assay the level of IgE in serum and also as the basis of the *in-vitro* assay of specific IgE antibodies, e.g. by the 'radio-allergosorbent test' (RAST). Raised levels of IgE, and of IgE class antibodies to the relevant antigens, have been detected in the serum and nasal secretions, etc., but such *in-vitro* tests have so far been applied mainly in cases where the results of skin tests are equivocal.

Role of mast cells and basophil leucocytes. Mast cells are widely distributed in most tissues, and are particularly numerous adjacent to small blood vessels. Basophil leucocytes resemble mast cells in appearance and function; like other leucocytes, they can respond to chemotaxins and migrate from the blood into the tissues. Both mast cells and basophils have large basophilic cytoplasmic vesicles (secretory granules) which can be discharged ('degranulation') by various stimuli, e.g. the various causal agents of acute inflammation, releasing histamine and other vasoactive compounds from the cell.

Many mammalian species are capable of developing immediate-type hypersensitivity reactions similar to atopic reactions in man, and studies on rodents have demonstrated that reaginic antibody binds firmly by its Fc component to surface receptors of mast cells and basophils. This leaves the Fab ends of the antibody free to react with the corresponding antigen, and when this occurs, degranulation results.

The mechanism by which binding of antigen activates mast cells and basophils sensitised by IgE antibody involves indirect cross-linking of the IgE receptors, for monovalent antigen (hapten attached to protein) does not induce activation, while (bivalent) antibody to IgE links adjacent IgE molecules bound to the cell

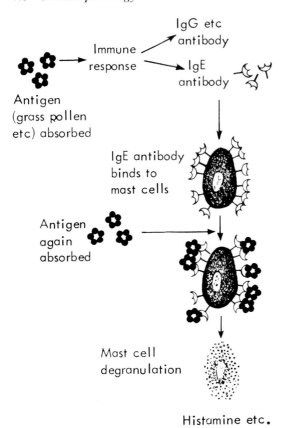

IgG etc antibody

Immune response

IgE antibody

Antigen (grass pollen etc) absorbed

IgE antibody binds to mast cells

Antigen again absorbed

Mast cell degranulation

Histamine etc.

Fig. 7.4 The mechanism of atopic reactions. IgE antibody to pollens, etc., binds by its Fc component to mast cells (and basophil leucocytes), and subsequently absorbed antigen triggers off the sensitised cells (by linking together antibody molecules on their surface) to release histamine, etc.

surface and activation results. Antibody to the IgE receptors has the same effect.

Atopy in man differs in certain respects from experimental immediate-type hypersensitivity in rodents, and human cellular studies have been performed mainly on basophil leucocytes because of the difficulty of obtaining human mast cells. Recently, however, fairly pure suspensions of mast cells have been prepared from proteolytic enzyme digests of surgically-removed human lung tissue. It has been shown that human IgE binds firmly to receptors on human mast cells and basophils, and that cross-linking by anti-IgE (see above) activates these cells. There is thus strong evidence that the mechanism of human atopy is that shown in Fig. 7.4.

The changes involved in activation of mast cells and basophils are highly complex. When cross-linked, the IgE receptors have been shown to activate enzymes at the inner surface of the plasma membrane. One effect is to increase the concentration of ionic calcium in the cell cytosol by ingress of calcium through the plasma membrane or from calcium-rich organelles within the cell. This is an essential feature of activation. The role of cAMP in activation is controversial. Activation is associated with a transient rise in cAMP, followed by a sharp fall, and β-adrenergic agents which activate adenylate cyclase, and thus increase cAMP, inhibit degranulation.

Cross-linked IgE receptors also activate phospholipase A_2 and this results in release of arachidonic acid from phospholipid of the cell membrane. The products of arachidonic acid metabolism may play a role in degranulation and also act as mediators of the atopic reaction (see below).

Endogenous mediators of atopic reactions. Localised atopic reactions are mediated by the products of activated mast cells. When the granules are discharged, they release *histamine*, *platelet activating factor*, and two tetrapeptides which are termed the *eosinophilic chemotactic factors of anaphylaxis* (*ECF-A*) because they are chemotactic to eosinophil leucocytes. In addition to these products of degranulation, activated human mast cells, as noted above, are active in synthesis and secretion of arachidonic acid metabolites. Cyclo-oxygenase activity results in production of prostaglandins, notably PGD_2 and lipoxygenase activity produces *leukotrienes*, notably LTC_4 and LTD_4. Before these components were identified, the mixture was known as the *slow-reacting substance of anaphylaxis* (*SRS-A*). The biological effects of most of these products of mast cell activation have been described in relation to the acute inflammatory reaction (pp. 4.19–20). Between them, they account for the major features of localised atopic reactions—congestion (vasodilatation), oedema due to vasodilatation and increased venular permeability, and infiltration with eosinophil leucocytes. They also explain the increased secretion of the mucosal glands in hay fever and asthma and the bronchospasm of asthma which results from contraction of bronchial smooth muscle.

It will be apparent that local atopic reactions

exhibit some of the features of an acute inflammatory reaction, but there are important differences, notably in the participation of eosinophil leucocytes instead of neutrophils, the absence of severe tissue injury and necrosis, and the contraction of smooth muscle, e.g. in the bronchi. These differences are explicable on the basis that acute inflammatory lesions result from tissue injury by bacterial toxins, physical or chemical agents. Atopic reactions do not result from such injury, but from the reaction of usually harmless antigens with sensitised mast cells, and represent the effects of mast cell activation without tissue injury.

The role of eosinophil leucocytes. These cells appear to modulate the intensity of the reaction induced by mast-cell products. Experimentally-induced immediate-type hypersensitivity reactions in rats are enhanced by injection of an anti-eosinophil serum which depletes the blood of eosinophils, and these cells not only secrete histaminase and arylsulphatase, which inactivate histamine and leucotrienes respectively, but there is also evidence that they may inhibit both mast-cell degranulation and restoration of degranulated mast cells. The eosinophil also plays a defensive role against parasitic worms (see below).

Other immunological factors. Atopic subjects show exaggerated immune responses to environmental allergens, and although atopic reactions depend mainly on production of IgE antibodies, other classes of antibody, and also cell-mediated immune responses, may also contribute to their hypersensitivity reactions. There is recent evidence that IgG4 antibody (p. 6.7) can mediate a complement-dependent form of immediate type hypersensitivity, although it has not yet been proved that this second mechanism plays a significant role in hypersensitivity reactions in man. In some atopic subjects the immediate reaction is followed by an Arthus (type 3) hypersensitivity reaction due to the formation of complexes of antigen with IgG antibody and possibly also by a delayed-hypersensitivity (type 4) reaction, due to primed T lymphocytes. These later reactions, which may cause difficulty in detecting the responsible antigen(s), have been demonstrated most readily by provocation tests.

Atopic hypersensitivity can sometimes be reduced, but seldom abolished, by subcutaneous injection of the responsible antigen in a slowly soluble (e.g. alum precipitated) form. The mechanism of such **hyposensitisation** is not known, but it has been widely assumed that it stimulates increased production of IgG and IgA antibodies to the atopy-inducing antigen, and that these intercept naturally-absorbed antigen and thus prevent it from reacting with the IgE antibody bound to mast cells. However, production of IgE, like other classes of antibody, is usually influenced by the T-cell response (p. 6.27) and hyposensitisation might conceivably either induce specific T-cell tolerance to the antigen or stimulate production of suppressor T cells (p. 6.26). Hyposensitisation is not always successful, and the outcome is not predictable. There is, moreover, a possibility that, by stimulating the production of IgG antibody, the procedure may predispose the individual to immune-complex disease (p. 7.16). The possible role of IgA antibodies in atopy is discussed below.

Agents which inhibit atopic reactions include: (1) adrenal glucocorticoids, which have multiple effects, including the stabilisation of membranes of mast cells; (2) disodium chromoglycate, which inhibits activation of mast cells following sensitisation by antigen; (3) β-adrenergic agonists, which increase mast-cell cAMP, and (4) antagonists to the products of activated mast cells, e.g. antihistamine drugs.

Acute systemic anaphylaxis occurs when sufficient antigen enters the body to produce a significant level in the plasma. This has the effect of activating the sensitised basophil leucocytes with consequent degranulation and secretion of arachidonic-acid metabolites. The mediators are similar to those secreted by mast cells, but the arachidonic-acid lipoxygenase pathway is much less active than in mast cells and leukotrienes are therefore produced in relatively small amounts. Circulating antigen does, however, leave the bloodstream and activates adjacent mast cells. The result is widespread peripheral vasodilatation, causing severe shock, together with intense contraction of non-vascular smooth muscle, notably of the bronchial tree, and urticaria. As noted earlier, severe systemic anaphylaxis is rare, but it can result from insect stings and from drugs, particularly penicillin. The severe condition is a medical emergency and prompt intravenous injection of adrenaline may be necessary.

Predisposition to atopy

The occurrence of atopy in several generations of some families suggests a genetic predisposition. In general, atopic subjects have higher total serum IgE levels, and produce more IgE antibody in response to antigenic stimulation, than control subjects. Accordingly, it seems likely that the genetic factor determines the intensity of IgE responses. Some support for this is provided by the finding that, within a particular family, the occurrence of atopy is associated with inheritance of particular HLA haplotypes. Population studies have not demonstrated that any particular HLA genes are associated with atopy, and the family associations may be due to linkage disequilibrium of HLA haplotypes with immune response genes (p. 2.13).

Although atopy is attributable to the reaction between antigens and IgE antibodies, there must be other important factors, for in some cases the skin tests do not correlate with provocation tests nor with the occurrence of clinical atopy. This may, however, be due to local production of IgE antibody by mucosal plasma cells without a significant release into the plasma. Related to this is the possible importance of the IgA antibody response and the secretion of IgA by mucous membranes. It has been shown that injection of IgA antibody into rats inhibits the absorption of inhaled or injected antigens. Most atopic subjects have normal serum IgA levels, but it has been reported that intranasal application of antigen results in the appearance of less IgA antibody and more IgE antibody in the nasal secretion in hay-fever subjects than in controls (Butcher, Salvaggio and Leslie, 1975). It is also of great interest that assay of the serum IgA levels of the infants of atopic parents has shown that those with a low level of IgA at three months of age are more liable subsequently to develop atopic eczema (Taylor et al., 1973) and probably also asthma (Soothill, personal communication). The same group of workers has also reported that avoidance of the environmental antigens which commonly cause atopy (including dairy products) during the first six months of life reduces the incidence of atopic eczema in infants with an atopic predisposition (Matthew *et al.*, 1977). There is, however, no general agreement on this observation.

It has also been reported that T cell depletion in rats enhances IgE antibody responses. In atopic subjects, there is no good evidence of a T-cell deficiency, although children with the rare Wiskott-Aldrich syndrome (p. 7.35), who have a congenital T-cell deficiency, are prone to develop atopy.

The importance of non-immunological factors in atopy is suggested by the lack of close correlation between serum levels of IgE antibody and the degree of hypersensitivity to the allergen, and also by the fact that, in asthmatic subjects, an acute attack may be brought on by various stimuli in addition to inhalation of the antigen, e.g. hyperventilation in cold air or inhalation of irritating fumes, and by emotional stress. The role of non-immunological factors is not fully understood, but asthmatic subjects are known to respond more strongly than others to β-adrenergic blockade or to cholinergic receptor agonists, both of which tend to induce bronchoconstriction (Townley, 1983). It thus seems possible that imbalance of autonomic control of the bronchial musculature is a significant factor. It has, however, also been shown that asthmatics are unduly responsive to agents which act directly on the bronchial smooth muscle, causing constriction, e.g. histamine.

Another possibility is that the mucosal surfaces affected in atopy are unduly permeable to macro-molecules, including allergens, but the evidence is not convincing.

It is noteworthy that in African communities with a high rate of infection with parasitic worms, IgE levels are also high, although atopy is uncommon. Infection with worms or injection of worm extracts has been shown in animals to increase the IgE antibody response to various antigens. IgE antibody is important in the defence against worms, and it has been suggested that, by binding to mast cells, antiparasitic IgE antibody, if present in relatively high concentration, excludes the binding of other IgE antibodies and thus protects against atopy. This would account for the higher incidence of atopy in populations with a low level of parasitic infestation, and it may be that elimination of most of our parasites has exposed us to the harmful effects of exaggerated IgE antibody responses to various otherwise harmless environmental antigens.

The very small amounts of IgE antibody produced by immune responses (e.g. to micro-organisms) in normal individuals may play a defensive role in microbial infections by activating mast cells and thus triggering off acute inflammation at the site of a subsequent infection.

Cytotoxic antibody (type 2) reactions

The only distinctive feature of this type of hypersensitivity reaction is that it is mediated by antibodies which cause injury to cells by combining specifically with antigenic determinants on their surface. With few exceptions, the targets of cytotoxic antibodies are the cells of the blood. Such injury has been investigated mainly in man, in whom it may occur in the following circumstances.

1. Auto-antibodies may develop which are reactive with normal antigenic constituents on the surface of cells. This unexplained breakdown of self-tolerance may occur in isolation or as a feature of systemic lupus erythrmatosus (p. 7.26) and is sometimes associated with a number of infections and also with neoplasia of lymphoid cells.

2. Drug-induced cytotoxic antibodies. Some drugs or their metabolites bind to the surface of one or other type of cell: if such a drug is haptenic, it induces an antibody response, and the reaction of antibody with the cell-bound hapten may bring about destruction of the cell.

3. Iso-antibodies can cause injury to cells of the blood following blood transfusion or transplantation of haemopoietic or lymphoid tissue. Maternal iso-antibodies of IgG class may also pass through the placenta and injure the cells of the fetus.

Cytotoxic antibodies to cells of the blood

Cytotoxic auto-antibodies. The classical example is *auto-immune haemolytic anaemia* in which red cell injury is brought about by auto-antibody reactive with the various antigenic determinants inherent in the surface of red cells. The antibody may be of IgG or IgM class, and can be detected on the red cell surface by the antiglobulin test (p. 6.11). When present in low concentration on the cell surface,

IgG may have little or no effect. In higher concentration, it promotes the binding of the red cells to the Fc receptors of macrophages; such binding may result in injury to the red cell membrane or to phagocytosis and destruction of the red cell by macrophages, mostly in the red pulp of the spleen and the hepatic sinusoids. IgG antibody can also activate complement and cause intravascular lysis of the cells; this requires the binding of pairs of IgG antibody molecules to closely adjacent antigenic sites on the red cell surface. IgM antibodies, even in low concentration, often cause red cell destruction by intravascular lysis because single IgM molecules binding to two or more antigenic determinant sites on the red cell surface are capable of activating complement. Complement activation also promotes binding of the red cells to macrophages (by the C3b receptors of the latter), while IgM antibody can also cause agglutination of red cells, particularly where the circulation is slow, as in the red pulp of the spleen; both these effects result in intrasplenic destruction of red cells.

Idiopathic thrombocytopenic purpura is caused by auto-antibody which reacts with the surface components of normal platelets, with similarly destructive effects. The frequency with which splenectomy is followed by a rapid rise in the platelet count indicates the importance of the splenic macrophages in the increased platelet destruction.

Auto-antibodies to leucocytes may be a cause of leucopenia (reduced numbers of leucocytes) but this is difficult to prove, partly because such auto-antibodies must usually be sought by testing the patient's serum with leucocytes from another individual, and iso-antibodies to leucocytes are a common snag. Secondly, leucocytes tend to bind IgG non-specifically and give a false-positive antiglobulin test.

Drug-induced cytotoxic antibodies. Some drugs or their metabolites are capable of binding to the surface of red cells, leucocytes or platelets, and acting as haptens. Antibody develops and binds to the hapten on the cell surface, and cell injury and destruction may then result, as in the case of auto-antibodies (see above). A good example of this is provided by penicillin, the benzyl-penicilloyl degradation product of which binds firmly to red cells. Most people who have received penicillin have some antibody (usually IgM) to the penicilloyl group, but after prolonged heavy dosage, high titres of IgG antibody develop in some patients and this brings about the destruction (mostly by splenic phagocytosis) of sensitised red cells. Some drugs, for example rifampicin, result in platelet destruction by an immunological reaction; this may be due to its binding to the platelet surface and acting as a hapten, as described above, but it seems more likely that it forms complexes with antibody in the plasma and that it is the binding of such complexes to Fc receptors of the platelets which causes their destruction (p. 7.23).

A very few drugs can induce the development of *auto-antibodies*; for example, patients receiving α-methyldopa for a few months often develop auto-antibodies to surface (notably Rh) antigens on their red cells, detectable by the direct antiglobulin test: there is no evidence that the antibodies react with drug-derived antigens, for they are true auto-antibodies and react with the patient's and other individuals' red cells. One explanation is that, by altering a protein constituent of the cell, α-methyldopa renders it immunogenic to T lymphocytes, which then act as helper cells in the production, by B lymphocytes, of antibody to a surface (e.g. Rh) antigen: In other words, the altered red cell protein acts as a 'foreign' carrier and thus promotes an antibody response to the antigenic determinant, just as antibody is produced to hapten attached to a foreign protein (p. 6.24). In most instances, there is insufficient antibody to cause significant red cell destruction, but approximately 1 per cent of patients develop a haemolytic anaemia which gradually disappears on withdrawing the drug.

Cytotoxic iso-antibodies. In blood transfusion, administration of red cells possessing the A or B surface iso-antigens to an individual whose plasma contains the natural anti-A or anti-B iso-antibodies usually results in rapid destruction of the donated red cells. These natural antibodies are of IgM class and so complement fixation and lysis of the incompatible red cells results. There are literally dozens of other red cell iso-antigens, but normally the corresponding antibodies appear in the plasma only after blood transfusion or pregnancy (see below). After the ABO groups, the Rhesus (Rh) system of iso-antigens is of most importance in man. Transfusion of red cells possessing Rh antigens which are not present in the recipient's red cells

often results in devlopment of the corresponding Rh antibody, following which the transfused cells are destroyed abnormally rapidly in the spleen. During labour (or abortion) some fetal red cells enter the mother's circulation, and, if Rh-incompatible (which depends on the father's Rh group) they sometimes stimulate development of Rh antibodies.

The Rh antibodies are particularly important in pregnancy, because they are usually mainly of IgG class, and so can cross the placenta. If the pregnant woman has developed Rh antibodies, as a result of a previous pregnancy or blood transfusion, they enter the fetal circulation and, if the fetal red cells possess the corresponding Rh antigens, abnormal destruction results in fetal death or anaemia (Fig. 7.5).

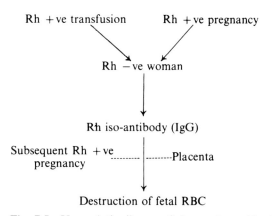

Fig. 7.5 Haemolytic disease of the newborn. Fetal red cell destruction is brought about by maternal iso-antibody which has developed as a result of previous Rh +ve pregnancy or transfusion of Rh +ve blood.

Once an individual has developed Rh antibodies, from either pregnancy or transfusion, subsequently transfused Rh-positive red cells are liable to be destroyed rapidly. The development of Rh antibodies can very often be prevented by injecting Rh antibody into the Rh-ve mother within 48 hours after the birth of an Rh-incompatible child (p. 17.31).

In common with tissue cells, the leucocytes and platelets have antigens belonging to the HLA system (p. 2.12). This is seldom of importance in blood transfusion unless the aim is to supply these cell types to a deficient recipient. Blood transfusion and pregnancy do, however, stimulate the development of HLA and other antibodies, and subsequently transferred platelets or leucocytes may be destroyed rapidly. Such iso-immunisation is of importance if subsequent transplantation, e.g. of a kidney, is performed (p. 7.31) and maternal iso-antibodies to platelets may also cause thrombocytopenia in the fetus.

Immune responses to HLA iso-antigens may also develop as a result of tissue transplantation, and are responsible for transplant rejection (p. 7.30).

Auto-antibodies to tissue constituents

Auto-antibodies which react with components of tissue cells *in vitro* are demonstrable in the serum of patients with various diseases (p. 7.24), but the available evidence suggests that they are not usually a major cause of cell injury. In some instances, this is because they react with intracellular, as opposed to surface constituents, of the target cells. A good example is antibody to deoxyribonucleoprotein, which is present in the plasma of patients with systemic lupus erythematosus: it can react with, and lead to destruction of, the nuclei of dead cells, but does not reach the nuclei of living cells.

There are, however, two important examples of auto-antibodies which react with cell surface receptors and have a profound effect on the target tissue cells. One is a thyroid auto-antibody, which reacts with the TSH receptor of thyroid epithelium and, like TSH itself, stimulates the cell to increased function and proliferation by activation of adenylate cyclase: this is the cause of *Graves' disease*, the common type of hyperthyroidism, and is sometimes termed *stimulatory hypersensitivity*. The other is an antibody to the acetylcholine receptors of skeletal muscle: it blocks the receptors and thus causes the muscle weakness of *myasthenia gravis* (p. 21.76). A third example of a harmful auto-antibody is found in a small proportion of sterile men; it reacts with spermatozoa and may be present in sufficient concentration in seminal fluid to impair their motility.

Although 'cytotoxic' implies injury to cells, type 2 hypersensitivity is generally extended to include antibody-induced injury to extracellular tissue elements. The best known example of this is a rare type of glomerulonephritis in which auto-antibody develops to glomerular capillary basement membrane. Union of this antibody with the inner surface of the basement membrane is followed by activation of complement, as in the Arthus reaction, and a destructive inflammatory lesion results in the glomeruli (p. 22.35).

Antibody-dependent lymphocyte cytotoxicity

When a suspension of living cells is treated with an IgG-class antibody which reacts with their surface membrane, and normal lymphocytes (e.g. from the peripheral blood of a normal individual) are added, some of the lymphocytes bind to the surface of the sensitised cells and bring about their destruction: this probably involves penetration of the target cell membrane by the lymphocyte (Reid *et al.*, 1979). The cytotoxic lymphocytes, sometimes called K cells (p. 6.33), do not have surface Ig, and so are not B lymphocytes: they may be a subset of T cells. The importance of this type of cell injury in man is not known, but there is evidence suggesting that it contributes to the destruction of tumour cells in experimental animals.

As noted above, the binding of antibody to surface constituents of cells may result in destrution of the target cells by complement or by phagocytes: their destruction by K cells is simply another effector mechanism of 'cytotoxic' antibody, and should not be regarded as a distinct type of hypersensitivity.

Immune-complex, Arthus-type (type 3) reactions

These result from formation of immune complexes by union of antigen with IgG or IgM antibody with consequent activation ('fixation') of complement. This leads, in turn, to acute inflammation with accumulation of polymorphs and aggregation of platelets. The polymorphs phagocytose the immune complexes and release lysosomal enzymes which cause tissue injury and aggravate the inflammatory response directly and by activating the kinin, clotting and plasmin systems (Fig. 4.21, p. 4.19). Depending on the distribution of antigen, the reaction may be *localised* to a particular tissue, and is then termed an Arthus reaction, or immune complexes may form in the blood, producing a *generalised* reaction commonly known as 'serum sickness' or circulating immune-complex disease.

The local or Arthus reaction

This was described in 1902 by Arthus, who injected rabbits repeatedly with horse serum. When the animals had developed high serum levels of antibodies to horse serum proteins, he noticed that a subcutaneous injection of horse serum induced a local acute inflammatory reaction, developing over a few hours and sometimes progressing to necrosis. It has since been shown that the reaction may be induced by local injection of a soluble antigen into various tissues in animals with a high level of the corresponding precipitating antibody in their blood. It can be induced also in animals immunised passively by intravenous injection of precipitating antibody (passive Arthus reaction). Localisation of the reaction depends on precipitation of the antigen in the tissues around the injection site, and thus on a high titre of precipitating antibody in the plasma.

Histological features. Microscopy of the Arthus reaction shows the typical changes of acute inflammation with congestion of small vessels, inflammatory exudation, and marked pavementing and emigration of neutrophil polymorphs. There may be aggregation of platelets in the small vessels and, depending on the severity, haemorrhages and thrombosis, and necrosis extending from the walls of small vessels to surrounding tissues.

Mechanism. Immunofluorescence techniques have demonstrated precipitates of antigen–antibody complexes in the lesion, particularly in the walls of venules. Fixed components of complement may also be detected in the precipitates. The Arthus reaction is largely suppressed in animals by depletion either of neutrophil polymorphs, e.g. by nitrogen mustard, or of complement, e.g. by cobra-venom factor; the intensity of the reaction is reduced by administration of corticosteroids. From such evidence, it has been deduced that the reaction is brought about as follows (see also Fig. 7.6). Immune complex formation and deposition in the walls of venules leads to activation of complement, the

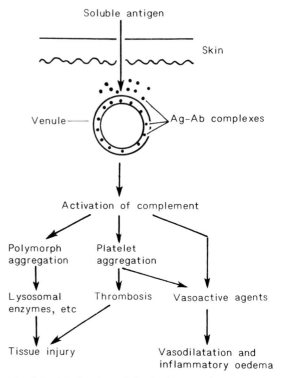

Fig. 7.6 Mechanism of the Arthus reaction.

products of which include **anaphylatoxins*** (C3a and C5a) which bring about acute inflammation both directly and by releasing histamine, etc., from mast cells. C5a, and possibly other complement products, are chemotactic for polymorphs, which consequently migrate into the vessel walls and surrounding tissues where they phagocytose the immune complexes. In so doing, they release lysosomal enzymes, including neutral proteases and cationic proteins which cause further tissue damage, digest proteins with production of kinins and other vaso-active peptides, and thus aggravate the inflammatory reaction. Platelet aggregation occurs in the damaged vessels and initiates thrombosis with consequent ischaemic necrosis.

The Arthus reaction in man was commonly seen in the days when crude preparations of horse antitoxic globulin or whole antitoxic serum was administered in the prevention and treatment of diphtheria, tetanus, etc. This resulted in the development of precipitating antibodies to horse proteins and a subsequent sub-

*The term *anaphylatoxin* is unfortunate, because products of complement fixation do not participate in classical anaphylaxis in man, which is due to IgE antibodies (p. 7.6).

cutaneous or intramuscular injection of horse globulin or serum elicited an Arthus reaction. More recently, it has been shown that the Arthus reaction is the basis of extrinsic allergic alveolitis, a good example of which is 'farmer's lung'. The farm worker inhales large numbers of the spores of bacteria growing in mouldy hay; bacterial antigen is absorbed via the alveolar walls and stimulates antibody production. Subsequent inhalation of the spores induces an acute Arthus reaction in the alveolar walls. Many farm workers develop precipitating antibody to the bacteria in mouldy hay and yet do not suffer from farmer's lung on subsequent exposure. The additional factors determining predisposition are not known, but there is some evidence suggesting that IgE antibody is also necessary, and that the Arthus reaction is triggered off by an initial atopic reaction which allows escape of antibodies of IgG class into the vessel walls. As in the rabbit, Arthus reactions in man are inhibited by administration of glucocorticoids.

Extrinsic allergic alveolitis also occurs in various occupations in which workers inhale dust containing proteins, fungi and other biological material (p. 16.62).

Circulating immune-complex disease: serum sickness

This occurs when antigen and antibody react in the plasma to form immune complexes which not only activate complement, neutrophil polymorphs and monocytes in the blood, but are also deposited in the walls of blood vessels, especially the glomerular capillaries, where they cause tissue damage.

Experimental basis. The basis of this form of hypersensitivity has been elucidated by Dixon, Cochrane and others (see Cochrane, 1973), mainly in rabbits. After a single injection of a large amount of antigen,, e.g. bovine serum albumin, no harmful effects occur until, after several days, antibody is produced. As it appears, it combines with antigen still present in the plasma, forming immune complexes. Initially antigen is present in relative excess and its union with antibody produces small soluble complexes (Fig. 6.4, p. 6.9) which are not readily phagocytosed and so persist in the circulation. As antibody increases, intermediate-

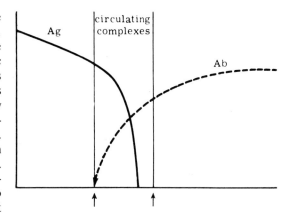

Fig. 7.7 The formation of antigen–antibody complexes in the circulation. Injection of antigen is followed after some days by the appearance of antibody in the plasma: during the next few days, the concentration of antigen falls sharply and antigen antibody complexes are present in the plasma.

sized soluble, and then large insoluble complexes are formed, and after a few days free antibody can be detected. Large aggregates of immune complex are rapidly taken up and destroyed by phagocytic leucocytes and by macrophages in the liver, spleen, etc. Accordingly, in a rabbit producing a lot of precipitating antibody, complexes disappear from the plasma in a few days (Fig. 7.7). During this period, however, in which soluble complexes formed in antigen excess are present in the circulation, their presence triggers off a series of reactions leading to release of histamine and other vasoactive agents, with consequent increase in vascular permeability. This in turn allows the soluble complexes, along with plasma proteins, to leak out between the endothelial cells of various blood vessels. At the sites of leakage, complexes are trapped and accumulate between the endothelium and basement membrane, where their presence results in vascular injury.

The mechanism of increase in vascular permeability, as in inflammation, is complicated, and varies in different species. In the rabbit, in which most of the reservoir of histamine in the blood is in the platelets, histamine release appears to be due mainly to union of antigen with IgE antibody bound to basophil leucocytes (i.e. a type 1 hypersensitivity reaction); this induces release of a platelet activating factor which causes the platelets to aggregate and discharge their histamine. Other mechanisms of release of histamine from platelets involve activation of complement by the complexes and participation of neutrophil polymorphs. Intravascular pressure is also important, for it provides the force which allows fluid to escape and so drives protein molecules through the endothelial 'gaps' which account for increased vascular permeability (p. 4.8).

In the experiment described above, in which rabbits are given a single injection of an antigen, immune complexes in the blood are deposited beneath the vascular endothelium, particularly in the glomerular capillaries, the small vessels in the joints, skin and the endocardium, and focally in various arteries. The deposited complexes continue to fix complement, and, except in the glomeruli, this triggers off an Arthus-type reaction, with acute inflammation, infiltration of polymorphs, and sometimes thrombosis and necrosis. The reaction is particularly intense in the arterial lesions, which may extend to involve the whole thickness of the wall. Activation of complement and polymorphs results in phagocytosis of the deposited complexes within 48 hours, so that, although intense, the reaction is brief. Like the local Arthus reaction, it can be suppressed by prior depletion of polymorphs or complement. In the glomeruli, complexes deposited within or on the epithelial side of the capillary basement membrane fix complement, and yet inflammation is relatively mild and polymorphs are scanty; an obvious explanation is the one-way flow of filtrate from the capillary lumen to the urinary space, which presumably washes away the anaphylatoxins and chemotaxins produced by complement activation. Complexes persist in the glomeruli for many days, and cause glomerular injury by some unexplained mechanism, with resultant proteinuria.

Chronic immune-complex disease can be produced in rabbits by giving daily intravenous injections of soluble antigen in amounts sufficient to provide a period of relative antigen excess over antibody in the plasma after each injection. In contrast to acute serum sickness, the complexes are deposited solely in the glomerular capillaries, where they give rise to lesions resembling various forms of progressive glomerulonephritis in man. Deposition of immune complexes is also influenced by the nature of the antigen and quality of the antibody. Unless there is gross antigen excess, precipitating antibody forms large insoluble complexes which, as stated above, are rapidly phagocytosed and cause little or no injury, so that antigen excess is necessary for formation of smaller, pathogenic complexes. Antibodies which can only react with very few determinant sites on the antigen molecule and have poor avidity (p. 6.7) also form pathogenic soluble complexes, even when the antibody is present in relative excess.

Circulating immune-complex disease in man results from injection of heterologous immunoglobulin (now an uncommon cause) and administration of potentially haptenic drugs. It also occurs naturally in systemic lupus erythematosus, in which auto-immune complexes are formed, and in various infections. The formation of immune complexes in the blood may induce a *general reaction*, and also lesions in the glomeruli and elsewhere resulting from *deposition of immune complexes in the walls of blood vessels.*

The acute generalised reaction. In its extreme form, for example when a large amount of foreign protein is injected into an individual with a high titre of the corresponding antibody in the plasma, the rapid formation of high concentrations of immune complexes in the plasma may induce a rapid collapse: this is attributable to intense activation of complement, release of polymorph lysosomal enzymes, etc., and activation of platelets and of the kinin, clotting and plasmin systems. The clinical features are similar to those of anaphylactic shock (p. 7.6). When a foreign protein is injected for the first time, classical serum sickness may develop 7–10 days later, i.e. when production of antibody results in the formation of immune complexes in the plasma. It is a short febrile illness characterised by intense itching of the skin and urticaria, swelling of peripheral joints, enlargement of lymph nodes and proteinuria. Histamine antagonists bring partial relief. Examination of the serum reveals abnormally low levels of complement components and the presence of products of complement activation. Immune complexes are also demonstrable, although the available techniques are not entirely satisfactory. The neutrophil polymorph count is at first low, but later raised. After recovery, free antibody appears in the serum. These features indicate that immune complexes form in the blood, activate complement, and trigger off the release of vaso-active agents, including histamine from basophil leucocytes. Ingestion of complexes by neurotrophils and monocytes is accompanied by secretion of lysosomal enzymes, etc. Phagocytosis of circulating complexes probably results in degeneration and disappearance of most of the polymorphs, and also in the release of endogenous pyrogen (interleukin 1) from monocytes, and thus the development of fever (p. 8.20).

The mechanism of release of histamine, etc. involves the anaphylatoxins of complement, release of polymorph lysosomes, activation of Hageman factor and production of kinins. Bronchospasm and occasionally severe circulatory collapse may be due partly to involvement of IgE-sensitised mast cells and basophils, as in the rabbit, while disseminated intravascular coagulation (p. 10.11) may result from activation of the clotting system.

The typical attack of serum sickness which followed injection of crude antisera is now uncommon, but similar reactions can follow administration of drugs which confer antigenicity to plasma proteins. The severe form of dengue, *dengue haemorrhagic fever* or *dengue shock syndrome*, is believed to result from a second infection in a child who has already developed antibodies to the virus. It is postulated that the second infection is caused by another strain of the virus and that the circulating antibody can cross-react with the virus without neutralising it, In consequence, viral antigen-antibody complexes are formed in the circulation, resulting in shock and thrombocytopenia with mucosal haemorrhages. If this explanation is correct, it carries the implication that dengue virus vaccines may predispose to this serious form of the disease. In spirochaetal infections, including syphilis, and in lepromatous leprosy and some other chronic bacterial infections, the first dose of treatment by an effective drug may kill very large numbers of micro-organisms and so release microbial antigen, which, depending on the level of circulating antibody and the amount of antigen released, either forms complexes in the blood or induces local Arthus reactions in the lesions. The features of the reaction (*the Jarisch–Herxheimer reaction*) suggest that both phenomena may occur.

Immune-complex deposition is an important cause of glomerulonephritis in man. The typical acute glomerulonephritis following a streptococcal throat infection resembles that of acute serum sickness in the rabbit. It develops when antibody to streptococcal antigen enters the blood and immune complexes are formed and deposited in the glomerular capillaries. Other infections and drug hypersensitivities can have the same effect, and more chronic glomerular injury occurs from prolonged or intermittent immune-complex formation in quartan malaria, lepromatous leprosy and some other chronic infections. In systemic lupus erythematosus, auto-antibodies develop which react with various cellular constituents, e.g. DNA, and complexes formed in the blood are deposited in small vessels in the skin, glomeruli and elsewhere. In most types of human immune-complex glomerulonephritis, however, the nature of the antigen is unknown: the various patterns of disease depend partly on the size of the circulating complexes and the duration and rate of their deposition, and there is also evidence that antigen may be deposited in the glomerular capillary walls, followed by the binding of circulating antibody to form complexes. It is not clear why glomerular capillaries are unduly susceptible to deposition of circulating antigens and immune complexes. Part of the explanation lies in the unusually high pressure of the blood within them. Their endothelium is fenestrated (p. 4.6) and thus differs structurally from vessels in the dermis and muscles, in which tissues most of the work on mediators of increased vascular permeability has been conducted.

Arterial lesions due to deposition of complexes are less common in man, and their nature is usually difficult to prove because, as in the rabbit, the immune complexes are phagocytosed rapidly by polymorphs. Nevertheless, the focal lesions of polyarteritis nodosa and some other forms of arteritis appear to be of this nature, and surface antigen of the hepatitis B virus has been implicated in some cases.

In many patients with immune complex disease, IgM antibodies develop which are capable of reacting with the Fc component of IgG. These '*rheumatoid factors*' react most avidly with the IgG which has already reacted with antigen and so is in the form of immune complexes. The binding of rheumatoid factors may cause circulatory disturbances by increasing the viscosity of the blood, or aggravate the injury caused by deposited immune complexes. The IgM–IgG complexes often precipitate in cooled serum, and are then termed *cryoglobulins*.

The lesions produced by immune complex deposition in the kidneys and elsewhere are described in more detail in the appropriate chapters.

Delayed hypersensitivity (DHS or type 4) reactions

Antibody production and cell-mediated immunity are both parts of the normal immune response to most antigens. The union of antibodies with antigens can result in the hypersensitivity reactions described above. Delayed hypersensitivity (DHS) does not involve antibody, but is mediated by the specifically-primed T lymphocytes produced in the cell-mediated immune response. By means of their specific surface receptors., these cells can bind to the antigen which has stimulated their production, and this results in tissue injury characterised by a slowly developing inflammatory reaction—hence *delayed* hypersensitivity.

The reaction of primed T lymphocytes with microbial antigens is an essential defence mechanism against many pathogenic bacteria, viruses and fungi, etc.: the DHS reaction promotes their destruction, and the accompanying tissue injury is the price which must be paid for this protection. Cell-mediated immunity to tumour-cell antigens is known to develop in some cancer patients, and is being intensively investigated in the hope that it may be utilised for the effective destruction of tumours by DHS reactions. So far, however, clinical results have been disappointing.

Cell-mediated immunity develops also against harmless foreign antigens, body constituents modified by foreign haptens, transplanted allogeneic cells or tissues, and sometimes even against the individual's own apparently normal tissue cells. In these circumstances, unwanted DHS reactions occur, resulting respectively in contact dermatitis, rejection of transplants, and auto-immune disease.

Strong cell-mediated immunity is induced experimentally by injection of antigen incorporated in complete Freund's adjuvant (p. 6.30), and a DHS reaction may then be induced by intradermal injection of the antigen. Immunising injections of the antigen alone or in incomplete Freund's adjuvant (i.e. lacking acid-fast bacilli) induces a weaker cell-mediated response, and intradermal antigen challenge then induces a briefer and milder inflammatory reaction, termed the *Jones-Mote* or *cutaneous basophil hypersensitivity reaction* (p. 7.22).

Morphological features

The DHS reaction can occur in any part of the body where primed T lymphocytes encounter the corresponding antigen. Its induction in the skin is used as a test for cell-mediated immunity to various antigens, the classical example being **the tuberculin reaction** in which a small amount of tuberculoprotein ('purified protein derivative' or PPD) is applied to the skin or injected intradermally as in the Mantoux test. This has no effect in non-immune individuals, but in subjects who have developed cell-mediated immunity to tuberculoprotein as a result of tuberculosis or immunisation with BCG (attenuated *Mycobacterium bovis*) the typical delayed inflammatory reaction appears in 12–24 hours and persists for 48 hours or more. The skin becomes reddened and a firm central nodule appears. In a highly sensitised individual, necrosis and ulceration may follow.

Microscopically, the features are microvascular congestion, accumulation of lymphocytes in and around small vessels, and swelling of the collagen due to inflammatory oedema. At the height of the reaction there is intense infiltration with lymphocytes and occasional macrophages, both in and around the capillaries and venules, particularly round the sweat glands and hair follicles (Fig. 7.8). There may also be transient accumulation of small numbers of neutrophil polymorphs. These are the features of the DHS reaction to a soluble protein in man. In animals, accumulation of polymorphs and macrophages, in addition to lymphocytes, is much more prominent. The morphological features of DHS reactions in infections are complicated by the injuries inflicted directly by the micro-organisms or their toxins and by other types of hypersensitivity reactions. A glance at the microscopic appearances of various inflammatory lesions in which DHS is a prominent feature will show considerable differences (e.g. tuberculosis, p. 9.17, tuberculoid leprosy, p. 9.25; typhoid fever, p. 3.31, and contact dermatitis, p. 7.23). In general, infiltration with macrophages, lymphocytes and lymphoblasts is prominent. The macrophages may also change to epithelioid cells, fuse to form giant cells and undergo necrosis.

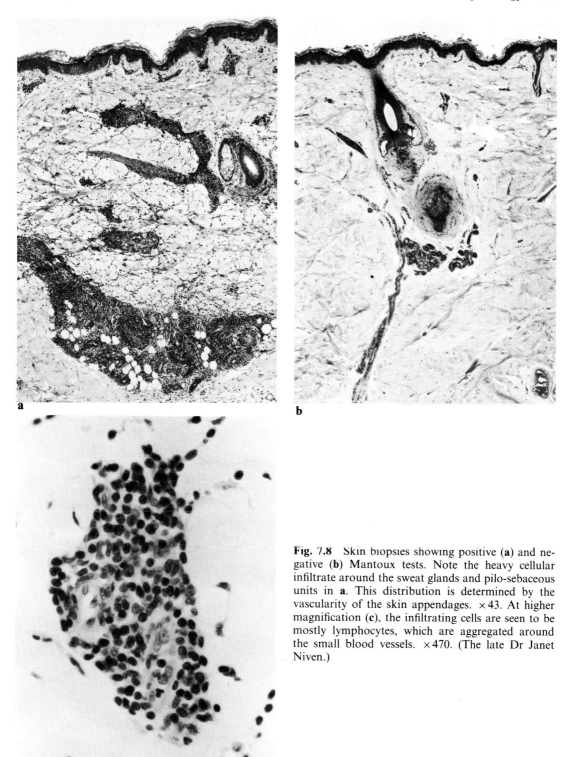

Fig. 7.8 Skin biopsies showing positive (**a**) and negative (**b**) Mantoux tests. Note the heavy cellular infiltrate around the sweat glands and pilo-sebaceous units in **a**. This distribution is determined by the vascularity of the skin appendages. × 43. At higher magnification (**c**), the infiltrating cells are seen to be mostly lymphocytes, which are aggregated around the small blood vessels. × 470. (The late Dr Janet Niven.)

The mechanism of DHS reactions

DHS reactions occur when specifically-primed T lymphocytes (mainly memory T lymphocytes) encounter antigen with which they can react. For this to occur in the tissues, specifically responsive T lymphocytes must leave the blood in the vicinity of the antigen, and the factors involved in such emigration are largely unknown.

There is no evidence to suggest that soluble antigen is chemotactic to specifically responsive lymphocytes. In animal experiments involving passive transfer of radio-labelled lymphocytes, it has been shown that the lymphocytes which aggregate at the site of a delayed hypersensitivity reaction are recently-divided cells and premitotic immunoblasts. In these experiments, it was also shown that only a small proportion of the cells accumulating at the test site were specifically primed to the antigen. It still remains undecided whether specifically-primed T lymphocytes are attracted preferentially to the antigen site, or whether a DHS reaction is initiated by a small number of specifically primed T memory cells which encounter the site of antigen by chance during their random recirculation through various tissues (p. 6.33).

The T-cell surface antigen receptors are more complex than the Ig type of receptor on B cells, and *most T cells will react with the corresponding antigen only when it is presented in association with HLA molecules on the surface of antigen-presenting cells: they do not react with free antigen*. This has important implications for T-cell immune responses, which have already been discussed (p. 6.22). It also means that the primed T cells induced by an immune response are mainly concerned with defence against intracellular micro-organisms, namely viruses and some fungi, bacteria and protozoa. Following phagocytosis by macrophages, such micro-organisms may resist killing and may even multiply within macrophages (p. 8.12). When this happens, their persistence is reflected in the development of microbial antigens in association with HLA molecules on the surface of the infected macrophages.

As noted on p. 6.21, there are at least three different types of T cells—helper, suppressor and cytotoxic cells. Primed helper T cells recognise antigen expressed on cell surfaces in association with class II HLA molecules, and

as the latter are expressed on macrophages, helper T cells can react with infected macrophages. This reaction results in blast transformation and proliferation of helper T cells and stimulates them to secrete an antigen-specific factor which in turn stimulates cytotoxic and suppressor T cells. The transformed helper cells also secrete interleukin 2 and proteins termed lymphokines which are responsible for most of the features of the DHS reaction (see below). The stimulated cytotoxic T cells recognise antigen in association with class I HLA molecules on cell surfaces, and since these are expressed on virtually all cell types, cytotoxic T cells can attack viral-infected cells of any type: the mechanism by which they kill the infected cells is not known, but having killed one cell, the cytotoxic cell can then attach to and kill others. When viruses enter cells, their antigens are incorporated into the cell surface and the cell thus becomes susceptible to killing by cytotoxic T cells even before the virus has had time to replicate within it. Since macrophages also express class I HLA molecules on their surface, macrophages infected with bacteria or fungi are killed by cytotoxic T cells, but this may result in release of the live micro-organisms and may thus not help to eliminate the infection. Activation of macrophages by lymphokines does, however, increase their capacity to kill ingested micro-organisms (see below).

Some suppressor T cells appear to be capable of recognising antigen alone, while others recognise antigen only in association with class II HLA antigens. With the help of transformed helper T cells, they suppress both helper and cytotoxic T cells by secreting antigen-specific suppressor factors and thus help to regulate both T and B cell immune responses and DHS reactions.

As noted above, DHS reactions can be induced by intradermal injection of a soluble antigen to which the individual has developed cell-mediated immunity, the classical example being the tuberculin reaction. In view of the apparent inability of helper and cytotoxic T lymphocytes to respond to antigens in the free state, it must be assumed that tuberculoprotein and other free antigens become bound to the surface of macrophages or tissue histiocytes, possibly in the form of antigen-antibody complexes which adhere to the macrophage Fc receptors, or by expression on the cell surface of phagocytosed antigen. It may also be that Langerhans cells (p. 6.36) can act locally as antigen-presenting cells.

Lymphokines. As noted above, most T lymphocytes react with the corresponding antigen on the surface of antigen-presenting cells. When helper cells react thus, they secrete lymphokines (Fig. 8.2, p. 8.10) which are proteins or glycoproteins of molecular weight 8000–20 000. The reaction may conveniently be elicited by adding antigen to a suspension of lymphocytes and macrophages and examining the supernate for lymphokines by a combination of *in-vitro* and *in-vivo* tests. Transformation to lymphoblasts and proliferation and secretion of lymphokines can also be induced by adding certain plant mitogens, e.g. PHA, to T lymphocytes (p. 6.32). By such means, the following properties of lymphokines have been demonstrated.

1. Induction of acute inflammation. Intradermal injection demonstrates a factor (inappropriately termed *skin reactive factor*) which induces congestion of small blood vessels and inflammatory oedema. This could account for these features in the DHS reaction.

2. Effects on mononuclear phagocytes. These are complex, but there is evidence for the following.

(*a*) *A chemotactic factor.* This induces chemotaxis of monocytes or macrophages *in vitro* and emigration of monocytes *in vivo*: it may account for accumulation of macrophages in DHS reactions.

(*b*) *A migration inhibition factor*, demonstrable by its inhibitory effect on the migration of macrophages, e.g. from the open end of a horizontal capillary tube. When the tube is immersed in tissue culture fluid, addition of this factor to the fluid inhibits migration. Secretion of the factor *in vitro* provides the basis for a test of cell-mediated immunity (p. 6.24). It may also play a role in the accumulation of macrophages in DHS reactions.

(*c*) *A macrophage activating factor*, which increases the metabolic activity of macrophages and enhances their mobility and capacity to phagocytose and kill micro-organisms. This microbicidal effect has been demonstrated *in vitro* and *in vivo*.

(*d*) *A specific macrophage-arming factor* (*SMAF*) has been demonstrated in experimentally-induced cell-mediated immunity to tumour cells. The DHS reaction between primed T cells and tumour cells releases a factor which confers on macrophages enhanced killing properties specific for the tumour cells. This factor differs from (*c*) above in that it is antigen-specific.

3. Other factors. Another factor released when primed T cells react with antigen is termed *lymphotoxin*. It is cytotoxic for tissue cells, and may contribute to the necrosis commonly seen in DHS reactions. This is distinct from the antigen-specific killing of target cells by cytotoxic T lymphocytes mentioned above, which requires close contact.

Interleukin 2 (IL-2) is secreted by antigen-stimulated helper T cells. It is also called *T-cell growth factor* and acts synergistically with antigenic stimulation on cytotoxic T cells, inducing proliferation and thus promoting the destruction of infected cells. Other lymphokines are chemotactic for lymphocytes and this may explain why so many of the lymphocytes in DHS reactions are not specifically primed to react with the antigen which has induced the reaction (see above).

Characterisation of these T-cell products is still at an early stage. Their importance as mediators of the changes seen in DHS reactions is suggested by their detection not only in reactions in test tubes, but also in extracts of DHS reaction sites.

Factors secreted by macrophages (Monokines). As in inflammatory lesions in general, activated macrophages in DHS reactions are capable of synthesising and secreting a large number of biologically-active substances. The known number exceeds fifty, and they include numerous lysosomal enzymes, prostaglandins, leukotrienes, platelet activating factor, complement components, cytotoxins, and factors which affect the proliferative activity of lymphocytes and fibroblasts and the formation of new blood vessels (angiogenic factor). Obviously, we are facing a situation in which, as in acute inflammation in general, there is a superabundance of potential mediators, the individual significance of which is not yet clear. However, one macrophage product, **interleukin 1**, is known to be important: not only does it act on the thermoregulatory centre to induce fever (p. 8.20) and promote increased production of acute phase proteins in the liver (p. 8.14), but it also enhances proliferation of antigen-stimulated T cells and thus amplifies immune responses and DHS reactions (p. 6.27). It also promotes differentiation of antigen-stimulated B cells.

Man and other primates show, in general, much stronger cell-mediated immune responses and DHS reactions than do lower animals. It is therefore unwise to assume that the findings for guinea-pigs, etc., are applicable to man. Lawrence's transfer factor (p. 6.24) may be important in cellular immunity and DHS reactions in man, although its nature is unknown and its role is controversial.

Until a few years ago, it was widely assumed that the presence of lymphocytes in a hypersensitivity reaction was a good indication of a DHS component, but B lymphocytes can and do migrate into sites of antigen (hence the presence of plasma cells in many infections): also it is now known that so-called K cells (p. 7.13), which have the appearances of small lymphocytes, may bind by surface Fc receptors to target cells sensitised with IgG class antibody and bring about their destruction. The *in-vivo* significance of this co-operative cytotoxic effect of antibody and K lymphocytes is not yet known. The presence of macrophages in hypersensitivity reactions is also not necessarily indicative of DHS, for they are attracted also by antigen-antibody complexes and by non-antigenic foreign and endogenous material (p. 4.35).

The Jones-Mote or cutaneous basophil hypersensitivity reaction is an inflammatory reaction developing after intradermal injection of antigen, and is seen in animals which have developed both antibody and weak cell-mediated immunity to the antigen. The reaction is characterised by developing and subsiding more rapidly than a typical DHS reaction, and by the accumulation of large numbers of basophil leucocytes in addition to lymphocytes and macrophages. It appears to be a combination of a weak DHS reaction and an immune-complex reaction, although the emigration of basophils has not been explained. The major known importance of this type of reaction lies in the danger of confusing it with an Arthus-type or a DHS reaction.

Systemic effects of DHS reactions

Although this account has concentrated on local DHS reactions, systemic reactions also occur. For example, injection of relatively large amounts of tuberculoprotein into an individual who has developed cell-mediated immunity to it results not only in a severe localised DHS reaction at the injection site but also fever, malaise, increase in acute phase proteins (p. 8.14) and a reduction in circulating lymphocytes. If the individual has active tuberculosis, the DHS reaction of the lesion is also aggravated, with extension of necrosis. These effects are known collectively as the *Koch phenomenon* after Robert Koch, the German bacteriologist who, in 1882, discovered the tubercle bacillus and showed it to be the cause of tuberculosis. They are probably attributable to the release of interleukin 1 by lymphokine-activated macrophages and also by necrosis of macrophages and tissue cells. The Koch phenomenon is not observed in individuals who have not developed cell-mediated immunity to tuberculoprotein.

Hypersensitivity to drugs and chemicals

Most drugs and chemicals which cause hypersensitivity reactions do so because they or their metabolic products combine with host proteins and act as haptens. At first sight, this seems to contradict the observation that haptens can only stimulate an immune response when combined with *foreign* carrier proteins to which the recipient develops cell-mediated immunity (p. 6.24). The explanation is that the many drugs and chemicals which cause hypersensitivity reactions not only act as haptens, but alter the configuration of the protein molecules with which they combine, thus rendering them 'foreign'.

The type of hypersensitivity reaction which results will then depend on the nature of the immune response, the particular cell or tissue constituent with which the hapten has complexed, the route of administration and dose, etc. In individuals with a tendency to atopy, reaginic antibodies may develop, and further administration of the hapten can then induce a **type 1 reaction**, e.g. asthma or hay fever if the hapten is inhaled as a vapour or airborne suspension, an immediate inflammatory reaction if it is applied locally, or a generalised anaphylactic reaction if a large amount of hapten is absorbed by any route. Anaphylactic reactions to penicillin and related compounds are not uncommon, and have resulted in a number of deaths: in most instances the hypersensitivity is directed towards the penicilloyl degradation product of penicillin. The development of IgG class antibody to a haptenic drug or chemical can give rise to **local reactions of Arthus type (type 3)** when the hapten is localised to one particular area within the tissues, or can lead to formation of complexes of hapten and antibody within the plasma, with the risk of circulating immune-complex disease (p. 7.16).

A number of drugs which act as haptens stimulate the production of antibodies which, although not cytotoxic, can bring about destruction of red cells, leucocytes or platelets. For reasons unknown, complexes of these drugs with antibody bind to cells of the blood, and although such binding is often loose, activation of complement by the drug-antibody complex results in lysis of the cell—'bystander' or 'reactive' cytolysis. The binding of immune complexes and complement components also promotes phagocytosis of the cells in the spleen. Drugs which form complexes with these effects include sulphonamides, phenacetin, chlorpromazine and rifampicin, but the list is long and differs for red cells, leucocytes and platelets.

Thirdly, binding of a haptenic drug or drug metabolite to red cells, leucocytes or platelets may render the cells susceptible to injury by antibody to the drug—**cytotoxic (type 2) antibody reaction** (p. 7.11). It is not known whether tissue cells are injured in this way.

Lastly, cell-mediated immunity may develop towards the hapten–protein complex, and, as described above, subsequent absorption of the haptenic compound gives rise to a **delayed hypersensitivity (type 4)** reaction. This is seen in **contact dermatitis** in which relatively simple chemicals behave as haptens; they are absorbed into the body, often through the skin, and combine with tissue proteins. Perhaps because of the antigen-presenting function of Langerhans cells (p. 6.27), the modified protein in the skin stimulates a strong cell-mediated immune response, and subsequent skin contact with the same chemical induces a delayed hypersensitivity reaction (Fig. 7.9), causing inflammatory lesions with cellular infiltration, predominantly lymphocytic, and oedema which affects both the dermis and epidermis and progresses to formation of vesicles. Very many substances can induce contact dermatitis, particularly chemicals which combine firmly with proteins, e.g. dyes, chrome salts, formalin and various der-

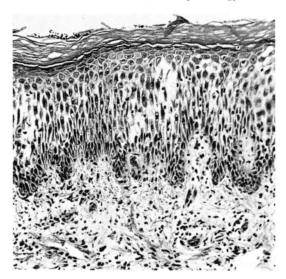

7.9 Contact dermatitis. Note oedema of epidermis and perivascular infiltration of lymphocytes in the dermis. The patient had developed hypersensitivity to chromium salts used as a hardener in cement. × 110.

ivatives of benzene. Reactions of this type occur commonly in women in relation to nickel fasteners on underclothes, some of the nickel being dissolved by acid sweat and absorbed as nickel salts which can combine with skin proteins. Contact with some plants, e.g. poison ivy and primulas, is another common cause, and cases also occur from the use of hair dyes, such as paraphenylene diamine, which, of course, bind firmly to keratin. Contact dermatitis results also from application of various medicaments to the skin. It is noteworthy that any individual can be sensitised to various chemicals, and contact dermatitis can thus be induced, but nevertheless some people appear to develop it more readily than others. This is seen in the use of various adhesive surgical dressings which usually produce no reaction but in some instances lead to contact dermatitis, and a similar effect may result from wearing rubber face masks.

It is important to appreciate that the above account is an oversimplification. In many instances, hypersensitivity to drugs or chemicals is extremely complex and the clinical features often conflict with the results of the various available tests for hypersensitivity. With the ever-increasing number of chemicals used therapeutically and in industry, it is not surprising that hypersensitivity reactions, particularly those manifested in the skin and mucous membranes, are becoming increasingly common. Apart from the possession of highly reactive groups by which they can bind to proteins, it is not yet known what properties of a substance are related to the likelihood of its stimulating the development of hypersensitivity. Individuals predisposed to atopy and patients with systemic lupus erythematosus are prone to develop drug hypersensitivities, but, apart from this, predisposition to drug reactions is quite unpredictable.

Auto-immunity and auto-immune diseases

Some confusion exists over the definitions of auto-antibodies and auto-immune diseases. *Auto-antibodies may be defined as antibodies which react with the individual's own normal body constituents* (which may accordingly be termed **auto-antigens**). This definition excludes antibodies which react only with body constituents which have been altered, for example by a haptenic drug, and so have become 'foreign' to the individual (see above). The definition does not, however, assume that normal body constituents have necessarily stimulated the production of the auto-antibodies. For example, *Streptococus pyogenes* possesses antigens similar to constituents of human myocardium and a streptococcal pharyngitis can induce antibodies which react with normal myocardium (p. 15.25): these qualify as auto-antibodies. Within this definition, *auto-antibodies to several cell products or constituents are quite commonly present in the serum of individuals both with and without clinical evidence of disease*: they include, for example, antibodies to thyroglobulin, to thyroid epithelial cells, to gastric parietal cells and to the deoxyribonucleoprotein of cell nuclei. These antibodies all react *in vitro* with the individual's own body constituents and with those obtained from others, so that they are acceptable as true auto-antibodies.

Although auto-immunisation occurs without clinical disease, it is strongly associated with a number of diseases. For example, most apparently normal individuals with thyroid auto-antibodies have been shown to have sub-clinical chronic thyroiditis, and patients with more severe, clinically apparent chronic thyroiditis usually have high titres of thyroid antibodies. Similarly, high titres of antibodies to deoxyribonucleoprotein occur especially in patients with the connective tissue diseases, and particularly in systemic lupus erythematosus.

Cell-mediated auto-immunity has also been demonstrated by in vitro tests in some diseases. For example, thyroid auto-antigens inhibit the migration of leucocytes (p. 6.24) of patients with chronic thyroiditis.

It is thus apparent that, in some diseases, there is evidence of auto-immunisation against particular body consituents. These are the so-called **auto-immune diseases**. In most, it has still not been proved that the lesions are due to immunological reactions against the target auto-antigens; in some instances this probability is supported by production of similar lesions by auto-immunisation of animals, or by investigations on naturally-occurring auto-immune diseases in inbred strains of animals.

There are also a number of examples in which auto-antibodies develop as a *result* of tissue injury and appear to be without pathogenic effect, an example being auto-antibodies to myocardial cells, which frequently develop following ischaemic necrosis of the myocardium: presumably antigen is released by the dead muscle cells and stimulates an immune response.

Auto-immune diseases may be classified into: (1) a group of organ-specific diseases affecting glandular tissues; (2) systemic lupus erythematosus and possibly the other connective tissue diseases; and (3) a number of miscellaneous diseases which do not fit readily into either of the above classes.

The organ-specific auto-immune diseases

These are characterised by chronic inflammatory destruction of a particular glandular tissue accompanied by the presence in the plasma of auto-antibodies which react specifically with normal cellular components of the target tissue. The tissues which may be affected include the thyroid, gastric mucosa, adrenal cortex, parathyroid glands and cells of the pancreatic islets of Langerhans. The main features are exemplified by **chronic auto-immune thyroiditis**, in which infiltration of the thyroid gland by lymphocytes, plasma cells and macrophages is accompanied by glandular epithelial destruction and fibrosis (Figs. 26.12–14, p. 26.20). These changes may be focal and are then sub-clinical and usually non-progressive, or they may be diffuse, giving rise to either thyroid enlargement (*Hashimoto's thyroiditis*), sometimes with hypofunction, or destruction and shrinkage of the gland with gross hypofunction (*primary hypothyroidism*). Auto-antibodies to normal thyroid constituents are detectable in the serum in virtually all cases of Hashimoto's thyroiditis and primary hypothyroidism and in most people with sub-clinical focal thyroiditis. They include antibodies reactive with: (1) thyroglobulin, often in sufficient concentration to give a precipitin reaction (Fig. 6.5, p. 6.9); (2) a second constituent of thyroid colloid; and (3) cell membrane constituents ('microsomes') of thyroid epithelium—the so-called thyroid microsomal antibody (Fig. 6.9, p. 6.11). Chronic thyroiditis occurs much more often in women than in men, and the incidence increases with age. Over 10% of middle-aged or elderly women have one or more thyroid antibodies and some degree of chronic thyroiditis. There is a general correlation between the presence and titres of the serum antibodies and the extensiveness and activity of the thyroiditis, but the correlation is by no means exact for any one antibody or any combination of antibodies.

A fourth thyroid auto-antibody reacts with the TSH receptors on the thyroid epithelial cells. It may have the same effect as TSH, and is the cause of thyroid hyperfunction in Graves' disease. Auto-antibody which blocks the TSH receptor without stimulating the cell has been demonstrated in patients with primary hypothyroidism and may explain why there is little or no regeneration of follicular tissue in this disease, as compared with Hashimoto's thyroiditis, in which the gland is enlarged.

Chronic auto-immune gastritis, affecting the acid-secreting mucosa of the gastric fundus, has many points of resemblance to chronic thyroiditis. It affects women more often than men, and the incidence increases with age. In most cases, the serum contains 'microsomal' antibody to gastric parietal cells and, in a minority of cases, antibodies to the intrinsic factor which is essential to absorption of vitamin B_{12}. The affected mucosa is infiltrated with lymphocytes, plasma cells and macrophages, and all grades of destruction of chief and parietal cells are observed. In most cases, the gastritis is mild and sub-clinical, and progresses very slowly, but in some cases it progresses more rapidly to diffuse atrophy of the mucosa (like the thyroid in primary hypothyroidism) and parietal cell deficiency then results in achlorhydria and lack of intrinsic factor, the latter leading in some cases to B_{12} deficiency and pernicious anaemia.

Auto-immune adrenalitis is a much less common condition; it is, however, the major cause of adrenal cortical atrophy and functional deficiency (Addison's disease). The serum commonly contains auto-antibody to a cell-membrane ('microsomal') constituent of adrenocortical epithelium. **Primary hypoparathyroidism** is rare: specific auto-antibodies are demonstrable in the serum in some cases, and the parathyroid glands are shrunken and extremely difficult to find at autopsy.

In addition to their morphological and serological similarities, each of these diseases tends to have a high familial incidence, and moreover the diseases tend to occur in association, both within affected families and in individuals. For example, patients with Hashimoto's thyroiditis have a high incidence of gastric antibody and a particular tendency to develop pernicious anaemia, while thyroid and gastric antibodies, sometimes associated with the corresponding clinical diseases, are unduly common in patients with auto-immune Addison's disease or primary hypoparathyroidism: even these two latter rare diseases have been found to be particularly associated with one another.

Insulin-dependent type (type I) diabetes differs from the other organ-specific auto-immune diseases in affecting mainly children and young adults, and there is evidence suggesting that it may be initiated by a viral infection. Auto-antibodies to cells of the islets of Langerhans are detectable in the serum in nearly all early cases, and in family studies their appearance has been shown to precede the onset of diabetes by months or even years. The islets at first show lymphocytic infiltration (Fig. 20.70, p. 20.63) and later become atrophic.

Pathogenesis. It has not been proved that these diseases are the result of autohypersensitivity reactions, an alternative explanation being that the glandular destruction is due to some other (unknown) agent, and that auto-

antibodies develop as a secondary phenomenon. In favour of an auto-immune pathogenesis, auto-antibodies do not, in general, result
from destruction of tissue. For example,
thyroid injury by large doses of radio-iodine or
viral thyroiditis does not initiate the production
of thyroid antibodies, although if antibodies are
aready present their titres increase a little; nor
does recurrent alcoholic gastritis result in gastric antibodies. Secondly, organ-specific lesions
resembling those of the human diseases, but
usually reversible, can be induced experimentally in animals by injections of homogenates of
the organ (e.g. thyroid or adrenal) incorporated
in Freund's adjuvant. The adjuvant enhances
immune responses, particularly those dependent on T lymphocytes (p. 6.30) and passive
transfer of lymphocytes and antibody suggest
that cell-mediated immunity is a more important cause of tissue injury than auto-antibodies
in these experimental conditions. There are,
however, exceptions, one being the chronic thyroiditis which develops spontaneously in an
inbred obese strain of chickens: it is accompanied by thyroid auto-antibodies and is more
severe in chickens rendered deficient in T cells
by thymectomy after hatching, but is prevented
by depriving the birds of B cells by early bursectomy (p. 6.14). The same results apply to
artificially-induced auto-immune thyroiditis in
ordinary chickens.

In man, the pathogenic significance of auto-
antibodies and cell-mediated immunity in the
organ-specific auto-immune diseases is not
known. It is noteworthy that in the two
examples of diseases in which the function of
tissue cells are known to be affected by auto-
antibodies (thyrotoxicosis and myasthenia
gravis—p. 7.13), the antigen is a receptor projecting from the surface of the target cell. Thyroid microsomal antibody has been shown, in
the presence of complement, to be cytotoxic for
thyroid epithelial cells in culture, but only if the
cells are first treated with trypsin, and it may
be that such treatment is necessary to expose
cell-membrane auto-antigen. There is no evidence of thyroid injury in the infants of mothers with Hashimoto's thyroiditis although in
some cases high concentrations of thyroid antibodies of IgG class are transferred to the fetal
circulation.

It is difficult to investigate the pathogenic
role of cell-mediated auto-immunity in man, for
while macrophage migration inhibition tests
(p. 6.24) suggest that this develops, it does not
necessarily follow that the tissue destruction
results from delayed hypersensitivity reactions.
The lesions are typically infiltrated with lymphocytes, which suggests a delayed hypersensitivity reaction, but could also represent an
antibody-dependent lymphocytotoxic reaction
(p. 7.13). Also, there are usually some, and
often many, plasma cells in the lesions, and a
high concentration of locally-produced antibody might have a cytotoxic effect. In spite of
the rather flimsy nature of the evidence, there
is fairly general belief that the lesions of these
diseases are mediated largely by delayed hypersensitivity reactions.

The possible mechanisms involved in the
development of auto-immunity are discussed
on pp. 7.27–29.

The connective tissue diseases

Systemic lupus erythematosus (SLE). This is
one of the connective tissue diseases. It is
characterised by acute and chronic inflammatory lesions in many organs and tissues, and by
the occurrence in the plasma of various auto-
antibodies, most of which react with normal
constituents common to most types of cell in
the body. The sites of lesions include the skin,
muscles, joints, glomeruli, heart and blood vessels, but the distribution varies greatly and may
be even wider. Auto-antibody to deoxyribonucleoprotein is nearly always demonstrable in the
serum by immunofluorescence tests (Fig. 7.10),
and antibodies to DNA, RNA and various
cytoplasmic cellular constituents are commonly
present. There may also be cytotoxic auto-
antibodies to red cells, platelets and leucocytes,
and to clotting factors in the plasma.

The auto-antibodies to nuclear and cytoplasmic constituents are not cytotoxic, and
many of them occur in other diseases and,
usually in low titre, in some normal subjects.
The corresponding auto-antigens may, however, be released by breakdown of cells, and
immune-complex (type 3) reactions can then
result. In fact, most of the pathological features
of SLE can be explained on the basis of deposition of circulating immune complexes in the
walls of small blood vessels. Disease activity
correlates fairly closely with the concentration
of anti-DNA in the plasma (measured by DNA

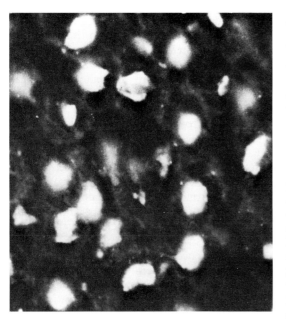

Fig. 7.10 Antibody to deoxyribonucleoprotein demonstrated by the immunofluorescence technique. Note the diffuse nuclear fluorescence technique. × 775. (Professor J. Swanson Beck.)

binding capacity of the serum) and low levels of serum complement. The glomerular lesions (p. 22.35) are due to deposition of immune complexes in the glomerular capillary basement membrane and subsequent complement fixation, and this process is responsible also for at least some of the lesions in the skin and elsewhere. Auto-antibodies to native (double-stranded) DNA are virtually specific for SLE and their complexes with DNA contribute significantly to the renal lesions. Antibodies to denatured (single-stranded) DNA occur also in other diseases and do not correlate so closely with disease activity.

Rheumatoid arthritis (RA). Because of its high incidence and disabling effects, this is the most important of the connective tissue diseases. The main feature is a destructive polyarthritis, in which the synovial membrane is infiltrated with lymphocytes, macrophages and plasma cells. Immune complexes and activated complement components are present in the synovial fluid and are deposited in the synovial membrane. In most cases, the serum contains **rheumatoid factors**: these are immunoglobulins (usually IgM) which behave as antibodies to auto-antigenic components of IgG. Rheumatoid factors react only weakly with native IgG, but strongly with IgG which has been heat-denatured, and with IgG antibody coupled with the corresponding antigen. Experimental evidence suggests that rheumatoid factors develop when IgG antibody forms immune complexes: binding with antigen alters the Fc of the IgG molecule and renders it auto-antigenic.

It appears that the inflammatory changes of RA are brought about as a result of activation of complement by antigen-antibody complexes. Initially such complexes might be provided by antibody reacting with a postulated infective agent. Subsequently, complexes are formed by IgG rheumatoid factor which reacts with its own Fc component (Fig. 23.62, p. 23.58). RA may thus be an Arthus (type 3) reaction, but there are other possibilities, including a delayed hypersensitivity (type 4) reaction between specifically primed T lymphocytes and synovial lining cells.

Polyarthritis is not uncommon in SLE, but is seldom so severe or destructive as rheumatoid arthritis. This and other associations do not necessarily indicate an auto-immune pathogenesis for rheumatoid arthritis, but merely suggest that common genetic and possibly environmental factors predispose to both conditions.

The other connective tissue diseases are dealt with in the relevant systematic chapters. Apart from the variable occurrence of anti-nuclear and other auto-antibodies, there is little evidence to suggest an auto-immune pathogenesis.

Other auto-immune diseases

Auto-immune destruction of red cells, leucocytes and platelets by cytotoxic antibodies (p. 7.11) may occur in isolation, or in association with systemic lupus erythematosus. The pathogenic effect of auto-antibodies in *Graves' disease* and *myasthenia gravis* have already been mentioned (p. 7.13).

Other diseases in which auto-immunity may be significant include *ulcerative colitis*, in which the intestinal epithelium may be the target cell of an auto-immune response, and some types of chronic liver disease, notably *primary biliary cirrhosis* and virus-negative *chronic active hepatitis*, in which there is evidence of auto-immunity to components of bile-duct epithelium and hepatocytes respectively. In skin diseases of the pemphigus group, auto-antibody to surface constituents of the cells of the epidermis and squamous epithelium of the oral cavity is demonstrable and correlates well with the activity of the disease (p. 27.15), while anto-antibody to the basement membrane of epidermis is a common finding in bullous pemphigoid. Various other diseases could be mentioned, but as the list lengthens, the evidence becomes progressively weaker.

Possible causes of auto-immunity. Regardless of the relative importance of auto-antibodies and cell-mediated auto-immunity in the pathogenesis of auto-immune diseases, we are still faced with the question of why some individuals develop auto-immune responses. Auto-antibodies react with tissue constituents possessing relatively few of the appropriate antigenic determinants, and it is unlikely that this can happen without the co-operation of helper T cells (p. 6.24). The auto-immune responses therefore appear to involve participation of both T and B cells. The lymphocytes of normal individuals have been shown to include B cells capable of binding and responding to particular auto-antigens, e.g. thyroglobulin or DNA, and also T cells which, when grown in culture with various autologous tissues and stimulating lectins, e.g. phytohaemagglutinin, become effector cells capable of reacting with cellular auto-antigens. The cells necessary for auto-immune responses are thus available and auto-immunity appears to develop from a disturbance of homeostasis which might result either from increased antigenic stimulation or from an abnormality of the regulatory mechanisms of immune responses.

Increased antigenic stimulation. In most of the auto-immune diseases, there is no evidence that the tissues affected are antigenically abnormal. Auto-antibodies react just as well with tissue constituents of normal individuals as with those of the individuals producing them. Auto-immunity can, however, result from treatment with certain drugs. For example, many patients treated for hypertension with methyldopa develop antibody which reacts with a rhesus antigen (e) in their own red cells, and this may result in increased red cell destruction (haemolytic anaemia). The most likely explanation is that methyldopa modifies the red cell membrane in such a way that it behaves like a foreign protein, stimulating a T-cell response,

and that the responsive T cells collaborate with B cells which are thus enabled to treat the antigen e as a hapten (p. 6.24). Similarly, patients treated with hydralazine, isoniazid or procainamide tend to develop antibodies to nuclear constituents and may develop some of the features of rheumatoid arthritis or SLE. The mechanisms of these drug-induced auto-immunities is, however, not clear, and they usually subside on stopping the drug.

It is also possible that environmental antigens may stimulate auto-immunity because they resemble normal tissue constituents and so induce the development of T cells and antibodies which can cross-react with cellular constituents. This occurs in rheumatic fever, which results from streptococcal pharyngitis: the antibodies to certain strepcococcal antigens cross-react with myocardium and may be responsible for the acute myocarditis of rheumatic fever (p. 15.25).

Increased availability of auto-antigens might result in auto-immunity, and in some tissues, e.g. the eye and the testis, potentially antigenic cells are normally sequestered, but are made available to recirculating lymphocytes by tissue injury. This might account for the strong immune reaction, in lens-induced uveitis (p. 21.80), to fragments of lens tissue left behind in removing the lens for cataract. In sympathetic ophthalmitis (p. 21.80) damage to the iris or ciliary body is followed by a chronic destructive uveitis in both eyes; the latter lesion appears to be of auto-immune nature. A third example is provided by the development of agglutinating auto-antibodies to spermatozoa following rupture of a retention cyst of an epididymal tubule. Other auto-antigens, e.g. thyroglobulin and cell nuclear material, are normally present in low concentration in the plasma and, as noted earlier, tissue injury has little or no auto-immunising effect for these auto-antigens. Nor does injection of tissue extracts alone induce auto-immunity in animals, although when the extract is incorporated in Freund's adjuvant (p. 6.30) its injection does result in auto-immunity and in self-limiting auto-immune disease. The role of the adjuvant in such experimental disease is not understood.

One of the most interesting recent discoveries relating to the aetiology of organ-specific auto-immune diseases is the observation that, whereas the class II molecules of the HLA system are normally expressed only on the surface of the macrophage series of cells and some subsets of lymphocytes, the follicular cells of the thyroid in patients with auto-immune thyroid disease display these molecules (Hanfusa *et al.*, 1983). This may be of great significance because helper T cells can only respond to antigens associated with HLA class II molecules on the cell surface (p. 7.20). The thyroid epithelium might thus, by displaying DR antigens, act as antigen-presenting cells for T cells, and stimulate an auto-immune response.

Abnormalities of the immunity system. A striking feature of auto-immune diseases is the large amounts of IgG auto-antibodies which are often produced. This suggests that both T cells and B cells are involved (p. 6.26), and that auto-immunity does not result from over-stimulation of B cells alone. In infectious mononucleosis (p. 18.10) B cells are infected by the EB virus, which induces polyclonal B-cell proliferation and enhanced antibody production. Various auto-antibodies are produced in this disease, but they are of IgM class and disappear after recovery from the infection. Auto-immunity also develops in lepromatous leprosy and in mycoplasma pneumonia, but in the latter this is a transient phenomenon with production of IgM antibodies.

There is some evidence of disturbance of the immunity system in the connective tissue diseases. For example, the lymphocytes of patients with SLE show a reduced transformation response when stimulated in culture by concanavalin A, suggesting a deficiency of suppressor T cells. This may explain enhanced production of auto-antibodies. There is also evidence of impaired thymic function in SLE patients, and in their healthy relatives, and this may be the cause of reduced suppressor T cell activity. In the F1 hybrids of NZB × NZW mice, which develop spontaneously a disease closely resembling SLE, thymic function is impaired and suppressor cell activity is reduced, and transfer of lymphocytes from a mouse with the disease to young mice who have not yet developed it results in persistent disease only if the suppressor T cells of the young mice are depressed by x-irradiation or by anti-lymphocyte serum.

The role of genetic factors is suggested by the tendency for auto-immune diseases, and their associated auto-antibodies, to develop in more than one member of particular families. HLA typing has also shown that particular HLA antigens are accompanied by an increased risk of developing auto-immunity (p. 2.13). There is little intra-familial and individual overlap in the occurrence of the organ-specific and non-organ-specific auto-immune diseases, and different genetic factors appear to be involved in the aetiology of the two groups of diseases.

In conclusion, the aetiology of the two major groups of auto-immune disease is obscure. There is no evidence of enhanced tissue auto-antigenicity apart from the recent discovery that thyroid epithelial cells express Ia antigens in patients with auto-immune thyroid disease. In SLE, there is evidence of thymic deficiency and impaired suppressor cell activity, and this may explain the development of auto-immune clones of T and B cells. Whatever the aetiology, it seems certain that genetic factors are involved in the organ-specific diseases, and very likely that they are involved in the connective tissue diseases. The aetiology of the latter diseases is further discussed on pp. 23.59–62.

Rejection of transplanted tissues

The treatment of burns by skin grafting is a well-established procedure. The epidermis of *autologous grafts* extends to cover the denuded area and survives indefinitely, while *allogeneic grafts* become established, but invariably undergo necrosis within two or three weeks. Evidence that this rejection process is mediated by an immunological reaction on the part of the host was first provided by Gibson and Medawar in 1943. In a series of important experiments, Medawar and his colleagues went on to lay the foundations of transplant immunology. They showed that skin grafts between syngeneic* mice were accepted permanently, while allogeneic grafts stimulated an immune response in the host and were consequently destroyed ('rejected') 1–3 weeks after grafting. They also showed that mice injected at birth with allogeneic cells would subsequently accept permanently a skin graft from the same donor strain and that this state of unresponsiveness— the first experimental demonstration of

* For terminology, see p. 6.4.

acquired immunological tolerance (p. 6.28)—could be abolished, with consequent rejection of the skin graft, by injection of host-strain lymphocytes from a normal mouse or from one that had previously rejected a graft from the allogeneic strain. Lymphocytes from the latter mouse induced more rapid and intense graft rejection, showing that, as a result of previously rejecting an allograft, it had developed persistent immunity, manifested by the reactivity of its lymphoid cells. This early work suggested the importance of cell-mediated immunity in allograft rejection. It is true that antibodies also developed in the recipients of allografts, but their injection into tolerant animals bearing an appropriate allograft did not result in rejection.

Medawar's major observations and conclusions have been confirmed in experiments involving transplantation of various tissues in many vertebrate species. The mechanism of rejection is complex, but in most situations cell-mediated immunity plays a major role and the graft is destroyed mainly by a delayed hypersensitivity (type 4) reaction. Specifically primed cytotoxic T lymphocytes bind to 'transplant' alloantigens on the surface of the graft cells and bring about their destruction. The mechanism of such cytotoxic activity is not known. Specifically-reactive T lymphocytes also release lymphokines (p. 7.21), which activate macrophages, and possibly also a specific macrophage-arming factor (SMAF) which enables macrophages to bind specifically to the transplant antigens of the graft cells and destroy them (p. 7.21). In organs such as the kidney, which are transplanted by connecting the major blood vessels of the graft to host vessels, injury may result also from a cytotoxic antibody (type 2) reaction (p. 7.11).

The alloantigens which stimulate an immune response to tissue transplants from another individual are mainly those determined by the major histocompatibility complex (MHC), i.e. HLA antigens in man and H-2 antigens in mice (p. 2.12). There are also, however, weaker 'transplant' alloantigens encoded by genes outwith the MHC region. The greater the genetic disparity between donor and recipient in MHC antigens, the stronger and more rapid will be the rejection reaction.

Graft versus host reaction. If normal lymphoid cells are injected into an allogeneic host,

they will be destroyed unless the host is immunologically deficient or tolerant and cannot mount a rejection reaction. In the latter circumstance, the grafted cells may survive and mount an immune response against the host, with a consequent **graft-versus-host (G.v.H.)** reaction. This occurs when allogeneic lymphocytes from an adult mouse are injected into neonates or into mice rendered immunodeficient, e.g. by thymectomy and x-irradiation, and when an F1 hybrid mouse is injected with lymphocytes of either parental strain. The G.v.H. reaction is complex and includes splenomegaly, lymph node enlargement, haemolytic anaemia and predisposition to infections. When induced in the neonate, these changes, together with impairment of growth, have been termed *runt disease*.

In man, a G.v.H. reaction develops when an immunodeficient patient, e.g. with severe combined immunodeficiency (p. 7.34) is treated by infusion of cells of the haemopoietic marrow. The transplanted cells include T lymphocytes and precursors, and some of these respond to the host's HLA antigens, with development of cell-mediated immunity to host cells. The B cells of the donor also develop an antibody response to the host's HLA antigens. Features of the G.v.H. reaction include fever, weight loss, exfoliative dermatitis, anaemia and thrombocytopenia, diarrhoea, intestinal malabsorption, pneumonia and hepatosplenomegaly. Some of these effects are due to infections. As in graft rejection, the intensity of the G.v.H. reaction depends mainly on the degree of HLA disparity between donor and recipient, and a strong untreated reaction is rapidly fatal.

A G.v.H. reaction is most readily minimised by transplanting marrow cells from an HLA-identical sibling (Fig. 2.11, p. 2.12). Failing this, parental marrow may be used, but only half of the HLA antigens will be identical with those of the recipient, and a G.v.H. reaction will result. The intensity of this may be reduced by destroying T cells in the aspirated donor marrow before infusion to the recipient. Recently, anti-T monoclonal antibodies have been used for this purpose, with improved results. Treatment of the recipient with cyclosporin A further diminishes the G.v.H. reaction.

Bone marrow transplantation is also performed in the treatment of aplastic anaemia and also in leukaemia following destruction of the patient's leukaemic (and normal haemo-poietic) cells by cytotoxic drugs and radio-therapy. In such cases, the purpose is to provide haemopoietic stem cells, but if the grafted cells are not rejected by the host, the G.v.H. reaction is a major problem and must be avoided or minimised by the methods outlined above. The T cells in blood may also cause a G.v.H. re-action when an immunodeficient individual is treated by blood transfusion, and this may also result from the presence of circulating T cells in transplanted solid organs.

Human renal transplantation

Many thousands of kidneys have been trans-planted in the past few years to patients with irreversible renal failure. The major obstacle is immunological rejection of the graft and, except for transplants between identical twins, it is es-sential to protect the graft by administration of immunosuppressive drugs such as glucocortic-oids, azathioprine or cyclosporin A. Initially, high dosage is necessary to prevent acute rejec-tion, but the dosage can gradually be reduced, in some cases to very low levels, without rejec-tion occurring. This indicates that the host be-comes increasingly less responsive to the graft antigens. One possible explanation is that the continued release of antigens by the graft, together with immunosuppression, results in specific immunological tolerance. Another is that the host develops 'enhancing' antibodies (p. 6.31) which protect the graft by suppressing the cell-mediated immune response or by com-bining with graft antigens and so concealing them from specifically responsive T lympho cytes. Administration of iso-antibodies reactive with antigens of the grafted tissue has been shown to prolong graft survival in animals, and patients who have developed HLA antibodies as a result of previous blood transfusion are less likely to reject a renal allograft than non-transfused patients. There is preliminary evi-dence that administration of HLA antibodies may have a similar enhancing effect in human renal transplantation, although such antibodies (presumably in larger amounts) can also cause immediate rejection (p. 22.46).

While on large doses of immunosuppressive drugs, transplant patients are very liable to develop infections, both with virulent patho-gens and with opportunistic micro-organisms such as *Cytomegalovirus*, *Pneumocystis carinii* and various fungi.

In spite of these problems, approximately 50% of the transplants have done well and are functioning some years later.

One of the most promising drugs for prev-enting graft rejection is cyclosporin A, which is particularly cytotoxic for antigen-stimulated T cells. Its toxicity for haemopoietic and other tissue cells is relatively low, and animal experi-ments have shown that it is capable of inducing long-lasting immunological tolerance to tissue transplants. It has less effect on secondary im-mune responses than on the primary response, and so its use does not result in the degree of susceptibility to infection encountered with drugs which have a more general immunosup-pressive effect.

The pathological features of rejection of renal transplants are described on pp. 22.45–47.

Tissue typing. At present, tissue typing is usually performed by a cytotoxicity test, using typing antisera and complement, upon cells of the individual to be typed: if the cells possess the corresponding iso-antigen, they will be killed (Fig 3.7, p. 3.4). All tissue cells, leucocytes and platelets (but not red cells) possess HLA antigens, and it is convenient to use blood lymphocytes for typing. HLA antisera are obtained from recipients of blood transfusions or previous transplants, or from parous women, some of whom have developed anti-bodies to HLA antigens of the fetus. By testing with a panel of lymphocytes of known HLA phenotypes, and suitable absorption to remove unwanted antigens, specific HLA antisera can be provided.

There is no doubt that renal allografts have a better chance of surviving when the donor and recipient are closely matched for HLA anti-gens. The effect is greatest in grafting between HLA-identical siblings and over 90% of kidneys are functioning well one year later. Even with close matching of HLA-A and -B antigens between unrelated donors and recipients, the figure is only about 60% because identity at the other HLA loci is unlikely. Matching for HLA-D or -DR antigens has not been exten-sively practiced, but it is likely to improve greatly the results of transplantation. In addi-tion to the HLA antigens, there are loci on other chromosomes determining weaker trans-plant antigens, and even grafts between HLA-identical siblings will be rejected unless the recipient receives immunosuppressive therapy.

For reasons explained on p. 22.46, it is essential to ensure ABO blood group compatibility in human renal transplantation, and to test the recipient's serum for cytotoxic antibody to the cells of potential donors.

Transplantation of other tissues

As noted above, infusion of **haemopoietic cells**, which include pluripotent stem cells (p. 6.15), is a logical treatment for infants with congenital deficiency of haemopoietic stem cells, for patients with certain forms of aplastic anaemia, and for children treated for acute leukaemia by cytotoxic drugs in doses which destroy their haemopoietic and lymphoid cells. The depressed immune responsiveness of such patients reduces the risk of rejection of the donated cells, but immunocompetent T lymphocytes in the donation are very liable to respond to transplant antigens of the host, causing a fatal graft-versus-host reaction.

Great technical advances have been made in recent years in **heart** and **liver transplantation** and use of cyclosporin A has contributed greatly to the survival of recipients.

Successful **corneal allografting** has long been practised without immunosuppression of the recipient. This is because the cornea is avascular and therefore a 'protected site' in which the graft does not induce an immune response in the recipient. If, as sometimes happens, blood vessels extend into the grafted cornea, then rejection occurs.

In allografts of **blood vessels** and **tendon**, the cells either die from ischaemia or are destroyed by a rejection reaction, but the collagen and elastic fibres persist, and are repopulated with host cells and vessels: thus the use of stored vessel or tendon is equally, if not more effective. Similarly, the cells of **bone grafts** die, but the matrix may provide the desired mechanical effect (p. 23.2). The use of **cartilage grafts** in plastic surgery is of considerable interest: both the cells and the matrix of allografts may survive for long periods without inducing a rejection reaction. This is due to the avascular nature of cartilage, and to the matrix, which allows diffusion of nutrients and metabolites between graft chondrocytes and host, but acts as an 'immunological barrier' between them.

Another exception to the general phenomenon of allograft rejection is provided by nature's allograft, **pregnancy**. The trophoblast, of fetal origin, is bathed in maternal blood, and yet it is tolerated for nine months, in spite of the presence of incompatible (paternal) transplant antigens in the fetal cells. There is slight depression of maternal immune responsiveness during pregnancy, but the mother does not develop specific immunulogical tolerance to the fetus. The most likely explanation of failure to reject the fetus appears to be that the cells of the syncytiotrophoblast are coated with a layer of mucopolysaccharide, which provides an 'immunological barrier'.

Immunodeficiency States

There are a large number of conditions in which the normal defence mechanisms against invasive micro-organisms are impaired. For most purposes it is useful to classify such deficiencies into two major groups. Firstly, **deficiencies of non-specific resistance**, as in diabetes mellitus, impaired function of neutrophil polymorphs (p. 17.14), etc. This miscellaneous group is dealt with under the appropriate diseases: it includes also lesions which impair resistance locally, for example obstruction of hollow viscera, e.g. the urinary tract or air passages, and ischaemia of the lower limb leading to gangrene.

In the second major group, which is discussed here, impaired resistance is due to **defects in specific immune responsiveness**. These are best classified into primary and secondary types, and also in relation to the type of immunological defect present.

In the group of *primary conditions*, the immunological deficiency becomes manifest usually, but not always, in early childhood, and in most of the conditions there is good evidence that the defect is genetically determined. Other abnormalities, e.g. thrombocytopenia in the Wiskott-Aldrich syndrome, or hypoparathyroidism in the DiGeorge syndrome, may accompany the immunological defect, giving rise to characteristic disease complexes, but the immunological deficiency is not secondary to the other parts of the syndrome. By contrast, the *secondary immunodeficiencies* occur at any age, are not genetically-determined, and the defects of immunity are the result of injury to the lymphoid tissues, either by various disease processes, particularly lymphoid neoplasia, or by immunosuppressive agents.

The type of immune defect present determines the clinical picture and form of therapy required. The division of lymphoid cells into two major classes—thymic-dependent (T) and thymic-independent (B)—has been dealt with in Chapter 6. Its validity in man is demonstrated by the occurrence of immunodeficiency states affecting mainly T-cell function, with depression of CMI and antibody responses, or mainly B-cell function, with depression of antibody production alone: combined deficiencies, affecting both T- and B-cell function, are also observed. Such well-defined immunodeficiencies occur as primary, congenital defects, but they are rare. Less serious and less clearly-defined deficiencies also occur as inherited and acquired conditions.

Primary immunodeficiencies

This group of conditions has contributed to our understanding of the functions of the various cells involved in immune responses. As noted above, they are rare, but diagnosis is important because they are life-threatening conditions, effective treatment for some of which is now possible. The classification used here is based on the recommendations of the World Health Organisation (1983).

(1) Deficiency mainly of B-cell function. This group is exemplified by **infantile sex-linked agammaglobulinaemia**, which was the first to be described and is sometimes known as the **Bruton type of agammaglobulinaemia** after its discoverer. The major abnormality is a virtually complete inability to produce the three major classes of immunoglobulins—IgG, IgM and IgA. In consequence, there is little or no antibody production in response to infections or immunisation procedures, and the normal blood group iso-antibodies are usually not detectable. The condition is observed in boys, being transmitted by a gene defect in the X chromosome (sex-linked recessive). Symptoms usually arise in the first or second years of life, protection before that being provided by maternal antibodies of IgG class transmitted to the fetus. The defect results in unusually frequent and serious bacterial infections, particularly those due to the pyogenic bacteria (p. 9.5), and including respiratory and pulmonary infections, meningitis and septicaemia and persistent diarrhoea due to intestinal infection with *Giardia lamblia* or rotaviruses. 'Opportunistic' infections (p. 8.1), e.g. pneumonia due to the protozoon, *Pneumocystis carinii*, also occur. The infections respond to appropriate antibiotics, and diagnosis depends upon the demonstration of the near-absence of serum IgG (below 0·5 g/litre), IgM and IgA (below 3×10^{-2} g/litre). Deficiency of IgG cannot be demonstrated until the maternal IgG has fallen to a low level—usually by about 8 months of age, although very low levels of the other two immunoglobulins are observed before this time, since they do not cross the placenta.

The condition is due to a failure of pre-B cells (p. 6.15) to differentiate into B lymphocytes. The haemopoietic marrow contains normal numbers of pre-B cells but the lymph nodes and tonsils are small, and biopsy reveals an absence of germinal centres and plasma cells, while rectal biopsy reveals absence of plasma cells in the mucosa. The blood lymphocytes are not greatly diminished, but B lymphocytes are virtually absent. The thymus is normal, and cell-mediated immune responses are not impaired. In spite of this, patients may suffer from prolonged fungal, parasitic and some viral infections and injection of poliomyelitis vaccine (attenuated poliovirus) may actually cause the disease. These features indicate that defence against viral and fungal infections is dependent partly on antibodies. Chronic polyarthritis, closely resembling rheumatoid arthritis, is of common occurrence. A family history of immunodeficiency is obtained in only a minority of cases, and rarely a similar disease is inherited as a recessive abnormality of an autosomal gene, when female infants may also be affected.

The effectiveness of regular injections of

human IgG in preventing infections has increased the importance of early diagnosis. It is important to distinguish the Bruton type of agammaglobulinaemia, which requires lifelong therapy, from **transient hypogammaglobulinaemia**. This latter condition presents similar clinical features and morphological changes in the lymphoid tissues, but is merely a delay, and not a permanent failure, of the capacity to produce immunoglobulins. It is familial, relatively common, and more frequent and severe in infants born prematurely because the fetus gains maternal IgG via the placenta mainly late in pregnancy. Transient hypogammaglobulinaemia affects both sexes, and the defect disappears within the first three years of life. Curiously, severe immunoglobulin deficiency is usually limited to IgG, and normal levels of IgM and IgA in the serum may help to distinguish it from the Bruton type.

There are a number of less-well-defined conditions which appear to fall within this group. In all of them, there is defective production of one or more classes of immunoglobulins, impairment of antibody production, and relatively normal cell-mediated immune responses. In some instances, there is apparently a failure to switch from IgM-class antibody production to IgG, IgA, etc. There is B-cell hyperplasia but virtual absence of immunoglobulins of classes other than IgM. Selective IgA deficiency is reportedly of relatively common occurrence, usually detected by scanning blood donors, but only a small proportion of those affected have any clinical abnormality—either frequent infections or auto-immune diseases. The evidence favouring a genetic predisposition, and a particular mode of genetic transmission, varies in the different types. Some forms of immunoglobulin deficiency do not become manifest until adult life, and yet tend to occur in families, and often exhibit a familial association with other disturbances of immunity, e.g. hypergammaglobulinaemia and systemic lupus erythematosus. Some patients with such late-onset immunoglobulin deficiency also develop auto-immune diseases such as pernicious anaemia and connective tissue diseases, but without demonstrable auto-antibodies.

(2) Deficiency of T-cell function. An example of this group is provided by the rare **DiGeorge syndrome**, in which there is almost complete failure of development of the thymus and the parathyroids from the third and fourth branchial arches.

In those infants who survive the neonatal period, immunoglobulin production appears normal, although antibody responses are impaired, probably because of lack of helper T cells. The lymph nodes contain plasma cells and germinal centres, but the paracortical (thymus-dependent) areas are deficient in small lymphocytes, and the number of circulating lymphocytes, although variable, is low in some cases. The condition may affect infants of both sexes, and there is no evidence for a genetic predisposition. Affected infants can deal perfectly well with pyogenic bacteria, but suffer from 'opportunistic' infections, e.g. by *Pneumocystis carinii* (p. 28.20) and fungi and also from severe virus infections. Impairment of cell-mediated immunity is demonstrable by failure to develop delayed hypersensitivity to agents such as dinitrochlorobenzene (p. 13.37) and immunisation with live vaccines is liable to give rise to fatal generalised infections. Less severe degrees, with reduced thymic lymphopoiesis, are more common than complete failure of T-cell production. When severe, the condition is fatal: in some instances life has been prolonged by transplantation of thymic tissue, but the problem here is to prevent rejection of the grafted thymus by the host T lymphocytes which generate under its influence. Thymic tissue from a closely matched HLA donor is less likely to be rejected.

(3) Severe combined immunodeficiency. In this condition, both the thymus-dependent and -independent immunity systems fail to develop. The thymus is hypoplastic and deficient in Hassall's corpuscles and small lymphocytes, the lymph nodes are extremely small and lacking in germinal centres, lymphocytes and plasma cells, and circulating lymphocytes are scanty. There is a near-absence of the three main classes of immunoglobulins from the serum, and both antibody production and cell-mediated immunity are grossly defective. The condition may be transmitted as either an X-linked or an autosomal recessive character, and affected infants show retarded growth, recurrent bacterial and virus infections and often candidiasis of the mouth, larynx and skin. Response to antibiotics and chemotherapy is poor. Immunisation with living viruses is likely to prove fatal, and the condition usually results in death during the first or second year. The basic defect appears to lie in the haemopoietic stem cells (p. 6.15), which fail to undergo lymphopoiesis.

In about half of the autosomal recessive patients, the defect is in a gene coding for adenosine deaminase, provision of which (by transfusing frozen irradiated red cells) affects temporary improvement. Marrow transplantation is, however, usually necessary.

Reticular dysgenesis is a severe combined immunodeficiency in which there is also greatly reduced production of cells of the granulocyte series.

In both these conditions, the deficiencies are restored by infusion of haemopoietic cells, which include stem cells, but unless the donor is an HLA-identical sibling there is a grave risk of fatal graft-versus-host reaction (p. 7.30). Recently, however, success has been achieved using parental ('hemi-identical') marrow cells from which T cells have been removed.

(4) Other primary immunodeficiencies are mostly of obscure nature. **Ataxia telangiectasia** results from an autosomal recessive gene defect which results in impairment of both T and B cell function. It is accompanied by cerebellar ataxia developing at about two years of age and subsequently the appearance of widespread vascular defects characterised by dilatation of small vessels (telangiectases). Immunodeficiency develops insidiously with depression of cell-mediated immunity and low levels of IgE and IgA in the blood. The IgG level is also low in some cases. Recurrent infections of the paranasal sinuses and lungs are the most common consequences of the defect of immunity. In some instances the thymus has been found to be poorly developed and lacking in Hassall's corpuscles. The condition is fatal, often from the development of a lymphoid tumour. There is no form of curative therapy.

Another condition in which immunodeficiency develops insidiously is the **Wiskott–Aldrich syndrome** in which the platelets are reduced in number and size. There is progressive depletion of lymphocytes in the blood and in the T-dependent areas of the lymphoid tissues and cell-mediated immunity gradually declines. The blood level of IgM is usually raised, IgG is about normal and IgA and IgE are low. Blood group iso-antibodies are absent. The condition is determined by a sex-linked genetic defect and affects boys: atopic eczema, attacks of diarrhoea and recurrent infections are common features. The thymus appears normal or is slightly diminished in size.

Reports suggesting that Lawrence's transfer factor (p. 6.24) brings about improvement have not been confirmed. Treatment by marrow transplantation following destruction of the patient's own haemopoietic and lymphoid cells by cytotoxic drugs or x-irradiation is, however, sometimes successful. This treatment does not restore the platelets and splenectomy may be necessary to relieve the thrombocytopenia. Without treatment, the disease is usually fatal in childhood from infections, haemorrhage, or development of a lymphoid tumour.

Secondary immunodeficiencies

These are conditions in which the immunity system develops and functions normally but becomes defective from the direct or indirect effect of various disease processes or immunosuppressive agents. Causal conditions include malnutrition, certain infections, various forms of cancer and renal failure.

Susceptibility to infections is a well-known feature of malnutrition, but is is only recently that **protein deficiency**, both experimental and in man, has been demonstrated to impair cell-mediated immune responsiveness. *Because of its prevalence in many parts of the world, this is probably the most important cause of immunodeficiency.*

Depression of cell-mediated immunity may be a feature of various **acute virus infections**, but has been demonstrated most clearly in measles and infectious mononucleosis, in both of which a temporary depression of cell-mediated immunity has been shown by skin tests (e.g. to tuberculoprotein) becoming negative, and by impaired responsiveness of lymphocytes to stimulation *in vitro* by antigens or phytomitogens (see below). The **acquired immune deficiency syndrome (AIDS)**, which appears to be caused by chronic infection with HTLV-III virus and has reached epidemic proportions in homosexual male communities in the USA, is described on p. 25.5.

Impaired cell-mediated immunity occurs also in some **bacterial and protozoal infections** in which there is extensive colonisation of the macrophage system, e.g. lepromatous leprosy and leishmaniasis. T cell function is depressed also in **sarcoidosis**, a condition of unknown cause characterised by tubercle-like granulomas of the lymphoid and various other tissues.

Patients with **advanced cancer** commonly have depression of both T and B cell function: without doubt, this is a result of cancer, although there is evidence that the incidence of cancer (of both the lymphoid and epithelial tissues) is increased in patients who survive with primary immunodeficiencies and in patients on long-term immunosuppressive therapy, e.g. following renal transplantation.

Immunodeficiencies are particularly common in patients with **lymphoid neoplasia (lymphoma)**. In chronic lymphocytic leukaemia, there is very often deficient T and B cell function; this may be due to crowding of the lymphoid tissues, marrow and blood with neoplastic (usually B) lymphocytes. It is, however, of interest that immunosuppression is an early effect of infection with the retroviruses which induce lymphomas in animals, and it may be that human chronic lymphocytic leukaemia (and some other lymphomas) are also virus-induced. Depression of antibody levels is a feature of multiple myeloma, a plasma-cell tumour usually confined to the bone marrow; the high levels of Ig secreted by the myeloma cells increase the rate of Ig catabolism and may also depress antibody responses.

In a third lymphoid neoplasm, Hodgkin's disease, the lymphoid tissues are often extensively infiltrated, and T-cell deficiency is then the usual result: tuberculosis or virus infection (e.g. herpes zoster) may prove fatal.

The immunodeficiency of **renal failure** affects T-cell, and probably also B-cell, function. This is important in renal transplantation because it helps initially to prevent rejection of the transplanted kidney.

With increasing use of immunosuppressive and cytotoxic drugs—cortisone, azathioprine, cyclophosphamide, etc., and also radiotherapy, infections due to immunodeficiencies are becoming common, and often limiting factors in renal transplantation and the treatment of various forms of cancer and other fatal diseases. Some of these agents destroy not only lymphocytes, but also haemopoietic cells, and thus depress resistance to infection in more than one way.

Assessment of immune function

In cases of suspected immunodeficiency, information can be obtained from examination of the blood to determine: (*a*) the levels of the various classes of Ig; (*b*) the presence and titres of ABO blood group antibodies; and (*c*) the proportions and numbers of T and B lymphocytes and the ratio of helper to suppressor T cells. The responsiveness of lymphocytes to stimulation by antigens, e.g. tuberculoprotein, and to phytomitogens, gives some indication of function. Blast-cell transformation occurs when normal blood lymphocytes are cultured in the presence of phytohaemagglutinin (PHA) or concanavalin A (con-A), both of which stimulate T cells, pokeweed mitogen (PWM) which stimulates both T and B cells, and bacterial endotoxin, which stimulates B cells.

Other tests include assay of antibodies against commonly encountered antigens, and cell-mediated immunity may be investigated by skin tests or *in vitro* techniques (p. 6.24). Finally, antigens may be administered and the responses measured, but live vaccines should not be used for this purpose in subjects who may not be able to eliminate even attenuated micro-organisms. The capacity to develop contact dermatitis to agents applied to the skin, e.g. dinitrochlorobenzene, is sometimes used to test cell-mediated immune responsiveness.

References

Butcher, B.T., Salvaggio, J.E. and Leslie, G.A. (1975). Secretory and humoral immunogenic response of atopic and non-atopic individuals to intra-nasally administered antigen. *Clinical Allergy* **1**, 33.

Cochrane, C.G. and Koffler, D. (1973). Immune

complex disease in experimental animals and man. *Advances in Immunology*, Vol. 16, pp. 186–264. Academic Press, New York and London.

Dale, M.M. and Foreman, J.C. (Eds.). (1984). *Textbook of Immunopathology* pp. 407. Blackwell Scientific Publications, Oxford. (Excellent reviews of the mediation of hypersensitivity reactions).

Franklin, E.C. (Ed.). (1981). *Clinical Immunology Update* pp. 427. Churchill Livingstone, Edinburgh. (Excellent reviews of many aspects of clinical immunology and hypersensitivity).

Gibson, T. and Medawar, P.B. (1943). The fate of skin homografts in man. *Journal of Anatomy* **77**, 299–310.

Hanafusa, T., Chiovato, L., Doniach, D., Pujol-Borrell, R., Russell, R.C.G. and Botazzo, G.F. (1983). Aberrant expression of HLA-DR antigen on thyrocytes in Graves' disease. Relevance to autoimmunity. Lancet, **ii**, 1111-4.

Ishizaka, K., Ishizaka, T. and Hombrook, M.M. (1966). Physico-chemical properties of reaginic antibody. V. Correlation of reagin activity with γE-globulin antibody. *Journal of Immunology* **97**, 840-53.

Ishizaka, T., Ishizaka, K. and Tomioka, H. (1972). Release of histamine and slow reacting substance of anaphylaxis (SRS-A) by IgE—anti-IgE reactions on monkey mast cells. *Journal of Immunology* **108**, 513–20.

Matthew, D.J., Norman, A.P., Taylor, B., Turner, M.W. and Soothill, J.F. (1977). Prevention of eczema. *Lancet* **i**, 111–13.

Reid, F.M., Sandilands, G.P., Gray, K.G. and Anderson, J.R. (1979). Lymphocyte emperipolesis revisited. *Immunology* **36**, 367–72.

Taylor, B., Norman, A.P., Orge., H.A., Turner, M.W., Stokes, C.R. and Soothill, J.F. (1973). Transient IgA deficiency and infantile atopy. *Lancet* **i**, 111–13.

Townley, R.G. (1983). Receptors and non-specific bronchial reactivity, pp. 197–203 in *Proceedings of the XI International Congress of Allergology and Clinical Immunology*. Eds, J.W. Kerr and M.A. Ganderton. Macmillan Press Ltd., London and Basingstoke.

Wilkinson, P.C., Parrott, D.M.V., Russell, R.J. and Sless, F. (1977). Antigen-induced locomotor responses in lymphocytes. *Journal of Experimental Medicine* **145**, 1158–68.

World Health Organisation (1983). Primary immunodeficiency diseases: report prepared for the WHO by a Scientific Group on Immunodeficiency. *Clinical Immunology* and *Immunopathology* **28**, 450–75.

Further Reading

Chandra, R.K. (1983) *Primary and Secondary Immunodeficiency Diseases.* pp. 303. Churchill Livingstone, Edinburgh.

Dixon, F.J. and Fisher, D.W. Eds. (1983). *The Biology of Immunologic Disease.* pp. 399. Blackwell Scientific Publications, Oxford, etc.

Holborow, E.J. and Reeves, W.G. (Eds.) (1983). *Immunology in Medicine.* 2nd edn., pp. 655. Grune and Stratton, London, etc. (A comprehensive account of the aetiological and clinical aspects of diseases with an immunological basis.)

Kerr, J.W. and Ganderton, M.A. (Eds.) (1983). *Proceedings of the XI International Congress of Allergology and Clinical Immunology*, pp. 560. The Macmillan Press Ltd., London and Basingstoke. (Brief reports on recent work, mostly on atopic hypersensitivity.)

Lachmann, P.J. and Peters, D.K. (Eds.) (1982). *Clinical Aspects of Immunology*, 4th edn., pp. 2495. Blackwell Scientific Publications, Oxford, etc. (Extensive reviews by leading workers.)

Roitt, I.M. (1984). *Essential immunology*, 5th ed., pp. 369. Blackwell Scientific Publications, Oxford, etc.

Rosen, F.S., Cooper, M.D. and Wedgewood, R.J.P. (1984). The primary immunodeficiencies. *The New England Journal of Medicine*, 311, 235–42 and 300–10.

Theofilopoulos, A.N. and Dixon, F.J. (1982). *Autoimmune* diseases: immunopathology and etiopathogenesis. *American Journal of Pathology*, **108**, 319–65.

See also Bibliography for Chapter 6 (pp. 6.39–40).

8

Host—Parasite Relationships

Throughout evolutionary development, many species have adapted to a parasitic existence, living in or on the surface of a host of another species from which they derive warmth, nourishment and mobility. The relationship is not necessarily harmful to the host, and may be advantageous. For example, various relatively harmless bacteria colonise the skin of man and help to exclude more harmful bacteria, while reabsorption of bile pigment from the gut and the production of vitamin K depend largely on the metabolic activities of the intestinal bacterial flora. These normal inhabitants of the skin and mucous membranes are called **commensals**. Other parasites, termed **pathogens**, are less well adapted and may, by injuring the host severely, endanger their own survival: they include many species of micro-organisms (microbes) including viruses, bacteria, fungi and protozoa, and also metazoa of various sizes. The terms **pathogenicity** and **virulence** are commonly used synonymously to indicate the capacity of a particular micro-organism to cause disease.

Although it is important to distinguish between commensals and pathogens, the distinction is not absolute, for many commensals are only harmless so long as they are kept at bay by the host's defence mechanisms. In immunodeficiency states, for example, various normally harmless microbes may cause 'opportunistic' infections. Similarly, a breach of local defence mechanisms, even in a normal individual, may allow commensals to cause severe infections, an example being *Escherichia coli*, which normally inhabits the gut: this bacterium may be introduced into the urinary tract by catheterisation of the bladder, and may then cause severe acute pyogenic infection, even extending into the kidneys. Local abnormalities in the host may also predispose to injury by commensals: for instance, heart valves which have been scarred

and distorted by rheumatic fever are readily colonised by *Streptococcus viridans*, a bacterium which lives in the mouth and finds its way into the blood following tooth extraction, or even when the teeth are brushed vigorously. In normal individuals, it is quickly eliminated, but it can settle and multiply in the distorted valve cusps, causing bacterial endocarditis. Because the distinction between pathogens and commensals is not sharp, it is helpful to use the term **infection** to indicate the presence of a particular type of micro-organism in a part of the body where it is normally absent, and where, if allowed to multiply, it is likely to be harmful, i.e. to cause **infective disease**.

As implied above, most infective diseases depend on penetration of the host's tissues by micro-organisms, and the factors concerned in such invasion provide the first major topic of this chapter. Following invasion, the microbes may be eliminated without causing obvious disease (sub-clinical infection) or clinical disease of any grade of severity may follow: the factors determining these events form a second major topic. Lastly, two important reactions to infection, neutrophil leucocytosis and fever, will be considered.

The subject of infective disease is extremely complex, involving as it does a consideration of the relationships between man and numerous species and strains of micro-organism. The following account is limited to a brief outline of the subject.

Factors determining invasion

The skin and mucous membranes are exposed to many different types of micro-organisms present in expired droplets in the air, in dust particles, and in food and water. The skin and various mucous membranes on which these organisms settle have properties which render them suitable for the survival and sometimes multiplication of certain organisms, but inhospitable to others. In some instances, the requirements of a particular microbe for growth *in vitro* help to explain its colonisation of particular parts of the surface of the body, but many of the factors determining such colonisation are still unknown, and indeed the predilection of certain bacteria for a particular host species is in most instances quite unexplained. Nevertheless, certain factors are known to be of great importance in limiting or preventing invasion by many types of microbes, and these must be considered briefly.

Barriers to invasion

(a) **Mechanical barriers.** The superficial keratinised layer of the epidermis is an excellent mechanical barrier to microbial invasion and provided it is kept clean and dry, direct invasion is extremely unlikely. Penetration may, however, occur when dirt is allowed to accumulate on the skin and particularly in moist warm areas subject to friction, such as the axillae and sub-mammary folds. In many skin diseases which result in exudation with loss or sogginess of the keratin layer, bacterial and fungal infections are common complications. The conjunctival, oral, respiratory-tract and gastro-intestinal mucosae, covered as they are by a film of mucous or serous secretion, also present a formidable barrier to many micro-organisms, although some can readily infect the epithelium, e.g. influenza virus and rhinoviruses.

Wounds and ulcers of the skin and mucous membranes open up pathways for bacterial invasion and are obviously important causes of infection. Burns are particularly liable to become heavily infected because the dead superficial tissue provides a good medium for coliform bacilli, staphylococci, *Pseudomonas aeruginosa* and many other bacteria. In the mouth, tooth extraction and tonsillectomy inevitably lead to bacterial invasion, and tonsillectomy has been shown to predispose to invasion by the virus of poliomyelitis in the postoperative period. Vitamin A and C deficiencies also impair the resistance of the mucous membranes and skin to bacterial invasion.

Some parasitic organisms have evolved a life cycle in which they multiply in insect vectors and are introduced to man and other hosts by the insect bite, thus penetrating the major barrier of the skin. Examples include the protozoa which cause malaria, the metazoan filarial worms, and the virus of yellow fever, all of which are transmitted by mosquitoes. *Yersinia pestis*, the cause of bubonic plague (the Black Death), is transmitted by the flea of the black rat, and the rickettsiae which cause typhus are spread by lice. Rabies virus enters the tissues by the bite of a rabid animal.

(b) **Glandular secretions.** The secretions of glands opening on to the skin surface play an important role by maintaining the integrity of the skin, and also by providing an environment in which many types of bacteria cannot survive for long. The acidity of the sweat and the long-chain unsaturated fatty acids produced by the action of commensal bacteria on sebaceous secretion both exert a selective bactericidal effect, and consequently the bacterial flora of the skin surface tends to be rather constant: it has been shown that some types of pathogenic bacteria, when placed on the skin, are virtually all destroyed within an hour or two. The secretions of mucous membranes possess similar qualities. **Lysozyme**, an enzyme which digests the mucopeptide of bacterial cell walls, is present in high concentration in the lacrimal gland secretion and probably exerts an important protective effect in the conjunctival sac: it is secreted also by the salivary and nasal glands but in much smaller amounts. **Antibodies of IgA class**, modified by addition of a 'transport piece' so that they are resistant to digestive enzymes, are present in saliva, tears, intestinal contents, respiratory tract mucus, milk and urine (p. 6.8). Provided that IgA antibody has developed against a particular organism as a result of previous infection, it will be represented in these secretions. This is of importance in preventing invasion by certain viruses, for the virus may encounter the antibody in the surface mucus and be neutralised by it: its significance in relation to bacterial invasion is less certain, although there is evidence that IgA antibody may render bacteria highly susceptible to the lytic action of lysozyme, and it also activates complement by the alternative pathway.

The acidity of the gastric juice is effective in killing most types of microbes ingested in food or water; but hypochlorhydria due to chronic gastritis is common, and minor illnesses and even emotional stresses can reduce temporarily the acidity of the juice. In general, those microbes which cause intestinal infections, such as the salmonellae, dysentery bacilli and enteroviruses, are relatively acid-resistant. *Entamoeba histolytica*, the cause of amoebic dysentery, produces cysts which resist the gastric juice and pass through the stomach before hatching out and invading the wall of the colon.

The normal acidity of the urine contributes to the defences of the urinary tract against infection, while some IgA is secreted by the urinary tract epithelium, and may help to eliminate bacteria.

(c) Secretion currents. The continuous flow of tears over the surface of the conjunctiva has an important effect in the removal of contaminating bacteria, which are carried rapidly into the nasopharynx. In the nose and mouth also, the secretions covering the mucosa flow towards the pharynx and hence to the stomach, carrying with them residual food particles, bacteria, etc. The importance of the saliva is illustrated by the oral infections and severe dental caries which accompany loss of salivary secretion in Sjøgren's syndrome (p. 19.9). The lacrimal secretion is also diminished, and conjunctival infections result. The importance of removal of contaminating bacteria by the saliva may explain the common occurrence of infection in the crypts of the tonsils and also in the periodontal sulci, for once bacteria gain entrance to these spaces, they are out of the main stream of salivary flow.

In the respiratory tract there is a continuous flow of mucus upwards over the surface of the bronchial and tracheal mucosa: inhaled particles are caught up and removed in this stream, and the air is almost sterile by the time it reaches the respiratory bronchioles. This defence mechanism is dependent on a normal production of mucous secretion and on the integrity of the ciliated respiratory epithelium. Most of the micro-organisms capable of invading the respiratory mucosa in spite of mucociliary flow are enabled to do so by having surface components which allow them to bind to respiratory epithelium: such organisms include influenza viruses, *Mycoplasma pneumoniae* and *Bordetella pertussis* (whooping cough). Other micro-organisms are less likely to cause respira-

tory infections unless the mucosa is first damaged. Such damage may be caused by the viruses of influenza which parasitise the respiratory epithelium and interfere with its protective function by destroying cilia: as a result, secondary bacterial infection invariably develops, and by extending into the alveoli may give rise to pneumonia. The integrity of the respiratory mucosa is also seriously impaired in chronic bronchitis, most commonly due to cigarette smoking but also to atmospheric pollution: this leads to metaplasia, the ciliated epithelium being replaced by goblet cells in the smaller bronchi. There is increase in the amount of secretion, which also becomes more viscous, and this tends to stagnate and become infected.

Intestinal pathogens, such as the salmonellae of 'food poisoning' and the shigellae of bacillary dysentery, induce an acute inflammatory reaction in the intestinal mucosa: diarrhoea results from the increased peristalsis and exudation, and repeated evacuation of the gut helps to get rid of the offending bacteria.

The flow of urine is of importance in preventing growth and spread of any bacteria gaining entrance to the urinary tract by the urethra, and any abnormality resulting in stagnation of urine or incomplete emptying of the bladder, particularly if chronic, e.g. obstruction by an enlarged prostate, predisposes to infection.

(d) Bacterial commensals. In spite of the defence mechanisms described above, the skin, mouth, nasal cavity, conjunctival sac and intestines are all colonised by bacteria of various types. The local environment provided by each of these various surfaces favours the survival of particular types of bacteria and thus each regional surface develops its own flora. In their usual site of colonisation, most of these commensals are non-pathogenic, and they tend to prevent the establishment of other types of microbes, including pathogens, by competing for nutrients and by release of metabolic products which are toxic to other organisms. Some bacteria secrete *bacteriocins*, which are proteins and are taken up by bacteria of closely related species: they mostly exert enzyme activities, e.g. nucleases, which cause the death of the recipient bacteria.

In normal circumstances, the bacterial florae of the various surfaces are remarkably stable, but if they are disturbed, colonisation by pathogens may result: hence the common occurrence of fungal infections of the pharynx in patients on antibiotic therapy, and the production of lesions by the toxin of *Clostridium difficile* in pseudomembranous colitis, which may arise when the normal flora is depressed by broad-spectrum antibiotics. 'Seeding' of the gut with non-pathogenic bacteria has achieved some success in preventing the overgrowth of pathogens in neonates and in patients treated by antibiotics.

(e) Phagocytes. There is evidence that phagocytic cells migrate on to the surface of various mucous membranes: for example neutrophil polymorphs pass through the thin epithelium lining the depths of the tonsillar crypts, and macrophages pass into the alveoli of the lungs. In both these sites the migrant cells have been shown to phagocytose particles on the surface of the mucosa and this may play a role in preventing invasion.

Invasive capacity of micro-organisms

Micro-organisms vary greatly in their capacity to invade the host's defensive barriers. Most bacteria cause injury only after they have invaded the host's tissues, but some are vitually incapable of invasion and yet can produce disease. For example, *Clostridium tetani*, the cause of tetanus, flourishes only in dead tissue, foreign material and exudate in wounds, but its toxin is absorbed and has serious effects on the nervous system. *Vibrio cholerae* does not invade the mucous membrane of the small intestine, but secretes a toxin which, by disturbing the control of fluid transport across the epithelium, causes severe dehydration. Other organisms, particularly viruses, are highly invasive and infect virtually all individuals who have not previously encountered or been immunised against them, e.g. the viruses of morbilli (measles) and rubella (german measles). Examples of highly invasive bacteria include *Yersinia pestis* (the cause of plague), *Salmonella typhi* (typhoid fever) and brucellae (undulant fever), all of which regularly invade the bloodstream. However, a great many bacteria lie intermediate between these extremes in their invasive capacity. This includes the more important pyogenic bacteria which are commonly present in the nose or throat or on the skin. Their presence is often harmless, but disturbances of defence mechanisms may allow them to invade and cause lesions.

In general, bacteria of high invasive capacity are also highly pathogenic, but there is little correlation between the invasive capacity and pathogenicity of viruses. For example, poliovirus invades readily but only a small proportion of infected individuals develop clinical disease, and non-pathogenic strains are administered orally to produce infection and immunity. Also, the protozoon *Toxoplasma gondii* is highly invasive and yet, apart from the lesions it causes in fetal life, it is of low pathogenicity.

Pathogenic effects of micro-organisms

Bacteria which have invaded the host tissues may be destroyed without causing clinically apparent disease, may promote a local inflammatory lesion, or may spread to other parts of the body and produce widespread lesions. The two major ways in which bacteria are known to cause pathological changes are firstly by the production of toxins, and secondly by promoting hypersensitivity reactions on the part of the host.

Viruses cause injury by invading the host's cells and utilising the cellular synthetic processes for their own replication. The infected cells may be destroyed directly by the replicating virus, by cytotoxic T cells, or possibly by lymphotoxin (p.7.21) secreted by T cells in the delayed hypersensitivity reaction.

Bacterial pili

Another factor which influences their pathogenicity is the capacity of micro-organisms to adhere to mucosal epithelial cells. Adherence is usually determined by bacterial fimbriae (pili) which are hair-like projections from the bacterial surface. Pathogenic strains of *Escherichia coli* may have pili of various types. Some, termed common pili, are the products of chromosomal genes, and bind to mannose residues on the surface of intestinal epithelium. Some strains have pili which are products of plasmid genes (p. 8.6): these are of various types, bind to various other sugar residues, and are distinguished by their antigenicity. The types of pili determine the mucosal surfaces to which *Esch.*

coli can adhere, e.g. to the small intestine or the urinary tract epithelium. Adherence by pili is a feature of many Gram − ve bacteria; they are of importance, for example, in gonococcal infection and determine the various parts of the urogenital tract and other mucosae which are colonised by particular strains of gonococci (Zak *et al.*, 1984). The fibrillae of Gram + ve bacteria play a similar role. For example, strains of *Streptococcus pyogenes* which cause rheumatic fever adhere strongly to the pharyngeal epithelium. In this instance, genetic host factors are also involved, and this has also been demonstrated in the adherence of *Esch. coli* to the urinary tract epithelium: individuals of blood group P1 are more prone than others to suffer from urinary tract infections with *Esch. coli*, presumably because a blood-group antigen on the surface of their urothelial cells binds certain strains of this micro-organism.

Bacterial toxins

These are of two main types, exotoxins and endotoxins.

Exotoxins are mostly secreted by living bacteria, although in some instances they are released only when the bacterium dies. They are simple proteins, are often extremely potent, and vary considerably in their biological effects upon the host. They are antigenically specific and their biological activity is usually neutralised by union with antibody. Many pathogenic bacteria produce a number of different exotoxins when cultured *in vitro*. Thus *Streptococcus pyogenes* and *Staphylococcus aureus*, two of the most important pyogenic bacteria, produce toxins which damage cell membranes and kill neutrophil polymorphs and macrophages. They also secrete hyaluronidases which digest hyaluronic acid of ground substance. Some strains of *Strep. pyogenes* secrete a toxin which lyses epidermal cells, while *Staph. aureus* secretes a coagulase which clots fibrinogen, and lipases which break down sebaceous secretions. The exudate in streptococcal infections is thin and watery because *Strep. pyogenes* produces an enzyme which digests nucleic acids. Some strains of *Strep. pyogenes* also produce erythrogenin, a toxin which causes vasodilation of the small blood vessels in the skin, and is responsible for the erythematous rash of scarlet fever. Intradermal injection of erythrogenin results in local erythema unless the subject has circulating antitoxin, and is used in the *Dick test* for immunity to *Strep. pyogenes*. Similarly, injection of antitoxin locally results in blanching of the skin in a patient with scarlet fever, and has been used as a diagnostic procedure (the *Schultz-Charlton test*). Some exotoxins are injurious to virtually all types of host cell and their effects thus depend on their concentration and distribution. *Corynebacterium diphtheriae*, the cause of diphtheria, secretes such a toxin and at the site of infection, usually the pharynx, it causes local tissue necrosis. Less florid but still severe cell injury is far more widespread and is reflected morphologically in fatty change and necrosis of the parenchymal cells of the various organs: in severe cases, death may result from its effect upon the myocardium (Fig. 8.1). The mechanism of injury by this particular toxin is known (p. 3.10): other toxins with a similarly widespread effect are produced by many of the pathogenic Gram + ve bacteria but in most instances the mechanism of toxic action is not known. Some have enzymic activity, e.g.

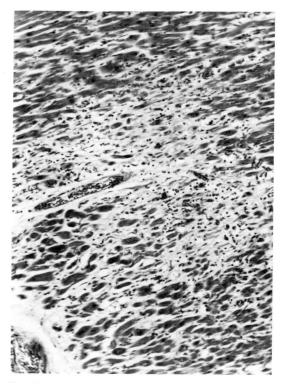

Fig. 8.1 Heart muscle in fatal diphtheria, showing destruction and disappearance of muscle fibres and a light inflammatory cellular infiltrate. × 115.

phosphatases, proteases, lipases. Some bacteria produce toxins which act specifically on one type of tissue. For example, the major toxin of *Clostridium botulinum* is absorbed from the gut, circulates in the bloodstream, and enters the motor nerve endings at neuromuscular junctions, where it inhibits the release of acetylcholine and thus causes a flaccid paralysis, usually fatal from respiratory failure. *Cl. botulinum* does not invade living tissues. Its heat-resistant spores contaminate preserved foods, in which the bacterium grows in anaerobic conditions and produces its toxin. Botulism is caused by eating preserved fruits, vegetables, meat, sausages, etc., containing the toxin, and is thus due to inadequate sterilisation of such foods. Another neurotoxin is produced by *Clostridium tetani*. This organism is a commensal of the intestine of various mammals, including domestic animals. Its spores thus contaminate the soil and infect dirty wounds, where the bacterium grows in anaerobic conditions in dead tissue and foreign material soaked with blood and exudate. The toxin is stored in the vegetative form of the organism and is released when it dies. The toxin enters nerve fibres and passes along the axons, both locally and generally (after dissemination in the blood), to reach the spinal cord, where it inhibits the release of glycine, the major inhibitory agent in nerve endings synapsing with the anterior horn cells. This results in increased tone of the skeletal muscles and a central excitatory state with attacks of generalised spasm of the voluntary muscles.

It is often difficult to determine the importance of particular bacterial toxins. Not only are many toxins produced by a single strain of bacteria but different samples of a toxin, even in highly purified form, may have different biological properties. Also, toxins vary greatly in their effects on hosts of different species, and experimental observations on animals are not necessarily applicable to man. Finally, production or non-production of toxin by bacteria growing *in vitro* does not necessarily indicate a similar behaviour *in vivo*. It is a feature of exotoxins that their biological effects are neutralised by the corresponding antitoxin, and in some instances, e.g. diphtheria and tetanus, prior administration of the antitoxin or active immunisation by injection of *toxoid* (inactivated toxin which maintains its immunogenicity) will protect animals against the effects of injection of the toxin and man against the disease. Thus in some instances, particular toxins have been incriminated beyond all reasonable doubt as the pathogenic agents responsible for the disease; in others, it seems most likely that toxins are responsible, but there remains the possibility that bacteria may have other pathogenic properties in addition to the toxins they are known to be capable of producing.

Some exotoxins are encoded by genes in the bacterial chromosome. Others are encoded by genes in **plasmids**, which consist of a ring of DNA separate from the bacterial chromosome. Plasmids also code for the sex pili of bacteria, formation of which is necessary for *conjugation*, i.e. sexual exchange of DNA between bacteria. This occurs between most Gram −ve and some Gram +ve bacteria, and during the process plasmids of the donor ('male') bacterium divide and one plasmid is transferred to the recipient ('female') bacterium, which thus becomes a transvestite 'male'. Part of the DNA of the bacterial chromosome may also be transferred. Conjugation can occur between bacteria of different species, and plasmid genes which confer greater pathogenicity may thus be acquired, resulting in bacteria of enhanced pathogenicity. Transfer of plasmids is also mainly responsible for the development of strains of bacteria resistant to antibiotics (see below).

Some toxins are encoded by genes transmitted to bacteria by bacteriophages ('phages'). When a bacteriophage inserts its DNA into a bacterium, replication of the phage DNA may occur, with assembly of phage particles which are released on the death of the bacterium. Phages which behave thus are termed *virulent*. Alternatively, one of the two strands of DNA which constitute the phage genome may be inserted at a specific site in the DNA of the bacterial chromosome, a process termed *transduction*. During bacterial division, the phage DNA is copied in the other DNA strand, and henceforth is transferred to the progeny as part of the chromosomal DNA. Phages which integrate into the bacterial genome in this way are termed *temperate phages*, the process of integration is termed *lysogeny* and the bacterium is then called *lysogenic*. When lysogenic bacteria proliferate, the phage DNA (*prophage*) usually remains in the chromosomal DNA, but in an occasional cell it is excised and replicates, and phage particles are assembled and released. Lysogenic bacteria express some of the prophage genes, and if these include genes coding for a toxic product, the bacterium produces and secretes the toxin. The outstanding example is *Corynebacteria diphtheriae*, the toxin of which is only produced by lysogenic bacteria containing the prophage toxigenic gene. Other examples include the erythrogenic toxin of some strains of *Strep. pyogenes* (see above) and the neurotoxins of some strains of *Clostridium botulinum*.

Pathogenicity of bacteria may be altered by a third genetic process, termed *transfection*, in which a fragment of DNA released by death of a bacterium is taken up by a living bacterium of the same or a closely-related species and incorporated into its DNA. This was first demonstrated by transformation of a gene coding for production of capsule material of *Streptococcus pneumoniae*: the capsule confers pathogenicity by inhibiting phagocytosis. Subsequently, it has been shown to occur with other species of bacteria, and while the fragment of DNA transferred is random, it may enhance pathogenicity by various means, depending on which genes become incorporated. Transformation has been shown experimentally to be capable of conferring resistance to various antibiotics.

Bacteria capable of transformation under natural conditions include streptococci, staphylococci, gonococci, meningococci and haemophilus.

Endotoxins are constituents of the cell wall of Gram −ve bacteria and are released mainly when bacteria die. They are complexes of phospholipid (lipid A), polysaccharide and protein and are often referred to as bacterial lipopolysaccharides (LPS). The endotoxins produced by different bacteria differ in their antigenicity but they all have the same biological effects, which are due mainly to lipid A.

Compared with many exotoxins, endotoxins are relatively weakly cytotoxic to cells in general, but in extensive Gram −ve bacterial infections they do cause injury to the parenchymal cells of the various organs. In addition, they induce the following changes.

1. Discharge of lysosomal granules from neutrophil polymorphs, with escape of their contents to the exterior. This is rapidly followed by death of the degranulated polymorphs.
2. Release of young neutrophil polymorphs from the marrow into the blood.

3. Activation of monocytes, with increased motility, phagocytic capacity and increased synthesis and secretion of their lysosomal enzymes.
4. Stimulation of monocytes and macrophages to synthesise and secrete endogenous pyrogen (interleukin 1).
5. Activation of Hageman factor with consequent triggering of the coagulation, kinin and fibrinolytic cascade systems of the plasma.
6. Aggregation of platelets and triggering of the platelet release reaction.
7. Activation of the complement system by the alternative pathway.

It will be apparent from Chapter 4 that these various activities result in the production of the many potential mediators of the acute inflammatory reaction, and when a small dose of endotoxin is injected locally, e.g. intradermally, it induces acute inflammation which lasts for a few hours. Presumably this reaction is triggered off by the cytotoxic effect of endotoxin. Once initiated, the reaction is augmented by the products of neutrophil polymorphs, macrophages and platelets, activation products of the cascade systems and enzymes released from damaged tissue cells.

When larger amounts of endotoxin are injected intravascularly, a systemic reaction results, characterised by fever, headache, vomiting and endotoxic ('septic') shock, the features of which are described on p. 10.42.

The state of shock is caused by peripheral vasodilation and the damaging effect of endotoxin on parenchymal cells, including the myocardium. There is an initial neutrophil leucopenia followed within a few hours by leucocytosis. Systemic activation of the coagulation system may result in disseminated intravascular coagulation (p. 10.11) followed by a bleeding state caused by thrombocytopenia, consumption of coagulation factors and activation of the plasmin system with consequent hypofibrinogenaemia. Death may result from either multi-organ or circulatory failure, which is aggravated by haemorrhage from mucous membranes. The kidneys are particularly severely affected by fibrin formation in the small blood vessels and renal tubular or cortical necrosis may develop. The adrenals also suffer from haemorrhage and necrosis (Fig. 26.23, p. 26.36) with consequent acute adrenocortical insufficiency—The Waterhouse-Friderichsen syndrome. These systemic effects of endotoxin occur in septicaemia or major local infections, notably peritonitis, caused by Gram—ve bacteria.

Slow infusion or repeated injection of small amounts of endotoxin intravascularly results in a refractory state, developing after a few hours and lasting for several days, during which many of the effects of endotoxin, including fever, are diminished, although larger doses still produce the usual effects.

If a small amount of endotoxin is injected intradermally into a rabbit, followed 24 hours later by an intravenous injection, the second injection is followed by haemorrhage and necrosis at the site of the intradermal injection, associated with local formation of platelet thrombi. This experimental phenomenon is termed the **local Schwartzmann reaction**. If both injections are given intravenously, a state of shock and disseminated intravascular coagulation develops after the second injection—the **generalised Schwartzmann reaction**. These changes can be induced by relatively small amounts of endotoxin, and it is not clear why two spaced injections should produce an exaggerated effect.

The presumably specific cell receptors for endotoxin have not been identified. Endotoxins also act as thymic-independent antigens (p. 6.24) inducing short-lived antibody production by B cells. They also act as polyclonal B cell activators and stimulate B cells to differentiate and secrete their specific antibodies, thus by-passing the need for helper T cells.

Hypersensitivity reactions to micro-organisms

Virtually all microbial infections stimulate immune responses by the host, and the reaction of the antibodies or primed T lymphocytes with microbial antigens can result in hypersensitivity of various types. Atopic (type 1) reactions, such as urticaria, are a common feature of infection by parasitic worms, even in individuals not otherwise predisposed to atopy, and microbial infections sometimes cause atopic reactions in individuals predisposed to this type of hypersensitivity. Cytotoxic antibody (type 2) reactions may, in theory, result from the cross-reaction of microbial-induced antibodies with host cells, a probable example being rheumatic fever, in which antibodies to *Strep. pyogenes* react with heart muscle. Immune-complex (type 3) reactions are important complications of some infections. Local Arthus reactions occur when microbial antigens in infected tissues react with antibodies in the plasma: immune complexes are deposited in the walls of small blood vessels. Circulating immune-complex disease occurs when microbial antigens enter the blood, immune complexes then being formed in the plasma, resulting in an acute febrile reaction and/or deposition of the complexes in small blood vessels, notably in the glomeruli where they are responsible for glomerulonephritis (p. 7.17). The acute generalised reaction is believed to be the cause of the dengue shock syndrome which, together with other examples of infections giving rise to immune-complex reactions, and the way in which lesions are produced, are described on pp. 7.15–17.

Cell-mediated immunity is an important defence mechanism in various infections. The lymphokines released when primed T cells react with microbial antigens (p. 7.20) contribute to both destruction of micro-organisms by macrophages and the tissue injury of delayed (type 4) hypersensitivity. Consequently, the two phenomena are commonly associated. The classical example is tuberculosis, in which cell-mediated immunity develops to tuberculoprotein, and is largely responsible for the lesions of this disease. *Myco. tuberculosis* has not been shown to produce toxins and can colonise macrophages in culture without causing apparent injury: addition of primed helper T lymphocytes reactive with tuberculoprotein on the surface of infected macrophages activates the macrophages and promotes killing of their ingested micro-organisms, although the infected macrophages may be destroyed by cytotoxic T cells. The morphological features of tuberculosis, described in the next chapter, can all be explained on the basis of delayed hypersensitivity. Leprosy is another disease in which delayed hypersensitivity is a decisive factor. In some cases, cell-mediated immunity is weak or absent and *Myco. leprae* multiply progressively, mostly within macrophages. Like tubercle bacilli, they cause little or no cell injury, and the lesions consist of enlarging nodules composed of macrophages containing large numbers of *Myco. leprae*. In other cases, strong cell-mediated immunity develops, and the bacteria are kept partly in check. Very few are demonstrable in the lesions, but delayed hypersensitivity results in tubercle-like granulomas and fibrosis (p. 9.24). This is a good example of the dual effect of cell-mediated immunity—it limits the numbers of micro-organisms, but also causes injury of host tissues.

Delayed hypersensitivity reactions are commonly prominent in fungal, viral and chronic bacterial infections. They are probably involved also in some of the skin lesions of chickenpox, measles, etc. but firm evidence on the pathogenesis of the skin rashes in these conditions is remarkably scanty.

Defence mechanisms in infections

When micro-organisms have invaded the tissues, there are three inter-related major defensive reactions which tend to limit their multiplication and spread, and bring about their destruction: these are the inflammatory reaction, phagocytic activity and specific immune reactions.

The inflammatory reaction

The acute inflammatory reaction. The defensive role of this reaction has been considered on p. 4.25. Without doubt, it is of considerable importance, and *those infections which are accompanied by acute inflammation at the site of invasion are more likely to remain localised than those in which invasion is accomplished without local injury or reaction.* The pyogenic bacteria are a common cause of the former type of infection, while silent invasion is illustrated by *Treponema pallidum*, the cause of syphilis, which spreads widely through the body before the appearance of a local lesion at the site of entry. Other bacteria which may enter the body silently and spread widely include *Neisseria meningitidis*, a cause of acute meningitis, and brucellae, the cause of undulant fever. Many of the parasites transmitted by biting insects, such as the plasmodia which cause malaria, produce generalised infection without a significant local reaction, and many viruses invade the body and produce viraemia without first producing a local inflammatory lesion at the site of initial infection.

Chronic inflammatory change also plays a defensive role by exposing the micro-organisms to phagocytes, antibodies and effector T lymphocytes, and by surrounding them with a layer of granulation tissue which has been shown to be an effective barrier to bacteria. In the more prolonged infections, such as tuberculosis, surviving micro-organisms may be effectively confined within a zone of dense fibrosis resulting from chronic inflammatory change.

Phagocytosis and killing of micro-organisms

A general account of phagocytosis has been given on p. 4.25, and we are concerned here with factors which determine the capacity of neutrophil polymorphs and macrophages to phagocytose and subsequently kill micro-organisms. Bacteria differ greatly in their resistance to these processes, and such resistance is often an important factor in their pathogenicity.

The inflammatory and immune responses are important host factors favouring phagocytosis and killing of micro-organisms. They help to provide an environment favourable to phagocytosis, render the micro-organism more susceptible to phagocytosis, and increase the phagocytic and killing activities of phagocytes. These factors are illustrated for macrophages in Fig. 8.2. Emigration of polymorphs and monocytes is part of the inflammatory reaction, and the inflammatory exudate opens up tissue spaces in which the emigrated phagocytes can move. Immunoglobulins and components of complement enter infected tissues in the inflammatory exudate; if specific antibodies are present, they may aid phagocytosis by rendering the micro-organisms more susceptible to phagocytic ingestion (opsonisation), or by neutralising toxins harmful to phagocytes. The reaction of antibodies usually activates complement, which may kill Gram −ve bacteria directly and favours the destruction of micro-organisms in general by enhancing the inflammatory reaction and chemotaxis of phagocytes (pp. 4.18–19).

Both polymorphs and macrophages have surface receptors for the Fc component of IgG antibodies, and this facilitates surface binding and subsequent phagocytosis of microbes sensitised with IgG antibodies (Fig. 8.2): they also have surface receptors for the C3b component

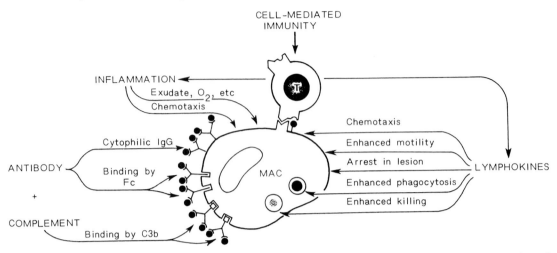

Fig. 8.2   The integrated effects of inflammation, cell-mediated and humoral immunity on the destruction of micro-organisms by macrophages (MAC). Note that helper T cells (T) are activated by reacting with a combination of class II HLA molecules (ʍ) and antigen (●) expressed on the surface of macrophages, and the delayed hypersensitivity reaction is thus triggered by macrophages which have phagocytosed micro-organisms (●).

of reacted complement but, surprisingly, while complement fixation by antibody-sensitised bacteria enhances binding to the phagocyte, it does not render the bound micro-organisms more susceptible to phagocytosis. IgM antibodies are opsonic, particularly for micro-organisms with a non-protein capsule. Their opsonic effect is not due to specific binding to phagocytes, which do not have surface receptors for Fc of IgM, although complement activation, binding by C3b receptors and phagocytosis are likely to follow.

Cell-mediated immunity is particularly effective in destroying microbes which invade host cells. The lymphokines released when primed T cells react with antigen on the surface of infected cells include factors which promote inflammation, accumulation of macrophages and lymphocytes, and enhance, both specifically and non-specifically, the phagocytosis and killing of ingested micro-organisms by macrophages (p. 7.20).

The mechanisms of killing of micro-organisms by phagocytes are complex. Unlike phagocytosis, which can occur readily under anaerobic conditions, killing is associated with increased oxygen uptake. In **polymorphs**, oxygen is converted by NADPH into superoxide ($^-O_2$) by removal of an electron; some of this is converted into hydrogen peroxide (H_2O_2) and singlet oxygen ($'O_2$), which has an

unstable distribution of electrons around the two nuclei, is also produced. All these forms of highly reactive oxygen are produced within the phagolysosome, the membrane of which protects the cell from their effects. They react with the wall of the phagocytosed micro-organism and are highly lethal to many bacteria, viruses and fungi. Hydrogen peroxide also co-operates with myeloperoxidase which, together with halogen ions, forms a system which attacks the microbial cell wall.

In addition to the above mechanisms, the low pH within phagolysosomes is unfavourable to many micro-organisms, and other lysosomal products exert a harmful effect, notably cationic lysosomal proteins which injure microbial cell walls, apolactoferrin (an iron-binding protein), and lysozyme, which has a synergistic lytic effect with complement.

Macrophages lack myeloperoxidase, cationic microbicidal proteins and apolactoferrin. They are, however, capable of producing microbicidal forms of oxygen and they are activated by bacterial products and by the lymphokines produced by T lymphocytes in delayed hypersensitivity reactions (p. 7.21); their motility, phagocytic activity, lysosomal enzymes and killing capacity are all increased as a result.

Microbial resistance to phagocytes. In general, those bacteria which develop a non-protein capsule, e.g. the anthrax bacillus or smooth strains of *Strep. pneumoniae* and *Haemophilus influenzae*, are not readily phagocytosed. Some bacterial products are chemotactic, but *Strep. pyogenes* and some other bacteria secrete toxins which injure phagocytic (and other) cells and so inhibit phagocytosis. Other bacterial products, e.g. the endotoxins of Gram −ve bacteria, enhance the phagocytic activity of polymorphs and macrophages in low concentrations, but inhibit it in higher concentrations. The pili of some Gram −ve bacteria inhibit phagocytosis, while *Staphylococcus aureus* secretes a factor ('protein A') which binds to the Fc of IgG, and thus interferes with the binding and phagocytosis of bacteria opsonised by IgG antibody.

A number of micro-organisms undergo phagocytosis but are able to resist the microbicidal activity of phagocytes and even multiply within them. A good example is provided by *Neisseria gonorrhoeae* (the cause of gonorrhoea) which is readily phagocytosed but may kill the polymorph and multiply within it (Fig. 8.3). Another factor of importance in infections is the requirement of bacteria for iron. Neutrophil polymorphs contain iron in the form of lactoferrin, i.e. bound to protein, but some bacteria produce iron-binding proteins (*siderophores*) which are capable of transferring iron from lactoferrin to the bacterium. It is of interest that *Neisseria gonorrhoeae* occasionally spreads by

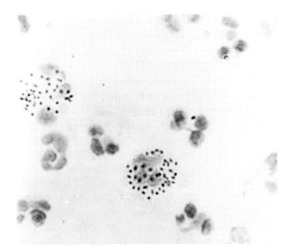

Fig. 8.3 Smear of urethral exudate in acute gonorrhoea. Two polymorphs contain large numbers of gonococci, and show degenerative changes. Other polymorphs contain few or no bacteria and appear relatively healthy. (Gram stain.) × 1200.

the blood and settles in joints, causing a septic arthritis. This is most likely to occur in women during menstruation and has been attributed to the increased availability of iron at that time.

Some viruses undergo phagocytosis by macrophages, but can bind to the phagosomal wall and pass into the cytosol of the host cell where they replicate. A number of organisms succeed in preventing the fusion of lysosomes with the phagocytic vacuole, and so protect themselves from lysosomal microbicidal products: this is observed with tubercle bacilli ingested by macrophages in culture and with the protozoon *Toxoplasma gondii* and the fungus *Aspergillus flavus*, all of which cause chronic infections in man. In other instances, the organism can flourish within phagolysosomes, e.g. the brucellae of undulant fever. Other organisms have a suppressive effect on cell-mediated immunity and persist within macrophages which are handicapped by lack of the enhancing effects of T-cell lymphokines on their microbicidal activity. They include the leprosy bacillus and some viruses and protozoa.

The immune response

The several ways in which antibodies and cell-mediated immunity help to destroy micro-organisms have been described in this and preceding chapters, and may be summarised as follows. **Antibodies** of IgA class are important in preventing the invasion of mucous membranes by viruses and probably by some bacteria (p. 8.2). IgM and IgG antibodies can neutralise bacterial toxins, agglutinate and immobilise micro-organisms (p. 6.7), and prevent cell invasion by viruses: by activating complement, they may cause lysis of microbial cell walls without the intervention of phagocytes (p. 7.4). Activation of complement also promotes the inflammatory reaction and attracts polymorphs by chemotaxis (pp. 4.13–18). Antibodies, particularly those of IgG class, also opsonise micro-organisms, thus favouring their ingestion and destruction by phagocytes (see above).

When the primed T lymphocytes produced by **cell-mediated immune responses** react with the surface of infected macrophages, they release lymphokines which induce the inflammatory and other changes of the delayed hypersensitivity reaction (p. 7.18). In addition to exerting chemotactic and immobilising effects on macrophages, lymphokines include a macrophage-activating factor which increases their killing capacity for ingested micro-organisms, and a second factor—the specific macrophage-arming factor—which enables macrophages to kill allogeneic target cells and may also mediate destruction of micro-organisms. Eventually the macrophages are converted to epithelioid cells, the functions of which are not known.

One of the main purposes of this summary is to emphasise the complex relationships and synergism by which *the inflammatory response, phagocytosis, and immunological reactions together provide a closely interwoven system of defence against micro-organisms.*

Interferons (p. 9.2) are probably mainly responsible for arresting virus infections, yet children with congenital T-cell deficiencies tend to develop progressive virus infections. This could be attributable to loss of the interferon (IFN-γ) which is produced by T cells responding to antigen. Many types of cell are capable of producing interferons when infected by viruses, but this does not appear to eliminate the infection unless it is accompanied by cell-mediated immunity and production of interferon-γ by T cells (p. 9.2).

Microbial resistance to the host's immune response. Micro-organisms which colonise host cells are protected from **antibody** in the plasma and tissue fluids, and can persist in spite of a strong antibody response. This is illustrated by the brucellae of undulant fever, the protozoon *Leishmania donovani* which causes leishmaniasis, and some fungi, all of which can survive in macrophages. This mode of protection is particularly successful for organisms which do not kill the host macrophage nor prevent its division. As obligatory intracellular parasites, viruses are protected from antibodies once they are inside a cell, but the presence of antibody in the blood normally protects the host from re-infection by the same virus.

To survive, intracellular micro-organisms must also protect themselves against the host's **cell-mediated immune response** and many of them do this by exerting a suppressive effect on cell-mediated immunity in general. This is observed in a number of viral infections, including measles, mumps, infection with the Epstein-Barr virus (the cause of infectious mononucleosis), and the animal leukaemia viruses which infect and transform lymphoid cells. It is also a feature of lepromatous leprosy (p. 9.23), leishmaniasis (p. 28.9) and malaria (p. 28.3).

In some infective diseases, the micro-organisms proliferate rapidly before the development of an effective humoral immune response. This is seen in severe acute cases of meningococcal septicaemia and meningtitis, in which free bacterial polysaccharide antigen can be detected in the serum and CSF (a test used in diagnosis), and also in acute pneumococcal pneumonia or septicaemia. Some persistent infections are associated with failure of the humoral immune response. An example is provided by the B hepatitis virus (p. 20.11) which replicates in the liver and produces large amounts of viral surface antigen: in carriers, free viral surface antigen can be demonstrated in the serum. The cell-mediated immune response may also be ineffective in extensive infections, for example in widespread tuberculosis or acute tuberculous broncho-pneumonia; in these conditions, cell-mediated immunity develops, but is insufficient to counter the large number of micro-organisms, and the skin test with tuberculoprotein, which is based on a delayed hypersensitivity reaction (p. 7.18), becomes negative.

Another ingenious method of circumventing the host's immune response is by **antigenic variation**. This is exemplified by relapsing fever, caused by *Borrelia recurrentis* and trypanosomiasis caused by flagellate protozoa. Both of these organisms stimulate an antibody response to which they are susceptible, but they possess a number of genes coding for the antigenically-distinct glycoprotein which forms their outer coat. Although the great majority are destroyed by the host's antibody response, occasional organisms express another gene for production of antigenically dissimilar outer coat and arise as resistant variants with consequent relapse, and so the diseases are characterised by successive relapses. The influenza virus is notorious for *antigenic drift*, in which the antigenicity of its surface haemagglutinating antigen changes gradually, and *antigenic shift* in which there is sudden change of the composition of the surface antigen.

Another elegant method of protection is illustrated by the group of parasitic trematodes termed *Schistosomes*. These parasites enter the body as a larval form (schistosomule), which stimulates an immune response in the host, but the larvae rapidly become coated with host blood-group substances and so provide themselves with an immunological cloak which they maintain during development and adult life. The immune response is partly effective in destroying schistosomules subsequently entering the body, before they become coated, and further infection is thus usually limited. Unfortunately many of the eggs produced by the adults are arrested in the host tissues and elicit a delayed hypersensitivity reaction resulting in a chronic inflammatory lesion, notably in the liver (p. 28.25).

Mention should also be made of the possibility of a micro-organism inducing in the host **specific immunological tolerance** to its own antigens. This occurs when mice are infected via the ovum with lymphocytic choriomeningitis virus. The virus induces tolerance and persists into adult life, notably in the ependyma and cells lining the meninges; little or no harmful effects result until tolerance partly breaks down and the development of antibodies is followed by deposition of antigen-antibody complexes in the glomeruli and elsewhere. If a mouse is first infected some time after birth, it develops choriomeningitis due to the development of cell-mediated immunity and a consequent delayed hypersensitivity reaction to viral-infected cells. A parallel in man has not been demonstrated. Tolerance might arise also from **molecular mimicry**, in which a micro-organism possesses surface antigens closely similar to host antigens. Some of the coliform bacilli in the gut have been shown to share a common antigen with colonic epithelium, and antibodies induced by various bacteria react with particular transplant (HLA) antigens of man. Such antigenic similarities have not been shown to influence infections, but individuals possessing particular HLA antigens have been found to be unduly prone to certain infections. For example, Reiter's syndrome (p. 25.2), due to a chlamydia, occurs especially in people with HLA-B27, and tolerance or genetically-determined inability to respond to a particular microbial antigen remain as possibilities. There is evidence that the capsular polysaccharide of group B strains of *Neisseria meningitidis* is antigenically similar to polysialic acid groupings present in normal brain tissue, and T-cell immunological tolerance to the latter may explain why antibody to group B *Neisseria meningitidis* polysaccharide following injection of vaccine or natural infection is of low titre and restricted to IgM class. In contrast, the antibody response to other groups of *Neisseria meningitidis* polysaccharide is much greater, includes IgG-class antibody, and provides effective immunity.

Antibacterial drug therapy

Antibiotic drugs are capable of killing bacteria or suppressing their multiplication, and often tip the balance in favour of the host and terminate the infection. Antibiotic therapy is not, however, without risk. Apart from their toxic side-effects and the induction of hypersensitivity reactions, antibiotics can, as already mentioned, encourage the multiplication of resistant strains of bacteria. Weak resistance may be determined by orthodox genetic bacterial inheritance, but strong resistance is usually determined by the products of plasmid genes and may be transmitted to bacteria (of the same or different species) by conjugation (p. 8.6). Bacteria may carry more than one type of plasmid, and the resistance (R) genes of plasmids are sometimes incorporated into lengths of DNA termed *transposons*, which are capable of transferring between different plasmids and also between plasmid and chromosomal DNA. Accordingly, the same plasmid may acquire separate genes conferring resistance for different antibiotic agents.

Antibiotic resistance has been observed to develop in virtually all species of bacteria causing disease in man, and multiple resistance to several antibiotics is becomoming increasingly common. There is no doubt that resistance has increased in frequency as a result of widespread use of antibiotic drugs, and it appears that, for every antibiotic drug used, there are corresponding R genes. This is perhaps not surprising, for effective antibiotics must interfere with vital bacterial matabolic processes, the integrity of which has been protected throughout evolution by the selection of various genes conferring the capacity to survive in adverse conditions.

Plasmid-conferred resistance to antibiotics has resulted in major epidemics, notably of bacillary dysentery and typhoid fever. Resistant strains of *Neisseria gonorrhoeae* have developed and are increasing, and resistant forms of many other bacteria are being encountered. Over 90%

of *Staphylococcus aureus* infections acquired in hospitals are resistant to penicillin, and often to other antibiotics, but plasmids carried by this species are incapable of inducing conjugation, and the R genes are transferred by transduction (p. 8.6). Hospitals are excellent breeding grounds for resistance because of their heavy use of antibiotics and the frequency of infections in hospital patients. It is noteworthy that R plasmids conferring resistance can occur and spread among commensal micro-organisms, e.g. *Escherichia coli* in the intestine. This provides a reservoir from which plasmids may be transferred to pathogens.

R plasmids have been detected in bacteria maintained in lyophilised state since before the introduction of antibiotics. The effect of widespread use of antibiotics has been to favour the spread of bacteria containing them and to encourage the proliferation of bacteria acquiring them. The problem requires the implementation of policies in the use of antibiotics, not only in treating patients, but also in animal husbandry, where antibiotics are sometimes incorporated as growth-promoting agents in animal foodstuffs. The spread of resistant bacteria by this practice is illustrated by an experiment in which two of fifty chickens were infected with *Esch. coli* carrying a plasmid conferring resistance to tetracycline. When tetracycline was included in the food, the resistant strain spread to all the chickens and also to those in a separate cage 15 metres away. Incorporation of tetracycline in the food was responsible for such spread, for without it the resistant strain was rapidly eliminated from the two infected chickens without spreading to others (Levy *et al.*, 1976).

Diminished resistance to infection

There is a wide range of individual 'natural' resistance to microbial infections among apparently normal individuals. This is largely unexplained, but it is apparent that variations in susceptibility to some infections are related to the individual's HLA type (p. 2.12). This does no more than indicate that genetic factors are involved.

Impaired resistance to infection can occur in many ways. Examples of defects in local barriers to invasion have been given earlier in this chapter. Normal phagocytic function, immune responsiveness and complement function are all essential factors contributing to the range of protective mechanisms. A serious fall in the number of polymorphs in the blood, as in agranulocytosis, predisposes to bacterial invasion and severe, spreading infections, e.g. of the pharynx and intestine, by both commensals and more highly pathogenic bacteria. Genetically-determined defects of polymorph function also predispose to bacterial infection. These polymorph abnormalities are considered on pp. 17.13-15. There are also many diseases which impair specific immune responses; they include the rare congenital immunodeficiency states and also acquired diseases which involve the lymphoid tissue and affect their immunological functions (pp. 7.32-36). Patients with immunodeficiency, especially of cell-mediated immunity, are unduly susceptible to viral infections and particularly to reactivation of latent infections, e.g. herpes zoster, cytomegalovirus infection, and progressive multifocal leucoencephalopathy (p. 21.37). Children with congenital T-cell deficiencies are also prone to develop giant-cell pneumonia when infected with measles virus.

In other diseases, predisposition to infection is well known but unexplained. A good example is diabetes mellitus, in which boils and urinary tract infections are common and there is a predisposition to tuberculosis: it may be that phagocytic activity, which requires the energy provided by glycolysis, is impaired by the defective carbohydrate metabolism of untreated diabetes.

C-reactive protein (CRP)

This is the best known of the acute phase reactants which are present mostly in low concentrations in the plasma and increase rapidly and dramatically following tissue trauma or development of an inflammatory reaction, and return to normal levels when the inflammation subsides. C-reactive protein is synthesised by hepatocytes and consists of a complex of five identical polypeptide chains arranged in a disc-like structure. It was discovered by its property of binding to and precipitating the C polysaccharide of the capsule of *Streptococcus pneumoniae* (hence the name) but it binds also to capsular polysaccharides of various other bacteria, to choline phosphatides and other constituents of the lipids of cell membranes. Such binding activates complement by the classical pathway and so promotes phagocytosis and enhances inflammation. Proteins showing sequence homology with CRP are present in the plasma of most if not all vertebrates, and have thus been preserved during evolution. Although its physiological role is not known, it is thought to aid in the phagocytic removal of cellular fragments and may also contribute to phagocytosis of bacteria.

Assay of CRP is used as a diagnostic aid in acute infections, in which the plasma level may rise by several hundredfold within a few hours of onset, and also in monitoring the activity of rheumatoid arthritis and Crohn's disease. Its production is mediated by endogenous pyrogen (p. 8.20) and by prostaglandin E_1. The only known vertebrate protein with a similar structure is the P protein of amyloid.

Two important reactions to infection are leucocytosis and fever, accounts of which follow.

Polymorphonuclear Leucocytosis

The number of neutrophil polymorphs in the blood, normally $2 \cdot 5 - 7 \cdot 5 \times 10^9$/litre (2500–7500/$\mu$l) in older children and adults, increases in various pathological conditions. The increase is a controlled reaction and when the cause subsides the leucocyte count returns to the normal level for that individual. This account deals with the causes and mechanisms of such a neutrophil leucocytosis and with the changes in the haemopoietic marrow responsible for increased leucocyte production. The proliferation of leucocytes in myeloid leukaemia is neoplastic rather than reactive and is described in Chapter 17.

Causes

Neutrophil leucocytosis occurs in association with acute inflammatory reactions, tissue necrosis, thrombosis, haemorrhage, acute lysis of red cells, and sometimes cancer. A mild polymorph leucocytosis occurs in pregnancy and also results from strenuous exercise, severe mental stress, and from injection of glucocorticoids, corticotrophin or adrenaline. By far the commonest cause in clinical medicine is inflammation due to bacterial infection, and in general the degree of leucocytosis correlates with the size of the inflammatory lesion and the intensity of polymorph emigration in the infected tissues. Pyogenic infections, due for example to virulent staphylococci, streptococci, pneumococci and coliform bacilli, are accompanied by a brisk leucocytosis, the height of which depends partly on the duration and partly on the extent of the infection. A boil or acute appendicitis may induce a moderate rise, e.g. to 10×10^9 polymorphs per litre, while a large abscess, acute bacterial pneumonia or general peritonitis are commonly accompanied by a count of 20×10^9/l or more. In some severe infections with pyogenic bacteria, e.g. streptococcal septicaemia or pneumococcal pneumonia, there may be absence of leucocytosis, or even leucopenia; this usually indicates overwhelming toxaemia and is a bad prognostic sign. In some severe acute infections, e.g. gas gangrene due to *Cl. welchii*, polymorph emigration is less intense, and the increase in polymorphs in the blood is less marked, while the acute inflammatory lesions of the intestine caused by the typhoid and paratyphoid bacilli are virtually devoid of polymorphs (Fig. 8.4) and there is actually a fall in the number of polymorphs in the blood. Some virus infections, particularly in the early stages, are also accompanied by a neutrophil leucopenia.

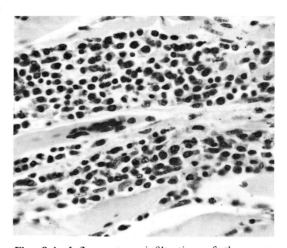

Fig. 8.4 Inflammatory infiltration of the muscular layer of the small intestine in typhoid fever, showing mononuclear cells and absence of polymorphs. × 150.

Necrosis of tissue, for example myocardial infarction, causes a slight or moderate neutrophil leucocytosis, and extensive thrombosis, e.g. in the leg veins, or severe haemorrhage, both have a similar effect.

Leucocytosis may develop within a few hours of the onset of a bacterial infection and is of diagnostic value. This early rise is due partly to release of many polymorphs which normally lie marginated in the venules of the lungs and elsewhere, and partly to release of young polymorphs lying in the sinusoids of the haemopoietic marrow. Soon, however, there is an increased rate of formation of polymorphs in the marrow and the leucocytosis is thus maintained. It appears from recent observations that the life of the neutrophil polymorph in the blood is probably not more than 12 hours, and since there are approximately 5 litres of blood containing about 4×10^9 polymorphs per litre, the normal daily production must be at least 4×10^{10}. In a suppurating infection, ten times this number may be lost daily for weeks or months in the pus discharging from an abscess, while at the same time the blood level may be maintained at 20×10^9/litre or more. It is thus apparent that the output of polymorphs is capable of enormous and sustained increase, and the process responsible for this is hyperplasia of the bone marrow, considered below.

Production of polymorphs (Granulopoiesis)

In the normal adult, production of the granulocyte or myeloid series of leucocytes is restricted to the haemopoietic marrow, where it occurs along with the production of red cells, platelets and monocytes. All these cells, and also lymphocytes (p. 6.14), originate from *haemopoietic stem cells*, which give rise to more stem cells and also to cells of more restricted potential: some are progenitors of red cells, other of megakaryocytes, while recent observations have demonstrated progenitor cells capable of giving rise to both polymorphs and monocytes (see below).

Because of their basic role in haemopoiesis, haemopoietic stem cells are dealt with in the chapter on blood (p. 17.2).

Stages of granulopoiesis. The earliest recognisable granulocyte precursor is termed a myeloblast: small numbers of these are present in normal haemopoietic marrow and they divide

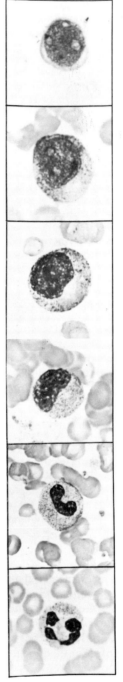

Myeloblast: non-granular (oxidase-negative), basophilic cytoplasm (rich in RNA); nucleus roughly spherical, with dispersed chromatin (euchromatin), and containing 2 or more nucleoli. 10–18 µm diameter.

Promyelocyte: a few primary (oxidase positive) cytoplasmic granules; basophilic cytoplasm; nucleus spherical, still with dispersed chromatin and nucleoli. 12–18 µm diameter.

Myelocytes: cytoplasm less basophilic; primary granules disappear and secondary granules develop—they are strongly oxidase-positive and specific (neutrophil, eosinophil or basophil). Nucleus spherical or ovoid with some condensation of chromatin (heterochromatin). Active mitosis occurs at this stage. 12–18 µm diameter.

Metamyelocyte: cytoplasm only faintly basophilic (poor in RNA), with many specific granules and no primitive granules. Nucleus becoming elongated, smaller and more condensed. 12–15 µm diameter.

Polymorphonuclear leucocyte: cytoplasm as in metamyelocytes; nucleus smaller, and chromatin more condensed, at first horse-shoe shaped, later lobulated. 10–15 µm diameter.

Fig. 8.5 Cells in haemopoietic marrow representing stages of granulopoiesis: from the myelocyte stage, only neutrophil cells are illustrated. Leishman stain × 1000. (Dr. R. Brooke Hogg.)

to give rise to a population of cells which undergo successive mitoses and form the largest cell population in the marrow. This proliferation is accompanied by a continuous process of differentiation up to the granulocyte stage: representative stages are illustrated in Fig. 8.5. Throughout the process the ratio of cytoplasm to nucleus increases and after initial enlargement up to the early myelocyte stage, diminution in size is a feature of differentiation. In the primitive stages the nucleus is large, ovoid or indented, and the chromatin is finely distributed. Gradually the nucleus shrinks, becoming more deeply staining, and eventually it becomes elongated giving the 'band form', followed by division into lobes, the number of which increases during the late stages of maturation of the polymorph in the marrow and in the blood. In preparations stained by a Romanowsky dye (e.g. Leishman's, Wright's, Jenner's or Giemsa stains), the cytoplasmic changes are as described in Fig. 8.5: from the myelocyte stage, there is not sufficient RNA to impart strong basophilia, and the cytoplasm is pale blue. Lysosomal granules appear in the cytoplasm in the promyelocyte stage: at first they are large and stained reddish-blue, but in the myelocyte stage these early granules are gradually replaced by granules specific for neutrophil, eosinophil or basophil polymorphs. In the neutrophil myelocytes the granules are small and are stained reddish or purple: in the eosinophil they are larger and bright orange, while those of basophils are large and dark blue. These characteristic granules persist in the three type of mature granulocytes or polymorphs. In an early neutrophil leucocytosis there is an increased proportion of young cells and even myelocytes may appear in the blood.

Leucocytosis is brought about by hyperplasia, (i.e. an increase in the number of cells), in the haemopoietic marrow, and the proportion of myeloid cells, and particularly of myelocytes, is increased. This is termed a *granulopoietic reaction* and is analogous to the

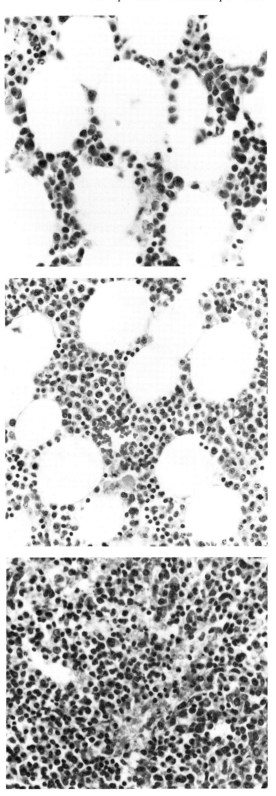

Fig. 8.6 Sections of haemopoietic marrow illustrating hyperplasia associated with neutrophil leucocytosis. *Top*, normal marrow. *Middle*, marrow showing increased cellularity in a patient with leucocytosis of short duration. *Bottom*, marked hyperplasia of marrow in a patient with prolonged leucocytosis: the fat cells have been replaced by haemopoietic cells. × 315.

erythroblastic reaction in response to an increased requirement of red cells, e.g. after haemorrhage. The fat cells normally present in haemopoietic (red) marrow diminish in number as the cellularity increases (Fig. 8.6) and also foci of haemopoietic tissue arising from stem cells appear in the yellow fatty marrow of the long bones. These foci extend rapidly and in a severe prolonged suppurating infection much of the yellow marrow in the shafts of the femur and other long bones may be replaced by red marrow, the change starting in the upper ends of the bones and extending downwards. All the cellular constituents of normal marrow are present in this newly formed haemopoietic tissue, but myelocytes and later forms predominate (Figs. 8.7, 8.8).

Factors controlling granulopoiesis. It has long been known that many substances promote a neutrophil leucocytosis when injected into animals: they include peptones, digestion products of nucleic acids, and metabolic products and extracts of bacteria. Such observations have not helped much in the elucidation of the mechanisms of leucocytosis, but investigations involving the culture of marrow cells *in vitro* have

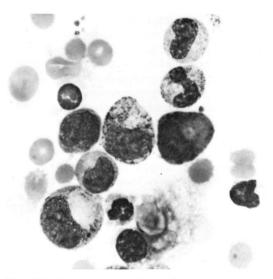

Fig. 8.8 Smear preparation of marrow showing finely granular myelocytes and transitions to polymorphonuclear leucocytes. × 1000.

proved more successful. When cultured in a suitable semi-solid medium, the growth of myeloid cells requires the presence of a factor (**colony stimulating activity** or **CSA**) which stimulates the proliferation of individual cells to form discrete colonies. At first, the proliferating cells are mainly or entirely granulocyte precursors but, as the numbers increase, some of the cells differentiate into polymorphs and others into monocytes. Since such colonies are derived from single cells, this is evidence of a common progenitor cell of polymorphs and monocytes. CSA can be extracted from most tissues (including haemopoietic marrow) and is present in the serum and urine. It is now known to be produced by monocytes, macrophages, vascular endothelium and stimulated lymphocytes. Assay of CSA by its effect on marrow culture is difficult and complex. This is probably because it is produced by monocytes in the culture, and in heavily seeded cultures sufficient CSA is produced to promote colony formation. It now seems likely that local production of CSA in haemopoietic marrow is important in the physiological production of neutrophil polymorphs and monocytes. Mature neutrophils produce a factor (possibly lactoferrin) which inhibits leucopoiesis and thus provides a negative feedback mechanism. Shortly after an injection of bacterial endotoxin, a **polymorph-releasing factor** appears in the plasma, and has the effect

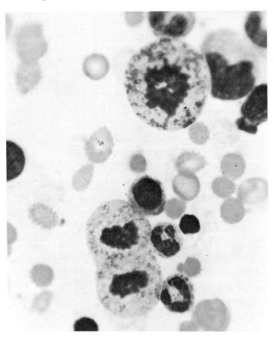

Fig. 8.7 Smear preparation of sternal marrow during a granulopoietic reaction. Note granular myelocytes in mitosis and various stages of transition to polymorphonuclear leucocytes. × 600.

of releasing mature neutrophil polymorphs from the marrow sinusoids into the blood. It may be that, by thus reducing the production of the neutrophil inhibitory factor in the marrow, this allows hyperplasia with production and release of more granulocytes. Bacterial endotoxin also increases the production of CSA by monocytes in culture and *in vivo*, and so it may reduce the negative feedback in the marrow and also directly stimulate leucopoiesis.

Other factors of possible importance include a lipoprotein present in normal plasma which,

when added to marrow cell cultures, is said to increase the production of monocytes at the expense of polymorphs. A factor is also produced by polymorphs in culture fluid which inhibits proliferation of early polymorph precursors in culture.

Although these observations promise considerable advances in our understanding of polymorph production, their relevance to natural neutrophil leucocytosis in man is still not known.

Disturbances of Body Temperature

Pyrexia (Fever)

In this account, *pyrexia* and *fever* are used synonymously to mean a rise in the internal temperature of the body ('core temperature') to levels above the normal range. Traditionally, *fever* is also used in the nomenclature of various diseases (usually infections) in which pyrexia is a prominent feature, e.g. typhoid fever, yellow fever and cerebrospinal fever. Doubtless both these usages will continue.

Body temperature is controlled partly by reflexes initiated by the thermo-sensory nerve endings in the skin, and partly by a central control mechanism in the hypothalamus.

The peripheral reflex control mechanism can be demonstrated simply by observing a fall in the temperature of the skin of the left hand when the right hand is immersed in cold water. This is brought about by impulses from the cold receptors in the chilled skin (of the right hand) which stimulate sympathetic vasoconstrictor fibres supplying the skin and subcutaneous tissues in general. The result is a reduction in heat loss and maintenance (or even rise) of the core temperature. This experiment works when the blood flow through the right arm is arrested by a pressure cuff, and so is not dependent on the temperature of the blood reaching the hypothalamus. In experimental animals, the reflex can be elicited even when the spinal cord has been transected at a higher level, and so is not attributable to sensory impulses reaching the brain.

The central thermo-regulatory mechanism

may, for practical purposes, be likened to a thermostat. The thermo-sensory centre, shown in animals to be in the anterior hypothalamus, responds to variations in the temperature of the blood flowing through it, and may be demonstrated experimentally by direct heating of the anterior hypothalamus, which results in a fall in the core temperature. Signals from the thermo-sensory centre influence the activity of other hypothalamic centres which regulate the physiological processes responsible for heat production and heat loss, thus controlling the core temperature. It is not known how the thermo-sensory centre responds to variations in local temperature. Experimental studies suggest that release of catecholamines and 5-hydroxytryptamine by nerve endings in the anterior hypothalamus are important in the control of temperature in extreme environmental conditions, and that there are marked species differences in the influence of these monoamines on body temperature. Under moderate environmental conditions, however, their depletion or inhibition does not seriously influence temperature control.

Fever accompanying infections and various other pathological conditions is attributable to a humoral effect on the hypothalamic thermo-sensory centre (analogous to the thermostat being set high). It is important to distinguish this from conditions in which the centre is functioning normally but, for various reasons, heat loss cannot keep pace with heat gain, and so the body temperature rises, e.g. during vigorous exercise in a hot, moist atmosphere.

Disturbances of the thermo-sensory centre

It has long been realised that injection of dead bacteria or bacterial products induces fever. A number of such products, termed **exogenous pyrogens**, have been detected in filtrates of cultures of various bacteria and fungi, but the **endotoxins** of Gram-negative bacteria have been most extensively investigated. On injection into rabbits, these phospholipid-polysaccharide-protein complexes (p. 8.7) induce fever in about 1 hour, and this is followed by a refractory period in which further injections of endotoxin are ineffectual. Following injection of small amounts of endotoxin or other exogenous pyrogen into rabbits, a second pyrogenic factor appears in the plasma; this causes fever in about 20 minutes following injection into a second rabbit, and differs from endotoxin in being pyrogenic in rabbits rendered refractory to endotoxin. This second pyrogen, known as **endogenous** (or **leucocyte**) **pyrogen (EP)**, has also been detected in the plasma of animals in the early stages of febrile bacterial and viral infections. It is produced when suspensions of human or rabbit monocytes are stimulated by endotoxin or by readily phagocytosed material such as dead bacteria or antigen–antibody complexes, and when macrophages are activated by lymphocytes in delayed hypersensitivity reactions (p. 7.21). Synthesis of RNA and protein is necessary for EP production. The only cells known with certainty to produce it are monocytes and macrophages. Its production by neutrophil polymorphs was formerly suspected, but this appears to have been a result of contamination of the cell suspension by macrophages. Macrophages obtained from inflammatory exudates produce EP *spontaneously* when incubated in culture medium, indicating that they have been stimulated *in vivo*.

These various observations suggest that many of the agents capable of inducing fever act by stimulating production of EP. In addition to its production by human monocytes *in vitro*, EP has been demonstrated in inflammatory exudates in man. Its detection in human plasma during infective fevers has proved difficult, but this is not surprising because fever can be induced in man by injection of amounts of EP too small to provide a detectable level in the recipient's plasma. EP has, however, been demonstrated in human plasma at the onset of a bout of malarial fever. Further investigations on EP will be greatly helped by a more sensitive method for its detection than that depending on production of fever in experimental animals. There is now evidence that EP consists of a group of proteins, and that it is identical with **interleukin-1** (p. 7.21). Its detailed composition is not known, but radioimmunoassay techniques are now becoming available.

While endotoxin and other microbial products stimulate monocytes and phagocytes to produce EP in acute infections, this cannot explain the fever which accompanies tissue destruction, e.g. myocardial infarction, or necrotic tumours. This is probably also mediated by EP released by macrophages in the inflammatory reaction to the necrotic tissue. Endogenous factors capable of inducing EP production by macrophages have not been demonstrated, but complement activation products have been suspected.

Effector mechanisms of fever (Fig. 8.9)

Although fever cannot be regarded as a physiological reaction, it is nevertheless brought about by stimulation of the physiological mechanisms for heat production and inhibition of those responsible for heat loss. For example, the shivering which accompanies a sharp rise of temperature is the normal response to a cold environment, and is associated with increased catabolic activity and heat production in the skeletal muscles. The coldness and pallor of the skin at the onset of fever are due to cutaneous vasoconstriction and, together with 'gooseflesh' (contraction of the arrector pili muscles) and inhibition of sweating, are part of the normal heat-saving reaction to cold. Heat production is also increased in fever, as it is in a cold climate, by increased metabolic activity, particularly in the skeletal muscles and liver. This is mediated in part by stimulation of the sympathetic system and increased catecholamine secretion, and eventually thyroid activity may increase. A high caloric diet is necessary to provide the fuel needed to maintain the body at temperatures above normal, failing which catabolism of endogenous fat and protein increases, resulting in a negative nitrogen balance and,

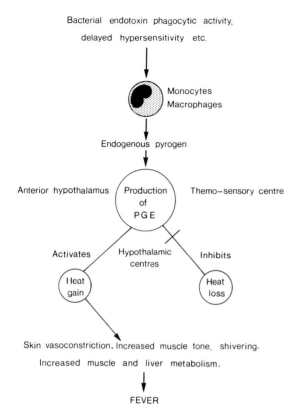

Bacterial endotoxin phagocytic activity, delayed hypersensitivity etc.

Monocytes Macrophages

Endogenous pyrogen

Anterior hypothalamus — Production of PGE — Themo−sensory centre

Activates — Hypothalamic centres — Inhibits

Heat gain — Heat loss

Skin vasoconstriction. Increased muscle tone, shivering. Increased muscle and liver metabolism.

FEVER

Fig. 8.9 The probable mechanism of fever in bacterial infections, etc.

especially in children, keto-acidosis. These catabolic activities account for the wasting commonly seen in patients with prolonged fever, and the metabolic status in fever is, in fact, closely similar to that following injury (p. 10.44): in both, a warm environment and a high caloric intake, including increased protein, are beneficial.

Not only is the 'thermostat set high' in fever, but it is unstable, so that the temperature commonly fluctuates, and is readily affected by environmental conditions. As described above, a rise of temperature is achieved by increasing heat production and reducing heat loss by physiological mechanisms. Conversely, a fall of temperature, either during or at the end of a fever, is accomplished by reduction in catabolism and by cutaneous vasodilatation and sweating. The skin is flushed, warm and moist, and the patient feels hot. During fever, the degree of increased metaboliic activity, etc. will depend largely on the environmental conditions

and, in a chilling environment, on the degree of insulation of the body by clothing.

Heat production and loss are regulated by centres in the posterior hypothalamus, including one which influences activity of the sympathetic system, and a second which appears to control muscle tone and induction of shivering. When injected into the anterior hypothalamus, EP induces fever within a few minutes. It now appears likely that EP does not act on the thermo-sensory centre directly, but by stimulating the production of prostaglandins of the E series (PGE) in various parts of the brain, including the anterior hypothalamus. This view is supported by the following observations. (1) High levels of PGE are present in the cerebrospinal fluid during fever induced by endotoxin. (2) Injection of minute amounts of PGE_1 or E_2 induces fever in various species when injected directly into the anterior hypothalamus or third ventricle. (3) Aspirin-like drugs, which inhibit the synthesis of prostaglandins (p. 4.20) prevent the induction of fever by endotoxin (and by EP) but have no effect on fever induced by PGE. In the cat, PGE_2 is mainly involved, but other prostaglandins may be concerned in other species.

The role of prostaglandins explains the fever associated with induction of labour in pregnant women by an infusion of PGE_2; it would account also for the antipyretic effect of aspirin and similar drugs.

Cortisone is also antipyretic, but its inhibitory effect on production of EP by monocytes stimulated by endotoxin, etc., probably accounts for this.

Effects of fever

Fever is usually accompanied by general malaise, anorexia and increased catabolism. If the temperature rises to 41·6°C (107°F), there is a danger of direct thermal injury to various tissues, and particularly to cerebral neurones. There is little clinical evidence that fever has a beneficial effect, and its reduction by antipyretic drugs or by cooling the body does not seem to influence significantly the course of infections. Beneficial effects may, however, by obscured by the individual variations in resistance to infecting micro-organisms. Apart from the spirochaete of syphilis and gonococcus (the cause of gonorrhoea), micro-organisms in culture do not appear to be adversely affected by moderate rises in temperature. It has been shown, however, that infection in poikilothermic vertebrates (e.g. lizards and fish) leads them to seek a warmer environment and that, by thus raising their body temperature, they become capable of a more rapid inflammatory reaction and overcome the infection more quickly (Kluger *et al.*, 1975). Evidence that fever is beneficial in infections in homeotherms is less impressive, although it has been shown that the antibody response by human lymphoid cells incubated with interleukin-1 is many times greater at 39°C than at 37°C, and that this is attributable to a greatly increased proliferation of T cells to provide helper cells (see Atkins, 1983).

The effects of fever on viral infections are complex, but most viruses replicate less well at temperatures above 37°C. The spontaneous movement of neutrophil polymorphs *in vitro* and their response to a chemotactic stimulus are most rapid at 40°C (104°F), and fever may thus enhance the defensive role of these cells in infections. It thus appears that interleukin-1 may increase the resistance to infection not only by enhancing immune responses by a direct action on T and B cells, but also by raising the body temperature (Duff and Durum, 1982).

Other causes of fever

Lesions of the hypothalamus may cause fever by interfering with the functioning of either the thermo-sensory centre or the hypothalamic areas which regulate heat loss and heat production. In experimental animals, injury of the anterior hypothalamus often causes pyrexia, while injury of the posterior hypothalamus may induce hypothermia. In man, haemorrhage in the pons is often accompanied by fever, and lesions between the hypothalamus and upper cervical cord interfere with tracts controlling heat loss and production, rendering the individual less able to respond to environmental temperature changes, etc.

Fever may occur in the absence of any disturbance of the thermo-sensory mechanism in conditions where the physiological mechanisms of heat loss cannot keep pace with heat production. This occurs in *thyrotoxicosis*, in which secretion of excess thyroid hormone stimulates general metabolism and physical activity and thus increases heat production. In normal subjects, vigorous exercise or a hot moist environment may both cause fever, and the combination is particularly likely to do so. Obviously, heat loss is influenced by the temperature and humidity of the atmosphere, air currents and insulation by clothing. These factors affect loss of heat by conduction, convection, radiation and evaporation, and also by the effect of breathing cold air. Sweating is a major mechanism of heat loss, but is only effective if the sweat evaporates on the skin surface, thus extracting the latent heat of vaporisation. Excessive sweating may, however, cause dehydration and, if water is restored, salt deficiency. Also, marked cutaneous vasodilation may impair the circulation. These various factors are associated in combinations which give rise to several clinical syndromes, the chief of which are as follows.

1. Heat exhaustion results from physical activity in a hot climate, particularly if the atmosphere is moist. Vasodilatation in the skin and skeletal muscles creates a relative hypovolaemia: filling of the enlarged vascular bed reduces the return of blood to the right side of the heart, and so cardiac output falls. Literally, there is not enough blood to go round. The heart rate increases and the blood pressure falls, giving a fast weak pulse, dyspnoea and other signs of circulatory insufficiency. The skin is hot and damp, and the subject feels tired and becomes confused. Rest and restoration of fluid usually bring rapid improvement.

2. Dehydration exhaustion. When dehydration due to excessive sweating, reduced fluid intake, etc., accompanies heat exhaustion, all the features of circulatory failure are exaggerated by actual, in addition to relative, reduction in the blood volume. Dehydration in a hot dry climate is also increased by loss of fluid through the epidermis, which is not entirely impervious. The core temperature may be very high and collapse and sudden death may occur.

3. Heat stroke. In the two conditions mentioned above, heat-losing mechanisms operate, but are inadequate. In heat stroke, exercise in a hot environment, with consequent fever, leads in some way to a breakdown of the control mechanisms, so that the heat-losing mechanisms remain inactive, and the termperature continues to rise and may reach 43°C (109°F). At this temperature, brain injury is accompanied by coma and convulsions, and death or permanent brain injury results.

4. Heat cramps. Painful cramps in the muscles are the result of salt deficiency. This is liable to occur when there is excessive loss of water and salt by sweating and only the water is replaced.

5. Malignant hyperpyrexia. This is an unusual complication of general anaesthesia, usually with suxamethonium but also with other agents. During the anaesthesia, muscle tone increases and the temperature rises rapidly, often to above 42°C (107·5°F). Cyanosis, shock and keto-acidosis develop and death may occur from cardiac arrest unless the condition is recognised and treated. The underlying metabolic predisposition is not understood, but in some instances has been shown to run in families, members of which have a raised level of plasma creatine phosphokinase.

Hypothermia

This may be defined as a fall in the core temperature of the body to below 35°C (95°F). It has no particular relevance to host-parasite relationships and is considered here simply because the processes involved in temperature control, described above in relation to fever, are equally important in hypothermia.

Hypothermia occurs when heat production fails to keep pace with heat loss. In robust adults, this occurs only in conditions of extreme heat loss, such as immersion in the sea or exposure on mountains. However, factors which interfere with heat production predispose to hypothermia in less rigorous environmental conditions. Because of their relatively large surface area and thin layer of insulating fat, infants, particularly if premature, are especially liable to it. Old people, especially women, living in cold surroundings on an inadequate diet, are particularly prone to develop hypothermia in winter. Predisposing diseases include hypothyroidism, generalised skin diseases, psychiatric disturbances and conditions which impair consciousness, metabolic or physical activity, e.g. alcoholism, narcotic drugs, paralysis, severe trauma and general states of disability.

Pathology. In general, metabolic processes decline rapidly below 33°C (91°F) and the cardiac output, blood pressure and respiratory rate fall. Fluid leaks from the microvessels with consequent haemoconcentration and increased blood viscosity. Blood flow to the tissues is further impaired by peripheral vasoconstriction; hypoxia and CO_2 retention increase and a combination of respiratory and metabolic acidosis develops. Below 25°C (77°F), the thermo-regulatory mechanism ceases to function, and death results from cardiac arrest.

The changes found at autopsy include venous thrombosis, multiple small infarcts in various organs, pulmonary haemorrhages and bronchopneumonia. Acute pancreatitis is a common complication in patients who survive.

Induction of hypothermia to reduce the metabolic requirements of the brain and other organs was formerly practised in surgical procedures involving interruption of the circulation, but it carries a risk of ventricular fibrillation and is now used only occasionally, in association with a pump to maintain the circulation.

References and Further Reading

Atkins, E. (1983). Fever—new prespectives on an old phenomenon. *New England Journal of Medicine* **308**, 958–60.

Duff, G.W. and Durum, S.K. (1982). Fever and immunoregulation: hyperthermia, interleukins 1 and 2 and T cell proliferation. *Yale Journal of Biology and Medicine*, **55**, 437–42.

Johnson. A.P. (1981). The pathogenesis of gonorrhoea. *Journal of Infection* **3**, 299–308.

Kluger, M.J., Ringler, D.H. and Anver, M.R. (1975). Fever and survival. *Science* **188**, 166–8.

Lancet (1982). Genetics of resistance to infection. (Editorial) *Lancet* **1**, 1446–7.

Levy, S.B. (1982). Microbial resistance to antibiotics. *Lancet* **ii**, 83–8.

Levy, S.B., Fitzgerald, G.B. and Macone, A.B. (1976). Spread of antibiotic-resistant plasmids from chicken to chicken and from chicken to man. *Nature* **260**, 40–2.

Mims, C.A. (1982). *The Pathogenesis of Infectious Disease*. 2nd edn., pp. 320. Academic Press, London.

Pepys, M.B. and Baltz, M.L. (1983). Actue phase proteins with special reference to C-reactive protein and related proteins (pentaxins) and serum amyloid A protein. *Advances in Immunology* **34,** 141–212.

Topley and Wilson's Principles of Bacteriology, Virology and Immunity (1983). 7th edn., Vol. 1, *Immunity and General Microbiology.* Sir Graham Wilson and Heather M. Dick (Eds.). Edward Arnold, London.

Zak, K., Diaz, J.L., Jackson, D. and Heckel, J.E. (1984). Antigenic variation during infection with *Neisseria gonorrhoeae*: detection of antibodies to surface proteins in sera of patients with gonorrhoea. *Journal of Infectious Diseases,* **149,** 166–74.

See also bibliography for Chapter 9 (p. 9.38).

9

Types of Infection

Within living memory, infective disease was the major cause of death throughout the world, and the elimination or reduction in the incidence of many important infections largely accounts for the greatly increased lifespan in technologically advanced communities. Various factors have contributed to this decline of serious infections: they include improved standards of community and personal hygiene, better nutrition and housing, prophylactic immunisation and antimicrobial therapeutic agents.

In spite of these great triumphs, infective disease is still of considerable importance: it remains the major cause of death in many tropical and subtropical countries where, in addition to bacterial and viral infections, protozoal and metazoal parasites account for a great deal of illness. Even in countries where infections have been greatly reduced, many problems remain. The common cold is as common as ever, and upper respiratory virus infections are the major cause of absenteeism from school, office and factory. The rise in the volume and speed of world travel has increased greatly the risk of epidemics of influenza, cholera, etc. Even anti-

biotics have not proved an unmixed blessing, for their use has resulted in the spread of resistant pathogenic bacteria, particularly in hospitals. There are, moreover, a number of important diseases which may eventually prove to be due to infections, for example rheumatoid arthritis, multiple sclerosis, ulcerative colitis and sarcoidosis. Viruses are probably important causal factors of various lymphoid neoplasms, the evidence being strongest in adult T-cell leukaemia/lymphoma and Burkitt's lymphoma. It is also very likely that the hepatitis B virus is a major causal factor of liver-cell cancer.

This chapter gives a brief account of the various types of infection and describes some of the more important examples. As with other forms of disease, the effects of infection depend not only on the nature of the lesion, but also on its site in the body, and for this reason the special features of infection of the lungs, kidneys, brain, etc., are described in the appropriate systematic chapters. Diseases caused by **protozoan and metazoan parasites** are described in Chapter 28.

Virus Infections

Of all the pathogenic organisms which affect man, viruses show the most extreme degree of parasitism. In the extracellular state, viruses are metabolically inert and depend absolutely on the metabolism of the host cell for their replication. Basically, all viruses consist of a protein shell or **capsid** surrounding and protecting the nucleic acid of the viral genome which may be either DNA or RNA. The **virion** or complete infectious particle of some viruses has an addi-

tional outer layer, or **envelope**, partially derived from the plasma membrane of the host cell. When a virus enters a susceptible host cell, the nucleic acid is released from the capsid and becomes functionally active: it is either transcribed into messenger RNA, or acts itself as messenger RNA, which re-directs the host-cell ribosomes to manufacture components for new virus particles. This involves the synthesis of enzymes involved in the replication of nucleic acid molecules and in the production of the structural proteins which make up the capsid of new virus particles.

Apart from the arboviruses, which enter the host by the bite of an insect (e.g. yellow fever), or in the case of rabies virus by the bite of an animal, all viruses must enter the host by invading the surface epithelial cells of some part of the body. In most instances the site of initial infection is in the respiratory or alimentary tracts.

In man, most virus infections are mild and are followed by complete recovery. Many infections are entirely symptomless and immunity to reinfection is acquired without serious disturbance at the time of primary infection. Although latent viral infection may continue for months or even years, viruses do not form a non-invasive flora in the way that some bacteria do. A few viral infections, such as rabies, always cause serious disease and even viruses such as herpes simplex or the enteroviruses, which generally cause mild or symptomless infections, may occasionally give rise to severe disease in an unusually susceptible host (Fig. 21.40, p. 21.35). Viral infections, especially of the upper respiratory tract, are both mild and extremely common in the community and are, in general, more frequent in childhood than in adult life.

Viruses are structurally simple parasites and do not produce disease by the elaboration of toxins as bacteria do. *Lesions in viral infections are caused by direct invasion of body tissues with subsequent cell damage due to the effect of viral replication in the host cells.* In most clinically-apparent virus infections, replication of the virus is accompanied by death of the infected cell (Fig. 9.1). Some viruses induce fusion between infected and adjacent non-infected cells, with the formation of multinucleated giant cells, for example measles (Fig. 18.7, p. 18.12), respiratory syncytial virus and some strains of herpes simplex. Such giant cells usually die, at least in tissue culture preparations, but their formation may be important in allowing virus to spread without entering the surrounding medium. There is increasing evidence that *the immune response of the host may sometimes play an important role in causing lesions of a hypersensitivity nature.* In arbovirus encephalitis, for example, it seems likely from animal experiments that the lesions are due to virus–antibody

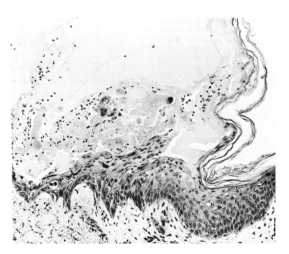

Fig. 9.1   Part of a vesicular skin lesion in varicella, illustrating virus-induced cell injury. The virus has replicated in the epidermal cells, resulting in cell death. The resulting epidermal defect has then become distended with inflammatory exudate, forming the vesicle. Note the swelling and hyperchromatic nuclei of the colonised epidermal cells, lying free in the vesicle and in the underlying epidermis. × 96. (The late Professor J.A. Milne.)

complexes inducing a type 3 hypersensitivity reaction rather than to the direct effect of the virus on the cells of the brain.

Unlike some bacterial infections, *virus diseases are not usually accompanied by a polymorphonuclear leucocytosis, but a lymphocytosis is common.* Most are associated with fever, and rash and lymphadenopathy are quite commonly seen. In the acute phase of virus infection a group of proteins termed **interferons** (IFN) can be detected in the blood and tissues. Interferon is released from cells in response to virus infection and when taken up by other cells makes them refractory to virus infection. Although the production of interferons is induced by virus, they are encoded by genes of the host cell genome. Interferons are currently classified into three types, α β and γ. The first two types are synthesised by viral-infected cells: the stimulus for their production is the presence in the cell of double-stranded RNA, formation of which is a feature of both DNA and RNA viruses. Cells can be induced to secrete interferon by double-stranded synthetic polyribonucleotides. IFN-γ is produced by T lymphocytes activated either in the reaction of specifically primed T lymphocytes with antigen on the surface of infected cells (p. 7.20), or experimentally by the action of T-cell mitogens, e.g. concanavalin A (p. 6.32).

Interferons do not protect the viral-infected cells producing them: they attach to receptors on adjacent uninfected cells and have the effect of inhibiting the translation of viral mRNA proteins. Interferons are species-specific, but inhibit virtually all viruses. *Interferon production is an important host defence mechanism against virus infection and is probably the major factor in bringing about recovery from acute virus infections.* Although specific neutralising antibody is responsible for immunity to re-infection, it begins to appear in the bloodstream only when the initial infection is subsiding. It is notable that infants with immunological deficiencies resulting in impairment of T-lymphocyte function (p. 7.34 *et seq.*) are prone to develop chronic progressive vaccinia (vaccinia gangrenosa) following vaccination, and giant-cell pneumonia following infection with measles virus (p. 16.43). This provides evidence that cell-mediated immunity plays an important role in limiting viral lesions in normal individuals.

Distribution of lesions in virus infections

In some instances, the main lesion is at the site of the initial infection. For example, the virus responsible for influenza gives rise to a localised infection which spreads rapidly throughout the epithelial lining of the larger air passages of the respiratory tract. This results in epithelial injury and necrosis of varying extent, and the cell injury and loss results in acute inflammatory oedema, which is the major clinical feature of influenza. The severity of the illness depends on the extent of epithelial necrosis, but secondary bacterial infection of the damaged mucosa is also of importance, especially in major epidemics. Influenza virus may enter the bloodstream, but appears unable to replicate successfully in the cells of other tissues. Other examples of virus infections which remain localised, and produce lesions mostly at the site of initial infection, are molluscum contagiosum virus (p. 27.6) and the common cold.

In many other instances, the initial infection is clinically silent, but the virus invades various other tissues and organs and produces characteristic lesions in them. Thus in childhood fevers such as measles and varicella, the initial infection is probably in the respiratory tract.

From there the virus spreads widely, invading the blood (viraemia) and many other tissues and organs. The characteristic vesicular lesions in the skin in varicella are due to invasion of the epidermal cells, and are one manifestation of the systemic infection. Suppuration of the skin lesions (pustulation) is due to secondary bacterial infection. Mumps and rubella are other examples of generalised virus diseases which follow initial infection via the respiratory tract.

Because of the mode of virus spread in these childhood fevers, the incubation period between initial infection and appearance of symptoms is 12–21 days. *Poliovirus* also spreads in a complex fashion within the body: following ingestion of the virus, there is an initial infection of the Peyer's patches in the small intestine. The virus then spreads to the regional lymph nodes, and in many instances produces viraemia. In a few individuals (e.g. about 1% of those infected with poliovirus type 1) the organism invades the anterior horn cells of the spinal cord (Figs. 21.40 and 21.41, p. 21.35), causing paralytic poliomyelitis. The intestinal infection is clinically silent, but it nevertheless results in the development of antibody in the blood and in the appearance of IgA antibody in the gastro-intestinal tract (p. 8.2): immunity is thus provided against subsequent infection with the same type of poliovirus.

Persistent virus infections are known to occur in man. Herpes simplex virus, for example, remains latent within the trigeminal ganglion but becomes activated from time to time, e.g. during pneumonia or other febrile illness, to produce vesicles around the mouth. Varicella virus also commonly remains latent, and may subsequently become active and replicate within the cells of the dorsal root ganglia to produce an attack of herpes zoster (Fig. 21.39, p. 21.33).

There is considerable interest at present in **slow virus infections**, which may be defined as infectious diseases caused by 'unconventional agents' and having a long incubation period, in some instances years, and a prolonged and progressive course. Such diseases have been demonstrated to occur in certain animals, e.g. Aleutian disease of the mink, and it seems very likely that kuru and Creutzfeldt–Jakob disease (p. 21.37) are examples in man. Scrapie, a widespread slow-virus disease in sheep, is most unusual in the remarkable resistance of its causal agent to heat and viricidal chemicals. The agents responsible for these diseases appear to be infectious, but they are smaller than the known viruses.

Active immunity can readily be produced by the administration of attenuated viruses, e.g. Sabin poliovirus vaccines, and also—although somewhat less effectively—by inactivated viruses, e.g. influenza and rabies vaccines. Naturally-acquired immunity after virus infection is generally life-long and is due to the development in the blood of antibodies which neutralise the infectivity of viruses. However, in a few virus diseases, reinfections or repeated infections are common. This may be due to the existence of numerous serologically distinct strains of virus, e.g. the common cold, or to the

virus undergoing antigenic variation, e.g. influenza. In the case of certain viruses, and especially herpes simplex and herpes zoster viruses, reactivation of virus, despite the presence of circulating antibody, is not uncommon. Such recurrences are due to the ability of these viruses to remain latent—probably in the form of integrated DNA as *provirus* within the neurons of sensory ganglia. Reactivation takes place, with axonal spread down sensory nerves, to produce vesicles in the area of skin supplied by the sensory nerves affected. The presence of antibodies in people who have experienced a virus infection can be demonstrated by various *in-vitro* tests for antibody such as complement fixation, immunofluorescence, ELISA, etc (pp. 6.10–13).

The possible role of virus infections in neoplasia is considered in Chapter 13.

Acute Bacterial Infections

The several processes which constitute the acute inflammatory reaction have been described in Chapter 4. They are basically the same in all acute inflammatory reactions, including those due to bacterial infections, but they differ in detail depending on the properties of the causal agent and the special features of the tissue involved. In some lesions, for example, inflammatory oedema may be unusually severe, while in others emigration of polymorphs or fibrin deposition may be predominant. In consequence of these variations, some acute inflammatory lesions due to infections present sufficiently characteristic appearances to warrant the use of such descriptive terms as catarrhal, pseudomembranous, serous, haemorrhagic and pyogenic (suppurating) inflammation (p. 4.28). Infections causing some of these types of inflammation, and also the special features of gangrenous infection, are considered below.

Catarrhal inflammation is characteristic of relatively mild infection of a mucous membrane, as occurs in most of the many viral infections of the nose or throat, including the common cold, and in the trachea and bronchi in mild cases of influenza (p. 9.3). Examples of catarrhal bacterial infection include 'food poisoning' caused by *Salmonellae* (excluding typhoid and paratyphoid fevers), in which the mucosa of the

stomach and intestine are involved (gastroenteritis) and the milder forms of bacillary dysentery, which is an acute colitis. Microscopically, there is some loss of surface epithelium, inflammatory oedema of the underlying connective tissue, and infiltration with polymorphs. Increased secretion of the mucosal glands, together with exudate, produces a thin, watery discharge from the mucosal surface, which in some instances, e.g. the common cold, becomes mucopurulent before the original infection and secondary bacterial infection are overcome (p. 4.22). After a single attack, the mucosa returns to normal, but repeated or chronic infection can result in metaplasia of the surface epithelium and scarring of the underlying tissue, as occurs in the paranasal sinuses and the larynx. **Pseudomembranous inflammation** occurs when infection of a mucous membrane is severe enough to cause superficial necrosis. The dead tissue becomes impregnated and coated with fibrin from the inflammatory exudate to form a pseudo- (i.e. non-living) membrane (Fig. 9.2). It is caused by bacteria which are of low invasive capacity but produce potent exotoxins, the classical examples are diphtheria (now uncommon in immunised communities), which may affect the nose, throat or larynx (p. 16.5), and severe forms of bacillary dysentery. Such

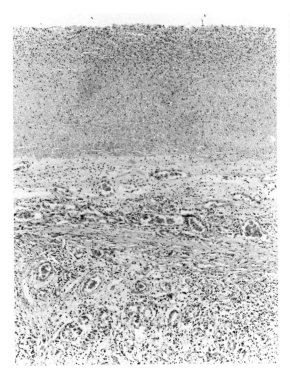

Fig. 9.2 Pharyngeal diphtheria. The mucosal surface (top) is coated with a false membrane composed of dead epithelium and fibrinous exudate. The underlying connective tissue shows acute inflammatory congestion. × 85.

changes occur in the more recently described pseudomembranous colitis caused by *Clostridium difficile* (p. 19.48). Polymorphs accumulate at the junction of the living and dead tissue, where their digestive enzymes result in detachment of the pseudomembrane leaving a raw surface which becomes re-epithelialised, sometimes with loss of mucosal glands and some scarring. **Serous inflammation** of the walls of coelomic cavities, and fibrinous and **haemorrhagic inflammations** (pp. 4.21–22) require no further description.

Pyogenic or suppurating inflammation (p. 4. 28)

This is caused by invasive bacteria which produce potent exotoxins affecting all types of cell, and promote considerable emigration of neutrophil polymorphs, resulting in formation of

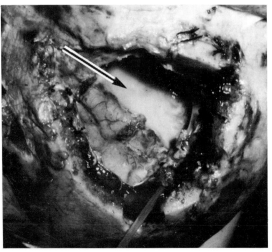

Fig. 9.3 Abscess of brain. Part of the skull has been removed surgically and a cavity containing pus (*arrow*) is seen in the brain. (Photographed at autopsy).

pus, either in a body cavity or in spaces formed by toxic necrosis of tissue and digestion of the dead tissue by neutrophil polymorphs (Figs. 9.3 and 9.4). The causal bacteria are termed pyogenic (pus-forming) and include *Streptococcus pyogenes, Streptococcus pneumoniae, Staphylococcus aureus, Neisseria meningitidis, Neisseria gonorrhoeae, Pseudomonas aeruginosa (Ps. pyocyanea), Proteus* ssp, *Bacteroides* and invasive

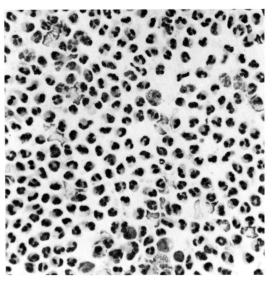

Fig. 9.4 Smear of pus. Most of the cells are neutrophil polymorphs: some are undergoing autolysis. × 400.

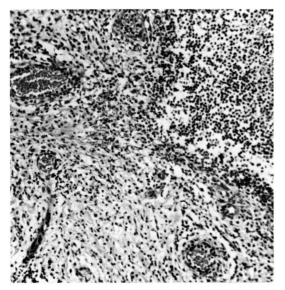

Fig. 9.5 Wall of an abscess. The abscess cavity is seen at the top right. The wall consists of vascular granulation tissue showing an inflammatory re-action. × 120.

strains of *Escherichia coli* (p. 8.4). Various species of *Bacteroides*, the anaerobic bacilli present in enormous numbers in the colon, are frequently present in pyogenic infections of the abdomen and female genital tract, commonly accompanied by *Escherichia coli*.

In past centuries, the term 'laudable pus' implied that abscess formation was a favourable development. At least it meant that infection was localised, which was better than dying from septicaemia. Suppuration does, however, indicate that infection has progressed to a stage where the defence mechanisms are rendered largely ineffective, because influx of exudate into an abscess gradually diminishes as the pressure rises and the beneficial effects of a continuous flow of exudate (p. 4.25) are thus lost. As a result, bacteria continue to multiply in the pus and their toxins cause necrosis of the surrounding tissue, with increase in size of the abscess. Accordingly, suppurating infection tends to persist, and even if the infection is eventually overcome, maturation of the large amount of granulation tissue formed (Fig. 9.5) may result in considerable scarring. Sometimes a hard mass results from calcification of inspissated pus. More often, the abscess eventually ruptures onto a surface and the pus is discharged. When this happens, the pressure is relieved and flow of exudate recommences with either elimination of the infection and healing with scarring, or a persistent sinus discharging

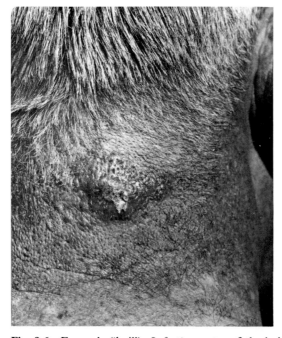 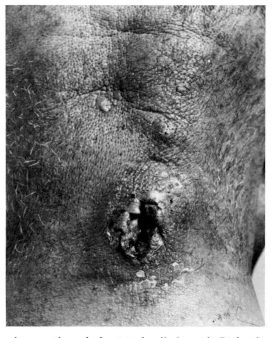

Fig. 9.6 Furuncle ('boil'). *Left*, the centre of the lesion is necrotic and about to be discharged. *Right*, the necrotic core has been discharged, leaving a ragged ulcer. × 1. (The late Professor J.A. Milne.)

pus. Antibiotic therapy may eliminate the infection in a small abscess, but in a larger one it may not be possible to achieve a sufficient concentration of antibiotic in the stagnant pus, and surgical drainage is usually necessary to promote elimination of the infection before extensive tissue destruction has occured.

Perhaps the commonest example of an abscess is a **boil (furuncle)**. It occurs most often in the dense dermal connective tissue at the back of the neck. The causal organism, *Staphylococcus aureus*, invades via the hair follicles or sebaceous ducts and sets up an acute inflammatory swelling. It spreads locally in the dermis, and necrosis of a patch of skin at the centre of the lesion results from toxic action: polymorphs migrate from the surrounding inflamed tissue and digest the periphery of the necrotic 'core', which thus becomes separated from the lining tissue by a layer of pus. When separation is complete, the core is discharged, leaving an ulcer (Fig. 9.6). This is usually followed by elimination of the staphylococci, and the ulcer heals, leaving a pitted scar. In some instances, particularly in individuals with impaired resistance to infection, e.g. untreated diabetics, the infection may spread extensively in the dermal and underlying soft tissue of the

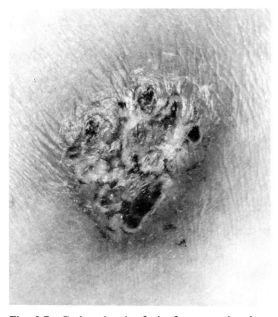

Fig. 9.7 Carbuncle: the foci of suppuration have extended to the overlying skin and discharged pus at several places. × 1. (The late Professor J.A. Milne.)

neck, giving rise to a **carbuncle** consisting of a complex loculated abscess, or several separate abscesses, with multiple discharging sinuses (Fig. 9.7).

Suppuration in a serous cavity presents the same general features as an abscess developing in a solid tissue, and the principles of treatment are the same.

Bacterial infection of the blood

It is customary to classify the presence of bacteria in the blood into **bacteraemia, septicaemia and pyaemia**. The distinction between the three is not sharp, but they are none the less useful terms. In bacteraemia, bacteria are present in relatively small numbers, but do not multiply significantly, in the blood. Septicaemia and pyaemia are much more serious conditions in which bacteria, usually of high pathogenicity, multiply in the blood.

Only very rarely are bacteria present in the blood in sufficient numbers to be detected by direct microscopy, blood culture being necessary for their detection.

Bacteraemia. Small numbers of bacteria of low virulence are present from time to time in the blood of normal subjects, or in individuals with minor, often subclinical lesions. *Streptococcus viridans* may be cultured from the blood after vigorous brushing of the teeth, particularly if there is dental sepsis. It is also likely that occasional intestinal bacteria enter the portal circulation. Because of its high content of antibodies and complement, and the large numbers of circulating phagocytes and sinus-lining macrophages in the liver, spleen, etc., the blood is a hostile environment to most micro-organisms, and although bacteria may multiply in local infections, those entering the blood are usually destroyed rapidly. Even in more serious and extensive localised infections, such as pneumococcal pneumonia, or *Escherichia coli* infections of the urinary tract, bacteria can sometimes be detected by blood culture, but usually they fail to multiply significantly in the blood and disappear from it when, or even before, the local infection subsides. This applies also to the bacteria which enter the bloodstream as a regular feature of certain diseases, for example typhoid fever and brucellosis (undulant fever).

Bacteraemia is of some importance, for whenever they enter the blood, bacteria may settle in various parts of the body and cause lesions, for example suppurative meningitis or arthritis in pneumococcal pneumonia, periostitis due to *Salmonella typhi* in typhoid fever and endocarditis by *Streptococcus viridans*.

Septicaemia means the presence and multiplication of bacteria in the blood, and is applied especially to the rapid multiplication of highly pathogenic bacteria, e.g. the pyogenic cocci or the plague bacillus, *Yersinia pestis*. The term thus implies a serious infection with profound toxaemia, in which the bacteria have overwhelmed the host defences.

In some instances it is difficult to distinguish between bacteraemia and septicaemia. For example, invasive strains of *Escherichia coli* cause infections of the peritoneal cavity, urinary and genital tracts: blood infection may occur, particularly as a complication of generalised peritonitis, but it is often not clear whether the bacteria are multiplying in the blood or are continuously entering it, e.g. from the infected peritoneum.

Multiple small haemorrhages may occur in septicaemia (Fig. 9.10), due either to capillary endothelial damage from the severe toxaemia or to multiple minute metastatic foci of bacterial growth. The number of neutrophil polymorphs in the blood may be raised, although in overwhelmingly severe septicaemia they may be diminished and show toxic granulation (p. 17.12). The spleen is often enlarged and congested, and may contain large numbers of polymorphs. If the septicaemia is not rapidly fatal, foci of suppurating infection may develop in various parts of the body as a result of local invasion by blood-borne bacteria.

Pyaemia. In localised pyogenic infections, toxic injury to the endothelium of veins involved in the lesion may result in thrombosis: bacteria may invade and multiply in the thrombus, which then becomes heavily infiltrated by polymorphs and broken down by their digestive enzymes. Small fragments of the softened septic thrombus may then break away and be carried off in the blood (*pyaemia*—literally, pus in the blood). Where they become impacted in small vessels, they cause local injury both by obstructing the vessels and by the release of toxins from their contained bacteria: a combination of necrosis, haemorrhage and suppuration results, with formation of multiple **pyaemic abscesses** in the various tissues, their distribution depending

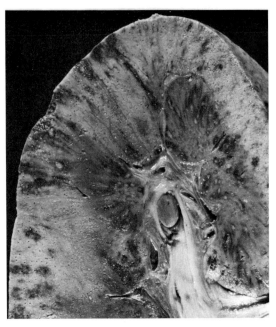

Fig. 9.8 The kidney in pyaemia, showing multiple small abscesses which are seen as pale areas surrounded by dark haemorrhagic zones.

on the site of the original septic thrombosis. Pyaemic abscesses are typically surrounded by a zone of haemorrhage (Fig. 9.8). Microscopy of an early lesion may show a central zone of necrosis (Fig. 9.9) often containing huge numbers of bacteria; this is surrounded by a zone of suppuration and an outermost zone of acutely inflamed, often haemorrhagic tissue. As the lesions progress, the necrotic tissue is digested, and apart from their multiplicity and widespread distribution, the lesions become indistinguishable from non-haematogenous abscesses. In septic thrombosis of major veins, larger fragments may be released into the circulation and impact in arteries, causing correspondingly larger foci of necrosis and suppuration (**septic infarcts**).

Septic thrombosis of systemic veins results especially, but not exclusively, in pyaemic abscesses in the lungs, while septic thrombosis in pulmonary veins results in pyaemic abscesses mainly in the systemic arterial distribution. In acute bacterial endocarditis, in which septic thrombus forms on the infected valve cusps, the distribution of pyaemic lesions depends on the particular heart valve(s) involved. Septic thrombus of a portal venous tributary, e.g. in acute

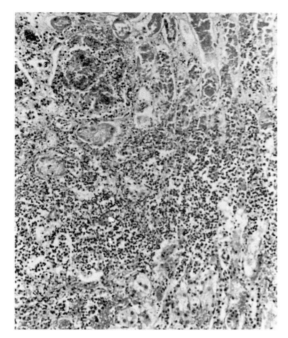

Fig. 9.9 Pyaemic abscess of kidney in a case of staphylococcal pyaemia. Infarcted tissue (*above*) is separated from congested living tissue (*below*) by a zone of suppuration. The dark patches in a glomerulus are masses of staphylococci, which have probably increased after death. × 65.

appendicitis, gives rise to **portal pyaemia**, with abscesses mainly in the liver.

Inevitably, bacteria are released from septic thrombus in pyaemia, and frank septicaemia commonly supervenes.

Septicaemia and pyaemia were formerly most often due to the pyogenic cocci. The incidence has, however, been greatly reduced by antibiotic therapy, and bacterial infections which are less readily eliminated by antibiotics have increased in relative importance, invasive strains of *Escherichia coli* with virulence factors conferred on them by plasmids (p. 8.6) now being the commonest cause of blood infections in general hospital practice. In states of lowered resistance to bacterial infection, e.g. agranulocytosis, immunodeficiencies and therapeutic immunosuppression, blood infection is a particular hazard. Because of impaired defence mechanisms, bacteria normally of relatively low resistance may cause septicaemia and pyaemia in these conditions.

The common pyogenic bacteria

Pyogenic infections in man are most commonly caused by *Staphylococcus aureus* and *Streptococcus pyogenes*. *Staphylococcus aureus* is the usual cause of boils, carbuncles and septic lesions of the fingers (*whitlows*): the infection usually remains localised, although suppurating lymphadenitis may occur in the local nodes, and unless treatment is effective, septicaemia and pyaemia may occasionally develop. Most strains of *Staph. aureus* causing hospital infections, and many encountered in general practice, are now resistant to penicillin and sometimes to other antibiotics: symptomless nasopharyngeal carriers of resistant types are commonly responsible for outbreaks of infection of surgical wounds, burns, etc., in hospital. Phage typing has proved of great value in tracing the source of such outbreaks: it is performed by testing the susceptibility of *Staph. aureus* isolated from various sources to the lytic effects of a panel of bacteriophages. Staphylococci are also a cause of pneumonia complicating influenza and other viral infections of the respiratory tract, and may produce a fulminating enteritis in patients receiving broad-spectrum antibiotics. The staphylococcal lesion shows the usual features of acute inflammation, and unless checked by antibiotic therapy it frequently progresses to suppuration and discharges a thick creamy pus.

Streptococcus pyogenes commonly produces acute pharyngitis and tonsillitis, 'whitlows', otitis media and mastoiditis and extensive inflammation of the subcutaneous connective tissues (*cellulitis*), *impetigo* (pustular lesions, usually of the face) and *erysipelas*, a spreading infection of the dermis producing a raised, red, painful lesion of the skin, usually of the face, with a well-defined margin. Before the introduction of antiseptics, *Strep pyogenes* was a very common and important cause of fatal peritonitis or septicaemia arising from infection of the genital tract following childbirth. It can also cause fatal septicaemia resulting from a minor injury, e.g. a finger prick sustained by the surgeon or pathologist dealing with a streptococcal infection. Aseptic and antiseptic techniques and the use of antibiotics have, however, greatly diminished the incidence of serious and fatal streptococcal infections. *Strep. pyogenes* has not been observed to develop resistance to penicillin. The organism does not readily withstand drying and is spread by droplet infection by nasal and throat carriers, who are usually symptom free. It also causes bovine mastitis and outbreaks of infection may result from infected milk.

Some strains of *Strep. pyogenes* produce a prophage-determined erythrogenic toxin and cause an acute pharyngitis accompanied by an erythematous skin rash (*scarlet fever*—p. 8.5). Streptococcal pharyngitis may be followed by *rheumatic fever*, which is believed to result from a hypersensitivity reaction (p. 15.25), and another sequel of *Strep. pyogenes* infections is *post-streptococcal glomerulonephritis* in which antibody reacts with streptococcal antigen deposited in the glomeruli (p. 22.22).

The differences between infections due to staphylococci and streptococci are partly explicable by their toxins (p. 8.5). Staphylococcal infections show a greater tendency to remain localised, possibly due in part to the production of staphylocoagulase which clots fibrinogen, producing a deposit of fibrin which may help to limit spread of the organisms and promote their phagocytosis. Streptococcal lesions tend to spread, possibly due partly to the production of hyaluronidase, which digests hyaluronic acid and thus liquifies the ground substance of connective tissues. *Streptococcus pyogenes* also produces fibrinolysins, and leucocidins which kill polymorphs.

Other pyogenic bacteria include: **(1)** *Strep. pneumoniae* which used to be the commonest cause of acute bacterial pneumonia. *Strep. pneumoniae* infections may be complicated by bacteraemia or septicaemia and metastatic blood-borne lesions, e.g. suppurative meningitis or arthritis. A major factor in the pathogenicity of *Strep. pneumoniae* is its capsular (C) polysaccharide which inhibits phagocytosis and is also released into the blood, where it combines with antibody and thus protects the organism from opsonisation. Non-capsulated (rough) forms of *Strep. pneumococci* are non-pathogenic. There are over sixty serotypes of this organism, classified by the antigenicity of their capsule. The most virulent is type 3, which has the thickest capsule. *Strep. pneumoniae* produces a relatively weak exotoxin which in blood-agar cultures causes partial lysis of red cells and a greenish discolouration due to reduction products of haemoglobin. **(2)** *Neisseria meningitidis* (meningococcus), which invades the nasopharynx,

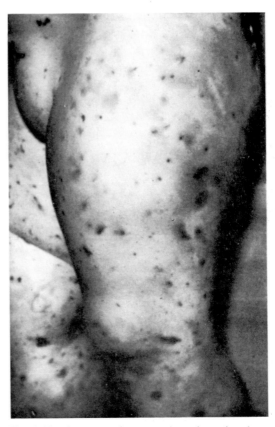

Fig. 9.10   Acute meningococcal septicaemia, showing the haemorrhagic rash.

often silently, and produces a septicaemia or bacteraemia with the subsequent development of meningitis. The septicaemia is often associated with a haemorrhagic rash (Fig. 9.10) and severe endotoxic shock with acute haemorrhagic adrenocortical necrosis (Waterhouse-Friderichsen syndrome (Fig. 26.23, p. 26.36). **(3)** *Neisseria gonorrhoeae* (gonococcus), which is transmitted by coitus and produces an acute urethritis, etc. (p. 25.2). The importance of plasmid-determined pili in the pathogenicity of *N. gonorrhoeae* is discussed on p. 8.5. **(4)** The intestinal commensals, which are important causes of pyogenic infections in the abdomen, e.g. appendicitis, diverticulitis and peritonitis, and in the lungs; they also infect surgical and other wounds, bedsores, burns, and ulcers of the skin. They include *Escherichia coli, Bacteroides, Streptococcus faecalis, Proteus, Pseudomonas aeruginosa* and *Klebsiella*, and may cause infections singly and in various combinations. These organisms are of particular importance in debilitated and immunosuppressed patients. All of them, but especially *Esch. coli* and *Bacteriodes*, give rise to septicaemia and pyaemia, with severe septic shock (p. 10.42). The factors involved in the pathogenicity of *Esch. coli* are discussed on pp. 8.1, 8.4 and 9.8.

Gangrene

Definition. The term gangrene means digestion of dead tissue by saprophytic bacteria, i.e. bacteria which are incapable of invading and multiplying in living tissues. Many types of bacteria, often present in various combinations, may participate, and breakdown of tissue proteins, carbohydrates and fat may result in simple end-products, including the volatile compounds and gases which give the foul odour of putrefaction, and the same changes are observed post mortem and in putrefaction of meat, etc. Gas production may give rise to emphysematous crackling on palpation. The changes in colour—dark-brown or greenish-brown and sometimes almost black—are due to changes in haemoglobin, and are most conspicuous when the dead tissue contains a lot of blood.

Gangrene may be either *primary* or *secondary*. The difference lies in the cause of the tissue necrosis. Primary gangrene is brought about by infection with pathogenic bacteria which both kill the tissue by secreting potent exotoxins and then invade and digest the dead tissue. In secondary gangrene, necrosis is due to some other cause—usually loss of blood supply from vascular obstruction or tissue laceration—and saprophytic bacteria then digest the dead tissue.

Primary gangrene

This includes *gas gangrene* which results from infection with specific bacteria, and gangrene brought about by various other bacteria.

Gas gangrene is caused by a group of anaerobic sporulating bacteria, the *Clostridia*, of which the three most important are *Cl. welchii*, (*Cl. perfringens*), *Cl. oedematiens* (*Cl. novyi*) and *Cl. septicum*. These organisms are intestinal commensals in man and animals; their spores are widespread in soil, and are liable to contaminate wounds. Being anaerobic and saprophy-

tic, they cannot multiply in living, oxygenated tissue, but they flourish in bloodsoaked foreign material and dead tissue in dirty puncture or lacerated wounds such as are caused by road accidents and by shrapnel. Given such a favourable environment, the *Clostridia* produce exotoxins which diffuse into and kill the adjacent tissues and these in turn are invaded, so that the process spreads rapidly, particularly along the length of skeletal muscles (Fig. 9.11). Gas

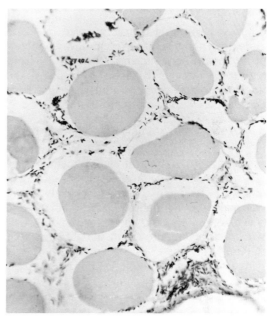

Fig. 9.11 Skeletal muscle in gas gangrene. The muscle fibres are necrotic and their nuclei have disappeared. Large numbers of *Cl. welchii* are present in the dead tissue, mainly in the endomysium. × 400.

gangrene is most often due to *Cl. welchii*. Before the muscle and other tissues are killed, they become intensely oedematous, are extremely painful, and appear swollen and pink. Microscopically, emigration of leucocytes is minimal. Among a number of toxins, *Cl. welchii* produces a lecithinase (α toxin) which by its action on phospholipids lyses cell and mitochondrial membranes, also hyaluronidase and collagenase, which digest ground substance and collagen respectively and may promote the rapid spread of infection. *Cl. welchii* ferments sugars, producing H_2 and CO_2 which collect as bubbles in the dead tissues, rendering them crepitant on palpation. The subcutaneous tissue and skin are also involved, and the affected part, often a limb, may burst open as a result of the swelling of oedema fluid and pressure of gas. The dead tissues are commonly invaded by a mixture of other organisms present in the original wound, and these may play a major role in putrefaction. Gas gangrene may complicate intestinal lesions, e.g. appendicitis or strangulation of the gut (p. 19.55), clostridia being present in the intestine; it occurs also as a puerperal infection of the uterus from contamination via the perineum.

In addition to the rapidly spreading local lesion, gas gangrene is accompanied by acute haemolysis and a severe toxaemia which affects all the internal organs, and death results from peripheral vascular collapse. Spread by the bloodstream may occur as a late, usually terminal event. In consequence, all the tissues at autopsy may contain large numbers of clostridia and show extensive digestive changes. When autopsy is performed after a body has remained a day or more in a warm environment, putrefactive changes, including bubbles of gas, may be seen in various tissues and especially in the liver and other abdominal viscera. This is due to agonal and post-mortem spread and growth of *Cl. welchii*, etc. present in the gut. It is seen especially in obese or oedematous subjects dying from any cause and must not be confused with gas gangrene.

If lacerated wounds are treated by early excision of the devitalised tissue, clostridial infections are unlikely to become established. Antibiotics have also contributed greatly to the prevention of gas gangrene by inhibiting the growth of clostridia. Once gas gangrene has developed, all the affected tissue must be excised. Antibiotic and antitoxic therapy alone is not effective.

Other effects of *Clostridium welchii*. The clostridia of gas gangrene may also cause infection of subcutaneous tissue (cellulitis) without affecting the underlying muscle, or may grow in dirty wounds, producing a foul discharge but without either severe toxaemia or invasion of the surrounding tissues.

There are five types of *Cl. welchii*, and gas gangrene in man is usually caused by type A. A strain of type A with particularly heat-resistant spores sometimes causes food poisoning in man: its spores are activated by heating to 75–80°C, after which they germinate and undergo vegetative growth, e.g. in foods kept at room temperature. When such food is eaten, the vegetative bacteria sporulate in the gut and in doing so produce an enterotoxin which is released with the spores and causes acute diarrhoea, apparently by stimulating adenylate cyclase activity in the intestinal epithelium. A necrotising enteritis, termed pig-bel, occurs in Papua New Guinea and is a result of eating pork and offal infected with type-C *Cl. welchii*, which produces a necrotising toxin. It occurs especially in the highlands, apparently because the diet consists largely of sweet potatoes which contain a protease inhibitor and prevent the destruction of the toxin in the intestine.

Other examples of primary gangrene. In gas gangrene, we have an example of primary gangrene caused by members of a group of clostridia whose toxins kill the tissue and, sometimes in association with other anaerobes, digest it. Primary gangrene can be caused by many other bacteria and mixtures of bacteria. For example, inhalation of dirty water in partial drowning, or of foul discharge from an ulcerated and infected cancer of the larynx, or from an oesophageal cancer which has ulcerated into the trachea, can each cause a gangrenous infection of the lungs in which various bacteria and fungi participate.

Gangrenous infection is particularly liable to develop in debilitated individuals and in those whose resistance to infection is lowered by various diseases; for example, gangrenous pharyngitis or colitis may develop in patients with agranulocytosis, who lack the defences provided by neutrophil polymorphs. Diabetics also, unless their carbohydrate metabolism is adequately controlled, are particularly susceptible to infections, and gangrene may supervene. The following two unusual forms of primary gangrene also deserve mention.

'Meleney's post-operative synergistic gangrene.' This is a slowly spreading infection of the skin and subcutaneous tissue of the chest or abdominal wall; it starts at the site of an operation wound and usually the operation has been perfomed to deal with a focus of sepsis in the chest or abdomen. The spreading edge of the lesion is acutely inflamed and appears red and swollen: as it spreads, the central zone becomes darker and finally gangrenous, followed by sloughing to leave an ulcerated area with a granulating base. The lesion may spread relentlessly to involve much of the trunk. It is usually caused by a synergistic combination of *Staphylococcus aureus*

and a streptococcus, but other combinations may have a similar effect.

Noma (*cancrum oris*) is a gangrenous condition occasionally seen in poorly .nourished children and tends to complicate debilitating infections; it begins on the gum margin and spreads to the cheek, where an inflammatory patch of dusky red appearance forms and then becomes darker in colour and ultimately gangrenous. The condition is caused by bacteria of the genus *Bacteroides* (which, in addition to being present in huge numbers in the intestine are also part of the normal flora of the mouth) together with *Borrelia vincenti*, another mouth commensal. Deficient intake of the vitamin B complex, especially of nicotinic acid, is a predisposing factor.

Secondary gangrene

This is usually the result of ischaemic necrosis (from loss of blood supply) followed by invasion and digestion of the dead tissue by putre-factive micro-organisms. It is seen most often in the foot and leg, and in the intestine. As explained below, it occurs in two forms—'wet' and 'dry' gangrene.

Gangrene of the leg. Infarction of toes, a foot, or the lower leg is not uncommon as the result of arterial occlusion (Fig. 3.33, p. 3.33), the collateral circulation being insufficient to keep the part alive. This is caused by arterial thrombosis complicating advanced atheroma (p. 10.14), which is very common in old people and tends to be particularly severe in diabetics (hence the terms '*senile*' and '*diabetic*' *gangrene*). It may result also from embolism of the leg arteries, e.g. from ulcerating aortic atheroma, or in early or middle adult life in patients with thrombo-angiitis obliterans, a disease which affects multiple arterial branches, expecially in the lower limbs. Another occasional cause is the symmetrical spasmodic contraction of arteries in primary Raynaud's disease (p. 14.34).

If there is much subcutaneous fat, and particularly when the limb is oedematous, as in congestive heart failure, **wet gangrene** commonly supervenes in the infarcted tissues, with blebs of fluid in the skin, sometimes gas production, and rapid putrefaction: there is no sharp line of demarcation between dead and living tissue, and indeed gangrene may spread proximally beyond the tissues originally affected. When infarction occurs in a non-oedematous leg, particularly when there is little subcutaneous fat and when gradual arterial occlusion has preceded the actual infarction, so-called **dry gangrene** is liable to ensue: the skin becomes cold and waxen, the haemoglobin diffuses out of the veins and produces reddish-purple staining of the dead tissues, which then become brownish-red and ultimately almost black, and the dead tissue gradually dries out and shrinks (*mummification*).

Use of the term dry gangrene is controversial. Commonly, mummification occurs with little or no putrefaction. Saprophytic organisms are, however, usually present in small numbers, particularly adjacent to the junction with living tissue, where the dead tissue remains moist. If amputation is not performed, putrefaction becomes established at this site, and a process of slow putrefactive ulceration penetrates the soft tissues, ultimately down to the bone.

Secondary gangrene of the intestine occurs when the blood supply to part of the intestine is arrested by thrombosis of the mesenteric arteries or when a loop of intestine becomes impacted in a hernial sac. In the latter case, secretion of fluid, and gas production by bacteria in the lumen, result in a rise of pressure in the entrapped loop, with consequent interference with blood flow. In both cases, the impaired blood flow results in necrosis of the wall of the intestine, which is then invaded by putrefactive bacteria from the lumen, becomes gangrenous, and ruptures unless removed without delay. While the intestine is dying, the wall becomes swollen and at first red and then black from fluid and red cells escaping from the small vessels. The features are thus those of wet gangrene. The lumen also becomes distended, partly as a result of exudation and partly from failure of the dying smooth muscle to maintain tone and pass on the contents, even when there is no mechanical obstruction.

Necrosis of other organs, e.g. the pancreas in acute pancreatitis,, may also progress to wet gangrene if it becomes infected with putrefying bacteria from the gut.

Anthrax

Anthrax is a fatal epizootic disease of animals, particularly cattle and sheep, caused by a large Gram-+ve sporulating bacillus, the spores of which can survive for many years in soil.

During the 1939–45 war, soil on the island of Gruinard, off the West Coast of Scotland, was experimentally seeded with the spores of *Bacillus anthracis*. They are still viable and the public is warned to keep clear of the island. In herbivores, the disease is contracted by ingestion of spores and causes a severe acute enteritis with a terminal septicaemia: the excreta and secretions are highly infective. More chronic, localised lesions can also occur in animals. In man, *B. anthracis* is of low infectivity, but acute lesions occur in the skin from direct contact with infected material, or more rarely internally from inhalation or ingestion of spores.

The factors determining the virulence of the bacillus include a capsular polypeptide rich in D-glutamic acid, which renders the organism resistant to phagocytosis, and a complex exotoxin which promotes increased vascular permeability, causing gross inflammatory oedema. Death can result from hypovolaemic shock due to local and generalised exudative loss of plasma fluid.

Cutaneous anthrax (malignant pustule) of man occurs from direct contact with animal material, e.g. carcasses, hides or bristles in shaving brushes. Although many imported hides are contaminated with spores, anthrax is rare among those handling them. The organism probably enters through a minor abrasion, and a painful papule forms and may develop one, and then many, small vesicles containing clear or, later, bloodstained fluid. As the lesion enlarges, it becomes necrotic and haemorrhagic and is covered by a dry, hard eschar which becomes black (Fig. 9.12), hence the name. A striking feature is the gross oedema which spreads well beyond the site of the lesion. The malignant pustule is usually less than 2 cm in diameter. The bacillus is readily detected in scrapings of the early lesion, and may be suspected from its microscopic appearance—a large Gram +ve oblong bacillus with sharp corners, often forming short chains, and with a demonstrable capsule. It grows readily in culture. Leucocytic emigration is usually scanty. Spread may occur to the regional lymph nodes, which become enlarged, oedematous and haemorrhagic. Although uncommon, the condition is an important example of a serious, sometimes

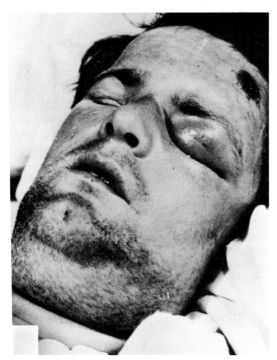
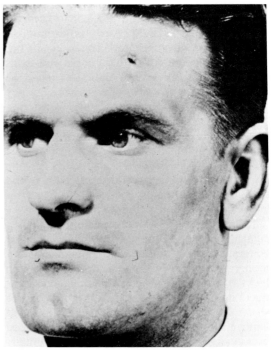

Fig. 9.12 Anthrax. *Left*, before treatment. The malignant pustule is seen on the forehead. Note the gross and extensive inflammatory oedema. *Right*, following treatment. (By kind permission of Dr W.M. Jamieson and the Editor of *Medicine*.)

fatal infection which can be effectively treated if diagnosed early.

Respiratory anthrax occurs from inhaling spores, usually from hides or wool. A localised lesion develops in the lower trachea or larger bronchi: it consists of a patch of haemorrhagic, ulcerated mucosa with intense oedema, involvement of hilar and mediastinal lymph nodes, extension to the lungs and haemorrhagic pleural and pericardial effusions: the prognosis is poor.

Intestinal anthrax is rare in man. It consists of one or more haemorrhagic foci in the wall of the upper small intestine, with central necrosis, gross oedematous swelling and involvement of the mesenteric lymph nodes.

Septicaemia and a haemorrhagic meningtitis may occur in man, but are rare.

Chronic Bacterial Infections (Infective Granulomas)

As stated on p. 4.32, there is an increasing tendency to restrict *granuloma* to inflammatory lesions consisting of aggregates of macrophages. I have preferred to use *macrophage granuloma* to describe such a lesion, and to retain the traditional usage of *granuloma* to mean any chronic inflammatory lesion.

Accordingly, under this heading are included the many infections which give rise to chronic inflammation. In most of these, the exudative reaction so prominent in acute inflammation is not a conspicuous feature. A more characteristic feature is the formation of granulation tissue which eventually progresses to fibrosis. The general features of chronic inflammation have been described on pp. 4.30–32 and a more detailed account of the production of granulation-tissue is given on pp. 5.4–9. The following account describes briefly some of the more important chronic infections. Because of its wide prevalence and tuberculous-like features, sarcoidosis is also included here, although there is no evidence that it is an infection.

Tuberculosis

Formerly one of the great killing diseases of temperate climates, tuberculosis is now much less common in most of the developed countries. It is, however, prevalent in communities with a poor standard of living, and still ranks among the world's most important infections. The disease illustrates well various basic features of bacterial infection, and in particular the importance of the reaction of the host in determining the nature of the lesions, and the spread of infection within the body. The causal organism, *Mycobacterium tuberculosis* or tubercle bacillus, is an aerobic Gram +ve bacillus with a waxy cell wall which renders it difficult to stain. Once the stain has penetrated the cell wall, however, it is also difficult to remove, and the mycobacteria are sometimes referred to as acid- and alcohol-fast bacteria, since they resist decolourisation by mineral acids and alcohol, as in the Ziehl-Neelsen stain. Tubercle bacilli grow slowly in culture; they are highly pathogenic for the guinea-pig, inoculation of which has been much used for their detection when present in small numbers in sputum, etc. In man, they usually cause chronic disease but can also produce a much more acute and even rapidly fatal infection. In addition to the tubercle bacilli, of which there are two major types causing human disease (see below), the mycobacteria include *Bacillus leprae* which causes leprosy, and there are also various ill-defined organisms, sometimes termed *anonymous* or *atypical mycobacteria*, which cause lesions in the skin, lymph nodes, lungs and elsewhere.

Epidemiology

The two types of tubercle bacillus mainly responsible for disease in man are the human type, *Mycobacterium tuberculosis*, and the bovine type, *Mycobacterium bovis*. The *human type* is the more important; infection with it is usually contracted by inhalation, and the initial or primary lesion is nearly always in the lungs. Patients with chronic pulmonary tuberculosis provide the reservoir of infection and spread the disease by exhaling infected droplets and by coughing up infected sputum. The organism is resistant to drying and can survive for long periods in dust, inhalation of which is the usual method of contracting the disease. Infection of the tonsils or of the intestine can also occur from swallowing the human type of tubercle bacillus in contaminated dust, or the bovine type of bacillus in contaminated milk from cows with tuberculous mastitis.

Several factors are responsible for the declining incidence of tuberculosis in Western Europe and North America. Firstly, the rising standard of nutrition and housing: there is no doubt that under-nourishment predisposes to tuberculosis and impairs the resistance of the individual who has contracted the disease. Overcrowding and inadequate personal and domestic hygiene are also of importance in spreading the disease in the home and in public transport and meeting places, etc. The environment of a subject coughing up the organism is likely to be heavily contaminated, and spread within families is especially common, giving rise to both pulmonary and alimentary infections.

Since the 1939–45 war, the use of specific chemotherapeutic bactericidal agents has also helped to reduce the incidence of the disease by diminishing greatly the infectivity of patients with chronic pulmonary tuberculosis. Mass miniature radiography has revealed unsuspected cases of tuberculosis in the community, and protection against infection has been provided by means of BCG vaccination.

In countries where the disease is rife, infants and young children are particularly at risk, and in this country the mortality rate in children contracting the infection before the age of 3 years was formerly very high. Those who overcome the infection develop partial resistance to the organism, but may become re-infected and develop chronic pulmonary tuberculosis in adult life. The bacteria may survive for many years in dormant lesions, without clinical manifestations, and these may become active as a result of malnutrition, as in war or famine, as a complication of other debilitating diseases such as diabetes mellitus, or from administration of corticosteroids or other immunosuppressive agents. In Western Europe, a high proportion of 'new' cases are middle-aged or old and have had dormant lesions for many years, i.e. from the time when the disease was much commoner. It is, however, relatively common among Asian immigrants, younger age groups being affected. *Mycobacterium bovis* causes mastitis in cattle, and is transmitted to man by consuming infected milk and milk products. Infection results usually by way of the gut or tonsils. In many countries, bovine infection in man has been eradicated by pasteurisation of milk, which kills the organism, and by tuberculin testing of cattle and elimination of infected cows. The avian tubercle bacillus (*Myco. avium*) is a rare cause of disease in man.

Hypersensitivity and immunity

The immune response to the tubercle bacillus provides the classical example of cell-mediated immunity, i.e. the production of specifically primed T lymphocytes which are capable of reacting directly with antigen derived from the bacterium on the surface of infected macrophages. The mechanism of this type of response (p. 6.19), and the state of delayed hypersensitivity which results from it (p. 7.17) have been described in earlier chapters. It is not understood why cell-mediated immunity is the dominant type of immune response to the tubercle bacillus, but it may be of significance that mycobacteria, living or dead, have a powerful enhancing effect on cell-mediated immune responses to antigens in general, and this forms the basis of their use in Freund's adjuvant (p. 6.30). Whatever the explanation of its adjuvant effect, infection with tubercle bacilli results, within two weeks or so, in the development of a high degree of cell-mediated immunity to proteins of the organism (tuberculoproteins) and the subsequent course of the infection and the features of the lesions are profoundly influenced by the development of a delayed hypersensitivity (type 4) reaction to these antigenic products of the tubercle bacillus. This state of hypersensitivity was demonstrated by Robert Koch (1891), using a crude preparation termed 'old tuberculin'. A more refined preparation is termed 'purified protein derivative' (PPD). The specifically primed T cells react with the surface of infected macrophages and release the various lymphokines described on p. 7.20. The results are both beneficial and harmful. *The tubercle bacillus has not been shown to produce any direct toxic effect, and can survive and multiply within macrophages in tissue culture without harm to the cultured cells. Indeed, it is likely that the tissue injury resulting from tuberculous infection* is due mainly or entirely to the delayed hypersensitivity reaction against the bacteria. Nevertheless, without an immune response, multiplication of the organism would presumably continue unchecked. The delayed hypersensitivity reaction is therefore to be regarded as protective in reducing or eliminating the infection, but at the same time injurious to the tissues. In the following account, the structural changes of the lesions of tuberculosis are interpreted in terms of a delayed hypersensitivity reaction.

Although antibodies to mycobacterial antigens develop in tuberculosis, they do not appear to influence the course of the infection, and have not provided the basis of a useful diagnostic test.

Tuberculin skin testing. This is carried out by intradermal injection of very small amounts of purified derivative (PPD), a mixture of tuberculoproteins, as, for example, in the *Mantoux test*. In individuals who are, or have previously been, infected, a delayed hypersensitivity reaction develops, the features of which are described on p. 7.18. In some patients with very severe tuberculosis, the test is negative, presumably because the large numbers of cells presenting antigen have fully occupied the available specifically primed T cells. Tuberculin skin tests give positive reactions in infections with both human and bovine types of tubercle bacillus, and with other types of mycobacteria. For this reason, they may be positive in individuals infected with *Mycobacterium leprae*. Positive tests are also observed in healthy inhabitants of tropical and sub-tropical countries, apparently as a result of previous sub-clinical infection with other mycobacteria.

Immunisation against tuberculosis. Protective immunisation requires the induction of cell-mediated immunity to tuberculoproteins, and this is most effectively achieved by injecting living mycobacteria. Attenuated strains of the bovine type, e.g. *bacille Calmette-Guérin* (BCG), or other non-human stains such as *Myco. muris* (the vole bacillus), are used for this purpose. Cell-mediated immunity develops, with consequent delayed hypersensitivity reactions at the site of injection and sometimes also in the draining lymph nodes which may become infected. The attenuated bacilli are destroyed and the lesions heal, but the cell-mediated immunity persists.

Structural changes

When a guinea-pig is inoculated with *Myco. tuberculosis* there is little reaction during the first day or so apart from local infiltration with neutrophil polymorphs, which soon disappear. During the next few days, macrophages migrate into the area and ingest the bacteria without bringing about their destruction. After ten days or so, lymphocytes begin to appear in the lesion, and macrophages derived mainly from monocytes of the blood aggregate in increasing numbers to form a minute nodule consisting of a macrophage granuloma. These very early stages of infection cannot, of course, be observed in man, but the subsequent changes are closely similar in man and the guinea-pig. The macrophages enlarge and change to **epithelioid cells** (p. 4.36). Small lymphocytes accumulate around the margin of the nodule, which is then termed a **tubercle** and becomes visible to the naked eye about 3 weeks after the onset. In the central part of the lesion, multinucleated **Langhans' giant cells** (p. 4.36) are formed by

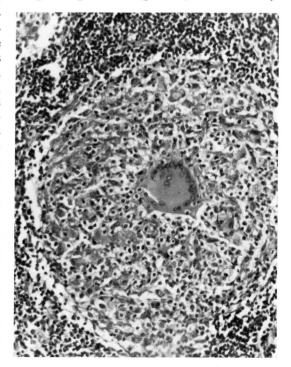

Fig. 9.13 An early tubercle, consisting mainly of epithelioid cells, some of which have fused to form a Langhans' giant cell. Lymphocytes are scattered among the epithelioid cells and are numerous around the periphery. × 174.

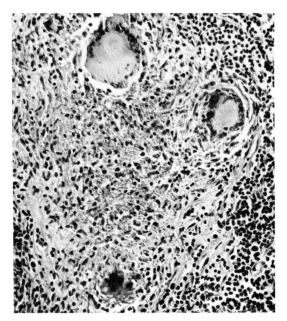

Fig. 9.14 A more advanced tubercle with three giant cells and early necrosis among the most centrally-placed epithelioid cells. × 150.

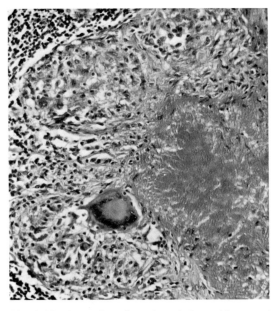

Fig. 9.15 Part of a tuberculous lesion with central caseation (*right*) and surrounding epithelioid cells with giant-cell formation. Note the structureless appearance of the caseous material. × 150.

fusion of epithelioid cells (Fig. 9.13). As the tubercle enlarges, the epithelioid and giant cells in the central part undergo necrosis (Fig. 9.14): the cells lose their outline and nuclear staining and become fused into a homogeneous or slightly granular material, which may also contain fibrin from vascular exudation. The tubercle thus comes to consist of a necrotic centre, surrounded by epithelioid and sometimes giant cells (Fig. 9.15), with a peripheral aggregation of small lymphocytes. The necrotic material is creamy-white, and resembles cream cheese in appearance and consistence—hence the terms **caseation** and **caseous material**.

The initial accumulation of macrophages and phagocytosis of tubercle bacilli occur before there is any immune response and are seen also in the reaction to particles of various non-antigenic foreign materials. Lymphocytic infiltration, however, follows the development of cell-mediated immunity and some of the cells are specifically primed T-cells which, by releasing various lymphokines (p. 7.20) contribute to the arrival of more macrophages by chemotaxis, and to their arrest around the tubercle bacilli by migration-inhibition factor: macrophage-activating factor may transform the macrophages to epithelioid cells, and may mediate the destruction of phagocytosed bacilli. Cytotoxic T cells and lymphokines presumably account for the necrosis of macrophages at the centre of the lesion, although the tubercle follicle is avascular and ischaemia may also be important. It has been shown in animal experiments that many of the lymphocytes in the tuberculous lesion are not specifically primed cells resulting from the cell-mediated immune response (pp. 7.19–20): they may be attracted to the site of infection by a chemotactic lymphokine, but their significance in the lesion is obscure.

The further course of the infection depends on several factors, including the infecting dose and virulence of the organism and also the degree of resistance of the host. What determines virulence in strains of tubercle bacilli is not understood, but the so-called virulent strains are those which are capable of relatively rapid multiplication *in vivo*. If bacterial multiplication is checked, tubercles are replaced by fibrous tissue. If the bacteria continue to multiply in the lesions, they may escape and gain a foothold in the surrounding tissues, with further tubercle formation. A cluster of tubercles may thus arise, and as these enlarge, they become confluent, and the central areas of caseous necrosis eventually unite to form a large caseous patch with tubercles around the periphery. Such lesions may reach several centimetres in diameter. When they arise in **the lungs**, they seldom reach this size without involving the wall of a bronchus, and the caseous material is then discharged via the bronchus, leaving a tuberculous cavity (Fig. 9.16). In

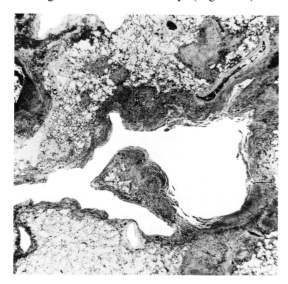

Fig. 9.16 Formation of a tuberculous cavity. The lesion has ulcerated into a bronchus and the caseous material is discharging. × 4.

other tissues, and particularly in the **kidneys** and in lesions of **bone** extending into the surrounding soft tissues, caseous material may be invaded by neutrophil polymorphs, with resultant liquefaction ('tuberculous pus'). Such a lesion used to be called a **cold abscess**, because it is not accompanied by the intense acute inflammation of a pyogenic bacterial infection. The softened caseous material may track through the tissues and may eventually reach a surface and discharge.

Some tuberculous lesions present more acute features than those described above. For example, rapid dissemination may occur by the air passages throughout the lung, resulting in multiple scattered lesions. Microscopy then shows extensive filling of the alveoli with large rounded macrophages and scattered lymphocytes (Fig. 9.17): the macrophages rapidly undergo fatty change and necrosis, and the lesions

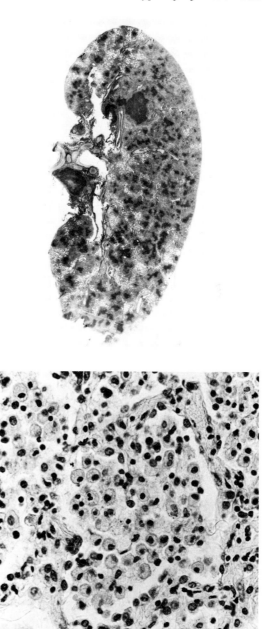

Fig. 9.17 Acute tuberculous bronchopneumonia. *Above*, Primary pulmonary tuberculosis in a child. The infection has spread by the bronchi and has caused widespread lesions which are becoming confluent and have undergone central caseation (dark areas). *Below*, the lesions consist initially of accumulations of macrophages and lymphocytes in the alveoli. The macrophages undergo fatty change and appear 'foamy': necrosis then supervenes. × 370.

enlarge and coalesce with little or no attempt at healing. If it infects the **subarachnoid space**, usually by way of the bloodstream, the tubercle bacillus multiplies rapidly in the cerebrospinal fluid and the meningitis is of acute exudative inflammatory type with deposition of fibrin and accumulation initially of neutrophil polymorphs and later of macrophages and lymphocytes. Tubercles are usually poorly formed, and involvement of the walls of arteries and veins lying in the subarachnoid space may cause severe narrowing of their lumina by endarteritis (Fig. 21.29, p. 21.27) or occlusion by thrombosis. The lesions which result from infection of the **pleural and peritoneal cavities** are also commonly exudative, with a serous or serofibrinous exudate, and when the **pericardium** is involved the exudate may be rich in fibrin and is often haemorrhagic, presumably as a result of the mechanical effect of the heart beat.

Primary and re-infection tuberculosis

Infection of an individual who has not been previously infected or immunised gives rise to the **primary lesion** at the portal of entry in the lung, tonsil or small intestine. This usually remains small, and commonly heals without becoming detectable. Early spread of bacteria to the *regional lymph nodes* is, however, the rule, and their rapid multiplication may occur in the affected nodes, i.e. at the hilum of the lung (Fig. 16.29, p. 16.45), in the neck or in the mesentery, depending on the site of the primary lesion. The combination of the primary lesion and enlarged, caseous regional lymph nodes is called the **primary complex.**

Re-infection or **chronic tuberculosis** results from infection of an individual who has overcome a primary infection or been immunised by BCG. The re-infection lesion is usually in the apex of one or other lung and may extend to give a large local lesion with one or more cavities (Fig. 9.18). There is usually little or no involvement of the local lymph nodes. Re-infection lesions occur also in the tonsils, small intestine, pharynx and skin, again without much involvement of the regional nodes, but these are relatively uncommon sites. Individuals with re-infection tuberculosis of the lungs may, however, develop lesions in the larynx, mouth and intestines as a result of endogenous infection by coughing up and swallowing sputum

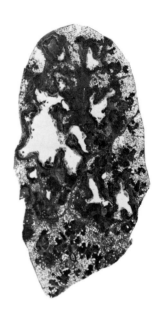

Fig. 9.18   Apical part of the lung showing chronic (reinfection) tuberculosis. The infection has extended to form coalescing lesions with central caseation and peripheral fibrosis. The caseous material in the larger lesions has discharged via the bronchi, leaving several cavities with fibrous walls.   × 0·7.

containing tubercle bacilli (Fig. 19.58, p. 19.47). These metastatic lesions resemble those of reinfection tuberculosis in spreading locally with minimal or no involvement of the local nodes.

The differences between primary and re-infection tuberculosis appear to depend mainly on the spread of the bacilli to the local lymph nodes and their multiplication there in the early stages of the primary infection, before the development of a high level of cell-mediated immunity.

Although the term 're-infection tuberculosis' is commonly used for chronic tuberculosis occurring usually in adults, it may well be that, in some cases, tubercle bacilli persisting in a latent healed primary lesion are eventually reactivated and produce the 're-infection'.

The spread of infection within the body is discussed below, but more detailed accounts of the resulting lesions are given in the chapters on regional pathology, e.g. pulmonary tuberculosis, pp. 16.44 *et seq.*

Amyloid disease (p. 11.1) is an important complication of chronic tuberculosis.

Spread of infection

Tuberculous infection is very prone to spread by lymphatics and to produce lesions in lymph nodes. This occurs especially in the early stages of the primary infection, with resulting involvement of the draining lymph nodes, and infection may spread from these to adjacent nodes or groups of nodes, e.g. in the mediastinum. In chronic (i.e. re-infection) tuberculosis, lymphatic spread is usually localised to the tissue immediately around the lesions, the draining lymph nodes seldom being severely involved. This limitation of lymphatic spread is probably attributable to the modified behaviour of macrophages which results from delayed hypersensitivity. There is experimental evidence that lymphatic spread results from ingestion and transport of *Myco. tuberculosis* by macrophages, and the T-cell factors, which enhance the bactericidal activity of macrophages and interfere with their migration from the lesion, are likely to limit such spread.

Spread also occurs by the bloodstream. This is seen notably in **acute miliary tuberculosis**, in which large numbers of bacteria enter the blood and give rise to multiple scattered tubercles in the various organs. The condition arises most commonly in primary tuberculosis and is due usually to involvement of a vein by the large caseating lymph-node lesions of the primary complex—in most cases the pulmonary hilar nodes: the caseating process extends into the wall of an adjacent vein, usually one of the pulmonary veins, and caseous material containing large numbers of mycobacteria is then discharged into the circulation. The resulting lesions are particularly numerous in the liver, kidneys and spleen. They consist of tubercles of fairly uniform size, and without specific therapy death usually results from tuberculous meningitis after about a month, at which time the tubercles are of approx. 1–2 mm diameter (Fig. 16.31, p. 16.48): they are rather poorly developed, often without giant cells, but with central necrosis (Fig. 9.19) and are termed **miliary tubercles** (latin *milium*—millet seed). In some instances, the bacteria escape into a systemic vein, either directly or by involvement of the thoracic duct, and as a result the number of miliary lesions in the lungs far exceeds those in other organs. When a relatively small number of tubercle bacilli gain entrance to the bloodstream, few tubercles are produced in the vari-

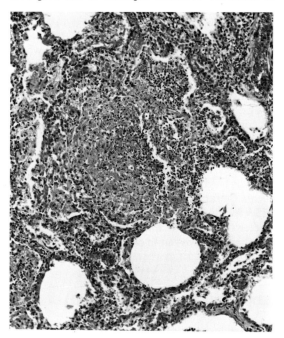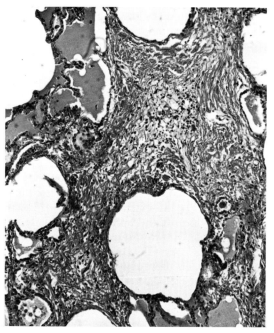

Fig. 9.19 On the left is shown a miliary tubercle of lung with central caseation and acute exudate in the surrounding alveoli from a patient with untreated miliary tuberculosis; on the right a fibrous scar containing a few lymphocytes, the remains of a miliary tubercle after specific chemotherapy. × 100.

ous organs, and since the patient may survive much longer than is the case in untreated acute miliary tuberculosis, the lesions may become larger. One or more large metastatic lesions may also occur, for example in the bones, joints, kidneys, epididymes or fallopian tubes, and less commonly in the brain. Although in heavily infected communities blood-borne lesions arise most commonly as a complication of the primary tuberculous complex in young children, in countries where the disease has been largely eradicated they are uncommon and are now seen mostly in older patients in the late stages of re-infection tuberculosis. Haematogenous lesions are also observed when chronic tuberculosis is complicated by other debilitating diseases, or as a result of corticosteroid or other immunosuppressive therapy.

Spread of tuberculous infection occurs also along hollow viscera and in body cavities. In the lungs, spread by the bronchi is of great importance. Mycobacteria coughed up in sputum may settle and give rise to lesions in the larynx and intestine. Spread may occur from the fallopian tubes to the endometrium, and from the kidney to the urinary tract, and dissemination may occur within the pleural, pericardial and peritoneal cavities and, in tuberculous meningitis, within the subarachnoid space and ventricles of the brain.

Healing of tuberculous lesions

The healing of tubercles or larger tuberculous lesions is dependent on the elimination or reduction in numbers of mycobacteria. Healing is brought about by formation, around the lesions, of reticulin fibres, progressing to more dense fibrosis. If caseation is slight or absent, as in early tubercles, the whole lesion may be gradually replaced by fibrous tissue, leaving a scar (Fig. 9.19), but extensive patches of caseation usually persist and become encapsulated in fibrous tissue. Slow progressive deposition of calcium salts commonly occurs in the caseous material, which eventually may become stony hard and clearly visible in radiographs: in some instances the calcified material may be replaced by bone, which may even develop spaces containing haemopoietic marrow. The course of the disease depends on the balance between bacterial multiplication, with extension and caseation of the lesions, and the reactive processes

involved in killing the bacteria, preventing their spread, and promoting a fibroblastic reaction. Tubercle bacilli may long remain alive in healed and even calcified lesions, and states of malnutrition, debilitation, etc., may allow re-activation of the disease.

The effects of drugs. The course and prognosis of tuberculosis have been radically changed by effective specific chemotherapy, which has also greatly modified the appearance of tuberculous lesions. When healing occurs naturally, i.e. without specific chemotherapy, large caseous lesions become walled off first by cellular tubercles and then by new-formed fibrous tissue, which penetrates the outer zone of tubercles and finally encapsulates the central caseous mass. Dense fibrosis and calcification complete the process: there is little resolution. Effective drug therapy is accompanied successively by resolution of the surrounding exudative lesions, increased vascularity, reversion of the epithelioid cells to foamy macrophages, formation of granulation tissue, absorption of necrotic and caseous material, and finally by healing with the production of minimal amounts of fibrous tissue. Combined therapy thus strikingly modifies the outcome; early lesions may clear up almost completely without residual effects and chronic caseous and fibrotic pulmonary lesions with excavation are transformed to smooth-walled cavities, which may become lined by epithelium.

Because of the spontaneous occurrence of mutant tubercle bacilli resistant to one or more drugs, it is now accepted practice to administer a combination of three drugs, usually isonicotinic acid hydrazide (isoniazid), rifampicin and ethambutol. Because the tubercle bacillus multiplies relatively slowly, it may take some months for the selective advantage conferred by drug therapy on a resistant mutant to be reflected in clinical deterioration, and repeated bacteriological examinations, e.g. of sputum, are therefore advisable during treatment.

Leprosy (Hansen's disease)

Leprosy is a chronic disease caused by infection with *Mycobacterium leprae* and affects primarily the peripheral nervous system and skin. As a result of nerve damage there may be paralysis, deformity and ulceration. About 12 million people in tropical and warm temperate climates are lepers although many more have been infected without developing the disease.

The leprosy bacillus has not yet been grown in culture. The mouse footpad supports growth and the nine-banded armadillo can become infected naturally and develop a disseminated form of the disease. *Myco. leprae* has a long dividing time of about 12 days. It colonises the cooler parts of the body.

Patients with the lepromatous form of the disease (see below) may excrete over ten million bacilli per day from the nose into the atmosphere and undiagnosed lepers are the main source of infection. The mode of transmission is not known. The bacilli probably enter via the respiratory tract, disseminate haematogenously and grow particularly in the dermal nerves.

The consequences of infection depend on the immune status of the host. Leprosy represents the best example of an infective disease that has a spectrum of clinical and histopathological manifestations which depend on the host's immune response. The bacillus is killed intracellularly by macrophages activated by specifically primed T lymphocytes, (p. 8.10); acquired resistance to *Myco. leprae* therefore depends on the cell-mediated immune response. Antibody has no protective effect. The bacillus itself is non-toxic and lesions are produced either by evoking a potentially destructive granulomatous reaction or by interference with the metabolism of cells (e.g. Schwann cells) by colonisation with huge numbers of bacilli.

Types of leprosy

The incubation period for clinical leprosy is measured in years. Most of those infected have innate resistance and the bacilli are destroyed in the skin by macrophages before they multiply significantly. Bacilli that survive and multiply in Schwann cells evoke initially a lymphocytic and macrophage response. Clinically, the disease usually presents as a hypopigmented, anaesthetic macule on the face or a limb. This early form is known as **indeterminate leprosy**. Bacilli are present, but very scanty, in dermal nerve twigs and most patients with this lesion eliminate the bacilli without treatment. About a quarter progress to **established leprosy**, the

bacilli continuing their multiplication and spreading beyond the dermal nerves.

The type of leprosy that results depends on the degree of immunity. A proportion of those infected fail to develop cell-mediated immunity (CMI) to *Myco. leprae* and this results in **lepromatous leprosy** in which bacilli are present in large numbers in the affected tissues. This defect of immunity is probably mediated by suppressor T-cells and is antigen-specific, so that lepers do not suffer from opportunistic infections. Conversely, those with a high degree of CMI develop **tuberculoid leprosy** with scanty bacilli in the tissues. A proportion of patients do not progress initially into typical tuberculoid or lepromatous leprosy but develop an intermediate, unstable form of disease, **borderline leprosy**. Without treatment, they move eventually along the immunopathological spectrum toward lepromatous or, less commonly, tuberculoid leprosy (Fig. 9.20).

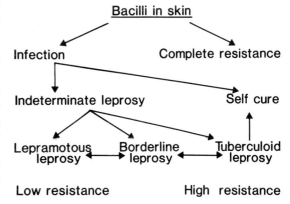

Fig. 9.20 Patterns of *Mycobacterium leprae* infection.

Lepromatous leprosy. The dermal lesions consist of symmetrical nodules and more diffuse coarsening and thickening of the skin over much of the body. The eyebrows are lost and the classical 'leonine facies' may develop. Pathologically, the dermis is filled with rounded macrophages stuffed with bacilli which often form clumps termed *globi* (Figs. 9.21, 9.22). An untreated case may have 10^7 bacilli per gram of skin, but most of the organisms are dead and fragmented. Lymphocytes are scanty or absent. The dermal nerves are infiltrated by bacilli-laden Schwann cells and macrophages, and eventually the nerves undergo fibrosis. Since this affects sensory nerves particularly, the

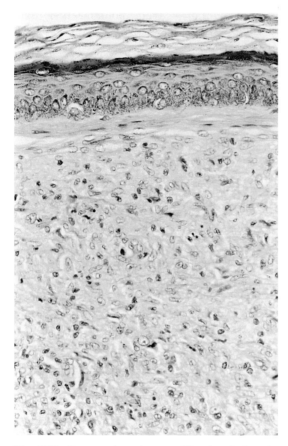

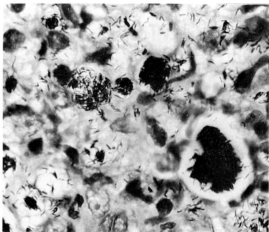

Fig. 9.22 Lepromatous leprosy. Stain for acid-fast bacilli on the same biopsy as Fig. 9.21. Abundant bacilli are seen, many of them in agglomerated clumps or 'globi'. (Wade-Fite stain) × 1000.

Fig. 9.21 Lepromatous leprosy. The dermis is uniformly infiltrated by rounded macrophages and very few lymphocytes. The unaffected zone between the epidermis and the infiltrate is typical for lepromatous leprosy. × 320.

extremities become anaesthetic in a glove-and-stocking distribution and are readily traumatised. This is the main reason for the atrophy and loss of digits and toes seen in advanced cases. Lepromatous leprosy is a systemic disease, the bacilli spreading by the bloodstream to the nasal mucosa, larynx, lymph nodes, liver, the eyes, bones and testes. These multibacillary lesions can cause iritis, osteitis and bone erosion, blocked nose, laryngeal mucosal thickening with hoarse voice and orchitis. In the testes, the lesions may heal with fibrosis resulting in hypogonadism, so that gynaecomastia is sometimes seen. In longstanding cases, secondary amyloidosis is often a serious complication. Lepromatous leprosy is stable in that, without treatment, the patient will not recover cell-mediated immunity and the bacilli multiply progressively.

Tuberculoid leprosy. This form is limited to the skin and peripheral nerves. The lesions are asymmetric and fewer and smaller than in lepromatous leprosy. They are annular, flat and anaesthetic, and peripheral nerves are often palpably enlarged, e.g. the median nerve at the wrist and the ulnar nerve at the elbow. Histologically, the lesions consist of tubercle-like epithelioid-cell follicles, with formation of Langhans' giant cells, in the dermis and cutaneous nerves (Figs. 9.23, 9.24). Lymphocytes are numerous at the periphery of the lesions and bacilli are scanty or cannot be found. Severe nerve damage results from the destructive effect of the fibrosing granulomas. The larger peripheral nerves may also be seriously damaged during leprosy reactions (see below), and the intraneural granulomas may undergo caseous necrosis (the only situation where leprosy granulomas become necrotic). Consequently, there is paralysis, claw hands, foot drop, claw toes and anaesthesia. Ulceration of the skin and secondary infection with cellulitis and osteomyelitis may follow. However, tuberculoid leprosy does not spread systemically, and patients with the polar form of tuberculoid leprosy, who have the strongest CMI, usually undergo self-cure even without treatment.

Borderline leprosy. Clinically and pathologic-

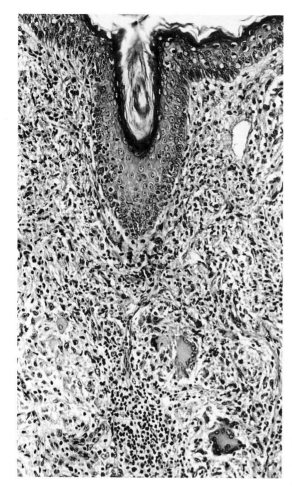

Fig. 9.23 Tuberculoid leprosy, showing non-caseating epithelioid-cell and giant-cell granulomas in the dermis and a lymphocytic infiltrate. The involvement of the basal layer of the epidermis by the inflammation is typical in tuberculoid leprosy. Leprosy bacilli were not found. × 200.

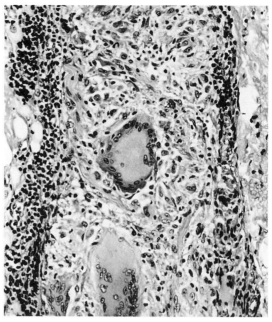

Fig. 9.24 Tuberculoid leprosy. A deep dermal nerve in the same biopsy as Fig. 9.23 shows infiltration by epithelioid cells and Langhans' giant cells and a peripheral lymphocytic infiltrate. This granulomatous reaction destroys the nerve and causes anaesthesia. × 250.

ally, this has mixed features of tuberculoid and lepromatous leprosy, with numerous erythematous skin papules containing moderate numbers of bacilli and a diffuse epithelioid-cell infiltrate in the dermis.

Some of the features of the different types of leprosy are shown in Table 9.1.

Diagnosis. 'Slit-skin smears' are used in the diagnosis of leprosy: fluid from an incised skin lesion is treated by a modified Ziehl-Neelsen stain for acid-fast bacilli. Many bacilli are seen in lepromatous and borderline cases, but very

Table 9.1 Features of the different types of leprosy

	Type of leprosy		
	LEPROMATOUS	BORDERLINE	TUBERCULOID
Type of macrophage infiltrate	simple macrophage diffuse	epithelioid-cell, diffuse	epithelioid- and giant-cell granuloma
Lymphocyte infiltrate	−	±	+ +
Number of bacilli	+ + +	+	±
Degree of nerve thickening	−	+	+ +
Degree of cell-mediated immunity to *M. leprae*	−	±	+ +

few or none in indeterminate and tuberculoid lesions. Scrapings from the nasal mucosa in lepromatous lepers also reveal abundant bacilli.

The lepromin skin test is an index of cell-mediated immunity to *Myco. leprae* and is performed by injecting heat-killed *Myco. leprae* intradermally. A positive reaction (*the Mitsuda reaction*) occurs within four weeks as an erythematous nodule in patients with tuberculoid or indeterminate leprosy. It consists of an erythematous nodule with the histological features of an epithelioid-cell granuloma. The reaction does not occur in lepromatous leprosy, and a positive result is of little diagnostic value because it may result from exposure to other mycobacteria and from self-cured sub-clinical *Myco. leprae* infections. In lepers, however, the test correlates well with *in vitro* tests for specific cell-mediated immunity, such as the lymphocyte transformation test (p. 6.24). In lepromatous leprosy, there is a raised serum IgG level, a high titre of antibody to *Myco. leprae* antigens, and often antinuclear auto-antibodies and a false-positive screening test for syphilis.

Leprosy reactions. Two types of acute immunologically-mediated reactions may be seen in leprosy patients, usually occurring after commencing microbicidal therapy.

1. Erythema nodosum leprosum occurs at the lepromatous end of the leprosy spectrum when initial drug treatment kills large numbers of *Myco. leprae* and releases antigenic material. As the antibody titre is usually high, immune complexes are formed locally and induce crops of painful inflammatory papules along with fever and malaise. Histologically, the tissues show oedema, polymorph infiltration and a mild vasculitis. The features are thus those of a mild Arthus-type reaction (p. 7.14). Circulating immune complexes may occur when there is relative antigen excess, and an acute generalised reaction, glomerulonephritis, polyarthritis or iritis may result.

2. Delayed hypersensitivity reactions occur in borderline patients, who are immunologically unstable. Their degree of cell-mediated immunity is liable to change, and, as treatment reduces the amount of *Myco. leprae* antigen, T-cell-mediated macrophage activation increases. There is cellular infiltration and oedema of the tissue granulomas so that swollen erythematous papules develop in the skin. The nerves become inflamed and may undergo necrosis and formation of 'cold abscesses' (p. 9.19), causing paralysis. Untreated borderline patients may spontaneously lose their cell-mediated immunity and undergo a clinically similar reaction, but with increasing bacillary load in the tissue granulomas and a loss of the epithelioid-cell pattern of infiltrate. They then move towards lepromatous leprosy and immune-complex reactions.

Relapse. Inadequate treatment or the development of drug resistance may permit the disease to relapse. This is seen as growth of the skin nodules, which then contain innumerable non-degenerate leprosy bacilli.

Causes of death. Many lepers die from other causes. The main fatal consequences of leprosy are renal failure from secondary amyloidosis and the glomerulonephritis arising from circulating immune-complex disease, which may rarely give rise also to severe or fatal acute systemic reactions (p. 7.17). Adequate drug therapy usually arrests the disease and very often cures it.

Sarcoidosis

This disease, which is of unknown causation, is characterised by multiple granulomatous lesions, and may affect lymph nodes, lungs, skin, spleen, eyes, salivary glands, liver and bones, particularly of the hands and feet. It is of world-wide distribution, but with great geographical variation in incidence. It occurs over a wide age range, but most commonly in young adults, and is much more common in negroes than whites in the U.S.A., and in immigrants than natives in Great Britain. The highest reported incidence is in Sweden.

The disease most commonly gives rise to enlarged mediastinal and pulmonary hilar lymph nodes, often without symptoms, but sometimes accompanied by fever. Other groups of lymph nodes are often affected and widespread minute lesions in the lungs may present an x-ray picture resembling that of miliary tuberculosis. Sarcoid lesions also occur in the skin and occasionally erythema induratum (p. 27.18) develops and may be the presenting clinical feature. Microscopically, the sarcoid lesions consist of tubercle-like follicles composed of epithelioid cells with occasional Langhans'

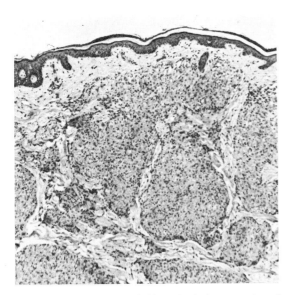

Fig. 9.25 Sarcoidosis of skin. The lesions consist of aggregates of epithelioid cells with relatively few lymphocytes. In contrast to tuberculosis, there is little or no necrosis. × 80.

giant cells but with fewer lymphocytes than in tubercles (Fig. 9.25 and Fig. 18.8, p. 18.13). The giant cells may contain curious calcium-rich star-shaped or conchoid inclusions (*asteroid* or *Schaumann bodies*). Unlike tuberculosis, the lesions do not undergo caseation although there may be a little central necrosis.

The course of the disease is unpredictable: it may be acute or chronic, and temporary or permanent remission may occur spontaneously. It can cause blindness by involving the uveal tract, and is occasionally fatal, usually as a result of fibrosis of the pulmonary lesions with consequent right ventricular heart failure, or as a result of intercurrent infections. Hypercalcaemia may develop with consequent renal damage.

Diagnosis. Non-caseating epithelioid-cell granulomas, with or without giant-cell inclusions, are not diagnostic of sarcoidosis: they occur in various conditions including tuberculosis, various fungal infections, syphilis, brucellosis and berylliosis. The diagnosis of sarcoidosis thus depends also on the clinical features, the distribution of the lesions, and on excluding the above possibilities. Sarcoid-like follicles are occasionally found incidentally in surgical and autopsy material and are of unknown significance.

Intradermal injection of a sterile suspension prepared from sarcoid lesions (**Kveim test**) leads to the development of a lesion becoming maximal in about six weeks and having the histological features of sarcoidosis. The test is positive in most cases of sarcoidosis, but conflicting results have been reported in some other conditions, notably Crohn's disease (p. 19.34). During the course of sarcoidosis the tuberculin test is negative in most cases, even in patients known to have been previously positive, and cell-mediated immunity in general is impaired in sarcoidosis. A fall in circulating T lymphocytes and a depressed response of T cells to PHA and other mitogens (p. 7.36) have also been reported. The capacity to produce antibodies however, is normal or even increased.

Aetiology. The significance of these immunological features is obscure. The sarcoid lesion, consisting of epithelioid cells and lymphocytes, is itself suggestive of a delayed hypersensitivity reaction, although no specific exogenous agent has been shown to be involved.

Subsequent development of tuberculosis has been observed in some patients, but sarcoidosis seems unlikely to be a modified form of tuberculosis, because depression of delayed hypersensitivity (as in sarcoidosis) would be expected to be associated with a florid form of tuberculosis with large numbers of *Myco. tuberculosis* in the lesions. Also, the condition is not aggravated, and is sometimes improved, by administration of steroids (c.f. tuberculosis). Various other aetiological factors have been suggested, but with little good supporting evidence.

Syphilis

Historical note

It is generally believed that syphilis was introduced into Europe on the return of the Spanish sailors of Columbus from America or the West Indies and that by the end of 1494 it had spread throughout Spain and along the Mediterranean coast into Italy. Within a century it had become widespread throughout Europe, having been carried everywhere by the mercenary troops returning to their own countries after the Siege of Naples (1495). At this time syphilis was clearly recognised as a new disease and its manifestations became so well known that Shakespeare was able to give a remarkably accurate (although anachronistic) account of them in *Timon of Athens* (Act IV, Scene 3). Absence of syphilis from the Old World is supported by the complete lack of evidence of the disease in skeletal remains dating back from 1494, whereas bones found in ancient tombs in Central America bear clear indications of the disease. The name comes from a poem composed in 1530 by Girolamo Frascatoro, a Verona physician, in which Syphilis, a swineherd, offended Apollo, who inflicted him with the disease.

General features

Formerly common, syphilis is now relatively infrequent in Western Europe: recent reports show some increase, particularly among homosexuals, but the rise is much less than for gonorrhoea. Syphilis is a **venereal disease**, i.e. it is usually contracted by coitus and the primary lesion then develops on the external genitals. Rarely, extragenital infection occurs on the lip, tongue or breast and also on the fingers from handling infective lesions. The causal agent is a small motile spiral micro-organism or spirochaete, *Treponema pallidum*, which is not stained by routine techniques, but may be detected by dark-ground illumination, immuno-fluorescence techniques, or in fixed tissue sections by silver impregnation techniques. It dies rapidly on drying and even if kept moist does not survive for long outside the body. Accordingly, infection is usually by direct contact. The organism appears capable of penetrating the intact skin or mucosa, although it is possible that minute abrasions facilitate invasion. The *primary lesion* develops in the skin or a mucous membrane at the site of infection, 2–12 (usually 3–4) weeks after infection, and heals in 2–4 weeks. In some, but by no means all cases, this is followed by the *secondary stage* in which multiple lesions develop in the skin and in most of the internal organs and tissues. The secondary lesions also heal in 2–4 weeks. In about 15% of cases, a *tertiary stage* develops after a *latent period* of 2–40 (average 10–15 years). This consists of one or more large lesions which may affect almost any tissue. Finally, in a small percentage of cases, *neurosyphilis* develops in the brain and/or the spinal cord. The infection can usually be arrested at any stage by adequate treatment with penicillin, although elimination of infection of the nervous system requires prolonged high dosage, and follow-up of treated patients is advisable.

Tr. pallidum has not yet been grown in culture. Inoculation of rabbits results in a primary and occasionally secondary lesions, and suspensions of *Tr. pallidum* can be prepared from infected rabbit testis. The organism synthesises acid mucopolysaccharide which forms its outer coat, and also produces a mucopolysaccharidase which may be associated with its attachment to host cells. It attaches by its distal end to cells in suspension: such attachment prolongs the survival of *Tr. pallidum*, but it does not appear to be of decisive pathogenic significance, for it occurs with the cells of many animal species which are resistant to infection.

It is convenient to give a general survey of the course of the untreated disease at this point. The special features of the individual lesions will be considered in the appropriate systematic chapters.

'Stages' of syphilis

The primary sore. The primary sore or **hard chancre** (Fig. 9.26) appears usually on the external genitals as a small, slowly growing, hard, pale brownish-red, usually painless nodule of about 1 cm diameter. The centre ulcerates and there may be some exudate which, in a skin lesion, is usually scanty and forms a crust. When the lesion is on a mucous surface and the part is not kept clean, there may be more ex-

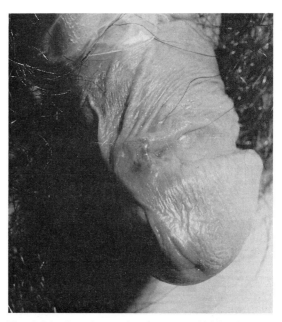

Fig. 9.26   An ulcerated primary syphilitic chancre involving the prepuce and frenulum of the penis.

tensive ulceration, and various organisms, sometimes including other spirochaetes, are present in addition to *Tr. pallidum*. The ulcer persists for some weeks, during which the inguinal lymph nodes, usually on both sides, become somewhat enlarged and hard. *Treponema pallidum* is usually detectable in the exudate of the ulcerated chancre, either by dark-ground microscopy or by use of fluorescein-labelled antibody: if this fails, it is usually demonstrable in fluid withdrawn by aspiration of the enlarged lymph nodes. *Dissemination by the blood takes place almost immediately after infection, long before the appearance of the primary lesion*, and syphilis has been accidentally transmitted by transfusion of blood withdrawn before the primary lesion had appeared in the donor.

The primary chancre subsides spontaneously after a few weeks, leaving a slight scar. In a significant proportion of cases, it does not develop or passes unnoticed.

Secondary lesions appear at a variable interval, usually 2–3 months after infection; they include multiple symmetrical lesions of the skin and squamous mucous membranes. The skin rash is macular or papular, but may become pustular, probably as a result of secondary bacterial infection. The palms of the hands and soles of the feet are commonly involved. Lesions of the hair follicles in the scalp lead to loss of the hair—*alopecia*. In the vulva, anus and perineum, flat raised papules sometimes develop—*condylomata lata*—and are intensely infective: they must not be confused with *condylomata acuminata*, the so-called venereal warts, which are of viral nature. The pharyngeal and buccal mucosa shows white, shining patches caused by thickening of the keratinised layer, and these break down, giving 'snail-track ulcers'. General slight enlargement of lymph nodes is also common and is most easily detected in the superficial nodes. Secondary lesions develop also in most of the internal organs and are usually accompanied by fever, anaemia and general malaise. After some weeks, all these features disappear spontaneously and the disease may subside permanently, or become latent and later cause tertiary lesions.

Tertiary lesions appear irregularly, especially in the internal organs, skin and mucous membranes; they are few in number but usually much larger than the primary and secondary lesions, and may lead to serious and permanent damage. They rarely appear in less than 2–3 years of onset, and sometimes only after many years. Tertiary lesions are characterised by extensive chronic inflammation with formation of granulation tissue and often with central necrosis. If necrosis is present, the lesion is termed a **gumma**. The central necrotic portion is dull yellowish, firm and rubbery and is surrounded by a more translucent zone of young connective tissue which has often a very irregular outline (Fig. 25.8, p. 25.12). Tertiary lesions occur most often in the aorta, liver, testes and bones. They cause extensive destruction, e.g. in the nasal bones with loss of the bridge of the nose and perforation of the palate, ulceration and destruction of the larynx, creeping ulcers in the skin and dilatation and sometimes rupture of the aorta. All tertiary lesions tend to heal eventually, but much distortion of the organs and interference with function may result from extensive scarring.

Neurosyphilis. Lastly, in a small proportion of cases there occur two important nervous diseases, *tabes dorsalis* and *general paralysis*.

The special features of syphilitic lesions of particular organs are described in the appropriate chapters.

Microscopic appearances

A conspicuous microscopic feature of the lesions of syphilis is accumulation of lymphocytes, plasma cells and occasional macrophages. These cells accumulate particularly around the small blood vessels, where the spirochaetes are most numerous. The vascular endothelial cells are enlarged and prominent and may proliferate, causing a reduction of the lumen. **Endarteritis** and **periarteritis** are thus important features of syphilis. Another feature is the accumulation of mucopolysaccharide material in the interstitial tissue, but this is demonstrable only by appropriate staining techniques.

In the **primary sore**, these changes occur in the dermis or submucosal connective tissue at the site of infection (Fig. 9.27). The involvement of small vessels is best seen at the periphery of the lesion. More centrally, the tissue is uniformly and heavily infiltrated with mononuclear cells, which together with mucopolysaccharide-rich oedema fluid, account for the

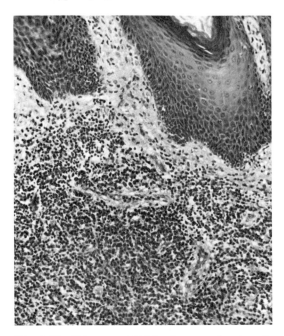

Fig. 9.27 Primary syphilitic chancre, showing the heavy cellular infiltration of the dermis. Most of the infiltrating cells (not readily identified at this magnification) are lymphocytes and plasma cells. × 120.

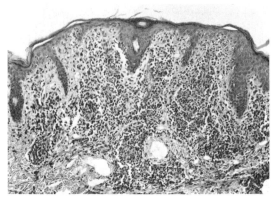

Fig. 9.28 Papular syphilitic rash, showing abundant cellular infiltration of the corium. × 115.

tion or fibrosis, often spreading extensively, and sometimes containing foci of gummatous necrosis. In the necrotic tissue, the structural outlines may be preserved for a long time, the cells not having the same tendency to fuse into amorphous material as is seen in tuberculous caseation. Multinucleated giant cells derived from macrophages may be present in the granulation tissue at the periphery, but they are usually smaller than in tuberculosis, and there are no well-formed epithelioid-cell follicles. Nevertheless, histological distinction between the two diseases is sometimes difficult. The important vascular lesions include **syphilitic mes-**

hardness of the lesion (p. 9.28). Later, ulceration occurs with exudative inflammation and formation of granulation tissue. *The histological features are not diagnostic without the demonstration of Tr. pallidum*, which requires special staining techniques. After a time, the cellular infiltration gradually diminishes and only a little thickening of the fibrous stroma remains. There is usually little or no residual scarring unless there has been much ulceration.

In the **secondary lesions** in the skin and mucous membranes the main changes are vascular engorgement and cell infiltration (Fig. 9.28), mainly of plasma cells, lymphocytes and macrophages. Cellular infiltration occurs also around and into the hair follicles, and the hairs may fall out. The disseminated lesions of the secondary stage usually heal without much scarring.

The **gumma** of the **tertiary stage** consists of parenchymal necrosis, surrounded by a layer of granulation and fibrous tissue showing the usual infiltration with mononuclear cells (Fig. 9.29). Eventual healing is accompanied by shrinkage, considerable scarring and distortion. Another common type of lesion is inflamma-

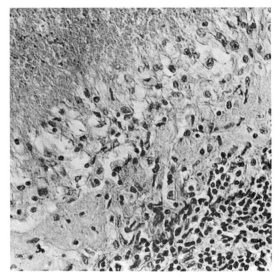

Fig. 9.29 Section of part of a gumma, showing the necrotic centre (*upper left*), bounded by connective tissue heavily infiltrated with lymphocytes. × 250.

aortitis, in which periarteritis and endarteritis of the vasa vasorum result in ischaemic damage to the media. The changes are described on p. 14.22. Involvement of cerebral vessels in syphilitic leptomeningitis (p. 21.28) results in infarction of the superficial neural tissue.

A non-venereal form, termed *endemic syphilis*, occurs in children in parts of Africa and India, and a similar condition, *bejel*, affects young children in Arab countries.

Congenital syphilis

Congenital syphilis is acquired by transplacental infection and its severity depends mainly on the duration of maternal infection. In the primary and secondary stages, the fetus becomes heavily infected and usually dies *in utero*, with premature birth of a macerated fetus. The parenchymatous organs contain very large numbers of spirochaetes and show diffuse proliferation of fibroblasts with minute foci of necrosis—miliary gummas—and there is severe damage to the liver, lungs, pancreas, etc. In subsequent pregnancies the effects are progressively less severe. If pregnancy occurs following the secondary stage, the child may be born alive with lesions of congenital syphilis, including a papular rash around mouth and nose, on the buttocks, palms of hands and soles of feet. Disease of the nasal bones and mucosa leads to 'snuffles' and interference with feeding. Syphilitic hepatitis with jaundice, splenomegaly, and lesions in the bones are also common. Later, a characteristic deformity appears in the incisor teeth, which are peg-shaped with notched edges (Hutchinson's teeth) and there is also pitting of the first permanent molars. Still later, neurosyphilis may develop and also intestial keratitis causing corneal opacity and blindness. The longer the interval between secondary syphilis and pregnancy, the more likely is the child to appear healthy at birth and to develop syphilitic lesions later, during childhood or adolescence.

Routine serological testing for syphilis in early pregnancy followed by effective treatment has greatly reduced the incidence of congenital syphilis in many countries.

Serological tests for syphilis

At least three distinct antibodies develop in syphilis, and their detection in the serum is of considerable diagnostic value. The older tests are based on the detection of antibody reactive with the diphosphatidylglycerol component of phospholipids of mitochondrial membranes. This antigen was first detected in the liver of congenital syphilitics, but is present in most normal mammalian, including human, tissues. It is thus an auto-antigen, but the antibody may develop in response to similar antigenic material in the cell membrane of *Treponema pallidum*. Alcoholic extract of beef heart muscle ('*cardiolipin*') is now used as antigen, but extracts of various mammalian tissues may also be used. Antibody is demonstrable by various precipitation (flocculation) techniques, e.g. the Kahn, Kline or VDRL (Venereal Disease Research Laboratory) tests, or by the Wassermann test which is based on complement fixation (p. 6.12). These are the so-called **standard tests for syphilis**: they are useful screening tests, antibody being detectable from an early stage, but are not specific for syphilis, **false positive reactions** occurring in various conditions, including many acute infections (e.g. malaria, infectious mononucleosis, mycoplasmal pneumonia) and in trypanosomiasis, leprosy and systemic lupus erythematosus. The tests are also positive occasionally in apparently normal individuals, particularly during pregnancy. Such false positive reactions may result from auto-immunisation as a result of tissue destruction from causes other than syphilis, with release of cellular constituents.

A second antibody, which reacts with group antigen common to various species of treponemes, may be detected by a complement-fixation test, using as antigen non-pathogenic treponemes which grow readily in culture; this is also used as a screening test but is not specific for syphilis.

Confirmatory tests for syphilis depend on the demonstration of antibody specific for *Tr. pallidum* by (a) the treponemal immobilisation test, in which the patient's heat-inactivated serum, together with guinea-pig serum as a source of complement, is added to a suspension of living *Tr. pallidum* obtained from infected rabbit testis: antibody is indicated by immobilisation of the treponemes, or (b) the fluorescent antibody technique in which binding of antibody to *Tr. pallidum* is demonstrated by means of fluorescein-labelled anti-immunoglobulin (p. 6.11). The immobilisation test is time-consuming and not now widely used. Antibody detected by these tests is distinct from anti-cardiolipin, which does not react with intact spirochetes.

Antibody tests usually become positive a week or so after the appearance of the primary lesion: they are virtually always positive in the secondary stage, following which the percentage of positives gradually falls. In neurosyphilis, antibody is more likely to be detected in the cerebrospinal fluid than in the serum.

Following cure, the antibody tests become negative, although the specific treponemal antibodies may persist for some years.

The pathogenesis of syphilitic lesions

The primary and secondary lesions of syphilis occur at sites of local proliferation of *Tr. pallidum*. The organism has not been shown to produce toxins and survives in macrophages in culture for several days without causing cytopathic changes. The early appearance of lymphocytes and plasma cells in the primary lesion is indicative of an immune response, but challenge of infected rabbits by inoculation of *Tr. pallidum* shows that solid resistance to re-infection takes about 12 weeks to develop. The immune response thus starts early, but resistance to re-infection builds up slowly. There is also evidence that resistance to re-infection develops slowly in man. Both humoral and cell-mediated immunity develop, but their respective importance in destroying the spirochaetes in the primary and secondary infections is not known. Nor is it understood why, following elimination of the primary infection, the spirochaete persists and sometimes proliferates in multiple foci to produce secondary lesions. A change in the surface antigenicity of the spirochaete, as in relapsing fever caused by *Borrelia*, would explain this, but so far no such change has been demonstrated. The long period of latency followed in some cases by the development of tertiary lesions is equally difficult to explain. Unlike the earlier lesions, the number of spirochaetes in tertiary lesions is small, and the histological appearances are suggestive of a delayed hypersensitivity reaction which, together with endarteritis and periarteritis, may account for the gummatous necrosis.

As noted earlier, *Treponema pallidum* synthesises an outer coat of acid mucopolysac-charide, which is continuously shed; in the secondary stage, this material can be detected in the plasma where, by combining with antibody, it may be the cause of the immune-complex glomerulonephritis observed in some patients. By diverting antibody, it may also interfere with antibody-mediated destruction of spirochaetes.

There are clearly many unsolved problems relating to syphilis and it may be that the success of penicillin therapy has discouraged further investigation of the disease.

Other treponemal diseases

Two other diseases caused by treponemes occur in tropical countries. One is **yaws**, which occurs in parts of Africa, India and South America. It resembles syphilis but is non-venereal and rarely causes cardiovascular or neurological disease. The causal agent, *Tr. pertenuae*, cannot be distinguished from *Tr. pallidum* and infection with either confers immunity to both: the distinction from syphilis is based on clinical features. The second condition is **pinta**, another non-venereal chronic disease of Central and South America somewhat resembling syphilis: it is caused by *Tr. carateum* which does not induce immunity to syphilis.

Other pathogenic spirochaetes

These include the **Borreliae,** which are transmitted by lice and ticks, and cause **relapsing fever** (p. 20.38) and the **Leptospirae** which infest rodents, etc., and cause febrile illnesses in man, the best known being Weil's disease (p. 20.37).

Actinomycosis

This disease is produced by organisms which are normal commensals in the mouth and gut and only occasionally invade the tissues to produce infection. The actinomyces are branching bacteria which grow in the tissues to produce characteristic radiate colonies, sometimes visible macroscopically. In man, the micro-aerophilic *Actinomyces israeli* is the chief pathogen, but occasionally aerobic organisms—*Nocardia*—are involved (p. 16.49), and also other genera, which grow more diffusely. In bovines, in which actinomycosis due to *Actinomyces bovis* is common, the lesions are localised and are large granulomatous masses which occur especially in and around the jaw. In man, the disease usually affects children and young adults, more often males than females, and agricultural workers appear to be particularly at risk. The lesions are of a more suppurative type, and in about 60% of cases are in the region of the mouth or jaws, the parasite gaining entrance commonly from a tooth socket following extraction or from a carious tooth. In 15% the infection is in the appendix or caecal region, from which spread by the blood stream to the liver may occur; in about 20% the initial lesion is in the lung and in 5% it is subcutaneous. The lesion is usually a chronic suppurative one, with formation of multiple abscesses, each containing one or more colonies of the organism—the so-called honeycomb abscesses. Fibrous septa between the abscesses are lined by granulation tissue which contains many foamy cells—macrophages laden with lipid—giving the lining of each abscess a yellowish colour. In the centre is pus containing actinomyces colonies (Fig. 9.30), which are sometimes visible by naked eye as small yellow or grey, gritty granules ('sulphur granules'). Lesions of the face and neck, originating about the jaw, may produce much granulation tissue in which many small foci of suppuration persist and discharge through the skin, resulting in multiple sinuses. The infection

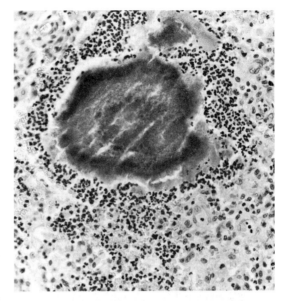

Fig. 9.30 Actinomycosis. A colony of *Actinomyces israeli* in a small abscess, the wall of which consists of granulation tissue heavily infiltrated with lipid-laden (foamy) macrophages. × 190.

spreads directly through the tissues but does not usually involve the regional lymph nodes; if untreated, it tends to invade the bloodstream, giving rise to pyaemia with secondary abscesses in the liver, lungs and other organs. Bacteria of the genus *Actinomycetes* are also responsible for some cases of mycetoma (p. 9.37).

Other Types of Infection

Rickettsial infections

The rickettsiae are micro-organisms of various shapes, smaller than bacteria but resembling them in their structural and metabolic features, including formation of a cell wall. They are obligatory intracellular parasites and infect many species including arthropods, birds and mammals. Several species of rickettsiae cause disease in man: in most instances they enter the body by the bites of infected ticks or mites, or from infected louse or flea faeces being scratched into the skin. The organisms enter and multiply in the endothelium of the capillaries and other small blood vessels; they are at first localised to the site of infection, but blood dissemination occurs during the incubation period and endothelial involvement then becomes widespread. Capillary obstruction occurs from endothelial swelling or thrombosis, with resultant necrosis in heavily involved tissues, and a mixed cell reaction develops, including polymorphs, macrophages, lymphocytes and plasma cells.

The rickettsial diseases include **endemic (murine) typhus**, caused by *R. mooseri* and transmitted by the rat flea; **epidemic typhus** (*R. prowazeki*) and **trench fever** (*R. quintana*) which are spread by the body louse: the **spotted fever** group (*R. rickettsi*, etc.) transmitted from various animals to man by the bites of infected ticks or mites, and finally **scrub typhus** (*R.*

tsutsugamuchi), transmitted from rodents to man by a mite. Epidemic and endemic typhus are of worldwide distribution: the epidemic disease occurs in crowded louse-infested communities, and is common in times of war, earthquakes and other major disasters. Man is the only known reservoir of infection of *R. prowazeki*, which can persist for years as a latent infection and cause relapse ('*recrudescent typhus*' or *Brill–Zinsser disease*): such cases are responsible for fresh outbreaks.

Various forms of spotted fever are related to particular localities.

The rickettsial diseases vary in their severity and pathological detail: in all, the small blood vessels are involved, and lesions tend to result especially in the brain, heart and skin. Infected material is particularly dangerous to laboratory workers, and diagnosis is usually made by demonstrating a rising titre of antibody, either in the patient or in laboratory animals inoculated with the patient's blood, etc. Only *R. quintana* has been cultured successfully in cell-free media.

Q fever is a typhus-like illness caused by the *Coxiella burneti* which closely resembles the rickettsiae but differs from them in its antigenicity and in being much more resistant to drying, etc. and in being capable of both intracellular and extracellular growth. It is a parasite of domesticated animals of worldwide distribution and man is infected by inhalation of droplets while attending to animal births or by drinking infected milk, etc. Q fever usually presents as a 'non-bacterial' pneumonia, although lesions may occur in the brain and other organs. *Cox. burneti* may also colonise the valves of the heart, producing a form of infective endocarditis.

Diagnosis is usually based on a rising titre of antibody, but demonstration of *Cox. burneti* in the blood by guinea-pig inoculation is sometimes necessary.

Mycoplasmal infections

Mycoplasmas are very small filamentous or coccobacillary micro-organisms which lack a cell wall but can be grown in cell-free media and are classed as bacteria. They are distributed widely and are pathogenic to many animal and plant species. In man only one species, *Mycoplasma pneumoniae*, has been shown conclusively to be pathogenic, although other mycoplasmas have been isolated from the lesions of various other diseases. A major difficulty arises from their ubiquity and the consequent contamination of culture media; they can pass through bacteria-retaining filters and are also liable to contaminate cell cultures used in virology and for other purposes.

Mycoplasma pneumoniae is the cause of one form of 'non-bacterial' pneumonia, which is endemic in most parts of the world and also occurs as outbreaks, particularly in children. The organism disseminates in the body and may cause a meningo-encephalitis. The immune response includes the production of an antibody which cross reacts at low temperatures with a human red cell antigen, and is responsible in some cases for acute haemolysis.

Chlamydial infections

The chlamydiae are a group of spherical micro-organisms intermediate in size between the larger viruses and bacteria. They are obligatory intracellular parasites, but otherwise resemble bacteria far more closely than viruses. The vegetative form multiplies by binary fission, and infection is spread by a smaller compact spore-like form (elementary body) which can survive, but not divide, extracellularly.

These organisms are enzootic in certain birds, including the psittacines (parrot family), and infect also sheep, goats and cattle. In man, they are responsible for sexually transmitted **urethritis** and **lymphogranuloma venereum**, for eye infections, the most important being **trachoma**, and pulmonary infection (**ornithosis**) which results from inhalation of the organism. The initial reaction to chlamydial infection is granulomatous, with accumulation of macrophages and lymphoid cells, necrosis, formation of granulation tissue and scarring. In lymphogranuloma venereum, a small ulcerating primary lesion develops in the genitalia, but the draining lymph nodes become grossly involved and prolonged suppuration and extensive scarring result. Similar lesions occur extragenitally in cat-scratch disease, but the nature of the causal agent is uncertain.

Both antibodies and cell-mediated immunity develop in chlamydial infections, the latter probably being the more important in the elimination of the infection. These diseases are considered more fully in the appropriate systematic chapters.

Fungal infections (Mycoses)

Fungi are primitive eukaryotic micro-organisms which are now usually classified as neither plant nor animal. They are mainly saprophytic and make an important contribution to the breakdown of dead animal and plant tissues. Only a few of the many known species are pathogenic to man, and most cause superficial, mild lesions.

Morphologically, most pathogenic fungi are dimorphic: that is, they may assume a *yeast-like* form (single rounded cells which multiply by budding) or a *hyphal* form (branching filaments that interlace to make a mycelium or mould, and produce spores). The form assumed depends on the environs of the fungus. In human tissues, the pathogenic species are usually either yeasts or hyphae, and this aids their histological distinction.

All fungal infections are environmental in origin, though some species are normally benign commensals, such as *Candida albicans* which is acquired at the time of birth. Broadly speaking, fungal diseases are classified into four groups, depending on the species of fungus and the parts of the body affected.

1. **Superficial mycosis**, e.g. *tinea nigra*. The fungus infiltrates the cornified layers of the skin, evinces little or no host reaction, and causes only a change in pigmentation or hair growth.

2. **Cutaneous mycosis**, e.g. *ringworm* and *muco-cutaneous candidiasis*. Fungus invades the epidermis, host reaction is marked and destruction of epidermis and skin appendages may be severe.

3. **Subcutaneous mycosis**, e.g. *mycetoma* and *sporotrichosis*. After inoculation by traumatic implantation from contaminated vegetation, the fungi may remain localised in the subcutis or slowly spread locally. Visceral dissemination is rare. The host reaction ranges from suppuration to epithelioid-cell granuloma formation.

4. **Systemic mycosis**, e.g. *systemic candidiasis, histoplasmosis, mucormycosis, aspergillosis* and *cryptococcosis*. These are basically respiratory diseases, inhalation of the fungus causing the primary lesion. Later, dissemination to lymph nodes, liver, bones, adrenals, etc., may occur, depending on host resistance. For example, histoplasmosis behaves analogously to tuberculosis, with a primary lung complex, healing and, in a proportion of patients, the development of chronic infection, often with caseous or ischaemic necrosis and foci of more acute, exudative reaction.

Resistance to invasive mycosis is effected mainly by cell-mediated immunity. In patients with a genetic immunodeficiency disease, or malignancy, or treated with immunosuppressive drugs, systemic infection by *Aspergillus* or by *Candida* is notably frequent.

In superficial infections, diagnosis can often be made from the clinical appearance of the lesions supported by microscopy of the skin or mucosal scrapings. For the subcutaneous and systemic infections, biopsy and culture of the tissue (and sometimes blood culture) are necessary. Histologically, some fungal infections appear similar and only culture can distinguish the species involved.

Some examples of fungal infection are described briefly below.

Candidiasis (Moniliasis)

Candida albicans is normally present in the mouth and intestines and on the surface of moist skin. Defective host defence permits the fungus to invade superficially or deeply: inherited immunodeficiency states, agranulocytosis, leukaemias, antibiotic administration, immunosuppressive therapy, diabetes mellitus and pregnancy are examples of states that predispose to candidiasis.

In **muco-cutaneous candidiasis**, the oral or vaginal mucosa is involved, with formation of white plaques (**thrush**) at sites of fungal growth. Pathologically, there is a characteristic combination of budding yeasts and hyphae in the epithelium with a polymorph and lymphocytic reaction beneath. During pregnancy, the lowered vaginal pH promotes the growth of the fungus, sometimes causing a vaginitis. At autopsy of patients dying of leukaemia, thick plaques of oesophageal candidiasis are frequently seen.

Cutaneous candidiasis is a destructive condition which may involve the entire skin surface, nails and mucous membranes. The fungus proliferates in the epithelium, which becomes hyperplastic and hyperkeratotic, and a chronic granulomatous inflammation is seen in the underlying tissues.

Severe immunodeficiency states can lead to **systemic candidiasis**. Blood culture may be positive and the heart valves, lungs and kidneys are commonly affected. In the kidney, there are multiple small abscesses resembling those seen in pyaemia and containing proliferating fungus in hyphal and yeast forms.

Aspergillosis

Spores of *Aspergillus* are ubiquitous in the atmosphere and many species infect man, although by far the commonest is *Aspergillus fumigatus*.

The spores are inhaled, and most people are resistant, but some with apparently normal immune responsiveness develop infection of the nasal sinuses characterised by granulomatous masses in which the branching hyphae of *Aspergillus* are seen microscopically.

The fungus causes four different types of pulmonary disease (p. 16.50): inhalation of spores may result in *bronchial asthma* from type 1 (atopic) hypersensitivity or *acute allergic alveolitis* from type 3 (immune-complex) hypersensitivity. The fungus can colonise old tuberculous or bronchiectatic cavities, in which it may form a large colony ('*mycetoma*'), or it may actually invade the lung tissue to produce a haemorrhagic and necrotising *pneumonia*. This last condition tends to occur in immunodeficient or immunosuppressed individuals, in whom the fungus may also invade the walls of the pulmonary veins, causing local thrombosis, and become disseminated by the bloodstream: infection of the heart valves may result in large vegetations. Invasion of the intestinal veins may also occur with consequent infarction.

Poisoning by aflatoxin, the mycotoxin of *Aspergillus flavus*, is fairly common in many developing countries where peanuts or maize, etc. is stored under unsatisfactory conditions. The fungus contaminates food and forms the toxin, which, if ingested in high concentrations, can cause fatal hepatic necrosis. Chronic ingestion of aflatoxin has been postulated to play a causal role in kwashiorkor and primary hepatocellular carcinoma (p. 13.20).

Histoplasmosis

Histoplasma capsulatum causes the commoner form of histoplasmosis and has a global distribution with particularly high prevalence in the southern USA. *Histoplasma duboisi* is restricted to Africa.

Histoplasmosis capsulati is primarily a pulmonary disease. The fungal spores are present in the soil and in the faeces of chickens and bats, and infection results from their inhalation. About 95% of infections are asymptomatic: as in tuberculosis, the primary lesion is a focal pulmonary granuloma that heals with fibrosis and calcification; the skin test (with histoplasmin) becomes positive. This test for cell-mediated immunity is positive in a high proportion of inhabitants of endemic areas.

A small proportion of infected people develop an acute symptomatic pneumonia or a chronic cavitating pulmonary disease—again similar to tuberculosis. Disseminated histoplasmosis, with a high mortality, is seen in the elderly and in those with defective immunity. The lymphoreticular system, bones and adrenals are involved, causing enlargement of the liver, spleen and lymph nodes. The adrenals may be destroyed by the process and histoplasmosis is a recognised cause of Addison's disease.

Microscopically, yeast-like bodies of 2–5 μm diameter are seen in macrophages (Fig. 9.31) and there are usually epithelioid-cell granulomas with or without caseation.

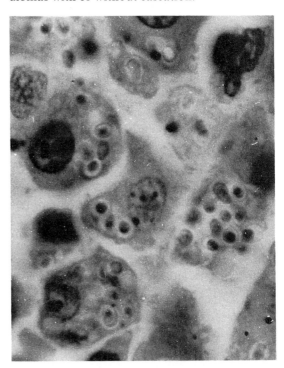

Fig. 9.31 Histoplasmosis. From the adrenals in a fatal case of disseminated histoplasmosis. The macrophages contain numerous small yeast-like cells of *Histoplasma capsulatum*. × 1500.

African histoplasmosis (*H. duboisi*) has larger fungal cells, again seen inside macrophages. The pulmonary phase of the infection is not commonly detected, and the disease usually presents clinically as skin nodules and lymphadenopathy.

Cryptococcosis

Cryptococcus neoformans is a ubiquitous fungus, most abundant in pigeon droppings. It is a yeast cell with a thick mucoid capsule. When inhaled, it can cause a diffuse or focal lung lesion. The diffuse (hypo-reactive) form is a mucoid pneumonia that grossly may be mistaken for a *Klebsiella* pneumonia or a bronchiolar cell carcinoma. It occurs particularly in immunodeficient patients. The focal lesion is often an incidental finding, seen on chest x-ray as a 'coin lesion'. The host reaction to cryptococci ranges from virtually nil to a necrotising granulomatous pneumonia. The mucoid nature of the lesion derives from the capsule of the fungus.

Occasionally the fungus disseminates by the blood to other organs, including bones, lymph nodes and particularly to the meninges where it causes a gelatinous meningitis with a variable slight or granulomatous reaction in which the budding cryptococci are seen. This form of the disease is also usually a complication of immunodeficiency.

Sporotrichosis

Infection by *Sporothrix schencki* is usually acquired from accidental inoculation into the skin, e.g. from the prick of a thorn. The organism lives in the soil and on plants. The initial lesion, usually in a limb, is a chronic subcutaneous nodule which ulcerates and discharges pus. The infection tends to ascend the limb via the lymphatics, producing a linear series of secondary nodules. Histologically, these deep dermal lesions are granulomas with central abscess formation and surrounding fibrosis. The fungal yeast cells are surprisingly sparse in the granulomas, and are often surrounded by eosinophil leucocytes—a Hoeppli reaction—which is atopic in nature. Systemic spread is rare.

Mycetoma (Maduramycosis)

This is a chronic suppurating infection of the subcutaneous tissues following traumatic implantation of a causative agent. The condition usually affects the limbs and results in gross swelling, fistulous tracks to the skin, and eventually invasion and destruction of bone. The causal agents of mycetoma can be either fungi (of which more than a dozen species are known, including *Madurella mycetomatis*) or members of the bacterial group *Actinomycetes*. These latter include *Actinomadura*, *Nocardia* and *Streptomyces* species. The aetiological distinction is important since drugs are effective in actinomycetomas but not in fungal mycetomas.

The lesions are similar to those of actinomycosis (p. 9.32). They consist of multiple intercommunicating abscesses and sinuses lined by granulomatous tissue heavily infiltrated with macrophages. They occur in the soft tissues and bones, usually of the foot and leg. The condition is chronic and massive subcutaneous fibrosis results. Grain-like colonies of the causal agent, visible to the naked eye, are present in the abscesses and in pus discharged from the sinuses. The hyphae of fungal colonies are often embedded in cement-like material which impedes the entry of antifungal drugs.

Mucormycosis

This is caused by *Rhizopus oryzae* (ex-*Mucor*), one of the zygomycete fungi which have characteristically wide, branching hyphae up to 25 μm across. Virtually all victims of mucormycosis are patients with uncontrolled diabetes mellitus in a state of keto-acidosis. The primary site of infection is the nasal turbinates, and the clinical features involve necrotising sinusitis, inflammation of the orbit with proptosis, and meningo-encephalitis. This last feature results from invasion of the fungus through the cribriform plate.

Rhizopus induces a florid acute inflammatory reaction and causes extensive necrosis. Further tissue damage results from its propensity to invade blood vessel walls with consequent thrombosis. Cavernous sinus thrombosis and pituitary infarction are commonly seen in fatal cases. Mucormycosis is the most fulminant of all mycoses, death usually occurring within a few days of diagnosis.

Further Reading

Christie, A.B. (1980). *Infectious Diseases: Epidemiology and Clinical Practice*, 3rd edn., pp. 1033. Churchill Livingstone, Edinburgh, etc. (A highly readable text, dealing with all aspects of infectious disease).

Chandler, F.W., Kaplan, W. and Ajello, J. (1980). *A Colour Atlas and Textbook of Histopathology of Mycotic Diseases*, pp. 336. Wolfe Medical, London.

Collee, J.G. (1981). *Applied Medical Microbiology* (Vol. 3 of *Basic Microbiology*), pp. 158. Blackwell Scientific, Oxford. (A short text for students.)

Davis, B.D., Dulbecco, R., Eisen, H.N., Guinsberg, H.S. and Wood, W.B. (1980). *Principles of Microbiology and Immunology*, 3rd edn., pp. 1584. Harper and Rowe, New York. (A comprehensive, well-written text.)

Duguid, J.P., Marmion, B.P. and Swain, R.H.A. (1978). *Medical Microbiology, Vol. 1*, 13th edn., pp. 666. Churchill Livingstone. Edinburgh. (A book for undergraduate and postgraduate students.)

Freeman, Bob A. (Ed.) (1982). *Burrow's Textbook of Microbiology*, 22nd edn. Saunders, Philadelphia, London and Toronto. (A multi-author text with a major contribution by the editor. Readable and well-illustrated.)

Jopling, W.H. (1984). *Handbook of Leprosy*, 3rd edn., pp. 160. Heinemann Medical, London.

Sleigh, J.D. and Timbury, M.C. (1981). *Notes on Medical Bacteriology*, pp. 354. (Churchill Livingstone, Edinburgh, etc. (A text for students and junior postgraduate trainees.)

Timbury, M.C. (1983). *Notes on Medical Virology*, 7th edn., pp. 155. Churchill Livingstone, Edinburgh, London and New York. (A short text for students.)

Tyrrell, David, A.J., Phillips, Ian, Goodwin, Stewart C. and Blowers, Robert (1979). *Microbial Disease: the use of the Laboratory in diagnosis, therapy and control*, pp. 340. Edward Arnold, London. (A clearly-written book which relates clinical problems with laboratory practice.)

Wilson, G.S. and Miles, A.A. (Eds.) (1984). Topley and Wilson's Principles and Practice of Bacteriology, Virology and Immunity, 7th edn. Edward Arnold, London. (A comprehensive text for practising bacteriologists.)

10

Disturbances of Blood Flow and Body Fluids

Disturbances of the flow of blood are intimately associated with lesions which affect the functioning of the heart and blood vessels: such lesions will be considered systematically in later chapters. Meanwhile it is useful to outline the main features of disturbances in total and local blood flow, the processes of thrombosis and clotting of the blood, and the disturbances in composition and volume of the body fluids. Accordingly, this chapter provides a general account of these phenomena.

Changes in Flow and Distribution of the Blood

Increase in total blood flow

This occurs when a sufficient number of arterioles relax to result in significant increase in the rate of passage of blood from the arterial to the venous compartment of the circulation. Physiological examples include the active hyperaemia in the skeletal muscles during physical activity and in the splanchnic circulation during digestion of a heavy meal. Pathological conditions causing an increase in total blood flow include the following.

(a) Hypoxia, which consists of a significant fall in the amount of oxygen delivered to the tissues. This occurs in anaemia, i.e. a reduction in the amount of haemoglobin in the blood. Cardiac output increases in severe anaemia, but not enough to compensate for the reduced oxygen-carrying capacity of the blood, and the tissues suffer from **anaemic hypoxia**.

Hypoxia occurs also when, as a result of abnormalities of pulmonary function, the arterial blood is not fully oxygenated (**hypoxaemic hypoxia**). In lesions which interfere with pulmonary ventilation, the situation is complicated by increased P_{CO_2} of the blood, which, together with lowered P_{O_2}, is termed **asphyxia**. Congenital abnormalities of the heart or great vessels which result in mixing of venous and arterial blood can also cause hypoxaemic hypoxia.

Increased cardiac output is a feature of these various conditions, but it does not, of course, occur when **ischaemic hypoxia** results from heart failure: this is due to failure of the heart to maintain an adequate circulation.

(b) Increased metabolic activity. The general body metabolism is increased in hyperthyroidism (thyrotoxicosis), in fever, and in convalescence from severe injury. The increased metabolism in these conditions is associated with an increased total blood flow.

(c) Arterio-venous shunts. A single large communication (fistula) between an artery and vein, such as sometimes results from trauma, allows the transfer of part of the cardiac output to the venous side of the circulation, and so reduces the amount of arterial blood available for tissue perfusion.

(d) Extensive active hyperaemia. In generalised inflammatory conditions of the skin, the active hyperaemia is sufficiently extensive to cause a significant increase in total blood flow. Similarly, a chronic increase in total blood flow occurs in extensive Paget's disease affecting several large bones. In this condition, the marrow cavity of the affected bones is replaced by vascular granulation tissue, with local increase in blood flow: also, there is persistent reflex active hyperaemia of the overlying skin and soft tissues, and the total blood flow is consequently increased (see Singer *et al.*, 1978).

(e) Liver failure. The cause of increased blood flow in liver failure is uncertain: it may be due to the vasodilator effects of accumulated metabolites, or of compounds absorbed from the gut, which are normally removed from the blood by the liver cells.

In these various conditions, increased cardiac output is associated with a lowering of arteriolar tone: the pulse is bounding (of high amplitude) and the skin is warm and pink. The mechanism of these changes is complex and not fully understood: the autonomic nervous system, vasomotor centres, adrenal cortex and medulla, local effects of tissue metabolites, baro- and chemo-receptors, are all involved. If long continued, as in untreated hyperthyroidism, the increased work of the heart is likely to lead to *'high-output' cardiac failure*, particularly in older people and especially if the heart is already handicapped, e.g. by coronary artery disease or thyrotoxicosis.

Locally increased blood flow

The outstanding example of a pathological increase in local blood flow is **acute inflammation**, in which arteriolar dilatation results in active hyperaemia and the characteristic warmth and erythema of the inflamed tissue. Active hyperaemia occurs also **following a period of temporary obstruction of the circulation**: this is important when the local circulation is arrested to facilitate a surgical operation, e.g. on a limb, for hyperaemia develops gradually, and small vessels which do not bleed immediately after the circulation is restored may subsequently do so.

Reduction in total blood flow

This is a feature of **heart failure**, in which the heart is incapable of maintaining the normal output. The condition may occur acutely, usually as a result of myocardial infarction, or chronic heart failure may result from in-

adequate function of the myocardium, usually due to coronary artery disease or to increased workload as in valvular lesions or pulmonary or systemic arterial hypertension. Chronic heart failure is often progressive; the heart is incapable initially of supplying the increased output required during physical activity, etc., but eventually it may fail to maintain an adequate circulation even at rest.

Reduced cardiac output is also the major feature of the acute condition of **shock**, in which grossly inadequate tissue perfusion can be fatal (pp. 10.38–44).

The cardiac output is also reduced in states of **general metabolic depression**, the commonest example being hypothyroidism, but in this instance it simply reflects the reduced requirements for tissue perfusion and is not of pathogenic importance.

The serious effects of heart failure are due very largely to **defective tissue perfusion**, which impairs the functions of all the organs. There are, however, two important structural effects: one is **general venous congestion**, from which the term **congestive heart failure** is derived: it is described below. The other is an increase in extravascular fluid, giving rise to **oedema**, which is described on pp. 10.30 *et seq.*

As mentioned above, conditions in which the total blood flow is increased predispose to heart failure: when this occurs, blood flow is reduced, but it may still be above normal.

Local reduction in blood flow (local ischaemia)

This is of extreme importance because it accounts for a high proportion of cardiac and cerebral disease. Reduction of flow is usually due to **arterial narrowing by disease of the vessel wall**, or **complete obstruction by thrombosis or embolism**. These latter processes are described on pp. 10.12–22, and local ischaemia on pp. 10.23–28.

Local ischaemia can result also from **venous obstruction**, usually by thrombosis: it is accompanied by local venous congestion, and commonly by oedema, of the tissue drained by the obstructed veins.

Venous congestion

When the heart fails to expel the normal amount of blood, arteriolar tone in general is increased by sympathetic stimulation and a greater proportion of the blood accumulates in the venous compartment, which is readily distensible. This, together with an increase in blood volume (the mechanism of which is poorly understood) causes the veins to become engorged with blood. **Systemic venous congestion**, i.e. engorgement of the systemic veins, is most severe when the failure is predominantly of the right ventricle, e.g. in narrowing (stenosis) of the pulmonary valve orifice and in various diseases of the lungs which interfere with pulmonary blood flow.

Pulmonary venous congestion develops when there is a raised pressure in the left atrium, and so in the pulmonary veins. It therefore occurs in left ventricular failure, as in many cases of coronary artery disease or systemic arterial hypertension: it occurs also when mitral valve stenosis restricts the flow of blood into the left ventricle. Chronic pulmonary venous congestion is complicated by the development of pulmonary arterial hypertension (pp. 16.23–26), often leading to right ventricular failure and systemic venous congestion.

Venous congestion may also be limited to parts of the systemic circulation as a result of a local obstruction to the venous outflow. Such **localised venous congestion** is commonly seen as a result of thrombosis of the leg veins, often extending up to and involving the femoral vein. It occurs in the spleen and gastro-intestinal tract when portal venous flow is obstructed, as in cirrhosis of the liver. Various other veins may be obstructed, either by thrombosis or by pressure or constriction by a tumour or by scar tissue.

Systemic venous congestion

As explained above, this usually results from right heart failure and, depending on the nature of the heart lesion, may be acute or chronic. In both instances, the outlook depends on the reversibility or otherwise of the cardiac failure: if this persists for long, the morphological changes of chronic venous congestion are striking, but it must be emphasised that *the conges-*

tive element is less important than the inadequate tissue perfusion of heart failure.

The systemic veins can dilate to accommodate more blood without an immediate rise of venous pressure, but as the congestion increases, the pressure rises. This may be demonstrated directly by venous catheterisation, but commonly it is apparent from pulsation of the veins in the neck when the patient is sitting or standing. Normally, the neck veins in these postures are partly collapsed and do not pulsate visibly, the pressure in them being slightly below atmospheric. When venous pressure rises, however, the veins in the lower part of the neck are distended, and they pulsate at about the level where the blood is at atmospheric pressure.

Because of the reduced blood flow in heart failure, the degree of oxygen dissociation in the capillaries is greater than normal, and in vascular tissues there may be sufficient reduced haemoglobin to impart a purple-blue colour known as **cyanosis**: this is seen, for example, in the lips and buccal mucosa. When there is also systemic venous congestion, the engorgement of the venules and capillaries with sluggishly-flowing oxygen-deficient blood increases the degree of cyanosis. Severe venous congestion is usually accompanied by oedema, particularly of the lower parts of the body (gravitational oedema); chronic hypoxia and the increased venular and capillary pressure are probably both contributory factors.

Structural changes of systemic venous congestion. Apart from generalised oedema (p. 10.32), the structural changes in systemic venous congestion are most obvious in the abdominal viscera. The **liver** may be moderately enlarged and is often tender and palpable. Microscopically, the centrilobular veins* are distended and the central part of each lobule consists of distended sinusoids, the hepatocytes having undergone atrophy and disappeared (Fig. 10.1). Macroscopically, this accentuates the lobular pattern, the dark, congested centrilobular areas contrasting with the paler, sometimes fatty peripheral lobular cells (Fig. 10.2). Because of its similarity to the surface of a nutmet cut longitudinally, this appearance has long been described by pathologists as 'nutmeg liver'. In some cases, and particularly when there have been recurrent periods of congestive

---

*The relationship between the traditional liver *lobule* and the *acinus*, the newer concept of the structural unit of the liver, is described on p. 20.1

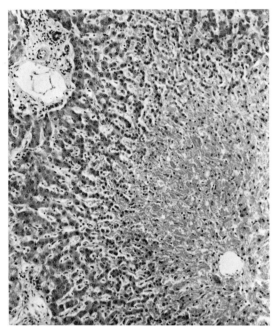

Fig. 10.1 The liver in chronic venous congestion, showing centrilobular atrophy and disappearance of liver cells accompanied by dilatation of sinusoids (rt. side of figure). × 105.

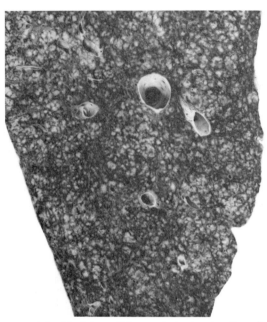

Fig. 10.3 Nodules of hyperplasia in the liver in chronic venous congestion, giving the irregular appearance of so-called cardiac cirrhosis. × 1.

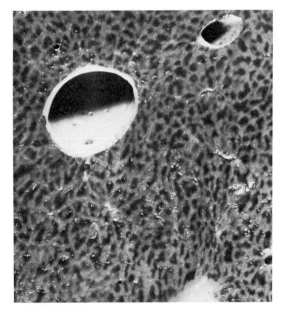

Fig. 10.2 The cut surface of the liver in chronic venous congestion. The congested centrilobular zones are dark, and contrast with the pale peripheral-lobular zones, giving the nutmeg-like appearance. × 1·8.

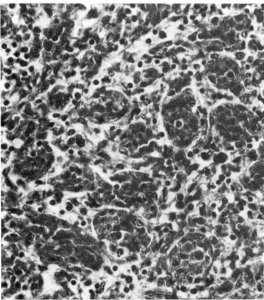

Fig. 10.4 Chronic venous congestion of the spleen. The dilated vascular sinuses are prominent, and the intervening medullary cords are relatively inconspicuous. × 250.

heart failure, centrilobular fibrosis occurs and nodules of hyperplastic parenchyma result from compensatory proliferation of surviving hepatocytes. The liver then appears diffusely irregular (Fig. 10.3): although commonly termed *cardiac cirrhosis*, these changes differ from true cirrhosis and do not progress to liver failure.

The **spleen** may be enlarged up to 250 g. It feels firm and maintains its firmness and shape on slicing, little blood escaping from the cut surface. The red pulp is congested and appears almost black: the Malpighian bodies may be visible as contrasting pale spots. Microscopy shows congestion of the venous sinuses in the red pulp, with some thickening of the reticulin framework and atrophy of the medullary cords (Fig. 10.4). More marked congestion of the spleen is seen in portal venous hypertension (p. 18.5).

The **kidneys** may be slightly enlarged and the medulla is particularly dark and congested; congestion is less obvious in the cortex, and appears as dark radial streaking (Fig. 10.5).

These structural changes in the abdominal viscera are without serious effects: there may be mild or sub-clinical jaundice, and some red cells and protein in the urine, but reduced blood flow and tissue hypoxia resulting from the underlying condition of cardiac insufficiency are far more important. Reduction in renal blood flow is at least partly responsible for retention of salt and water with increase in blood volume and oedema (p. 10.33).

Pulmonary venous congestion

In venous congestion of the **lungs**, the pulmonary venules and alveolar capillaries are engorged with blood (Fig. 10.6). The pulmonary veins react to the increased venous pressure by muscular thickening of the media and come to resemble pulmonary arteries. They also show intimal fibrous thickening. Red cells escape into the alveoli, sometimes resulting in bloodstained sputum, but many of them are broken down by alveolar macrophages, which come to contain large amounts of haemosiderin. The macrophages accumulate in the alveoli around respiratory bronchioles (Fig. 11.10, p. 11.12) and may appear in radiographs as a 'snow storm' effect. As haemosiderin is gradually released, the reticulin and elastic fibres in the walls of alveoli and blood vessels

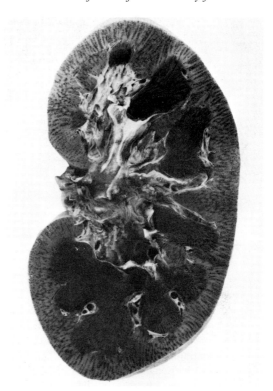

Fig. 10.5   The kidney in chronic venous congestion, showing intense vascular engorgement, particularly of the medulla.   ×0·7.

become encrusted with it and fibrous thickening occurs. These changes result in increased firmness and give the lung a brown appearance (*brown induration*). The fine structural changes of pulmonary venous congestion are described on p. 16.20.

Many patients with chronic pulmonary venous congestion suffer from attacks of pulmonary oedema. They also develop pulmonary *arterial* hypertension which, if prolonged, causes structural changes in the pulmonary arterial tree (pp. 16.23–26). The iron-laden macrophages may be found in the sputum: they have been termed 'heart failure' cells, but are often present in pulmonary venous congestion, e.g. in mitral stenosis, for years before heart failure supervenes.

Local venous congestion

As mentioned above, this results from mechanical interference with the venous drainage of blood from an organ, limb, etc. The effects

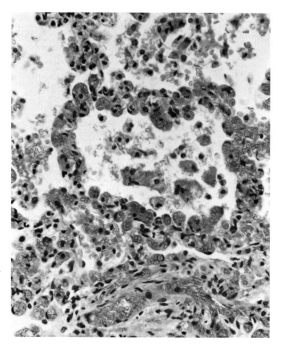

Fig. 10.6 Chronic pulmonary congestion, showing thickening of the alveolar walls, capillary congestion, and iron-containing macrophages lying free in the alveoli. × 210.

depend on the rapidity, degree and duration of obstruction and also on the local vascular arrangements.

Acute venous obstruction, e.g. by thrombosis or by a ligature, does not usually cause complete arrest of blood flow because in most parts of the body there is sufficient venous anastomosis to carry the blood away from the drainage area affected. In a few places, e.g. in the intestine, venous anastomosis is inadequate: the tissue becomes swollen, engorged with blood, and haemorrhagic due to rupture of small vessels. Ischaemic necrosis (venous infarction, p. 10.26) then develops.

In most sites, acute venous obstruction has less serious effects, and acute congestion either subsides or becomes chronic. This is illustrated by thrombosis of the deep veins of the leg, which is the commonest example of local venous obstruction, and often extends up to the femoral vein and even beyond. The limb may become cold, cyanosed and oedematous, but there is nearly always sufficient anastomosis to prevent infarction. The effects tend to subside gradually, partly because the anastomotic veins dilate and eventually become enlarged in

response to the increased blood flow through them, and partly because the size of the thrombus is reduced by contraction and by digestion by fibrinolysin. The lumen of the occluded vessel is often largely restored, and blood flow increases. Eventually, organisation and recanalisation of residual thrombus may further restore blood flow, but in spite of these changes, deep vein thrombosis, if extensive, sometimes results in chronic venous obstruction and persistent oedema of the limb. The valves present in veins play an important role in blood flow, particularly from the lower parts of the body: they may be obliterated if caught up in an organising thrombus or be rendered incompetent by dilatation, as in varicosity of the veins of the legs.

Chronic venous obstruction may result occasionally from obliteration of veins by organisation of thrombus, from compression or invasion of a vein by tumour, or constriction by fibrous tissue. When obstruction develops

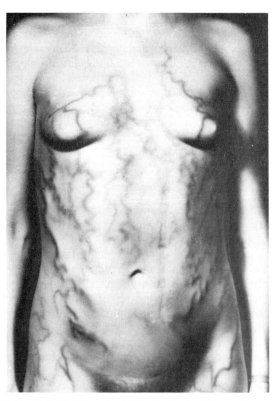

Fig. 10.7 Infra-red photograph showing enlargement of superficial veins to establish collateral circulation in a patient with obstruction of the inferior vena cava. (Dr G. Watkinson.)

gradually, however, collateral veins enlarge (Fig. 10.7) and drainage is often well maintained.

In chronic portal venous obstruction, which is an important effect of cirrhosis of the liver, the veins connecting the portal venous tributaries with systemic veins become enlarged and help to drain the portal system.

Haemostasis and Thrombosis

It is essential that the blood should remain fluid within the cardiovascular system, and yet should be capable of *local haemostasis* by forming a solid adherent plug to prevent excessive bleeding from an injury to a vessel wall. The vital importance of these properties of blood is reflected in the complexity of the systems involved.

The repair of vascular injury

Injuries of vessel walls can be classified as major when tissue is torn or cut and blood vessels are severed, and as minor 'wear-and-tear' defects which result from normal activities. **The minor defects** are presumably due to injury or loss of individual endothelial cells with consequent exposure of collagen, elastin, etc. Such lesions are repaired almost instantaneously by adherence of platelets, followed by growth of endothelium over the adherent platelets to restore the integrity of the vessel wall. The importance of platelets is illustrated by the spontaneous haemorrhages which occur from the microvessels in severe thrombocytopenia (a reduction in the number of platelets). The role of fibrin deposition is illustrated by the haemorrhages into joints (haemarthroses) in severe haemophilia, in which **coagulation** or **clotting** of blood (formation of solid fibrin) is defective. Evidently the small vessels in the joints are normally exposed to degrees of injury which, although minor, cannot be repaired by platelets alone.

More severe injury results in partial or complete severance of blood vessels. Bleeding is diminished temporarily by **vasoconstriction**: within seconds, platelets stick to the collagen fibres of the torn edge of the vessel wall and, together with deposition of fibrin strands, gradually build up to form a mass—the **haemostatic plug**, which may close the gap in the vessel and prevent further bleeding. Vascular endothelium extends to cover the haemostatic plug, which is then gradually removed by the process of organisation, the sub-endothelial gap thus being permanently repaired.

The factors involved in haemostasis

As explained above, vascular defects are repaired initially by formation of a haemostatic plug. This is an example of **thrombosis** (intravascular formation of solid material or **thrombus** from the constituents of the blood). In order to understand such beneficial haemostasis, and also disorders which upset the normal balance between the fluidity of the blood and its capacity to undergo thrombosis, it is necessary to consider in more detail the major factors involved: these are the *platelets, vascular endothelium*, the *clotting* or *coagulation process*, which leads to deposition of fibrin, and the *plasmin* or *fibrinolytic system*, which digests fibrin.

Platelet function

In normal blood, platelets circulate as single disc-shaped fragments of cytoplasm lined by a plasma membrane. They do not adhere to normal endothelium but, as stated above, if endothelium is lost they adhere to the exposed collagen fibres.

Adhesion is accompanied by conformational changes in which platelets become irregular in shape and throw out pseudopodia. This is followed by other features of platelet activation, notably adherence to one another (**aggregation**), as in the formation of the haemostatic plug. During these events, platelets also become actively secretory (the **release**

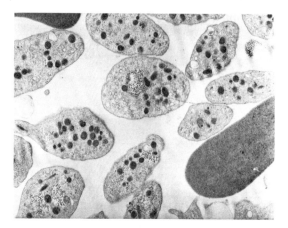

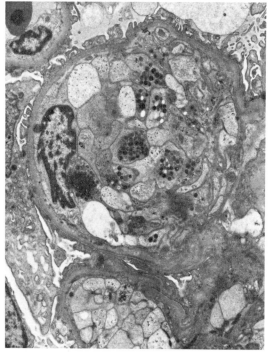

Fig. 10.8 Electron-micrographs of platelets. *Above,* free platelets in suspension, showing the dense storage granules. × 8000. *Below,* two glomerular capillaries plugged by aggregated platelets, most of which have discharged their granules. × 3000.

reaction): they discharge the contents of their granules (Fig. 10.8), including ADP, 5-HT, platelet factor 4 (see below) and various lysosomal enzymes, and synthesise and secrete arachidonic acid metabolites, notably stable prostaglandins and thromboxane A2 (see below). They also synthesise a phospholipid, platelet factor 3, which is a component of the clotting system.

These platelet products have important local effects on the walls of the small blood vessels, on the clotting system, and on the platelets themselves. Some stable prostaglandins, e.g. PGE_2, cause vasodilatation, while others, e.g. PGF_1, are vasoconstrictive. 5-HT and thromboxaneA2 are also vasoconstrictive and promote further aggregation of platelets and the release reaction, as does ADP. Platelet factors 3 and 4 play a role in coagulation (the latter by inhibiting the anticoagulant effect of heparin) and thus promote deposition of fibrin in the haemostatic plug. As noted above, some of the platelet products formed or secreted during the release reaction activate additional platelets, and thrombin, a factor produced during co-agulation, is also a platelet activator. A number of positive feedback mechanisms thus tend to enhance platelet activation.

Prostacyclin and thromboxaneA2. Arachidonic acid is released from the phospholipid of cell membrane by the hydrolytic action of phospholipase A2, and is metabolised by the cyclo-oxygenase pathway to produce cyclic endoperoxides, or by a lipoxygenase pathway to produce leukotrienes (p. 4.20). Cyclic endoperoxides are converted by specific enzyme systems into the stable prostaglandins (PGE_2 etc.), thromboxanes or prostacyclin (Fig. 10.9). The major arachidonic acid metabolites formed by activated platelets are stable prostaglandins and thromboxaneA2 (TxA2). As noted above, TxA2 induces further platelet activation and contracts small blood vessels, thus playing an important part in haemostasis. If unopposed, the positive feedback mechanisms which are activated by the platelet release reaction would cause an uncontrolled and progressive enlarge-

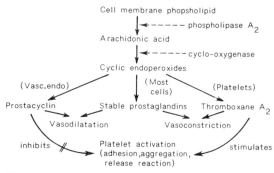

Fig. 10.9 The products of arachidonic-acid metabolism by the cyclo-oxygenase pathway and their effects on arterioles and platelets.

ment of the haemostatic plug. This is partly prevented by the instability of TxA2, which has a half life of 30 seconds. Another important controlling mechanism is exerted by vascular endothelium, which converts arachidonic acid to prostacyclin (PGI$_2$). The amount of PGI$_2$ produced by normal vascular endothelium is very small, but even slight endothelial injury results in greatly increased local production. The effects of PGI$_2$ are antagonistic to those of TxA2: it inhibits platelet aggregation and relaxes vascular smooth muscle. It is thus apparent that endothelial injury has two opposing effects. Platelets adhere to exposed collagen with subsequent platelet aggregation, the platelet release reaction, deposition of fibrin and vascular contraction. These haemostatic mechanisms are limited by increased endothelial production of PGI$_2$ which, like TxA2, is unstable (half life approximately 2 minutes), a feature which allows rapid regulation of the haemostatic mechanism.

A systemic role has been postulated for prostacyclin, which is released continuously in very small amounts from vascular endothelium into the blood. Control of the activity of circulating platelets is, however, obscure, and loose platelet aggregates do sometimes form in the blood and are believed to be responsible for transient neurological symptoms, known as *transient ischaemic attacks*, in old people.

The elucidation of the properties of TxA2 and PGI$_2$ has led to attempts to reduce the risk of coronary artery thrombosis by administration of aspirin. Several clinical trials have been reported, but so far the results have been disappointing. Aspirin and related drugs inhibit the cyclo-oxygenase pathway of arachidonic acid metabolism. When given in a daily dose of 1 gram, aspirin inhibits production of both TxA2 by platelets and PGI$_2$ by vascular endothelium, and is likely to have little overall effect on platelet function. This may account for the disappointing results of the clinical trials, in which the dosage of aspirin was of this order. It is possible that, by inhibiting TxA2 synthetase predominantly, much smaller dosage of aspirin might reduce the activity of platelets, and thus the tendency to thrombosis, but this awaits further trials.

It has been proposed by Moncada and Vane (1979) that prostacyclin may exert both a local and systemic control on platelet function. Its production by vascular endothelium may be of importance in preventing adhesion of platelets to normal endothelium. Mild physical or chemical injury to endothelium stimulates prostacyclin synthetase and so production of prostacyclin. Such injury may be sufficient to allow platelet adhesion to the damaged wall, thus effecting repair, but without the building up of a platelet aggregate, which is prevented by very low levels of prostacyclin.

Apart from the initial change in shape, all the features of platelet activation appear to be induced by a rise in the level of Ca^{++} in the platelet cytosol, and this effect, with consequent platelet activation, may be induced by the binding of agonists, e.g. adrenaline, to α-adrenergic platelet receptors. Platelet activation is also associated with a fall in cytosol cAMP, but it appears very likely that Ca^{++} is the important second messenger (p. 7.5) of platelet activation and that the cAMP system plays a modulating role.

Activation of platelets is usually assessed by measuring changes in the transmission of light through a stirred suspension of platelets following addition of platelet activators e.g. ADP. The initial change in shape is associated with increased transmission and this is followed by reduced transmission caused by aggregation, which increases as further aggregation is promoted by the products of the release reaction (ADP, thromboxaneA2, etc), with further diminution in transmission of light. By this means, the responsiveness of platelets to various activating agents can be assessed.

The above account is concerned mainly with the role of platelets in haemostasis, but they may be involved in other pathological processes, for example in acute inflammation (p. 4.20) and in the pathogenesis of atheroma (p. 14.13). The products of the platelet release reaction vary depending on the circumstances of their activation, and each of the three types of platelet granules (dense granules, α granules and lysosomes) may be discharged independently. In acute inflammation, platelet adhesion is not a prominent feature of vascular injury, but release of their cationic proteins and lysosomal acid hydrolases may contribute to the inflammatory reaction, while release of platelet-derived growth factor appears to be of importance in stimulating the proliferation of arterial smooth muscle cells, which is an important early feature of atheroma.

Platelet activating factor (PAF). This was discovered in investigations on hypersensitivity reactions in rabbits, in which species the union of antigen with IgE antibody bound to basophil leucocytes induces aggregation of circulating platelets and the release reaction. This effect is induced by PAF secreted by basophil leucocytes. PAF has since been shown to be a glycerophospholipid and has been obtained recently in fairly pure state. It is produced in other species (including man) by neutrophil polymorphs and macrophages during chemotaxis and phagocytotoxic activity. It has been detected in relatively high concentrations in human saliva and is produced also in the renal medulla. Its production by human basophil leucocytes is controversial.

PAF has been shown to activate platelets of human and various other species, is itself chemotactic for neutrophil polymorphs, and causes contraction of non-vascular smooth muscle. Injection locally causes erythema and inflammatory oedema and in larger amounts it induces short-lived systemic hypotension, a rise in pulmonary arterial pressure and bronchospasm: these effects do not appear to depend on activation of platelets.

Clearly, PAF is of considerable interest in relation to platelet function, acute inflammation and shock, but further work is required to assess its importance.

The coagulation (clotting) mechanism

By clotting is meant the conversion of fibrinogen to solid fibrin. This is the result of a complex series of reactions involving sequential activation of a large number of clotting factors, many of which are pro-enzymes and are activated by conversion to enzymes. Not only is the system complex, but most of the major factors have been numbered I to XIII (Table 10.1) in the order of their discovery, and not in the order of their participation. The clotting process up to the activation of factor X can occur by two main routes, the *intrinsic* and *extrinsic pathways*. After this stage, there is a *common pathway* leading to the formation of fibrin. The complexity of the process can be gathered from Fig. 10.10, which is a simplified scheme.

The intrinsic pathway results in clotting without the participation of factors released from injured tissues. It occurs when blood is withdrawn and placed in a tube and is probably involved in minor vascular injury and when blood stagnates in a blood vessel. It is initiated by contact of factor XII (Hageman factor) with a foreign surface or with collagen. Activated factor XII (termed XIIa) is an esterolytic en-

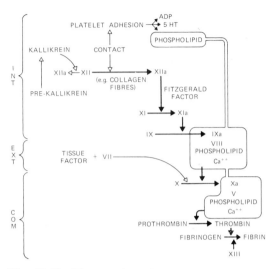

Fig. 10.10   The reactions involved in the clotting mechanisms. INT, intrinsic pathway; EXT, extrinsic pathway; COM, common pathway. Activated factors are indicated by the suffix 'a'.

zyme which, together with another factor (Fitzgerald factor), converts factor XI to XIa; this, in turn, activates factor IX. Factor X is then activated by a reaction involving IXa, Ca^{++}, factor VIII (antihaemophilic factor) and phospholipid (platelet factor 3) derived from activated platelets.

Table 10.1 International classification of the plasma coagulation factors (Roman numerals), together with their commonly-used names. There are a number of additional controlling factors, some of which are mentioned in the text.

Factor I	Fibrinogen
Factor II	Prothrombin
Factor III	Tissue factor
Factor IV	Calcium
Factor V	Pro-accelerin
Factor VII	Proconvertin
Factor VIII	Antihaemophilic globulin
Factor IX	Plasma thromboplastin component or Christmas factor
Factor X	Stuart–Prower factor
Factor XI	Plasma thromboplastin antecedent
Factor XII	Hageman factor
Factor XIII	Fibrin stabilising factor (plasma transglutaminase)

The extrinsic pathway is activated by tissue injury. It is triggered by a lipoprotein complex derived from damaged tissue cells (tissue factor 3 or thrombokinase), which activates factor VII: this in turn activates factor X.

The common pathway. Factor Xa, produced by either of the above routes, is a serine esterase which forms a complex with factor V and phospholipid in the presence of Ca^{++}: this complex converts factor II (prothrombin) to IIa (thrombin) which, in turn, converts fibrinogen to fibrin monomer. Factor XIII then polymerises fibrin monomer to form insoluble fibrin.

The clotting process is influenced by a number of *amplifying and inhibiting reactions*. For example, in the intrinsic system activated Hageman factor (XIIa) converts prekallikrein (a component of the kinin system— p. 4.18) to kallikrein, which activates more Hageman factor, while factor VII, which participates in the extrinsic pathway, is activated by a number of other factors—thrombin, XIIa, kallikrein, IXa and plasmin (see below). For the various activation steps there are specific inhibitors which modulate the clotting process and help to prevent inadvertent thrombosis.

The fibrinolytic (Plasmin) system

This is shown in outline in Fig. 10.11. Normal plasma contains the pro-enzyme *plasminogen* and a low concentration of *plasminogen activator* which is synthesised by vascular endothelium and can convert plasminogen to *plasmin,* a potent fibrinolytic enzyme. Conversion of plasminogen to plasmin is normally slow because plasminogen activator has a low affinity for free plasminogen. What little plasmin is formed in the plasma is inactivated almost instantaneously, mainly by α_2-antiplasmin. If, however, fibrin is formed intravascularly, as in thrombosis, plasminogen and its activator both bind avidly to it: this brings them into close contact and alters them in such a way that plasminogen is rapidly converted to plasmin, which digests the fibrin. In the bound form, plasmin is protected from degradation by α_2-antiplasmin, but as the fibrin is dissolved the released plasmin is degraded. The major activity of plasmin is thus ingeniously concentrated at the surface of deposited fibrin.

The control of synthesis and secretion of plasminogen activator is not understood. The plasma level is increased by deposition of fibrin and is raised after surgical operations or trauma. It is also increased by physical exercise, by administration of vasopressin or stanozolol and by catecholamines. Activated Hageman factor and kallikrein can both convert plasminogen to plasmin and plasmin can activate components of the complement system (p. 4.19).

$$\text{Plasminogen (pro-enzyme in plasma)}$$
$$\text{Activators} \rightarrow \downarrow$$
$$\text{Plasmin (fibrinolytic enzyme)}$$
$$\downarrow$$
$$\text{Fibrin} \rightarrow \text{soluble products}$$

Fig. 10.11 The fibrinolytic enzyme system.

The fibrinolytic system is probably in dynamic equilibrium with the clotting system, the two acting together to maintain an intact and patent vascular tree. According to this hypothesis, the coagulation and fibrinolytic systems may both be continuously active, the former augmenting adherence of platelets by laying down fibrin where needed on the endothelium to seal any deficiencies which may occur, and the latter removing such fibrin deposits after they have served their haemostatic function.

In *disseminated intravascular coagulation* (p. 17.68), massive conversion of plasminogen to plasmin occurs and the α_2-antiplasmin may be used up, leaving free plasmin which digests not only the intravascular fibrin but also plasma fibrinogen. The blood becomes incoagulable from lack of fibrinogen and because some of the peptides released by digestion of fibrin and fibrinogen have anticoagulant properties: in consequence, a haemorrhagic state develops. Agents which convert plasminogen to plasmin, for example streptokinase (a streptococcal product) and urokinase (a constituent of urine), can also cause a similar haemorrhagic state by converting circulating plasminogen to plasmin, an affect which is largely uncontrollable and which seriously limits the use of such agents to promote digestion of fibrin.

As explained in earlier chapters (e.g. p. 4.19) there are complex inter-relationships between the clotting, kinin, plasmin and complement systems, none of which can now be regarded in isolation.

Pathological Thrombosis

Thrombosis is defined as the formation of a solid or semi-solid mass from the constituents of the blood within the vascular system during life. Coagulation, i.e. deposition of fibrin, is involved in the formation of all thrombi except perhaps the minute deposits of platelets which maintain vascular integrity (p. 10.7).

Appearances and composition of thrombi

As already noted, the composition of thrombus is determined very largely by the rate of flow of the blood from which it forms. As a general rule, thrombus forming in rapidly flowing blood, e.g. in an artery, consists mainly of aggregated platelets (Fig. 10.8), with some fibrin; it enlarges slowly and, because few red cells are entrapped, is firm and pale, varying from greyish white to pale red, and is commonly called *pale thrombus*. The proportion of fibrin deposited in pale thrombus depends partly on the rate of blood flow, to which it has an inverse relationship. At the other extreme, thrombus forming in stagnant blood, e.g. adjacent to a complete occlusion of a blood vessel, is indistinguishable from blood which has been allowed to clot *in vitro*: the thrombus is soft, dark *red,* gelatinous and consists of a meshwork of strands of fibrin in which are entrapped red cells, leucocytes and platelets (Fig. 10.12). Contraction of fibrin may express fluid from the clot, causing it to shrink away from the vessel wall, revealing a smooth, shiny surface (Fig. 15.6 p. 15.10). Between these two extremes we have *mixed thrombi*, which form in slowly flowing blood, usually in veins, and consist of alternating layers of platelet aggregates and a network of fibrin entrapping red and white cells (Fig. 10.13). In other instances, veins may be filled with columns of red thrombus but with platelet aggregates at points of anastomosis. The formation of such thrombi is explained on p. 10.16. Except in recently formed thrombi, it is not easy to recognise aggregated platelets by conventional light microscopy, for they soon lose their outlines, presenting microscopically a granular or structureless appearance. Immunofluorescence studies and electron microscopy (Fig. 10.8) have, however, helped in their recognition.

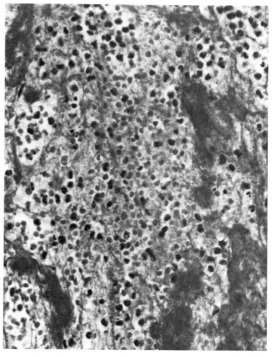

Fig. 10.12   Red thrombus, consisting of strands of fibrin lying among red cells, leucocytes and platelets. In this instance the proportion of entrapped red cells is much lower than in blood clot, indicating that there has been some flow of blood during thrombosis. × 305.

Predisposing factors of thrombosis

The three major predisposing factors are:

(*a*) *local abnormalities in the walls of blood vessels or of the heart.*

(*b*) *slowing and other disturbances of blood flow.*

(*c*) *changes in the composition of the blood favouring platelet aggregation and fibrin formation.*

The roles of these three factors in the formation of thrombi in the heart, arteries and veins are considered below.

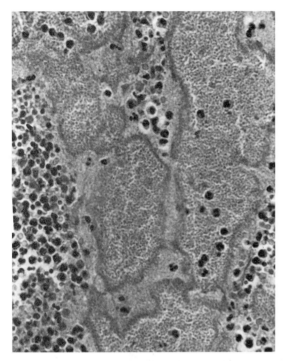

Fig. 10.13 Mixed thrombus, about 12 hours old, showing dense masses of granular material, composed mainly of platelets, with deposition of fibrin strands and collections of leucocytes. × 336.

(a) Cardiac thrombosis

Thrombi may form on the walls of any of the chambers of the heart, and also on the valve cusps.

In the atria, thrombosis is commonest in the appendices, especially that of the right atrium, in cases of heart failure or mitral stenosis with atrial dilatation (Fig. 15.26, p. 15.27). Slowing of blood flow, which is most marked in the atrial appendices, is the important causal factor and this is accentuated by atrial fibrillation, which commonly occurs in such patients and is very liable to be complicated by atrial thrombosis: the thrombus is usually red and is moulded to the irregular wall of the atrium.

Rarely, small flattened globular thrombi form in either the atria or ventricles. They are pale, composed mainly of platelets and may show central softening. In mitral stenosis, the left atrium may become almost filled by red thrombus (Fig. 15.27, p. 15.27), or rarely a large round thrombus forms and may plug the mitral valve ('ball-valve thrombus'). Thrombi

may also form **on the heart valves** in certain diseases and are termed *vegetations*: in rheumatic fever, the valve cusps are damaged along the line of apposition, and deposition of platelets and fibrin results in the formation of minute pinkish-grey bead-like vegetations (Fig. 10.14). In infective endocarditis, the cusps are colonised by micro-organisms and mixed thrombus forms larger, softer and more friable vegetations (c.f. Figs 15.22, p. 15.21 and 15.33, p. 15.35). **In the ventricles**, mural thrombosis commonly occurs on the endocardium overlying an infarct, i.e. a patch of ischaemic necrosis of the heart wall (Figs 10.15 and 15.10, p. 15.11). Depending on the size of the infarct, the thrombus may be large or small. It forms a flat reddish— or, if older, a brown—patch attached to the endocardium. Probably the important factors in its formation are the disturbances in blood flow caused by lack of pulsation in the dead muscle and also diffusion of factor III (tissue thromboplastin) from the dead tissue.

Clots formed after death are usually to be found in the chambers of the heart at autopsy. They are soft and dark red with a glistening surface and are not firmly adherent to the endocardium. Occasionally the red cells settle before coagulation occurs and the

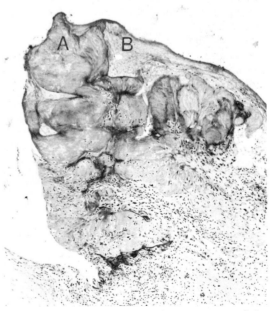

Fig. 10.14 Rheumatic vegetation on a cusp of the mitral valve. The vegetation consists mainly of dense hyaline material (A) composed of fused platelets, and fibrin coagulum (B). × 60.

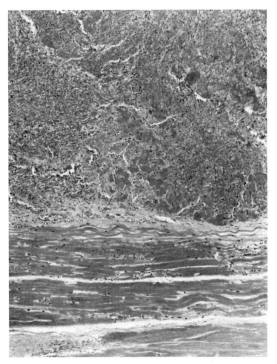

Fig. 10.15 Mural thrombus (*above*) which has formed on the ventricular endocardium over a myocardial infarct. Note the necrotic myocardium (*below*). × 120.

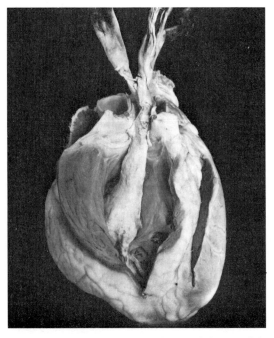

Fig. 10.16 Agonal thrombus in the right ventricle, extending along the pulmonary artery. × ½.

upper (usually anterior) part of the clot is then yellow and gelatinous. Thrombi may form rapidly as the circulation is failing immediately before death. They are yellow or pinkish with a glistening surface and have a somewhat stringy appearance (Fig. 10.16). Such **agonal thrombi** originate at the apex of the ventricle, to which they are attached, and may extend through the exit valve orifice. They are composed mainly of fibrin, which separates out from the sluggishly moving blood before death, and may occur in either or both ventricles.

(b) Arterial thrombosis

Probably because of the rapid flow of blood, arterial thrombosis is uncommon in the absence of a local lesion of the vessel wall. In affluent communities, **atheroma** is by far the commonest predisposing local lesion. It consists of multiple patches of fibrous thickening and lipid deposition in the intima of arteries of various sizes. *In the aorta*, atheroma is commonly severe and results in gross distortion and unevenness of the wall. When blood is flowing smoothly in a normal vessel, the particulate elements are separated from the vascular endothelium by a layer of cell-free plasma, but atheromatous plaques, by causing irregularities of the wall, result in turbulent flow, and platelets can then impinge on the wall. This alone probably predisposes to deposition of platelets, but because of the rapid flow of blood, deposition of fibrin is minimal. Frequently, however, atheromatous patches ulcerate, and large thrombi composed mainly of platelets and fibrin form on the ulcerated surface. In the aorta, such thrombi are usually mural, i.e. they do not occlude the lumen (Fig. 10.17), but thrombosis complicating atheroma of smaller arteries, notably those of the heart and brain, often occludes the lumen with consequent ischaemic necrosis of the deprived tissue. This is described later in the section on infarction and in the appropriate systematic chapters.

When there is gross *localised dilatation (aneurysm)* of the wall of the heart, aorta or other arteries, eddying of the blood usually results in some thrombosis. The thrombus may have a laminated appearance and may come to fill the aneurysmal sac (Figs 10.18 and 15.15, p. 15.15). **Inflammatory lesions** in the walls of arteries (pp. 14.21–28) also cause thrombosis: contributory factors may be irregularities of the wall, injury to or loss of the vascular endo-

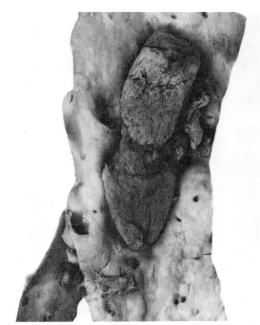

Fig. 10.17 Part of the abdominal aorta opened up to show a large thrombus which has formed over atheromatous patches. The dull, pale, shaggy thrombus consists mostly of fibrin and platelets.

thelium, and release of tissue thromboplastin. In **severe arterial hypertension**, necrosis of the walls of small arteries and arterioles is commonly followed by thrombosis.

(c) Venous thrombosis (Phlebothrombosis)

Apart from varicosity of the leg veins, diseases of the veins are uncommon, and although venous blood flow is slow, occlusion of veins in general occurs less frequently, and is usually less serious, than occlusion of arteries. The most important exception is *thrombosis of the veins of the lower limbs*, which is very common in bedridden patients, and is the usual cause of serious or fatal pulmonary embolism (see below): less often, thrombosis occurs in the *pelvic veins*, and this also may cause pulmonary embolism.

Thrombosis of leg veins usually starts in deep veins of the leg, most often within the calf muscles (Fig. 10.19), from where it may extend progressively to the posterior tibial, politeal, femoral (Fig. 10.20) and iliac veins, and occasionally to the inferior vena cava. In some instances, it may start more proximally than the calf, or several thrombi may form in the calf and thigh veins.

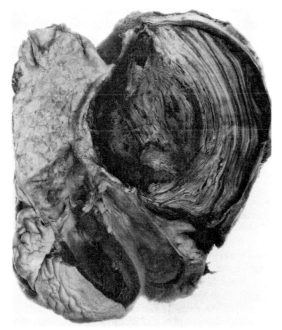

Fig. 10.18 A large aneurysm of the aortic arch (c.f. size of heart). The aneurysmal sac has become largely filled by laminated thrombus.

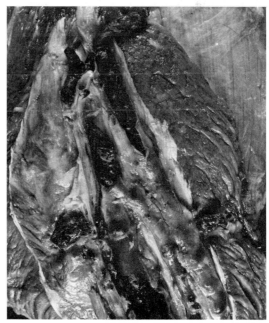

Fig. 10.19 Recently-formed red thrombus in the deep veins in the muscles of the leg.

Extension of the thrombus is sometimes very rapid: this probably occurs when flow of blood is very slow, and the thrombus resembles blood clot, being soft, red and friable, and is readily detached from the vessel wall to reveal a red glistening surface or a paler, dull appearance due to deposition of platelets and fibrin. In other instances, probably where the blood flow is less sluggish, thrombosis extends by stages, as depicted in Fig. 10.21. The initial thrombus formed in the calf veins occludes the lumen and, for some distance proximal to the occlusion, flow is virtually arrested. This column of stagnant blood is rapidly converted into red thrombus, largely by coagulation, up to the level of the next venous tributary, blood flow from which arrests further formation of red thrombus for a while. Platelets in the moving column of blood coming from the tributary are, however, deposited on the proximal end of the red thrombus, which thus becomes capped with more slowly formed pale thrombus consisting mainly of platelets and strands of fibrin. This may eventually occlude the entrance of the tributary, again producing stagnation, and so red thrombus forms and extends proximally to the next tributary. So the process continues with thrombus extending into larger, more proximal veins. Once the mouth of a tributary has been occluded, red thrombus also forms in the stagnant blood within it and so the thrombus in the main venous trunks comes to have branches extending into the tributaries: this feature is useful in recognising the embolic nature of thrombus which has become detached and lodged in the pulmonary arterial bed (see below).

Thrombosis of the deep leg veins (DVT) tends to occur especially in patients lying immobile in the supine position, and impairment of blood flow by pressure on the calves appears to be an important predisposing factor. It is particularly common after an abdominal operation, severe injury, myocardial infarction, and in patients with congestive heart failure. There is also an increased risk during pregnancy and following childbirth. Venous return from the lower part of the body is normally aided by muscular movements of the legs and by the pumping action which ensues from use of the abdominal muscles and diaphragm in breathing. In the above conditions, leg movements are reduced while those patients who have had

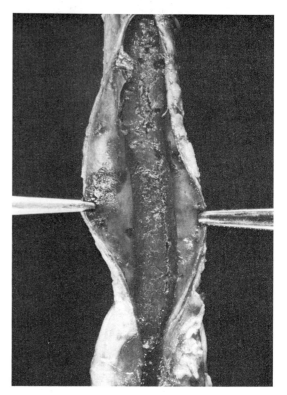

Fig. 10.20 Recent thrombosis of the femoral vein.

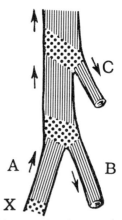

Fig. 10.21 Diagram showing the mode of extension of venous thrombosis. Thrombus occludes a small vein (A) at point X, and red thrombus (lined areas) rapidly extends in the stagnant column of blood up to the entrance of the next tributary (B), where platelet deposition forms a cap of pale thrombus (dotted areas): when this occludes the junction of A and B, red thrombus extends rapidly up to the entrance of the next tributary (C), and so on. Red thrombus also forms in each tributary as its entrance to the major channel is occluded. (Arrows show direction of spread of thrombosis.)

abdominal surgery tend to use mainly their thoracic muscles to breath and so avoid the pain of abdominal movements. In consequence, the pumping action of contraction of muscles is reduced and venous flow from the legs is slowed. For the two weeks or so after surgery, trauma or myocardial infarction, the clotting system is enhanced by increase in the number and adhesiveness of the platelets and raised levels of some of the clotting factors. This may help to explain why DVT extends so rapidly to major veins during this period. However, in surgical patients DVT appears to start during or very shortly after the operation, before these changes in the blood have developed.

DVT and consequent pulmonary emboli are very common autopsy findings, particularly in middle-aged and old people: in many instances they have not been suspected clinically, although extensive DVT often causes some oedema of the affected leg(s). Intravenous injection of ^{131}I-labelled fibrinogen has been used to detect DVT, the radioactivity being concentrated at sites of thrombosis.

The incidence of DVT and pulmonary embolism (p. 10.19) in high risk patients is reduced considerably by infusion or repeated small doses of heparin: in surgical patients this is most effective if started at the time of operation, the dosage being controlled by appropriate laboratory tests. It is partly to prevent DVT that patients are encouraged to get up and walk as soon as practicable after operation, childbirth, etc. and, while bedridden, to carry out muscular exercises and breathe with the abdominal muscles. The use of aspirin to reduce thromboxane production (p. 10.9) and thus inhibit thrombosis has not, so far, reduced the risk of DVT.

Individuals who have experienced DVT tend to have recurrences, sometimes after months or years and without obvious immediate predisposing factors. The incidence is increased in young women taking oral contraceptives.

Thrombosis of pelvic veins after operation, etc., is less common than leg-vein thrombosis. It is seen especially after childbirth, when the uterine blood flow diminishes considerably, predisposing to thrombosis in the hypertrophied uterine veins. Puerperal sepsis is also a predisposing factor in some cases. Pelvic venous thrombosis may also originate in haemorrhoids or in the prostatic venous plexus and is a complication of operations on the pelvic organs, particularly if there is sepsis. Extension to large veins, including the internal and common iliacs, may complicate pelvic venous thrombosis and fatal pulmonary embolism may follow.

Other causes of venous thrombosis include *malnutrition, severe debilitating infections* and *wasting diseases* such as cancer. When associated with these conditions it is sometimes called **marantic thrombosis** and in severely debilitated infants and young children may affect the superior longitudinal sinus (Fig. 10.31, p. 10.27). Venous thrombosis is also prone to occur in **some disorders of the blood**, for example leukaemia and polycythaemia rubra vera (in which there are excessive numbers of red cells, leucocytes and platelets). **Inflammation of veins (phlebitis)** also promotes thrombosis: this may occur as a *migrating thrombophlebitis*, affecting various veins throughout the body: it is usually of obscure aetiology (p. 14.37), but is sometimes associated with cancer of the internal organs, particularly the pancreas. Thrombophlebitis also occurs in various forms of vasculitis in which arteries and/or capillaries are also affected (p. 14.21–28). The thrombi are usually firmly adherent and embolism is unusual. In *septic venous thrombosis*, however, fragments of infected thrombus may break away and give rise to pyaemia (p. 9.8).

(d) Capillary thrombosis

Thrombosis in capillaries and venules commonly occurs in tissues involved in severe *acute inflammatory lesions*. It is due partly to endothelial damage and partly to haemoconcentration, the thrombi being composed mainly of packed red cells. Capillaries may also be occluded in those forms of vasculitis which affect particularly the small vessels (p. 14.28).

In the *Arthus reaction*, in which thrombosis of small vessels is often prominent, the endothelial injury is attributable mainly to release of enzymes by neutrophil polymorphs (p. 7.14).

Fibrin thrombi can be found in the capillaries in some patients dying of *disseminated intravascular coagulation* (p. 10.11), although in some cases they are absent as a result of fibrinolytic activity.

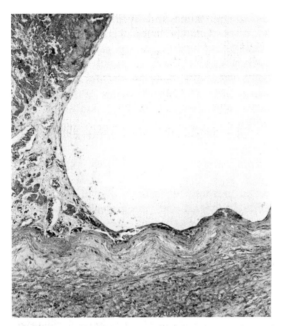

10.22 Endothelium has grown over the surface of this partially organised thrombus adherent to an artery wall. × 40.

The fate of thrombi

Like other abnormal digestible material deposited in the body, thrombus is removed by enzymic action, and the degree of restoration of the lumen of a thrombosed vessel depends on the success of such removal.

The processes involved in removal of thrombus are (a) shrinkage of the thrombus by contraction of fibrin, (b) digestion by plasmin and the proteolytic enzymes of neutrophil polymorphs and (c) organisation, involving digestion by macrophages and ingrowth of fibrovascular tissue. The relative importance and effects of these processes depend on the type of thrombus and the site of its formation.

Occlusive venous thrombi are usually formed mainly of soft red thrombus which contracts well. Where it remains attached to the vessel wall, it becomes invaded by fibroblasts and macrophages, along with capillaries which are probably derived from the vasa vasorum.

This ingrowth of granulation tissue does not often occur around the whole circumference of the vessel, usually being confined to sites where thrombosis has caused secondary damage to the intimal endothelium. Elsewhere, fluid-filled pockets may form where thrombus has re-tracted from the vessel wall or has been digested by the local action of plasmin. This is particularly prominent in the vicinity of the valve cusps of the vein. The cells of the intimal endothelium migrate and proliferate rapidly to cover the free surface of the thrombus, and also penetrate into it. This results in both fragmentation of the thrombus into tiny endothelial covered nodules and in the formation of small capillary channels, many of which are probably blind-ending, while a few link up with capillaries growing into the thrombus from the vein wall. The thrombus is also partially resorbed by the action of macrophages and sometimes the centre is softened by the enzymes from groups of dead polymorphs which have migrated from the newly formed thin-walled vessels. In this way, by the joining up of pockets, by fragmentation, resorption and softening of thrombus, a lumen may be restored leaving a thickened fibrovascular intimal plaque or a meshwork of fibrous strands marking the site of granulation tissue ingrowth with subsequent fibrosis. Occa-

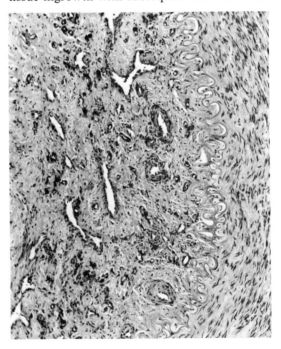

Fig. 10.23 Part of an artery showing the results of organisation of thrombus. The lumen was originally to the left of the internal elastic lamina, which runs vertically near the right margin. The lumen is now filled with vascular fibrous tissue in which some of the new capillaries have enlarged and acquired muscle to become arterioles. × 115.

sionally, however, and perhaps when the thrombus is especially dense and slowly formed, it remains adherent to the whole circumference of the vein; pockets are not formed and significant recanalisation fails to occur. The thrombus is then replaced by granulation tissue which becomes increasingly collagenous, the vein eventually being reduced to a solid, shrunken cord without a lumen.

Occlusive arterial thrombi are usually formed more slowly and are more dense than venous thrombi; they contain a higher proportion of platelets and fibrin and are less readily digested. Also, arterial endothelium is a relatively poor source of plasminogen activator and, possibly because of these factors, formation of pockets between the thrombus and arterial wall occurs much less than in veins. Consequently, the thrombus remains largely in contact with the artery wall and its removal takes place mainly by organisation. Macrophages migrate into the margin of the thrombus and gradually digest it. This is accompanied by invasion by fibroblasts from the intima and by new capillaries which develop from the arterial endothelium, including that which grows over the ends of the thrombus (Fig. 10.22). The vasa vasorum probably play no part if the internal elastic lamina is intact. The thrombus is thus gradually replaced by fibrovascular tissue and the length of vessel affected may eventually become a fibrous cord. The newly-formed capillaries anastomose and may develop into larger vessels extending through the length of the occlusion (Figs. 10.23; 15.7, p. 15.10), but such **recanalisation** does not often restore effective blood flow.

Mural thrombus. Thrombus may form on a part of the wall of a vessel (or of the chambers of the heart) without extending to fill the lumen. Such mural thrombi are rapidly covered with endothelium from the surrounding intima. Fibrinolysis, fragmentation, resorption and enzymatic breakdown probably all play a part in removing some of the thrombus, while granulation tissue grows in from the underlying wall and organises the remainder.

Embolism

By embolism is meant the transference of abnormal material by the bloodstream and its impaction in a vessel. The impacted material is called an **embolus.** In most cases it is a fragment of thrombus **(thrombo-embolism)** although fragments of material from ulcerating atheromatous plaques of the aorta quite commonly form emboli in distal arteries. A fragment of a tumour growing into a vein may also break off and form an embolus, and there may be embolism of the capillaries by fat globules, bubbles of air or nitrogen and even groups of parenchymal cells. The site of embolism will, of course, depend on the source of the embolus. Thus embolism of the pulmonary arteries and their branches is secondary to thrombosis in the systemic veins or in the right side of the heart. Rarely, where there is a patent foramen ovale, an embolus may pass from the right side of the heart to the left atrium and thus be carried to the systemic circulation; (*crossed* or *paradoxical embolism*). With this rare exception, emboli occurring in the systemic circulation are derived from thrombi formed in the left side of the heart, e.g. thrombotic vegetations on the aortic and mitral valves, and from thrombi or detached portions of atheromatous plaques in the aorta or large arteries. Emboli carried from tributaries of the portal vein lodge, of course, in the portal branches in the liver.

Effects of embolism

Systemic arterial emboli. The results are simply those of mechanical plugging and vary according to the site of the embolus, as described in pp. 10.23 *et seq.*

Pulmonary thrombo-embolism is a very common event in patients with acute or chronic debilitating disease. In most instances it results from detachment of thrombus formed in the veins of the lower limbs or much less commonly in the pelvic or other systemic veins or the right side of the heart. The predisposing causes and features of leg vein thrombosis are described on p. 10.16. Detached thrombus is carried in the venous blood through the right side of the heart and impacts in the pulmonary arterial bed.

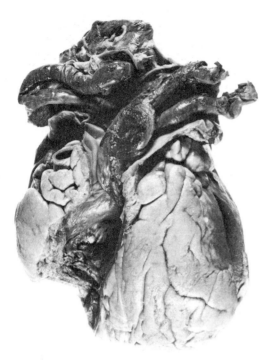

Fig. 10.24 Massive pulmonary embolism. Thrombus from the femoral vein has become detached and impacted in the pulmonary trunk and its right and left branches, causing sudden death.

The effects of pulmonary embolism depend mainly on the degree of occlusion of the pulmonary arterial bed and on the state of the pulmonary circulation. A large thrombus, extending up to the femoral or iliac vein, may become detached *en masse* and block the main pulmonary trunk (Fig. 10.24) or both of its branches, causing almost instantaneous death by arresting the circulation. Less massive but considerable embolism causes acute right ventricular failure by increasing the resistance to pulmonary blood flow. This usually results from occlusion of more than half the pulmonary arterial bed in previously healthy individuals, but is precipitated by lesser degrees of embolism in patients with pulmonary hypertension or incipient heart failure. Occlusion of medium-sized or small pulmonary arteries is usually without effect on the pulmonary circulation unless many vessels are occluded by a shower of smaller emboli. Multiple small emboli over a period of months or years very occasionally cause chronic pulmonary arterial hypertension.

The effects of pulmonary embolism on the lung tissue supplied by the occluded artery depend very largely on the general state of the pulmonary circulation. If this is normal, obstruction of medium-sized pulmonary arteries does not result in infarction, but if the circulation is impaired, e.g. by heart failure, infarction may result. This and other factors determining the effect on the lung tissue are discussed in detail on pp. 16.27–29.

Experimental studies have shown a remarkable capacity for removal of pulmonary thrombo-emboli. Emboli are partly digested and partly removed by organisation (as in the removal of venous thrombi—p. 10.18), leaving a patch of fibrous thickening of the vein wall. In man also, there is evidence that many pulmonary thrombo-emboli are removed with little loss of pulmonary vascular bed. Apart from the rare development of pulmonary hypertension due to recurrent small emboli, the main dangers are the immediate obstructive effects of large emboli and the tendency for venous thrombosis, and thus pulmonary embolism, to recur.

The incidence of pulmonary embolism at autopsy depends on the care with which the lungs are examined (p. 16.27). In most cases the emboli are small, and were often unsuspected clinically. Without doubt, most of them originate from thrombi which have formed as a terminal event, and would have undergone fibrinolysis had the patient survived.

Septic emboli. With the widespread use of antibiotics, septic emboli, containing pyogenic bacteria, have become relatively uncommon.

Large septic emboli originate usually from septic thrombosis in a vein involved in a suppurating infection or from the valves of the heart in bacterial endocarditis. Where such an embolus impacts, the effects are due to local ischaemia and sepsis, and a combination of tissue necrosis and suppuration result (p. 9.8). The wall of the artery at the site of impaction is weakened by suppuration and may become locally dilated (*mycotic aneurysm*): it may subsequently rupture. In various septicaemic and pyaemic conditions, the plugging of arterioles and capillaries by minute fragments of septic thrombus or aggregates of bacteria produces small haemorrhagic lesions (Fig 9.10, p. 9.10) which may suppurate.

Fat embolism. Entrance of globules of neutral fat into the circulation probably occurs after all

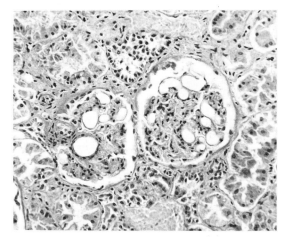

Fig. 10.25 Fat embolism of glomerular capillaries in a case of decompression sickness. Fat globules (dissolved out in processing the tissue) have impacted in glomerular capillaries and caused great distension. × 170. (Professor A.C. Lendrum.)

bone fractures. Most of the fat is arrested in the small vessels in the lungs, where the globules fuse to form columns of fat. In most cases this is symptomless and the fat is removed, but in a small proportion of patients with major fractures of the long bones or limb girdles, and particularly when fatty tissue is lacerated, a large amount of fat enters the circulation and the **fat embolus syndrome** may develop during the following three days. Its main features are mental confusion, fever, dyspnoea and tachycardia, a petechial rash and sometimes cyanosis, haemoptysis, coma and death. The symptoms are attributable largely to hypoxia resulting from pulmonary fat embolism which is complicated by pulmonary oedema and haemorrhages. Some of the fat passes through the pulmonary circulation and impacts in capillaries throughout the systemic circulation, where it causes widespread petechial haemorrhages in the skin and various tissues. In fatal cases, fat emboli are seen in the capillaries in many tissues (Fig. 10.25) and pericapillary haemorrhages and minute infarcts are often found in the brain, principally in the white matter. Thrombocytopenia develops in some patients and may contribute to haemorrhages. However, most patients recover without residual disability.

Fat embolism may also complicate trauma of fatty tissue and of a grossly fatty liver, severe burns, major surgery, acute pancreatitis, and in decompression sickness (see below).

Air embolism. The pressure in veins situated above the level of the right atrium (e.g. in the head and neck when upright) is below that of the atmosphere and when a wound involves the wall of such a vein, air may be sucked into it and pass into the circulation. This is particularly liable to happen in neck wounds involving the major veins and is a danger in cardiothoracic surgery. It may happen also where positive pressure is used in venous or arterial catheterisation and in venous infusion of blood or fluids. Small volumes of air entering the circulation are rapidly absorbed without ill effect, but volumes of over 100 ml may cause acute distress and 300 ml or more may be fatal. Such large volumes become churned up with blood in the right side of the heart: the froth is not easily expelled and blocks the pulmonary arterial circulation.

Decompression sickness

The amounts of inhaled gases which pass into solution in the body fluids and tissues are proportional to the atmospheric pressures, and when this is reduced rapidly, some of the dissolved gases come out of solution (just as a fizzy drink effervesces on opening the bottle) and form bubbles in the blood and tissues. This may occur when divers are brought to the surface too quickly, when workers in compressed air, e.g. tunnels and caissons, are restored rapidly to atmospheric pressure, and following rapid ascent to high altitudes in an unpressurised aircraft or sudden loss of pressure in a pressurised aircraft at high altitude.

With the increasing popularity of scuba diving as a sport and increase in naval and industrial diving, decompression sickness has increased in importance. If air has been breathed, the gas bubbles consist largely of nitrogen, which is less readily re-absorbed than oxygen and carbon dioxide. Bubbles form in the blood, body fluids and tissues, and particularly in fatty tissue, which can absorb a high concentration of nitrogen. The bubbles of gas enlarge and may coalesce and, in addition to their mechanical effect, those in the blood may induce important changes at the gas/blood interface. These latter include denaturation of plasma proteins with consequent sludging of the red cells and increased viscosity of the blood. Hageman factor may be activated at the interface and platelet aggregation and the release reaction (p. 10.7) may occur, followed by activation of the clotting, fibrinolytic, kinin and complement systems. In severe cases, these changes can lead to disseminated intravascular coagulation, thrombocytopenia and release of vaso-active agents which increase vascular permeability, causing leakage of fluid and proteins from the small vessels, haemoconcentration and a state of shock.

Symptoms of decompression sickness may develop during ascent of a diver to the surface or at any time up to 36 hours after completing a dive. In most cases, the onset is within 12 hours, and there is a general inverse correlation between the latent period and the severity of symptoms, although there are individual variations within this relationship.

Symptoms vary greatly, depending on where the gas bubbles accumulate. The commonest (and mildest) form consists of asymmetrical cramps of limb muscles (the 'bends') and pain around one or more large joints, usually the shoulder or knee. Skin manifestations include itching, patchy erythema, cyanosis and oedema. Accumulation of bubbles in the lungs may result in dyspnoea, cough and chest pain (the 'chokes'). Almost any neurological symptom may develop, but the thoracic spinal cord is often mainly affected, and paresthesia or weakness of a limb may develop and may extend and progress to paraplegia. After early death, the brain and cord are congested at autopsy, and in later deaths small haemorrhagic infarcts are seen in the white matter of the cord. It is not understood why the cord is predominantly affected. It is an uncommon site of emboli in general, and it has been suggested that increased respiratory effort impedes the drainage of the epidural vertebral venous plexus and that nitrogen bubbles accumulate there, followed by platelet aggregation and thrombosis with consequent obstruction of the drainage of blood from veins of the spinal cord into the plexus. There is some experimental and clinical evidence to support this view.

Muscle cramps are frequently the only symptom, but they may be accompanied or followed by skin, pulmonary or neural involvement, each of which may occur alone or in any combination. A haemorrhagic condition may result from thrombocytopenia and/or fat embolism (see below) and shock may develop and dominate the clinical picture.

Fat embolism (p. 10.20) occurs in some cases of decompression sickness, but is not usually a major feature. The fat probably enters the circulation as a result of the tearing of fatty tissue by formation of nitrogen bubbles in it. Denaturation of the protein of plasma lipoproteins also releases lipid which may coalesce and form emboli.

The amount of nitrogen dissolved in the body depends on the length and depth of the dive, but is influenced also by age, obesity, water temperature and degree of physical activity during the dive. In addition, there are individual variations in the susceptibility to decompression sickness which are not accounted for by the above factors and are of unknown nature. Reliable tables are available, indicating the duration of decompression required, depending on the duration and depth of the dive, and compliance with them should minimise the risk of decompression sickness.

The best treatment of decompression sickness is recompression in a hyperbaric chamber to a pressure which relieves the symptoms, followed by gradual decompression. Success depends on avoidance of delay between the onset of symptoms and recompression, and a delay of less than 30 minutes is associated in most cases with complete recovery. Other forms of treatment include administration of oxygen and, if necessary, treatment for shock.

Bone necrosis is of common occurrence in divers and compressed-air workers. It tends to be associated with a long diving experience, although it has occurred following a single dive. It also appears to be associated with a history of decompression sickness, although in some cases the history is negative. In most cases, the lesions affect part of the shaft of the femur, humerus or tibia, and are symptomless, being diagnosed radiologically. In a minority, however, juxta-articular necrosis results in collapse of a joint, most often the shoulder or hip joint. Radiological changes do not develop in less than three months, and necrosis is usually more extensive than the radiological changes. The decision on whether divers with symptomless bone lesions should continue to dive is a difficult one, but it seems likely that they have an increased risk of developing disabling juxta-articular lesions.

Decompression barotrauma. This occurs when decompression results in tissue damage from expansion of air in a body cavity. It is not dependent on dissolved gases and thus is unrelated to the duration of a dive. It is likely to occur when a diver holds his/her breath during ascent. Rupture of lung tissue may occur, leading to pneumothorax, interstitial emphysema (escape of air into the tissues) of the mediastinum and neck, and entry of air into pulmonary veins. This last may result in air embolus, usually of the brain, in which case neurological symptoms develop immediately, although symptoms of interstitial emphysema or pneumothorax may be delayed. Neurological features of decompression sickness differ in not usually being immediate and affect predominantly the cord.

Local Ischaemia

Complete arterial occlusion

Ischaemia means deficient supply of blood and is applied to tissue in which blood flow has ceased (complete ischaemia) or is abnormally low (partial ischaemia). Ischaemia localised to an organ, a part of the body, or a patch of tissue, is usually due to obstruction to arterial blood flow.

By far the commonest and most important causes of complete arterial occlusion are thrombosis and embolism; other causes include proliferative changes in the intima of small arteries, and also arterial spasm as in Raynaud's disease or ergot poisoning.

When an artery is obstructed, the result depends on the extent of **collateral circulation**, *i.e. alternative vascular routes by which blood can reach the deprived tissue*. The arterial anastomoses in the limbs are such that blockage of any one artery does not usually result in severe ischaemia provided that the other arteries are not seriously diseased. Similarly, there are effective collateral arteries in the integument and muscles of the trunk. When an artery of a limb is suddenly obstructed in a healthy subject, there is an immediate drop in the blood pressure beyond the obstruction, and the circulation is brought almost to a standstill; the arteries then contract and the part contains less blood than normally. Soon, however, the anastomotic arteries dilate and blood thus bypasses the obstruction to enter the vessels of the affected part, through which a flow of blood is gradually established and increased until ultimately it may approach normal. Thus in a subject with a healthy cardiovascular system the femoral artery may be ligated without permanent damage resulting. The limb becomes cold and numb, and some days may elapse before the pulse returns at the ankle, while restoration of full muscle power takes much longer. The collateral vessels remain dilated and maintain the circulation, and eventually they become permanently enlarged, with thicker walls (p. 14.2). Such hypertrophy in response to increased workload is illustrated dramatically by the rare congenital localised stenosis (*coarctation*) of the aorta beyond the arch, in which the vessels linking the arteries of the head and neck with those of the trunk and legs become enormously enlarged during life and supply most of the blood to the lower part of the body.

The development of an efficient collateral circulation often depends on dilatation of healthy anastomotic arteries, and on a healthy heart. If, however, the collateral arteries are diseased, e.g. atheromatous, fibrosed or calcified, they are unlikely to dilate sufficiently to supply the necessary amount of blood to the ischaemic part, and a varying amount of necrosis will follow. Accordingly, in middle-aged or old people with atheroma, etc., blockage of the main artery of a limb, or even of a large branch, may be followed by death of the tissues supplied by the obstructed vessel, the condition of 'senile' gangrene resulting (p. 9.13). Multiple emboli in the arteries of the lower limbs (usually resulting from aortic atheroma) or spreading thrombosis, as in thromboangiitis obliterans (p. 14.24), may also lead to ischaemia and gangrene, even in young adults.

Infarction

Tissue necrosis resulting from reduction or loss of blood supply is termed **infarction** and the dead tissue is called an **infarct**. It is usually caused by obstruction of one or more arteries by thrombosis or embolism. As noted above, the blockage of even a major artery supplying the skeletal muscles and integument of the body does not usually result in infarction because anastomosis with other arteries, beyond the point of obstruction, is sufficient to maintain the circulation. In the internal organs, however, anastomosis is less adequate, and blockage of a single artery is commonly followed by infarction. Such arteries are termed **end arteries**. In some tissues, infarction may also result from arterial narrowing without complete occlusion.

The term infarction literally means 'stuffing in', and originally it was applied to infarcts because in some of them the blood vessels become engorged with blood and extensive haemorrhage occurs into the dying tissue. In other instances, however, the dead tissue appears mostly pale with few or no haemorrhagic patches. The factors determining distinction between red and pale infarcts is of significance only because it affects their appearances.

General features. The size of an infarct depends upon the amount of tissue rendered ischaemic, the severity and duration of the ischaemia, and the susceptibility of the component cells of the tissue to ischaemic injury. Apart from whether it is red or pale, the appearances of an infarct depend on the nature of the subsequent changes in the dead tissue and in particular on whether it undergoes coagulative or colliquative necrosis (p. 3.32). In the days following infarction, the vessels in the surviving tissue around the infarct are congested and products of the dead cells diffuse out and promote an acute inflammatory reaction at the margin, with inflammatory oedema and accumulation of polymorphs and macrophages, which migrate into the dead tissue. The acute reaction soon subsides, and the infarct is replaced by the process of organisation (p. 5.23): macrophages continue to migrate into and digest the dead tissue, followed by capillaries which sprout from the adjacent vessels, and by proliferating fibroblasts which lay down collagen fibrils. A layer of granulation tissue thus forms at the margin and gradually replaces the infarct. As it ages, the granulation tissue matures into denser fibrous tissue and eventually the site of the infarct is marked by a fibrous scar.

These features are illustrated by the following examples of infarction.

Myocardial infarction is extremely important because it is a very common cause of disability and death from heart failure. It usually results from occlusive thrombosis supervening on atheroma of a major coronary artery and involves a patch of ventricular myocardium. The dead myocardium undergoes coagulative necrosis (Fig. 3.32, p. 3.32) and gradually becomes pale (Fig. 15.10, p. 15.11), but often with scattered haemorrhages. The size and site of the infarct depend on which artery is occluded and on the degree of collateral circulation from other coronary arterial branches. Polymorphs infiltrate the margin of the infarct and by digesting the dead tissue may increase the risk of rupture of the wall of the ventricle. In patients who survive, granulation tissue gradually grows in to replace the dead tissue (Fig. 15.11, p. 15.12) and eventually a fibrous scar is formed (Fig. 15.12, p. 15.12). Less commonly, infarc-

tion involves the inner parts of the wall of the left ventricle throughout its whole circumference (Fig. 15.16, p. 15.16): this is commonly associated with severe narrowing of the lumen of both coronary arteries or their major branches by atheroma, but without superadded occlusive thrombosis. Myocardial infarction may cause death from ventricular fibrillation, or heart failure may ensue from loss of part of the myocardium, and is sometimes aggravated by arrhythmias.

Cerebral infarction. Blood supply to most parts of the brain is dependent on end arteries, occlusion of any one of which results in infarction. Such occlusion usually results from thrombosis over an atheromatous patch or from embolism and affects the territory supplied by the occluded artery, but there is some collateral circulation between the major arteries and the size of the infarct varies depending on the state of the other arteries, and in particular whether they are narrowed by atheroma. The brain tissue is remarkably susceptible to ischaemia and parts of it, termed boundary zones, lie at the junction of territories supplied by the major arteries (p. 21.17). These zones are particularly susceptible to a more general reduction in blood flow to the brain, for example in a severe hypotensive episode, as in shock. Severe reduction of flow by lesions proximal to the circle of Willis, usually by a combination of atheroma and occlusive thrombosis of the vertebral and internal carotid arteries, can also cause infarction in the boundary zones.

Cerebral infarcts may be pale or haemorrhagic. The dead tissue undergoes autolytic digestion and breaks down to form a soft pulpy mass (Fig. 21.17, p. 21.18) which has popularised the term 'softening' for a brain infarct. In contrast to other tissues, the infarct is not removed by organisation: the debris is gradually taken up by macrophages (Fig. 21.3, p. 21.6), leaving a cavity (Fig. 21.18, p. 21.18) which eventually comes to contain clear fluid. Around the infarct there is a zone of brain tissue in which partial ischaemia at the time of infarction causes necrosis of the highly susceptible neurons, while the glial cells survive and the astrocytes apparently increase in number and provide a layer of 'gliosis' which, together with a little fibrous tissue, forms around the cavity. The effects of cerebral infarction depend on the part of the brain involved. At first there may be

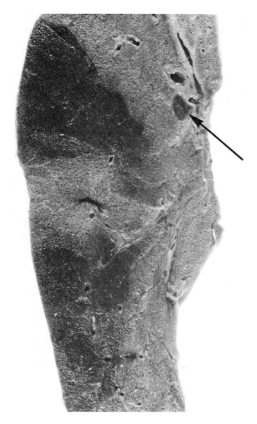

Fig. 10.26   Two haemorrhagic infarcts of lung, seen on section as dark wedge-shaped areas, widening towards the pleural surface (*left*). Note a pulmonary artery occluded by thrombus (*arrow*) beyond the apex of the upper infarct. × 1·3.

marked oedema around the infarct, and disability often diminishes as this subsides. The commonest sites of infarction are within the tissue supplied by the middle cerebral artery; the internal capsule is often involved, causing hemiplegia.

Infarcts of the **lung** are typically wedge-shaped, with the base projecting slightly on the pleural surface (Fig. 10.26). They are firm and haemorrhagic (Fig. 10.27). In some instances, pulmonary arterial occlusion results in a wedge-shaped haemorrhagic patch without necrosis and resolution may then occur. When there is necrosis, i.e. infarction, organisation follows, leaving a depressed scar in those who survive for more than a few weeks. Blockage of even a major pulmonary artery, which is usually caused by thrombo-embolus from the leg veins (p. 10.19), is not followed by infarction

provided the general pulmonary circulation is normal, and pulmonary infarction occurs particularly in subjects with pulmonary hypertension or heart failure. The factors involved are, however, complex, and are discussed on pp. 16.27–28.

When an infarct extends to a coelomic surface, e.g. the pericardium, pleura or splenic capsule, there is often deposition of a fine layer of fibrin on the surface and escape of clear or slightly turbid fluid exudate from it. The fibrin deposit may give rise to pain and a 'friction rub' may be heard on auscultation when the affected organ slides over the parietal coelomic surface, e.g. during beating of the heart or the pulmonary movement of respiration.

Splenic infarction. Thrombosis of the splenic artery is uncommon and leads to virtually complete splenic infarction. More commonly a branch of the splenic artery is occluded by an embolus and a wedge-shaped infarct results (Fig. 10.28). At first the infarcted tissue is dark red from congestion, but it soon changes to pale yellow, and is slowly organised to leave a depressed scar.

Renal infarction. Unless there is an additional aberrant artery, thrombosis of the renal artery leads to almost complete ischaemic necrosis of the kidney. Occlusion of a branch of the renal artery results in a wedge-shaped infarct (Fig. 10.29) the size of which depends on the artery

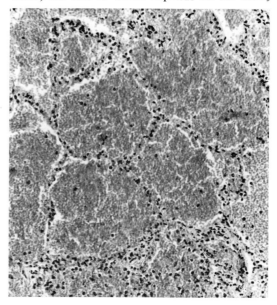

Fig. 10.27   Haemorrhagic infarct of lung, showing alveoli filled with red cells. × 115.

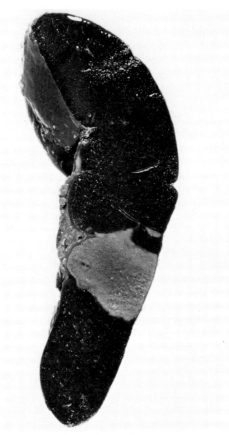

Fig. 10.28 Pale infarct of the spleen.

occluded. The margin of the infarct is haemorrhagic and the central part is usually pale.

Infarction of the intestine may result from occlusion of a major artery, usually the superior mesenteric, or from mechanical obstruction of the blood supply by twisting of a loop of the gut (volvulus—p. 19.58) or impaction in a hernial sac. The infarcted intestine ceases to contract and the effect is the same as mechanical obstruction.

The necrotic wall is congested, oedematous and haemorrhagic. Micro-organisms in the lumen proliferate and invade the dead tissue and bacterial toxins diffuse through it, causing severe toxaemia. Finally, the necrotic wall is likely to rupture and its contents escape. The condition is usually fatal from these various effects unless the infarcted length of gut is removed surgically without undue delay.

In the **liver,** obstruction of a branch of the portal vein is not followed by infarction, owing to the supply of blood from the hepatic artery.

The obstruction does, however, reduce the blood flow sufficiently to cause atrophy and loss of hepatic parenchymal cells, and the sinusoids become dilated, so that the lesion appears dark red and shrunken (Fig. 10.30) and is sometimes termed a 'red infarct'. Obstruction of the hepatic artery or of its branches may result in infarction of the liver (p. 20.4).

'Venous infarction'. Obstruction of a vein is an uncommon cause of arrest of blood flow through the tissue it drains, partly because in most tissues there is sufficient anastomosis to maintain venous drainage, and partly because thrombosis of veins in internal organs is relatively uncommon, and emboli cannot, of course, impact in veins (except in portal venous systems, as in the liver). When venous infarction does occur the infarct is intensely engorged, oedematous and haemorrhagic. Marantic thrombosis of the superior longitudinal sinus sometimes occurs in severely debilitated children: the engorged cerebral cortical veins may rupture (Fig. 10.31), and there may be patches of haemorrhagic infarction of the cortex. Thrombosis of the mesenteric veins extending down to the smaller tributaries causes infarction of the intestine, which progresses to gangrene. Venous infarction is also seen occasionally in the liver as a result of extension of carcinoma involving the hepatic veins. The best examples of venous infarction are, however, seen in the adrenals, which have several arteries but drain through a single large vein.

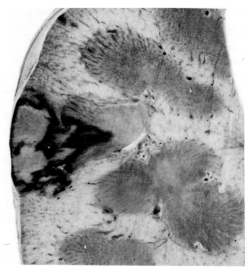

Fig. 10.29 Infarct of kidney, showing pale necrotic centre with haemorrhagic margin. × 1·2.

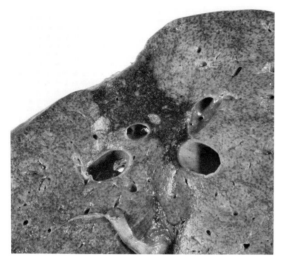

Fig. 10.30 A depressed red patch in the liver due to loss of parenchymal cells and sinusoidal congestion following thrombosis of a portal venous branch (not shown).

The susceptibility of tissues to ischaemia. The extent of infarction is usually less than that of the tissue supplied by the occluded artery, collateral circulation supplying the tissue at the periphery of the area. The size of the infarct resulting from occlusion of a particular artery may thus vary greatly, depending on whether the collateral arteries are healthy and capable of dilatation. The extent of necrosis is determined also by the capacity of the tissue to withstand ischaemia. As a general rule, *the parenchymal cells of the internal organs, which operate at a high metabolic rate, are relatively susceptible to ischaemia, whereas the supporting tissues—fibrous and fatty tissue and bone, are much less susceptible.* The neurons of the central nervous system are perhaps the most susceptible cells of all, and cannot withstand deprivation of blood supply for more than a very few minutes. Glial cells are somewhat less demanding in their requirements, and accordingly at the margin of a brain infarct there is a zone in which partial ischaemia is followed by restoration of the circulation by collaterals; this results in death of the neurons, while the glial cells persist and undergo reactive proliferation. Hepatic parenchymal cells are also highly susceptible to ischaemia and, as described above, thrombosis of a portal venous branch is commonly followed by atrophy and loss of liver cells with survival and dilatation of the sinu-

soids. The renal tubular epithelium has also a low resistance to ischaemia, and while in the central part of a recent renal infarct all the cells are dead, at the periphery there is a zone in which the glomeruli and intertubular capillaries have survived while the tubular epithelium has died.

Septic infarction. As noted above, an infarct of the intestine rapidly becomes gangrenous, and could appropriately be termed a septic infarct. The same applies to infarction of the foot or leg, particularly when the 'wet' form of gangrene supervenes (p. 9.13). The term septic infarction is, however, usually restricted to infection resulting from a septic embolus in which the bacteria in the embolus invade the dead tissue and bring about suppuration at the margin (Figs 10.32 and 9.9, p. 9.9): the infarct thus becomes surrounded by a layer of pus and is converted to an abscess.

The effects of infarction. The effects of infarction on function depend largely on the location and size of the infarct. In organs such as the kidneys, which have a large functional reserve, extensive or multiple infarctions of both kidneys are necessary to bring about any serious disturbance of function. Single infarcts of the myocardium are commonly sufficiently large to cause heart failure; infarcts involving the conducting system of the heart may cause heart block, and occlusion of a coronary arterial branch not uncommonly causes sudden death from ventricular fibrillation before infarction has become apparent. Infarction of brain tissue is the commonest cause of a 'stroke', and even

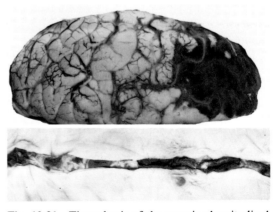

Fig. 10.31 Thrombosis of the superior longitudinal sinus (shown below), resulting in intense engorgement of the cerebral cortical veins and haemorrhage over the frontal lobe.

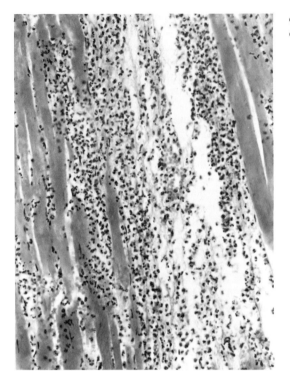

Fig. 10.32 Suppuration at the margin of a septic infarct of the heart. The necrotic myocardium (*right*) is becoming separated from the adjacent living tissue (*left*) by a purulent exudate. × 175.

a small one involving the internal capsule is followed by hemiplegia. As already explained, infarction of lung tissue tends to occur especially in association with embarrassment of the pulmonary circulation, and for this reason recent pulmonary infarcts are very commonly observed at autopsy of patients dying of heart failure.

The effect of infarcts in particular organs are considered more fully later, in the systematic chapters.

Partial arterial obstruction

Chronic narrowing of the lumen of arteries is very common, and is usually caused by **atheroma** (p. 14.3). It brings about the serious effect of ischaemic atrophy of specialised cells with accompanying overgrowth of fibrous tissue, for example in the *myocardium*, and is the usual cause of angina pectoris (spasms of pain from myocardial ischaemia). Atheromatous narrowing of the arteries which supply the *brain* predisposes to focal loss of neurons or to actual infarction (p. 21.17): these events are particularly liable to occur during hypotensive episodes and no doubt contribute to intellectual deterioration in old age. The high prevalence of atheroma in the elderly is an important cause of senile mental changes. Multiple or extensive patches of atheromatous narrowing of the lumen are common in the arteries of the *lower limbs*, and the resulting chronic ischaemia brings about various trophic changes, and also limping, and cramp-like ischaemic pain, induced by walking (*intermittent claudication*). Narrowing of the smallest arteries and arterioles—**arteriolosclerosis**—occurs commonly in the abdominal viscera and central nervous system as an ageing effect, and results particularly from arterial hypertension: it is usually most severe in the afferent arterioles of the *glomeruli*, where it brings about glomerular sclerosis. These regional changes are, however, more appropriately considered in relation to the various systems and organs.

Disturbances of Water and Salt Balance

Water and salt deficiency

The water content of the average male body, estimated by the deuterium method, is about 62%, and that of the female about 52%, the sex difference being accounted for by the higher fat content in females. A man weighing 70 kg contains about 42 litres and this is distributed as 30 litres of *intracellular* water and 12 litres of *extracellular* water; the latter is subdivided into about 3 litres of *intravascular* fluid, the plasma, and about 9 litres of *interstitial* fluid which is distinguished from the intravascular and intracellular fluids by its very low protein content.

The extracellular fluids contain practically all the sodium (except for that associated with collagen and that forming part of bone mineral), balanced chiefly by chloride and bicarbonate ions, whereas the intracellular fluid is almost devoid of sodium and chloride, its proteinate, sulphate and phosphate anions being balanced by potassium and magnesium. It is essential that the interstitial fluid should remain isotonic with the intravascular and intracellular fluids, and it contains a higher concentration of electrolytes which balances the colloid osmotic pressure of their proteins. Reductions in the water and salt content of the body are generally associated, but disproportionate depletion of either water or salt causes disturbances of the normal equilibrium which require different treatment. Deficiency of water tends to cause hypertonicity of the extracellular fluids so that water is withdrawn from the cells, which thus share in *primary dehydration*. Conversely, in relative salt depletion the extracellular fluids tend to become hypotonic, but this effect is minimised partly by increased renal excretion of water and partly by diffusion of water from the interstitial fluid into the cells with maintenance of isotonicity. Thus in salt deficiency the extracellular fluids are reduced in volume, but the administration of water or glucose solution without salt is actually harmful as it merely dilutes further the extracellular fluids and increases the diffusion of water into cells. *It is curious that whereas the need for water is normally indicated by thirst, in man there appears to be no urgent warning sensation when salt is lacking.*

Dehydration may be brought about in various ways and in minor degrees is very common. In hospital patients it is seen most often as a result of insufficient intake owing to physical weakness, coma and pyrexia. The urine is reduced in volume (500 ml) and is highly concentrated, the specific gravity rising to 1·04 or more. The plasma levels of Na^+, Cl^- and urea increase, probably as the result of diminished renal filtration, although the plasma volume is maintained relatively well by withdrawal of intracellular water and by active retention of Na^+ and excretion of K^+ under the influence of the renin–angiotensin–aldosterone system (p. 10.35) which is stimulated by the diminished blood volume—the so-called reaction of dehydration. More severe dehydration occurs under exceptional conditions, e.g. in people shipwrecked or

lost in the desert, and then the deficiency of body water may ultimately reach over 12% of body weight and amount to nearly 10 litres. Death is thought to be due to rise in the osmotic pressure of the cells. In children, the ratio of body surface to weight is higher than in adults so that cutaneous losses of water are proportionately greater; also children cannot produce such a high concentration of urine as can adults. As a result, lack of fluid has a more severe effect in infants and young children than in adults.

Salt depletion is a commoner cause of serious effects than is water depletion, and also is more liable to remain unrecognised. Excessive loss of sodium chloride from the body occurs in various conditions and is commonly only one factor in complex fluid and electrolyte disturbances. Loss of salt alone results from excessive sweating when water is consumed freely, e.g. in the tropics or when working in a very hot atmosphere. It gives rise to a state of 'heat exhaustion' which necessitates the administration of salt as well as water, the consumption of water alone being liable to produce severe cramps. Clinically, vomiting and diarrhoea are the most important causes of combined water and salt depletion: vomiting is complicated by alkalosis due to loss of H^+, and diarrhoea by acidosis from loss of the alkaline secretions of the small intestine. If water alone is restored, the picture of pure salt depletion follows: lowering of the osmotic pressure of the extracellular fluid leads to renal excretion of water and to increased osmotic absorption of water by the tissue cells. In consequence, there is severe depletion of both interstitial and intravascular fluid, and circulatory collapse (*shock*) supervenes. The effects of this *secondary extracellular dehydration* are actually more serious than those of the disturbed acid–base balance which may develop from disproportionate loss of sodium or chloride ions. The symptoms of salt depletion when water is consumed freely include lassitude, weakness, giddiness, fainting attacks and cramps; also anorexia, nausea and vomiting occur and tend to set up a vicious circle. Marked loss of weight and mental confusion may occur also. The plasma concentration of sodium, normally about 137–148 mmol/litre, falls to 130–120 mmol/litre or less. The chloride and bicarbonate concentrations are also reduced but their ratio varies with the presence of complicating acidosis or alkalosis. The blood is concentrated, with a rise of haemoglobin, haematocrit value and in plasma proteins. The urine contains little or no sodium or chloride except when the salt depletion is due to excessive renal loss, as in adrenocortical hypofunction (Addison's disease) or diabetic ketosis. The blood urea rises, often to over 17 mmol/litre (100 mg per dl), owing mainly to reduced renal blood flow and diminution in the volume of glomerular filtrate: this is known as *pre-renal uraemia* (p. 22.8).

Combined deficiency of water and salt is more common clinically than of either separately. Vomiting and diarrhoea are probably its most frequent cause. If water is ingested and retained, salt deficiency will predominate, as described above, but without fluid intake water loss exceeds salt loss. In such combined deficiency, the extracellular fluid therefore tends to become hypertonic and consequently fluid is withdrawn from the cells; this leads to symptoms like those of salt depletion and unless corrected may cause acute circulatory failure. The rise in blood urea often leads to the erroneous diagnosis of uraemia due to renal failure, but the administration of water and salt in adequate amounts may completely relieve the symptoms.

Regulation of the water content of the blood and urine is normally carried out by the kidneys, which in turn are controlled largely by secretion of antidiuretic hormone by the neurohypophysis: this regulates resorption of water in the distal renal tubule. The neurohypophysis is so highly sensitive to the osmotic influence of sodium chloride that an alteration of 1% in the osmotic pressure of the arterial blood can bring about a tenfold variation in the excretion of water, and the osmotic pressure of the extracellular fluids is thus very precisely controlled. Failure of this mechanism is seen in diabetes insipidus (p. 26.12), in which there is intense polyuria approaching maximum water excretion. An analogous situation in respect of excessive salt excretion results from failure of the secretion of adequate amounts of aldosterone by the adrenal cortex, e.g. in Addison's disease, in which the cortex is largely destroyed. Uncontrolled sodium loss in the urine leads to fall of the plasma sodium to far below the level at which it normally ceases to be excreted. In consequence, serious depletion of the body's store of sodium is brought about and this, if uncorrected, contributes greatly to the severe crises of Addison's disease and the tendency to acute circulatory collapse (p. 26.36). Other hormones also play minor parts in the regulation of water and salt excretion, e.g. ovarian hormones can cause a distinct retention of water, as is seen in the late phase of the menstrual cycle and in pregnancy.

The pathology of generalised oedema has to be viewed against this background of water and salt balance. Maintenance of osmotic equilibrium is more important for life and is therefore regulated more exactly than the total volume of fluid in the body or within any of its compartments. Most importance was formerly attached to the Cl^-, but it is now recognised that the Na^+ is even more significant in regulating the amount of body fluid in the extracellular compartment of the tissues, and that sodium is intimately concerned in the pathogenesis of oedema.

Water and salt retention: oedema

Oedema is an abnormal increase in the amount of interstitial fluid. It may be localised, e.g. in an organ, limb, etc., or more generalised. In generalised oedema there is usually accumulation of fluid also in the serous cavities (hydrothorax, ascites, etc.). When oedema affects the skin and subcutaneous tissue, swelling may be obvious, and momentary pressure will produce a depression ('pitting') which disappears in a few seconds as the oedema fluid returns to the tissue.

Control of interstitial fluid. It is widely accepted that the capillary endothelium has the physical properties of a semipermeable membrane, and that the passage of fluid across the walls of small blood vessels is determined by differences in hydrostatic and osmotic pressures of the fluid on either side of the wall. In 'resting' conditions, fluid is expelled from the arterial end of capillaries and re-enters at the venous end and in venules (Fig. 4.6, p. 4.7). Increase in the capillary hydrostatic pressure or rise in the osmotic pressure of the interstitial fluid will increase the net flow of fluid from the blood vessels into the interstitial space. A third factor of importance is the removal of interstitial fluid by the lymphatics, which can increase to several times the 'resting' rate of flow.

These factors are subject to both local and generalised variations, the causes of which are different. Accordingly, oedema may be localised to a part of the body, or it may be generalised.

Local oedema

This is caused by increased net loss of plasma fluid into the interstitial tissue or by obstruction of the lymphatic drainage.

Increased escape of plasma fluid can result from increased blood flow or from a rise in venous pressure. Increased blood flow occurs physiologically in metabolically active tissue, e.g. the leg muscles when running or the gastro-intestinal tract after a large meal. In these conditions, the arterioles are relaxed and capillary pressure rises, with increased net loss of fluid from the plasma. Oedema does not, however, develop, for the lymphatics are able to remove the increased amount of interstitial fluid.

In the **acute inflammatory reaction,** increased blood flow is accompanied by abnormal permeability of the endothelium of venules and capillaries, with escape of plasma proteins. Accordingly, not only is the vascular hydrostatic pressure raised, but the difference in osmotic pressure between the plasma and interstitial fluid is reduced. The result is greater loss of vascular fluid and diminished return of interstitial fluid to the vessels. The amount of fluid leaving the vessels is very often greater than can be removed by the lymphatics, and inflammatory oedema develops.

Oedema is thus a prominent feature of acute inflammatory lesions, including those caused by infections and also some hypersensitivity reactions. These have been described in previous chapters.

Hereditary angio-oedema is an uncommon condition characterised by acute attacks of localised oedema and pain, occurring most often in the skin of the face and trunk, but sometimes in the larynx, causing difficulty in breathing, and in the intestine, causing attacks of colicky abdominal pain and vomiting or diarrhoea.

In some cases, the condition is caused by a genetically-determined (autosomal dominant) defect of the inhibitor of the activated first component of complement (Cl-INH). This factor also inhibits activation of the kinin system, and inflammatory oedema probably results mainly from increased productions of kinins. Transfusion of fresh normal plasma has a temporary beneficial effect in preventing and treating attacks.

Similar conditions, apparently not genetically determined, occur in which local oedema results from pressure or exposure to cold, but their aetiology is obscure.

Another puzzling condition is *urticaria*, in which erythema, itching and wealing (sharply localised oedema) occurs in the superficial dermis. It is very common, and while in most cases attacks are occasional and mild, there may be frequent and severe attacks affecting much of the skin. In some patients, attacks occur after eating a particular food or taking certain drugs, notably aspirin. There is, however, very little firm evidence of an immunological hypersensitivity mechanism other than an increased incidence in individuals prone to atopic reactions. Histamine antagonists are sometimes beneficial, but in many cases the cause is unknown. Unless it is associated with a generalised anaphylactic reaction, urticaria is seldom a serious condition.

Local venous congestion and oedema. By raising the capillary pressure in the drainage area, venous obstruction predisposes to the development of oedema. The commonest example is the temporary oedema of the feet or ankles which develops, especially in old people, on sitting still for a long time, e.g. in travelling long distances. Leg movements help to pump the venous blood towards the heart, but if the legs are kept still, the valves of the leg veins do not alone interrupt the venous pressure gradient and oedema commonly results. Why this should occur more often in middle-aged and old people has not been explained.

The commonest cause of pathological venous obstruction is thrombosis of the deep leg veins (p. 10.15). In some cases, this is asymptomatic, but in others the affected leg becomes oedematous, and this occurs more often when the general circulation is impaired, e.g. by myocardial infarction. Experimentally, ligation of a major limb vein does not usually cause oedema in a healthy animal unless the draining lymphatics are also obstructed.

Venous obstruction is not a common lesion in internal organs, but when it does occur, ischaemic atrophy of the parenchyma is often a more prominent feature than oedema. Obstruction of the portal vein outside the liver does not usually cause oedema of the gastro-intestinal tract, but oedema with accumulation of fluid in the peritoneal cavity (*ascites*) is an important late feature of **cirrhosis of the liver.** In this condition, however, portal blood flow is impeded by fibrosis of the liver and in the late stages the hepatocytes fail to maintain adequate synthesis of plasma albumin, so that the osmotic pressure of the plasma falls. As noted below, a low plasma albumin level is an important cause of generalised oedema. A third feature of hepatic cirrhosis is the increased production of aldosterone in some cases: the cause of this is not known, but retention of sodium and water results, with aggravation of the ascites.

Chronic lymphatic obstruction. Although normal vascular endothelium is a largely effective barrier to macromolecules, small amounts of plasma proteins do escape from small blood vessels (p. 4.7). Such escaped protein cannot pass back directly into the blood vessels, and is removed by the lymphatics. In chronic lymphatic obstruction, fluid containing plasma protein (mainly albumin) therefore accumulates in the affected tissues. For unknown reasons, its presence is associated with growth of connective tissue, and the swollen tissue becomes firm and does not 'pit' on pressure.

Oedema from lymphatic obstruction is sometimes seen in the skin of the chest wall in breast cancer and is caused by extensive permeation of the lymphatics by cancer cells. 'Radical' surgery for breast cancer, including removal of the axillary lymph nodes and connective tissue, is sometimes followed by persistent and severe oedema of the whole of the arm and hand as a result of lymphatic obstruction, and radiotherapy may have a similar effect.

Lymphatic obstruction may also occur from involvement of lymphatics or lymph nodes in inflammatory conditions. For example, lymphogranuloma venereum (p. 25.3) may destroy the inguinal lymph nodes and cause oedema of the vulva. The filarial worm *Wuchereria bancrofti* lives in the lymphatic vessels. When it dies, it induces a chronic inflammatory reaction which obliterates lymphatics and may be followed by chronic oedema, most often in the lower limb and external genitalia. Overgrowth of the skin and connective tissue in the affected zone may be considerable, producing the condition known as **elephantiasis.**

Generalised oedema

It is important to appreciate that, regardless of its cause, generalised oedema represents retention of water and does not arise from a mere redistribution of the body fluids. In an adult, an increase of weight of about 5 kg invariably precedes the appearance of clinically recognisable generalised oedema, a fact utilised in the attention paid to the weight during pregnancy. Indeed, generalised oedema can be regarded as a method of disposing of excess fluid which cannot be discharged by the usual channels, in order to regulate the blood volume. The body appears to tolerate badly an increase in the volume of the intravascular fluid; the excess is shunted into the interstitial spaces where its presence requires the simultaneous retention of a sufficient quantity of electrolytes, chiefly salt, to equalise the osmotic pressure of this fluid with that of the cells and of the plasma. The osmotic effect of the intracellular and plasma proteins is balanced by a higher concentration of electrolytes—chiefly salt—in the interstitial fluid. It is unlikely that increase of capillary permeability to macromolecules plays any major part in the common forms of generalised oedema, for the protein content of oedema fluid is not sufficiently high to suggest this possibility. Also, there is no gross fall in the blood volume, as might be expected if exudation of protein-rich plasma fluid was an important factor. In rare cases, cyclical oedema has been accompanied by hypovolaemia, and it has been suggested that the oedema of hypothermia may be related to an increase of factors such as bradykinin, which increase capillary permeability.

Cardiac oedema is apt to develop in cases of **right ventricular failure** with longstanding systemic venous congestion. It appears first in the most dependent parts of the body and gradually extends upwards. Thus it is usually noticed first round the ankles, and pitting may be elicited by pressure over the lower end of the tibia. When the condition is advanced, the limbs become greatly swollen, the skin is tense and vesicles may form. Accumulation of fluid may occur also in the serous cavities. Distribution of the fluid depends on which parts of the body are most dependent, and in bedridden patients it collects particularly in the legs and backs of the thighs and lower trunk and in the scrotum.

As indicated above, increased transudation

from congested, dilated capillaries is not sufficient to produce oedema experimentally because the excess fluid is removed by the lymphatics. When, however, heart failure becomes severe, the diminution in cardiac output adversely affects renal function which depends upon normal renal blood flow. The kidneys can compensate to some extent for reduced blood supply by increasing the proportion of fluid filtered off in the glomeruli; this is probably mediated by increased tone in the efferent arterioles. The volume of urine is reduced and it is highly concentrated, indicating that there is excessive tubular re-absorption of water. The mechanism of this excessive re-absorption is not fully understood, but the reduced renal blood flow may stimulate the juxta-glomerular cells to secrete excess of renin, and this in turn will enhance the secretion of aldosterone by the adrenal cortex, with consequent re-absorption of sodium by the renal tubules. The effect of sodium retention is to stimulate secretion of anti-diuretic hormone by the neurohypophysis, and so more water is re-absorbed in the renal collecting tubules. This mechanism has been demonstrated to play a role in some, but not all, cases of cardiac oedema (p. 10.37). The stimulus to this secondary aldosteronism is not fully understood, as it occurs among patients with heart failure of both low and high cardiac output types. The great increase in body weight confirms the enormous amount of fluid retained in the oedematous tissues in cardiac failure, and the importance of water and salt retention is shown by the effect of diuretics in diminishing the oedema. Reduction in the intake of sodium chloride in the diet has also sometimes a markedly diuretic effect, water being eliminated with preservation of the isotonic state of the oedema fluid.

Other factors may play a part in the genesis of cardiac oedema, e.g. the accumulation in the tissues of waste products which, by their osmotic action, will tend to attract more water from the blood. There is also evidence that chronic hypoxia increases capillary permeability, although this view is not supported by the protein content of the oedema fluid, which is usually about 0·5% or less. The fundamental cause of cardiac oedema appears, however, to lie in the faulty elimination of fluid consequent upon the effect of the circulatory changes on renal function. The gravitational distribution of the retained fluid in the tissues is probably due to the greater venous pressure, and possibly greater reduction in blood flow, in the dependent parts of the body. Also, oedema fluid may gravitate along tissue spaces to reach the dependent parts. The distribution of oedema fluid is influenced also by the degree to which different tissues can be distended without a significant rise in tissue pressure.

In **failure of the left ventricle** of the heart, venous congestion occurs mainly in the lungs so long as the right ventricle continues to beat forcibly: pulmonary oedema may then develop without generalised oedema (p. 15.3).

Renal oedema. Generalised oedema occurs in various diseases which affect the glomeruli, including some types of glomerulonephritis, and also in acute renal failure due to injury to the renal tubules. The pathological changes in these conditions are described in Chapter 22. However, an understanding of the factors likely to be involved in the production of the various types of renal oedema depends not so much on a knowledge of the detailed structural changes but rather on the associated functional disturbances. Accordingly, renal diseases which give rise to oedema may be classified into the following three groups.

(1) Conditions in which all the glomeruli are affected, with reduction in renal blood flow and in glomerular filtration. This group is exemplified by *acute diffuse glomerulonephritis* and *rapidly progressive glomerulonephritis*. There is usually a rise in blood pressure and blood urea level, and production of a diminished amount of concentrated urine containing moderate amounts of protein. The oedema in these conditions is not influenced by gravity to the same extent as is cardiac oedema and is often noticed first in the loose connective tissues, e.g. of the eyelids and face: in ambulant patients, however, gravity is seen to have some effect. The protein content of the oedema fluid is usually less than 0·5% and the oedema therefore cannot be attributed to increased capillary permeability. Also, the proteinuria is usually only moderate and the loss does not result in any significant reduction in the levels of the plasma proteins. The blood volume is normal or increased, and the oedema seems likely to be due to excessive re-absorption of salt and water in the renal tubules. The factors responsible for this excessive reabsorption are not, however, clearly defined.

The renin–angiotensin–aldosterone system (p. 10.35) may be implicated, but even this is uncertain.

(2) *The nephrotic syndrome.* In some renal diseases, there is persistent and heavy loss of plasma proteins, particularly albumin, in the urine: when this exceeds about 10 g daily, the plasma albumin level falls considerably and this is accompanied by generalised oedema which often becomes very severe. This condition is known as the nephrotic syndrome. As in other types of renal oedema, the distribution of the tissue fluid is not so dependent on gravity as in cardiac oedema. In patients with nephrotic syndrome, the blood pressure is often not raised and there is commonly no rise in the blood urea, indicating that total renal blood flow and glomerular filtration rates are approximately normal. The nephrotic syndrome may arise in a large number of conditions: in some it is regularly present, for example in *glomerulonephritis* of *minimal-change* and *membranous* types (q.v.). It is a common result of *amyloid disease* involving the glomeruli; it occasionally complicates other types of glomerulonephritis and the glomerular lesions of diabetes mellitus and various other diseases. *In all these conditions, its development is dependent on excessive loss of plasma albumin into the glomerular filtrate.*

Glomerular leakage of protein exhibits a molecular sieving effect, the amount of plasma albumin which escapes being disproportionately great because of its relatively small molecular size. Also because of its small size and its relatively high concentration in the plasma, albumin is the protein mainly responsible for the osmotic pressure of the plasma, and consequently, in states of severe hypoalbuminaemia, the amount of fluid leaving the capillaries and venules throughout the body greatly exceeds the amount drawn back into them by osmosis. Accordingly, the plasma volume tends to fall and this brings into play the renin–angiotensin–aldosterone mechanism, resulting in increased re-absorption of sodium and water from the renal tubules: this tends, in turn, to dilute the plasma protein still further and so transudation into the tissues remains excessive; a vicious circle is set up and continues to operate so long as gross albuminuria persists. The involvement of the renin–angiotensin–aldosterone system is confirmed by the very high level of plasma aldosterone in the nephrotic syndrome. As would be expected, the oedema fluid has a very low protein content, and there is no evidence of general increased capillary permeability for macromolecules.

The importance of protein loss and hypoalbuminaemia is confirmed by the appearance of similar gross oedema in protein-losing enteropathy (p. 19.51) in which the kidneys are normal and there is gross loss of plasma protein into the gut.

(3) In *acute tubular injury*, the tubules lose their capacity for selective re-absorption and concentration of the glomerular filtrate. Consequently, most of the filtrate is re-absorbed and the small amount of urine produced approximates in its composition to a protein-free filtrate of plasma. There is retention of water and electrolytes and a progressive rise in blood urea. Apart from loss by sweating, vomiting, etc., most of the fluid taken by mouth is retained in the body, and, unless fluid intake is carefully controlled, gross oedema develops.

Acute tubular injury may result from shock or certain chemical poisons (p. 22.8). In some cases of acute renal failure following shock, the tubules show no convincing evidence of necrosis in a renal biopsy, and hyperactivity of the renin–angiotensin–aldosterone system appears to be involved (p. 22.11).

In the various forms of renal disease which are complicated by arterial hypertension, cardiac failure is liable to develop with consequent generalised or pulmonary oedema.

Nutritional (Famine) oedema

Generalised oedema is a feature of malnutrition. Protein insufficiency seems to be the main factor, and the extreme example is termed kwashiorkor (p. 20.8). Examination of the plasma shows a marked fall in glucose, lipids and proteins, the last being sometimes reduced to half the normal. Fall in osmotic pressure of the plasma is a factor in the production of the oedema, but no strict parallelism has been found, some cases failing to become oedematous in spite of severe depletion of serum albumin, while others show gross oedema with plasma protein levels within normal limits; also, if the state of nutrition is improved, the oedema may disappear before there is any significant rise in the colloid osmotic pressure of the plasma. Loss of fat, with consequent laxity and low tissue tension in the subcutaneous tissues, may also be a factor. Nutritional oedema is commonly associated with xerophthalmia, a condition in which opacity with ulceration of the cornea results from deficiency of the fat-soluble vitamin A; possibly lack of the vitamin B complex is also concerned, and the 'wet' (oedematous) form of beri-beri is perhaps related. A similar form of oedema has been observed in infants when there has been excess of carbohydrates in the diet with marked deficiency in other foodstuffs. In all such examples of nutritional oedema, the problem is a complex one, and the relative importance of the various factors outlined above varies in individual cases.

Oedema may occur in patients with chronic wasting diseases, e.g. cancer, tuberculosis, etc., and is due mainly to cardiac failure, although fall in the plasma proteins and the laxity of the connective tissues may also be contributory factors.

Pulmonary oedema

The osmotic pressure of the plasma (25 mm Hg) is substantially greater than the normal hydrostatic pressure in the pulmonary capillaries (8–10 mm Hg). Consequently, the development of oedema of the lungs usually requires a considerable rise in the hydrostatic pressure. As elsewhere, this occurs, together with increased vascular permeability, in acute inflammatory lesions, and inflammatory oedema is pronounced in severe influenza and lobar pneumonia, etc.

Pulmonary oedema can be produced readily in healthy dogs by interfering with the flow of pulmonary venous blood, for example by compressing the left atrium or ventricle, or constricting the aorta. Similarly, in man, it occurs in left ventricular failure, as in some cases of myocardial infarction and in systemic hypertension. In this latter condition, acute pulmonary oedema comes on especially when the patient is lying down, probably due to improved venous return from the legs, and perhaps also to increase in the blood volume by reabsorption of oedema fluid from the legs when recumbent. The attack is usually relieved by sitting up. Chronic pulmonary congestion, as, for example, in stenosis of the mitral valve,

is not alone sufficient to produce pulmonary oedema in man. This is probably because increase in tone of the hypertrophied pulmonary arterioles protects the pulmonary capillary bed from excessive rise in pressure. However, the situation is precarious, and pulmonary oedema is prone to result from physical exertion or other factors which increase the pulmonary blood flow. Chronic pulmonary oedema may occur as part of generalised renal oedema, particularly when there is, in addition, systemic hypertension, as in acute glomerulonephritis. Another important cause is overloading of the circulation by rapid transfusion of blood to patients with severe anaemia. Finally, pulmonary oedema occurs in some cases of increased intracranial pressure, most commonly in head injury or intracranial haemorrhage.

Apart from the above causes, oedema of the posterobasal parts of the lungs is a very common finding at autopsy, particularly in old people and where death is due to a toxic condition or has been preceded by coma. The oedema fluid is very prone to become infected by a mixture of bacteria, usually of low virulence, producing *hypostatic pneumonia* which, if untreated, is likely to be the immediate cause of death.

Depending on the causal factors, pulmonary oedema may be confined within the alveolar walls, i.e. interstitial oedema, or the fluid may pour into the alveolar spaces. The factors concerned are considered on pp. 16.19–20.

The renin–angiotensin–aldosterone system

The major components of this system (Fig. 10.33) are renin, angiotensin II and aldosterone. Renin is a proteolytic enzyme secreted by the kidney. It releases angiotensin I, an inactive decapeptide, from angiotensinogen, an α_2-globulin in plasma and tissue fluids. Angiotensin I is converted to the octapeptide angiotensin II by enzymes which are widely distributed in the tissues. Angiotensin II causes peripheral vasoconstriction and thus has a potent pressor effect. Conversion of angiotensin I in the plasma to angiotensin II occurs mainly in the pulmonary circulation, but conversion also occurs in the kidney and probably has an

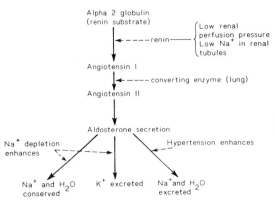

Fig. 10.33 Mechanisms involved in the renin-angiotensin-aldosterone system.

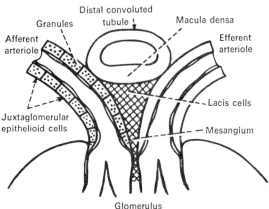

Fig. 10.35 Diagram of the juxta-glomerular apparatus.

important local effect. Angiotensin II is mainly responsible for stimulating the secretion of aldosterone by the adrenal cortex. Aldosterone increases re-absorption of Na^+ in the renal tubules and in some circumstances causes a rise in blood pressure, probably by increasing blood volume and cardiac output.

Renin is thus the main regulator of the system, the effects of which are mediated by angiotensin II and aldosterone.

Renin is synthesised, stored and secreted mainly by the granular cells in the walls of the distal part of the afferent glomerular arterioles (Fig. 10.34), which form part of the juxtaglomerular apparatus. Some renin-secreting cells are

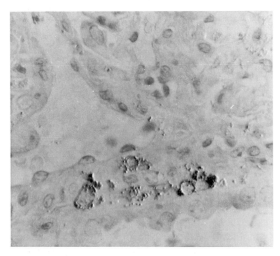

Fig. 10.34 Renin in the granular cells of an afferent glomerular arteriole (cut longitudinally). Renin was stained by the immunoperoxidase technique, using a polyclonal antibody.

also found in the walls of the efferent arterioles and arteries within the kidney. Most of the renin is secreted into the interstitium rather than into the lumen of the vessel, and probably passes into the blood via the peritubular capillaries. Secretion of renin is stimulated by a fall in pressure in the afferent arteriole. Another component of the juxtaglomerular apparatus, the macula densa, is a group of specialised tubular epithelial cells lining that part of the distal convoluted tubule adjacent to the glomerular arteriolar axis (Fig. 10.35): this is probably a sensor mechanism which regulates the release of renin in response to changes in the composition of the fluid in the tubular lumen. Release of renin is probably stimulated by a low Na^+ concentration in the tubule.

The systemic effects of renin have been studied more fully than its local action within the kidney, and will be considered first.

Systemic effects of renin. By releasing angiotensin, renin has three principal actions:

(a) Stimulation of the adrenal to secrete aldosterone.

(b) A pressor effect, mediated mainly by the vasoconstricting action of angiotensin II.

(c) A direct renal effect, in which angiotensin II modifies the urinary output of water and electrolytes.

Other actions, which hitherto have been less fully studied, are the central stimulation of thirst and release of catecholamines and vasopressin.

The relative dominance of the three principal actions mentioned above is much modified by the prevailing sodium status. Sodium deprivation, for example, enhances the aldosterone-stimulating effect of angiotensin II, while minimising its pressor action, so that marked increase of circulating renin, angiotensin II, and aldosterone occur with little or no rise in arterial blood pressure.

The direct renal effects of administered angiotensin vary widely according to the dosage, the prevailing sodium status, arterial pressure, and species. At most doses which can safely be given to normal man, angiotensin *reduces* renal excretion of sodium and water, and this effect is enhanced by severe sodium depletion, as in untreated Addison's disease. By contrast, in hypertension, irrespective of aetiology, and also in hepatic cirrhosis with ascites, angiotensin usually *increases* water and sodium loss.

Secondary hyperaldosteronism. The renin-angiotensin-aldosterone system is stimulated, and high circulating levels of all three components may be found, in sodium depletion, whether due to dietary sodium restriction, sodium-losing renal disease, diuretics or purgatives: haemorrhage and shock produce a similar response. In these situations the increase in aldosterone is in response to a rise in renin, and is termed 'secondary' hyperaldosteronism.

Secondary hyperaldosteronism develops in some but by no means all, cases of *untreated congestive heart failure*, in *hepatic cirrhosis with ascites*, and in *the nephrotic syndrome*. It may seem paradoxical that patients with these oedematous states, with their retention of sodium and water, should react as though sodium-deprived. The explanation is probably that the excess sodium and water is principally extravascular, and thus not capable of recognition by the kidney. The kidney therefore responds as in sodium deprivation; hence plasma renin and angiotensin, and in consequence, aldosterone, are elevated.

Renal artery stenosis. The old belief that renal artery constriction, by leading to increased circulating renin and angiotensin, is simply and directly responsible for hypertension via the pressor effect of angiotensin (p. 14.21) is a considerable oversimplification. It is clear, however, that in many cases of severe renal artery stenosis with hypertension, both renin and aldosterone are increased. A similar mechanism—possibly multiple intrarenal arterial lesions—may be the cause of the secondary hyperaldosteronism which accompanies malignant hypertension in which, irrespective of aetiology, the plasma levels of renin and angiotensin II are often very high. Similarly, in some cases of chronic renal failure, the level of angiotensin II is sufficiently high to have a direct pressor effect. However, angiotensin II also raises blood pressure by a slower-developing mechanism: infusion of angiotensin II at a rate too low to have a direct vasoconstrictor effect raises the blood pressure gradually and sometimes markedly. Some workers consider that this second effect is more important in renal artery stenosis than the direct vasoconstrictor effect of angiotensin II.

In pregnancy, there is a physiological increase in the plasma levels of renin, renin-substrate, angiotensin II and aldosterone.

A particularly interesting form of secondary hyperaldosteronism is found in the rare condition of benign juxta-glomerular-cell tumour, which occurs mainly in young patients.

Other patterns of variation in circulating renin and aldosterone are readily predictable. Sodium loading, or the administration of sodium-retaining substances such as DOC, fluorocortisone, carbenoxolone or liquorice, depress circulating renin and aldosterone.

Primary hyperaldosteronism. An adrenocortical adenoma secreting an excess of aldosterone leads to sodium retention, and thus to the combination of renin suppression with elevated aldosterone. This is known as '*primary*' *hyperaldosteronism* (p. 26.34). The same combination will also be seen in any situation where excess aldosterone secretion is stimulated by mechanisms other than the renin–angiotensin system.

Hypoaldosteronism. In Addison's disease, the sodium deficiency stimulates marked secretion of renin, but aldosterone production remains deficient despite this stimulus, because the diseased adrenal cortex is unable to respond appropriately.

Primary renin deficiency, found mainly in elderly patients, is accompanied by selective aldosterone deficiency, cortisol secretion being normal.

Direct effects of renin and angiotensin on the kidney. There are extrarenal renin-angiotensin systems in various tissues. Since they do not contribute to plasma hormone levels, they probably act locally. Renin also acts locally in the kidney where its release generates angiotensin II in the interstitium. The kidney is thus affected by both angiotensin in the plasma and that which is generated locally. The direct renal effects of angiotensin II have proved difficult to study in isolation from its pressor and aldosterone stimulating effects.

As mentioned earlier, a small proportion of angiotensin I can be converted to angiotensin II in the interstitial fluid around the efferent arteriole, and may play a part in autoregulation of renal blood flow. In addition, it may modulate the glomerular filtration rate of individual nephrons in response to a signal from the macula densa. Glomeruli have receptors for angiotensin II and under its influence the mesangial cells cause glomeruli to contract. Locally-generated intrarenal angiotensin II may also affect the handling of sodium by tubules in addition to its effect as a circulating hormone. These postulated local effects are under active investigation.

Many years ago Goormaghtigh suggested that a renal effect of renin might be responsible for the reduced renal blood flow and oliguria of acute renal failure (see p. 22.10). This is now supported by the demonstration that very large doses of angiotensin II can produce acute renal failure with tubular necrosis in experimental animals. A wide variety of stimuli causing increases in renin secretion predispose to acute renal failure with or without renal tubular necrosis. These include cardiac failure, sodium depletion, pregnancy, haemorrhage, Addison's disease and renal artery occlusion. Conversely, sodium loading and renal denervation reduce renin levels and are thought to protect against acute renal failure.

Shock

Definition and nature of shock. Shock is the name given to the complex series of changes which result from an acute fall in cardiac output.

These changes include regulatory mechanisms which are beneficial in that they tend to maintain the blood supply to those organs with the most vital and urgent perfusion requirements—the heart and the central nervous system. This is, however, achieved only by severe reduction in the circulation through most of the other tissues, and unless cardiac output can be restored without undue delay, ischaemic injury to the specialised cells of the various organs results in multi-organ failure.

A clear distinction should be made between shock and the *fainting* or *vaso-vagal* attack. The latter is immediate, can result from all grades of injury, from severe pain, or from psychogenic stimuli such as a fright or witnessing an accident or surgical operation. Fainting is characterised by pallor, sweating, weakness, sometimes vomiting, a slow pulse, marked fall in blood pressure due to widespread arteriolar dilatation and loss of consciousness from cerebral ischaemia: convulsions may also occur. These changes last only a few minutes and recovery is rapid. The fainting attack is mentioned here because it used to be known as 'primary shock'. In fact, it is quite distinct from shock, and should not be confused with it.

Causes and types of shock

The three major causes of shock are:
1. Reduction of blood volume, which induces **hypovolaemic shock**: examples include *severe haemorrhage*, *extensive vascular exudation* as in burns, and conditions which cause *dehydration*.
2. Acute cardiac insufficiency, i.e. severe fall in cardiac output caused by an acute cardiac lesion, usually myocardial infarction. This is termed **cardiogenic shock.**
3. Severe infections, usually with bacteriaemia or septicaemia, which induce **septic shock**.

Although all three major types have many features in common, they also differ in important ways. It is also necessary to emphasise that the longer shock persists, the more complicated it becomes, and in advanced shock all three factors—hypovolaemia, cardiac insufficiency and bacterial infection—are often combined. It is convenient to give first an account of hypovolaemic shock, and then to describe the special features of the other types.

The features of *anaphylactic shock* (p. 7.6), the shock-like state of *acute immune-complex disease* (p. 7.16), and shock arising in decompression sickness (p. 10.21) are described elsewhere.

Hypovolaemic shock

This results most commonly from **acute severe haemorrhage,** due to trauma, to involvement of blood vessels in disease processes, or to a haemorrhagic disorder. Another important cause is **severe burning**, in which hypovolaemia results from inflammatory exudation of plasma fluid from the damaged small blood vessels in the vicinity of extensive burns. Thirdly, hypovolaemic shock can develop in **severe acute dehydration**, for example in severe gastroenteritis or cholera.

Clinical features

The shocked patient is often restless and confused, has a pale, cold, sweaty skin, often with peripheral cyanosis, a rapid weak pulse, a low blood pressure, increased rate and depth of respiration, and may become drowsy and confused and finally comatose.

Haemorrhagic and traumatic shock

A normal healthy adult can lose 550 ml of blood, i.e. about 10% of the blood volume, without any significant disability; the blood volume is almost restored within a few hours, although replacement of plasma proteins takes a day or two, and restoration of red cells takes much longer. Loss of 25% of the blood (about 1250 ml) results in significant hypovolaemia over the next 36 hours, while a rapid loss of about half the blood so reduces the circulation that death is likely unless the blood volume is restored therapeutically.

Early changes. Acute hypovolaemia results in a reduced central (systemic) venous pressure and so a diminished flow of blood into the right atrium. The stroke volume is thus lowered and the cardiac output and arterial blood pressure fall. These haemodynamic changes trigger off peripheral and central baro-receptors with consequent sympathico-adrenal stimulation, and there is a huge increase in the levels of catecholamines in the plasma, sometimes by over 200 times. As a result of impaired renal perfusion, there is also intense secretion of renin and therefore great increase of angiotensin II and aldosterone levels in the plasma (p. 10.37).

The combined effects of these massive amounts of vasoactive agents include an increase in the tone of the systemic veins so that, in spite of their reduced content of blood, central venous pressure and right atrial filling are partially restored, the heart rate increases, and the effect of hypovolaemia on the circulation is minimised. Put more simply, increased venous tone reduces the total size of the vascular compartment, favouring the continued circulation of the reduced volume of blood within it. The high levels of catecholamines and angiotensin also cause constriction of the arterioles and venules in the skin, splanchnic area, and indeed most of the tissues of the body, so that peripheral resistance is increased, and even without treatment *the blood pressure may be partially or fully restored, although tissue perfusion is low.* The heart and central nervous system do not suffer to the same extent as the other tissues because they can autoregulate their own perfusion: their small blood vessels do no contract in response to noradrenaline, etc., but have an inherent property of relaxing when the blood pressure falls and contracting when it rises. In consequence of this autoregulatory mechanism, *cerebral and coronary blood flow are maintained close to normal levels at blood pressures down to 50 mm Hg.* At this pressure, arteriolar relaxation is maximal and perfusion rapidly falls off at lower pressures.

This, then, is the haemodynamic status in early shock. Compensating changes have tended to keep up the cardiac output and blood pressure, and the brain and heart are preferentially supplied with blood at the expense of diminished perfusion of the other tissues. If less than 25% of the blood has been lost, and if there are no serious complicating factors (see below), the blood volume will rise naturally: vasoconstriction of the arterioles is greater than in the venules, so that the pressure in the capillaries is low and extravascular fluid passes into them (p. 4.7), and the high level of aldosterone in the plasma promotes retention of salt and water. The circulation is nevertheless precarious, and further bleeding, major surgery to deal with the causal injury or bleeding vessel, severe pain, or the development of infection, will all tend to increase the circulatory deficit. *It is therefore important, in all save the mildest cases, to restore the blood volume by intravenous administration of fluid.* The nature of the fluid is not so important as the avoidance of delay: buffered saline or macromolecular solutions (plasma, dextran, etc.) are both effective initially, but macromolecular solutions have the advantage of maintaining the osmotic pressure of the plasma, thus tending to hold fluid in circulation, and are usually used for losses of around 25% or more of the blood. It is also important to maintain the haematocrit at around 30% in order to minimise tissue hypoxia, and matched blood (or in an urgent situation Group O Rh-negative blood) are normally administered if haemorrhage has exceeded 25% of the blood. Some estimate of the volume of fluids required can be made from the amount of blood lost, the clinical state, and the severity and nature of injury, but account must also be taken of internal haemorrhage, e.g. into the gastro-intestinal tract or around a fracture. The haemoglobin and haematocrit levels are not reliable guides to the degree of hypovolaemia during the first 36 hours. In the absence of cardiac insufficiency, a low blood pressure is an indication of hypovolaemia in early shock, but because of the compensatory mechanisms described above, it may be normal or nearly so in patients with serious hypovolaemia. A low central venous pressure is often, although not always, a useful indication of hypovolaemia, and if possible this should be monitored in all except mild cases of shock.

Although the peripheral vasoconstriction of shock serves a compensatory function, it is also harmful by reducing tissue perfusion of abdominal viscera and it may, by increasing peripheral resistance, induce heart failure (see below). In some cases, the blood pressure may rise above normal, and the vasoconstriction may persist in spite of restoration of the blood volume. Drugs which promote vasodilatation (e.g. thymoxamine, sodium nitroprusside) are therefore sometimes beneficial, but only when steps have been taken to restore the blood volume: in the hypovolaemic patient they are liable to cause further circulatory collapse.

The changes of advanced shock. If shock persists, the widespread arteriolar constriction gradually passes off, but venular constriction is more persistent and capillary pressure rises with consequent loss of fluid into the extravascular space and further fall in blood volume. At this late stage of shock, the capillaries are congested with slowly-flowing blood, and *cyanosis* may be apparent. The general reduction in blood supply to the tissues is aggravated by a number of complex factors brought about by changes in the blood itself and by the injury to vascular endothelium and tissue cells caused by perfusion failure. Some of the changes are as follows:

(*a*) *Viscosity of the blood* is increased by the haemoconcentration resulting from loss of plasma fluid. This leads to sludging of the red cells and rouleaux formation and these effects are increased by the rise in plasma fibrinogen which follows haemorrhage.

(*b*) *Release of thromboplastin* (clotting factor III) from hypoxic endothelium and tissue cells results in the production of thrombin, which promotes aggregation of platelets and occasionally leads to disseminated intravascular coagulation (p. 10.11).

(*c*) *Neutrophil polymorphs* adhere to the injured vascular endothelium of small vessels.

(*d*) *Hypoxic injury* results in release of lysosomal enzymes and secretory products into the blood. Proteolytic enzymes, e.g. trypsin from the pancreas, may activate the kinin system and thus further embarrass the circulation by causing vasodilatation and increased permeability. Production of prostaglandins may also be increased: those of the E group have a kinin-like effect, while the F group may increase the resistance to pulmonary blood flow.

Metabolic disturbances. The hypoxia of shock interferes profoundly with cell metabolism. It prevents the entrance of pyruvic acid into the citric acid cycle and in consequence lactic acid accumulates and glucose passes out of the hypoxic cells, leading to insulin-resistant hyperglycaemia and increased glycogenolysis. These metabolic disturbances, together with high levels of catecholamines, result in a rise of fatty acids and amino acids in the plasma. Impaired carbohydrate metabolism results in a fall in production of adenosine triphosphate and so energy is not available for many cell functions, including the sodium pump: *potassium leaves the cells and sodium and water enter and cause swelling: these effects, sometimes termed the 'sick cell syndrome' may, by lowering the level of blood sodium, lead to inappropriate administration of salt.*

Metabolic acidosis, with rise in blood lactic acid, contributes to the increased respiratory effort observed in patients with shock.

Organ function in shock. While all the organs are affected in shock, respiratory and cardiac failure are commonly of life-threatening importance. Quite apart from cardiogenic shock (see below), **acute heart failure**, first of the left and then of both ventricles, may develop in severe hypovolaemic or septic shock, and is particularly common in older patients with pre-existing coronary artery disease. The increased load on the heart resulting from peripheral vasoconstriction and its treatment with vasodilator drugs have been considered above. A factor which reduces myocardial contractility (*myocardial depressant factor*) has been detected in the plasma of shocked patients who subsequently died of cardiac failure: it is believed to be released from the pancreas. The impaired blood flow of severe shock, together with activation of the clotting mechanism, predispose to coronary thrombosis in patients with coronary artery disease. If operation is necessary, anaesthetic drugs may also impair cardiac function. Monitoring of the cardiac filling* and systemic

---

* The central venous pressure is used as a measure of the right heart filling pressure and the pulmonary artery 'wedge' pressure as an indication of the left heart filling pressure.

arterial pressures, and particularly of changes in them during intravascular administration of fluid, helps to distinguish between hypovolaemia and cardiac insufficiency in shock. In some cases, drugs such as dopamine or digitalis, which increase myocardial contractility, are beneficial.

Disturbance of gas exchange in the **lungs** is another important complication of shock, and can be assessed by comparing the mixed venous and arterial oxygen tensions. Improvement usually follows restoration of the blood volume, together with intermittent positive-pressure ventilation if necessary, but in some cases pulmonary function continues to deteriorate due to a combination of causes—pulmonary oedema, alveolar collapse, intravascular fibrin formation, embolism, infection, etc., known collectively as **shock lung** (p. 16.22), and death is then likely to result largely from the additional burden of respiratory failure.

Perfusion of the **kidneys** in shock is directly proportional to the blood pressure. Production of urine ceases at about 50 mm Hg and if the pressure remains low for some hours, focal hypoxic injury to the tubular epithelium may be associated with acute renal failure which persists for days or weeks after recovery from shock (p. 22.10). Renal damage is particularly common in shock associated with crush injury, childbirth, incompatible blood transfusion or severe infection.

Because of its autoregulatory mechanism, blood flow to the **brain** is relatively well-maintained unless the blood pressure falls below 50 mm Hg. Even a brief period of more severe hypotension can cause severe ischaemic brain damage (p. 10.24). Ischaemic centrilobular necrosis of liver cells may also occur, although liver failure is seldom prominent.

Other causes of hypovolaemic shock

Burns. In burning or scalding, necrosis of the more superficial tissues is accompanied by a lesser degree of injury to the underlying tissues, the reaction to which is acute inflammation, with increased vascular permeability and exudation of protein-rich fluid. When the area involved is extensive (10% or more of the skin surface), the loss of fluid is severe enough to induce hypovolaemia and shock. The changes are similar to those following haemorrhage but hypovolaemia develops more slowly, haemoconcentration is more pronounced, with attendant sludging and rouleaux formation. There is usually a marked leucocytosis, and the state of shock may recur or increase on the second or third days as a result of infection or absorption of breakdown products from the necrotic tissue. The principles of treatment of burn shock are the same as for haemorrhagic shock, but the loss is of plasma rather than whole blood, so that plasma transfusions are used initially. Some destruction of red cells does however, occur in the burned area, and in very extensive burning severe anaemia may develop, necessitating blood transfusion. Another important complication of burning is bacterial infection, the dead tissue providing a good culture medium from which bacteria commonly invade the underlying tissue and bloodstream. Streptococci and staphylococci were formerly the most important invaders, but with antibiotic therapy, Gram-ve bacilli, and especially *Pseudomonas aeruginosa*, now predominate. The features of septic shock commonly supervene, and sepsis is now the major cause of death from burns.

Dehydration, if severe, causes hypovolaemic shock, although the blood volume is reduced relatively less than the extravascular fluid, and the effects of cellular dehydration are regarded as the usual cause of death (p. 10.29).

Cardiogenic shock

Acute lesions of the heart may severely reduce cardiac output and the subsequent haemodynamic and other changes are similar to those in hypovolaemic shock. The cardiac filling pressures are, however, raised, and although the clinical features—pallor, weak rapid pulse, sweating, etc.—are the same as in hypovolaemia, intravenous administration of fluids, which is beneficial in selected cases, must proceed with caution.

The commonest cause is myocardial infarction, and although only a small proportion of patients with this condition develop the full picture of shock, the mortality from this complication is very high even in highly competent coronary care units. Other conditions which can cause cardiogenic shock include rupture of a valve cusp, major arrhythmias, and cardiac tamponade due to haemopericardium (resulting from direct trauma or as a complication of a ruptured myocardial infarct). Although not strictly cardiogenic shock, acute obstruction to blood flow by pulmonary emboli can result in a similar condition. As already indicated, cardiac insufficiency can develop as a complication of hypovolaemic and other types of shock.

Septic (Endotoxic) shock

Some patients with septicaemia or extensive localised infections, e.g. generalised peritonitis, pass into a state of shock which resembles that of hypovolaemia, but is often more prolonged, with a higher incidence of serious complications, and an overall mortality exceeding 50%.

Septic shock is a common complication of infected burns, and of surgical operations, manipulations or instrumentation on an infected urogenital or biliary tract or on the gastrointestinal tract. It occurs also in patients with immunodeficiency states, such as leukaemia and lymphomas, and as a complication of cytotoxic drugs or immunosuppressive therapy. Many such patients are dehydrated, and this is an important predisposing factor.

In a patient with known sepsis, high fever and symptoms and signs of shock, the diagnosis is not difficult, but in many patients, especially the elderly and following surgical procedures, septic shock develops insidiously, often without fever, and there may be an initial 'hyperdynamic' stage in which cardiac output is increased, the blood pressure reduced, peripheral resistance low, and the skin warm: these features may be due to bacteria-mediated release of kinins and other vaso-active agents. More often circulatory changes are similar from the onset to those of hypovolaemia, with pallor, sweating, cold extremities, increased peripheral resistance and reduced cardiac output, etc. Septic shock is particularly difficult to reverse and, as with other forms of shock, the longer it persists the more refractory it becomes. Tissue hypoxia results in widespread derangement of cell function, and features of multi-organ failure often develop. **Respiratory failure** due to 'shock lung' is often combined with **cardiac failure** and

arrhythmias. **Acute renal failure** is also very common, although (as in hypovolaemic shock) many of its serious effects develop after recovery from shock.

Disseminated intravascular coagulation (p. 17.68) is more prone to develop in septic than in hypovolaemic shock. It interferes further with organ perfusion and may greatly aggravate pulmonary failure, or may, by consumption of clotting factors and activation of the plasmin system, progress to a bleeding state with widespread haemorrhage, e.g. from the gastrointestinal mucosa.

Treatment of septic shock is based on elimination of the causal infection, restoration of the circulation, and correction of hypoxaemic metabolic acidosis and electrolyte imbalance. Antibiotic therapy cannot usually await the results of bacteriological culture of the blood etc. and tests for sensitivity, although it may need to be modified subsequently depending on the bacteriological findings. The choice and rate of administration of intravascular fluids will depend on the results of monitoring procedures and haematological and biochemical tests. These include monitoring the cardiac filling and systemic arterial pressures, and frequent assay of the blood gases and pH, plasma electrolytes and osmolality, platelet counts and haematocrit. It may also be necessary to assay the status of the coagulation and plasmin systems. Intermittent positive-pressure ventilation, instituted at an early stage, has been shown to decrease the risk of the development of pulmonary failure, and drugs which increase cardiac output and tissue perfusion may be of value. The prognosis depends very much on the availability of experienced staff and facilities.

Aetiology. The microbial factors responsible for septic shock are by no means fully elucidated. With widespread use of antibiotics, the aerobic Gram-ve bacilli have replaced the pyogenic cocci as the major cause of septicaemia and bacteraemia. The organisms most commonly responsible include *Esch. coli, Proteus, Klebsiella* and, in cases of burns, *Pseudomonas aeruginosa*. About 50% of patients with blood infection by these bacteria develop septic shock. Bacteroides (the anaerobic non-sporing bacilli which constitute over 99% of the faecal flora) are now recognised as an important cause of blood infection, and about 30% of cases are complicated by shock. All these Gram-ve bacteria release endotoxins when they die, and there is a widespread belief that endotoxin is a major cause of the manifestations of septic shock. Animals injected with endotoxin present many of the features of septic shock, including disseminated intravascular coagulation (the so-called *Schwartzmann reaction*, p. 8.8), and endotoxin is detectable in the blood of shocked patients with Gram-ve septicaemia by means of the limulus test (in which endotoxin is detected by its property of clotting a lysate of the blood amoebocytes of *Limulus polyphemus*, the horse-shoe crab). The limulus test is, however, time-consuming and, unless performed by an expert, can be misleading.

The properties of endotoxins (p. 8.7), which are thought to induce septic shock include activation of Hageman factor, with consequent triggering of the complement, coagulation, kinin and fibrinolytic systems, activation of platelets, activation of complement by the alternative pathway and stimulation of neutrophil polymorphs to release cationic proteins, etc.

Although septic shock is a particularly common complication of extensive Gram-ve infections, a similar condition occurs less commonly in severe Gram +ve bacterial infections, and is presumably induced by exotoxins.

In the past few years a serious but rare condition known as the *toxic shock syndrome* has been described in women. It occurs during menstruation and is associated with the use of highly absorbent tampons. It is caused by absorption of toxins produced by *Staphylococcus aureus* growing in the menstrual blood in the tampon. Clinical features include headache, dizziness, myalgia, conjunctivitis, nausea, abdominal pain, vomiting and diarrhoea and skin rashes. In severe cases, shock, disseminated intravascular coagulation and respiratory distress may prove fatal. The incidence has been reduced by use of less highly absorbent tampons (see Shepherd, 1982).

Severe shock sometimes develops in patients with fungal or acute viral infections, and in some instances immune-complex formation may be involved.

Other causes of shock

Some cases of shock do not fall into any of the three major types described above. For example, escape of gastric or duodenal juice into the peritoneal cavity, via a perforated peptic ulcer, causes severe shock, and so does acute haemor-

hagic pancreatitis (which is non-bacterial), and ingestion of many poisons. In these conditions, it is likely that shock is chemically induced, but there may also be severe pain which, without doubt, aggravates shock.

Severe shock results from transfusion of strongly incompatible blood to which the recipient has iso-antibodies; also in acute circulating immune-complex disease (p. 7.16) and acute generalised anaphylaxis (p. 7.6).

Morphological changes in shock

The morphological changes in patients dying from shock are often inconspicuous. In spite of the fundamental disturbances of cell function, the parenchymal cells in general usually show only swelling and sometimes fatty change. In addition to the causal changes—injury, haemorrhage, coronary thrombosis, septicaemia, etc.—there may be various pulmonary changes, including oedema, congestion, hyaline membrane formation, collapse and bronchopneumonia (p. 16.22). The kidneys usually show the pallor and cortical swelling of acute tubular injury (p. 22.9) and there may be centrilobular hepatic necrosis. If the patient has survived sufficiently long for its recognition, there may be acute ischaemic necrosis in the 'boundary' zones of the brain (p. 21.17). Features of disseminated intravascular coagulation include widespread haemorrhages, and microscopy may reveal fibrin thrombi in the small vessels, especially in the lungs and kidneys (Fig. 10.36). The adrenals show the lipid depletion of the 'stress' reaction (p. 26.31), but occasionally there is a combination of haemorrhage and necrosis, particularly in septic shock associated with meningococcal septicaemia.

Metabolism after injury

The metabolic disturbances associated with shock (p. 10.40) include incomplete carbohydrate catabolism, metabolic acidosis, disturbed protein and fat metabolism and a rise in the blood levels of glucose, amino acids and fatty acids. These changes were demonstrated experimentally by Cuthbertson, who termed

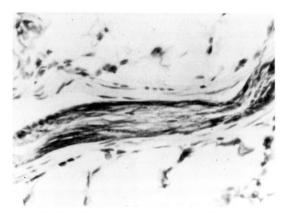

Fig. 10.36 Fibrin thrombus in a small pulmonary vessel in a case of disseminated intravascular coagulation. × 200.

them the '*ebb phase*'. Energy production is consequently depressed, and there is a general disorder of cellular metabolic processes. These changes are liable to develop in the first days following a severe injury, burn or surgical operation. Following the period of shock (or 2–3 days after such injury when shock has been prevented), the metabolism changes to a '*flow phase*' in which there is increased energy (and heat) production, due largely to breakdown of depot fat and protein, with consequent loss of weight and a negative nitrogen balance. During this period, which may persist for days or months depending on the severity of the injury, carbohydrate catabolism is complete and there is no metabolic acidosis unless carbohydrate intake is low. The mechanism of the increased metabolic activity, which resembles that in fever, is uncertain, but weight loss can be minimised by a high calorie, high protein diet, and a warm environment.

Blood Groups and Blood Transfusion

Before administering a blood transfusion, it is essential to make sure that the donor's red cells are compatible to the patient, and in particular that the patient's plasma does not contain iso-antibodies reactive with surface antigens on the donor's red cells. The ABO blood group system is of outstanding importance, for iso-antibodies are normally present in the plasma (see Table 10.2) and their reaction with incompatible transfused red cells usually causes a severe haemolytic reaction with fever, shock, often acute renal failure and sometimes death. The rhesus (Rh) blood group system comes next in importance. Unlike the ABO system, Rh iso-antibodies are not usually present in the plasma, but they sometimes develop as a result of an Rh-incompatible blood transfusion or pregnancy.

For blood transfusion, the patient's ABO and Rh types should be determined and blood of the same type should be selected for transfusion. In addition, it is necessary to perform a *compatibility* or *cross-matching* test in which the donor's red cells are incubated in the recipient's serum at 37°C, and the cells are then examined for agglutination and also by the antiglobulin test (p. 6.11) to detect non-agglutinating (IgG) antibodies in the recipient's serum. The purpose

Table 10.2   The four ABO blood groups

Blood group	Red cell antigens	Iso-antibodies in serum	Can accept blood of group	Can donate to patients of group	Incidence in Britain* (%)
AB	AB	nil	all groups	AB	3
A	A	anti-B	A, O	A, AB	42
B	B	anti-A	B, O	B, AB	8
O	O	anti-A + anti-B	O	all groups	47

*The frequencies of the four groups vary greatly between different races.

of this procedure is to detect (1) technical or clerical errors in grouping and in collection and storage of the donor's blood, and (2) the presence of unusual iso-antibodies in the recipient's plasma.

As a life-saving measure, it may be appropriate to transfuse Group O, Rh–ve blood to a patient of unknown group, but it is usually preferable to administer plasma while grouping procedures are being performed, and in any case the direct matching procedure should always be performed.

Incompatibility can also arise when a donor's blood contains high-titre antibodies reactive with the patient's red cells. Transfusion reactions from this cause are not usually severe because the donor's plasma (and thus the antibody) is diluted *in vivo* by the recipient's plasma. If donor and recipient are of the same ABO and Rh type the danger is largely excluded.

The ABO group

Individuals can be classified into four groups by the presence or absence of A and B antigens on their red cells and of anti-A and anti-B antibodies in their plasma (or serum). Table 10.2 shows the features of the four groups.

Standardised anti-A and anti-B serum (from selected subjects of group B and A respectively) are used to determine the group to which any individual belongs. If the red cells are agglutinated by both sera the blood belongs to group AB, if agglutinated by group B serum alone the blood belongs to group A, if by group A serum alone to group B, and if by neither serum, it belongs to group O. Since the serum of group AB does not agglutinate the red cells of any of the groups an individual of group AB can receive the red cells of any other group and is thus a 'universal recipient'. The cells of an individual of group O are not agglutinated by the serum of any group; the red cells can be transfused into an individual of any group and such persons are known as 'universal donors'.

The three blood group substances A, B and O are determined by allelic genes, one from each parent, so that there are six genotypes (AA, BB, AB, AO, BO and OO). O substance, however, is for practical purposes non-antigenic, and accordingly grouping is based on the presence or absence of A and B, giving the four phenotypes, which were first detected by Landsteiner. The natural iso-antibodies are mainly of IgM class, and develop after birth, apparently as a result of exposure to bacterial and other substances antigenically similar to A and B. Group A (or B) individuals are immunologically tolerant to A (or B) antigens and so do not develop the corresponding antibodies.

The Rhesus (RH) groups

The Rh blood group system was discovered by Landsteiner and Wiener (1940), who were interested in the antigens of human and animal red cells, and noted that guinea-pig or rabbit antisera to the red cells of *Macacus rhesus* monkeys agglutinated the red cells of 84% of white Americans; accordingly, these 84% were called Rh-positive, and the 16% of non-reactors, Rh-negative. The human Rh system is, however, more complex, and further elucidation has come from the use of iso-antibodies which, unlike the ABO antibodies, are not routinely present in human serum, but develop in about 50% of Rh– subjects transfused with Rh+ blood, and in about 5% of Rh– women as a result of an Rh+ pregnancy (p. 7.12). Once Rh antibodies have developed, a subsequent Rh+ blood transfusion is likely to cause an acute reaction with immune destruction of the transfused red cells by a cytotoxic antibody (type II) reaction, while an Rh+ fetus is liable to suffer from haemolytic disease of the newborn (p. 17.30).

Rhesus iso-antibodies may be of either IgM or IgG class: their demonstration requires incubation with appropriate red cells at 37°C. IgG antibodies sensitise the red cells without agglutinating them, and are usually detected by the antiglobulin reaction (p. 6.11), by methods which render red cells agglutinable by Rh antibodies, e.g. treating the red cells with papain or suspending them in a concentrated albumin solution.

Rh sub-groups. In simple terms, Rh blood group antigens are determined by three pairs of allelic genes, one of which codes for antigens C or c, one for D or d and the third for E and e. As the genes are closely linked, they are transmitted as haplotypic 'sets' which may be expressed as CDe, cde, etc., or by a set of symbols (R_1, r, etc.). The frequency of the eight possible

Table 10.3 The major Rh haplotypes and their frequency in Britain.

Haplotype	Abbreviation	Frequency*†
CDe	R_1	0·420
cde	r	0·389
cDE	R_2	0·141
cDe	R_0	0·026
cdE	r″	0·012
Cde	r′	0·010
CDE	R_z	very rare
CdE	r_y	very rare

* The frequency varies greatly in different peoples.

† The frequency of any given *genotype* is obtained by multiplying together the frequencies of the two haplotypes as given here: thus CDe/cde occurs in 0·420 × 0·389 = approx. 16% of the population of Britain, and cde/cde in 0·389² = 15%. Reversing the calculation gives an estimate of gene frequency.

haplotypes varies considerably in different peoples: their frequency in this country, together with the alternative symbols, are shown in table 10.3.

Each individual inherits one of these sets from each parent, and his red cells may thus have from 3 to 6 different Rh antigens. In practice, iso-immunisation develops mainly when an individual of genotype cde/cde receives red cells which are D-positive. Accordingly, individuals whose red cells possess D are termed *Rh-positive* and those without D (i.e. with dd) are termed *Rh-negative*. In Caucasian stock, about 15% of individuals are cde/cde (hence the

frequency of cde as calculated in the table is $\sqrt{\frac{15}{100}} = 0.389$). Rh−ve individuals with other genotypes are comparatively rare.

There is also a significant risk of the development of anti-C when C + cells are transfused to an Rh−ve individual, and it is common practice to use a mixture of anti-C and anti-D for Rh grouping. Iso-immunisation may also result when c + or e + blood is transfused to CC or EE individuals respectively, but d + blood does not iso-immunise DD individuals.

The Rh system is, in fact, much more complex than has been suggested above: a fourth antigen, G, is closely associated with C and D, and further antigens, determined by variants of the common allelic genes or joint products of the genes, also occur.

Other blood group systems

In addition to the ABO and Rh groups many other blood group systems are known but, as in the Rh system, natural iso-antibodies are absent, and the sera that detect these groups are obtained mostly from persons immunised by transfusion or by pregnancy. These groups only rarely bring about iso-immunisation. Nevertheless the greatly increased use of blood transfusion necessitates their consideration and identification when a cross-matching test reveals an unexpected antibody. Use is now being made of monoclonal antibodies (p. 6.17) for grouping.

References

Moncada, S. and Vane, J.R. (1979) Arachidonic acid metabolites and the interactions between platelets and blood-vessel walls. *New England Journal of Medicine* **300,** 1142–7.

Sevitt, S. (1973). The mechanisms of canalisation of deep vein thrombosis. *Journal of Pathology* **110,** 153–65.

Sevitt, S. (1973). The vascularisation of deep vein thrombi and their fibrous residue: a post-mortem angiographic study. *Journal of Pathology* **111,** 1–11.

Shepherd, J.H. (1982). The toxic shock syndrome. *British Journal of Hospital Medicine* **28,** 234–6.

Singer, F.R., Schiller, A.L., Pyle, E.B. and Krane, S.M. (1978). Paget's disease of bone. In: *Metabolic Bone Disease*. Vol. 2. pp. 548–9. Ed. Avioli, V. and Krane, S.M. Academic Press, New York, London and San Francisco.

Further Reading

Cuthbertson, D.P. (1976). *Metabolism and the response to injury.* Ed. Wilkinson, A.W. and Cuthbertson, D.P. pp. 1–34. Pitman Medical, London.

Ledingham, I.McA. (1979). The pathophysiology of shock. *British Journal of Hospital Medicine* **22**, 472–82.

Mollison, P.L. (1982). *Blood Transfusion in Clinical Medicine.* 7th edn. pp. 1010. Blackwell Scientific, Oxford.

Moncada, S. (Ed.) (1983). Prostacyclin, thromboxane and leukotrienes. *British Medical Bulletin* **39**, No. 3. (Excellent reviews).

Ogston, D. (1983). *The Physiology of Haemostasis* pp. 378. Croom Helm, Beckenham, Kent.

Race, R.R. and Sanger, Ruth (1975). *Blood Groups in Man.* 6th edn. pp. 682. Blackwell Scientific, Oxford.

Rennie, M.J. and Harrison, R. (1984). Effects of injury, disease and malnutrition on protein metabolism in man. *Lancet,* **i,** 323–5.

Sevitt, S. (1974). *Reactions to Injury and Burns and their Clinical Importance.* pp. 256. Heinemann Medical, London.

Smith, R. and Williamson, D.H. (1983). Biochemical effects of human injury. *Trends in Biochemical Science* **8,** 142–6.

Thomas, D. (Ed.) (1977). Haemostasis. *British Medical Bulletin* **33**, 118–288. (Reviews by leading workers).

11

Miscellaneous Tissue Degenerations and Deposits

The degenerative changes which result from cellular injury, and the intracellular accumulation of lipids and glycogen resulting from certain disorders of metabolism, have been dealt with in Chapter 3. In the present chapter we describe a group of changes which, although heterogeneous, consist of either the accumulation in the tissues of various substances—amyloid material, mucus, pigmented compounds, calcium deposits and urates—or tissue degenerations which usually affect the stroma of supporting tissues, and are recognised by their microscopic appearances but are ill-defined chemically.

Amyloidosis

This consists of extracellular deposition of amyloid, an abnormal protein. Amyloid is insoluble and is resistant to digestion by proteolytic enzymes. Accordingly, deposits are persistent, and may increase until they cause disability by interfering with exchange of solutes between the blood and tissue cells, cause pressure atrophy of cells, or interfere mechanically with the contraction of myocardial and smooth muscle.

Amyloid is deposited in the walls of small blood vessels, on reticulin fibres and basement laminae. Extensive deposits cause enlargement and firm elasticity of the affected tissue and give it a waxy, slightly transparent macroscopic appearance (Fig. 11.1).

In histological sections stained by haematoxylin and eosin, it appears as homogeneous, refractile pale pink material, and can be distinguished from other hyaline deposits (p. 11.7) only by its characteristic distribution in some tissues.

The major component of amyloid is a fibrous protein which forms fibrils of 10–15 nm diam. visible by electron microscopy (Fig. 11.2). At higher magnification, the fibrils are seen to consist of two or more fine filaments twisted around each other.

Methods of demonstrating amyloid

The wide variety of methods currently used to demonstrate the presence of amyloid is an indication of their lack of specificity. Large deposits of amyloid are usually demonstrable by all the methods. If the

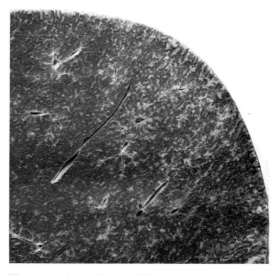

Fig. 11.1 Amyloidosis of liver. The amyloid material renders the organ firm, and gives it a dark, homogeneous appearance. × 1.

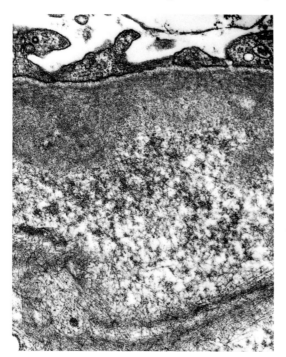

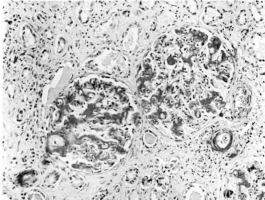

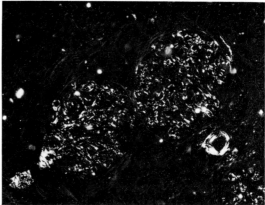

Fig. 11.2 Electron micrograph showing renal amyloidosis. The field shows glomerular capillary basement membrane on the outer side of which (above) the foot processes of the epithelium have fused to form a continuous layer. The inner part of the basement membrane is irregularly permeated by amyloid which also occupies the sub-endothelial space (lower half of the field) and is seen as fine filaments. × 39 000.

Fig. 11.3 The kidney in amyloidosis, stained by Congo red. The glomerular capillaries and the arterioles are affected. *Above*, viewed by ordinary light: the amyloid is seen as homogeneous material. *Below*, viewed through crossed polarising films, showing bi-refringence of the amyloid. × 105.

amount of amyloid present is small, however, the results with each method vary from case to case and identification is correspondingly difficult; for this reason it is usual to use several methods, the best known of which are as follows.

1. Lugol's iodine. Amyloid has a strong affinity for iodine (hence its name) and this forms the basis for a useful macroscopic test (Fig. 22.52, p. 22.41). When Lugol's iodine solution is poured over tissue, the amyloid is stained deep brown in contrast to the normal tissue which is only lightly stained. Congested tissues should first be rinsed free of excess blood as this obscures the test.

2. Congo red. This stain may be used on gross specimens and sections for microscopy. In polarised light, amyloid stained by congo red shows a green bi-refringence; this is the most reliable of the traditional techniques for demonstrating amyloid (Fig. 11.3).

3. Rosaniline dyes. These include gentian violet, methyl violet and crystal violet; they stain amyloid reddish, while other tissue elements appear purple.

This phenomenon of a dye reacting with a tissue constituent and undergoing a colour change is called *metachromasia*: it is believed that in this instance it is due to selective binding of impurities in the dyes by amyloid fibrils.

4. Fluorescent dyes. Thioflavine-T binds to amyloid and its presence is demonstrated by fluorescence microscopy. The reaction is not, however, entirely specific for amyloid.

5. Use is now being made of antibodies to amyloid proteins to identify amyloid and distinguish between the different types by **immunohistological techniques** (see p. 11.6).

The deposition and effects of amyloid

Amyloid is deposited extracellularly, and first appears in the walls of small vessels, both arterial and venous, in relation to the basement membrane of capillaries, vascular sinusoids, and epithelial structures, e.g. the renal tubular basement membrane.

When present in small amounts, amyloid has little effect on the organs, with the exception of the kidneys in which quite early glomerular deposition may result in proteinuria (see below). Involved small vessels tend to be susceptible to trauma and to bleed readily, giving rise to petechial haemorrhages.

In greater amounts, amyloid induces the changes and effects described above. The major features of involvement of the individual organs are as follows.

The **liver** is firm and elastic and may be palpable during life. Amyloid appears to be deposited first in the space of Disse (between the sinusoidal endothelium and the hepatocytes) and, as it increases, forms a continuous network between the sinusoids and columns of liver cells. The change usually begins in the sinusoids of the intermediate zones of the lobules: it may become very extensive and produce marked atrophy of the liver cells (Fig. 11.4). Even at an advanced stage, liver function is not usually severely impaired.

The **spleen** shows two distinct patterns of involvement. In one, the Malpighian bodies are changed to translucent globules by amyloid deposition in their reticulum (Fig. 11.5); hence the term 'sago spleen'. In this form, splenomegaly is not marked. In the diffuse form, the change affects reticulum of the red pulp, walls of venous sinuses, and many of the small arteries; the spleen may be palpable and weigh up to 1 kg. The explanation of the two distributions is not known.

Amyloidosis of the **kidneys** is particularly important because of its effect on renal function. Deposition occurs upon the basement membranes of the tubules and in the walls of arterioles (Fig. 11.3) and venules, but the most important site is in relation to the glomerular capillary basement membrane (Figs. 11.2, 22.50 and 22.51, p. 22.41): amyloid is deposited initially on the endothelial side of the basement

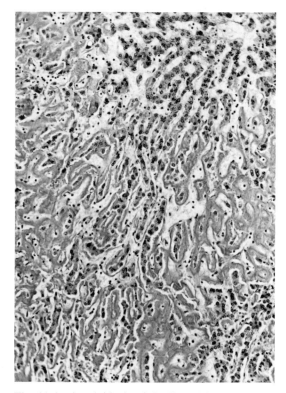

Fig. 11.4 Amyloidosis of the liver. The pale homogeneous amyloid has been deposited around the walls of the sinusoids, enclosing the columns of liver cells, which are undergoing atrophy. The zone around the central vein (*top right*) is least affected. × 115.

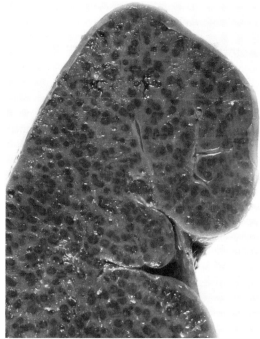

Fig. 11.5 Amyloid spleen of 'sago' type, i.e. affecting the Malpighian bodies.

membrane, but extends through it to accumulate also on the epithelial side. The glomerular capillaries are rendered abnormally permeable to macromolecules, with consequent heavy proteinuria and nephrotic syndrome (p. 10.34).

Eventually many of the glomerular capillaries are obliterated, the kidneys become scarred and shrunken and chronic renal failure develops.

In the **stomach** and **intestines**, amyloid deposits may be widespread and this leads to atrophic changes in the mucosa. Diarrhoea may result from severe involvement of the gut but, even when symptomless, amyloid material is very often demonstrable in rectal biopsy material, providing a useful diagnostic measure. Gingival biopsy is also useful, although less often diagnostic than rectal biopsy.

Other organs. Deposits of amyloid may also be found in the adrenals, heart, thyroid, skin and lymph nodes, and indeed in almost any tissue.

In the **heart**, it is deposited sub-endocardially and irregularly between myocardial fibres. Even when it has caused heart failure, there may be nothing to suggest its presence on naked-eye examination, but sometimes the ventricular myocardium is thickened and firm.

Classification of amyloidosis

Amyloidosis may be systemic, involving various organs and tissues, or localised to a single organ, e.g. the heart, skin or an endocrine gland.

Systemic amyloidosis is traditionally sub-divided into two major types, primary and secondary. Analysis of amyloid fibrils has shown that they differ in the nature of their constituent amino-acid chains, and classification is now usually based on the nature of the fibrous protein.

Apart from eliminating predisposing conditions, there is no way of arresting amyloid deposition, nor of removing deposited amyloid. Accordingly, the effects of amyloidosis depend on its distribution in the tissues, the amount deposited and the rate of deposition. Classification into primary and secondary types is of some practical importance because they differ in the distribution of the deposits, and secondary amyloidosis frequently complicates chronic infections which can often be eliminated. However, there is considerable overlap in the distribution of amyloid in the two types, and cases in which distribution is typical of neither. Classification based on the type of amyloid deposited has greater scientific merit. Moreover, the fibrils of primary amyloidosis usually consist of immunoglobulin (Ig) light chains, (**amyloid L or AL protein**) and the fibrous protein of secondary amyloid is of a different type (**amyloid A or AA protein**). To a large extent, the two methods of classification thus correlate with one another and, because of the many cases that are atypical in the distribution of deposits, neither is of great practical value.

AA amyloidosis occurs mostly as a complication of chronic infections or chronic inflammatory diseases of obscure aetiology, notably rheumatoid arthritis. It may complicate chronic suppurative infection continuing for years, such as chronic osteomyelitis, bronchiectasis, or chronic suppurative pyelonephritis, and also non-suppurating conditions such as tuberculosis, leprosy or syphilis. Hodgkin's disease (a neoplastic condition of the lymphoid tissues) and less commonly carcinomas are sometimes complicated by AA amyloidosis. In most of the developed countries, the commonest cause is now rheumatoid arthritis, in which amyloid deposits may be found in about 20% of cases at autopsy, although only a small proportion of these have had clinical evidence of amyloidosis. In chronic infection of many years duration, amyloidosis is very commonly present, perhaps in almost 50% of cases, although it is sufficient to cause symptoms in only about 5%. In countries where tuberculosis is still common, it is the major cause of amyloidosis.

Typically, the deposits in secondary amyloidosis are greatest in the solid abdominal viscera—the liver, spleen, kidneys and adrenals, although lesser deposits are much more widely distributed and rectal biopsy is positive in about 80% of cases. The major cause of death is renal failure.

AL amyloidosis. This occurs most often in old people, in some cases without predisposing disease, in others as a complication of multiple myeloma or other monoclonal gammopathy (see below).

Amyloid deposition is often severe in the heart, alimentary tract (including the tongue), skin, skeletal muscles, and sometimes also in the solid abdominal viscera. The tongue may be enlarged, and disability and death may result from cardiac or renal failure. Involvement of the gastro-intestinal tract may cause persistent diarrhoea, malabsorption, chronic obstruction and haemorrhage, and a haemorrhagic (purpuric) rash may occur on slight trauma or spontaneously as a result of involvement of small vessels in the dermis. Rectal biopsy is positive in most cases.

Amyloid of immunoglobulin origin is often atypical in its staining reactions, and when present in small amounts it may be difficult to demonstrate convincingly.

Localised amyloidosis, restricted to one organ or tissue, is relatively common in the larynx, where it gives rise to small tumour-like nodules. It may be restricted to the skin, bronchi, lungs, heart or urinary bladder, and is a rare cause of enlargement of the thyroid. It occurs also in the pancreatic islets in many diabetics, and as a feature of certain tumours, e.g. medullary thyroid cancer, islet cell pancreatic tumours and phaeochromocytomas of the adrenal medulla. Amyloid is also present in the core of the senile (Alzheimer) plaques which occur in the cerebral grey matter in senile dementia and Alzheimer's disease (p. 21.45).

Genetically-determined amyloidosis. Several familial forms of amyloidosis have been described. The best known are familial mediterranean fever and primary familial amyloidosis.

Familial mediterranean fever is found principally in Sephardic Jews and Armenians and is inherited as an autosomal recessive disease. In its most typical form, recurrent fever is associated with pain in the chest, abdomen, joints and skin; amyloidosis supervenes, causing death by renal involvement, but affecting also the spleen, lungs and liver. Variants of the disease are recognised in which the amyloidosis becomes apparent before the other features.

Primary familial amyloidosis. This is least rare in parts of Portugal and is inherited as an autosomal dominant. The disease presents in the 3rd and 4th decades with increasing leg weakness and loss of reflexes. Subsequently sphincteric disturbances and malabsorption from intestinal involvement lead to death within 10 years.

Many other rare syndromes have been described in individual families, each with a particular distribution of amyloid deposition.

The nature and aetiology of amyloidosis

Amyloid is composed mainly (over 90%) of a fibrous protein, of which there are two major types, and a non-fibrous protein (P protein) which is the same in all cases.

The fibrous proteins of systemic amyloidosis are, as noted above, of two major types: AL and AA proteins. In addition, there are other types in the rare genetically-determined systemic amyloidoses.

A characteristic feature of all types of amyloid fibrous protein, revealed by x-ray diffraction analysis, is that their polypeptide chains are arranged in sheets in which they lie at right angles to the long axis of the filaments. This is termed a *β-pleated configuration* to distinguish it from the usual α or helical arrangement of amino-acid chains in virtually all other fibrous proteins of vertebrates. The unusual β-pleated structure of amyloid is responsible for its insolubility, high resistance to vertebrate proteolytic enzymes, staining reactions and rather weak antigenicity.

AL amyloid. AL protein consists of whole light chains and parts of light chains which include the N-terminal (variable) region. In any particular case, the protein is made up of either λ or κ chains (λ being twice as common as κ), and amino-acid sequencing has shown that the amino-acid chains are homologous in any one case. AL amyloidosis develops usually after the age of 50, and in about 20% of cases is a complication of multiple myeloma, occurring in about 15% of patients with this disease. Multiple myeloma is a malignant growth of plasma-cell type and in most cases the tumour cells secrete significant amounts of immunoglobulin (usually IgG) and/or light chains.

The light chains pass into the glomerular filtrate and can be detected in the urine as Bence-Jones protein. As the tumour cells represent a clonal proliferation, the Ig and light chain molecules are homogeneous ('monoclonal') and a sharp band of IgG can often be detected on serum electrophoresis (Fig. 17.44, p. 17.61). Free light-chain molecules are secreted by virtually all myelomas complicated by amyloidosis, although many myelomas secrete light chains without producing amyloidosis. The sequences in the variable regions of light chains in multiple myeloma are specific for the individual case, and in cases developing amyloidosis, are identical with those of the AL protein. There is thus no doubt that AL amyloid is derived from myeloma light chains. The mechanism of conversion of light chain molecules to amyloid is not known, but partial enzymic digestion of light chain produces fragments which tend to combine in a β-pleated configuration resembling AL protein in its physical, chemical and staining properties, and a similar mechanism is suspected *in vivo*. A β-pleated structure is assumed more rapidly by λ than by κ light chain fragments.

In 80% or so of cases of AL amyloidosis without multiple myeloma, the AL protein also consists of 'monoclonal' light chain and fragments. A few of these cases have a less highly malignant plasmacytic tumour—*Waldenstrom's macroglobulinaemia*. The remainder have an excess of plasma cells in the marrow and in about half of them, free 'monoclonal' light chains can be detected in the urine. They are mostly examples of the non-progressive monoclonal plasma-cell proliferation which occurs in about 1% of old people.

Antibody to light chain does not stain AL amyloid, presumably because of its peculiar structure. Antibody to the light chain obtained from the urine of a case of AL amyloid will react with that individual's amyloid in immunohistological tests, but not with AL amyloid from other individuals. This is explained by the individual-specificity of the variable regions of the light chain constituents of AL protein.

AA amyloid. AA protein consists of polypeptide chains made up of 76 amino acids. These show sequence identity with the N-terminal end of a plasma protein (serum amyloid A or SAA protein) which is normally present in trace amounts but is an acute-phase reactant, the plasma level rising considerably in inflammatory and traumatic conditions (p. 8.14). AA amyloidosis occurs in chronic conditions accompanied by a persistent rise in SAA protein, and it seems likely that AA amyloid is formed by assumption of a β-pleated structure by proteolysis fragments of SAA protein.

Antibody to SAA protein reacts with AA amyloid from both the same individual and from other cases, and thus can be used in immunohistological techniques to detect AA amyloid and to distinguish it from AL amyloid. The fibrous proteins of amyloid complicating familial mediterranean fever is of AA type.

Other types of systemic amyloid. The fibrous protein of the amyloid deposits in *primary familial amyloidosis* (AF protein) consists of plasma pre-albumin, and can be demonstrated by immunohistology, using an antibody to pre-albumin.

The fibrous protein of localised amyloidosis. In amyloidosis localised to the myocardium, the fibrous protein (ASc_1) is apparently derived from plasma pre-albumin. In amyloid localised to an endocrine gland, the fibrous protein has been shown in some instances to be a product of a hormone or pro-hormone. For example, the amyloid deposits in thyroid medullary carcinoma (which secretes calcitonin) consist of a part of the calcitonin molecule, while that of insulin-secreting islet-cell tumours is thought to be derived from insulin. These and other polypeptide hormones have been shown to assume a β-pleated structure following partial proteolytic digestion. The nature of the fibrous proteins in localised amyloidosis of the skin, and of the brain in senile dementia and Alzheimer's disease is not known.

P protein. Amyloid contains a second protein ('P') which constitutes about 5% of all types of amyloid with the possible exception of the amyloid in senile cerebral plaques. It is readily soluble and is removed from amyloid during processing of tissue; *in vitro* it forms pentamers with a ring-like structure which become stacked (like red cells in rouleaux) to form rods with periodic cross-marking. It is identical with a trace plasma protein, serum amyloid P (SAP) protein which binds to amyloid fibrils: this presumably explains its presence in amyloid.

Amyloid also contains mucopolysaccharides, lipoproteins and fibrin in trace amounts, but it is likely that these have either been trapped by amyloid as it is deposited or are plasma constituents which have permeated it.

Amyloid of AA type is readily induced in animals by prolonged antigenic stimulation or oral administration of casein, and its deposition is enhanced by thymectomy and by immunosuppressive agents. Although human AA amyloid is associated with conditions which involve the immunity system, there is no common immunological disturbance: for example, in lepromatous leprosy cell-mediated immunity is depressed, whereas in tuberculosis it is normal or enhanced. This does not accord with the suggestion that amyloidosis results from T-cell depression and B-cell stimulation (Scheinberg and Cathcart, 1976).

There is some evidence that amyloid may be resorbed following effective treatment of the causal disease, but renal amyloid is persistent and steroid therapy has not, in general, proved beneficial.

Hyaline and Fibrinoid Changes

The term *hyalin** is applied to material of homogeneous, refractile, usually eosinophilic appearance seen on microscopy of stained tissue sections. It is purely descriptive, and many different formed tissue elements, as well as cell cytoplasm, may assume a hyaline appearance. In most instances the chemical basis of hyaline change is not known, although fibrin and amyloid both have a hyaline appearance. The collagen and ground substance of old dense fibrous tissue and the walls of aged blood vessels are often hyaline and because of its association with age this is often called *hyaline degeneration*. In the kidney and other organs, the walls of arterioles usually become thickened and hyaline in arterial hypertension (Fig. 22.6, p. 22.5), and glomeruli injured by chronic ischaemia became converted to hyaline balls (Fig. 22.7, p. 22.5). These vascular changes, which occur also in diabetic nephropathy, are believed to be due to accumulation of substances leaking out from the blood—*plasmatic vasculosis* (see below). There are many conditions in which abnormal amounts of plasma proteins leak into the glomerular filtrate; part of the protein is resorbed by the tubular epithelium where it is seen as eosinophil refractile droplets (Fig. 22.26, p. 22.26) commonly termed *hyaline droplets*. Protein may also coagulate in the tubular lumen and is then secreted in the urine as cylindrical *'hyaline casts'*. In viral hepatitis, damaged liver cells may appear hyaline (Fig. 20.14, p. 20.15) and *'Mallory's hyalin'* appears in the hepatocyte cytoplasm in alcoholic and certain other forms of liver cell injury. In Cushing's syndrome, hyaline material is seen in the basophil cells of the pituitary (*Crooke's hyaline change*—Fig. 26.3, p. 26.10). Necrotic tissue, e.g. myocardium, and fused platelets in thrombi (Fig. 10.14, p. 10.13) may also appear hyaline.

These examples serve to show that hyaline material and its pathological associations are widely heterogeneous. It is nevertheless sometimes of diagnostic value, as will be seen from the many examples which crop up in the systematic chapters.

A second term, **fibrinoid change**, has long been used to describe impregnation of tissues with hyaline material which is brightly eosinophilic and has other staining properties similar to those of fibrin. The term 'fibrinoid' was originally applied by German pathologists who doubted that the material was fibrin in spite of its staining reactions. It became popular in the 1940s when fibrinoid change (incorrectly regarded as diagnostic of hypersensitivity reactions) was noted to be a common feature of the so-called collagen or connective-tissue diseases. More recently, immunofluorescence staining, and to a lesser extent electron microscopy, have provided more specific techniques for identifying fibrin in tissue sections, and have shown fibrin to be present in some, but not all, 'fibrinoid' lesions: in some instances the eosinophilic hyalin is due to ground-substance mucopolysaccharides; in others its nature remains unknown.

Deposition of fibrin in the tissues results from vascular exudation of fibrinogen, which is converted to fibrin by the action of tissue thromboplastin. If the injury causing the exudation is severe, there may also be death of tissue cells, and the changes are then traditionally known as *fibrinoid necrosis*. Examples of this are seen in many acute inflammatory lesions including the Arthus reaction (Fig 14.27, p. 14.27), in some infarcts (in which plasma exudes from the ischaemic blood vessels) (Figs. 3.30, p. 3.31 and 3.32, p. 3.32), in the arteriolar lesions of malignant hypertension (Fig. 14.19b, p. 14.18) and in the necrotic base of peptic ulcers. Fibrin is detectable in some fibrinoid lesions of the connective-tissue diseases, e.g. in some examples of the subcutaneous nodules of rheumatoid arthritis (Fig. 23.52a, p. 23.46).

Deposited fibrin is usually removed by the action of plasmin or by phagocytic cells. It has, however, been demonstrated in slowly developing, permanent hyaline changes in the walls of arterioles and glomeruli in plasmatic vasculosis, and this supports the view of Lendrum (1969) and others that such hyaline change results from an exudative process (see also p. 14.17). Recognition of the fibrin in such vascular lesions was long delayed because, as it ages, it loses the staining properties of fibrin and stains more like collagen.

---

* From the Greek *'hyalos'*, meaning glass.

Corpora amylacea. Under this term are included a number of rounded or ovoid hyaline structures, which may stain deeply with iodine, hence the name. They sometimes show concentric lamination and may undergo calcification. Such structures form in various situations and they cannot be regarded as all of the same nature. They are often a prominent feature within the acini of the prostate in the elderly; they occur also in the lungs, and sometimes in tumours.

In the nervous system they are very common; e.g. in old age, in chronic degenerative lesions, and in the region of old infarcts and haemorrhages. They vary greatly in size, the smallest being spherical and homogeneous, and these usually stain deeply with haematoxylin. They appear to form simply by a deposition, in the intercellular spaces, of organic material containing acid mucopolysaccharides in globular form, but their exact composition is not known. They are of no importance except as a manifestation of the degenerative condition with which they are associated.

Mucins and Myxomatous Change

Mucins consist of complexes of proteins with carbohydrates and mucopolysaccharides. They are characterised by their slimy nature and histologically by their affinity for basic dyes and metachromasia with thiazine dyes such as toluidine blue. Most mucins are precipitated by acetic acid.

Mucins are secreted by various glandular epithelia and also by fibroblasts, osteoblasts and chondroblasts as important constituents of the ground substance of the various connective tissues. Both epithelial and connective tissue mucins are mixtures of *glycoproteins*, which are rich in hexose polymers and are stained pink in the PAS method, and *mucoproteins* in which the mucopolysaccharide is rich in hexosamines and which stain metachromatically with toluidine blue at low pH.

Disturbances of epithelial mucin secretion are not of much pathological importance except in *cystic fibrosis of the pancreas* (p. 20.60) in which an abnormality of mucus secretion occurs in the glands of the intestine, pancreas, bile ducts, bronchi and sweat glands. The mucin is abnormally thick and obstructs the ducts, with subsequent gland atrophy and loss of function.

Obstruction of the ducts of small mucus-secreting glands, e.g. in the mouth, results in the development of mucin-filled cysts, and obstruction of the cystic duct may result in distension of the gallbladder with mucin—the so-called *mucocele* (Fig. 20.58, p. 20.51). Chronic irritation of a mucous membrane may result in increase in the number and activity of mucin-secreting cells, as in chronic bronchitis, in which there is abundant mucous sputum. Some epithelial tumours secrete mucin, and its detection in relation to tumour cells is sometimes of help in determining the origin of the tumour.

The mucopolysaccharides of **connective tissue mucins** include hyaluronic acid, chondroitin, chondroitin sulphates and other sulphated compounds. They form the ground substances of fibrous tissue, cartilage and bone, and also joint fluid. In the soft tissues, the ground substance is largely in the form of a gel, but in acute inflammatory lesions the mucopolysaccharides are depolymerised, with conversion mainly to a fluid phase, which is more readily permeable to exudate and cells of the inflammatory reaction. Some bacteria also secrete hyaluronidase and other enzymes which may facilitate their spread in the tissues.

Some connective tissue tumours secrete abundant mucin, which appears as a pale basophilic stroma; they are called *myxomas* (p. 23.65). An increase in mucoid ground substance of connective tissue, so that it comes to resemble myxoid tissue of the fetus and umbilical cord, is termed **myxomatous** or **myxoid change**. It occurs in the aortic media in *Erdheim's medial degeneration* (Fig. 14.33, p. 14.32), and also, together with similar changes in other connective tissues, in *Marfan's syndrome*: in both conditions the inner part of the weakened aortic wall may rupture and blood may track along the media (dissecting aneurysm). Myxomatous change is also seen in the valve cusps of the heart and sometimes results in stretching and incompetence of the valves.

Production of ground substance is influenced by hormones; there is a generalised increase, for example, in *hypothyroidism*, giving rise to the term **myxoedema**: the bloated appearance of the face is due to myxomatous change in the dermis, and the croaky voice is due to the same change in the larynx. Curiously, myxomatous change is seen in the pre-tibial region in some cases of thyrotoxicosis (hyperthyroidism).

The mucopolysaccharidoses. These result from a number of rare genetic defects of mucopolysaccharide metabolism. Excess mucopolysaccharides accumulate in various types of cell, and are excreted in the urine. The conditions are distinguished by the chemical nature and/or distribution of the material. The two least rare are *Hurler's syndrome* (gargoylism) and *Hunter's syndrome*. The features of **Hurler's syndrome (MPS I)** include dwarfism, skeletal deformities, a characteristic facies, mental deficiency, corneal opacities and hepatomegaly. It is due to an autosomal recessive tract, causing deficiency of the enzyme α-L-iduronidase, which is necessary to catabolise excess of demetran and heparan sulphates. These compounds are deposited in brain, blood vessel walls, liver and spleen, etc., and are excreted in the urine. Nasopharyngeal involvement causes recurrent respiratory infections and death usually occurs in the first decade from pneumonia or coronary artery occlusion. In **Hunter's syndrome (MPS II)** the same substances accumulate: the symptoms are similar but develop later and corneal opacities do not occur. The condition is caused by an X-linked recessive trait, and so occurs only in males: the changes result from a deficiency of iduronate sulphatase, which is also necessary for the metabolism of demetran and heparan sulphates.

A third condition, **Morquio's syndrome (MPS IV)**, is probably a heterogeneous group of variable severity and inherited as an autosomal recessive trait. Excess keratan sulphate is demonstrable in the urine in only some cases, and the specific enzyme deficiency has not yet been determined. In contrast to Hurler's syndrome, these dwarfed patients are of normal intelligence, and without facial abnormality or corneal clouding. The joints are lax rather than stiff, but the vertebral changes are similar. In some patients, atlanto-axial instability results from failure of a hypoplastic odontoid process to fuse with the body of the axis so that intubation for anaesthesia is dangerous. A few patients later develop spinal cord compression. Death usually occurs before the age of 20 from respiratory or cardiac problems.

Melanin Pigmentation

The melanins are iron-free sulphur-containing pigments varying in colour from pale yellow to deep brown. They are formed intracellularly from colourless precursors—melanogens—and are very stable substances, resistant to acids and many other reagents, but soluble in strong alkalis; they can be bleached by powerful oxidising agents such as potassium permanganate or hydrogen peroxide. They are related to the aromatic compounds, tyrosine, phenylalanine and tryptophane, and may be formed from such substances by oxidation. On treating sections of skin with dihydroxyphenylalanine (dopa), 'dopa-positive' cells in the epidermis oxidise this substance by means of an enzyme like tyrosinase and become blackened in consequence. The only cells in the skin which are 'dopa-positive' *in vivo* are the *dendritic cells*, or *melanocytes*, which lie extended between the basal cells of the epidermis (Fig. 11.6). They are the only melanin-producing cells in the skin and fine granules of melanin in their dendrites are taken up, by pinocytosis of the tips of the dendrites, into adjacent epidermal cells and also into macrophages in the dermis which may become laden with coarse pigment granules and are then called *melanophores*. Melanin granules can reduce certain silver salts, e.g. ammoniacal silver nitrate, with consequent deposition of metallic silver; melanin can thus be blackened in histological preparations, scanty or light-coloured granules being rendered conspicuous. This property is widely used histochemically. It is now known that the dendritic cells are of neuro-ectodermal origin, being derived from the cells of the embryonic neural crest, as are also the melanocytes of the squamous mucous membranes, the meninges, choroid and adrenals. This view harmonises well with the evidence about the origin of the naevus cells of pigmented moles from neuro-ectodermal cells and also accords with the experimental work of Billingham and Medawar on the behaviour of melanocytes in skin autotransplants. This work seems to have rendered untenable the alternative view that melanocytes are modified basal epidermal cells. The Langerhans cells of the epidermis are now regarded as modified macrophages and may play a part in the

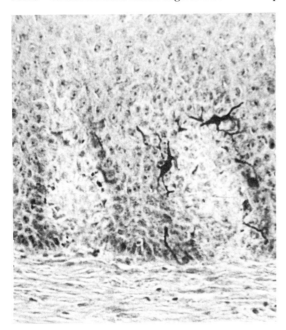

Fig. 11.6   Dendritic cells (melanocytes) in the basal part of the epidermis. (Dopa reaction.) × 220.

control of keratinisation. Darkening of the skin on exposure to ultraviolet radiation is brought about first by migration of the melanin granules and subsequent darkening of their colour; later there is increased formation of pigment, apparently by the activity of the dendritic cells, which under further stimulation may increase in number.

In **Addison's disease**, which results from destruction of the adrenal cortex (p. 26.37), there occurs a general increase in melanin pigmentation of the skin, especially in areas exposed to light and in areas normally pigmented. There may also be pigment deposition on the inner surface of the cheeks on a line corresponding to the junction of the teeth, and on the sides of the tongue, the position being apparently determined by mild irritation. In the skin, the pigment is in the form of very fine brownish granules in the deeper layers of the rete Malpighii, and is present also as coarser granules, chiefly within macrophages in the underlying cutis, the appearance and distribution resembling those in the negro skin. The pigmentation in Addison's disease represents an increase of normal pigment, and occurs under the influence of corticotrophin and β lipotrophin which is released in excess from the adenohypophysis in the absence of inhibition by adrenocortical hormones (p. 26.6).

Chloasma is a condition observed principally during pregnancy, and occasionally in association with ovarian disease, in which pigmented patches occur in the skin of the face, and other pigmented areas, e.g. the nipples, may become darker, under the influence of oestrogenic and melanocyte-stimulating hormones. A similar condition has been described in women taking oral contraceptives.

Leukoderma (vitiligo) denotes patchy depigmentation of skin and is sometimes accompanied by increase of pigment in the intervening areas. In the affected areas the dendritic cells are of abnormal structure and have lost their capacity to oxidise dopa to form pigment.

Irregular pigmentation of the skin is common in chronic arsenical poisoning and in neurofibromatosis. In haemochromatosis also, the colour of the skin is due partly to deposition of haemosiderin in the dermal fibrocytes around sweat glands (p. 11.17), and also to increase in melanin. A striking degree of melanotic pigmentation of the oral and labial mucosa occurs in association with familial multiple polyposis of the small intestine, especially the jejunum (Peutz-Jeghers syndrome): the disorder is transmitted as a Mendelian dominant. The control of pigment metabolism in the skin is obscure, but it is known to be affected by exposure to light, chronic irritation and increased vascularity, activity of endocrine glands, including the adrenals, pituitary and ovaries, and nervous influences.

Pigmented tumours. Melanin pigment is formed in large amount in the melanotic tumours which arise in the skin and in the pigmented coats of the eye, and most chemical analyses of melanin have been carried out on the pigment from such tumours. The urine of patients suffering from extensive melanotic tumours occasionally contains a melanogen which darkens on exposure to the oxygen of the air.

Melanosis coli. This is a rather uncommon condition, characterised by varying degrees of brownish to black pigmentation of the mucosa of the colon, beginning in the caecum and ascending colon, and sometimes extending to the anus. The pigment is contained mainly in macrophages in the lamina propria; it is absent from the epithelial cells. The condition is commonest when there has been intestinal stasis or chronic obstruction, and it is now recognised to be the result of absorption of aromatic products from the gut. This is commonly associated with the prolonged use of anthracene-derived purgatives, e.g. cascara, and the pigment consists of derivatives of anthraquinone combined with products of protein decomposition. The pigment resembles melanin in its reactions, but differs from it in being autofluorescent, weakly PAS-positive, and weakly sudanophilic. The cells containing pigment are dopa-negative.

Ochronosis. In this very rare condition, cartilages, capsules of joints and other soft tissues assume a dark brown or almost black colour, owing to pigment deposition. The pigment resembles melanin in some of its properties but does not reduce silver nitrate. In virtually all cases of ochronosis, alkaptonuria is present, a condition in which homogentisic acid (2,5-hydroxyphenylacetic acid) is excreted by the kidneys and causes the urine to blacken on standing owing to oxidation, especially alkaline urine. Homogentisic acid is formed from tyrosine and phenylalanine. Normally it is converted to malylacetoacetic acid by homogentisic acid oxidase in the liver and kidneys, but alkaptonurics lack this enzyme, and consequently homogentisic acid is not metabolised normally, but is oxidised into pigment and deposited in the tissues, producing ochronosis. The metabolic defect in alkaptonuria is inherited as an autosomal recessive trait. In the early days of antiseptic surgery, exogenous ochronosis occasionally followed the prolonged use of carbolic dressings for a long time, and the pigment is believed to have been formed from the absorbed carbolic acid.

Breakdown Products of Haemoglobin

At the end of their lifespan, red cells are taken up and destroyed by macrophages in the spleen, marrow, etc. Intracellular breakdown of haemoglobin (Hb) begins with opening of the porphyrin system of haem, the four pyrrole nuclei and globin now forming a long-chain molecule (choleglobin). The globin and iron are then split off and the residual *biliverdin* pigment, consisting of four pyrrole rings, is reduced to *bilirubin* and passes into the plasma, where it is bound mainly to albumin. The bilirubin is taken up by the hepatocytes, dissociated from albumin, conjugated with glucuronic acid and excreted as bilirubin glucuronides in the bile. The iron which is split off from haem is stored mainly as *ferritin* and *haemosiderin* and re-used.

Breakdown products of Hb may accumulate in the body in the following circumstances: (*a*) local deposition results from haemorrhage into the tissues; (*b*) more generalised accumulation of bilirubin occurs when there is excessive red cell destruction, i.e. in haemolytic anaemias; (*c*) increase in bilirubin or its glucuronides occurs when there is some defect along the metabolic or excretory pathways by which the iron-free part of haem is delivered into the intestine as bilirubin glucuronide; (*d*) accumulation of iron-containing compounds occurs when the amount of iron entering the body exceeds significantly the small amount which is lost physiologically. The effects of these abnormalities are described below.

Local accumulation of pigments

When haemorrhage into tissues occurs, many of the red cells in the escaped blood undergo lysis; their Hb diffuses away and is taken up and catabolised in macrophages in the draining lymph nodes, spleen, etc. However, some of the red cells are phagocytosed locally by macrophages derived from monocytes which migrate into the lesion, and bilirubin and iron compounds are produced as described above. This process is illustrated experimentally in Figs. 11.7 and 11.8: in man it is reflected in the changing colours of a 'black eye' or any other superficial bruise. Most of the bilirubin diffuses away and is eventually dealt with by the liver,

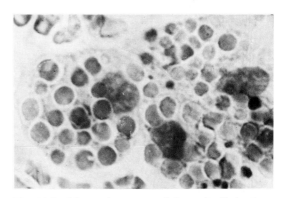

Fig. 11.7 Macrophages containing red cells in phagocytic vacuoles. From the subcutaneous tissue of a mouse six days after an injection of red cells. × 1200.

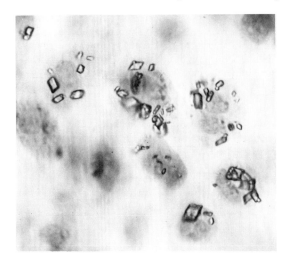

Fig. 11.8 Intracellular formation of bilirubin crystals in macrophages, 16 days after subcutaneous injection of haemoglobin into a mouse. × 1200. (From preparations by the late Dr. Janet S.F. Niven.)

but some of it may persist locally in crystalline form around an old haemorrhage, particularly in the brain (Fig. 11.9): this may be due to the absence of lymphatics in brain tissue. Some of the iron released may also be retained locally as the pigment haemosiderin (see below), either within macrophages or as an encrustation on collagen and other tissue components.

Localised accumulation of haemosiderin may

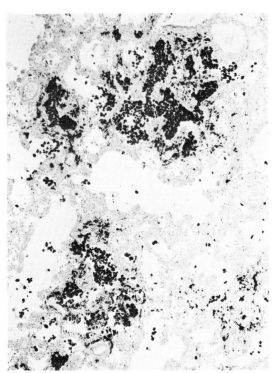

Fig. 11.10 The lung in mitral stenosis. Red cells escaping from the congested pulmonary capillaries are ingested by alveolar macrophages which become engorged with haemosiderin. The macrophages accumulate in the alveoli adjacent to respiratory bronchioles and are thus seen as aggregates. Prussian blue reaction. × 50.

occur in the **lungs** as a result of haemorrhages in pulmonary venous congestion, e.g. in *mitral stenosis* (Fig. 11.10) and also in the rare *idiopathic pulmonary haemosiderosis*, in which it is accompanied by fibrosis. Haemosiderin deposition also occurs in the **renal tubular epithelium** when intravascular haemolysis results in release into the plasma of haemoglobin, which leaks into the glomerular filtrate and is taken up by the tubular cells (p. 17.34).

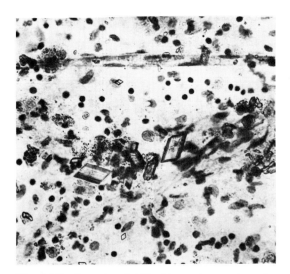

Fig. 11.9 Crystals of bilirubin and granular pigment, some of which is in phagocytes, at the site of an old cerebral haemorrhage. × 500.

Bile pigments

A rise in the level of **bilirubin** in the plasma results from increased breakdown of red cells in the haemolytic anaemias, or from failure of the liver cells to remove and conjugate it with glucuronic acid. Lesions of the liver or biliary tract which prevent excretion of **bilirubin glucuronide** result in its regurgitation into the plasma. When the levels of either compound exceed 2–3 mg per 100 ml (35–50 μmol/l), **jaundice** develops, i.e. the skin, sclera and various other tissues become distinctly yellow. In adults, jaundice itself causes little disability, but in infants a rise of unconjugated bilirubin in the plasma to over 15 mg per 100 ml (250 μmol/l) carries a risk of toxic brain injury. The types of jaundice and their causes and effects are, however, dealt with in Chapter 19.

Disorders of iron storage

Iron is essential to all forms of life, and micro-organisms and multicellular plants and animals have all developed mechanisms of obtaining the element from the environment. Compared with other mammals, man (and especially woman) is in a precarious position for acquiring sufficient iron, and it has been estimated that about 800 million people throughout the world suffer from some degree of iron deficiency. This is mainly because the human mechanism of iron absorption developed when man was a hunter and is attuned to the absorption of haem iron. The growing of grass crops and change to a more mixed diet rich in carbohydrate only occurred 10000 years ago and has resulted in a diminution of dietary haem iron (derived from fish and meat) and an increase in less readily available ferrous iron from cereals and green vegetables. Another factor, which predisposes women to iron deficiency, is the monthly menstrual cycle with loss of iron in the menstrual blood.

Paradoxically, man is also the only species in which disease is known to result from excessive absorption of iron. This is because the amount of iron which can be excreted is much smaller in man than in other mammals, and disturbances in the regulation of the absorption mechanism can result in accumulation of excess iron which cannot be excreted.

About 70% of the 3–4 g of iron in the body is incorporated in the haem of haemoglobin: 5% is in myoglobin, and small but important amounts are incorporated in cellular cytochrome, respiratory and metallo-flavo-enzymes. The remainder (0·3–1·4 g) is mostly in storage form in macrophages of the spleen, bone marrow, etc. and in various tissue cells, particularly hepatocytes.

Iron absorption is by way of the epithelial cells lining the gut, mainly those of the villi of the duodenum and proximal jejunum, absorption decreasing progressively more distally. Dietary iron consists of both haem which is absorbed as metalloporphyrin, and non-haem iron which is absorbed mainly as ferrous salts, ferric salts being very poorly absorbed. The mechanism of uptake of iron by cells of the villi is not clear. Some workers consider it likely that specific receptors for ferrous and haem iron are involved, and that receptor-bound iron is taken into the cells by endocytosis. The amounts of iron taken up by the epithelium depend mainly on two factors: the body's total storage iron and the amount of available iron in the diet. *The amount taken up bears an inverse relationship to the total storage iron in the body* (Fig. 11.11) *and, within limits, varies directly with the amount available in the diet.* It may be that the number of postulated iron receptors on the cells of the villi can be varied, or some other mechanism may be involved. The regulatory mechanism does not conserve fully the amount of iron stored in the body, for a significant increase in absorption is induced only by a large reduction of storage iron. Other dietary factors also influence iron absorption. For example, absorption of **non-haem iron** is aided by ascorbic acid, citric acid and amino acids, all of which form monomeric complexes with iron and prevent the formation of non-absorbable polymers. Gastric HCl also favours absorption by preventing polymer formation, and alcoholic drinks increase iron intake, possibly by stimulating gastric secretion but also because some drinks are rich in iron. Reduction of ferric to ferrous iron by ascorbic acid and other reducing agents also promotes absorption of non-haem iron. Formation of non-absorbable polymers is favoured by gastric achlorhydria and by the presence in the diet of certain compounds, e.g. phytate from cereals, tannates,

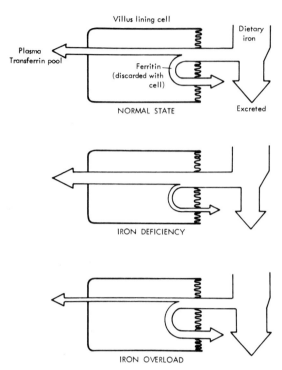

Fig. 11.11 The effect of the total iron store on absorption of dietary iron by intestinal epithelium. Only a fraction of the available dietary iron is normally taken up by the epithelium (*upper*): the fraction taken up is increased when total storage iron is depleted (*middle*) and decreased when the iron store is increased (*lower*). Of the iron taken up by the epithelium, the proportion transferred to the plasma transferrin pool is similarly affected by the total iron store.

phosphates and ethylenediamine tetra-acetic acid (EDTA) used as a food preservative. These factors do not, of course, regulate iron absorption but influence the proportion of non-haem iron available for absorption, which may vary from 1% to 20%. They explain why iron deficiency is particularly common and often severe among people living on a largely vegetable diet. **Haem** is a particularly important source of iron because, although it represents only a small part of the total dietary iron, the proportion absorbed is relatively high (up to about 40%): its absorption is favoured by amino acids and is not inhibited by dietary factors (or achlorhydria) which inhibit absorption of non-haem iron. Overall, individuals who are not iron-deficient absorb about 10% of the iron in a good mixed diet.

Within the mucosal epithelial cells, haem iron is broken down and forms a common pool with the absorbed non-haem iron. Part of this pool is rapidly transferred through the epithelial cells to enter the plasma. The remainder is incorporated into intracellular ferritin (see below), much of which is lost when, within a few days, the cell exfoliates. The amount of epithelial-cell iron transferred to the plasma increases with the concentration of iron in the lumen of the gut, but the *proportion* transferred diminishes. Over a wide range of iron concentrations in the lumen, *the proportion of iron transferred is greater in subjects with iron deficiency, i.e. with depleted iron stores,* and is diminished when the iron stores are large (Fig. 11.11). It is possible that this regulatory effect is exerted by plasma ferritin, the concentration of which is directly proportional to the total iron stored in the body (see below).

Iron loss amounts to approximately 1 mg daily, most of it in the form of ferritin in the epithelial cells desquamated from the skin (0.2–0.3 mg) and gut (0.6 mg). Only a small proportion is lost in the bile, sweat, etc., and most of that lost by gut epithelium has been absorbed from the lumen by the cells and incorporated into ferritin; it has never really entered the body's iron store. In women of reproductive age, menstruation accounts for an average loss of an additional 0.6 mg daily, although there is great individual variation. Pregnancy, childbirth and lactation represent a rather greater loss than this.

From the above, it will be apparent that *iron balance depends largely on the control of absorption from the gut: iron loss is small and can only be increased significantly by haemorrhage.*

Plasma iron. The plasma of normal adults contains an average of about 1.2 mg of iron per litre, although the range is large. Over 95% of this is in the form of **transferrin**, which consists of ferric iron bound to a specific transport protein, a β-globulin termed **apotransferrin**, which is synthesised by the liver cells. Transferrin possesses two binding sites for iron and is normally only about 30% saturated in the plasma. *Although transferrin makes up only a very small percentage of total body iron, it is very important, for it is the form in which iron is transferred between the intestinal epithelium, macrophages, hepatocytes and red cell precursors* (Fig. 11.12). In fact, the plasma iron is provided

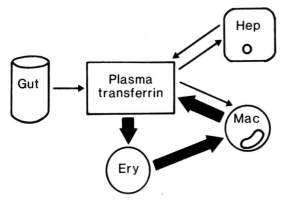

Fig. 11.12 The central role of plasma transferrin in carrying iron between the gut, macrophages (Mac), hepatocytes (Hep) and the red cell precursors and red cells (Ery). The heavy arrows indicate the major flow.

mainly by macrophages of the spleen, haemopoietic marrow, liver, etc., which break down red cells and both store iron and pass it to the plasma transferrin pool. Plasma transferrin is taken up by red cell precursors and used for haemoglobin synthesis.

The plasma also contains **ferritin** which differs from intracellular ferritin in being partly glycosylated and almost iron-free. The normal concentration varies with age and sex. In children and women of reproductive age, it is approximately 30 µg/l. The level in boys rises after puberty to about 100 µg/l at the age of 30 and remains at this level. A similar rise occurs in women after the menopause. The function of plasma ferritin is not known, but the level is increased during pregnancy and by infection and inflammatory lesions in general, and particularly those involving the liver. Apart from such fluctuations, the concentration of plasma ferritin parallels the total iron stored in the body, 1 µg/l representing approximately 8 mg of stored iron.

Haemoglobin synthesis. Red cell precursors have surface receptors for transferrin, which they take up avidly by endocytosis. Uptake is proportional to the concentration of transferrin in the plasma and its percentage saturation with iron. Within the cell, iron is split off and used in haem synthesis, while the apotransferrin is returned to the plasma. With increasing maturity, the number of transferrin receptors on the erythroid cell diminishes, the mature red cell having none.

Storage iron. Iron is stored in macrophages in the spleen, marrow, etc., and in parenchymal and other tissue cells in general. Most of the parenchymal store is normally in the hepatocytes and for practical purposes the store may be regarded as the iron in these two cell types. Most if not all cells synthesise apoferritins and store iron as **ferritin**, which consists of micelles of ferric oxide and phosphate enclosed in a protein molecule which is water-soluble. Ferritin is capable of incorporating approximately 4500 atoms of iron per molecule, but it is never fully saturated and provides a readily available reserve of iron. It is located in the cytosol where it is not detectable by light microscopy and does not give a prussian blue reaction (see below) but has a characteristic electron-microscopic appearance. Iron is stored also in lysosomes, in which the protein of ferritin is degraded and the iron is in a highly concentrated form known as **haemosiderin**, which may have an iron content up to 50%. Haemosiderin is insoluble and if present in large amount is seen microscopically as golden-yellow intracytoplasmic granules, while macroscopically the tissue looks brown. It gives the *prussian blue reaction* on treatment with hydrochloric acid and potassium ferrocyanide, the intense blue colour being due to formation of ferri-ferrocyanide.

If the size of the iron store is normal, macrophages in the marrow contain sufficient haemosiderin to give a positive prussian blue reaction. In the hepatocytes, iron is normally stored mainly as ferritin, although if the total store is large there may be sufficient haemosiderin in the hepatocytes to give a faint prussian blue reaction. In states of increased storage, the proportion of iron in the form of haemosiderin increases, and in gross iron overload it may be present in enormous amounts, its distribution between macrophages and parenchymal cells depending on the cause of the iron overload (see below).

In states of negative iron balance, iron is transferred readily from the intracellular ferritin and haemosiderin of macrophages and hepatocytes to the plasma transferrin pool, and *anaemia does not develop until after the stores are depleted.*

Iron deficiency

This is the commonest disturbance of iron metabolism. It results first in depletion of storage iron and then in anaemia and fall of the iron-containing enzymes of tissue cells. The most obvious effects of iron deficiency are due to anaemia, which is dealt with in Chapter 17. The effects of deficiency of iron-containing enzymes in man are not well understood. In experimental animals, they have been shown to include impaired muscle metabolism with lactic acidosis and undue fatigability and, in pregnancy, delay or arrest in fetal development.

Iron deficiency is particularly common, and often severe, in many of the developing countries, the main factors being an inadequate diet and loss of blood from hookworm infection.

Iron overload

This can result either from absorption of excessive amounts of iron from the gut or from administration of parenteral iron, for example by multiple blood transfusions.

The outstanding example of naturally occurring iron overload is provided by the disease termed **idiopathic haemochromatosis**, in which storage occurs predominantly in the parenchymal cells of the internal organs where it causes cell injury, probably by catalysing peroxidation of cell membranes. By contrast, when multiple transfusions are administered over a period of years to patients with aplastic anaemia (due to marrow aplasia), iron accumulates mainly in macrophages, where it causes little injury. The effects of iron overload thus depend not so much on the amount of iron stored, as on its distribution between macrophages and parenchymal cells.

In iron overload due to excessive dietary iron or oral iron therapy, and in certain disorders of haemoglobin or red cell production, the distribution of stored iron, as explained later, is more complex.

States of increased iron storage are conveniently termed **haemosiderosis** or **siderosis**.

Idiopathic (Primary) haemochromatosis

This is characterised by excessive absorption of dietary iron, from birth onwards. The total iron in the body gradually increases until, by the age of 40 years or so, it may exceed 20 g instead of the normal 3–4 g. Erythropoiesis is normal and the excess of iron is stored as haemosiderin, mainly in the parenchymal cells, particularly in the liver (Fig. 11.13), pancreas and myocardium, but also in many other organs.

The condition occurs mainly (80–90%) in men. Iron-induced hepatocyte destruction with accompanying fibrosis leads to cirrhosis, which is often the cause of presenting symptoms. The toxic effect of iron on the myocardial cells commonly leads to congestive heart failure and cardiac arrhythmias, while heavy deposition in the pancreas results in cell loss and fibrosis. Over 50% of patients develop diabetes, probably due to a combination of liver and islet-cell injury. Macroscopically, the liver, pancreas, etc. appear brown and give an intense prussian blue reaction. Microscopy shows heavy deposition of haemosiderin in the parenchymal cells. Death of damaged cells results in release of haemosiderin, which is seen in the adjacent stroma and is ingested by macrophages in the

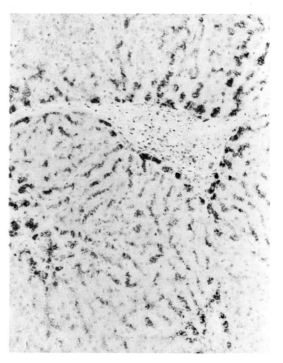

Fig. 11.13 Needle biopsy of the liver in haemochromatosis. The excess iron is stored mainly as haemosiderin in the hepatocytes, and is seen as dark granules. Prussian blue reaction. × 150.

affected organs and their draining lymph nodes. Apart from this, the amount of haemosiderin in macrophages in general, e.g. in the spleen and bone marrow, is not greatly increased. The skin develops a bronzed appearance (hence the term **bronzed diabetes**) due to excess melanin production, which is unexplained; in some cases, however, the skin appears more leaden owing to iron deposition, mainly in fibrocytes adjacent to the sweat glands. Other features include the polyarthritis of pseudo-gout, due to the formation in the joint tissues and spaces of calcium pyrophosphate crystals; this may result from the inhibitory effects of iron on pyrophosphatase. Hypogonadism, probably due to iron-induced injury to the cells of the adenohypophysis, is common, and also vague neurological symptoms of unknown cause.

Aetiology. The nature of the metabolic defect responsible for excessive iron absorption is unknown. The plasma transferrin is not increased but is almost fully saturated with iron (over 80% in men and over 70% in women, c.f. normal 30%), and the plasma ferritin level is over 700 μg/l). Tests of iron absorption have given conflicting results, but if the iron stores are depleted by venesection etc., absorption can then be demonstrated to be increased. If the iron stores are allowed to re-accumulate, absorption falls, sometimes to normal. The inverse relationship between total iron store and absorption is thus maintained, but *the proportion of dietary iron absorbed at all levels of iron storage is abnormally high*: as noted by Bothwell *et al.* (1979), the 'absorbostat' is set too high.

Although the nature of the defect is unknown, it has been suggested that macrophages are incapable of storing excess iron as haemosiderin, and that in consequence the plasma transferrin becomes near-saturated and so excess iron is taken up by the parenchymal cells of the liver, etc. Because transferrin is approaching saturation, iron absorbed from the gut and transferred to the plasma may be transported by the portal blood in a form which is more readily taken up by the liver cells, thus explaining why the liver is particularly severely affected.

Genetic predisposition for haemochromatosis has long been suspected, and has recently been confirmed by the demonstration of associations with HLA types. The strongest is with HLA-A3, over 70% of patients being positive (c.f. 27% in general population) and there are weaker associations with HLA-B14 and B7. This suggests involvement of a genetic factor closely linked with the HLA-A locus on chromosome 6 and family studies of HLA haplotypes suggest strongly that the disease is inherited as a recessive trait. The frequency of the abnormal gene appears to be about 0·05 in Sweden and the USA, giving an estimated incidence of homozygotes of 1 in 275. In fact, the observed incidence of the disease is much less, partly because homozygous women are protected against gross iron-overload by loss of menstrual blood, and partly because the clinical features of haemochromatosis develop from the age of 50 onwards, and many homozygotes may die from other causes before it becomes apparent.

Within a family, homozygous siblings of a patient with haemochromatosis can sometimes by identified by HLA haplotyping and are commonly found to have excessive iron storage and other features suggestive of a pre-clinical stage of the disease. Heterozygotes may also show minor degrees of iron-overload.

Removal of excess iron prevents or slows down tissue injury. This may be achieved by repeated withdrawal of blood or, if the patient becomes anaemic, by injection of the iron-chelating agent desferrioxamine, which promotes greatly increased excretion of iron in the urine.

Iron-overload in other diseases. Iron deficiency is the commonest cause of anaemia, but in some types of anaemia due to other causes there may be greatly increased iron storage. For example, in *aplastic anaemia*, in which haemopoiesis fails and the marrow becomes hypocellular, life can be maintained only by regular blood transfusions and since each unit of blood contains 200–250 mg of iron, gross iron overload can develop over a number of years. In contrast to haemochromatosis, most of the iron accumulating as haemosiderin is stored in macrophages in the spleen, liver (Fig. 11.14), marrow and elsewhere. There is some increase of iron in the hepatocytes; initially it is relatively slight, but later may increase as a result of redistribution of iron.

The situation is different in patients in whom anaemia is due to defective red cell production in spite of hyperplasia of the erythropoietic tissue, i.e. in which there is *'ineffective erythropoiesis'*. A good example is provided by the *thalassaemias* (p. 17.28), in which there is

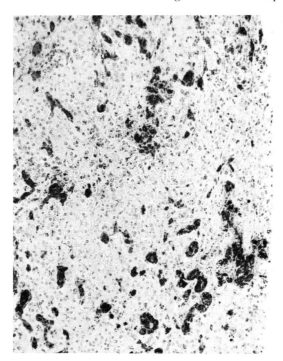

Fig. 11.14 Needle biopsy of the liver in a case of aplastic anaemia with haemosiderosis resulting from multiple blood transfusions. Haemosiderin is present in groups of enlarged Kupffer cells and macrophages in the portal areas. The patient suffered from chronic renal failure and had been maintained on haemodialysis. × 150.

defective haemoglobin synthesis, and in the familial form of *sideroblastic anaemia* (p. 17.42) in which incorporation of iron into haemoglobin is defective. In such conditions, immature erythroid cells are destroyed in the marrow. In some unknown manner, increased but ineffective erythropoiesis increases iron absorption and thus causes overload, which, as in haemochromatosis, results in deposition of iron in parenchymal cells. If the condition is inherited and so present from birth onwards, a picture similar to haemochromatosis may develop. Multiple blood transfusions are usually necessary in these conditions and add greatly to the storage iron, which then accumulates in both parenchymal cells and macrophages.

In anaemia with increased but *effective* erythropoiesis, e.g. chronic haemolytic anaemia, in which circulating red cells are destroyed abnormally rapidly, and in which compensatory increase in erythropoiesis occurs, there is some increase in iron absorption but gross overloading does not usually occur unless multiple transfusions are administered. Increased iron absorption and haemosiderosis occur as a complication of various liver diseases, including cirrhosis. Apart from alcohol, the causal factors of over-absorption are not apparent.

Dietary iron overload

It is rare for serious iron overload to occur from increased iron intake in the diet, partly because in most diets with a high iron content much of the iron is in unavailable form, and partly because any increase in iron stores inhibits absorption of dietary iron. There is, however, one outstanding example of overload resulting from dietary factors, and that is in South Africans of the Bantu tribe. Their intake of iron is very high, partly because iron pots are used in cooking, but mainly from drinking beer brewed in iron containers. Because of its low pH, the brew dissolves iron and as much as 50–100 mg of iron may be ingested daily in a few litres of the (rather weak) beer. The distribution of iron varies: in many cases, however, it accumulates both in macrophages and in the parenchymal cells in the liver and sometimes other organs, and the picture of haemochromatosis with hepatic cirrhosis and sometimes diabetes may develop. In such cases, the degree of liver injury has been shown to correlate partly with the amount of iron in the hepatocytes. A striking difference from haemochromatosis is the deposition of haemosiderin in the lamina propria of the villi of the proximal small intestine. In other individuals, storage of iron is predominantly in macrophages and without serious effects. It is not known why iron deposition is parenchymal in some and in macrophages in others, but it has been reported that, in the former, there is a high degree of saturation of plasma transferrin. With the increasing use of commercially prepared beverages, the incidence of haemosiderosis in the Bantu has declined considerably. The alcohol in the beer also doubtless contributes to the hepatic injury and in some cases the picture is that of alcoholic cirrhosis with excess iron deposition.

The risk of serious iron overload from prolonged taking of medicinal iron by mouth appears to be slight, for although there are reports of haemochromatosis developing, in many other cases the iron stores do not appear to have been very greatly increased. Acute iron poisoning can, however, result from gross overdosage with iron.

Tests for iron overload

The level of plasma ferritin is rasied to over 200 μg/l in nearly all cases of iron-overload, regardless of the distribution of the iron, and in haemochromatosis the level is over 700 μg/l. The plasma transferrin is highly saturated in haemochromatosis and other forms of parenchymal overload, but not usually in macrophage overload. Excretion of 4 mg or more of iron in the urine during the 24 hours following an injection of desferrioxamine (see above) is strongly suggestive of haemochromatosis, less than 3 mg being excreted in macrophage overload. Finally, needle biopsy of the liver is usually necessary to confirm and assess parenchymal overload and to determine the presence and degree of liver damage.

Malarial pigmentation

In malaria, the parasites within the red cells produce from the haemoglobin a dark brown pigment, haematin, in the form of very minute granules, which accumulates within the parasites. When the adult divides into young forms (merozoites), the red cell disintegrates and the pigment is released to be taken up by monocytes (Fig. 17.12, p. 17.16) and by macrophages, especially in the spleen, liver and haemopoietic marrow, where it remains practically unchanged for many years. In chronic malaria these tissues appear dark brown. Malaria pigment does not give the prussian blue reaction and resembles closely the artefact pigment derived from formalin acting on blood. In severe cases of malaria, significant amounts of haemosiderin may be deposited in the organs in addition to the malarial pigment.

Lipofuscin: Age Pigment

In the later years of life a fine brownish-yellow pigment tends to appear in various types of cell, notably in the heart muscle, smooth muscle and various parenchymal cells. This accumulation of pigment is more marked in people with wasting diseases. In some cases of malabsorption syndrome, for example due to coeliac disease, it is present in the smooth muscle of the small intestine and oesophagus, and in smaller amounts in that of the stomach and colon: experimental studies suggest that vitamin E deficiency may be responsible.

In the heart muscle, the pigment accumulates in the central part of the cells around the poles of the nucleus, and when this is associated with wasting of the muscle, the term *brown atrophy* is applied. Similar pigment occurs in the liver cells in the central parts of the lobules, in the cells of the testis, and in the nerve cells of the cortex of the brain. Heavy deposits of pigment are seen in the cortical neurons in senile dementia and allied conditions and must be distinguished from that which occurs normally in the pigmented neurons of the locus caeruleus and substantia nigra, which belongs to the melanin group. In brown atrophy, the pigment is believed to be chiefly lipid, as it reduces perosmic acid and is usually coloured by the sudan stains. It is often called *lipofuscin*, but differs in its chemical and staining reactions in the various organs, some being fluorescent, doubly refracting or acid-fast in varying degree, e.g. *ceroid*, an acid-fast pigment found in the liver in certain forms of experimental cirrhosis. In electron micrographs, it is seen as *residual bodies* (p. 3.14), which result from incorporation of cell constituents into phagosomes, e.g. in the process of apoptosis, the lipofuscin persisting as indigestible residues of cellular lipids.

Exogenous Deposits

Inhaled compounds. A certain amount of soot, stone dust, etc., enters and accumulates in the lungs of all individuals living in an atmosphere polluted by smoke and dust, and the accumulation becomes excessive in those exposed occupationally to an atmosphere heavily contaminated by various dusts. The lungs may be infiltrated by foreign particles of various kinds—coal, silica, asbestos, iron and other ores and various organic substances. The resulting pathological changes will be described later with the diseases of the lungs.

The entrance of such particles into the lungs is favoured by the presence of chronic bronchitis or other conditions in which there is interference with the action of the ciliated epithelium, but even in normal health, particles of less than 5 μm gain access to the pulmonary alveoli if the concentration in the inspired air is great. The dust particles are quickly taken up by macrophages in the pulmonary alveoli (Fig. 11.15). Some of the macrophages with the ingested particles are expelled via the bronchi, some enter the interstitial tissue of the lungs and pass into the lymphatics, while some settle in the alveoli alongside respiratory bronchioles and the pigment is eventually incorporated into

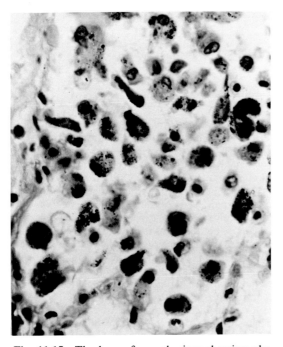

Fig. 11.15 The lung of a coal-miner showing phagocytosis of inhaled particles of coal dust by alveolar macrophages. × 520.

the respiratory bronchiolar walls. Much of the pigment is, however, carried into the lymphatics and is deposited mostly in the hilar nodes, but also in the pleura. The degree of tissue injury resulting depends on the nature of the particles. Large collections of carbonaceous particles (*anthracosis*) may provoke little or no cell injury or overgrowth of connective tissue. The bronchial lymph nodes become pigmented and enlarged, the accumulation within their phagocytic cells being virtually permanent. Some of the pigment which has accumulated in the lungs may be removed by macrophages which appear in the sputum for a long time after removal of the individual from the dusty atmosphere. Inhalation of silica particles in stone dust causes persistent destruction of macrophages (p. 3.14) with consequent low-grade inflammation and formation of nodules of dense fibrous tissue in the lungs—**silicosis**. Asbestos (fibrous silicates) is similarly irritating and not only causes more diffuse pulmonary fibrosis but also predisposes to cancer.

Ingested compounds. Deposition of brownish granules of **silver compounds** (*argyria*) was a common result of taking medicines containing silver preparations. The granules are formed by reduction of silver albuminate and are seen especially in the skin (giving a dusky appearance), the gut wall, and the basement membranes of the glomeruli and renal collecting tubules. It is now rare. In **chronic lead-poisoning**, an albuminate is produced in a similar way, and around the teeth hydrogen sulphide reacts with it to produce the characteristic blue line on the gums. **Melanosis coli** (p. 11.10) is now the commonest example of pigmentation resulting from ingestion of chemicals.

Tattooing. In tattooing, fine particles such as india ink, ultramarine, cinnabar (mercuric sulphide), etc., introduced through the epidermis, are taken up by macrophages and lodge in small spaces or clefts in the connective tissue of the cutis. Some particles are carried also by the lymph stream to the regional lymph nodes and then are conveyed by phagocytes into the lymphoid tissue. Both at the site of introduction and in the lymph nodes, the pigment remains for life.

Pathological Calcification

Pathological calcification of soft tissues occurs most commonly without any general disturbance of calcium metabolism: the level of plasma calcium is normal, and deposition is due to local changes in the affected tissue. This is termed *dystrophic calcification*. Less commonly, pathological calcification is a result of an increase in the level of ionic calcium in the plasma, and occurs in normal soft tissues: this is termed *metastatic calcification.*

In both dystrophic and metastatic calcification, the deposits resemble in composition the minerals of bone, but show much greater variations in the proportions of calcium to magnesium and phosphate to carbonate.

Identification of calcium salts in tissues. Calcium salts have an affinity for haematoxylin, and the earliest sign of calcification is given by the appearance of hyaline or finely granular material of a deep violet tint. Later, the calcium salts form irregular and somewhat refractile masses: they are, of course, readily soluble in weak acids, and small bubbles of carbon dioxide are released from the carbonates. When treated with dilute sulphuric acid, the characteristic crystals of calcium sulphate separate out. This occurs more readily when the sections are in 50% alcohol, in which the solubility of the crystals is low. When carbonate or phosphate (which are nearly always deposited as calcium salts) are treated with silver nitrate, yellow silver phosphate is formed, and this quickly undergoes reduction on exposure to light and turns black (von Kossa's method). Neither the affinity for haematoxylin nor von Kossa's method is specific for calcium. Silver nitrate is reduced by other substances, e.g. iron, and the reaction with haematoxylin is given by a substance formed before the deposition of calcium, and is positive after the tissue is decalcified. The best reagent is alizarin, the staining principle in madder, or its derivatives. Alizarin stains calcium salts red, but the reaction may not be given by very old deposits. When injected *intra vitam*, alizarin colours growing bone (but not fully formed bone) and also pathological deposits of calcium unless they are very old.

Calcification is often accompanied by diffuse or granular deposition of iron compounds which give a prussian blue reaction (p. 11.15).

Dystrophic calcification

This consists of the irregular deposition of calcium salts in altered or necrotic tissues and formed elements such as thrombi. Deposition is irregular and may be sufficiently heavy to render the part chalky or even stony hard.

Predisposing changes. The local changes which predispose to dystrophic calcification are as follows.

1. Hyaline change in fibrous tissue. This occurs as an ageing change in arteries. Increase in calcium in hyalinised artery walls is usual, and it may be sufficient to convert the vessel to a rigid tube, as in Monckeberg's sclerosis (Fig. 14.38, p. 14.35). Calcification is also common in dense connective tissues, for example tendons, the dura mater, and the scarred heart valves following rheumatic endocarditis. It occurs in some tumours, for example in fibromas (Fig. 11.16) and in uterine myomas which become

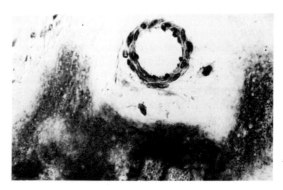

Fig. 11.16 Dystrophic calcification of hyaline connective tissue adjacent to a small blood vessel in a fibroma. The calcified tissue is stained by haematoxylin (even after decalcification), and presents a dark granular appearance. × 500.

atrophic and hyaline after the menopause. The 'brain-sand' bodies of some meningiomas consist of concentrically arranged cells which undergo hyaline change followed by calcification.

2. Tissue death. Calcification commonly occurs in (a) the necrotic lipid debris in atheromatous patches, (b) fat necrosis (usually around the pancreas or in the breast), (c) old infarcts (d) caseous patches in tuberculosis, necrotic foci in histoplasmosis and other chronic infections, (e) necrotic foci in malignant tumours, and (f) dead parasites (e.g. *Trichinella spiralis* and echinococcal cysts). Calcification of such dead tissue is a slow process, and occurs only when necrotic material persists for a long time without undergoing organisation.

3. Inspissated pus and *organic material in ducts, etc.* A large collection of pus, unless discharged, may eventually become inspissated, then calcified, and even ossified. Organic material accumulating in the ducts of salivary glands, or in the appendix, may become calcified, forming 'stones' in these sites. Calcium deposition in the urinary tract, both as discrete stones and as soft, crumbling material, is caused by urinary infections, but stone formation occurs also as a result of increased calcium excretion (see below).

4. Thrombi. Calcification occurs very commonly in old venous thrombi which have not undergone organisation: hard masses are thus formed in veins, e.g. in the legs, and show up on x-ray as *phleboliths.*

The chemical reactions involved in dystrophic calcification are not understood. Factors which may be involved include the following. (*a*) Local changes in pH of hyaline or necrotic tissue, etc.: calcium is deposited more readily from an alkaline medium. (*b*) Breakdown products of cells or tissue elements to provide a nucleus with an affinity for calcium salts. Release of phosphate from nucleoprotein breakdown is a possible example. The strong tendency for calcification of necrotic fatty tissue was formerly explained by the affinity of fatty acids for calcium, forming insoluble calcium salts. This suggestion lacks supporting evidence, and, in particular, subcutaneous injection of fatty acids does not lead to calcification. (*c*) Local enzyme changes: the normal process of calcification of growing bone occurs in the presence of high local concentrations of alkaline phosphatase. In experimentally-induced lesions, some correlation has been observed between high levels of alkaline phosphatase and deposition of calcium salts, but the correlation is not a very good one, and this is not a convincing factor in dystrophic calcification in man.

Calcinosis circumscripta. This is a condition in which irregular nodular dystrophic calcification occurs in the skin and subcutaneous tissues, especially of the fingers. The overlying skin becomes ulcerated and the chalky material is discharged or may be scraped out. This appears to consist chiefly of calcium carbonate, as shown by solution with effervescence in hydrochloric acid. Microscopically, a mild chronic inflammatory reaction with giant cells surrounds the nodules. The causation of the lesion is obscure. The deposits are easily distinguished from gouty tophi by their dense opacity to x-rays and by histochemical tests (see also tumoral calcinosis, p. 23.56).

Occasionally calcium deposition is more widespread, involving also muscles and tendons—this is known as **calcinosis universalis.**

A number of other diseases, including scleroderma and dermatomyositis, are occasionally complicated by calcification of the dermis or subcutaneous tissues.

Metastatic calcification

This occurs in the following conditions.

1. Excessive absorption of calcium from the gut, seen most commonly in infants with hypervitaminosis D due to over-fortification of infant foods with vitamin D and calcium (p. 23.16). Similar experimental changes can be produced readily in the rat (Fig. 11.17).

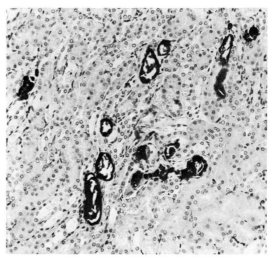

Fig. 11.17   Rat kidney in hypervitaminosis D. Note calcified small vessels and renal tubules. × 120. (From preparation kindly lent by Dr. J.R.M. Innes.)

Excessive intake can result also from taking very large amounts of calcium by mouth, for example milk and calcium carbonate, formerly a very common treatment for peptic ulcer, sometimes results in hypercalcaemia and alkalosis (the milk-alkali syndrome).

2. Excessive mobilisation of calcium from the bones. This occurs in patients with *widespread bone destruction*, as, for example, in multiple myeloma or metastatic carcinoma. *Prolonged immobilisation* in bed for any reason is also of importance, the bones undergoing disuse atrophy. Excessive mobilisation of bone calcium is also brought about by *primary hyperparathyroidism*, usually due to a parathyroid adenoma (p. 26.27), but a more common cause is *secondary hyperparathyroidism* associated with parathyroid hyperplasia and resulting from chronic renal failure with retention of phosphate (p. 26.29).

Metastatic calcification occurs especially in the walls of arteries and in the kidneys. It is occasionally seen in the myocardium, acid-secreting gastric mucosa and the alveolar walls of the lungs. It may be that the sites of metastatic calcification are determined partly by a relatively high pH, e.g. around the renal tubules and the acid-secreting gastric glands. Deposition is seen initially on the surface of elastic fibres, basement membranes and other formed elements.

The **kidneys** and **urinary tract** are the commonest and most important sites of metastatic calcification. In the kidney, deposition of calcium occurs in the tubular epithelium and may be seen by electron microscopy in relation to mitochondria. More gross calcium deposition

may occur in the tubular basement membranes and the interstitial tissue, and calcified concretions may form in the tubular lumen, usually of the collecting tubules. These changes are accompanied by impaired function, and by the development of coarse scars involving segments of the cortex and medulla (possibly due to obstruction of individual collecting tubules). Chronic renal failure may result. The renal arteries may also be calcified but, as with other arteries, their patency is little affected.

Another important feature of hypercalcaemia is the formation of calcium carbonate/phosphate stones in the renal pelvis (p. 22.60).

Nephrocalcinosis and stone formation are particularly liable to occur when there is increased intake of calcium associated with alkalosis and an alkaline urine, as in the milk-alkali syndrome; they occur also in renal tubular acidosis (p. 22.45).

Deposition of Uric Acid and Urates

Uric acid is formed as the final breakdown product of purine bases, and is thus derived from catabolism of nucleic acids. Normal plasma urate levels depend greatly on the assay technique, but levels above 7·0 mg/100 ml (0·42 mmol/l) for men and 6·0 mg/100 ml (0·36 mmol/l) for women are abnormally high. Adults produce 400–700 mg of endogenous uric acid daily and dietary purines contribute 300–600 mg. Most of this uric acid is excreted by the renal distal convoluted tubules, which can normally increase the rate of excretion, as necessary, to maintain homeostasis.

Hyperuricaemia is not uncommon, particularly in men over 40. It tends to be familial, but sporadic cases occur. The metabolic abnormalities concerned are not clearly understood. In some instances, increased production of uric acid results from a deficiency of the phosphoribosyl-transferase enzyme which is necessary for the re-utilisation of hypoxanthine for purine synthesis. This deficiency results in increased breakdown of hypoxanthine into uric acid. Other enzyme deficiencies with similar effect have been detected in some instances of hyperuricaemia. In others, there is a defect of unknown nature in renal excretion of uric acid.

These defects account for at least some cases of *primary hyperuricaemia* in which nucleic acid breakdown is normal. *Secondary hyperuricaemia* results from increased nucleic acid breakdown, as in chronic granulocytic leukaemia (p. 17.54).

There is considerable variation in the effects

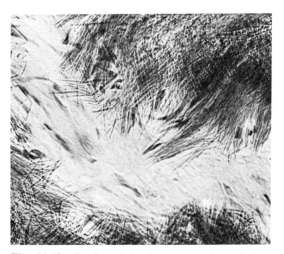

Fig. 11.18 Section through gouty nodule of skin, showing deposit of needle-like crystals of monosodium urate. × 370.

of hyperuricaemia. In most instances, there are no associated pathological changes. In others, there is deposition of uric acid or urate in the collecting tubules of the kidneys, seen macroscopically as brown-yellow streaking of the medulla: this may have little or no effect, or may be followed by formation of uric acid stones (p. 22.59). Uric acid streaking of the medulla is a common autopsy finding, particularly in children, and appears to be associated with a state of dehydration before death. The most important complication of hyperuricaemia is **gout** (p. 23.51), in which crystals of monosodium urate are deposited in and around the joints, in the skin (Fig. 11.18) and elsewhere. It is always accompanied by hyperuricaemia, and yet the relatives of patients may have equally high plasma levels of uric acid without developing gout. As indicated above for hyperuricaemia in general, a number of individual abnormalities of purine metabolism can result in gout.

Further Reading

Bothwell, T.H., Charlton, R.W., Cook, J.W. and Finch, C.A. (1979). *Iron Metabolism in Man*, pp. 576. Blackwell Scientific, Oxford, London, Edinburgh and Melbourne. (A comprehensive review by four leading experts, with an extensive bibliography.)

Finch, C.A. and Huebers, H. (1982). Perspectives in iron metabolism. *New England Journal of Medicine* **306**, 1520-8.

Goodwin, F.J. (1982). Hypercalcaemia. *British Journal of Hospital Medicine*, **28**, 50-8.

Gorevic, P.D. (1981). The amyloid diseases: clinico-pathological and biochemical correlations. pp. 1-30 in *Clinical Immunology Update*. Ed. E.C. Franklin. pp. 427. Churchill Livingstone, Edinburgh.

Hind, C.R.K. and Pepys, M.B. (1984). Amyloidosis: Classification and pathogenesis. *Hospital Update*, 593-8. (An excellent brief review).

Lendrum, A.C. (1969). The Validation of Fibrin and its Significance in the Story of Hyalin. In *Trends in Clinical Pathology*, pp. 159-183. British Medical Association, London.

Pepys, M.B. and Baltz, M.L. (1984). Amyloidosis. In *Copeman's Textbook of the rheumatoid diseases*, 6th ed. pp. Ed. Scott, J.T. Churchill Livingstone, Edinburgh.

Scheinberg, M.A. and Cathcart, E.S. (1976). Comprehensive study of humoral and cellular immune abnormalities in 26 patients with systemic amyloidosis. *Arthritis and Rheumatism*, **19**, 173-82.

12

TUMOURS: I.   General Features, Types and Examples

What is a tumour?

In previous chapters we have seen examples of cell proliferation and growth of tissue in the processes of regeneration and repair and as a hyperplastic response to increased workload or hormonal stimulation. Such growth is both purposeful and beneficial and occurs as a response to physiological stimuli: its control is dependent on the fact that normal cells will only divide if they receive the appropriate stimulus, and complex feedback mechanisms, which are not fully understood, regulate the stimulating factors and thus control cell proliferation. By contrast, *tumours (neoplasms) develop by a process of pathological proliferation of cells which is both excessive and purposeless. It continues indefinitely in the absence of physiological stimuli and without regard to its effect on the surrounding tissues or the requirements of the individual.* The nature of the change which makes tumour cells behave thus is not fully understood, but it is irreversible and persists after removal of the causal factors which have induced the changes leading to the development of a tumour from what was originally a normal cell. Such neoplastic change is also heritable in the sense that when a tumour cell divides, it produces more tumour cells of the same type.

Because they exhibit various degrees of uncontrolled proliferation, tumours are sometimes termed *autonomous*, but they are, of course, dependent on the host for their blood supply, nutrition and supporting stroma. Also, their escape from the mechanisms which control proliferation of normal cells is not always complete, for the growth of some tumours can be retarded or arrested by changes in their hormonal environment.

The proliferation of tumour cells (*neoplastic cells*) usually results in a lump consisting of the tumour cells and their products, e.g. mucin, collagen, and they also contain blood vessels and supporting stroma. In some instances, however, the tumour cells may infiltrate diffusely, causing more general enlargement of the affected organs and tissues: this is seen particularly in neoplasms of the haemopoietic and lymphoid cells in which large numbers of tumour cells may also circulate in the blood (*leukaemia*). With these reservations, a tumour may be defined as follows.

A tumour is a mass of tissue formed as a result of abnormal, excessive and inappropriate proliferation of cells, the growth of which continues indefinitely and regardless of the mechanisms which control normal cellular proliferation.

The importance of tumours

The division of tumours into **benign** and **malignant** types is fundamental in any consideration of their importance. **Benign tumours remain localised, forming a single mass which is often symptomless and can usually be excised completely.** When they do give rise to symptoms, these are usually due to pressure on adjacent structures or to excessive production of hormones. By contrast, **malignant tumours, known collectively as cancer, invade the surrounding tissues and their cells spread by lymphatics and blood vessels to other parts of the body where they give rise to secondary tumours or metastases.** In most instances, complete excision provides the only hope of cure of cancer, and while this can often be achieved for cancers developing in conspicuous sites, e.g. in the skin, those originating in the internal organs and deeper tissues have all too often spread beyond the possibility of complete excision by the time they

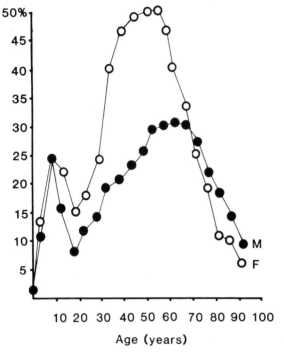

long. Although much less common in younger people, the incidence of cancer is, however, by no means negligible at any age (Fig. 12.1): in one form or another it is second only to accidents as a cause of death below the age of thirty years. After this, the incidence of cancer increases, at first gradually and then more sharply (Fig. 12.2).

The stage at which metastasis occurs varies greatly for different types of cancer, and even for cancers of similar type arising at a particular site. For example, cancer of the breast may grow to a large size without metastasising to other sites, or it may spread widely before the primary tumour has become large enough to be detected. The outlook for individual patients thus varies greatly.

Fig. 12.1 Deaths from cancer in males and females in England and Wales expressed as a percentage of all deaths in five-year age groups. In childhood and young adult life, the incidence of accidental deaths is relatively high in males, and between the ages of 40 and 65 males have a relatively high incidence of deaths from ischaemic heart disease. These factors account largely for the lower percentages of male deaths from cancer up to the age of 65. (Mortality Statistics, (1983) HMSO, London.)

are detected. This is why screening procedures have been set up in many countries to detect early cancer, or better still, to detect precancerous (*premalignant*) changes, e.g. in the cervix uteri, which often precede the development of cancer by several years. The importance of malignant tumours does not require emphasis, for **cancer accounts for about 20% of deaths in most of the developed countries, being second only to ischaemic heart disease.** Nor is cancer dreaded solely as a major cause of death, but also because many patients with it are condemned to a long and often painful terminal illness. One slightly consoling feature is that the great majority of cancer patients are elderly: this is one reason why it is so common in the developed countries where life expectation is

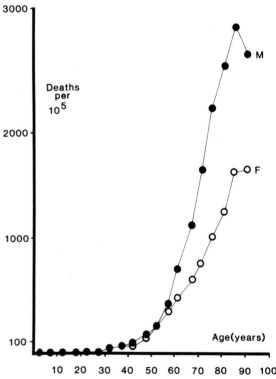

Fig. 12.2 Death rates from cancer in males and females in England and Wales expressed as the number of deaths per 100 000 in five-year age groups. The differences between men and women are attributable mainly to the higher incidence of bronchial carcinoma in men. (Mortality Statistics (1983) HMSO, London.)

The origin, diversity and classification of tumours

The available evidence suggests that most tumours arise by clonal proliferation of a single cell. The evidence for this has been provided largely by the demonstration that most types of tumour occurring in women who are heterozygous at the locus on the X chromosomes coding for glucose-6-phosphate dehydrogenase iso-enzymes produce only one type of enzyme, indicating their origin from a single cell (p. 2.11) (Fialkow, 1976). Evidence of the monoclonality of tumours of B lymphoid cells is provided by the production by their cells of immunoglobulin molecules of single light chain type, either κ or λ (p. 6.15). *Tumours can arise from the cells of virtually all types of tissue*, and this diversity of origin is largely responsible for the great variety of structural appearances of tumours, for **the cells of most tumours show some degree of differentiation towards the adult cell type of the tissue of origin**. For example, the cells of tumours arising from squamous epithelium tend to undergo some degree of keratinisation, while those derived from osteoblasts frequently produce bone matrix. Many other examples of tumour differentiation are illustrated in this chapter, but the important point to note here is that *the tendency for the cells of a tumour to differentiate along a particular pathway usually allows recognition of the type of tissue cell from which it is derived, and this forms the basis of the histogenetic classification of tumours*. Thus, most tumours can be recognised to be of epithelial or connective-tissue nature: epithelial tumours may be further classed as squamous-cell, glandular, etc., and connective tissue tumours as derived from fibroblasts, smooth muscle cells, cartilage cells, etc. The histogenetic classification of tumours is in universal usage, together with the important classification into benign and malignant tumours. The major classes of tumours are shown in Table 12.1. Meanwhile, it is convenient here to note that the word **neoplasm** is applied to all types of tumour; **cancer** includes all types of malignant tumour, while malignant epithelial tumours are termed **carcinomas** and malignant connective-tissue tumours, **sarcomas**. **Neoplasia** or **neoplastic change** are terms applied to all kinds of tumour. **Oncogenesis** means the changes involved in the development of any kind of tumour and **carcinogenesis** means the

changes involved in the development of all types of malignant tumours. The suffix **-oma**, as in carcinoma or sarcoma, is of Greek origin and means a tumour or swelling. It is also used for individual types of tumour, for example a tumour of liver cells is a hepatoma and a tumour of lymphoid cells is a lymphoma. Unfortunately it is used for some non-neoplastic swellings, for example granuloma and tuberculoma, both of which are inflammatory lesions.

Our knowledge on which type of cell in any

Table 12.1 Histogenetic classification of tumours

Cell or Tissue Type	Benign	Malignant
Epithelial tumours		
surface	papilloma	carcinoma (various types)
glandular	adenoma	adenocarcinoma
Non-epithelial and mixed tumours		
Connective tissues		
adipose	lipoma	liposarcoma
fibrous	fibroma	fibrosarcoma
cartilage	chondroma	chondrosarcoma
bone	osteoma	osteosarcoma
smooth muscle	leiomyoma	leiomyosarcoma
striped muscle	rhabdomyoma*	rhabomyosarcoma
Neuro-ectodermal		
glial cells	—	gliomas
nerve cells	ganglioneuroma	neuroblastoma medulloblastoma
melanocytes	pigmented naevus*	malignant melanoma
meninges	meningioma	malignant meningioma
nerve sheaths	schwannoma neurofibroma	neurofibrosarcoma
Haemopoietic and lympho-reticular		leukaemias myeloproliferative disorders lymphomas
Blood vessels and lymphatic vessels	haemangioma* glomangioma lymphangioma*	haemangiosarcoma ?Kaposi's disease lymphangiosarcoma
Germinal and embryonal cells	benign teratoma	malignant teratoma dysgerminoma ($\female$) seminoma ($\male$)
placenta	hydatidiform mole†	choriocarcinoma

* Tumour-like lesions which are probably hamartomas (see p. 12.47).

† Neoplastic nature doubtful (see p. 12.42).

particular tissue can become neoplastic relates mainly to malignant tumours, and is based on the fact that transformation from a normal to a cancer cell is a prolonged process involving several stages, including mitotic divisions. Accordingly, end-stage cells, which cannot divide, for example mature red cells, granulocytes and neurons, cannot become transformed to tumour cells. The surface epithelial cells of the skin and mucous membranes exfoliate after a limited lifespan. Only the stem cells of these epithelia persist, and they divide repeatedly to produce stem cells and cells destined to differentiate and exfoliate. For example, the stem cells of stratified squamous epithelium lie in the basal layer. When they divide, their daughter stem cells remain in the basal layer while differentiating cells move into the next layer and, as the stem cells continue to divide, differentiating cells progress towards the surface and are eventually exfoliated as squames. The mechanics are different for surface epithelia of single-cell thickness, as in the gastrointestinal tract, but the principle is the same: only the stem cells are retained. Accordingly, oncogenesis occurs only in the stem cells of these tissues,

the successive cellular changes involved being inherited by successive generations of stem cells arising from the stem cell in which the initial change—the first step towards a cancer cell—occurs.

The epithelia of the liver and renal tubules and various glandular and connective tissues consist of stable cells (p. 5.1) which normally divide infrequently and only to compensate for cell death or in response to increased workload. Such cells act as both stem cells and fully differentiated functional cells, and are capable of developing into tumour cells.

As will be explained in the next chapter, carcinogenesis is almost certainly caused by changes in the nuclear DNA. Any changes in the base sequences of the DNA of a stem cell will be transmitted by mitosis to the daughter stem cell so that, over the years, such damage will be cumulative, and may eventually result in the development of a cancer cell. In general, cancers develop most frequently in tissues with a high rate of cell turnover, and they originate in many instances from repeatedly dividing stem cells.

Differentiation, growth rate and spread of tumours

As explained above, tumours vary greatly in their structure and behaviour. These variations depend upon the type of cell from which a tumour has originated, the degree of differentiation achieved by the tumour cells, and on whether the tumour is benign or malignant. *As a general rule, benign tumours are highly differentiated: their cells are usually uniform, grow slowly and, by definition, remain localised, neither invading the adjacent tissues nor giving rise to metastases elsewhere in the body. Malignant tumours are usually less well differentiated; their cells tend to grow rapidly, to show differences in size and shape and, by definition, invade the tissues locally and metastasise to distant sites.* These important features require more detailed description.

Differentiation

A tumour is said to be highly differentiated when its structure bears a close resemblance to that of the tissue of origin. This requires that the tumour cells should resemble the adult cells of the tissue of origin in their morphology, in their arrangement in relation to one another and to the stroma and blood vessels, and in their functional activities. For example, a well-differentiated tumour of thyroid epithelium forms follicles, produces and stores thyroglobulin (Fig. 12.3), and, may secrete thyroid hormone. To take another example, a well-differentiated tumour of fat cells (a lipoma) is remarkably similar both grossly (Fig. 12.4) and microscopically to normal adipose tissue. In both these examples, the tumours are readily distinguishable from non-neoplastic thyroid or adipose tissue only because they form a discrete mass. Even benign tumours, however, are often

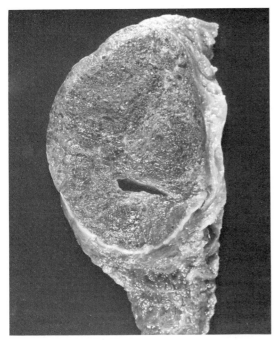

Fig. 12.3 An adenoma of the thyroid gland. The tumour is partly enclosed in normal thyroid tissue and is enveloped in a fibrous capsule, most clearly seen around the lower margin. The cut surface of the tumour resembles thyroid tissue. × 1·5.

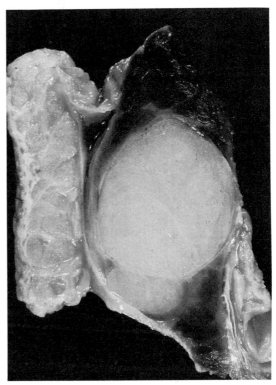

Fig. 12.4 Lipoma in skeletal muscle, consisting of one large and two small nodules which are sharply defined from the surrounding muscle. The tumour tissue resembles the subcutaneous fat seen on the left. × 3.

imperfectly differentiated, for example the thyroid adenoma shown in Fig. 12 5.

At the other extreme, some malignant tumours show no recognisable attempt at differentiation, and are termed **anaplastic**: the individual tumour cells have a primitive, undifferentiated appearance, producing a highly cellular mass in which little attempt at forming special structures or cell products can be discerned (Fig. 12.6), so that it is often not possible to determine their histogenesis. Anaplastic tumours are nearly always highly malignant, but most malignant tumours show some evidence of differentiation, even though it is usually much less perfect than in benign tumours. For example, a malignant tumour of colonic epithelium, i.e. a carcinoma of the colon, usually shows some formation of glandular structures (Fig. 12.7), the cells of which secrete mucous fluid, while the cells of malignant tumours derived from lipoblasts (adipose tissue stem cells) often produce and store droplets of fat (Fig. 12.8).

Not only do the cells of malignant tumours fail to differentiate fully, but they also vary ab-

normally in size and shape (in the same tumour), in their arrangement in relation to one another, in having relatively large, sometimes distorted nuclei and a high nuclear/cytoplasmic ratio. These changes and also mitotic activity (see below), are sometimes collectively termed **cellular atypia**. They are, in general, most pronounced in highly malignant, poorly differentiated cancers, in which cellular variability (**pleomorphism**) is sometimes extreme. This is seen in Fig. 12.9, a tumour in which some of the cells are enormous and contain a single very large nucleus or multiple nuclei: such cells have arisen by replication of the cellular DNA without the completion of mitosis. Abnormal mitoses, e.g. with unequal division of DNA between the daughter cells or with formation of three mitotic spindles instead of two, are also observed in highly malignant tumours.

Some of the above features of malignant tumours are also observed in cells which have not yet formed a tumour, for example in the

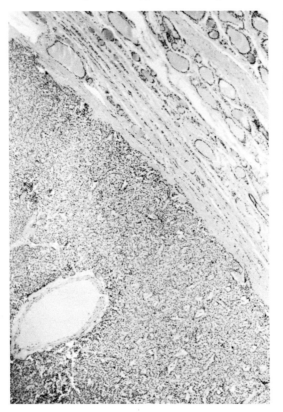

Fig. 12.5   Part of a thyroid adenoma of the 'solid' or micro-acinar type, which contrasts in appearance with normal thyroid tissue. Note the fibrous 'capsule' which is composed largely of residual stroma of compressed, atrophic thyroid surrounding the tumour. × 40.

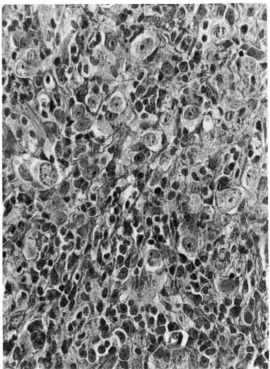

Fig. 12.6   An anaplastic malignant tumour, the histogenesis of which is not obvious. Immunohistology using monoclonal antibodies to epithelial cell markers showed it to be a carcinoma. × 300.

squamous epithelium of the cervix uteri, a common site of carcinoma. The abnormal cells are still confined by the basement membrane of the squamous epithelium, i.e. they have not invaded the underlying tissue, but show various types of atypia. This non-invasive cellular change is commonly termed **dysplasia**, and is found also in other sites (Fig. 12.10). It is often accompanied by chronic inflammatory change and carries a greatly increased risk of the development of invasive carcinoma. In some instances, however, the cellular changes of dysplasia are reversible (p. 24.4). **Tissue pleomorphism** is a feature of some tumours, and notably of teratomas, which are tumours whose cells, like those of the embryo, can differentiate into various tissues (Fig. 12.56, p. 12.41).

Some tumours show a high degree of cell specialisation, but do not resemble the tissue of origin. For example, the ovarian tumour, mucinous cystadenoma, is highly differentiated (Fig. 12.11) but is unlike any normal ovarian structure: the tumour cells have differentiated in a different direction from those of the parent tissue.

Rate of growth

The rate of increase in the number of tumour cells depends on the rate of cell production and the rate of cell loss. The **rate of cell production** depends on the number of cells undergoing mitosis and on the time they take to complete the mitotic or cell cycle (Fig. 5.15, p. 5.11). The proportion of cells seen to be in mitosis in histological sections of tumours (**the mitotic index**) is a useful guide to the rate of cell production, but it can be misleading for it does not take account of the cell cycle time, which varies con-

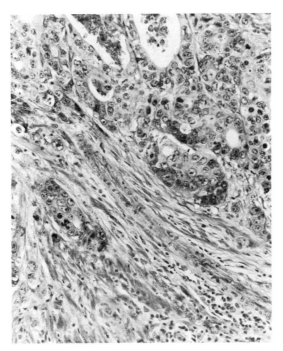

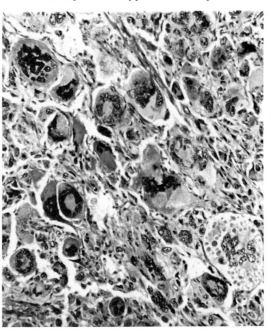

Fig. 12.7 Adenocarcinoma of bowel invading the muscle coat. *Below*, nearly solid strands of tumour are invading smooth muscle on each side of the arteriole which runs up from the bottom right corner. *Above*, the older tumour strands have developed gland-like lumens. × 160.

Fig. 12.9 A malignant connective-tissue tumour (sarcoma) showing considerable variation in the shape and size of the tumour cells and of their nuclei (pleomorphism). × 200.

siderably for different tumours. For example, mitoses are usually numerous in basal cell carcinoma of the epidermis (Fig. 12.32) and yet this tumour grows very slowly, partly because

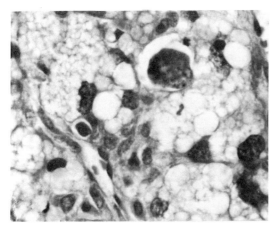

Fig. 12.8 Pleomorphic liposarcoma, consisting of very large cells with large pleomorphic nuclei, and with much fat in the cytoplasm. × 450.

the cell cycle time is long. The use of micro-densitometry or microfluorimetry to measure the nuclear DNA of individual cells in suitably stained preparations gives an indication of the number of cells in the S and M phases of the cell cycle, but in pleomorphic tumours a high DNA content does not necessarily mean that a cell is in the mitotic cycle and this introduces an error. Much more accurate estimates of cell production can be made experimentally by administration of colchicine or vincristine (which arrest mitotic cells in metaphase) and counting the mitotic figures in serial biopsies of the tumour obtained at subsequent fixed intervals. Alternatively, radio-active (tritiated) thymidine may be administered and autoradiography performed on sections prepared from subsequent biopsies: the thymidine is incorporated into newly synthesised DNA as thymine and auto-radiographs thus demonstrate the proportion of cells in the S phase of the cycle. These latter methods indicate the proportion of cells entering a particular phase of the cell cycle in a given time (**the mitotic rate**). By use of these techniques, it has been shown that malignant tumours in experimental animals show logar-

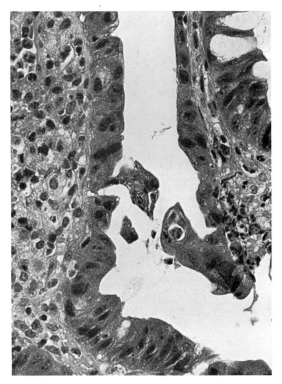

Fig. 12.10 Dysplasia of the colonic epithelium in ulcerative colitis. The cells are pleomorphic, with large irregular nuclei, cytoplasmic basophilia and mitoses. The patient refused colectomy and developed colonic carcinoma. × 350.

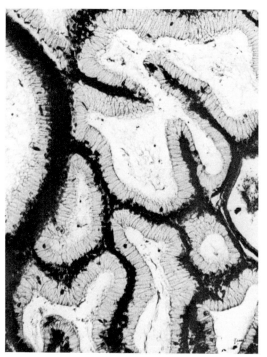

Fig. 12.11 Mucinous cystadenoma (Cystic adenoma) of ovary. The cysts (small in this case) are lined by tall mucin-secreting epithelium. The nuclei, situated at the base of each cell, form a continuous line hardly distinguishable in this picture from those of the next cyst. × 150.

ithmic growth at first but, as the tumour enlarges, cell loss increases and the rate of growth gradually slows down. This increase is due partly to the cells of malignant tumours being abnormal and having a rather short average lifespan, which varies for individual tumours. Another cause of cell loss is ischaemia: as a tumour enlarges, it tends to outgrow its blood supply, particularly if growth is rapid, as in many malignant tumours. Ischaemia inhibits mitosis and causes death of individual cells and groups of cells. In some rapidly growing tumours, extensive necrosis is seen macroscopically in the central part of the tumour (Fig. 12.12) and microscopically in those cells which lie furthest from small blood vessels (Fig. 12.13). By the time a human cancer is discovered, it has usually passed the initial period of logarithmic growth and the rate has slowed down considerably because of increasing cell loss. It follows that, even if the present rate of growth can be accurately assessed, it cannot be

used to calculate the age of the tumour. In some cancers, for example, basal-cell carcinoma of the epidermis, many of the cells undergo shrinkage necrosis (*apoptosis*—p. 3.29) and the high rate of loss is another reason why this tumour grows very slowly in spite of a high mitotic index.

Another method of studying the cell kinetics of tumours is by **clonogenic assay,** which indicates the proportion of tumour cells capable of indefinite clonal proliferation. It may be performed by injecting given numbers of tumour cells intravenously into immunosuppressed, (e.g. x-irradiated) animals and counting the numbers of tumours which develop in the lungs, or by culturing a suspension of tumour cells in a sloppy agar medium and counting the number of colonies which develop. It has been shown by these methods that the proportion of tumour cells which give rise to clones is often small. It thus appears that tumours, like normal tissues, contain a proportion of 'stem' (clon-

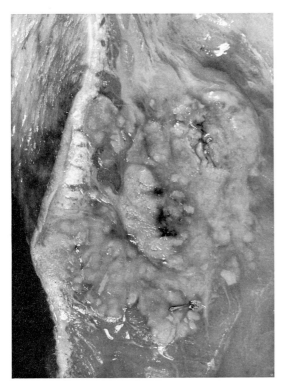

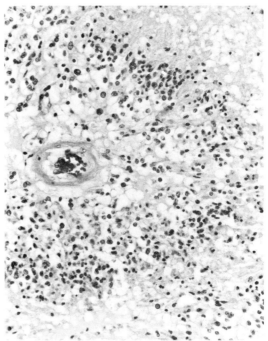

Fig. 12.12 Carcinoma of the breast. Foci of necrosis with breakdown of tumour tissue seen in the central mass (which happens to be shaped like a fetus) and also in the deep upper part of the tumour. Haemorrhage is also apparent. Note the irregular invasion of the breast at the tumour margin. ×1.5

Fig. 12.13 Ischaemic necrosis in a tumour. In this example, the tumour is a rapidly growing anaplastic astrocytoma of the brain, composed of cells with a round dark nucleus. The tumour cells immediately around a small blood vessel have survived, forming a cuff which occupies most of the picture. More peripherally the tumour has undergone ischaemic necrosis with loss of nuclear staining. ×190. (Dr A. M. Lufty.)

ogenic) cells and that the other cells can undergo, at most, a few mitoses before becoming resting cells and developing various degrees of differentiation.

The above features of tumour cell kinetics are potentially important for, short of complete removal, effective treatment of a malignant tumour must depend on the elimination of its stem cells by irradiation or cytotoxic drugs, and since cells in mitosis are most susceptible to these agents, information on the kinetics of the stem cells, and particularly the duration of their G1 phase, should be useful in planning the course of treatment likely to be most effective. In addition, there is now some evidence that the sensitivity of clonogenic tumour cells in tissue culture to various cytotoxic drugs correlates with the clinical response to drug therapy, a finding which, if confirmed by more extensive investigations, should contribute greatly in selection of the appropriate drugs.

Spread of tumours

Benign tumours grow by expansion: they compress the surrounding tissue, causing atrophy and disappearance of its cells. The stroma of the surrounding tissue is more resistant and becomes condensed to form a fibrous capsule around the tumour (Figs. 12.3, 12.5) and this may increase in thickness as a result of a desmoplastic reaction stimulated by the tumour. Some benign tumours have little or no capsule and yet the margin between tumour and surrounding tissue remains sharp, without evidence of local invasion.

Malignant tumours grow both by expansion and by infiltrating the surrounding tissues: their cells also invade the walls of lymphatics and blood vessels in and around the tumour and are carried away to other parts of the body where

Table 12.2   Contrasting features of benign and malignant tumours

	Benign	Malignant
(a) *Evidence of rapid growth*		
Mitoses	Few and normal	Numerous and often abnormal
Nuclei	Little altered	Enlarged, often vary in size (pleomorphic)
Nucleoli	Little altered	Usually large
Cytoplasmic basophilia	Slight	Marked
Haemorrhage and necrosis	Unusual	Often extensive
(b) *Differentiation*		
Naked-eye resemblance to tissue of origin	Often close	Variable: from close to none
Microscopic resemblance to tissue of origin	Usually close	Usually poor
Function, e.g. secretion	Usually well maintained	May be retained, lost, or abnormal
(c) *Evidence of transgression of normal boundaries*		
Capsule intact	Frequent	Rare (usually none)
Local invasion	Absent	Very frequent
Metastases	Absent	Frequent

they may give rise to **secondary tumours** or **metastases.** This aggressive behaviour of malignant tumours presents the major obstacle to their complete removal. The nature of the changes in cancer cells which make them invasive is not known, but abnormal motility and secretion of enzymes which digest formed tissue elements and damage cell membranes may be involved (p. 12.11).

Although there are exceptions, it is a general rule that malignant tumours which are poorly differentiated tend to grow rapidly, invade extensively and metastasise early. More highly differentiated malignant tumours tend to behave less aggressively, but individual types of tumour show differences in their behaviour, and a detailed knowledge is necessary to draw conclusions from the histological features on the likely behaviour of each particular type of tumour.

The anatomical features of the spread of carcinomas and sarcomas are described on pp. 12.22–28 and 12.32 respectively. The contrasting features of benign and malignant tumours are summarised in Table 12.2.

Other features of cancer cells

The features by which tumours are recognised—the morphological abnormalities of their cells, uncontrolled growth and, in the case of malignant tumours, their invasiveness—have been emphasised in the preceding sections. Tumour cells differ from normal cells also in their metabolism and particularly in the features of their plasma membrane. These differences are observed mainly in the cells of malignant tumours, but carcinogenic agents damage cells in many ways and it is difficult to determine which of the changes are responsible for the characteristic behaviour of cancer cells and which are incidental to the process of carcinogenesis. The most important changes are as follows.

Plasma-membrane changes. An important feature of cancer cells is their reduced adhesiveness to one another. In the case of carcinoma cells, this seems likely to be due to diminished formation of **spot desmosomes** (p. 12.11) which are important points of adhesion between normal epithelial cells. Lack of adhesiveness may be an important factor in the infiltration of surrounding tissues by the cells at the periphery of a cancer, and in their penetration of the walls of blood vessels and lymphatics.

The cells of some cancers also show impaired formation of gap junctions. When normal cells of the same type come into contact, they form junctions through which molecules of up to about 1500 daltons pass from cell to cell. The functional importance of such intercellular communication is not known, but it may have a controlling effect on cell motility and mitosis.

Another feature of cancer cells is their increased **negative surface charge.** The negative charge of normal cells is attributable mainly to the sialic acid residues of their surface glycoproteins. Sialic acid residues are not increased in cancer cells, but cancer cells lack surface proteins which in normal cells obscure some of the sialic acid residues. This may have an important effect on control of mitosis, for enzymic removal of surface protein from normal cells in culture results in a temporary increase in mitotic activity and disordered growth resembling that of cancer cells in culture (p. 13.5). There is also evidence that the binding of lectins (plant proteins) to sialic acid residues on the surface of cancer cells results in temporary inhibition of their disordered proliferation in culture.

Biochemical features of cancer cells. It has long been known that cancer cells rely more than normal cells on **anaerobic glycolysis** as a source of energy. The availability of oxygen suppresses anaerobic glycolysis in normal cells but much less so in cancer cells. The significance of this difference is, however, obscure.

Another feature of cancer cells is a relatively low level of **intracellular cAMP**. The level of cAMP in normal cells is diminished during mitosis, and provision of cAMP to cancer cells in culture tends to reduce their proliferative activity.

Discharge of **lysosomal enzymes** is a feature of cancer cells and occurs also in normal cells during mitosis. Release of collagenase and various other proteinases, lipases, etc. may contribute to the invasiveness of cancer cells by damaging the surrounding cells and digesting stromal elements. It could also explain the loss of surface protein from cancer cells (see above).

Production of oncofetal antigens and hormones by tumours and other 'paraneoplastic' effects are described on pp. 12.43–45.

Vascularisation of tumours

Unless it derives a blood supply from adjacent host tissues, a tumour cannot grow beyond 1–2 mm in diameter. When small fragments of various human and animal malignant tumours are implanted in the cornea or anterior chamber of the eye of experimental animals, they stimulate a rapid growth of capillaries from the adjacent vascular tissues, and the new vessels penetrate and supply the tumour. Most benign tumours and non-neoplastic tissues are much less actively angiogenic. Evidence that this property of malignant tumours is attributable to diffusible products of the tumour cells has been provided by implanting tumour enclosed in millipore membranes, and by the demonstration that cell-free extracts of malignant tumours also promote capillary formation *in vivo* and stimulate proliferation of vascular endothelial cells in culture. Work in this field has been handicapped by lack of a simple quantitative test for tumour angiogenic factors (TAFs), the chemical composition of which is not known. Macrophages and lymphocytes, both of which are commonly present in malignant tumours, are also capable of producing angiogenic factors.

Two aspects of tumour angiogenesis are of particular interest. First, there is now good evidence that TAFs are produced from an early stage of the transformation between normal and cancer cells, and indeed their production may precede any obvious morphological change (Jensen *et al.*, 1982). Development of sensitive and reliable methods of detecting TAF might therefore provide an early warning of pre-cancerous change. Secondly, the growth of implanted tumours and new blood vessels in mice has been reported to be inhibited by systemic injection of extracts of cartilage, a tissue which is non-vascular and relatively resistant to invasion by cancer. This raises the possibility of treatment of cancer patients by agents which inhibit tumour angiogenesis.

Epithelial tumours

Epithelium has two essential characteristics which are retained by its tumours, both benign and malignant.

(a) Epithelial cells form sheets or groups in which they are closely apposed and are attached to one another, notably by **spot desmosomes** (Fig. 12.14). This is true of epithelia lining surfaces or ducts and also of glandular epithelia. Even in anaplastic malignant epithelial tumours, in which most other special features of epithelium fail to develop, and in which cell adherence is weak, spot desmosomes can still

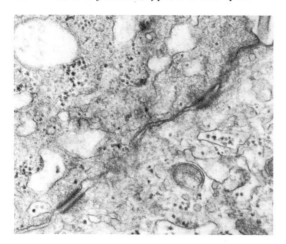

Fig. 12.14 The junction between two epithelial cells showing their close apposition. Two zones of adherence (spot desmosomes) are seen as double lines of increased density of the cell membranes. Desmosomes are observed in the cells of malignant epithelial tumours, but are reduced in number or defective with consequent weakening of cell adhesion. × 40 000.

be detected, although in reduced numbers. By contrast, connective tissue cells are largely surrounded by ground substance, collagen, etc., and where they are in contact with one another do not usually form desmosomes.

(b) Epithelium requires a fibrovascular stroma for its support and nutrition. This is equally necessary for neoplastic epithelium and all epithelial tumours appear capable of stimulating the local fibroblasts and blood vessels. In benign tumours, this **desmoplastic reaction** is usually well controlled, the stroma resembling that of the corresponding normal epithelial tissue. In malignant epithelial tumours, it is more variable (pp. 12.17–18). Connective-tissue tumours also stimulate the growth of blood vessels, but the tumour cells, like their normal counterparts, provide their own supporting stroma.

Benign Epithelial Tumours (Papillomas and adenomas)

Papillomas

These develop in epithelium covering a surface, for example the epidermis, and they project above the surface. For a tumour to develop,

proliferation of tumour cells must exceed cell loss, and since the tumour is benign its cells do not invade the underlying connective tissue, e.g. the dermis, and must be accommodated in the epithelial layer. Apart from some epithelial thickening, which is limited by the extent to which nutrients can diffuse from the underlying capillaries, the neoplastic proliferation causes a local increase in *area* of the epithelium, with the result that it becomes raised up into a mass of folds, each of which is covered by neoplastic epithelium and has a fibrovascular core derived from the underlying connective tissue (Fig. 12.15). Such a tumour is termed a *papilloma* and its constituent elevations are termed *fronds* or *papillae*. As each papilla is compressed by those around it, they tend to grow by increasing in length, extension of the fibro-vascular core being promoted by a desmoplastic reaction. In some instances, as in Fig. 12.16, the papillae arise directly from a broad base and the tumour is termed a **sessile papilloma***; in others, the papillae grow from an elongated stalk (pedicle or peduncle—Fig. 12.17) and the tumour is termed a **pedunculated papilloma**.

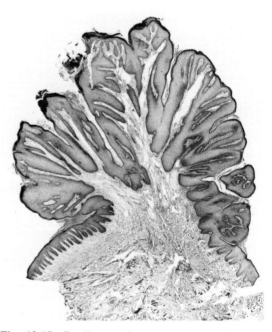

Fig. 12.15 Papilloma of muco-cutaneous junction of lip, showing branching processes of connective tissue covered by stratified epithelium. × 10.

* *Sessile*: sitting, low-growing.

major injury or sepsis (p. 10.44), notably increased protein synthesis and catabolism, increases in gluconeogenesis and oxidation of fatty acids, and raised resting metabolism.

As already noted, the cells of some cancers secrete excessive amounts of hormones, oncofetal proteins, etc. Because of their biochemical abnormalities, it would not be surprising if they were to produce also substances which interfere with the metabolism of the cells of various tissues. However, search for such products has so far been disappointing. Necrosis of non-neoplastic tissue, e.g. in myocardial infarction or mechanical trauma, can result in pyrexia and disturbances of general metabolism. The necrosis which is so common in malignant tumours may therefore contribute to malignant cachexia, even when bacterial infection does not supervene.

Occasional effects of tumours

Apart from the mechanical and general effects described above, and in some instances the excessive production of various hormones, some cancers are complicated by ill-defined **neuropathies** or by **myopathies** of the skeletal muscles: these effects are very likely caused by release of undefined humoral factors by the cancer cells. Other necrotic effects include **multiple venous thromboses** (which are especially common with pancreatic carcinoma—p. 14.37), various **skin rashes,** e.g. acanthosis nigricans (p. 19.30), **micro-angiopathic haemolytic anaemia** (p. 17.32) and a low-grade form of **disseminated intravascular coagulation** (p. 17.68). **Renal disturbances**, notably the nephrotic syndrome (p. 10.34), occasionally result from the deposition of tumour antigen/antibody complexes in the glomeruli.

These and other effects of tumours are illustrated in the appropriate systematic chapters.

Staging and grading of cancers

A quantitative measure of the factors which are known to influence the prognosis of a particular type of malignant tumour is often required. Sometimes it is used in deciding on the best method of treatment for a particular patient but it is also very useful in statistical studies, notably in the comparison of the effects of different forms of treatment. Suppose, for example, it is required to compare the success rate of radical excision of a cancerous breast, together with the axillary lymph nodes, with local excision of the cancer followed by radiotherapy. It is essential to ensure that the group of patients treated by one method does not contain a higher proportion with smaller, earlier or better-differentiated tumours than does the group treated by the other method. It is difficult to establish firm criteria, applicable to cancers in general, for this purpose, and elaborate sets of criteria have been set up for most of the common individual forms of cancer. It is, however, generally agreed that there are two major factors, the **grade** and **stage** of the tumour.

Grading is based on histological examination of the degree of differentiation of the tumour cells and the mitotic index. There is no precise system of grading, for assessment of the degree of differentiation is empirical and subjective. Also, different parts of the same tumour vary in the degree of differentiation and mitotic activity, and a biopsy specimen may not be representative of the whole tumour. In general, tumours are graded by the pathologist into well, moderately and poorly differentiated: the system is most useful if the criteria used place about 25% of tumours into the good group, 50% into the middle group and 25% into the bad group.

Staging provides an estimate of the degree of spread of the tumour. Many systems use four or more stages, the criteria being modified to suit cancers of various sites. For example, squamous-cell carcinoma of the uterine cervix might be staged as follows

Stage	Extent of spread
0	Carcinoma in situ (no invasion)
I	Confined to the cervix
II	Limited local spread
III	Greater local spread, e.g. to the lower vagina or pelvic wall
IV	Lymph-node or distant metastases

Alternatively, the **TNM system** may be used, in which staging depends on the size of the primary tumour, graded as T1–4, absence of lymph-node involvement (NO) or involvement of few (N1) or many (N2) nodes, and distinct metastases absent (MO), few (M1) or many (M2), e.g. T2, N1, MO.

Assessment of the extent of spread of a tumour will depend on the methods used in its detection. The simplest but least precise method of staging is based on clinical examination and has the advantage that it can be applied to all patients. More accurate staging is provided by combining clinical examination and imaging techniques, including lymphangiography, or by surgical exploration. Whatever methods are used, it is, of course, essential that they should be applied to all the groups of patients involved in clinical trials of different forms of therapy.

In some conditions, accurate staging is of great clinical importance to the individual patient. For example, in Hodgkin's disease, radiotherapy is commonly used when the disease is localised, and drug therapy when it has spread to one or more distant sites. Where distant spread is not evident on physical examination or radiographically, it is common practice to perform a laparotomy and, if necessary, excise the spleen and examine it histologically for evidence of the disease.

Not surprisingly, tumours of high grade (i.e. poorly differentiated and with a high mitotic index) are likely to have spread more extensively than low-grade tumours at the time of diagnosis, so that there is some correlation between grade and stage.

Immunohistological diagnosis of cancer

Improvements in the treatment of various forms of cancer are dependent on the accuracy of diagnosis of the presence and type of tumour and the extent of its spread. The information provided by routine histological techniques is by no means always precise and increasing use is being made of the detection of markers on tumour cells by means of monoclonal antibodies.

The technique of preparing monoclonal antibody (MAB) is outlined on p. 6.17. It has the advantage of being technically simple, for the antigen need not be obtained in pure form, and once an MAB has been shown to be useful, it can be prepared in very large amounts from the producer cell line and so can be distributed as a standard reagent. Because they are pure antibodies, MABs give clear-cut results when used to stain tissues by the immunohistological techniques described on p. 6.11. Faint reactions are, of course, observed where the cellular antigen is scanty or where there is a weakly cross-reacting antigenic determinant, but there is virtually none of the non-specific background staining which is a problem when polyclonal antibodies are used.

Hopes of producing an MAB which reacts with all malignant neoplastic cells or with all carcinoma cells, and not with any other types of cell, have not been realised. Such an antibody would be of great value in those cases in which the pathologist has difficulty in deciding whether the changes in a biopsy are indicative of cancer or of a chronic inflammatory or dysplastic reaction. However, immunological studies (p. 13.34 *et seq.*) have not provided evidence for the existence of tumour-specific antigens common to all forms of cancer or to all carcinomas, and the ideal MAB for the detection of cancer cells may prove to be illusory. There are, however, an increasing number of MABs which react with the cells of some types of cancer and with a limited range of non-neoplastic cells, and their value in the detection of cancer in biopsy material is at present being explored.

The use of MABs in accurate diagnosis of tumour type has already achieved considerable success, and is, indeed, revolutionising histological diagnosis. This is illustrated by the common problem of distinguishing between an anaplastic carcinoma and a lymphoma, which can now often be resolved by immunohistological staining with a panel of MABs, some of which react with constituents of epithelial (including carcinoma) cells, others with constituents of lymphoid (including lymphoma) cells (Gatter *et al.*, 1984). The antigenic epithelial constituents to which useful MABs are available include cytokeratin filaments, human milk-fat globule antigen, carcino-embryonic antigen and keratin, while antibodies to common leucocyte antigens are available which react with lymphoid cells. Lymphomas and lymphoid leukaemias can also be classified more accurately by means of cell-marker studies, including the use of MABs to various sub-sets of T cells. Some B-cell lymphomas can be recognised by demonstrating immunohistologically, that their cells produce immunoglobulins of a single light-chain type (κ or λ).

There are many more examples of MABs which are of value in precise diagnosis. For example, antibody to neuron-specific enolase stains the cells of all types of apudoma (p. 12.43), while antibody to thyroglobulin stains some carcinomas of the thyroid and anti-myoglobin and anti-desmin are of value in the diagnosis of rhabdomyosarcomas (sarcomas of striped muscle).

The choice of treatment for a patient with cancer often depends on the presence or absence of metastases. It is easy to detect large metastases by imaging techniques, but the detection of single or small groups of carcinoma cells, e.g. in aspirates of bone marrow, may require prolonged microscopic examination of multiple sections. The search is greatly facilitated by immunohistological staining with an MAB which has been shown to react with the cells of the primary tumour. This procedure is particularly helpful in seeking for carcinoma cells in tissues such as marrow or lymph nodes, which do not contain any non-neoplastic epithelial cells.

Immunohistological techniques have already provided the most important advance in histopathology since staining methods were first introduced. As the numbers of useful MABs increase, histopathological diagnosis in general, and particularly of tumours, will become progressively more accurate. It is also apparent that immunohistological examination of sections of fresh tissue will become increasingly important, for fixation of tissue destroys many of the antigenic constituents which are useful as cell markers.

Tumour-like Lesions and Cysts

There are a number of lesions which resemble tumours but have distinctive features which cast doubt on their neoplastic nature. Examples already described in this chapter include the fibromatoses (p. 23.64), haemangiomas (p. 14.39) and monstrosities. Among such tumour-like lesions, those termed *hamartomas* merit further description. *Cysts* are not tumours and are described here for want of a better place.

Hamartoma

This is a convenient term for an ill-defined group of lesions which have some resemblance to tumours but are not neoplastic. They usually appear before or soon after birth, grow with the individual and cease to grow when general body growth ceases. They may consist of a single type of cell, e.g. pigmented naevi, composed of a collection of melanocytes (p. 12.36), a particular type of tissue, e.g. haemangioma (p. 14.39), or a mixture of tissues, e.g. cartilage, epithelial-lined clefts, adipose and fibrous tissue in the so-called adenochondroma of the lung (p. 16.65). Those in the internal organs form lumps which can be mistaken grossly for tumours, while in the skin they may be nodular or may present as a patch of discolouration, e.g. the capillary haemangioma and some pigmented naevi. Hamartomas can best be understood as arising from a localised disorder of the relationships of normal tissues leading to overproduction of one or more elements but without the property of progressive growth characteristic of tumours. There are many varieties, and some have a tendency to progress to true neoplasia, for example pigmented naevi (although the risk is small) and osteocartilaginous exostoses (p. 12.31) arising from the metaphyseal region of bones.

Cysts

The term 'cyst' properly means a space containing fluid and lined by epithelial cells. In most cysts the epithelial lining is not neoplastic and such cysts are neither tumours nor parts of tumours: they are included here only for convenience. Nearly all cysts arise by the abnormal dilatation of pre-existing tubules, ducts or cavities, though a cyst may lose its cell lining due to inflammatory or other change, and come to be lined by granulation or denser fibrous tissue. The term is, however, often applied in a somewhat loose way to other abnormal cavities containing fluid. For example, the term 'apoplectic cyst' is applied to a space in the brain containing brownish fluid, which has resulted from haemorrhage. Many tumours develop ischaemic necrosis or slow degeneration in their most central parts. In some, e.g. gliomas, the degenerate centre is replaced by an accumulation of fluid, and the term 'cystic change' is often used even when no true cyst is formed.

The cysts peculiar to each organ will be described in the later chapters: we shall give here only a classification of their causes. True cysts also occur in some tumours, the lining epithelium being neoplastic, e.g. in *cystadenomas* (p. 12.14) and *cystadenocarcinomas* (p. 12.20) and also in teratomas (p. 12.40). Apart from these, cysts fall naturally into two main groups: (1) those due to congenital abnormalities, and (2) acquired cysts, i.e. those produced by lesions in post-natal life.

(1) Congenital cysts

These may also be grouped into two types:

(a) They may arise *within otherwise normal organs or tissues*, as a result of the presence of epithelium of a type not usually present at that site after birth, either as a result of some minor displacement of an embryonal tissue or (more often) the failure to disappear of some embryonic duct or cleft. The commonest site of cysts derived from vestigial ducts is the genito-urinary tract, where the disappearance of the mesonephros and its duct in both sexes, and of the Wolffian ducts in females and Müllerian ducts in males, often leaves behind a variety of persistent epithelial remnants: small cysts are very common among these, and larger ones (**parovarian cycsts**) are not uncommon in the broad ligaments (p. 24.29).

Other embryonic ducts which may persist and give rise to cysts include the thyroglossal duct (mid-line of neck, usually near the hyoid), and the urachus (usually at the umbilicus). A similar mechanism operates with the branchial clefts; **branchial cysts** are produced at the side of the neck and are lined by squamous epithelium, usually with a rim of lymphoid tissue.

A different mechanism produces the **sequstration dermoids** which result from imperfect fusion of embryonal skin flaps. They are lined with squamous epithelium and filled with keratin, and are found mostly in the mid-line of the chest and neck or at the angles of the eye.

The 'pearly tumour' of the meninges, etc. (actually a squamous-epithelium-lined cyst, p. 21.63) is an example of a simple displacement of squamous epithelium into the meninges at the time of neural tube closure.

(b) Cysts arising as *part of a major congenital abnormality of an organ*. Examples are (1) **polycystic disease of the kidneys** (p. 22.66), in which a major maldevelopment of the renal tubules (of several possible types) results in the formation of cysts in great numbers; (2) the **meningocele** and other types of cystic swelling that complicate some cases of spina bifida, failure of normal closure of the neural tube being the basic defect (p. 21.47).

(2) Acquired cysts

These are of several varieties, the three following being the most important:

(a) **Retention cysts.** These are formed by retention of secretion produced by obstruction of the lumen of a duct. A single cyst, sometimes large, may be produced by the obstruction of the main duct, e.g. of a salivary gland or of a part of the pancreas. Obstruction of the orifice of a hair follicle gives rise to a cyst-like swelling filled chiefly with breaking-down keratin—the **epidermal** or **'sebaceous' cyst**, seen especially in the scalp. Numerous small cysts may result from obstruction of small ducts, an occurrence which is not uncommon in fibrosing lesions of the kidney.

(b) **Distension cysts** are formed from natural enclosed spaces. They occur in the thyroid from dilatation of the follicles, and occasionally also in the pituitary: cystic dilatation of graafian follicles in the ovaries is also common. Distension of spaces lined by mesothelium is also seen; for example, a bursa may enlarge to form a cystic swelling, and there is the common condition of hydrocele due to an accumulation of fluid in the tunica vaginalis.

Occasionally in the adult an **implantation cyst** occurs by the dislocation inwards of a portion of epidermis by injury. The epithelium grows and comes to line a space filled with degenerate epithelial squames (Fig. 12.59); rarely hair follicles are present in the wall. Implantation cysts may result also from wounds of the cornea.

(3) Parasitic cysts. These are cystic stages in the life cycle of cestode parasites. The most striking examples are the **'hydatid' cysts** produced in man, usually in the liver, by the dog tapeworm *Taenia echinococcus*, though small cysts may be produced in the brain and other parts by the cysticerci of *Taenia solium*.

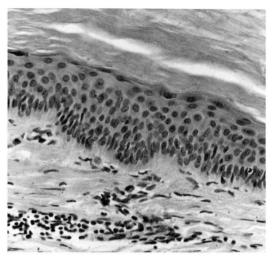

Fig. 12.59 Implantation cyst in the subcutaneous tissue, showing a lining of stratified squamous epithelium and keratin in the lumen (*top*). × 200.

References

Bagg, H.J. (1936). Experimental production of teratoma testis in the fowl. *American Journal of Cancer*, **26**, 69–84.

Fialkow, P.J. (1976). Clonal origin of human tumours. *Biochimia et Biophysica Acta*, **458**, 283–321.

Gatter, K.C., Fahmi, B. and Mason, D.Y. (1984). The use of monoclonal antibodies in histological diagnosis. pp. 37-67 in *Recent Advances in Histopathology, No. 12*. Ed. P.P. Anthony and R.N.M. MacSween. Churchill Livingstone, Edinburgh.

Jeevanandam, M., Horowitz, G.D., Lowry, S.F. and Brennan, M.F. (1984). Cancer cachexia and protein metabolism. *Lancet*, i, 1423–6.

Jensen, H.M., Chen, I., De Vault, M.R. and Lewis, A.E. (1982). Angiogenesis induced by 'normal' human breast tissue: a probable marker for precancer. *Science*, **218**, 293–5.

Further Reading

Ashley, D.B. (1978). *Evans' Histological Appearances of Tumours*, 3rd edn., pp. 857. Churchill-Livingstone, Edinburgh, London and New York. (An account of the behaviour and appearances of human tumours based on a considerable experience.)

Rosai, J. (1981). *Ackerman's Surgical Pathology*, 6th edn. Two vols. pp. 1702. The C.V. Mosby Company, St. Louis. (A practical text with extensive sections on tumours.)

Sobin, L.H., Thomas, L.B., Percy, Constance and Henson, D.E. (Eds.) (1978) *A Coded Compendium of the International Histological Classification of Tumours*, pp. 116. World Health Organisation, Geneva. (A widely accepted system of classification, coding and nomenclature of human tumours.)

Willis, R.A. (1973). *The Spread of Tumours in the Human Body*, 3rd edn., pp. 417. Butterworths, London.

American Journal of Surgical Pathology. Masson Publishing, New York. A monthly publication containing many well-illustrated articles on the pathology of human tumours).

Atlas of Tumour Pathology. US Armed Forces Institute of Pathology, Washington, DC. (Numerous 'Fascicles' on tumours of particular organs, tissues and regions. A valuable source of detailed information on the histology and behaviour of individual tumours.)

13

TUMOURS: II. The Aetiology of Cancer

The mechanisms involved in the conversion of a normal cell into a cancer cell pose one of the biggest problems facing medical science. The first major advance was made in 1777 when Sir Percival Pott*, a London surgeon, observed a high incidence of cancer of the scrotum among chimney sweeps. An example is shown in Fig. 12.24, p. 12.17. He attributed this correctly to lodgement of soot in the rugose scrotal skin, and chimney sweep's cancer was virtually eliminated by personal hygiene. This was the first indication that the development of cancer might not be a 'spontaneous' process, but rather the result of contact with **carcinogenic chemicals**. The demonstration that coal tar contains chemicals capable of causing cancer in animals was not achieved until early in this century. Subsequently, very large numbers of chemicals have been shown to be carcinogenic and chemicals are now routinely examined for possible carcinogenicity before being used as drugs or in foodstuffs. Similar precautions are taken to protect workers from exposure to cancer-inducing chemicals.

The induction of cancer by exposure to **ionising radiation** became apparent from the high incidence of cancer of the skin of the hands in early radiologists, who used to calibrate their machines by exposing their own hands. Subsequently, a high incidence of leukaemia was observed in radiologists, and it also became obvious that fair-skinned people living outdoor lives in a sunny climate very commonly develop cancer on the exposed skin, an affect shown to be caused by **ultraviolet rays**.

In 1911, Rous described investigations on a sarcoma which occurred naturally in chickens and showed that it could be transmitted by inoculating chickens with a cell-free extract of the

*Percival Pott's name is still applied to Pott's fracture and Pott's disease of the spine.

tumour. It was subsequently shown that the Rous sarcoma was caused by infection with a virus, and that many viruses are capable of inducing sarcomas, leukaemias, carcinomas, etc. in various species of animals: these are termed *oncogenic viruses*. There is now good evidence that **viruses** may be involved in the aetiology of a limited number of types of tumour in man, but the great majority of human tumours do not appear to be caused by viruses. Virological studies have, however, contributed to important recent discoveries on the role of oncogenes in the aetiology of human tumours (see below).

It has long been suspected that **genetic factors** influence the risk of developing cancer, and strains of mice with a high or low incidence of particular cancers have been produced by selective breeding. In man, genetic factors clearly play a major role in some uncommon tumours, e.g. retinoblastoma. Many of the common cancers have a high incidence in some families but no clear mode of inheritance is apparent, and multigenic factors may be involved.

The discovery of **cellular oncogenes** in the past few years and recent evidence that they are likely to play a major causal role in human and animal cancers has had an enormous impact on theories of carcinogenesis. This recent work on oncogenes has not diminished the importance of the causal factors mentioned above—chemicals, radiations, viruses and genetic factors—but it does provide, for the first time, an acceptable basis for an explanation of how the environmental factors induce cancer.

The discovery of cellular oncogenes resulted from investigation of a group of RNA viruses, the oncornaviruses, now widely called oncogenic retroviruses, which can induce cancer in animals. The features of these viruses will be described first, followed by an account of the cellular oncogenes and their role in carcinogenesis, and finally the parts played by other types of viruses, chemical and physical agents and genetic factors.

Viruses and cancer

Both RNA and DNA viruses have been shown to be capable of causing cancer in various vertebrate species. Virus infection plays a part in the development of some tumours in man but investigations on oncogenic viruses, and particularly on retroviruses, have contributed greatly to our understanding of the molecular biology of the common forms of cancer in man.

A knowledge of some of the more important techniques used for the investigation of viral and cellular genes is essential to the understanding of recent developments of the molecular biology of carcinogenesis. These include nucleic acid hybridisation, transfection, DNA cloning, use of restriction endonucleases, the Southern blot technique and the use of cell cultures to investigate the effects of viruses and genes. Brief accounts of these topics are included in the following sections.

Retroviruses

The name 'retrovirus' derives from **reverse transcriptase**, an enzyme associated with this group of viruses and essential for their mode of replication.

When a retrovirus infects a host cell, the envelope fuses with the plasma membrane and the nucleocapsid enters the cell cytoplasm, where the RNA genome is freed. Reverse transcriptase is also released from the virion. This enzyme is an **RNA-dependent DNA polymerase** and catalyses the synthesis of a strand of DNA complementary to the RNA viral genome (which acts as a template). Note that this is the reverse of the orthodox process of gene expression in which DNA is transcribed into mRNA—hence the term *reverse transcriptase* used to describe the enzyme. The new strand of DNA synthesised on the viral genome is converted to a double-stranded helix of DNA by synthesis of a complementary DNA strand, and one or more copies of the double strand, termed a provirus, are inserted into the DNA of the host genome (Fig. 13.1). In this state, the virus is said to have integrated and the proviral 'genes' (appropriately termed progenes) can be transcribed, like the host-cell genes, into mRNA which is then translated to provide the constituents of the viral capsid and envelop and reverse transcriptase. The whole provirus is also transcribed, to produce new copies of the viral RNA genome. In this way, all the constituents of the virion are provided and new virions are assembled at the plasma membrane of the cell. Most retroviruses insert envelope glycoprotein into the plasma membrane of the host cell and during their release by budding off from the cell (Fig. 13.2) the virions become coated in an envelope which consists of modified plasma membrane: the retroviruses which adopt this procedure are known as *C-type viruses*.

Cells which support the replication of an integrated retrovirus are termed *permissive cells*. In non-permissive cells, replication of the integrated virus does not occur, but there may be limited expression of the proviral genes with production of viral gene proteins which may thus be detectable in, or on the surface of, the non-permissive cell.

When a cell containing an integrated virus divides, copies of the integrated provirus are transmitted, as part of the cell genome, to the daughter cells. Some retroviral proviruses have integrated into the germ cells of the host and are therefore transmitted to the offspring and subsequent generations as stable Mendelian genes (vertical transmission). Such viruses and their proviruses are termed **endogenous** and are

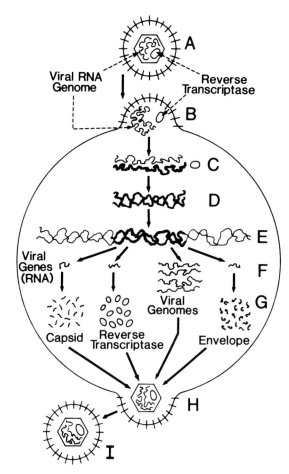

Fig. 13.1 Integration and replication of a retrovirus in the host cell. The virion (**A**) consists of an outer envelope and a capsid enclosing the viral genome (two identical strands of RNA) and reverse transcriptase. The envelope fuses with the host-cell plasma membrane (**B**) and its contents are released into the cytosol where reverse transcription provides a strand of DNA complementary to the viral RNA genome (**C**). A second strand of DNA, complementary to the first, is formed (**D**) and the two strands are integrated into the host-cell genome as the provirus (**E**). Transcription of the proviral genes provides mRNA (**F**) which is translated into viral capsid and envelope proteins and reverse transcriptase (**G**), while transcription of the whole proviral strand provides new viral RNA genomes. These viral constituents are assembled at the plasma membrane (**H**) and new virions (**I**) are released. Note that integration of the provirus is necessary for viral replication.

widely distributed in various species of vertebrates, possibly including man.

Detection of integrated viruses

A replicating retrovirus can be detected by orthodox virological techniques. The detection of integrated virus in a non-permissive cell is more difficult, but is of great importance in viral oncology. In some instances the virus can be induced to replicate in cell cultures. One method is to fuse the cells to be examined with non-infected permissive cells to form hybrid cells in which viral replication may occur, thus demonstrating the presence of the integrated provirus in the cells under investigation. As noted above, an integrated provirus in a non-permissive cell may express one or more of its progenes, so that, for example, viral envelope antigen may be detected at the host-cell surface

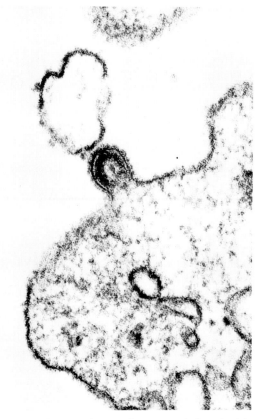

Fig. 13.2 A part of a cell from a cat infected with feline leukaemia virus, showing formation of a virion by budding from the cell surface. Note that the envelope is formed from the plasma membrane, and that the virus particle becomes coated with an outer spiky layer. The section happens to include part of another cell immediately above the virion. × 80 000. (Dr Helen Laird.)

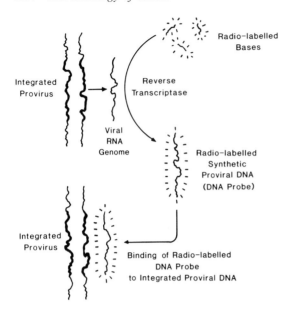

Fig. 13.3 Production of a nucleic-acid probe. In this example, a DNA probe is assembled from bases (some of which are radio-labelled) using reverse transcriptase and the whole or part of the RNA genome of a retrovirus as a template. The radio-labelled probe is capable of hybridising with the integrated provirus, thus demonstrating its presence.

or reverse transcriptase may be detected in the cell. A number of other manipulations, including exposure of cells in culture to ionising radiation or chemical carcinogens, are used to enhance expression of viral progenes, or even induce viral replication, in non-permissive cells. The detection of serum antibody to viral proteins also provides evidence of infection with integrated viruses.

Nucleic acid probes. If viral-specific RNA can be obtained from infected cells, reverse transcriptase can be used to catalyse *in-vitro* synthesis of strands of DNA complementary to the viral RNA genome (or parts of it). In other words, the provirus or parts of it can be synthesised *in vitro*. The synthetic proviral DNA will, under suitable conditions, bind to ('hybridise' with) DNA complementary to the provirus, and if radio-active bases are used in the *in vitro* synthesis, such **hybridisation** can be detected by autoradiography in DNA extracted from infected cells or in the nuclei of cells in tissue sections. In this way, **radioactive probes**

can be constructed to detect the presence of integrated provirus in cellular DNA (Fig. 13.3).

Transfection is the process by which free DNA is taken up by, and incorporated into, the genome of animal cells or micro-organisms. This occurs when DNA fragments are added under suitable conditions to cells in culture. By this technique, it has been shown that certain genes isolated from tumours are capable of immortalising or transforming cultured cells (see below).

DNA cloning is a technique used to obtain large amounts of a particular DNA sequence of bases. It is important because it allows the synthesis of genes and groups of genes in sufficient quantity to determine their base sequences, to investigate their effects after transfection into cellular DNA, and to study the properties of their products. Isolated cloned genes can also be inserted into the DNA of micro-organisms in such a way that they are expressed and large amounts of their products can thus be obtained. Such techniques of genetic engineering are currently being used for commercial production of insulin, growth hormone, etc.

To clone a particular gene, the fragment of DNA containing it is recombined with the DNA of a plasmid (p. 8.6) or a bacteriophage. Recombinant plasmids or phages containing the additional gene are then grown in suitable bacteria. When the bacteria divide, their plasmids divide with them and are transferred to both of the daughter cells, so that large numbers of plasmids, each containing a copy of the inserted gene, are thus produced. These can be isolated and the inserted fragments of DNA obtained in pure form. DNA cloning by bacteriophages is somewhat similar. The transfected phages are seeded into cultures of bacteria in which they are capable of replicating (p. 8.6). The DNA fragment is then isolated from the large numbers of phage particles produced. The rapidity with which plasmids and phages multiply in bacterial cultures, and the relatively small size of their genomes (from which the cloned gene can be isolated fairly simply) makes them well suited as vehicles for DNA cloning.

Use of restriction endonucleases. Intact DNA extracted from cells or organisms can be digested with enzymes termed **restriction endonucleases** which break the strand up into specific smaller fragments of various lengths. Restriction endonucleases are bacterial enzymes which cleave DNA at points where a short sequence of a few (4–6) particular bases occurs, thus breaking it up into fragments ('**restriction fragments**'), the lengths of which differ depending on the distribution of the cleavage sites attacked by the particular enzyme used. Restriction endonucleases differ in the particular sequence of bases they digest and a wide choice is available. The number and average size of the restriction fragments obtained will depend upon the endonuclease used to digest the DNA: by suitable choice of enzyme, fragments containing whole genes can be prepared.

Restriction fragments can be separated according to their sizes by electrophoresis in an agarose gel. The fragments obtained from the relatively small genomes of plasmids or bacteriophages separate into discrete bands, but the immensely greater number of fragments obtained from the much larger genome of vertebrate cells form a continuous smear along the electrophoretic track (Fig. 2.4, p. 2.4).

The Southern blotting technique. This is used for detecting and isolating particular fragments of DNA separated by electrophoresis on an agarose gel as described above. A sheet of cellulose acetate paper is laid on the electrophoretic track of the agarose gel so that restriction fragments distributed along the gel are transferred to the paper. The fragments can then be 'baked' onto the paper and specific fragments can be detected by hybridization with suitable radioactive probes (see above). After washing the paper to remove the free (unhybridised) copies of the probe, the position of the hybridised fragments can be detected by autoradiography (Fig. 2.4, p. 2.4). The part of the electrophoretic gel containing the wanted fragments is then excised and the DNA fragments in it are subjected to further electrophoretic separation. In this way, the fragment required can be enriched sufficiently to simplify cloning it as described above (Fig. 13.4).

Cell transformation. When normal cells from mammalian tissues are cultured, they usually die after a limited number of mitotic divisions. In some instances, however, one or more of the cells develops into a clone of cells which continue to divide indefinitely. Such **immortalisation** indicates a change in the cell, and can be induced by certain viruses and by various manipulations. The immortalised cells are not can-

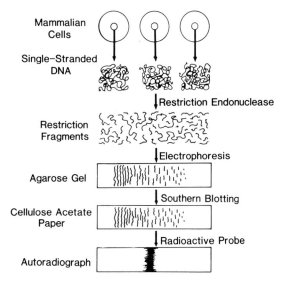

Fig. 13.4 Isolation and detection of specific sequences of DNA. The DNA is obtained from mammalian cells, converted to single-stranded form by heating, and broken up into fragments of various lengths by a restriction endonuclease. The restriction fragments are subjected to electrophoresis in agarose gel, which separates them according to fragment length, and copies of the the DNA on the electrophoretic strip are made on cellulose acetate paper (Southern blotting technique). The position of particular DNA fragments can be determined by use of radioactive probes and the fragments can then be obtained from the appropriate part of the agarose gel and subjected to further purification.

cer cells and will not grow into tumours when injected into histocompatible animals. In culture, they spread out on the surface of the culture dish, proliferate until they form a continuous monolayer, and then stop dividing, a phenomenon termed **density-dependent inhibition** (formerly *contact inhibition*—p. 5.10). Such immortalised cell lines, and particularly NIH3T3, a cell-line derived from mouse fibroblasts, have been widely used to study the capacity of viruses and chemicals to induce **transformation** to malignant cells. The transformed cells show an altered growth pattern: they become rounded in shape and grow to high density, heaping up on one another to form irregular masses (Fig. 13.5). Other features of transformed cells include the capacity to grow in soft agar—loss of 'anchorage dependence', and to grow in medium containing only low concentrations of serum. However, the best criterion for malignant transformation is the capacity to form tumours when the cells are injected into suitable animals.

At some stage in carcinogenesis, which is widely regarded as a multi-step process, immortalisation must occur, and the capacity of a virus or other agent to induce immortalisation is an indication that it may contribute to carcinogenesis. It must be distinguished, however, from malignant transformation. It is also important to note that immortalised cells, such as NIH3T3, have already undergone part of the change involved in carcinogenesis, and that cell lines are more readily transformed to cancer cells than are cells in primary culture (i.e. non-immortalised cells).

Oncogenic retroviruses

These are of two distinct types: some induce the development of tumours in animals within a few weeks after injection, while others produce tumours only after a long 'incubation period', usually of some months. The 'acute' oncogenic viruses can also induce malignant transformation of most of the cells in cell lines established in tissue culture. The 'slow' oncogenic viruses do not transform cells in culture.

The slow oncogenic retroviruses include leukaemia viruses, which induce leukaemias and lymphomas in various species, e.g. mice (murine leukaemia virus—MLV), cats (FeLV) and bovines (BLV). Others induce sarcomas. They are transmitted horizontally, i.e. by contact between infected and non-infected animals. Transmission also occurs vertically (i.e. via the germ cells) to the offspring but feline leukaemia, which has been extensively investigated by Jarrett and his colleagues in Glasgow, appears to spread naturally by horizontally-transmitted infection. *Integrated retroviruses do not require to replicate within a cell to transform it to a cancer cell, the important factor being integration of one or more copies of the provirus into the host cell genome.* Its presence can be detected by nucleic-acid hybridisation, using a DNA probe (p. 13.3). Integrated viruses may also express structural proteins of the viral capsid or envelope, and the latter may be detected on the surface of infected host cells by use of a suitable

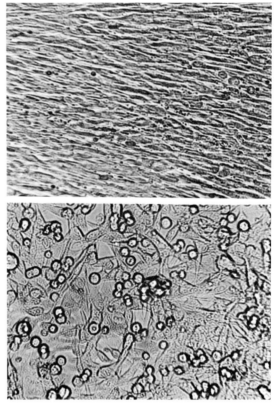

Fig. 13.5 Cultures of hamster fibroblasts. The upper culture shows formation of a regular monolayer. The lower culture is infected with polyoma virus and shows cellular pleomorphism and loss of contact inhibition, the cells being piled on top of one another.

antibody, or reverse transcriptase may be detected within the cells by means of antibody or enzyme assay. Infection can also be detected by demonstrating, in the serum, antibodies to viral capsid or envelope constituents.

Not only is there a long incubation period between infection and the development of leukaemia with this type of oncogenic retrovirus, but many infected animals do not develop leukaemia. Some cats infected with FeLV develop auto-immune phenomena, while others remain symptomless for life. Leukaemia is most likely to develop in animals receiving a large infecting dose while still young. There is evidence that, in these circumstances, the virus has an immunosuppressive effect which is an important factor in the subsequent development of leukaemia. Immunisation of cats against the virus by a vaccine is protective against feline leukaemia, even when performed after the cat has become infected with the virus.

There is now strong evidence that a human adult leukaemia/lymphoma syndrome (ATLL) is caused by infection with a human retrovirus termed human T-cell leukaemia virus, type I (HTLV–I) (Gallo, 1984). This condition is described on p. 18.28. Epidemiological studies performed by testing for antibodies have shown that infection with HTLV–I is endemic in certain populations, e.g. in the Caribbean islands and in the islands of Kyushu and Shikoku in South-west Japan, where at least 12% of the population shows serological evidence of infection. The human adult leukaemia/lymphoma syndrome has a relatively high incidence in these endemic areas and occurs among antibody-positive members of the community. In other parts of the world, both the tumour and serological evidence of infection with HTLV–I are rare.

The acute oncogenic retroviruses, which transform all the cells they infect when added to a cell culture and induce tumours rapidly *in vivo*, differ from the slow oncogenic retroviruses in having one or more genes termed **viral oncogenes (v-oncs)**. The slow oncogenic retroviruses have only three genes, termed Gag, Pol and Env, which code respectively for the capsid protein, reverse transcriptase and glycoprotein of the viral envelope (Fig. 13.6). Rous sarcoma virus, the first acute oncogenic retrovirus to be discovered, was shown by Rous in 1911 to induce sarcoma in chickens. It has been found to contain an additional gene, v–*src* (an abbreviation of viral sarcoma gene), which is responsible for its acute oncogenic properties. Strains of Rous sarcoma virus in which, as a result of mutation, v–*src* is not expressed, are not acutely oncogenic, while other mutants, in which v–*src* is functional only at lower temperatures, will only transform chicken cells in culture at the appropriate temperature and transformation is reversed by raising the temperature.

Many acute oncogenic retroviruses have now been identified and investigated. Each is oncogenic for a particular species (chickens, turkeys, mice, rats, cats or monkeys) and each usually produces a particular type of tumour (sarcoma, leukaemia or carcinoma), depending on the particular v–onc in its genome. Rous sarcoma virus is unique among the acute oncogenic retroviruses in being a '**complete**' **virus**. Its gen-

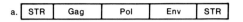

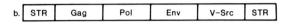

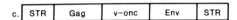

Fig. 13.6 Retroviral genomes. The genome of slow oncogenic retroviruses contains three genes, Gag, Pol and Env (**a**). The genome of Rous sarcoma virus (**b**) contains, in addition, the viral oncogene, v–*src* while in other acute oncogenic viruses (**c**) the viral oncogene (v–onc) has replaced part of the genome—in this case Pol. The genome also contains short terminal repeat sequences (STR) at each end.

ome contains v–*src in addition to* Gag, Pol and Env, and it thus possesses the genetic material necessary to replicate, invade host cells and induce malignant transformation in them. All the other members of the group so far discovered are **defective viruses** in which the v–onc has *replaced* other essential genetic material (usually Pol and often adjacent parts of Gag and Env—Fig. 13.6). In consequence, these viruses cannot replicate unless the host cell is infected also with a second ('helper') virus which can provide products of the missing or defective genes. Helper viruses are usually slow leukaemia viruses.

Because they are defective, the acute oncogenic retroviruses are not infectious under natural conditions and do not become endemic in the host population. They have been detected in tumours in individual animals and have been transmitted experimentally. Under natural conditions, they usually die out when the tumour they have induced kills the host animal. Although acute oncogenic retroviruses have not been detected in any human tumour, the origin of their v–oncs is of considerable interest and is discussed below.

Proto-oncogenes

The investigations on acute oncogenic retroviruses, described above, provided DNA probes

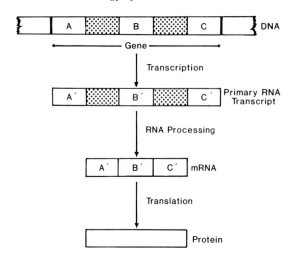

Fig. 13.7   Diagram of a vertebrate structural gene consisting of three exons (A, B and C) interrupted by two introns (stippled). The whole gene is transcribed into a primary RNA transcript, from which the sequences transcribed from the introns are excised and the exon transcripts (A', B' and C') are spliced, providing mRNA which is then translated into protein.

capable of detecting the DNA reverse-transcribed from the v–onc and inserted into the host cell DNA as part of the provirus. When the DNA of normal human cells was tested with v–onc probes, hybridisation was observed with probes for each of the 20 or so known v–oncs, and when restriction fragments of normal human DNA were tested, it was found that each v–onc probe hybridised specifically with particular DNA fragments. This indicated that all the known v–oncs, or closely similar DNA sequences, are present in the normal human genome. The same surprising result was obtained with the DNA of other animal species, even as far apart in evolution as *Drosophila*, the fruit fly. This leads to the striking conclusion that *genes closely resembling the cancer-inducing v–onc genes of acute oncogenic retroviruses are present at specific sites in the genomes of a very wide range of animal species, including man.* These normal genes are called **proto-oncogenes**.

Some of the proto-oncogenes in the genome of man and other animal species have been isolated, cloned in bacterial plasmids or bacteriophages (p. 13.4) and obtained in pure form. Analysis of their base sequences has shown that they code for mRNA with sequence homogene-

ity close to that of the corresponding v–oncs. There is, however, a striking difference. Proto-oncogenes consist of sequences termed exons, which code for peptides of the protein product, interrupted by intervening sequences termed introns. The introns are transcribed into mRNA, but their transcripts are excised from the mRNA which is then spliced and comes to consist of a sequence of bases corresponding to the exons, and translation of this processed mRNA provides the protein product of the gene (Fig. 13.7). By contrast, all the bases in the DNA of v–onc progenes are transcribed into mRNA, and the entire sequence of mRNA is translated to provide the product. This difference holds for genes in general, vertebrate genes consisting of exons and introns, and most retroviral progenes consisting of a continuous 'exon' uninterrupted by introns. *The presence of introns in proto-oncogenes is interpreted as indicating that they have developed by the normal evolutionary processes, and have not been acquired by integration of acute retroviral proviruses.* Accordingly, they are also known as **cellular oncogenes (c-oncs)**. Because of the close similarity of c–oncs and v–oncs, it follows that *v–oncs have been acquired by the acute oncogenic retroviruses in the form of processed host mRNA transcribed from c–oncs.* It is thus assumed that, by an error of transcription, RNA transcribed from an integrated retroviral provirus has included also a transcript of a proto-oncogene, which has thus become incorporated into the viral genome, converting the virus to an acute oncogenic virus. As noted above, in the case of Rous sarcoma virus, v–*src* has been thus acquired in addition to Gag, Pol and Env genes, and it has become a complete acute oncogenic retrovirus (Fig. 13.6). With other acute oncogenic retroviruses, the acquired v–onc has replaced part of the original viral genome and a helper virus is necessary for their replication.

It has also been shown that v–oncs are not exact copies of the processed mRNA of the normal host proto-oncogenes. They exhibit point mutations or greater differences, including loss of a part of the base sequence or gain of an unrelated base sequence.

Activated proto-oncogenes and cancer

Although the acute oncogenic retroviruses have been shown to induce tumours in various species of animals, there is, as already noted, no evidence that these viruses are responsible for any form of cancer in man. However, when DNA from human and other animal cells was digested with restriction endonucleases, and the fragments were used to transfect a cell-line in culture, it was observed that the DNA from normal cells did not transform the cells, while DNA from human tumours and from animal tumours induced experimentally (e.g. by chemical carcinogens), did effect transformation. The responsible genes were isolated by ingenious techniques (see Weinberg, 1983) and cloned by the genetic engineering techniques already described. Surprisingly, they were found to resemble closely proto-oncogenes and their related v-oncs. The oncogene most often detected in the DNA of human tumours belong to the *ras* family, for example the cells derived from a human cancer of the urinary bladder were found to contain a gene resembling v–Ha-*ras*, the v–onc of the Harvey murine sarcoma virus, while a colonic carcinoma contained a gene similar to v–Ki-*ras*, the v–onc of Kirsten murine sarcoma virus. To date, nine oncogenes resembling individual v–oncs have been detected in the DNA of various human tumours, including carcinomas, sarcomas, leukaemias, lymphomas, etc.

It has also been found that the same transforming oncogenes are present in various human tumours. For example Ki-*ras* has been detected in carcinomas of the lung, colon, bladder, chronic lymphocytic leukaemia cells and rhabdomyosarcoma. Some of the transforming genes isolated from human tumours are not related to any of the known v-oncs, perhaps because these genes have not been acquired by any known virus.

Sequence analysis of the bases in the human tumour oncogenes has confirmed the close similarity of some of them to v-oncs, but has shown that they have the structure of vertebrate genes, consisting of exons and introns, and it is thus apparent that they are derived from proto-oncogenes. The startling conclusion is that *the normal proto-oncogenes, which do not transform cells, can be converted to tumour oncogenes which are capable of transforming cells—**activated c–oncs**. Analysis of the normal and tumour *ras* genes has shown minor differences—in one instance a change in a single base. It therefore appears possible that a point mutation in a proto-oncogene can render it carcinogenic. Before accepting this possibility, however, it should be noted that the cells used to test the genes for transforming activity were a cell line, NIH3T3, derived originally from mouse fibroblasts and cultured over a considerable period. Although not frankly malignant, these cells differ from primary cultures of normal cells in being capable of indefinite proliferation. As already explained, such 'immortalisation' is observed as a stage in carcinogenesis (p. 13.5) and suggests that the fibroblasts have already progressed part of the way towards becoming cancer cells. There is some evidence that when the transforming genes, e.g. *ras* genes, obtained from the human tumours, are tested on primary cultures of cells obtained from tissues, they are not by themselves capable of malignant transformation, a second oncogene being necessary. Nevertheless, there is no doubt that the human tumour *ras* genes are capable of inducing part of the change towards malignancy in cultured cells.

Transforming genes have been sought in the DNA of various human tumours, but have been found in only a minority. This is possibly because the NIH3T3 mouse fibroblast cells used in most of these experiments may be an unfavourable target for human oncogenes, although they are readily transformed by many of the 20 or so v-onc progenes from retrovirally-induced animal tumours. The results of further experience, preferably with a range of tests cells, is awaited with considerable interest.

Activation of proto-oncogenes

As noted above, some oncogenes isolated from human tumour cells have been shown to transform a cell line in culture, whereas the corresponding proto-oncogenes in normal human cells are non-transforming. By cleaving a proto-oncogene and a tumour c-onc and uniting the fragments, a series of recombinant hybrid genes have been prepared and tested for oncogenic (transforming) properties. The capacity of a tumour c-*ras* gene to transform mouse fibroblasts was found to reside in a fragment of the gene differing from the corresponding segment of the proto-oncogene by a single **point mutation** (Fig. 13.8a) which would result in a single amino-acid difference in the protein

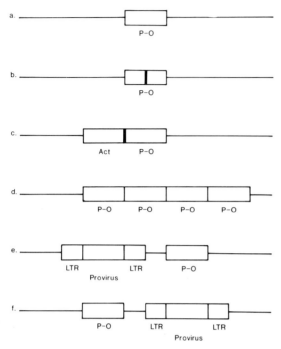

Fig. 13.8 Mechanisms by which proto-oncogenes may become actively oncogenic. **a** shows a proto-oncogene (P-O) in the cell genome. Activation may be induced by the following changes: occurrence of a mutation in the proto-oncogene (**b**); chromosomal translocation resulting in approximation of the proto-oncogene to an activating sequence (Act) (**c**); amplification of the proto-oncogene (**d**); insertion of a retroviral provirus either upstream (**e**) or downstream (**f**) from the proto-oncogene.

encoded by the gene. It thus appears that a specific point mutation converted the normal c-*ras* gene into a transforming oncogene.

Other mechanisms by which a proto-oncogene can become actively oncogenic have recently been described. For example, a human B-cell tumour, Burkitt's lymphoma, exhibits **chromosome translocations** in which a particular part of chromosome 8 is translocated to another chromosome, usually 14, but sometimes 2 or 22. These latter three chromosomes carry structural genes coding for immunoglobulin chains, and it has been demonstrated that a proto-oncogene c-*myc*, located near the break point of chromosome 8, is transferred to the vicinity of the immunoglobulin gene locus on one of the other three chromosomes. In this position, it is probable that expression of the translocated c-*myc* comes under the control of

the genetic mechanism responsible for expression of the adjacent immunoglobulin gene, and in B cells, whose function is to produce immunoglobulins, it will be expressed more actively than in its normal position on chromosome 8 (Fig. 13.8b). In some Burkitt's lymphoma cell lines, the translocated c-*myc* gene differs from the normal c-*myc* but in one cell line c-*myc* is reported to be identical with its normal counterpart.

A third method of activation of proto-oncogenes is by **gene amplification**, in which extra copies of the c-onc are inserted into the genome (Fig. 13.8c). Several human tumour cell lines have been shown to have up to 70 extra c-*myc* genes in the genome. Such amplification of c-*myc* has been detected in human neuroblastomas, and cell lines from lung cancers and other human tumours, and c-onc amplification has been detected in animal tumours. However, there is not a consistent relationship between proto-oncogene amplification and oncogenesis.

Inappropriate expression of a proto-oncogene may also result in oncogenicity. A remarkable example is provided by the proto-oncogene c-*sis*, which appears to code for platelet-derived growth factor (p. 5.10). This gene is normally expressed by platelets. It is, however, consistently expressed by the cells of some human sarcomas and glioblastomas and by T-cell lymphomas associated with HTLV–I virus (p. 13.7). It is not known if expression of v-*sis* is sufficient to account for these cancers, but production of a growth factor by tumour cells which can respond to its mitogenic properties is a possible mechanism of oncogenesis.

Finally, **integration of viral DNA** into the host cell genome may activate a proto-oncogene in the adjacent host DNA. The slow oncogenic retroviruses do not themselves possess a v-onc, but they have, at each end of their proviral DNA, a long terminal repeat (LTR) sequence which is formed by replication of the STR sequence (Fig. 13.6) and contains 'promoters' and 'enhancers'. Promoters initiate transcription of the genes in a 'downstream' position (i.e. in the direction in which DNA is transcribed), while enhancers can increase transcription of genes over 1000 bases distant, both 'upstream' and 'downstream'. These activation mechanisms are illustrated for an avian leukosis virus (ALV) which is a slow oncogenic retrovirus and produces neoplasia of lymphoid cells in chickens. Insertion of the proviral DNA in the tumour cells was regularly found to occur close to a c-*myc* proto-oncogene. In some instances the c-*myc* was upstream, in others downstream from the site of insertion of ALV proviruses (Fig. 13.8e, f), and it may be activated by the promoters and enhancers in the proviral LTR.

In summary, proto-oncogenes may be converted to active oncogenes by the occurrence of point mutations or major alterations in their base sequence, and by changes which result in altered expression. Such changes may include gene amplification, in which the number of copies of a c-onc per cell is increased; translocations, resulting in the approximation of a c-onc to an activating site, and integration of viral DNA sequences which increase transcription of the neighbouring host proto-oncogenes.

How do oncogenes induce cancer?

Twenty or so proto-oncogenes have so far been identified: they have been highly conserved during evolution, for example proto-*ras* is found in species as disparate as insects and man, indicating that it must have developed early, probably over 600 million years ago. The persistence of proto-oncogenes throughout this long period, in relatively unchanged form, implies that they must serve vital functions. For this reason, and because their altered expression appears to be an important factor in oncogenesis, the functions of their protein products are of intense interest.

Investigations on these proteins are at an early stage, and have involved mainly the products of v-oncs, but as the v-oncs of acute oncogenic viruses are similar to normal proto-oncogenes, it is likely that the proteins encoded by both types of gene have similar functions. The products of seven of the twenty or so known v-oncs have been shown to be protein kinases which phosphorylate the tyrosine residues of proteins. This is in contrast to most of the normal cellular protein kinases, which phosphorylate proteins at threonine and serine residues. The products of these seven v-oncs have been found to share a common sequence of about 250 amino acids and this sequence appears to be responsible for their tyrosine-specific protein kinase activity. Tyrosine-phosphorylated proteins are present in normal cells in very small amounts, and the amount in cells

transformed by the appropriate v-oncs may be increased tenfold. Because of the changes in shape and motility of cancer cells, it seemed likely that the proteins of the cytoskeleton might be altered in cancer cells, and one cytoskeletal protein isolated from normal cells, vinculin, has been found to contain phosphorylated tyrosine residues. Vinculin is thought to anchor actin fibrils to the cell membrane. In cells of the Rous sarcoma, which have been transformed by v-*src*, (p. 13.7), the oncogene product, a protein kinase termed p60*src*, is located adjacent to the plasma membrane of the sarcoma cells, and so is in the right place to phosphorylate vinculin, and tyrosine-phosphorylation of vinculin is increased by twenty times in the sarcoma cells. It may be that excessive phosphorylation of vinculin reduces its capacity to anchor actin filaments and that this explains the disorganisation of actin filaments in cancer cells.

By growing non-transformed cells and cells transformed by v-oncs in medium containing radio-labelled phosphate, it has been found that several proteins are phosphorylated at tyrosine in the malignant cells. The protein-kinases produced by the seven v-oncs tend to phosphorylate the same proteins, the functions of which, however, are not known. One of them is associated with sites of insertion of actin filaments in the mucosal surface of epithelial cells lining the intestinal villi, and could be involved in the changes in the cell membrane of cancer cells. Of the several proteins phosphorylated by v-onc protein kinases, only vinculin has been detected in tyrosine-phosphorylated form in normal cells, and v-onc protein kinases may therefore produce their oncogenic effects by phosphorylating inappropriate proteins. The enzymic nature of the products of oncogenes offers a solution to the problem of why cancer cells differ in so many ways from normal cells, for enzymes can have multiple effects on cell metabolism. It is of interest, for example, that p60*src*, the product of v-*src*, is capable also of phosphorylating phosphatidylinositol, a plasma membrane constituent whose breakdown products have been shown very recently to be involved in the major intracellular systems of messengers (p. 7.4). Modification of phosphatidylinositol alone could thus have profound effects on the activities of cells. Evidence on the functions of v-onc products is clearly fragmentary, and as v–oncs are similar to, but not identical with, activated c–oncs, there is no guarantee that the products of the latter behave like the corresponding v–onc products. Little is known about the products of the v–oncs which have not been shown to be protein kinases, but there are two additional findings relating to growth factors. One is the production of platelet-derived growth factor, or a similar substance, by v–*sis* (p. 13.10). The other concerns v–*erb*B, a v–onc of avian erythroblastosis virus which causes leukaemia and sarcomas in fowls. The product of v–*erb*B resembles closely that part of the receptor for epidermal growth factor (p. 5.11) which traverses the plasma membrane and projects into the cytoplasm. It does not code for the external part of the receptor, which binds epithelial growth factor. Binding of epidermal growth factor to its receptor normally stimulates cellular proliferation, probably by inducing a conformational change in the receptor protein, resulting in the activation of a tyrosine-specific protein-kinase activity at the inner surface of the plasma membrane. The product of v–*erb*B may provide a similar stimulus without involvement of epidermal growth factor.

Mouse mammary tumour virus (MMTV)

This is an oncogenic retrovirus which is described here because it illustrates how a cancer which appeared to be determined genetically was found to be induced by viral infection.

By selective breeding, strains of mice were developed in which nearly all the females developed breast cancer, and other strains in which breast cancer was rare. When mice of two such strains were crossed, the incidence of breast cancer in the daughters was the same as that of the maternal strain. A high-cancer strain mother produced daughters with a high incidence and a low-cancer strain mother, daughters with a low incidence. The strain of the father was unimportant. It was further shown that the incidence of breast cancer depended not on the strain of the mother, but on the strain of the mouse which suckled the litter. A high-cancer strain foster mother transmitted the high incidence to her charges. The causal agent was then shown to be present in high-strain mouse's milk ('*Bittner milk factor*') and proved to be a retrovirus which colonises cells of the mammary glandular epithelium. The genetic factor determines the susceptibility of the mice to the virus. Infection persists in a high-cancer strain but dies out in a low-cancer strain.

There is some evidence that human breast cancer may be associated with a virus similar to MMTV. For example, antibodies that react with MMTV are found in some individuals and have been reported to have a higher incidence in women with breast cancer and their relatives than in controls. Particles resembling MMTV have been detected in the milk of a proportion of women but the evidence of their relationship to a family history of breast cancer is conflicting. Sequences which hybridise with nucleic-acid probes for MMTV have been detected in the RNA of the cells of some breast cancers, suggesting that they are infected with a closely related virus. In spite of these findings, there is no evidence that avoidance of breast feeding of infants reduces the risk of breast cancer. Nor is there evidence that genetic factors play a role in the great majority of breast cancers in women, although there is a high incidence in some families (p. 13.28).

Oncogenic DNA viruses

Infection of a cell by a DNA virus may have two results. The virus may replicate with consequent lysis of the cell and release of virions, or the viral DNA genome may integrate into the host-cell DNA (Fig. 13.9). As with the retroviruses, oncogenesis has been found to be associated with viral integration in all instances where the oncogenic virus has been sufficiently investigated. Unlike the retroviruses, the oncogenic DNA viruses cannot both replicate and induce cancer in the same cell, for their replication leads to death of the cell.

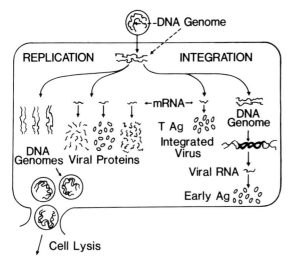

Fig. 13.9 Replication and integration of a DNA virus in the host cell. In replication, copies of the whole viral genome are produced by means of cellular DNA polymerase and the viral genes are transcribed into mRNA, translation of which provides the protein constituents of the virus. These processes, and assembly of new virions, take place in the cell nucleus. Release of the new virions so-formed is accompanied by cell lysis. Integration of the viral genome into the host-cell genome requires the production of an 'early' viral antigen (T antigen, which is necessary also for viral replication). Some genes of the integrated viral genome may be transcribed, providing mRNA coding for viral 'early' antigens, the detection of which is one method of revealing the presence of the virus. Note that persistence of virus in integrated form can only occur in non-permissive cells, for replication results in cell death.

The oncogenic DNA viruses include the group of papovaviruses, some herpes viruses, hepatitis B virus and some adenoviruses. Although none of these viruses has yet been clearly proved to induce cancer in man, there is evidence that some of the papovaviruses, herpes viruses and adenoviruses do so in animals and there are some strongly suggestive associations with certain human cancers.

A feature of oncogenic DNA viruses is that they code for proteins termed T (tumour) antigens which are virus-specific. T antigen is expressed soon after infection of the host cell, and observations on mutant viruses lacking the appropriate gene have shown that the presence of functional T antigen is necessary for transformation of the host cell. Despite extensive investigations, however, the detailed mechanisms of oncogenesis by the DNA viruses in many cases is unclear.

Papovaviruses

This group includes the papilloma viruses, which are known to cause warts, and the polyoma viruses, including simian vacuolating virus, SV40.

The papilloma viruses (PVs)

These viruses replicate in the differentiating layers of stratified squamous epithelium—the stratum spinosum and stratum granulosum. They cause benign warts of the epidermis and squamous mucous membranes in man and animals, which may be papilloma-like or flat plaques. Papilloma viruses do not replicate in cell cultures but some have been shown to transform mouse cells in culture. Detailed analysis of the genomes of papilloma viruses has been achieved by cloning their DNA (p. 13.4) and by using as probes radio-labelled fragments resulting from specific digestion with restriction endonucleases (p. 13.4). In this way, the viruses can be classified and it has been shown that there are at least 23 related human papilloma viruses (HPVs) and six bovine papilloma viruses (BPVs).

Most warts produced by PVs remain benign and in many cases regress spontaneously. However, some types of warts may progress to squamous carcinoma.

PVs were first discovered by Shope in papillomas of the skin of cottontail rabbits. These lesions are infectious because, although the virus does not replicate in the proliferating cells, it does so in cells which have stopped proliferating and are differentiating. Approximately one third of the Shope papillomas become malignant, and when extracts of the papillomas were introduced into the skin of domestic rabbits, the resulting papillomas were observed to become malignant much more often.

The PVs of cattle produce lesions in various anatomical sites. One bovine PV, type 4, produces papillomas of the stratified squamous epithelia of the mucosa of the upper alimentary tract, and it was shown by Jarrett *et al.* (see Jarrett 1981) that these lesions have a very high incidence (80%), and are often multiple, in cattle in upland areas of Britain. Transition to squamous-cell carcinoma was observed in up to 5% of these cattle. Virus was detected in the keratinising cells of the papillomas, while the carcinoma cells did not contain infective virus but probes prepared from BPV-4 DNA demonstrated viral DNA in their nuclei. The high incidence of alimentary papillomas and transformation to cancers was shown to occur in places where the cattle grazed on land contaminated by the bracken fern. Bracken contains a number of chemical carcinogens and also an unidentified factor which is capable of immunosuppression, and it was concluded that there might be synergism between the effects of the virus and these constituents of bracken.

Human papilloma viruses (HPVs) are responsible for the common form of skin warts which often regress spontaneously and do not become malignant. They are also responsible for the widespread warty lesions which occur in the very rare condition, *epidermodysplasia verruciformis*, which affects children with a genetic defect of cell-mediated immunity. By analysis of restriction fragments, 15 HPV types have been detected in patients with this condition and as many as 12 have been detected in one patient. In approximately one third of patients, invasive squamous-cell carcinoma develops, but rarely metastasises. Such malignant change has been associated with HPV of types 5, 8, 12 and 14.

HPV 6 and 11 are responsible for juvenile papillomas of the larynx, which occur in children, are usually multiple, and sometimes regress spontaneously at puberty. These papillomas rarely progress to squamous-cell carcinoma of the larynx. HPV 6 and 11 have also been found in some solitary laryngeal papillomas of adults, which have a greater tendency to progress to carcinoma. The same two virus types are usually responsible for the genital warts, *condylomata acuminata*, although other types of HPV have also been detected in these lesions. They occur in the penis, vulva, perineum and anus, and rarely become malignant. A second type of genital wart, a very small, flat lesion of the vagina and cervix uteri, is also caused by HPV, mostly types 6 and 11. The cervical lesions have usually been reported as mild dysplasia. Many of these lesions regress, but about 10% progress through the stages of dysplasia (CIN—p. 24.4) to invasive carcinoma. By

hybridisation studies, HPV 16 and 18, and also unclassified viruses, have been detected in cervical carcinomas, and also in some vulvar and penile carcinomas. The roles of these various viruses, and also of herpes simplex virus (p. 13.15) in cervical carcinoma are not clear, but the association with HPVs is particularly strong. Lesions associated with HPV 11 tend to regress, while those associated with HPV 16 and 18 tend to progress to carcinoma.

Elucidation of the role of PVs in carcinoma has been handicapped by lack of a method of growing these viruses in cell cultures. There is, however, no doubt that they produce monoclonal proliferations of cells, and that some types of these lesions can progress to carcinoma. The molecular state of the virus in the proliferating cells is obscure. In the past it has been assumed that PVs can transform cells without becoming integrated into the cellular DNA. Although the proliferating cells of the warts and squamous-cell carcinomas do not contain virus particles, PV DNA can often be detected in them, and in some instances has been found to be in the form of a circular molecule, i.e. in free viral form. Such molecules have been found in some cervical carcinomas, the viral DNA being apparently in the form of oligomers, separate from the cellular DNA. In others, however, the viral DNA was apparently covalently linked to cellular DNA.

Polyoma viruses

Polyoma virus infection occurs naturally in mice. It causes a wide range of tumours when injected into neonatal mice, other rodents and rabbits, and can transform cells in culture into cancer cells. Although many wild mice are infected, the virus seldom causes tumours in them because under natural conditions infection is acquired later in life and the mice develop an effective immune response and eliminate the virus and infected cells. The immunity system of neonatal animals cannot respond strongly or quickly enough to eliminate the virus and tumours develop after inoculation. Tumours can be induced in immunodeficient (nude) mice by infection at any age.

A virus of this group. *JC virus*, infects man and in immunosuppressed patients can cause progressive multifocal leukoencephalopathy, a fatal demyelinating disease. There is, however, no evidence that any of the polyoma viruses play a causal role in human tumours. Infection with JC and the related BK virus is widespread in man.

SV40

This is a vacuolating virus of monkeys which can induce tumours when injected into neonatal rodents and can transform human and other cells in culture. Many of the early vaccines for poliomyelitis were grown in monkey kidney cells and were subsequently found to be contaminated with SV40. However, there have been no adverse consequences, and there is no evidence that it plays any part in causing human tumours.

Adenoviruses

The human adenoviruses cause pharyngitis and upper respiratory tract infections. There is no evidence that they cause human tumours though some human adenovirus types have been shown to induce tumours when injected into neonatal rodents and can transform rodent cells in culture.

Herpes viruses

Herpes simplex virus (HSV), Epstein-Barr virus (EBV) and cytomegalovirus are candidates for oncogenicity in man: they are oncogenic in other species, are capable of inducing indefinite proliferation (immortalisation) of mammalian cells in culture, and epidemiological studies have shown that they are associated with certain human cancers. Following the primary infection, all the herpes viruses which infect man are capable of persisting, probably for life, in a latent state in which infectious virus is usually undetectable, but re-activation may occur at intervals, characterised by shedding of virus and sometimes by clinical disease.

The molecular biology of immortalisation of cells by these viruses is obscure and may differ for viruses within the group. DNA of HSV-1 and 2 has been shown to contain sequences which induce mutations in host cells, and both inactivated HSV and HSV DNA fragments have been shown to activate an endogenous retrovirus in murine cells.

HSV-2 and cervical carcinoma. Epidemiological studies have shown that the proportion of seropositive individuals and titres of antibody to HSV-2 are higher in patients with cervical carcinoma than in controls in the same population. In prospective studies, the presence of antibodies to HSV-2 has been found to be associated with an increased risk of subsequently developing cervical carcinoma. A significant proportion of patients with cervical carcinoma do not, however, have HSV-2 antibodies.

The results of attempts to detect specific HSV-2 DNA or its products in human cervical carcinoma or cell lines derived from this tumour are not clear cut. In a minority of cervical carcinomas investigated, nucleic acid probes for HSV-2 DNA have been found to hybridise with the tumour cell DNA and the hybridising sequences have been reported to correspond with immortalising sequences in the HSV-2 genome. Some of the positive tumours have been adenocarcinomas, others of squamous-cell type.

The evidence for an oncogenic role of HSV-2 in man is not strong. HSV-2 is transmitted venereally (p. 25.4) and the incidence of squamous-cell cervical carcinoma is particularly high in sexually promiscuous women. HSV-2 infection and cervical carcinoma may therefore be independent consequences of promiscuity. It has, however, been shown that repeated inoculation of HSV-1 or HSV-2 into the vagina of mice results in a high incidence of squamous-cell carcinomas and adenocarcinomas of the cervix and also endometrial carcinoma.

Infection with human papilloma virus (p. 13.14) is now more strongly suspected of a causal role in cervical carcinoma.

Cytomegalovirus (CMV) and human cancer. CMV is probably a heterogeneous group of viruses. Infection is transmitted between individuals by sexual and other contact, and to the fetus via the placenta. Infected cells have a characteristic appearance: they are very large and have a conspicuous intranuclear inclusion body (Fig. 13.10). Like other herpes viruses, CMV may establish latency. Re-activation in the salivary glands and kidneys results in virus being shed in the saliva and urine. Most adults have been infected and have antibodies to CMV, but the age at which infection is acquired varies in different communities and socio-economic groups. Infection of the fetus can result in various congenital abnormalities. Infection after birth is usually symptomless, but sometimes causes an illness similar to infectious mononucleosis (p. 18.10). Latent infection is commonly activated by conditions or drugs

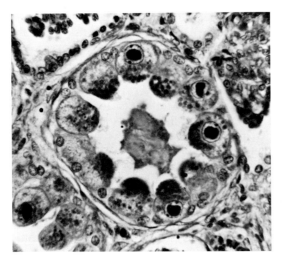

Fig. 13.10 Renal tubules, showing intranuclear and cytoplasmic inclusion bodies in the lining cells in cytomegalovirus disease in an infant. × 400.

which cause depression of cell-mediated immunity, and may result in severe and widespread infection.

Like HSV, CMV is oncogenic in some animal species and can induce proliferation of rodent fibroblasts and human embryonic cells in culture. The mechanism involved is obscure, but transforming sequences have been demonstrated in the viral genome and possess some similarity to those of HSV–2.

Cytomegalovirus infection has been considered as a possible cause of *Kaposi's sarcoma* (p. 14.41). This is a rare tumour occurring particularly in equatorial Africa, where its geographical distribution is similar to that of Burkitt's lymphoma. There is also a very high incidence of CMV infection and of an aggressive form of Kaposi's sarcoma in the acquired immunodeficiency syndrome (AIDS), which occurs principally in male homosexuals (p. 25.5).

Herpes virus particles identified as CMV have been detected in a cell line derived from a case of Kaposi's sarcoma and CMV DNA has been detected in some other Kaposi cell lines. Patients with Kaposi's sarcoma have a very high incidence and higher titres of CMV antibodies than controls, and it is likely that the high incidence of the tumour in AIDS is a result of immunodeficiency following HTLV–III infection (p. 25.5). Kaposi's sarcoma in Africa, like Burkitt's lymphoma, may be attributable in part to immunodeficiency, possibly resulting from chronic malaria or some other cause. This does not exclude a causal role of CMV in Kaposi's sarcoma, but AIDS patients suffer from many types of infection as a result of their immunodeficiency, and the association between CMV and Kaposi's sarcoma may be incidental.

Epstein-Barr (EB) virus. This virus was discovered in cell lines grown from Burkitt's lymphoma, a distinctive neoplasm of B lymphoid cells with a relatively high incidence in children in sub-Saharal parts of Africa. Subsequently, EB virus was shown to be the cause of infectious mononucleosis (p. 18.10) and to have a close association with anaplastic nasopharyngeal carcinoma (p. 16.5), a tumour with a high incidence in South-east China.

Most individuals throughout the world are infected with EB virus. Infection in childhood is usually asymptomatic, while in adolescents and adults it sometimes causes infectious mononucleosis. After infection, EBV persists in latent form, being present in occasional B lymphocytes, and 20% of adults shed infective virus intermittently in the saliva.

EB virus infects human B lymphocytes and stimulates them to proliferate. If human peripheral blood lymphocytes from an EBV-seronegative individual are grown in culture, they die within a few days. If EB virus is added to the culture, the B lymphocytes are transformed into large lymphoblasts which proliferate indefinitely. The virus has the same effect *in vivo*, but the infected B cells expressing EBV antigens are mostly eliminated by the T cells produced in the cell-mediated response to the infection. Antibodies also develop against three viral antigens, and two of them, antibody to EBV nuclear antigen (EBNA) and antibody to viral capsid antigen (VCA) continue to be produced indefinitely (p. 18.11). In spite of the immune response, a very small proportion of infected B cells survive, and when lymphocytes from an EBV-seropositive individual (who has been infected previously) are set up in culture, the infected cells proliferate indefinitely just as when lymphocytes are infected with the virus *in vitro*. The cell lines induced by EB virus have copies of the viral genome integrated into the cellular DNA and express viral antigens. The proliferation is polyclonal and differs in other respects from the neoplastic proliferation of Burkitt's lymphoma (see below). In very occasional cells, the virus replicates and destroys the cell.

The features of **Burkitt's lymphoma** are described on p. 18.26. Following the isolation of EB virus from Burkitt lymphoma cell lines, it was established that African children with this tumour virtually always have high titres of EB virus antibodies. The nuclei of the tumour cells contain (usually multiple) copies of the EB viral genome, demonstrable by nucleic-acid probes, and also EBNA (see above) demonstable by the immunofluorescence technique. Very occasional African cases of Burkitt lymphoma are negative for these EB viral markers, and of the rare cases in Europe and North America, 50–80% have been reported as negative. In a prospective investigation in Uganda, serum from 40 000 children up to 8 years old was stored and the children were kept under surveillance. Fourteen of them developed Burkitt's lymphoma from 7–54 months later: all were found to have EB viral antibodies in their stored serum, and the viral infection had clearly preceded the development of the tumour, in some cases by years. Analysis of the serological findings showed that high titre of antibody to VCA (see above) was associated with a thirty-fold increase in the risk of subsequently developing Burkitt's lymphoma.

G-6-PD iso-enzyme studies (p. 2.11) have shown Burkitt's lymphoma to be a monoclonal proliferation. A regular finding in the tumour cells is a chromosomal translocation in which part of chromosome 8 is transferred to chromosome 14 or, less commonly, to chromosomes 2 or 22. As noted on p. 13.10, these translocations result in the transfer of a proto-oncogene, c-*myc*, from chromosome 8 to the vicinity of immunoglobulin structural genes on the three recipient chromosomes, and it is thought that this may result in altered expression of the c-*myc*. The lymphoblastoid cell lines induced in culture by EBV infection (see above) do not show any chromosomal translocations, and, in addition to being polyclonal, they do not induce tumours when injected into immunodeficient (nude) mice. Burkitt's lymphoma cells appear more primitive, and grow into tumours in nude mice.

The above observations do not prove that EB virus plays a causal role in Burkitt's lymphoma, but this seems highly probable. The capacity of the integrated virus to induce lymphoblastic transformation, its ability to cause tumours in monkeys and its presence in Burkitt lymphoma cells all suggest an oncogenic role. However, the long interval between EB viral infection and development of the tumour, and the high incidence of EB viral infection throughout the world indicate that other causal factors are also involved, one of which is the specific chromosomal translocations described above. Another is believed to be an immunosuppression induced by chronic falciparum malaria (p. 18.26), although other immunosuppressive agents could be responsible, for example HTLV–III, the virus suspected of causing the acquired immune-deficiency syndrome (p. 25.5). The occasional occurrence of Burkitt's lymphoma in non-infected individuals indicates that the postulated oncogenic role of EB virus can be effected in other ways.

In immunodeficient individuals, EBV infection may flare up and cause polyclonal proliferation of B lymphocytes, which may be lethal. The polyclonal proliferation results in masses of B lymphoblasts carrying EBV DNA and expressing EBNA. In these cases, the proliferating B cells are not eliminated, as in normal individuals, because of the deficient T-cell response.

A second known tumour with a close association with EB virus infection is **anaplastic nasopharyngeal carcinoma**, which is rare in most parts of the world but common in South-east China, Greenland and North and Central Africa The cells of this epithelial tumour always carry EB virus DNA and express EBNA: they do not grow readily in culture and permanent cell lines have not been established. When injected into nude mice, the epithelial tumour cells grow and have been shown to contain EBV DNA and to express EBNA. Individuals with this tumour have high titres of antibodies to EB viral antigens. These findings suggest strongly that EB virus plays a causal role in this tumour. The high incidence of particular HLA types in patients with the tumour (p. 13.29) indicates that genetic factors are also involved.

Hepatitis B virus (HBV)

This virus is responsible for an acute hepatitis in man, and also causes a chronic carrier state in which the hepatocytes are persistently infected, resulting in some cases in chronic hepatitis which may progress to fatal cirrhosis. Hepatic cirrhosis can result from other causes, notably chronic alcoholism, and is a predisposing cause of hepatocellular carcinoma, but the incidence of carcinoma is much higher in cirrhosis caused by HBV.

HBV replication requires free viral DNA in the infected hepatocyte, but alternatively the viral DNA can integrate into the cellular DNA and in chronic B viral hepatitis, replication tends to diminish and integration increases. Integrated viral DNA is present in the cells of hepatocellular carcinoma developing in individuals with prolonged HBV infection, but there is no strong evidence that the development of carcinoma is associated with integration at specific sites in the cellular genome.

Cell lines which grow in continuous culture have been established from hepatocellular cancers in patients with chronic HBV infection and have been shown to contain multiple HBV genomes integrated into the cellular DNA. Related viruses have been isolated from animals and birds, for example the woodchuck, in which they also cause chronic hepatitis sometimes progressing to hepatocellular carcinoma, the cells of which contain copies of the viral DNA.

The epidemiological evidence that HBV is a major causal factor in hepatocellular carcinoma, described on pp. 20.39–40, is strong, and its integrated state is a feature of oncongenic DNA viruses. It has not, however, been possible so far to grow HBV in cell cultures, nor does it transform cells in culture. Its aetiological role in liver cell carcinoma is therefore uncertain, and is likely to be elucidated only by observing the effects of an effective HBV vaccine on the incidence of hepatocellular carcinoma.

Chemical carcinogens

The list of chemical compounds shown experimentally to cause cancer in animals is a long one, and there is strong epidemiological evidence that a number of compounds cause cancer in man. This account deals briefly with those carcinogens which have been most thoroughly investigated and with those known or suspected to be of importance as human carcinogenic agents. Methods of testing chemicals for carcinogenicity are outlined on p. 13.23.

Polycyclic hydrocarbons. Although the first evidence of chemical carcinogenesis was provided over 200 years ago (p. 13.1), it was only in 1917 that Yamagiwa and Itchikawa reported the production of cancers by repeated painting of the skin of rabbits with a solution of coal tar. A few years later, Kennaway and his colleagues sought to identify the carcinogenic factors in the complex mixture of chemicals in coal tar: they came to suspect benzanthracene compounds and demonstrated that synthetic 1 : 2, 5 : 6 dibenzanthracene, a polycyclic hydrocarbon, was indeed strongly carcinogenic. Subsequently 3 : 4 benzpyrene was isolated from coal tar and was also shown to be carcinogenic, and many other (but not all) polycyclic hydrocarbons are now known to be carcinogens. These compounds are formed in the combustion of most organic materials, including fossil fuels and tobacco leaf. They are also present in mineral oils and are detectable in significant concentrations in the atmosphere of cities and industrial areas.

Like most chemical carcinogens, polycyclic hydrocarbons are not directly carcinogenic: they are **procarcinogens,** which are metabolised to form carcinogenic compounds (**ultimate carcinogens**). Such activation depends on hydroxylation at specific carbon atoms of the ring structures, converting them to electrophilic reactants with positively charged sites which react with electron-dense sites in protein molecules and nucleic acids of the target cells. The carcinogenicity of a polycyclic hydrocarbon thus depends on whether it is convertible by mixed-function oxygenases to an ultimate carcinogen, and also whether it is susceptible to various other enzymes capable of inactivating it. Host factors are also important. For example, there is some evidence that smoking is more liable to cause cancer in those individuals in whom aryl carbohydrate hydroxylase is readily induced (a genetic characteristic) than in those with a poor enzyme response.

There is no doubt that many polycyclic hydrocarbons can induce cancer in man.

Because their conversion to ultimate carcinogens can occur in most types of cell, cancer develops at the site of exposure, for example in the skin of individuals exposed to direct contact, e.g. shale oil workers and cotton spinners tending machinery lubricated by mineral oils.

Aromatic amines and related compounds. An unusually high incidence of carcinoma of the urinary bladder was noticed almost a century ago in workers in the aromatic dye industry. The development of cancer at a remote site is in sharp distinction to the local development of cancer in the tissues exposed to the polycyclic hydrocarbons. The reason for bladder cancer in dye workers is that the carcinogen mainly involved—β-naphthylamine—is not itself carcinogenic, but is converted to an ultimate carcinogen, 1-hydroxy-2-naphthylamine, mainly in the liver. The liver also inactivates this latter compound by converting it to a glucuronide, in which form it is excreted partly by the kidneys. In some species, including dog and man, the urotheliumn splits off the glucuronide by means of a glucuronidase enzyme, and is thus exposed to the carcinogen. This explains the failure to induce bladder cancer in other species (which lack the glucuronidase enzyme) by administration of β-naphthylamine. Cancer of the bladder in workers in the rubber industry (e.g. motor tyre manufacture) and in the dying of textiles, printing and gas industries, has also been attributed to β-naphthylamine.

Related compounds which induce bladder cancer in man include **benzidine** and certain of its derivatives, which were formerly used without strict precautions in industry, and in medical laboratories to test for occult blood in faeces. Some **azo-derivatives of aromatic amines**, including dyes such as dimethylaminoazobenzene ('butter yellow') are also carcinogenic. Butter-yellow was formerly used to colour margarine until it was shown experimentally to produce cancer of the liver in animals. The **aminofluorenes**, notably 2-acetylaminofluorene, formerly used as an insecticide, induce cancer of the liver and urinary bladder in animals.

As with the polycyclic hydrocarbons, hydroxylation is an essential step in converting these compounds into ultimate carcinogens, but other changes are also involved.

Alkylating agents are another important group of compounds with carcinogenic properties for experimental animals. They include nitrogen mustards and the related compound cyclophosphamide, procarbazine and the nitrosoureas, all of which are used in the treatment of some forms of cancer. These compounds are directly carcinogenic and do not require to be converted to ultimate carcinogens within the body, and there is increasing evidence that they induce acute non-lymphoblastic leukaemia in man, although the risk appears to be relatively small.

Although the above major groups of chemical carcinogens differ considerably in their structure, they produce their effects on DNA by being, or giving rise to, electrophilic reactants. As noted above, these react with electron-dense sites on macromolecules. For example, they react with guanine in DNA and either form links between two guanines in adjacent DNA strands or become inserted between guanine and the next base in the same strand. Such changes can result in pairing of the altered guanine with the wrong base (adenine or thymine instead of cytosine) during DNA synthesis, thus causing a point mutation in the other strand. Insertion of the reactant between two bases can result in the loss or addition of a pair of bases into the two strands with the result that the wrong base triplets are transcribed and translated (*frame-shift mutation*) and a 'nonsense protein' is produced.

Asbestos, which consists of various fibrous silicates, has long been used for heat insulation, as brake linings for vehicles and for roofing materials, etc. It has become apparent, however, that, in addition to the well-known asbestosis (pulmonary fibrosis) which results from prolonged exposure, inhalation of asbestos fibres, particularly crocidolite ('blue asbestos'), can result in the otherwise rare malignant mesothelioma of the pleura or peritoneum and also in bronchial carcinoma. As with all chemical carcinogens, these cancers occur years after exposure to asbestos dust. Asbestos and cigarette smoking are synergistic in inducing bronchial carcinomas: the combination leads to a very high incidence.

Another industrial cancer, of quite recent recognition, is haemangiosarcoma of the liver in workers exposed to **vinyl chloride monomer**, used in the preparation of polyvinyl chloride.

Arsenical compounds, both organic and inorganic, cause chronic inflammation of the skin and epidermal hyperplasia if administered orally or parenterally (or absorbed through the skin) over a long period. In some cases, carcinoma of the epidermis, most often of basal-cell type, develops. The use of arsenicals as drugs has, however, diminished greatly.

Exposure to chemical carcinogens is not solely an occupational hazard. For example, **cigarette smoking** is very largely responsible for the world-wide high incidence of bronchial carcinoma: in the UK it accounts for the death of approximately 10% of men over 45 years old, i.e. 40% of male deaths from cancer. A number of carcinogenic hydrocarbons are present in small amounts in cigarette smoke and their effects may be additive. Another habit, the chewing of **betel leaves** mixed with tobacco leaves and slaked lime, has been associated with a high incidence of carcinoma of the oral mucosa in Southern India and South East Asia.

Dietary factors also appear to be of importance, particularly in carcinoma of the alimentary tract. The incidence of carcinoma of the large intestine is relatively high in developed countries with a high standard of living. Genetic factors do not appear to be of importance, for the incidence in migrant groups who have adopted the dietary habits of their new country is similar to that of the indigenous population and not to that of their country of origin. The incidence shows a positive correlation with the amount of meat, animal fat and protein in the diet, and a negative correlation with the amount of vegetable fibre. There is evidence that bacteria present in the gut can produce carcinogenic metabolites from various substances present in the diet or produced by digestion in the gut, e.g. from tryptophane, tyrosine, methionine, cycasin and cholesterol. So far, there is no strong evidence that bacterial action on such compounds is an important causal factor in colonic cancer, but the possibility remains.

The incidences of carcinoma of the oesophagus and stomach show marked geographical variations. Oesophageal cancer is relatively common in parts of Russia, China and Central and South America. The causes for this are likely to be dietary, but a combination of alcohol consumption and smoking appears to be associated with an increased risk. Gastric cancer has a very high incidence in Japan but much lower in Japanese in Western countries. In Europe and the USA, the incidence is much lower than in Japan and has declined during this century. Here again, the causal factors are unknown, but are likely to be dietary.

The addition of preservatives, colourants, etc. to foodstuffs is another possible cause of alimentary cancers. For example, nitrites are present in preserved meat, sausages, etc. and are converted by hydrochloric acid in the gastric juice to nitrous acid. This reacts with secondary amines to form **nitrosamines**, many of which have been shown to be carcinogenic in animals. There is, indeed, experimental evidence that addition of nitrites and secondary amines to the diet can cause alimentary cancers in animals, but the role of nitrosamines in human cancer is not known. It has also been suggested that cancer of the liver may result from ingestion of **aflatoxins**, metabolites of the fungus *Aspergillus flavus*, which contaminates peanuts. Aflatoxins are highly potent carcinogens, causing carcinoma of the liver when administered to animals, and the possibility exists that they may have a causal role in the very high incidence of this form of cancer in man in Kenya and some other parts of Africa. The demonstration of a close relationship between cancer of the liver and chronic infection with the hepatitis B virus (p. 20.40), regardless of the amount of aflatoxin ingested with contaminated peanuts, suggests that the latter is not an important factor, but the metabolism of aflatoxin is complex, and is made more so by the effects of malnutrition, particularly when this is seasonal, as in parts of Africa. Aflatoxin may still play a contributory role (Enwonwu, 1984).

Progress in the detection of carcinogenic chemicals in industry, in the atmosphere and in the diet has been slow, and there are many unsolved problems. The reasons for this will be appreciated by considering some of the more important features of chemical carcinogenesis.

Principles of chemical carcinogenesis

Epidemiological studies on individual forms of cancer in man and experimental work on animals have revealed the following important features of chemical carcinogenesis.

1. The induction of cancer by chemical carcinogens is a prolonged process. In man, cancer develops several (and often more than twenty) years after the commencement of exposure to a carcinogen. In experimental animals, the process is shorter, but still takes months, and varies with the species and strain of animal. Individual susceptibility is also apparent in man. Only a minority of those exposed to a carcinogen in industry develop cancer, and although dosage is important (see below) the total dose required to induce cancer varies greatly in different individuals. This is well illustrated by cigarette smoking: the risk increases with the total smoked, but some light smokers develop cancer and some heavy prolonged smokers do not. This variability may depend on genetic factors, e.g. the level of aryl hydrocarbon hydroxylase induced in the target cells (p. 13.18), and also on exposure to additional carcinogenic agents, e.g. the polluted air of industrial cities.

As will be seen later, *the prolonged period taken for a chemical carcinogen to induce cancer is a feature of carcinogenesis in general: it applies also to physical carcinogens and also to most of those human cancers in which viral infection appears to play a causal role.*

2. Chemical carcinogenesis involves at least two distinct and sequential effects on the target cell—**initiation** and **promotion**. Chemical carcinogens are initiating agents. They may also be promoting agents, but some agents which are not themselves carcinogenic can nontheless promote the development of cancer in cells that have been initiated. To give an example, a single application of a chemical carcinogen such as methylcholanthrene to the skin of mice does not usually cause cancer, but subsequent repeated applications of croton oil (itself not carcinogenic) will result in the development of cancers. Repeated applications of methylcholanthrene (and most other chemical carcinogens) alone will often result in cancer because most carcinogens act also as promoting agents (**complete carcinogens**).

Initiation involves two stages, the first being a change induced in the cell by the active (ultimate) carcinogen. The nature of this change is uncertain: as noted above, carcinogens can react with multiple sites in proteins and nucleic acids, but it now seems most likely that initiation is essentially an alteration in the DNA of the genome (p. 13.30). The second stage of initiation is mitosis. Initiation is an irreversible process, the initiated cells remaining susceptible to promoting agents virtually throughout life: this irreversibility is conferred by a single mitotic division. If, as suggested above, initiation involves the alteration of DNA, the important effect of mitosis might be to introduce a consequent abnormality in the *complimentary* strand of DNA which is synthesised during the S phase of the cell cycle, using as a template the altered strand.

In most instances, the only way that initiation can be detected is to demonstrate that the cells are responsive to promoting agents.

Promotion. Application of a promoting agent (**co-carcinogen**) results initially in a selective proliferation of initiated cells, producing thickenings and papillary projections when the skin is involved, or formation of hyperplastic nodules in solid tissues. The number of such lesions reflects the number of cells which have been initiated and thus the dose and potency of the carcinogen. At this stage, the proliferated cells are not neoplastic, for most of the focal proliferations subsequently disappear. Some, however, persist. It is from these persistent hyperplasias that a focus of malignant cells eventually develop (see below). The number of stages involved in promotion is not known. The next distinctive stage is the development of foci of dysplasia (p. 12.6) within those hyperplastic lesions which have persisted. This arises from the development of cells which have the morphological features of malignant cells and undergo spontaneous proliferation. Further changes are ill-defined, but the dysplastic cells may eventually give rise to frank cancers.

When the total dose of initiating carcinogen (which is usually also a promoter) is sufficiently large, cancers will develop without further manipulation, but subsequent application of a promoting agent will increase the numbers of cancers developing (in a group of animals) and will hasten their appearance. Unlike initiation, promotion is reversible, at least in its earlier stages. This follows from the well-established observation that repeated application of promoting agents to initiated cells is most effective if the promoter is applied at short intervals. The longer the intervals between applications, the less likely is promotion to be induced, even though the total dose of promoter may be well above that which is effective when applications are closely spaced. Ex-smokers become progressively less likely to develop bronchial carcinoma over the years until eventually the risk is only slightly greater than in non-smokers. This is presumably because tobacco smoke acts as a complete carcinogen and its promoting effects are reversible.

For obvious reasons, initiation and the early stages of promotion cannot be studied in man, and investigation of human carcinogenesis is very largely restricted to the late stages of promotion in which the pre-malignant changes can be recognised as dysplastic lesions. Such lesions are known from biopsy procedures to precede many carcinomas, for example carcinoma developing in the uterine cervix, the breast, the cirrhotic liver, the skin (e.g. following prolonged exposure to ultraviolet light), the colon (in ulcerative colitis) and the urinary bladder following exposure to β-naphthylamine. Excision of tissues in which carcinoma has developed frequently shows areas of dysplasia in addition to the carcinoma, although by the time they are removed, many cancers have invaded extensively and destroyed the surrounding tissue.

Although these dysplastic lesions in man represent relatively late stages of carcinogenesis, one of them, dysplasia of the uterine cervix (Fig. 24.3, p. 24.4) appears in some cases to be reversible: it may regress, remain static or progress to frank malignancy.

Nearly all investigations of carcinogenesis by initiation and promotion have been performed on rodents and much of it has employed croton oil in the promotion of skin tumours. Various other organic compounds have, however, been shown to be promoters and the effectiveness of a promoter has been found to vary for different tissues. The promoting agents in croton oil are phorbol esters. They are cytotoxic compounds and initiated cells appear more resistant to their toxic effect than normal cells, with the result that normal cells are lost and replaced by proliferation of initiated cells. Some other promoting agents, (and complete carcinogens) also promote by a similar toxic effect, but some promoting agents stimulate proliferation without injuring normal cells. For example, excessive oestrogen stimulation increases the risk of carcinoma of the endometrium and administration of oestrogen or prolactin to rodents following administration of a carcinogen promotes the development of carcinoma of the breast. There are a number of examples where chronic tissue injury, with continued proliferation to replace lost cells, predisposes to carcinoma. For example, in schistosomal infection of the urinary bladder, in chronic inflammatory lesions of the large intestine, notably ulcerative colitis, and in cholelithiasis (formation of stones in the gall-bladder). Indeed, carcinoma occurs most commonly in tissues where cells have a high rate of mitotic activity to replace cell loss (e.g. the epidermis and epithelium of mucous membranes). In tissues with a low mitotic activity, such as the liver, promotion may depend partly on continuous or repeated destruction of cells with consequent compensatory hyperplasia of the remainder. This is a feature of cirrhosis, in which the development of cancer is often associated with chronic destruction of hepatocytes, e.g. by the hepatitis B virus (p. 13.17). It thus appears that proliferation is an important feature of promotion, and that promoting agents either increase the rate of proliferation in tissues with labile cells or induce cell proliferation in those tissues where cells are normally stable (p. 5.1). However, the most effective promoting agents are those which stimulate disproportionate proliferation of initiated cells.

3. The relationship between the rate of administration of a chemical carcinogen and the duration of carcinogenesis has been investigated very largely by repeated administration of complete carcinogens alone rather than by separate administration of carcinogen and promoter. In such experiments, the effective initiating and promoting doses cannot be assessed. With this reservation, some carcinogens have been shown to have a total effective carcinogenic dose which depends on the particular carcinogen used and the strain of experimental animal. In such cases, halving the interval between individual doses, e.g. applications to the skin, or doubling the dosage, will half the time taken for cancer to develop. For other carcinogens, the duration of carcinogenesis is less dose-dependent so that halving the interval between individual doses, or doubling the dosage, will reduce the duration, but not by half.

4. As noted above, most chemical carcinogens are metabolised to ultimate carcinogens. Where such activation is a property of cells in general, tumours will develop among the cells exposed to the carcinogen. In some instances, activation occurs mainly in a particular organ, usually the liver, which may then be the site of cancer regardless of the route of administration of the carcinogen. The metabolic changes involved in the production of ultimate carcinogens may be more complex, as in the case of β-naphthylamine which, for reasons explained on p. 13.19, induces cancer of the urinary bladder.

The physical properties and chemical reactivity of a carcinogen are also important, for they determine whether it diffuses widely or stays mainly at the site of administration.

The contribution of chemically induced cancer to the understanding of carcinogenesis in general is discussed on pp. 13.29–31.

Testing chemicals for carcinogenicity

The traditional method of testing a chemical compound for carcinogenicity is to administer it to laboratory animals, e.g. mice or other rodents, by whatever route and in whatever form seems most appropriate. A solution of the chemical may be painted onto the skin, or it may be given orally, by parenteral injection, or by inhalation as a dust, vapour or aerosol. Administration must be prolonged and the animals must be kept under observation for many months and careful autopsies performed. Even when the dosage and route of administration are varied, and tests are carried out with and without promoting agents in large numbers of animals of various species, the results obtained are not necessarily applicable to man, for there is considerable species variability in the susceptibility to particular carcinogens, e.g. β-naphthylamine (p. 13.19). A negative result does not, therefore, exclude completely the possibility that the chemical is carcinogenic for man, nor does a positive result necessarily indicate carcinogenicity for man, although it means that the chemical must be regarded as potentially carcinogenic and suitable precautions taken in its use.

Traditional testing for carcinogenesis is an expensive and prolonged procedure. More recently, rapid tests for mutagenicity have been introduced. An ingenious method of testing involves the use of mutant strains of *Salmonella typhimurim* which cannot synthesise histidine. They will not grow in histidine-free medium, but addition of a mutagenic chemical increases the rate of reversion to the 'normal' histidine-synthesising strain. The chemical under test is therefore added to histidine-free agar medium to which the mutant bacteria are applied, and the number of mutations is reflected in the number of colonies which develop. This technique can be further exploited by using strains sensitive to different kinds of mutation, and enzyme systems can be added to the medium to convert procarcinogens to ultimate carcinogens.

The correlation between mutagenesis is not absolute but it is sufficiently close for chemicals found to be mutagenic to be regarded as potentially carcinogenic, and the technique is therefore of value principally as a method of screening chemicals.

The care with which a chemical or mixture of chemicals requires to be screened depends on their intended use. Proposed ingredients of foodstuffs, cosmetics, insecticides, etc. require to be tested with extreme care. Drugs for use in conditions not likely to be fatal require equally careful testing, but it is of little relevance that a drug to be used only in treating patients with advanced cancer may itself cause cancer some years later in a few of the recipients. Indeed, alkylating agents known to be carcinogenic are used with beneficial effect in treating patients with inoperable cancers of various types.

Hormones and carcinogenesis

As a general rule, cancer is more likely to develop in cells which undergo proliferation than in non-dividing cells. This is illustrated by tissues which are under the control of known hormones: cancer is more likely to develop in them if hormonal stimulation is increased. In the absence of the normal hormonal stimulation, such tissues become atrophic, and the development of cancer in the target organs is unlikely. There are, however, exceptions to this general rule, which is illustrated by the following examples.

Oestrogens can undoubtedly cause tumours in susceptible strains of mice: their administration in high dosage leads to an increased incidence of cancer of the breast in females and to the occurrence of breast cancer in males. Reduction of natural oestrogen levels by oophorectomy inhibits the development of cancer of the breast in susceptible female mice. It might seem that the excessive proliferation of breast ducts induced by oestrogen, carried to excess, has been the actual cause of the cancer, but, as noted on p. 13.12, oestrogens appear to induce cancer especially in female mice infected with a mammary tumour virus. In virus-free mice, and in other species, the effect is much harder to demonstrate. In tissues other than the breast the position becomes somewhat anomalous. The most obvious oestrogen target cells, the endometrial glandular epithelium, rarely develops tumours in oestrogen-treated animals, though connective-tissue tumours of the uterus are often produced and tumours result also in organs not usually regarded as oestrogen-responsive, for example the kidney in hamsters, and the Leydig cells of the testis in mice. These effects appear to depend only on the hormonal activity of the various oestrogens, and not on their precise structure.

It now seems likely that there is an increased risk of carcinoma of the endometrium in women receiving prolonged oestrogen therapy and in patients with an oestrogen-secreting granulosa-cell tumour of the ovary. In the past, the risk has been exaggerated by confusion between endometrial hyperplasia and carcinoma.

A striking example of hormone-induced cancer is provided by the development of adenocarcinoma of the vagina in adolescents or young adult females. This is a very rare tumour, but its incidence is greatly increased in girls whose mothers have received oestrogen therapy during pregnancy. It appears in this instance that oestrogen acts as an initiator of the vaginal epithelium during fetal life.

Contraceptive hormonal preparations. Considering the very large number of women taking oral contraceptive pills, there is little evidence of any carcinogenic effect, but for reasons given on p. 24.46, further experience and investigation are necessary before a possible carcinogenic effect on the breast can be excluded. There is a small increase in benign tumours of the liver, which correlates with dose and duration of therapy, while the incidence of benign breast lesions is decreased. An early type of 'pill', in

which different hormones were administered sequentially, was associated with an increase in endometrial carcinoma, and has now been withdrawn.

Androgenic/anabolic steroids. These hormones, notoriously used by athletes to increase muscle mass, may be involved in the development of cancer of the liver.

Experimental endocrine disturbances and tumours. Experimental procedures which induce an increased output of trophic hormones by the adenohypophysis have been shown to result in cancer in the target organs, although trophic hormones have not been shown to induce cancer in man.

Examples of this mechanism of tumour induction include the following. (a) If the ovaries of a rat are removed and pieces are implanted into the spleen, they continue to secrete oestrogen, but this passes via the portal vein to the liver, where it is mostly inactivated. In consequence, there is increased secretion of FSH by the adenohypophysis and a granulosa-cell cancer eventually develops in the stimulated follicular tissue of the transplanted ovaries. (b) If rats are treated with a drug such as thiouracil, which blocks the production of thyroid hormone, increased secretion of TSH by the adenohypophysis causes hyperplasia and eventually cancer of the thyroid follicular epithelium. Cancer develops more rapidly, and with more certainty, if a carcinogen. e.g. 2-acetylaminofluorene or radio-iodine (which is taken up by the thyroid epithelium) is administered to the experimental animals.

Another example of functional hyperplasia leading to neoplasia is provided by removing the thyroid gland in mice, or destroying it with a large dose of radio-iodine. In the absence of thyroid hormone, the TSH-secreting cells of the adenohypophysis undergo hyperplasia and in some strains of mice this progresses to neoplasia. It is of interest in relation to the following section that initially the tumour cells can be suppressed by thyroxine, but eventually they may continue to grow when transplanted serially into mice with normal thyroid function.

Hormone-dependent tumours in man. The experimental pituitary and thyroid tumours just mentioned may both be hormone-dependent in the sense that they may regress if the excessive hormonal stimulation that invoked them is removed. Related phenomena in man are few, but the following three carcinomas deserve mention. (1) Many **prostatic carcinomas** are sufficiently dependent on a normal male hormonal environment to be slowed down, arrested, or even to regress for long periods, if oestrogens are administered. (2) Some differentiated **thyroid carcinomas** are partially dependent on TSH, and their rate of growth and spread may be reduced or arrested by continued administration of thyroxine, which suppresses secretion of TSH by the pituitary. (3) Some **breast carcinomas** regress under various hormonal manipulations—treatment with male hormones, oophorectomy, adrenalectomy or hypophysectomy (p.24.46). Treatment by these methods has been largely empirical, but the cells of some

breast cancers have receptors for oestrogens and sometimes also for progesterone. When hormone binds to the receptors the hormone-receptor complex enters the cell and is passed to the nucleus where it affects nucleic acid metabolism. The clinical significance is that patients with tumours consisting of receptor-positive cells are more likely to respond to withdrawal of the hormone.

Just as the experimentally-induced hormone-dependent pituitary tumours become independent after serial transplantation (see above), hormone-sensitive tumours in man practically always resume growth eventually, though with thyroid and prostatic carcinomas the period of arrest or partial regression is often long.

Physical agents and carcinogenesis

The most important physical agents with carcinogenic effects are ionising and ultraviolet (UV) radiations. Mechanical injury to the wall of the gallbladder or urinary tract has been suggested as the cause of the increased risk of carcinoma in these tissues in individuals with gallstones or urinary stones. Acute physical injury has also been suspected of predisposing to cancer in the injured tissues, but the evidence is not convincing. Cancer does, however, arise more often than would be expected in scars resulting from repair of burns and various other forms of tissue injury. The mechanisms of carcinogenesis in these non-radiation forms of injury are obscure.

Ionising radiation. A detailed account of the effects of ionising radiation on cells is given on pp. 3.23–29. The various forms of ionising radiation—x-rays, α, β and γ rays—can all induce cancer in animals and man. They injure the cells through which they pass by dislodging electrons from water and other molecules, with formation of ionised molecules highly reactive with nucleic acids, proteins and other cellular constituents. As with other carcinogenic agents, cancer develops in man some years after the first exposure and the effects of repeated doses are cumulative, features which suggest strongly that, of the many cellular injuries caused by ionising radiations, the carcinogenic effect is due to damage to the DNA. This includes: (1)

changes in single bases (point mutations) and consequent change of an amino acid in the protein product of the affected gene: (2) breaks in one or both strands of the double helix, producing fragments which are liable to re-unite in the wrong order. This results in transfer of sequences of various lengths, sometimes visible microscopically as translocations and other chromosomal abnormalities (Fig. 3.28, p. 3.28) including the appearance of fragments of chromosomes which remain separate.

Very large doses of ionising radiation result in cell death by the changes produced by free radicals in DNA, proteins, etc. either immediately or when the injured cell attempts mitosis. Cells exposed to sub-lethal doses may have permanent changes in the DNA which predisposes then to malignant transformation. The amount of such injury depends on the total dosage to which the cells are exposed.

The effects of ionising radiation on different tissues depend on the type of radiation, which determines the depth of tissue penetration, and also on the nature of the tissues irradiated. Because of its density, bone tissue absorbs and scatters ionising radiations more than soft tissues and as a consequence haemopoietic tissue is severely damaged. Accordingly, leukaemias are among the commoner types of cancer resulting from ionising radiations. The thyroid, breast and lung are relatively common sites of radiation-induced carcinomas. The sites of cancer induced by radio-isotopes depend on their distribution. Insoluble radio-active dusts cause carcinoma of the lung, while osteosarcoma is the commonest tumour induced by radio-isotopes of those elements which are deposited in bone tissue. The latter include radium, strontium and plutonium. Radio-strontium released into the atmosphere in nuclear weapon tests is eventually deposited by rain and is absorbed by plants and secreted in the milk of cows feeding on contaminated grass. The risk to man by ingestion of radio-strontium from this source is not known, but as the effects of radiation are dose-dependent and cumulative, there is probably no safe dose. Any additional radiation is likely to increase the total incidence of cancer in the individuals or populations exposed to it. Administration of radio-iodine to rodents causes cancer of the thyroid, the main site of iodine storage. Therapeutic doses of radio-iodine have not been shown to cause thyroid cancer in man, but are usually used in patients over 45 years old. Accidental exposure to radio-iodine released by a nuclear bomb test has been observed to cause thyroid cancer in children, and x-irradiation of the neck in infancy or childhood carries a significant risk of the development of thyroid cancer in adolescence or early adult life.

A much-quoted example of radium-induced cancer occurred about 60 years ago in the USA. Girls employed to paint the dials of watches with luminous paint containing radium were in the habit of pointing the brushes with their lips, and they ingested enough radium to cause a high incidence of osteosarcoma. The early radiologists knew nothing of the risk of calibrating their machines by exposing their arms, forearms and hands. As the early x-rays were 'soft' and did not penetrate deeply, squamous-cell carcinomas occurred in the exposed skin. After the hazard of irradiation was appreciated and 'safe' practices introduced, the use of more penetrating x-rays still resulted in an increased incidence of deeper tumours in radiologists, notably *chronic granulocytic leukaemia* from exposure of the haemopoietic marrow. Further improvements in safety procedures have now virtually abolished this hazard.

Therapeutic x-irradiation is used mainly to treat various forms of cancer, most often in patients over 50 years old, and many of those treated nevertheless die of the tumour. For these reasons, a second form of cancer arising as a result of the irradiation is seldom observed in such patients. However, therapeutic x-ray treatment of the spine was formerly used to treat ankylosing spondylitis, a chronic condition which causes disability but seldom death. Follow-up showed that the x-ray treatment resulted in an increased incidence of leukaemia. The atom bomb explosions at Hiroshima and Nagasaki in 1945 were followed by a considerable increase in the incidence of leukaemia, peaking at about 6 years, in heavily exposed survivors, and smaller increases in the incidences of carcinomas of the thyroid, breast and bronchus have since been detected. These findings are based on sound statistical analysis and there is no doubt that ionising radiations induce cancers of various types. The contribution of radiation-cancer to the understanding of carcinogenesis in general is discussed on pp. 13.29–31 and the role of radiation in leukaemogenesis on pp. 17.55, 56.

Ultraviolet (UV) radiation and cancer. In contrast to ionising radiations, UV radiation penetrates tissues and clothes poorly and its effects are limited to the exposed skin. The main source of exposure is the sun and it has long been known that *light-skinned people whose occupation or life style involves heavy exposure to sunlight have a high incidence of basal-cell and squamous-cell carcinomas and malignant melanomas of the exposed skin.* This is well illustrated by the very high incidence of these skin tumours among white Australians, especially those with a fair complexion who do not tan readily in response to sunlight. The incidence is very high among farmers and other outdoor workers. The dark-skinned races are protected by absorption of UV rays by melanin in the superficial layers of the epidermis, a good example of evolutional selection. For the white-skinned races, who lived in less sunny climates, protection against UV was less necessary, and a white skin was advantageous in allowing absorption of UV to provide sufficient vitamin D. The benefits of these evolutional adjustments to the environment are illustrated by the development of skin cancers in white people who have migrated to a hot sunny climate, and vitamin D deficiency in those dark-skinned people who now live, for example, in the cloudy West of the British Isles.

UV rays injure cells directly and acute over-

Radio-labelled
Synthetic
Proviral DNA
(DNA Probe)

Binding of Radio-labelled
DNA Probe
to Integrated Proviral DNA

dosage produces the inflammatory changes of sunburn. It also induces clinically silent changes in the DNA of epidermal cells, the best known of which is the linking of pyrimidine bases, particularly thymine, to form dimers. The carcinogenic effect of these changes is strongly suggested by the high incidence of multiple skin cancers at an early age in individuals with *xeroderma pigmentosum*, a rare inherited condition in which there is a defect of an enzyme which excises abnormal segments of DNA as part of the process of repair (see below). Sufferers from this disease can only avoid skin damage and cancers by protecting themselves from exposure to UV light.

Inheritance of susceptibility to cancer

Changes in the DNA of somatic cells are now widely regarded as playing a major role in the transformation of a normal cell to a cancer cell. The occurrence in the germ-cell line of one or more changes in the DNA which occur during carcinogenesis would be expected to increase the incidence of cancer in those individuals inheriting the change. This is indeed observed in a number of cancers which show strong genetic inheritance, but such cancers are rare, and epidemiological studies of cancer in general, and of the common types of cancers, have not revealed any strong genetically-determined predisposition. It still remains possible that predisposition to cancer is influenced by multiple genes, giving a pattern of inheritance which is not readily detected or analysed.

Rare genetically-determined cancers

Genes which carry a strong predisposition to the development of cancer are likely to result in the development of cancer at a relatively early age. Accordingly, such cancer-predisposing genes are likely to confer a survival disadvantage and to be sustained in the population only by chance mutation. This accounts for the rarity of cancers with a strong inherited predisposition. Examples include retinoblastoma, adenomatosis (polyposis) coli and xeroderma pigmentosum.

Retinoblastoma is a highly malignant tumour of the eye which occurs in childhood and has an incidence of about 1 in 20 000. In a minority of cases, the tumour occurs in families and is often bilateral. Such cases are caused by a deletion in chromosomes 13. There is evidence that inheritance of this abnormality is not alone sufficient to induce the development of a retino-blastoma and it has been postulated that the tumour results from a somatic mutation in the chromosome 13 from the other parent with a normal genome. Mechanisms whereby a heterozygous inherited abnormality predisposes to a change in the corresponding normal gene are known to exist and their involvement has been suggested in the development of familial retinoblastoma. The tumour also occurs sporadically, but is usually unilateral and develops a few years later, features which are consistent with the requirement for two somatic mutations.

Xeroderma pigmentosum is a rare disorder with an autosomal recessive inheritance in which there are defects in a gene pair coding for an enzyme essential for the repair of some forms of DNA injury. The enzyme excises abnormal sequences of DNA which are then replaced by the normal sequence of bases. The deficiency results in failure to repair the change induced in the DNA of epidermal cells by UV light, and in patients with xeroderma pigmentosum the skin becomes dry and scaly and multiple skin cancers develop in childhood. In some cases, there is also progressive neurological disease and most patients die in childhood from this or from skin cancers. Seven sub-types of the disorder have been defined, each of which appears to have a different defect in the excision mechanism. Patients are also unable to repair DNA injury caused by many chemical carcinogens, and the disease is an example of a more general predisposition to cancer which manifests only in the skin because it is the only tissue subjected in the early years of life to the sort of DNA injury which these individuals are unable to repair.

Adenomatosis (Polyposis) coli. This condition

is inherited as an autosomal dominant trait. Affected individuals are normal until adolescence, when they develop very large numbers of adenomatous polyps of the mucosa of the small intestine. Cytological features of malignancy develop in many of the polyps and eventually one or more progress to invasive adenocarcinoma. This progression occurs so regularly that prophylactic excision of the large intestine is necessary. Skin fibroblasts from these patients are readily immortalised in culture by a chemical cancer promoter, suggesting that the abnormal gene in some way mediates initiation, but it is not known why the effects of the disease are confined to the large intestine.

Polygenic factors in carcinogenesis

A number of types of cancer, and particularly carcinoma of the breast, have been observed to occur relatively early, and with an unusually high frequency, in particular families. This suggests that genetic factors are involved but there are two other possible explanations. One is that any sporadic disease will, by sheer chance, occur more often than usual in groups of related individuals. Accordingly, the occurrence of clustering of cancers in families must be subjected to complex statistical analysis to determine if it is of any significance. Secondly, members of a family share much the same environment, and environmental factors may influence the occurrence of a particular cancer. This second problem can sometimes be overcome by comparing the incidence of cancer in groups of monozygotic and dizygotic twins. Monozygotic twins are genetically identical, whereas dizygotic twins have half their genes in common. If a cancer is determined partly by genetic factors, it should exhibit concordance (i.e. occur in both or neither of a pair of twins) more often in monozygotic than in dizygotic twins: put the other way round, discordance (occurrence of cancer in only one of a pair of twins) should be observed more often in dizygotic than in monozygotic twins. Results of such analyses are somewhat conflicting. In one of the most extensive investigations to date, use was made of the Danish Twin Register, which recorded all twin births in Denmark, and the Danish Cancer Registry, which includes all malignant tumour patients diagnosed in Denmark. The occurrence of leukaemia and of car-

cinomas of the breast, colon and rectum was investigated in pairs of twins of like sex born between 1881 and 1920. The findings indicated little if any difference in concordance for these cancers between monozygotic and dizygotic twins, and therefore gave no support for genetically-determined causal factors.

It must be emphasised that family and twin studies are not sensitive methods of detecting genetic predisposition for cancer unless the predisposition carries a high risk of cancer. As Bodmer (1982) has pointed out, a dominant gene might increase the risk of cancer by ten times, e.g. from 1 in 1000 to 1 in 100. In spite of this major difference, the chance of development of cancer in two sibs (or twins), both of whom possess the gene, would be 1 in 10 000— —so low that it would only be revealed by an enormous investigation. Because of this, it must be concluded that, while family and twin studies have not demonstrated the involvement of genetic factors predisposing to the common forms of cancer, they have not excluded this possibility.

Genetic markers

Genes which lie close together on the same strand of DNA are passed together from parent to offspring, and many closely linked allelic genes show linkage disequilibrium, which means that particular alleles are associated in the population more often than one would expect from their incidences. To give an example, CDe, cDE and cde are unduly common combinations of the three pairs of allelic genes (C,d; D,d, and E,e) of the rhesus blood group system (p. 10.45). The discovery of the HLA system (p. 2.12) and the availability of HLA typing have provided genetically-determined markers which, if closely linked to a gene predisposing to a disease, might demonstrate the existence of the predisposing gene. To give an example, over 90% of individuals with ankylosing spondylitis have the HLA allele for B27, which has an incidence of less than 10% in the population. This suggests either that the gene for B27 in some way predisposes to ankylosing spondylitis or that there is a predisposing gene close linked with the B27 allele on chromosome 6.

Investigations on inbred strains of mice have shown that specific H-2 types (H-2 is the murine equivalent to the human HLA system) are associated with susceptibility or resistance to leukaemia induced by particular murine leukaemia viruses. This was shown to be attributable to Ir genes (included in the Class II HLA genes in man) which determine the intensity of specific immune responses. It was further shown that resistance to leukaemia depended on the (Ir-dependent) intensity of the immune response to the leukaemia viruses. The incidence of spontaneous pulmonary tumours also differs greatly between congenic strains of mice of different H-2 types.

Very few associations between HLA types and cancers have been observed. There appears to be a slight but significant association between acute lymphoblastic leukaemia and HLA-A2, while in Hodgkin's disease (a form of malignant lymphoma) HLA-A1 has a relatively high frequency. Anaplastic nasopharyngeal carcinoma in South China, a tumour with a strong association with Epstein-Barr viral infection (p. 13.17), is associated with HLA-A2 and Bw46, while HLA-Bw35 appears to have an association with breast cancer. Associations with some other tumours have been reported, but confirmation is required. The commoner types of carcinoma, e.g. of the bronchus, colorectum, stomach, prostate, endometrium, urinary bladder and oesophagus, have all been investigated and no associations with HLA types have been observed. This holds also for the leukaemias other than acute lymphoblastic, and for the lymphomas other than Hodgkin's disease.

The absence of HLA associations does not, of course, provide any evidence against genetic predisposing factors, for only cancer-predisposing genes closely linked to the HLA region would be revealed by HLA typing. It should also be noted that many of the reported investigations did not test for associations at the HLA-C or -D loci, and association with Ir genes was therefore not tested directly.

The above findings were based on population studies. HLA typing of families with two or more cases of a particular form of cancer have also provided useful information. Family studies have the advantage that HLA haplotypes of parents and children can often be determined. In Hodgkin's disease, pairs of affected sibs are far more often HLA-identical (i.e. have inherited the same parental haplotypes) than the 25% expected (p. 2.12). Family studies also suggest HLA associations in malignant melanoma, adenomatosis coli and renal carcinoma, but the evidence is not strong and more extensive investigations are required.

On present evidence, it must be concluded that genetic differences between individuals have not been shown to have a strong influence on the risk of developing any of the commoner forms of cancer.

Theories of carcinogenesis

Three theories merit consideration. The multi-step theory regards carcinogenesis as a series of cellular changes. This is now widely accepted. The other two theories—the genetic and epigenetic theories—are concerned with the nature of the series of changes leading to the development of cancer: both of them are consistent with the multi-step theory.

The multi-step theory. With the exception of tumours caused by infection by viruses possessing oncogenes, e.g. the acute oncogenic retroviruses, the change from a normal cell to a cancer cell is a prolonged process, involving many generations of cells. This is clearly established in experimental carcinogenesis in small animals, in which months elapse between exposure to carcinogenic agents and the development of cancer. In man, it is never possible to be sure that exposure to a known or suspected carcinogenic agent is responsible for the development of cancer in any particular individual. However, most of the cancers caused among groups of individuals by exposure to a carcinogenic agent (e.g. inhaled cigarette smoke, β-naphthylamine in the dye industry or ionising radiations in the atom bomb explosions in Japan) have a peak incidence at least several years after exposure. There is very good evidence that changes in the exposed cells occur during this latent period, terminating in the final stage of invasive cancer. The early stages of carcinogenesis have been studied in experimental animals and by cell culture. In man, only the later stages can be recognized.

The features of initiation and promotion have been described on p. 13.21. An essential feature of promotion is the induction of proliferation of initiated cells. Initiation must be a rare event, occurring in only occasional cells among those exposed to the carcinogen, because promotion causes a few focal proliferations, each of which is monoclonal and derived from an initiated cell. Many of the foci of proliferation regress, but some persist and it is in these persistent foci that a second rare event occurs: this consists of a further change in a cell which causes it to proliferate more rapidly, producing a new focal proliferation. Each new focal proliferation tends to extend and replace the surrounding cells, so that the picture becomes confused, but an unknown number of rare events, each giving the changed cell a growth advantage over its neighbours, results in successive focal monoclonal proliferations. Eventually this process gives rise to a clone of cells which exhibit the morphological dysplasia of cancer cells (p. 12.28), the appearances then being those of cancer in situ. One of the dysplastic cells undergoes a final change which concerts it into a frankly malignant cell, and this gives rise to the invading and metastasising tumour.

Some of these multi-step changes are observed when cells in culture are subjected to oncogenic viruses or chemical carcinogens, for example *immortalisation, transformation and loss of anchorage dependence* and of *density-dependent inhibition* (p. 13.5), but comparison of the *in vivo* and *in vitro* changes is difficult and the total number of necessary events is unknown. There is no doubt, however, that carcinogenesis is a multi-step process.

Genetic and epigenetic theories of carcinogenesis. An essential feature of the cancer cell is that it 'breeds true'. In other words, the changes which make a cancer cell behave as it does are transmitted to its daughter cells when it divides. There are two possible explanations. The first is *the genetic theory*, which proposes that the essential changes are mutations, including such major abnormalities as chromosomal translocations. The second possible explanation is that the essential changes are not mutations, but other effects which influence the control of expression of genes—*the epigenetic theory*.

When normal cells, e.g. hepatocytes or fibroblasts divide, the daughter cells are of the same specialised type: they also 'breed true' and yet the specialised features of these cells are not attributable to intrinsic changes in the DNA, but to specialised patterns of expression of their genes. The epigenetic theory proposes that a cancer represents an abnormal form of differentiation.

The genetic theory of carcinogenesis is now widely accepted. Much of the evidence favouring it has been written into the preceding sections on the role of viruses, chemicals, physical agents, etc. in carcinogenesis. Some of the more important points are summarised below.

1. Physical agents which cause cancer, and most chemical carcinogens, bring about mutations in the cells exposed to them, and most mutagenic chemicals have been shown to be carcinogenic.

2. In some forms of cancer, notably the leukaemias and lymphomas, specific chromosomal transformations are associated with particular types of neoplasia. The outstanding example is the Philadelphia chromosome translocation which precedes the development of chronic granulocytic leukaemia, but specific chromosomal changes are associated with other types of leukaemia (pp. 17.49–55).

3. In the common types of carcinoma, specific chromosomal abnormalities are not associated with particular types of tumour, but chromosomal abnormalities are found in many tumours and the same abnormalities are observed in all the cells of a particular tumour. The DNA of malignant tumours is, however, unstable, and additional abnormalities develop within the individual cells of a tumour, giving rise to sub-clones of cells within it.

4. In the rare condition, xeroderma pigmentosum (p. 13.27), there is a defect in the mechanism of repair of the damage caused to DNA by ultraviolet rays. The high incidence of skin cancers at a relatively early age in patients with this condition suggests strongly that the carcinogenicity of ultraviolet light is due to its effects on DNA.

5. Sarcomas, leukaemias, etc. are induced in animals by integration of viral DNA into the host-cell genome.

6. Some rare forms of human cancer, e.g. retinoblastoma, arise in individuals with an inherited abnormality of a particular chromo-

some (p. 13.27). In other inherited cancers, a chromosomal abnormality has not been detected but genetic studies indicate a Mendelian form of inheritance, which can therefore result from abnormality of a single gene, a change which cannot be detected by studying the morphology of chromosomes. An example is provided by adenomatosis coli, which is inherited as a Mendelian dominant trait (p. 13.27).

7. Recent work on oncogenes (pp. 13.7–12) suggests strongly that changes in the DNA which result in modification of proto-oncogenes, or in their altered expression, are important causal factors in many forms of human cancer, including the common types of carcinoma.

8. The enzyme nature of the products of some oncogenes (p. 13.11) would provide an acceptable explanation of why cancer cells differ in so many ways from normal cells.

The genetic theory of cancer is thus well supported. By contrast, direct evidence for **the epigenetic theory** is flimsy. Two lines of research, are, however, of interest. The first involves experiments in which cells derived from mouse embryonal carcinomas (malignant teratomas) are inserted into mouse embryos at the blastocyst stage. In a minority of instances, the malignant cells differentiate normally and appear as normal cells in the various organs and tissues of the animal. The production of 'normal' chimeric mice in these experiments means that, when they come under the influence of the micro-environment of the mouse embryo, cancer cells are induced to behave like normal cells, and it therefore appears that the changes involved in carcinogenesis can be overruled by the factors responsible for normal differen-

tiation of cells. There is also recent evidence that mouse neuroblastoma cells injected into embryos at the somite stage sometimes differentiate normally into neurons. The explanation of these findings is obscure, but both these tumours have unusual features, and are capable of a degree of differentiation most unusual for malignant tumours. The cells of other types of malignant tumours of mice continue to grow as tumours when inserted into mouse embryos.

The second interesting topic concerns the effects of retinoids on carcinogenesis. Retinoids are closely related to retinal (vitamin A), which has important controlling effects on proliferation and differentiation of cells. There is some evidence of an inverse correlation between dietary intake of β-carotene, or serum level of vitamin A, and the risk of developing carcinoma of the bronchus, but the results of large scale trials are awaited. Some retinoids have been shown to inhibit the development of cancer in experimental animals exposed to chemical carcinogens. This effect is apparently not exerted on the carcinogen itself, for retinoids can apparently reverse pre-malignant changes, including actinic keratosis induced in the skin of man by sunlight. Retinoids have also been used successfully to treat basal-cell carcinomas of the skin, but these effects require local application of high concentrations of retinoids. The amounts of retinoids which can be given orally are limited by their toxic effects, and appear to have been beneficial to only a small percentage of patients with advanced cancers.

Until the mechanisms of these effects of retinoids have been elucidated, their significance in relation to theories of carcinogenesis cannot be assessed.

Host reactions in cancer

The natural history of cancer is not determined solely by the characteristics of the tumour cells, but also by the host's reaction to them. As indicated below, there is good evidence that protective host mechanisms exist, and that although these are very often unsuccessful in preventing the growth and spread of malignant tumours, and only very rarely bring about their complete destruction, they may nevertheless re-

strict the rate of tumour growth and spread and contribute to the degree of success achieved by various forms of treatment.

The nature of the host defences is largely unknown, but it has been shown that the cells of human and animal tumours possess surface antigens which are sufficiently foreign to the host to stimulate an immune response. This important property of tumour cells raises the possibility of immunotherapy, and in consequence there is considerable interest in the immunology of cancer, some of the major features of which are summarised below.

Experimental animal studies

Much of the experimental work has involved transplantation experiments. Before the importance of 'transplant' alloantigens was appreciated, rejection of transplanted tumours was frequently observed, but this early work has been invalidated by the discovery by Gorer of the importance of alloantigens in mice. The provision, by close inbreeding, of syngeneic strains of mice and rats has greatly facilitated experimental cancer research, not only by eliminating the 'transplant' antigens as a cause of rejection, but also by excluding other genetically-determined variables.

Specific immune responses to tumours

The elimination of cancer cells by a specific immune reaction on the part of the host requires (1) that cancer cells exhibit antigens to which the host is capable of mounting an immune response, and (2) that the products of the host immune reponse—antibodies and/or specifically reactive T lymphocytes—are capable of effecting destruction of the tumour cells. If these conditions are fulfilled, it must further be asked why tumours grow and spread in spite of the host's immunity, and whether the balance can be tilted in favour of the host.

Tumour-cell antigens. To render a tumour cell susceptible to an immune reaction, the tumour cell antigens must be exposed on the cell surface, and must also be sufficiently foreign to stimulate an immune response; this excludes those surface antigens which, although present on tumour cells, occur also on the host's normal cells. Thus species- and organ-specific antigens, 'transplant' antigens (e.g. those of the H2 system in mice and the of the HLA system in man) and blood-group antigens are all found (although often in reduced concentration) on tumour cells, but none of them is tumour-specific. There are, however, surface antigens on tumour cells which cannot be detected on normal cells: they are capable of eliciting immune responses and reactions and are sometimes called tumour-specific transplantation antigens (TSTA). In experimental carcinogenesis, these apparently tumour-specific surface antigens are largely dependent on the agent which has induced the tumour. *The cells of all tumours produced by any one oncogenic virus have been found to share relatively strong common surface antigens.* These include antigens which, although coded for by the viral genome, are not necessarily a structural component of the virion, and also, in the case of some viruses, antigens of the virus envelope which consists of modified host-cell membrane (p. 13.2). It follows that antibody or primed T-lymphocytes reactive with these virus-coded antigens on a particular tumour are reactive with the cells of all tumours produced by the same virus.

In sarcomas induced in mice by chemical carcinogens, strong TSTAs can be detected on the surface of the tumour cells, and are different for each tumour. This applies even for two tumours of the same type, induced in a mouse by the same carcinogen. When mice are immunised by injection of cells of such a tumour which have been rendered incapable of proliferation by x-irradiation, they develop an immune response and become capable of rejecting implants of the same tumour. Even the mouse in which a tumour has grown and been excised can be effectively immunised in this way. Resistance was further shown to be transferred by injection of T lymphocytes from an immunised mouse. These encouraging results led to considerable efforts to detect similar cell-surface antigens, specific for individual tumours, in human cancer cells, but the results have been disappointing and it now seems likely that the mouse tumour antigens are the products of endogenous retroviruses (p. 13.2) which are a feature of the mouse tumours, but are rarely found in tumours of man. As mentioned above, however, human cancers do have cell-surface antigens, and these are associated with particular types of tumour. For example, melanomas share common cell-surface antigens and so do colorectal carcinomas and many other forms of cancer. The cell-surface antigens of lymphoid leukaemias and lymphomas have been shown to be characteristic of various stages of differentiation. They occur also on the surface of non-neoplastic lymphocyte precursors at various stages of differentiation, and thus are not tumour-specific. This is important, because any immune responses to these antigens which results in destruction of the neoplastic cells is likely to destroy also the normal lymphocyte precursors. There is now evidence that the tumour antigens of melanomas, colorectal carcinomas, etc. are also 'differentiation antigens' (see Feizi, 1985).

Immune responses to tumour-specific antigens. Both antibodies and cell-mediated immunity have been demonstrated, by *in-vitro* techniques, to develop in animals bearing tumours. In general, these responses are more readily demonstrable when the tumour is small, and as it enlarges and spreads they tend to diminish and disappear. They are readily demonstrable after excision of the tumour and then gradually diminish unless the tumour recurs or is re-introduced into the animal.

Effects of the immune response to tumours. Although tumours grow in spite of the host immune response, under experimental conditions a protective effect can sometimes be demonstrated. For example, when tumour cells are injected into a histocompatible animal, a large number of cells (which varies with the particular tumour and with the age of the animal) is required to produce a tumour. This alone shows that the animal can destroy a limited (sub-threshold) number of tumour cells. Moreover, in an animal already bearing a tumour, the number of tumour cells of the same type which must be injected to produce a second tumour is often considerably greater than the threshold dose for a normal animal. This apparent paradox—that the animal can destroy an oncogenic dose of injected tumour cells while its original tumour continues to grow—is also a feature of allografts of normal tissue. An animal bearing a skin allograft may be only partially tolerant to the donor strain and yet may retain the graft. If, however, a second piece of skin of the donor strain is applied, it may be rejected before vascularisation has occurred. It thus appears that newly grafted tissue (and presumably tumour) is more highly susceptible to weak host immune defences than is a well-set graft (or established tumour).

The relatively strong cell-surface antigens of tumours induced by oncogenic viruses (p. 13.32) are capable of stimulating protective immunity under experimental conditions. Animals can be immunised by injection of x-irradiated cells of such a tumour, or by immunisation against the virus itself. Either procedure renders the animal resistant to subsequent challenge by the cells of a tumour induced by the same virus. This explains why virus-induced tumours are most readily induced when the virus is administered to immunologically immature, neonatal animals or to immunologically deficient animals, e.g. nude mice (p. 13.14).

Experiments in which immunity has been conferred passively by transfer of antibody or T lymphocytes from an animal immunised against a tumour indicate that protective immunity or subsequent tumour challenge is conferred mainly by T lymphocytes, and is thus attributable to cell mediated immunity.

The mechanism of destruction of tumour cells by specifically primed T lymphocytes (Fig. 13.11) may be a direct cytotoxic effect requiring contact between the lymphocyte and target cell (p. 7.20) or may be mediated by lymphokines, including those which attract, immobilise and enhance the phagocytic and killing capacities of macrophages (p. 7.21).

There is also some evidence that tumour cells are destroyed by natural killer (NK) cells (p. 7.13), but experiments involving inbred strains of mice which differ in the number of circulating NK cells suggest that, at least in this species, their role is not an important one.

As already noted, antibodies are probably capable of killing free tumour cells in the blood and in exudates in the peritoneal cavity etc. This may result from the susceptibility of antibody-sensitised cells to the lytic effect of complement, to phagocytosis and destruction by macrophages, and to the cytotoxic effect of K (antibody-dependent cytotoxic) cells (p. 17.13). Antibodies may thus play a role in reducing the number of metastases produced by cancer cells gaining entry to the blood, serosal cavities, etc. However, as explained below, in some circumstances antibodies may actually enhance the growth of tumour cells.

Enhancement and 'blocking' factors. The injection into animals of antibody to the surface antigens of tumour cells has been observed, under certain conditions, to reduce the dose of the tumour cells necessary to cause a tumour, and to enhance the growth of a previously-implanted tumour. This experimental enhancement of tumour growth is antigen-specific; it is closely similar to the protection of tissue allo-

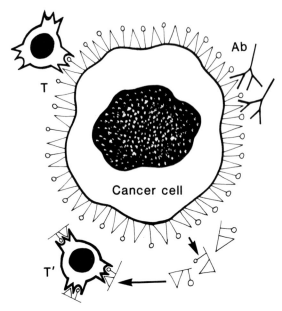

Fig. 13.11 Cell-mediated immunity to cancer cells and possible blocking factors. Specifically primed T lymphocytes (T) bind to a combination of HLA molecules (♀) and tumour antigens (Λ) expressed on the surface of the cancer cell. Binding of antibody (Ab) to tumour antigen may block the binding of T lymphocytes, and it is possible that a combination of HLA molecules and tumour antigen is released by the cancer cell and that it blocks the specific receptors on T lymphocytes (T′).

grafts by antibody (p. 7.31) and appears to be due to the antibody combining with antigen on the surface of the tumour cells and thus protecting them from attack by specifically primed lymphocytes. In other words, the antibody blocks the reaction of T lymphocytes with the tumour cells. In animals with large and progressing tumours, **blocking factors** have been detected in the serum; they have been shown to interfere with the killing of tumour cells *in vitro* by specifically-primed lymphocytes. It now seems unlikely that these are antibodies, for they disappear rapidly from the blood after excision of the tumour, at a time when the level of antibody increases. Other possibilities are that the blocking factors are free antigen molecules shed by the tumour cells as part of the normal turnover of plasma membrane constituents, or such antigens combined with antibody, i.e. immune complexes. Helper T cells are believed to react only with antigens presented on the surface of cells in association with HLA

molecules (p. 7.20), and tumour antigen, whether free or complexed with antibody, would not be expected to prevent specifically primed T cells from reacting with the tumour cells. It is possible, however, that tumour antigen is released from tumour cells in association with HLA molecules. Immune complexes might, in addition, bind to the Fc receptor sites of 'K' lymphocytes or macrophages, thus inhibiting their antibody-dependent cytotoxic activity for the tumour cells. These phenomena are shown diagramatically in Fig. 13.11.

Immunology of cancer in man

Once a cancer has spread beyond the possibility of excision, it usually progresses, and eventually proves fatal. Radiation and drug therapy may destroy many of the tumour cells, but are seldom curative. This applies to most types of carcinomas and sarcomas, but chemotherapy has advanced greatly in recent years and is often effective in some types of leukaemia and lymphoma, and in some testicular tumours (p. 25.13) and rare forms of cancer.

Quite apart from the effects of treatment, there are considerable variations in the rate of growth, even for tumours of the same type and histological appearances. In patients with carcinoma of the breast, for example, surgical excision is sometimes followed by many years of normal health, but with subsequent reappearance and relatively rapid growth of tumour in the operation scar or of metastases: this is sometimes observed also with some other cancers. Very rarely, complete spontaneous regression of a cancer occurs. Partial regression is more common, and it is not very unusual for patients with metastatic melanoma to have no obvious primary tumour. Examination sometimes reveals an area of skin depigmentation which on histological examination shows evidence of a regressing malignant melanoma.

Observations of the sort outlined above suggest that defence mechanisms against cancer can develop in the host, and that in some instances these are partially (and rarely fully) effective. The nature of host defence in these instances is unknown, but there is circumstantial evidence that specific immune responses may influence the course of some tumours. In the rapidly growing form of breast cancer termed encephaloid cancer, for example, a favourable prognosis following excision has been reported to show some correlation with lymphocytic infiltration of the cancer, and this suggests that a delayed hypersensitivity reaction, or possibly antibody-dependent lymphocyte cytotoxic activity, is involved. Seminoma, a rapidly growing carcinoma originating in the germinal epithelium of the testis, is very commonly infiltrated with large numbers of lymphocytes and may also contain tubercle-like macrophage granulomas, both of which are consistent with a delayed hypersensitivity reaction. This may help to explain why the cure rate is unusually high for such a rapidly progressing cancer; even when there is extensive metastasis, chemotherapy or radiotherapy is often curative. A third example of a cancer which is often highly susceptible to therapy is choriocarcinoma arising from the placental trophoblast. Although it grows and spreads very rapidly, this tumour can often be destroyed by cytotoxic drug therapy. It is however, unique among human cancers in being a tumour of fetal tissue which grows in the mother; the tumour cells may thus have HLA or other alloantigens which are inherited from the father and are foreign to the maternal host, so that allograft rejection is likely to contribute to the success of therapy. This is supported by the relative resistance to chemotherapy of choriocarcinoma which sometimes develops in testicular tumours, in which it is derived from the host's own cells.

Immune responses. *As in animal studies, antibodies and lymphocytes which react specifically with tumour cells have been demonstrated by in-vitro techniques in patients with various types of cancer.* They react with the patient's own tumour cells, with the cells of other tumours of similar type, and with cell lines derived from such tumours. Antibodies and cell-mediated immunity to the tumour cells are most often detectable in patients with early cancer, and tend to diminish as the tumour enlarges and spreads. Blocking factors, similar to those in animals (see above) also appear in the blood, particularly when the cancer is advanced. The tumour-specific antigens have not yet been fully characterised. Like HLA antigens, they have been reported to contain a β_2-microglobulin chain.

Oncofetal antigens (p. 12.44) are so called because they were first detected as products of cancers and of fetal tissues. Carcino-embryonic antigen, α-fetoprotein and other less thoroughly investigated oncofetal antigens are, however, secreted by the cells of those cancers which produce them and are present in the plasma. Accordingly, immunity to them would not be likely to result in the destruction of the tumours.

Immunological surveillance

The concept of immunological surveillance was advanced by Burnet, who postulated that one function of T lymphocytes is to monitor host cells and respond immunologically against any which have developed surface antigens foreign to the host. By this means, it is conceivable that many (perhaps most) malignant cells are destroyed before they are capable of developing into a tumour. As regards **experimentally-induced tumours**, there is little evidence that this hypothesis applies to those caused by chemical carcinogens, for such tumours are produced no more readily in immunosuppressed animals, or in congenitally immunodeficient (nude) mice than in normal animals. Immunological surveillance is, however, of considerable importance in preventing tumours induced in animals by retroviruses or DNA viruses. This is illustrated by the ease with which such tumours can be induced in neonatal mice, which are immunologically immature, and in adult immunosuppressed or immunodeficient mice (p. 13 33) Protection of neonates or immunodeficient mice is also afforded by transfer of syngeneic lymphocytes from an animal immunised against the virus-induced tumour. Indeed, immunosuppression by the oncogenic virus itself, as in the case of feline leukaemia virus (p. 13.6), predisposes to tumour production.

As regards **cancer in man**, there is some evidence favouring immunological surveillance, for children with certain congenital immunodeficiencies, and renal transplant recipients receiving long-term immunosuppressive therapy, have an increased incidence of cancer. However, the tumours arising in such patients do not reflect the natural incidence of cancer in the general population. Immunosuppressed recipients of a renal transplant have about a fifty-fold increase in the risk of developing certain types of non-Hodgkin's lymphoma, and these tumours develop surprisingly early, sometimes within a few months of commencing immuno-suppressive therapy. Many of them occur in the central nervous system, an otherwise rare site for lymphomas; this may be due to the blood-brain barrier, which affords some protection to the tumour cells against the products of the host's immune response. The rare tumour, Kaposi's sarcoma, has also been observed to occur with unexpected frequency in transplant recipients and this is of interest in relation to its very high incidence in patients with AIDS (p. 25.5) in which cell-mediated immunodefi-ciency is a prominent feature. A third tumour, which is about 40 times commoner in trans-plant recipients, is hepatocellular carcinoma. There appears also to be an increase in the incidence of malignant melanoma and squamous-cell carcinoma of the skin. The inci-dence of the commoner forms of carcinoma appears to be increased slightly, but they tend to occur after a much longer period of therapy. Immunosuppression predisposes to virus infec-tions, and it seems likely that tumours showing a marked increase relatively soon after trans-plantation are induced by oncogenic viruses. This might explain the high incidence of lym-phomas, which commonly result in animals from oncogenic viral infections, and also the greatly increased risk of hepatocellular carci-noma, which is strongly associated with the he-patitis B virus (p. 13.17).

Patients with immunodeficiency diseases, or receiving long-term immunosuppressive drugs for reasons other than renal transplantation, also have an increased incidence of cancers, with a pattern similar to that described above for transplant patients. Alkylating agents are both carcinogenic and immunosuppressive and their use carries an additional increased risk of acute non-lymphoblastic leukaemia.

The most likely example of effective immuno-logical surveillance in man is provided by infec-tion with the Epstein-Barr virus (p. 13.16) which in normal individuals induces a strong immune response on the part of T cells, and does not cause cancer. In African children who may be immunosuppressed by chronic malaria or some other infective agent (p. 13.17), infec-tion with EB virus is associated with the de-velopment of the Burkitt lymphoma, and in the Southern Chinese, in whom genetically-deter-mined immunological responsiveness may play a role, the virus is associated with naso-pharyngeal carcinoma.

It may be significant that most cancers occur in old age, for there is no doubt that immune responsiveness declines in the elderly, but the prolonged period required for development of cancer in man following exposure to environ-mental carcinogenic factors probably accounts for the age incidence. Tests for immune respon-siveness to various antigens have not, in general, revealed immunodepression in patients with early cancer as compared with age-matched control subjects. Advanced cancer patients commonly show evidence of immuno-depression, but this is most obvious in those with tumours which invade and destroy the lymphoid tissues, and is likely to result also from malnutrition and general debility caused by the cancer and by cytotoxic drugs.

The prospect of immunotherapy. The ad-vances in tumour immunology outlined above have demonstrated that, in spite of the occur-rence of anticancer immune responses in many patients, their tumours still progress and cause death. To be effective, the immune response to a tumour must kill the tumour cells more quickly than they are produced, and it remains possible that boosting the immune reponse might have this effect. The administration of immunological adjuvants, e.g. BCG, *Coryne-bacterium parvum* and Levamisole, has been attempted following chemotherapy and/or sur-gery in various neoplastic conditions. BCG has been claimed to have some effect in acute lym-phoblastic leukaemia but others have failed to confirm this, and in other neoplastic conditions the results have so far been disappointing. Vari-ous attempts have also been made to stimulate active specific immunity by implanting pieces of tumour which have been excised and treated with x-irradiation to prevent the cells from div-iding. Such a procedure is not very hopeful, for if the patient's tumour does not stimulate effec-tive immunity it seems unlikely that the im-planted cells will do so, but it remains possible that, by increasing the antigenicity of the im-planted cells, e.g. by coupling with a foreign antigen, or by using homologous tumour with its 'foreign' transplant antigens, the immune re-sponse to the relevant tumour antigens might be augmented. Immunity to tumour cells has been shown to be enhanced, for example, by immunising an animal with BCG and injecting it with tumour cells with tuberculin attached to their surface. Attempts have also been made to provide passive immunity by transplanting tumour to a volunteer hoping that therapeutically effective antibody will be produced. On at least one occasion, the volunteer failed to reject the transplanted tumour, which proved fatal. The therapeutic value of lymphocyte products and interferons (p. 9.2) are also being investigated.

Immunotherapy of cancer patients faces at least three major difficulties. Firstly, excision of an early cancer may effect a cure. It is not possible, at present, to identify those patients who will develop recurrences, and it therefore seems unjustifiable to apply to early cancer patients a form of therapy which is of unknown value. Accordingly, attempts at immunotherapy have mostly been made on patients with advanced cancer, when it is likely to be too late. Secondly, there is no guarantee that active immunisation will induce immune responses which contribute to the destruction of the tumour. There is, in fact, a risk of inducing the production of 'enhancing' antibody (p. 13.33) and thus increasing the rate of tumour growth. Thirdly, problems in assessing the results of any form of cancer therapy arise from the natural individual variations in the rate of growth and spread of cancer. In consequence, any trial of therapy must usually be extensive.

Attention has also been given to the possibility of vaccines to prevent cancer. This has been achieved in feline leukaemia (p. 13.6) and in Marek's disease, a lymphoma of chickens caused by an oncogenic herpes virus which occurs in epidemic form with a high mortality among flocks of birds. Immunisation of chickens either with a related but non-pathogenic virus, or with x-irradiated cells transformed by the virus, has been successful in eliminating the disease in the immunised flocks.

The types of human cancer most likely to be preventable by use of vaccines are those which appear to be induced by viruses. A vaccine for hepatitis B virus infection has recently become available and may reduce greatly the incidence of liver cell cancer in countries where the incidence is high. Tumours associated with EB virus—Burkitt's lymphoma and anaplastic nasopharyngeal carcinoma—are rare except in parts of Africa and China respectively. A vaccine for EB virus infection is not yet available, but might be of great benefit to the communities at special risk. Finally, the adult T-cell leukaemia/lymphoma (ATLL) common in parts of Japan and some other parts of the world appears almost certainly to be due to a human oncogenic retrovirus (p. 13.7) and so might, like feline leukaemia, be preventable by a vaccine.

Induction of a delayed hypersensitivity reaction at the site of a tumour has been used as a method of tumour destruction. This has achieved some success in the treatment of epidermal tumours, notably basal cell carcinoma. The patient is sensitised by application to the skin of an agent which induces cell-mediated immunity, e.g. dinitrochlorobenzene (DNCB) and subsequently DNCB is applied to the tumour and surrounding skin: a delayed hypersensitivity reaction develops, and may be successful in destroying the tumour. Two mechanisms may be involved: firstly, the delayed hypersensitivity reaction, if intense, causes necrosis of normal cells (as in tuberculin skin testing—p. 7.18) and may similarly induce necrosis of the tumour. Secondly, macrophages accumulate and become more actively phagocytic and cytotoxic for foreign cells (including cancer cells) unrelated to the antigen which has induced the delayed hypersensitivity reaction. Similarly, attempts have been made to destroy tumours by immunising the patient with BCG (p. 9.17) and injecting either BCG or tuberculoprotein into the tumour. It is scarcely possible to destroy all the tumour cells by this method and, whenever possible, surgical removal of the tumour is preferable.

Targetted cytotoxins. Monoclonal antibodies have now been prepared against many human tumours. They usually react not only with the tumour used in their production but also with other tumours of the same type, e.g. adenocarcinomas of the colon or breast carcinomas. Such antibodies, labelled by radio-isotopes, are at present being tested for their value in labelling tumours *in vivo* and aiding their detection by scanning techniques. Monoclonal antibodies can also be rendered cytotoxic by attaching to them highly toxic molecules such as ricin or diphtheria toxin. Such antibody-targetted cytotoxins have been shown to be capable of killing tumour cells in culture and the possibility of using them *in vivo* is being investigated.

References

Bodmer, W.F. (1982). Cancer genetics. *Cancer Surveys* 1 (No. 1), 1–15.

Enwonwu, C.D. (1984). The role of dietary aflatoxin in the genesis of hepatocellular cancer in developing countries. *Lancet* **ii**, 956–8.

Feizi, T. (1985). Demonstration by monoclonal antibodies that carbohydrate structures of glycoproteins and glycolipids are onco-developmental antigens. *Nature*, **314**, 53–7.

Gallo, R.C. (1984). Human T-cell leukaemia-lymphoma virus and T-cell malignancies in adults. *Cancer Surveys* **3**, 113–59.

Jarrett, W.F.H. (1981) Papillomaviruses and cancer, pp. 35–48. In *Recent Advances in Histopathology*, No. 11. Ed. P.P. Anthony and R.N.M. MacSween. Churchill Livingstone, Edinburgh.

Weinberg, R.A. (1983). A molecular basis of cancer. *Scientific American*, **249**, 102–16.

Further Reading

Advances in Cancer Research. Academic Press Inc., New York. (Detailed reviews of oncological topics of major importance—mostly excellent. Usually one volume published annually since 1953.)

Becker, F.F. (1981). Recent concepts of initiation and promotion in carcinogenesis. *American Journal of Pathology*, **105**, 3–9.

Cancer Surveys. A review journal published quarterly since 1982 under the auspices of the Imperial Cancer Research Fund. (The topics extend over a wide range of clinical, epidemiological and laboratory oncology.) Oxford University Press.

Collier, R.J. and Kaplan, D.A. (1984). Immunotoxins. *Scientific American*, **251**, 44–52.

Farber, E. (1982). Chemical carcinogenesis: a biologic perspective. *American Journal of Pathology*, **106**, 269–96.

Hunter, J. (1984). The proteins of oncogenes. *Scientific American*, **251**, 60–9.

Lachmann, P.J. (1984) Tumour immunology: a review. *Journal of the Royal Society of Medicine*, **77**, 1023–29.

Medline, A. and Farber, E. (1981). The multistep theory of neoplasia. pp. 19–34 in *Recent Advances in Histopathology*. No. 11. Ed. P.P. Anthony and R.N.M. MacSween. Churchill Livingstone, Edinburgh.

Paul, J. (1984). Oncogenes. *Journal of Pathology*, **143**, 1–10.

Symington, T. and Carter, R.L. (Eds.) (1976). *Scientific Foundations of Oncology*, pp. 690 and Supplement (1980). Heinemann, London. (Authoritative reviews on many aspects of oncology.)

14

Blood Vessels and Lymphatics

Arteries

Introduction

Normal structure of arteries. The walls of arteries are composed of three coats (Fig. 14.1): the innermost, or **intima**, consists of the endothelium separated by a thin layer of loose connective tissue from the internal elastic lamina— a thick fenestrated cylinder of elastic fibres which appears in histological sections as a wavy line but is kept taut in vivo by the blood pressure. The **media** consists of a tight spiral of smooth muscle cells which lie in a stromal meshwork of elastic and collagen fibres. The amount of stroma increases with vessel size: in the arterioles and smallest arteries it is very scanty, while in the aorta and larger 'elastic' arteries its volume exceeds that of the smooth muscle component. An external elastic lamina

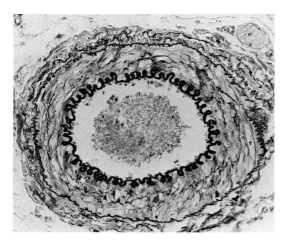

Fig. 14.1 Transverse section of a normal medium-sized artery, stained to show elastic tissue. The internal and external elastic laminae are seen as black wavy bands. × 10.

separates the media from the *adventitia*, a thin layer of loosely arranged collagen and elastic fibres, rich in lymphatics and traversed by the nerves which supply the medial smooth muscle.

All layers of the smallest arteries and arterioles are supplied with oxygen, etc., by diffusion from the lumen but larger arteries have small vessels, the *vasa vasorum*, which supply the adventitia and outer part of the media, the inner part of the wall depending on diffusion from the lumen.

The differences in structure of the media of arteries of various sizes are reflected in their functions. The larger elastic arteries absorb part of the force of left ventricular systole and their recoil helps to sustain the pressure for continued blood flow during diastole. The smaller arteries and arterioles (*resistance vessels*) regulate the overall arterial pressure and the blood flow to individual organs and tissues: this function is reflected in the predominance of smooth muscle in the media with its rich autonomic innervation which, together with circulating levels of vasoactive hormones, controls the calibre.

Effects of ageing. The structure of arteries of all sizes changes progressively with advancing age, the changes becoming prominent in the elderly when they are known as **senile arteriosclerosis**. The intima becomes thickened and fibrosed, sometimes with reduplication of the internal elastic lamina and medial smooth muscle and elastic fibres are partly replaced by collagen. These changes result in increased rigidity and stretching of the walls, both in diameter and in length, features well seen in the prominent and tortuous temporal and brachial arteries of some elderly people. Senile arteriosclerosis is of little consequence, although the increased rigidity contributes to the age-related increase in systolic and pulse pressures.

The walls of arterioles become thickened and hyaline in appearance with advancing age, probably as a result of plasmatic vasculosis (p. 11.7). The change is termed **hyaline arteriolosclerosis** and is particularly prominent in the arterioles of the spleen and the afferent arterioles supplying the glomeruli. If severe, it may result in narrowing of the lumen with consequent ischaemic effects.

Changes similar to those of ageing occur in the arteries and arterioles in persistent hypertension, but in arteries they are preceded by hypertrophy (see below) and they develop earlier in life and progress more rapidly.

Compensatory changes. The muscular and elastic nature of the arterial wall readily allows it to adjust to blood flow requirements. If, however, functional requirements for blood flow through an artery are *persistently* increased or decreased, structural changes occur. Examples of the effects of increased blood flow are seen in the uterine arteries during pregnancy, and in the collateral arteries when blood flow through a major artery is reduced by atheroma or arrested by occlusive thrombosis. The lumen of the affected arteries dilates and the wall undergoes **hypertrophy** by increase in elastic fibres and hyperplasia of the medial smooth muscle cells. In effect, the arteries undergo a compensatory increase in size which persists as long as there is increased demand for blood flow. Hypertrophy of the arterial walls occurs also in hypertension (p. 14.15).

Persistent reduction in blood flow requirements, for example in the uterine arteries following pregnancy or the menopause or in the arteries in the stump following amputation of a limb, result in a process of **involution**. The artery wall becomes partially collapsed and smooth muscle and elastic tissue is reduced and partially replaced by hyaline collagen. The lumen is further reduced by gross thickening of the intima by a process termed **endarteritis obliterans**: medial smooth muscle cells migrate into the intima and proliferate to form a thick layer which gradually becomes fibrosed (Fig. 14.2). This latter change is also commonly seen in arteries exposed to chronic inflammation, for example in the base of a peptic ulcer (Fig. 14.3) or in the wall of a tuberculous cavity in the lung: in these situations, the obliteration of ar-

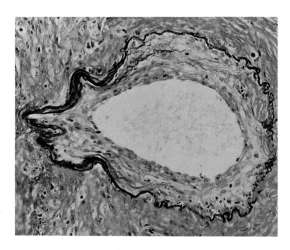

Fig. 14.2 Endarteritis obliterans in a leg artery proximal to an old amputation. The internal elastic lamina (black) marks the outer limit of the thickened fibrous intima. × 15.

teries often prevents serious haemorrhage, but the endarteritis obliterans of tuberculous meningitis, (21.29, p. 21.27) or syphilis, or following radiotherapy (p. 3.29) can cause serious effects due to ischaemia.

Diseases of arteries. The disease known as **atheroma** or **atherosclerosis** occurs in some degree in virtually all adults in most of the developed countries, where it causes more deaths than any other condition. The lesions are multiple and consist of gradually enlarging patches of thickening of the intima of arteries,

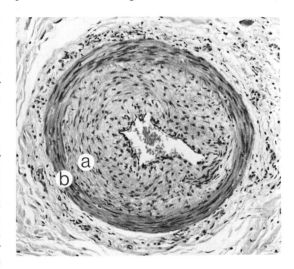

Fig. 14.3 Endarteritis obliterans in the base of a chronic peptic ulcer, **a** = intima, **b** = media.

each patch being composed of a layer of dense fibrous tissue beneath the endothelium and overlying a deposit of lipids in the outer part of the intima. Atheromatous patches in the arteries supplying the heart, brain and legs commonly narrow the lumen of these vessels with consequent chronic ischaemia of the tissues supplied by them, and complete occlusion is very liable to result from superadded thrombosis with consequent infarction, e.g. of the myocardium. Atheromatous patches in the aorta tend to form around the mouths of its abdominal branches and may reduce their lumen. Aortic atheroma may also ulcerate and release lipid or become coated with thrombus, both of which can give rise to emboli, notably in the arteries of the kidneys, intestines and legs.

Another extremely important disease, particularly in developed countries, is **systemic arterial hypertension**, often termed simply 'hypertension'. It is a state of elevated blood pressure in the systemic arteries and is sustained by increased peripheral resistance and increased force of left ventricular contraction. Hypertension is very common in middle and late adult life and in most cases the cause is not apparent (*'essential hypertension'*). If untreated, it commonly causes death from heart failure or cerebral haemorrhage due to rupture of a cerebral artery, while in its most severe form (*malignant hypertension*) it causes severe damage to the kidneys leading to renal failure. Fortunately, in most patients the blood pressure can now be controlled and its serious effects reduced. Inflammation of the walls of arteries (**arteritis**), is less common, and presents a complex and heterogeneous group of diseases, most of which are of unknown cause: in some, capillaries and veins may also be involved. Known causes of arteritis include deposition of immune complexes, heavy cigarette smoking, and syphilis, while infected emboli, e.g. in bacterial endocarditis, may cause localised acute arteritis. Complications of arteritis include occlusive thrombosis, aneurysm formation and rupture (see below), and chronic ischaemia.

Thrombosis and **embolism** of arteries have been dealt with on pp. 10.14, 10.19. The walls of arteries are built to withstand pressure: their strength lies mainly in the media and when this is weakened (usually by atheroma or arteritis), dilatation and rupture may occur, particularly if there is associated hypertension. Localised dilatation of an artery is termed an **aneurysm**, and is seen most commonly in the aorta and in the arteries at the base of the brain. The media is often weakened at the site of atheromatous patches, and this is the commonest cause of aneurysm of the abdominal aorta, while aneurysms of the thoracic aorta usually result from syphilitic aortitis. Aneurysms of the vessels at the base of the brain are attributable to a combination of gaps in the medial smooth muscle (of unknown cause) and hypertension, and are very liable to rupture and cause haemorrhage into the subarachnoid space.

Developmental abnormalities of blood vessels include the major malformations of the aorta and main pulmonary trunk, and also the **vascular hamartomas** including **haemangiomas**. **Tumours of blood vessels** are rare, the commonest being the benign *glomangioma*, a small painful superficial lump which occurs usually in the fingers and toes.

Atheroma (Atherosclerosis)

In most of the developed countries this is responsible for more deaths than any other disease. It causes narrowing of the lumen of arteries, is often complicated by occlusive thrombosis, and is the major cause of disability and death from heart disease, cerebral infarction and ischaemia of the lower limbs. It is virtually always present in some degree in middle-aged and old people in most industrialised Western countries.

Definition. The lesions of atheroma consist of patches ('plaques') of intimal thickening of the walls of arteries, due mainly to accumulation of lipids, proliferation of smooth muscle cells, and formation of fibrous tissue. The alternative term **atherosclerosis** is used because the lesion has a soft, lipid-rich part (athere = porridge) and a hard (sclerotic) fibrous component. The shorter term, **atheroma**, has historical priority and will be used in this account.

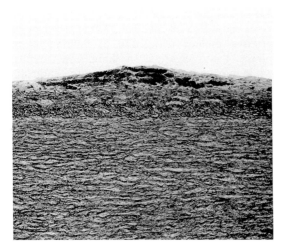

Fig. 14.4 Section of the aorta of a child showing a fatty streak. (Frozen section: lipid stained black). × 20.

Naked-eye appearances

The earliest deposits of lipid in the intima of the aorta and large arteries are seen predominantly in childhood and adolescence and are known as *fatty streaks*. They appear as yellow, slightly raised spots in the luminal surface, which enlarge and coalesce to form irregular yellow streaks. Microscopy shows them to consist of accumulations of lipid droplets beneath the endothelium, both free and in aggregates of macrophages lying beneath the endothelium (Fig. 14.4). Fatty streaks are almost invariably present at autopsy in the aortas of children and adolescents, and their presence and extent bear no relationship to the incidence of atheroma in older members of the community: they are not seen commonly in adults and so must regress, but it is possible that some of them persist and progress to atheroma in communities with a high incidence of this disease. By contrast, the incidence and extent of the more persistent fatty streaks in the coronary arteries of young people correlate with the amount and severity of atheroma in the community and they may represent the early stage of this disease (McGill, 1968). Other lesions which may possibly precede atheroma include foci of intimal oedema and increase in ground substance, termed *gelatinous patches*, and small intimal thickenings composed of smooth muscle cells, collagen and ground substance (*intimal cushions*). The role of these lesions in atherogenesis is, however, unknown.

The earliest recognisable atheromatous lesions are seen commonly from young adulthood onwards in atheroma-prone communities. They consist of small disc-like yellowish, slightly raised patches of intimal thickening with a smooth glistening surface. As the condition progresses, the patches enlarge and thicken by further deposition of lipid deep in the intima and by fibrosis more superficially (i.e. adjacent to the lumen): the patches become distinctly raised and when viewed from the intimal surface they may appear yellow or white depending on the amount of white fibrous tissue overlying the yellow lipid deposits. In any one individual, the patches vary in size and thickness, reflecting their development and slow growth throughout adult life.

Aorta. Atheroma occurs mainly in the abdominal aorta, often developing first around the origins of the intercostal and lumbar branches (Fig. 14.5). The patches vary in size up to several centimetres diameter and may in places become confluent. If a sizeable patch is cut across, lipid-rich paste-like material can

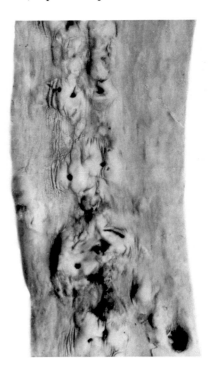

Fig. 14.5 Mild atheroma of the abdominal aorta. The lesions are seen as raised patches and are located mainly around the origins of the arterial branches. × 0·8.

sometimes be expressed from its deeper part, and fibrous thickening is seen as a white layer overlying this. The proportions of lipid and fibrous tissue vary considerably. When lipid is abundant and the fibrous layer is thin, *ulceration* may occur, and *mural thrombus* is then likely to be deposited on the ulcerated surface; another common change is *deposition of calcium salts* which may convert the plaque to a hard brittle plate. Plaques showing ulceration, calcification or thrombus deposition are commonly referred to as **complicated atheroma**, and may produce great irregularity of the luminal surface of the aorta (Fig. 14.6). Other important features of aortic plaques are *thinning of the overlying media*, and in some instances *extension of the plaque into the adjacent media*: the wall is thus weakened and an *aneurysm* may develop, with the danger of rupture (p. 14.29). Plaques developing adjacent to the origin of the splanchnic or renal arteries may seriously diminish the ostia of these vessels and cause ischaemic effects.

Severe atheroma of the thoracic aorta is unusual except in diabetics and in association with syphilitic mesaortitis.

Other arteries. Atheroma occurs in arteries of all sizes down to approximately 2 mm diameter and is seen occasionally in even smaller arteries. The general features are similar to those seen in the aorta except that the plaques are necessarily smaller, often involve the whole circumference of the intima, and can cause all degrees of *luminal narrowing* down to virtual occlusion (Figs 14.7, 14.8, 14.9). Atheroma tends to affect especially arteries supplying the heart, brain and lower limbs. There is considerable individual variation in its distribution, in some instances the aorta being mainly affected, in others the arteries at the base of the brain and/or the coronary arteries. The coronary arteries are often severely affected and are more often involved at a relatively early age than any other arteries. The cerebral arteries also are subject to severe atheroma, but this is found chiefly in elderly persons. Apart from diabetics, in whom atheroma is often extensive and severe, the renal arteries are not usually involved and only the first few centimetres of the main splanchnic arteries are affected. Aortic atheroma may, however distort and narrow the ostia of these and other branches.

In the thin-walled arteries at the base of the brain the patches are visible from both inner and outer aspects of the vessels, and their yellow opaque appearance contrasts with the reddish translucency of the normal parts of the vessel wall (Fig. 14.10).

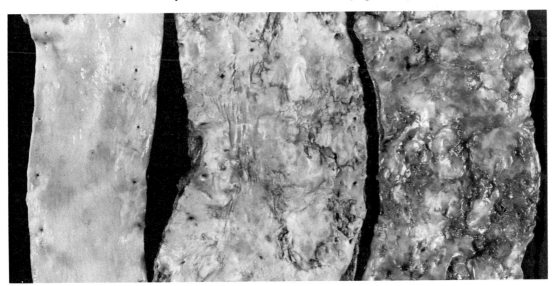

Fig. 14.6 Lengths of the abdominal aorta: *left*, minimal atheroma; *middle*, severe atheroma with cracking and early ulceration of patches; *right*, very severe atheroma with ulceration and mural thrombosis. Note also that the two atheromatous aortas have lost their elasticity and stretched; this may be due to atrophy of the media beneath the extensive atheroma, but could also be the result of arteriosclerosis.

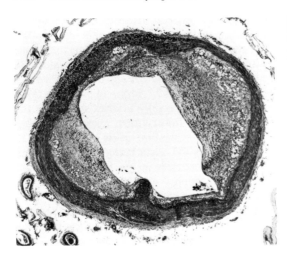

Fig. 14.7   Atheroma of a coronary artery causing moderate narrowing of the lumen. The spaces in the deep part of the plaque represent lipid accumulation. × 10.

Complications include: (*a*) **haemorrhage into a plaque**, which increases the degree of luminal narrowing (Fig. 15.3, p. 15.7); (*b*) **rupture or ulceration of a plaque** (Fig. 15.2, p. 15.7); and (*c*) **occlusive thrombosis** (Figs 14.9 and 15.6, p. 15.10) which is a major cause of infarction in

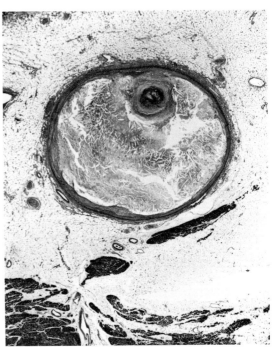

Fig. 14.9   Severe atheroma of the left coronary artery in a patient with myxoedema. The lumen has been greatly reduced by atheroma and occluded by recent superadded thrombus, which appears dark. × 10.

the heart, brain and intestine, and of ischaemia of the legs.

Microscopic appearances. The early changes are due to accumulation of lipids in proliferated spindle cells, shown by electron microscopy to be smooth muscle cells, lying in the intima (Fig. 14.11) and derived by proliferation and migration of medial smooth muscle cells (p. 14.13). Lipids also accumulate between cells deep in the intima (i.e. close to the media), particularly in relation to elastic fibres and the internal elastic lamina. As the patch develops, thin laminae of connective tissue appear between the lipid-rich smooth muscle cells in the more superficial (i.e. sub-endothelial) parts of the intima and form the fibrous part of the lesion. Areas of necrosis then develop in the deeper (outer) part of the lesion, converting it to a structureless accumulation of lipids, tissue debris (Fig. 14.12) and sometimes altered blood, and the necrosis gradually extends into the overlying fibrous tissue. Calcium deposition may be visible microscopically. Infiltration of neutrophil

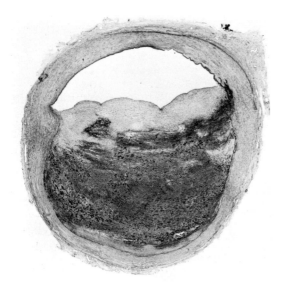

Fig. 14.8   Severe atheroma of the superior mesenteric artery, causing marked reduction of the lumen. Frozen section, stained with Scharlach R, showing the large amount of fatty material in the patch. × 15.

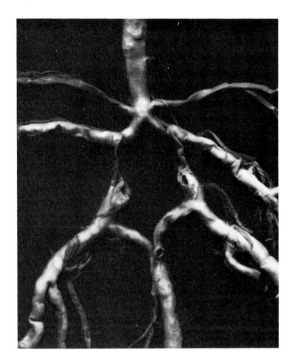

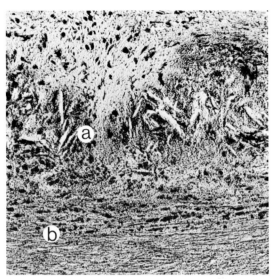

Fig. 14.12 Section showing part of an atheromatous patch of the aorta. In the deep part of the intima there is degenerate lipid-rich material **a**, the spindle-shaped spaces being due to cholesterol crystals. Lipid accumulation stops fairly abruptly at the junction with the media **b**. × 110.

Fig. 14.10 Circle of Willis and branches, showing marked patchy atheroma.

leucocytes and other inflammatory cells is common, and lipid-laden macrophages—'foamy cells'—may appear around the lipid deposits, which usually contain crystals of cholesterol, represented in paraffin section by the typical elongated clefts (Fig. 14.12). The internal elastic lamina deep to the plaque is usually disrupted and lipid deposition, necrosis and fibrosis may then extend into the adjacent media. Quite apart from this, the media deep to the plaque becomes thinned and atrophic (Fig. 14.13).

Small blood vessels grow into the atheromatous patch from vasa vasorum in the media of the affected vessels and sometimes also from the intimal surface. These may be the source of the haemorrhage which commonly occurs in the patch, although rupture of the overlying fibrous patch, which is often very thin, is a commoner cause of haemorrhage, the blood entering the plaque from the lumen.

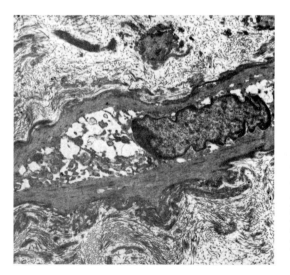

Fig. 14.11 Electron micrograph of part of a smooth muscle cell in an atheromatous plaque. The cytoplasm is made up largely of myofibrils, and contains globules of fat, shown as light spaces. The fine fibres on either side of the cell are collagen. × 7500.

Effects

Although the changes of atheroma are essentially the same in all arteries, their effects vary in arteries of different sizes.

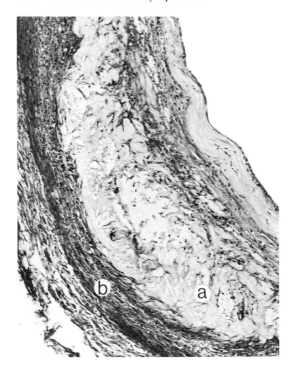

Fig. 14.13 Atheroma of a cerebral artery. The intima is greatly thickened with accumulation of lipid in its deeper part **(a)** and dense overlying fibrosis. The media **(b)** shows local atrophy over the patch. × 110.

Large arteries. Uncomplicated atheroma of large arteries, such as the aorta, very often have no clinical effect because usually it does not substantially reduce the lumen or seriously weaken the wall. In advanced cases, however, an *aneurysm* may form in the abdominal aorta (p. 14.29) or occasionally in a common iliac artery. *Thrombi* which form on ulcerated plaques in the aorta seldom cause complete occlusion, probably because the rapid flow limits platelet adhesion. Fragments of thrombi and atheromatous debris from ulcerated plaques may break away and form *emboli* in the arteries of the lower limbs and abdominal organs such as the kidneys. Occasionally thrombus forming on atheromatous plaques may occlude the whole lumen of the aorta, usually at or near the bifurcation, where it can result in gangrene of the legs unless adequate collateral circulation has developed, in which case there may be merely coldness and weakness of the legs with muscle wasting and sexual impotence but without ischaemic pain or gangrene (*Leriche syndrome*).

Smaller arteries. By far the commonest important effects of atheroma are due to involvement of smaller arteries, the lumen of which may be progressively narrowed by an atheromatous patch or suddenly occluded by superadded thrombosis (Fig. 14.9). These effects are well seen in the coronary arteries. Atheroma is the chief cause of *ischaemic heart disease*, the largest single cause of death in the developed countries (p. 15.6). *Ischaemic brain damage* is also very common and is usually the result of atheroma of the carotid, vertebral and basilar arteries, vessels of the circle of Willis and cerebral arteries (p. 21.17). Aneurysm formation is not a feature of atheroma of the smaller arteries, except occasionally in the basilar artery, but the two are often both present in the vessels of the circle of Willis.

Arteries supplying the legs are often severely atheromatous, with consequent progressive diminution in blood supply. Eventually the collateral circulation becomes inadequate: relative muscle ischaemia can then be induced by the increased metabolic demands of exercise, which produces severe pain in the leg, relieved by rest. This is the clinical syndrome of *intermittent claudication*. In time, ischaemia may be so severe as to cause *gangrene*, which usually starts in the toes (Fig. 3.33, p. 3.33) and spreads proximally. Examination of legs amputated for gangrene usually shows narrowing or obliteration and calcification of the major arteries. Because atheroma is often widespread, patients with severe involvement of the arteries of the lower limbs frequently suffer also from ischaemic heart disease.

For reasons unknown, the arteries of the arms (like the renal arteries) are seldom affected severely by atheroma.

Aetiology

Atheroma has been the subject of an enormous amount of investigation. Approaches to elucidating its aetiology are difficult, for it has usually been present for many years before symptoms develop. Investigations have been mainly along the following lines.

(1) *Epidemiological studies* have been used to detect risk factors, i.e. factors which increase or decrease the risk of developing atheroma. (2) *Intervention trials* have been conducted to

determine whether altering the risk factors, for example by modifying the diet or stopping cigarette smoking, reduces the subsequent incidence of severe atheroma and its complications. (3) *Biomedical laboratory research*, including the experimental production of atheroma-like lesions in animals, have aimed at detecting the mechanisms involved in the development and growth of atheromatous plaques.

Epidemiological studies—risk factors

Epidemiological investigations require some grading of atheroma in communities and individuals, but there is no simple method of detecting the disease unless it gives rise to symptoms, and in studying communities it is customary to regard ischaemic heart disease (IHD) as an indicator of the degree of atheroma in the community and to search for factors associated with the age-adjusted mortality rates from IHD, which are known for many countries. IHD is admittedly a crude index of atheroma, for death can result from a single atheromatous plaque in a coronary artery, while many people with severe and extensive atheroma are symptom-free. Also, IHD is commonly caused by occlusive thrombosis supervening on atheroma of the coronary arteries and when its risk factors are identified it is difficult to determine whether they have influenced the development of atheroma, superadded thrombosis, or both. In spite of these difficulties, autopsy experience indicates that there is a good general correlation between IHD, both fatal and non-fatal, and the severity of atheroma (Strong *et al.* 1968). Accordingly, IHD affords a good practical indication of the incidence and severity of atheroma in a community, and elucidation of its risk factors is of great importance.

Age-adjusted mortality rates from IHD vary greatly in different countries (p. 15.6), and epidemiological studies have investigated dietary, social, occupational and other environmental factors in different countries and communities in attempts to detect risk factors. Certain risk factors have been demonstrated by these epidemiological studies, and are discussed below.

Age and sex. Atheroma is a chronic disease which progresses slowly throughout adult life. It is not an inevitable accompaniment of ageing, but all the evidence suggests that the causal factors exert their effects over a long period, and that duration of exposure to them is of major importance. A lower incidence of IHD in women until after the menopause has been observed in all communities studied. It reflects the slower progress of atheroma in premenopausal women than in men, and is likely to have a hormonal basis, but the nature of this has not been elucidated.

Plasma lipids. Mean adult levels of total plasma cholesterol (TC) vary in different communities throughout the world from about 3.9 mmol/l (150 mg/dl) to over 7 mmol/l (275 mg/dl). When community levels are compared with IHD mortality rates, a striking correlation is observed (Keys, 1970). In countries with a mean TC level around 4 mmol/l IHD is rare, while those with means of 5·2 or more invariably have high rates of IHD. The correlation is not perfect, indicating that high TC levels are not the only risk factor, but it is sufficiently strong to indicate that the relationship is of major importance. The International Atherosclerosis Project (McGill *et al.*, 1968), which investigated autopsy material from over 20 000 individuals in various cities throughout the world, demonstrated also a strong association between the mean TC levels for various communities and the prevailing severity of atheroma.

In prospective studies *within* communities TC levels have been shown to be predictive of the risk of developing IHD. Many reports are now available, including that of the Pooling Project Research Group (1978) in which the results of eight investigations in separate areas in the USA showed that individual TC levels in middle-aged men were related to the subsequent development of IHD over the following ten years.

In considering further the importance of plasma lipids, it may be recalled (p. 3.12) that about 70% of the cholesterol is carried in the low density lipoproteins (LDL), about 20% in the high density lipoproteins (HDL) and only a small percentage in the very low density lipoproteins (VLDL), which carry most of the plasma triglyceride fats. The levels of LDL relate closely to TC levels, and prospective studies which have included lipoprotein assays have demonstrated that LDL levels are predictive of the risk of IHD (Kannel *et al.*, 1979). High VLDL levels are also of some predictive value, possibly because LDL are derived from metabolism of VLDL in the plasma and there is a correlation between the levels of the two groups of lipoproteins. By contrast, a number of prospective studies within communities have demonstrated that plasma levels of HDL are related *inversely* to the risk of IHD (Lancet, 1982) and HDL levels have been reported as being of greater predictive value than TC or LDL levels within, but not between, communities. The factors which determine HDL levels are, however, obscure.

Diet. Analysis of the habitual diets in various communities has shown that diets rich in saturated fatty acids and cholesterol are associated with high mean plasma levels of TC, LDL and VLDL, while diets with a high content of unrefined carbohydrate and low in saturated fats and cholesterol are associated with low TC, LDL and VLDL levels. The dependence of these lipids on diet has also been clearly established by observing the effects of dietary changes in individuals.

Prospective studies in middle-aged men in various communities have demonstrated that the risk of IHD is related directly to the percentage of calories derived from saturated fats, to high ratios of saturated/polyunsaturated dietary fats and to dietary intake of cholesterol. The risk of IHD has also been reported to bear an inverse relationship to the amount of dietary vegetable fibre and to the amount of polyunsaturated fats in the diet. It is also suspected that refined sugar increases the risk of IHD.

Blood pressure. In developed countries, systolic and diastolic systemic blood pressures increase with age, but the degree of increase shows considerable individual variation, and the *range* of pressures in the population therefore increases with age. The mean blood pressure differs considerably for different communities, and the mean levels have been shown to correlate with the community incidence of IHD and atheroma. The distribution of blood pressures also differs between communities, those with a high incidence of IHD having more people well above the mean, i.e. with systemic hypertension. A number of prospective studies within communities have shown a direct relationship between individual levels of blood pressure and the risk of IHD, in some instances the risk in the 20% with highest pressures being four times that for the lowest 20%.

Cigarette smoking. The incidence of IHD in different communities has been shown to be related directly to the average numbers of cigarettes smoked, and prospective studies within communities have shown that the relationship holds for individuals and that the risk is reduced by giving up smoking. Little is known of the influence of cigars and pipe smoking on IHD.

Alcohol consumption. In communities with a high incidence of IHD, consumption of about five or more drinks daily is associated with an increased risk of IHD. Alcohol consumption carries associations with obesity, smoking and raised blood pressure, but when allowance is made for these factors alcohol still appears to be a risk factor.

It is of interest that those who drink a little appear to have a lower risk of IHD than total abstainers, but the evidence for this is not strong and provides only a small grain of comfort.

Other risk factors. The concentrations of **calcium in water supplies** have been shown to bear an inverse relationship to mortality rates from IHD in the urban areas in the UK. The relationship is not strong, but the risk appears to be about 15% lower in communities with a hard water supply (Pocock *et al.* 1980). **Habitual physical exercise** is also associated with a reduced risk of IHD. It is likely that this is an indirect effect, due to the favourable effect of exercise on blood lipids and blood pressure. **Oral contraceptives** appear to be a risk factor, possibly by increasing the risk of thrombosis and by their adverse effect on blood pressure and plasma lipids: the risk is slight but appears to be greatly increased by smoking. **Behavioural patterns and stress** also appear to influence the risk of IHD, perhaps by increasing the output of catecholamines. People classified as having type A behavioural pattern, who are ambitious, aggressive, bustling, impatient and short-tempered are particularly at risk. Finally, there is an increased risk of atheroma and IHD in **diabetes mellitus**, perhaps because of its effects on plasma lipids and the increased incidence of systemic hypertension in diabetes. There is no good evidence on whether the risk is reduced by careful therapeutic and dietary control.

The risk factors considered above have been shown to be synergistic, each adding to the risk of developing IHD. They have also been shown to contribute to the risk of developing cerebral infarction and ischaemia of the lower limbs, both of which are nearly always complications of atheroma.

Genetic predisposition. The various environmental risk factors considered above are likely to account for the differences in the IHD rates between communities, but they do not predict accurately which members of a given community will develop IHD: they merely indicate the degree of risk within groups of individuals classified by their mean levels of risk factors. This lack of accurate prediction indicates that there must be additional risk factors, and the fact that there is a greater degree of concordance for IHD in monozygotic twin pairs than in dizygotic twins of the same sex suggests that genetic factors are involved. There is at present considerable interest in the various groups of lipoproteins and their apoproteins, which are much more complex than suggested above, and it may be that polygenically determined variations will prove relatively common and of aetiological importance in atheroma. Support for polygenically determined predisposition has been provided recently by the demonstration that the levels of plasma TC in members of a community show small but significant associations with ABO blood groups, Gm factors (allotypic factors in the Fc of IgG), haptoglobin patterns and secretor status (Orr *et al.*, 1981). This does not, of course, mean that these factors are directly involved with lipid metabolism, but rather that they are linked with genes which do influence TC levels.

Intervention trials

To prove a *causal* relationship between an associated or risk factor and a disease, it is usually necessary to show that modification of the factor influences the incidence or severity of the disease. To this end, a number of large trials have been carried out in which the risk factors have been modified in a community, or in selected high-risk individuals within it, and the incidence of IHD has been determined in succeeding years. For example in the Oslo trial (Hjermann *et al.*, 1981) men of 40–49 years were assessed for risk factors and those at high risk (based on blood pressure in the upper part of the 'normal' range, high TC and smoking habits) were divided into intervention and control groups. The intervention group were ad-

vised to stop smoking and adopt a diet rich in polyunsaturated fats and vegetable fibre and low in saturated fats and cholesterol. Compared with the control group, a significant fall in TC and smoking was achieved, and after five years the incidence of myocardial infarction and sudden cardiac death (which is usually due to IHD) was reported to be 45% lower in the intervention group than in the controls. In the World Health Organisation European Collaboration Trial (1982) reduction of risk factors was encouraged in workers in selected factories, and workers in other factories were used as control groups. Preliminary results show a reduction in IHD in those factories achieving the greatest reduction in risk factors.

Biomedical investigations

In 1852 Rokitansky suggested that atheromatous plaques resulted from repeated formation of mural thrombi which became covered by endothelium and replaced by fibrous tissue to form a plaque of intimal thickening. The lipid of the plaque was presumed to be derived from constituents of the thrombi. Four years later, Virchow proposed that atheroma was initiated by an 'irritation' (inflammatory lesion) of the arterial intima with insudation of plasma into the injured zone and subsequent fibrosis and 'fatty degeneration'. This **insudation theory** gained wide acceptance, but in 1946 Duguid independently reintroduced Rokintansky's **thrombogenic** or **encrustation theory** and the subject has since been controversial.

In support of the thrombogenic theory, platelets and fibrin are commonly detectable by electron microscopy as a fine layer on the surface of the plaque and by immunohistological techniques in the plaque itself. However, the amount of lipid in most plaques is greater than could be derived from such thrombi and there is now strong evidence that much of the accumulated lipid is derived by insudation of plasma lipoproteins into the intima. Accordingly, it is now widely accepted that both mural thrombosis and insudation of plasma lipids through the endothelium are involved in atherogenesis. It is also believed that these processes, and also the proliferation of smooth muscle cells seen in the early lesion, are the result of **endothelial injury**. The evidence for these views is presented briefly below.

Insudation of lipid. The predominant lipid in atheromatous lesions is cholesterol, which occurs in the plaque in free form and also esterified with linoleic and other fatty acids. Investigations involving injection of radio-labelled cholesterol suggest that most of the cholesterol in the plaque is not synthesised locally but is derived from the plasma. Since the vasa vasorum of normal arteries supply only the outer part of the wall, lipid entering the intima must do so by crossing the endothelial lining, and animal studies have shown that plasma proteins and some lipoproteins normally enter the intima by this route. Such influx is greater in certain sites, notably around the mouths of arterial branches of the aorta. When pieces of fresh aorta are incubated in culture fluid rich in plasma lipoproteins, both LDL and HDL (but not VLDL) pass through the endothelium, but LDL accumulate in the intima in much greater amounts than HDL, suggesting some form of clearance mechanism for the latter (see below). Assay of plasma lipoproteins in the human aortic intima has demonstrated disproportionately high concentrations of LDL and examination of pieces of coronary artery and aorta obtained during vascular surgery from patients previously injected with a radiolabelled subfraction of autologous LDL has shown that the net influx of LDL into the intima is proportional to the plasma level of LDL (Niehaus *et al.*, 1977).

Apart from increased insudation through the endothelium, the factors which determine deposition of lipids in the intima of arteries are unknown. LDL are the major source of the cholesterol required by cells for production and maintenance of cell membrane although, if necessary, cells can synthesise their own cholesterol from acetate. Uptake of LDL by cells is facilitated by surface receptors which bind LDL, following which they are ingested by pinocytosis.

Receptor-dependent uptake of LDL by arterial smooth muscle cells is not essential to the development of atheroma, for individuals with the rare homozygous form of hyperbetalipoproteinaemia, who lack cellular LDL receptors, develop severe atheroma in childhood and die in youth from IHD. In this condition, failure of cell uptake of LDL results in very high plasma LDL levels and this is probably the explanation of the early development of severe

atheroma. Failure of receptor-dependent uptake of LDL by smooth muscle cells may contribute to the accumulation of cholesterol in the atheromatous plaque. Individuals who are heterozygous for the defective gene (about 1 in 500 of the population) have reduced numbers of LDL receptors: they too have high plasma LDL levels and usually die relatively early of IHD.

The inverse relationship between plasma levels of HDL and the risk of IHD suggests that HDL may protect against atheroma. It is also known that HDL can accept and incorporate free cholesterol from the surface of various cell types in culture, including smooth muscle cells, and it has been suggested that HDL provide a clearance system for cellular cholesterol and prevent its accumulation in the tissues. This is supported by the demonstration of a negative correlation between HDL levels and the cholesterol content of human tissues but proof of a clearance function for HDL is likely to be much more difficult, for it is now known that there are many different lipid apoproteins and that HDL and other classes of lipoproteins are complex mixtures, the metabolism and functions of which are at an early stage of investigation.

The role of endothelial injury. The patchy nature of atheroma suggests that there is either focal increase in the amount of lipid entering the intima, i.e. increased endothelial permeability, or focal impairment of metabolism or removal of intimal cholesterol. There is substantial evidence to suggest that increase in permeability is important, and that it is induced by endothelial injury. Much of this evidence has come from the experimental production of lesions bearing some resemblance to human atheroma in various species of mammals by feeding them on a diet which raises the level of plasma cholesterol (TC). The earliest changes observed are retraction of endothelial cells with the appearance of gaps between them and loss of occasional cells. These changes are accompanied by oedema of the intima and subsequently by the formation of plaques resembling those of atheroma (see Ross, 1981). It thus appears that a high level of plasma lipids may itself cause injury to arterial endothelium, although the mechanism is obscure.

The experimental atheroma-like lesions associated with dietary-induced hyperlipidaemia have been shown to be enhanced by various forms of endothelial injury, including (a) *mechanical abrasion* by balloons or indwelling catheters, (b) *immunological injury* resulting from circulating immune complexes, (c) *chemical injury*, e.g. by inhalation of cigarette smoke or administration of nicotine or homocystine (see below) and (d) *physical injury* by excessive heat or cold or by x-irradiation. Each of these forms of injury has been shown to accelerate the development of dietary-induced experimental 'atheroma', and in some instances persistent injury alone has resulted in similar lesions.

An acceptable theory of atherogenesis should explain why the lesions are localised plaques. None of the risk factors seems likely to act focally and it is likely that susceptibility to injury varies in different sites in arteries. One possibility is shearing stress, which might be expected to be greater at certain sites, including the arterial wall around the mouths of branch arteries (where atheroma is particularly common). This is supported by the demonstration of an increased rate of turnover of endothelium at these sites in normal guinea-pigs (Wright, 1971). Mechanical stress injury to the endothelium would be expected to be related to blood pressure, and might help to explain the increased incidence of atheroma and IHD in people with chronic systemic hypertension. Evidence of increased platelet consumption in hypertension is, however, conflicting.

Cellular proliferation. The cells which accumulate in the intima in early atheroma have been shown to be smooth muscle cells (see Fig. 14.11), most of which are provided by migration and proliferation of cells in the inner media. There is evidence that this occurs as a result of endothelial injury.

Aortic smooth muscle cells in culture are stimulated to proliferate by a factor which is present in the storage granules of platelets and is discharged by the platelet release reaction (p. 10.7). Normal vascular endothelium produces prostacyclin, which inhibits platelet adhesion, but mechanical or other injury to the endothelium results in adhesion of platelets to the collagen exposed by loss or retraction of endothelial cells, and the platelet release reaction ensues. This appears to play a role in migration and proliferation of smooth muscle cells, for accumulation of smooth muscle cells in the intima following injury is inhibited by suppressing platelet function by dipyridamole or by inducing thrombocytopenia by injecting antiplatelet antibody.

Study of iso-enzymic forms of glucose-6-phosphate dehydrogenase enzymes in the proliferated smooth muscle cells of atheromatous plaques has produced interesting results. These iso-enzymes are determined by genes in the X-chromosome, and approximately 30% of American female blacks are heterozygous so that, as a result of lyonisation (p. 2.11) half of their cells produce one type of enzyme (A) and the remainder produce a second type (B). Analysis of early atheromatous plaques from such heterozygous women have shown that the smooth muscle cells of some plaques produce only iso-enzyme A, while those of other plaques (from the same individual) produce only B. This suggests that the cellular proliferation in each plaque is *monoclonal*, although there are other possible explanations (Benditt, 1974). It has since been reported that the cells in organised thrombi from heterozygotes also appear to result from a monoclonal proliferation (Pearson *et al.*, 1979), while the fibroblasts in healed skin wounds consist of the expected mixtures of A and B iso-enzyme producers. The features of atheromatous plaques and organising thrombi do not resemble those of neoplasia, and the significance of Benditt's observations remains unexplained.

Other features of atheroma have not helped to elucidate its aetiology. The collagen and elastic fibres and ground substance of the superficial fibrous part of the plaque are products of the smooth muscle cells, but the stimulus for their production is unknown. The necrosis which is often observed in the deeper parts of the plaque may be due to ischaemia, although this part of the lesion is supplied by extension of vasa vasorum through the media. Another possible factor is the presence of small amounts of lipids shown to be capable of causing tissue injury. Dystrophic calcification of the plaque may be favoured by intake of calcium, e.g. by a hard water supply, and this may explain the lower incidence of IHD observed in hard water areas, for calcification may render the plaque less likely to rupture and so reduce the risk of superadded occlusive thrombosis of the coronary arteries (p. 15.7).

Conclusions

There is no doubt that a high level of plasma LDL is an important factor in the development and progression of atheroma. Indirect evidence suggests that continuous or repeated endothelial cell injury over a long period is also a causal factor, and that it operates by increasing the endothelial permeability to plasma lipoproteins and also promotes platelet adhesion and deposition of fibrin. These elements contribute to the growth of the plaque by adding to its bulk and possibly also by providing a platelet factor which may explain the observed smooth muscle proliferation. There are, however, endothelial and other factors which may influence the growth of smooth muscle cells. The postulated endothelial cell injury is most likely due to haemodynamic stress aggravated by some of the known risk factors such as systemic hypertension, high levels of LDL and inhalation of cigarette smoke. However, these and other risk factors have complex effects, and may influence the disease in various ways, including effects on the plasma levels of the various types of lipoproteins, and by affecting the function of platelets and other components of the clotting and fibrinolytic systems.

It must be emphasised that there are other, undiscovered risk factors, that the role of genetic factors has not been elucidated, and that much of the evidence on which conclusions are based is derived from the experimental production of atheroma-like lesions in animals. Most of these animal experiments are of relatively short duration, and in some of them the lesions bear more resemblance to fatty streaks than to atheroma.

Although the aetiology of atheroma remains unclear despite considerable investigation, there is no doubt that the present epidemic of ischaemic heart disease (IHD), atheroma's most important effect, has accompanied the increasing exposure to known risk factors and that individuals with high levels of risk factors are most prone to develop or die from IHD. During the past 20 years or so, age-corrected death rates from IHD have fallen by 30% in the USA and falls have also been observed in Australia, Canada and some European countries (p. 15.6). In the British Isles there is little evidence of a fall, except in the higher socio-economic classes. The reasons for these improvements are not known with certainty, but they do appear to have occurred among communities who are particularly conscious of the risk factors and therefore likely to have had opportunity to take steps to reduce them. It is thus likely that physical exercise, control of hypertension and avoidance of smoking, excessive alcohol, overeating and a diet which induces hypercholesterolaemia, would further reduce the incidence and mortality of IHD, and probably of atheroma, in the developed countries.

Systemic hypertension

Definition. In the developed countries, mean blood pressure increases with age, but there is considerable individual variation in the increase, and recordings of the blood pressures in a general adult population show a wide range. Any definition of hypertension must therefore be arbitrary, and there is no general agreement on the level of blood pressure to be regarded as pathological. Indeed, there is good evidence, for example from insurance companies' statistics, of a general inverse relationship between the height of the blood pressure, including variations within the 'normal range', and the expectation of life. This applies to both the systolic and diastolic pressures, although the latter is of greater predictive value.

Classification. In about 85% of cases of hypertension the cause is not apparent and these patients are said to have **primary, essential** or **idiopathic** hypertension. In the remaining 15% hypertension is **secondary** to other disease processes: nearly always diseases of the kidneys are responsible (**'renal hypertension'**) but occasional cases result from certain functioning adrenal tumours or as a feature of Cushing's syndrome (see Table 14.1). Coarctation of the aorta (p. 15.41) is accompanied by hypertension in the arteries arising proximal to the constriction. It is likely that, as diagnostic techniques improve, further causes of hypertension will be identified, and the proportion of patients with so-called essential hypertension will thus become smaller.

Regardless of the aetiology, hypertension may be divided into **chronic** or so-called '**benign**', and **malignant** (sometimes called **accelerated**) types. In benign hypertension the rise of blood pressure is usually slow, progressing over

Table 14.1 Classification of systemic hypertension

I. Essential   { benign (90%)
    (85%)   { malignant (10%)
II. Secondary   { benign (80%)
    (15%)   { malignant (20%)
  (a) of renal origin ('renal hypertension'), due to:
      chronic pyelonephritis
      glomerulonephritis
      diabetes
      polycystic disease of the kidneys
      renal amyloidosis
      connective tissue diseases, particularly polyarteritis
      urinary tract obstruction (occasional cases)
      renal artery disease
      radiation nephritis
      some renal tumours
      some congenital malformations of kidney, possibly by predisposing to pyelonephritis
  (b) adrenal-mediated hypertension.
      Conn's syndrome (primary hyperaldosteronism)
      Cushing's syndrome
      phaeochromocytoma
  (c) coarctation of the aorta.

many years, and usually the level is only moderately raised (below 200/110) although in some patients it is higher. Many patients with benign hypertension lead active lives for many years with few or no symptoms, and die of some independent disease. Unless the blood pressure is controlled by antihypertensive drugs, however, it frequently causes disability and death from heart failure, and greatly increases the risk of myocardial infarction and cerebrovascular accidents.

Malignant hypertension is characterised by a very high blood pressure, by eye changes which include retinal haemorrhages and exudates and sometimes papilloedema, by rapidly progressive renal injury terminating in uraemia, and by hypertensive encephalopathy. The pathological hallmark of this state is fibrinoid necrosis of arterioles (see later). These special features appear to depend on the rapid development of a very high blood pressure. Unless treated, patients with malignant hypertension usually die within a year or so, but frequently the blood pressure can be reduced by anti-hypertensive drugs, and the outlook is then greatly improved.

Benign and malignant hypertension should not be regarded as unrelated conditions. Malignant hypertension supervenes in a small proportion of cases of benign essential hypertension although more often it arises apparently *de novo*, i.e. without evidence of preceding benign hypertension.

Changes in the blood vessels

Changes develop in arterial vessels of all sizes as a result of hypertension. In the larger arteries, from the aorta down to vessels of about 1 mm diameter, the changes are widespread, and are termed **hypertensive arteriosclerosis**. Changes in the vessels below this size, i.e. in the smallest arteries and arterioles, tend to affect especially the small vessels of the viscera, and in particular those of the kidneys. The changes occurring in the larger arteries are of the same nature in all types of hypertension, but those in the smaller vessels, particularly the arterioles, are different in benign and malignant types of hypertension, and require separate descriptions.

Large and middle-sized arteries. The vascular changes in hypertension, uncomplicated by the arterial lesions common in the aged, are most readily studied in young patients with high blood pressure secondary to renal disease. **In the early stages** they consist mainly of hypertrophy, with increase of smooth muscle cells and elastic fibres. In the aorta, there is increase in both of these elements in the media. In muscular arteries the increase is mainly in the smooth muscle of the media (Fig. 14.14) but the internal elastic lamina becomes thickened, and very often new laminae are formed towards the intima (Fig. 14.15). **In longstanding hypertension,** which is usually of benign essential type, these hypertrophic changes give way to fibrous replacement of muscle and the elastic tissue may break up and undergo partial absorption. The arterial walls are thickened and of increased rig-

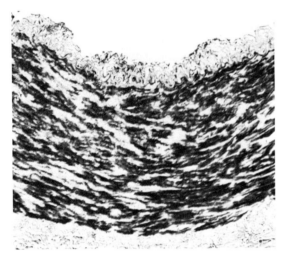

Fig. 14.14 Section of hypertrophied radial artery, from a case of systemic hypertension in a young subject, showing hypertrophy of the media. (Smooth muscle appears black.) × 140.

idity, the lumen is dilated (Fig. 14.16) and the vessels are often elongated and tortuous. In the aorta, there is increase in the elastic and fibrous tissue of the media. In the muscular arteries, the media is thickened and fibrosed with patchy loss of smooth muscle cells, and there may be fibrous thickening of the intima (Fig. 14.17).

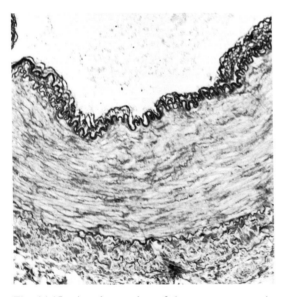

Fig. 14.15 Another section of the same artery as in Fig. 14.14, showing increase of elastic tissue formed by replication of the internal elastic lamina. (Elastic tissue appears black.) × 120.

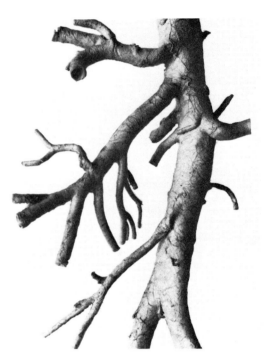

Fig. 14.16 Arteriosclerosis of the aorta and its branches in a patient with hypertension who died aged 36 from chronic renal failure. The walls of the vessels are thickened and rigid: they are also dilated, although this is not readily apparent. × 0·35.

These changes are widespread, and vary in degree. They are mostly without important effects.

The arteriosclerotic changes described above are similar to those observed in normotensive elderly subjects (*senile arteriosclerosis*—p. 14.1) but in the absence of hypertension they are usually less pronounced, and the media, although fibrosed, is often not thickened.

Hypertension predisposes to the development and rupture of the 'berry' aneurysms which occur in the arteries at the base of the brain in some individuals (p. 14.32), and is the usual cause of *subarachnoid haemorrhage*.

Atheroma tends to be particularly severe in individuals with chronic hypertension, and there is no doubt that prolonged elevation of the blood pressure aggravates this condition.

Hypertension thus results at first in hypertrophy of the arterial walls, with increase in muscle and elastic fibres, followed by arteriosclerosis and a tendency to severe atheroma. The early hypertrophic changes are usually observed only in young hypertensive subjects: in older patients

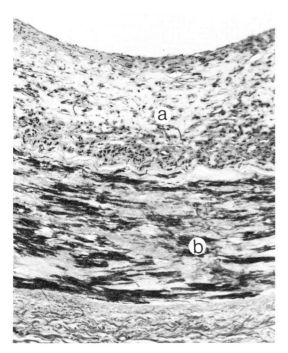

Fig. 14.17 Part of a transverse section of an arterio-sclerotic artery. The intima (**a**) is thickened, while the muscle (shown as black) of the media (**b**) is partly replaced by fibrous tissue. (Compare with Fig. 14.14) × 200.

with chronic hypertension, arteriosclerosis and atheroma predominate.

Small arteries and arterioles. In arteries of 1 mm diameter or less, and in the arterioles, the changes differ from those in the larger vessels, and they differ also in benign and malignant hypertension.

(*a*) *Benign hypertension.* The small arteries show the medial thickening seen in the larger vessels, but a more pronounced degree of intimal thickening, due to concentric increase in connective tissue; in the smallest arteries the intimal change predominates, and may result in narrowing of the lumen in contrast to the dilatation seen in the larger arteries.

The *arterioles* undergo *hyaline thickening* of their walls (*hyaline arteriolosclerosis*), which consists at first of patchy deposition of hyaline material, often beneath the endothelium, but sometimes more peripherally: the hyaline change gradually extends to involve the whole circumference, and when severe it replaces all the normal structures of the wall except the endothelium. This change occurs also apart from hypertension, and is seen especially in old age. In both normotensive and hypertensive subjects it is observed most commonly in arterioles in the spleen, then in the afferent glomerular arterioles of the kidneys (Fig. 14.18), and in the pancreas, liver and adrenal capsules. In all these sites, the change is appreciably commoner and usually more severe in hypertensives than in normotensive subjects of corresponding ages. Hyaline arteriolosclerosis is uncommon in the arterioles of the brain, gastro-intestinal tract, pituitary, thyroid, heart, skin and skeletal muscles (Smith, 1956). The nature of the change is not fully understood: initially, the hyaline material resembles fibrin in its staining properties, but later it stains like collagen. It also contains lipid material, and there is evidence that it is due, at least partly, to *plasmatic vasculosis* (p. 11.7). Apart from its occurrence as an ageing process and in hypertensive subjects, hyaline arteriolosclerosis is often severe and extensive in diabetes mellitus (pp. 20.64, 22.39).

In benign essential hypertension, hyaline arteriolosclerosis causes chronic ischaemia of individual nephrons and thus increases the normal loss of nephrons which occurs with age. It does not usually cause renal failure but decreases the reserve of the kidneys and increases

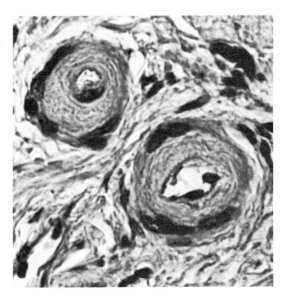

Fig. 14.18 Hyaline arteriolosclerosis of afferent glomerular arteriole in chronic systemic hypertension. The arteriole is not only thickened, but also tortuous, and so has been cut twice in cross-section in the same plane. × 1500.

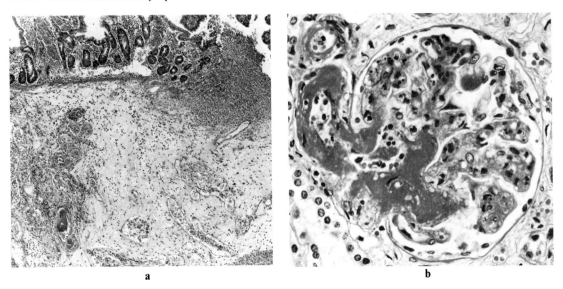

Fig. 14.19   Arteriolar lesions in malignant hypertension. **a** Ulceration of the colonic mucosa due to fibrinoid necrosis and thrombosis of arterioles: one such vessel is seen (*lower left*) in the submucosa. **b** Fibrinoid necrosis of a glomerular afferent arteriole and part of the tuft.

the danger of renal failure if and when heart failure develops.

(*b*) *Malignant hypertension*. The characteristic early change of malignant hypertension is **fibrinoid necrosis** (p. 11.7) of the walls of arterioles and the smallest arteries. The lesion consists of necrosis of the vessel walls and gross thickening due to permeation of the necrotic tissue by plasma constituents. The affected vessel wall appears eosinophilic and refractile and can be shown by immunohistological techniques to contain fibrin, immunoglobulins, complement components and other plasma proteins: there may also be red cells, singly and in small groups, lying in and around the vessel wall and sometimes visible by naked eye as small haemorrhages. Nuclear debris and occasional polymorphs may also be seen in the wall. The lesion commonly involves the whole thickness and circumference over various lengths of arteriolar walls, while the lesions in small arteries tend to be more patchy. The main effect is to reduce the lumen, obliteration of which is often completed by thrombosis, resulting in small infarcts (Fig. 14.19). The passage of blood through such a damaged arterial bed causes red cell fragmentation—*micro-angiopathic haemolytic anaemia* (p. 17.32) which is caused by the intravascular deposition of fibrin.

There is good evidence that hypertensive

fibrinoid necrosis is due to focal failure of the vessel wall to resist a rise in intraluminal pressure to abnormal levels, and both clinical and experimental evidence suggests that the rate of rise is more important than the level reached. Intravascular thrombosis may contribute to the vascular damage, for morphologically similar changes are seen in conditions where thrombosis occurs without hypertension.

In patients with established or treated malignant hypertension, fibrinoid necrosis is often inconspicuous or even absent and the characteristic lesion is a concentric 'onion-skin' thickening of the intima of small arteries, a form of **endarteritis obliterans** best seen in the interlobular arteries of the kidney (Fig. 22.10, p. 22.7). The intimal thickening consists initially of concentrically arranged smooth muscle cells lying in a matrix rich in mucopolysaccharides but later this is replaced by collagen. When severe, endarteritis causes local ischaemia from reduction of the lumen.

These vascular changes are widespread in malignant hypertension: they are conspicuous in the internal organs, and notably in the brain, gut and pancreas, but the small vessels of the kidneys are usually most severely affected. They are not specific for malignant hypertension and appear to be induced by various kinds of injury, including renal allograft rejection, progressive systemic sclerosis and high dosage x-irradiation (see also p. 3.29).

Cerebral haemorrhage in hypertensives is probably due to rupture of micro-aneurysms of the small arteries within the brain (p. 14.33).

Course and clinical features

Chronic ('benign') essential hypertension. As already stated, this is much the commonest type of hypertension. The blood pressure rises very gradually over a period of years, in most cases to moderately high levels, e.g. 180/100 mm Hg, but occasionally much higher. The increase nearly always starts before the age of 45 years, and individuals with a resting blood pressure consistently below 140/85 at this age are very unlikely to develop essential hypertension. The diastolic pressure is less subject to physiological variations than the systolic pressure, and a diastolic pressure persistently exceeding 90 mm Hg is generally regarded, on an arbitrary basis, as abnormal. However, the disease develops very slowly, and it may be years before the rise in pressure clearly exceeds that which occurs normally with age.

The condition may be symptomless, and many cases come to light during routine medical examination for insurance or other purposes. *Common symptoms* include palpitations, audible pulsation in the head, headaches, attacks of dizziness particularly on stooping, and reduced exercise tolerance.

Without treatment, about 60% of patients with benign essential hypertension die of heart failure; this is due to the increased work load thrown on the left ventricle and to the commonly associated severe coronary artery atheroma. About 30% of untreated patients die from cerebral haemorrhage or infarction, and 10% from various causes unrelated to the hypertension. Although changes occur in the kidneys as a result of the vascular lesions, renal failure is uncommon in benign essential hypertension. When heart failure develops, however, there is usually a moderate rise in the blood urea level. In those patients who progress from chronic to malignant hypertension, renal failure commonly supervenes.

Malignant ('accelerated') essential hypertension. This develops in approximately 10% of patients with chronic essential hypertension. In those cases not preceded by chronic hypertension, the onset is usually between 30 and 45 years. It can result in heart failure or cerebral haemorrhage, but *without effective treatment renal injury is severe and usually causes death within a year* (p. 22.6).

Eye changes are an important feature in malignant hypertension: lesions in the small arteries in the retina result in oedema, haemorrhages, infarcts and exudates, and blindness may ensue. Papilloedema, associated with cerebral oedema, is often present. *Hypertensive encephalopathy*, characterised by epileptiform fits and transient paralysis, is not uncommon, and is caused by cerebral oedema resulting from failure of the resistance vessels of the brain to withstand the increased blood pressure. The small arteries and arterioles become focally and then more diffusely overdistended with a consequent rise in capillary pressure and oedema. This has been observed directly in rats with experimental hypertension and the fits have been shown to cease when the blood pressure is lowered.

Secondary hypertension. Hypertension is a feature of **chronic renal failure**, and is more often of malignant type than is the case in essential hypertension. The superadded imposition of further renal injury from hypertensive vascular lesions, whether benign or malignant, aggravates and accelerates renal failure.

Aetiology of hypertension

The blood pressure depends upon the cardiac output and the peripheral vascular resistance, and hypertension is attributable to an increase of one or both of these factors. There is evidence that the cardiac output is increased in the early stages of essential hypertension in man and of experimentally-induced renal hypertension in rats, but in established hypertension cardiac output is normal, and maintenance of the high blood pressure is therefore attributable to increased peripheral resistance. In normal circumstances the peripheral resistance is controlled by the muscular tone in the arterioles throughout the body, and the major aetiological problem is the elucidation of the factors which, by increasing arteriolar tone, bring about the various types of hypertension. The possibility that the structural changes of arteriolosclerosis initiate the hypertensive state is unlikely, for such changes are sometimes absent, particularly in early cases, and moreover structural changes are not present in arterioles which are protected from hypertension by occlusive changes in the larger arteries supplying them. Accordingly, the observed structural changes in the resistance vessels are widely regarded as the result of hypertension, and not the cause. It is likely, however, that structural changes in the arterioles and small arteries of the kidneys impair renal blood flow, and this may play a part in *maintaining* hypertension once the vascular changes have become pronounced.

Essential hypertension

Sodium intake. The prevalence of hypertension in different populations has been shown to correlate well with their average salt intake. Communities who do not add salt to food not only have minimal hypertension but also have no age-related rise in blood pressure, while the prevalence of hypertension in adults can reach 40% in populations with a high salt intake. Sodium balance studies have failed to show an individual correlation between blood pressure and salt intake but there could be many explanations for this, and it is noteworthy that hypertension is readily induced in animals by a high salt intake and that sodium retention is responsible for the hypertension of chronic renal failure. It therefore seems likely that excessive salt intake is an important aetiological factor in essential hypertension.

Other environmental factors. *Stressful stimuli* cause a rise in blood pressure, but chronic stress is difficult to assess. In several countries blood pressure levels are higher in inner cities than in urban areas. *Obese individuals* have higher mean blood pressures than others, although it does not correlate closely with degree of obesity. *Alcoholics* are often hypertensive and there is a direct correlation between alcohol intake and blood pressure in nonalcoholics.

Genetic factors. Essential hypertension often runs in families and studies of the blood pressure in twins and adopted children further suggest that genetic factors play a major part in this familial tendency; however its mode of inheritance remains controversial. Several inbred strains of rats develop a condition similar to essential hypertension in man, and so far inheri-

tance has proved to be polygenic. In developed countries, essential hypertension is commoner in negroes than in caucasians.

There is recent evidence of an increase in intracellular sodium in red and white blood cells of untreated patients with essential hypertension and their first degree relatives, suggesting the possibility of a fundamental metabolic defect of sodium and potassium handling by the cell membrane. Such an abnormality could have important effects on the excitability and tone of vascular smooth muscle and therefore on peripheral vascular resistance.

Humoral vasoconstrictive factors. In patients with hypertension due to a phaeochromocytoma, the large amounts of catecholamines released by the tumour into the blood (see p. 26.39) are very likely to be the cause of the hypertension.

The vasoconstrictor substances renin and angiotensin (p. 10.35) are believed to be of importance in the pathogenesis of malignant hypertension secondary to renal disease: plasma concentrations of both renin and angiotensin are increased in this disorder. By contrast, their levels in most patients with benign essential hypertension are normal, and in patients with Conn's syndrome (primary aldosteronism, p. 26.34) plasma renin concentration is actually reduced. Nevertheless, it cannot be concluded that renin and angiotensin are not involved in the raised blood pressure of benign essential hypertension, for sensitivity to the pressor effects of injected angiotensin is known to be increased in hypertensive patients, and thus the normal or subnormal amounts of angiotensin in the blood might conceivably raise the blood pressure to abnormal levels.

Search for other vasoactive substances in the blood of patients with hypertension has failed, but there is considerable interest in the possible role of the recently discovered regulatory peptides (p. 12.43), and also in the kallikrein–kinin system and prostaglandins, all of which may be involved.

Neural factors. The possibility that neural factors may play a role in essential hypertension deserves consideration. There is evidence that in both human and experimental hypertension the threshold of the vascular receptors is elevated, so that abnormally high pressures are necessary to initiate neurogenic anti-pressor reflexes. It may also be that variations in sensitivity to pressor agents, possibly genetically determined, are involved.

Effects of treatment. The use of effective antihypertensive drugs has greatly improved the prognosis in benign essential hypertension. Lowering of the blood pressure reduces greatly the incidence of heart failure, cerebral haemorrhage and transition to malignant hypertension, although the risks of developing ischaemic heart disease and cerebral infarction are not greatly reduced and myocardial infarction has now become the commonest cause of death in treated benign hypertension.

Aggressive therapy has also improved the outlook in malignant hypertension, but the severe endarteritis of the small renal arteries commonly causes death from uraemia some years later: almost equally common causes of death in treated patients are myocardial infarction and cerebrovascular accidents.

Secondary hypertension

A firm experimental basis for renal hypertension was provided in 1934 by Goldblatt and his colleagues, who showed that partial clamping of the renal arteries produced hypertension in dogs. This has been confirmed repeatedly in several species and it has been shown that hypertension can be produced in the rat by partial clamping of one renal artery. Vascular hypertensive changes have been produced by this method, and it is of interest that they do not affect the kidney which is protected by the clamp from hypertension. At first, the experimental hypertension is abolished by removing the clamp or excising the clamped kidney, but if the clamp is removed after some months, the hypertension persists because of arteriolar changes produced in the unclamped kidney.

Renal hypertension in man is similar in many ways to the experimental condition. The diseases which cause it are listed in Table 14.1 on p. 14.15 and are described in Chapter 22: because of their relatively high incidence, *chronic glomerulonephritis* and *chronic pyelonephritis* are the most important ones. Release of excess renin from the abnormal kidney or kidneys may be an important factor in producing hypertension in such diseases, but the original view that the hypertension is due simply to the pressor effect of excessive renin production by the ischaemic kidney is now known to be an oversimplification. High levels of renin have usually been found only in malignant hypertension with underlying renal disease, and even in these the importance of renin is not fully established.

Secondary hyperaldosteronism in hypertension. In some patients with severe hypertension, particularly those with malignant hypertension, secondary hyperaldosteronism develops. Plasma renin concentration is invariably increased and this leads to stimulation of aldosterone secretion which in turn produces potassium depletion (see p. 26.34). The condition is recognised usually by a decrease in the concentration of potassium, and often of sodium, in the plasma. It must be distinguished from primary hyperaldosteronism (Conn's syndrome) in which the hypertension and hypokalaemia are associated with *increased* sodium and *decreased* plasma renin concentration.

Pulmonary hypertension

In contrast to systemic hypertension, a rise in blood pressure in the pulmonary arterial system is usually explicable on the basis of disease of the lungs, heart or major vessels. These causes, and the effects of pulmonary hypertension, are described on pp. 16.23–26.

Arteritis

This term covers a heterogeneous group of conditions in which there is focal or more extensive inflammation of the walls of arteries and/or arterioles. In some of these, arteritis is a component of a more extensive *vasculitis* in which veins and capillaries are also affected. In severe arteritis there may be necrosis of the artery wall, which may result in occlusive thrombosis, rupture or aneurysm formation. The healing phase of arteritis often causes severe permanent narrowing of the lumen, resulting either from organisation of thrombus or from endarteritis obliterans, and chronic ischaemia is likely to result.

In most cases of arteritis the aetiology is obscure, and there is thus no satisfactory aetiological classification. However, apart from some forms of infective arteritis, which can affect vessels of any size, arteritis falls into patterns depending on the size of arteries mainly affected, and this provides a useful basis for classification which accords with the clinical features. It must be emphasised, however, that there is considerable overlap in the lesions of the various conditions and that the same aetiological agent may be associated with different patterns of arteritis (see Mitchison, 1984).

Infective arteritis. The arteries are relatively resistant to bacterial invasion and in acute infections the arteries in the inflamed tissues are usually spared unless suppuration or gangrene occur. Infected emboli, for example in bacterial endocarditis (p. 15.37) may cause an acute arteritis at the site of impaction: if severe, this may result in necrosis and rupture or development of a mycotic aneurysm (p. 14.32). More widespread invasion of arterioles, capillaries and venules by micro-organisms can give rise to a vasculitis causing necrosis and thrombosis of the vessels. This occurs in the *rickettsial diseases* e.g. typhus (p. 9.33) and Rocky Mountain spotted fever. In immunosuppressed patients the *fungal infections* such as aspergillosis and mucormycosis promote increased tissue destruction due to their ability to invade veins and arteries, causing thrombosis and infarction.

Tuberculosis most often causes endarteritis of the arteries in an infected area, but occasionally caseation can involve the media, causing aneurysm formation or rupture and haemorrhage, e.g. into a tuberculous cavity in the lung.

Arteritis of the aorta and large arteries

Syphilitic arteritis

Syphilis causes lesions in the small vessels involved in primary, secondary and tertiary lesions, and also affects the aorta and rarely its larger branches. The lesions of small vessels are

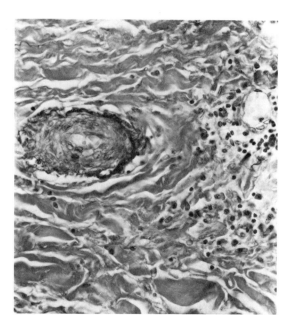

Fig. 14.20   Syphilitic aortitis, showing severe endarteritis of an arteriole in the adventitia of the aorta, and infiltration by plasma cells and lymphocytes around two small vessels (*right*). × 330.

described on p. 9.29: they consist of fibrous thickening of the intima and adventitia and perivascular infiltration of lymphocytes and plasma cells (*endarteritis* and *periarteritis*). Their effect is to reduce the calibre of the small vessels, thus causing local ischaemia. These changes may occur in the vasa vasorum of the thoracic aorta, appearing first where these vessels traverse the adventitia of the aorta (Fig. 14.20) and extending into the media (Fig. 14.21): they provide the first evidence of **syphilitic mesaortitis**. Whether due to ischaemia from the changes in the vasa vasorum or to a hypersensitivity reaction to the spirochete, there follows an irregular patchy loss of the musculo-elastic laminae of the media and replacement by collagenous tissue. In places, the patches may coalesce and involve the whole thickness of the media (Fig. 14.22): their effect is to weaken the media with consequent diffuse dilatation and localised bulges in the affected aortic wall (Fig. 14.23) which may progress to aneurysm formation. Dense fibrous intimal thickening develops in areas of medial involvement and is seen on the intimal surface as smooth grey-white areas, which extend and fuse and become irregularly contracted to

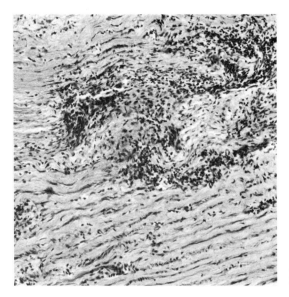

Fig. 14.21 Section of a syphilitic aorta, showing cellular accumulations around the small vessels in the media, with destruction of the laminae. × 160.

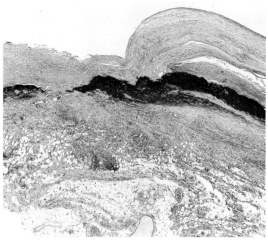

Fig. 14.22 Syphilitic aortitis; elastic tissue appears black. The section shows part of a thickened intimal plaque (*upper right*) and irregularity, thinning and interruptions in the elastic tissue of the media, which has also lost most of its muscle and is grossly thinned: the paler tissue below is the adventitia and adjacent fatty tissue. × 10.

produce a wrinkled 'tree-bark' appearance (Fig. 14.23) and stellate scars.

Syphilitic mesaortitis usually develops 20 or so years after contracting the disease, and is often associated with severe atheroma (which is otherwise unusual in the thoracic aorta) and yellow atheromatous patches complicate the picture. In younger patients, e.g. with congenital syphilis, the mesaortitis is seen in pure form. The first few centimetres of the aorta are often involved first, but the aortic arch is by far the commonest, and sometimes the only, site affected. The abdominal aorta is rarely involved.

Occasionally the lesions in the aorta are more florid, with formation of microscopic gummas in the media, or rarely more extensive gumma formation extending inwards from the adventitia.

Although a common and dreaded complication of untreated syphilis, mesaortitis, like other late manifestations of the disease, has become rare in countries where early diagnosis and treatment have been achieved.

Effects. *Aneurysm formation* is an important complication of syphilitic mesaortitis and is due to weakening of the vessel wall from loss of medial elastic and muscle tissue: the effects of aneurysm are described on p. 14.29.

Aortic incompetence. The dilatation of syphilitic aortitis may involve the root of the aorta, with consequent incompetence of the aortic valve. The cusps become stretched, thickened and distorted (p. 15.31).

Coronary artery narrowing due to involvement of their orifices by mesaortitis is now a rare cause of myocardial ischaemia.

Other forms of aortitis

Aortitis resembling syphilitic mesaortitis occurs in some patients with *ankylosing spondylitis* (p. 23.47), *Reiter's syndrome* (p. 23.48) and *psoriatic arthritis* (p. 23.48). It affects mainly the root of the aorta and, as in syphilis, dilatation of the valve ring gives rise to aortic incompetence. The aetiology is unknown.

Giant cell arteritis may affect the aorta and its branches, but more often medium-sized arteries, and it is dealt with below.

Rheumatic aortitis. The aorta and large arteries may be affected in rheumatic fever. The adventitia and outer media are inflamed, with formation of typical Aschoff bodies. The wall is not sufficiently weakened to produce aneurysms or any clinical effect. Arteritis in rheumatic fever is occasionally more extensive and may affect arteries of any size.

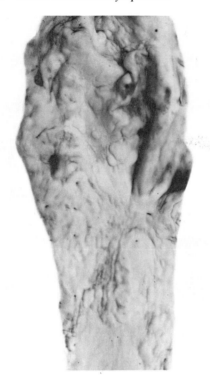

Fig. 14.23 The thoracic aorta in syphilitic aortitis. The arch of the aorta is stretched, with localised bulgings, thickened intimal patches and irregular wrinkling and scarring. In this example the changes stop abruptly below the arch. × 0·5.

Aortitis of unknown aetiology has been described in various countries, notably in Africans in Uganda.

Takayasu's disease. This is a rare condition, first reported from Japan, in which the aorta and the large arteries arising from the aortic arch are affected by an arteritis which may resemble syphilitic aortitis, caseating tuberculosis or temporal arteritis. Intimal thickening, sometimes with superadded thrombosis, severely narrows or occludes the subclavian, carotid and innominate arteries (hence the term *pulseless disease*), with resulting ischaemia of the head and arms. The disease affects mainly young women, and the aetiology is unknown.

Arteritis of medium-sized and small arteries

Thromboangiitis obliterans (Buerger's disease)

Definition. Buerger's disease is an inflammatory condition of arteries and veins, with throm-

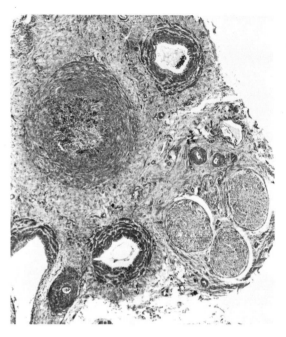

Fig. 14.24 Thromboangiitis obliterans. Occlusion of the posterior tibial artery (*upper left*) and surrounding fibrosis extending around the adjacent veins and nerves. × 32.

bosis, organisation and recanalisation of the affected vessels. It occurs almost exclusively in men, and affects mainly the vessels of the lower limbs, but sometimes also those of the upper limbs, giving rise to severe pain and progressive ischaemic changes.

Pathological changes. The early changes are not often available for histological examination. They consist of occlusion of the affected vessel by thrombus which contains foci of intense polymorph infiltration. The whole thickness of the vessel wall is also infiltrated with polymorphs. These acute changes give way to chronic inflammation, and the thrombus is replaced by granulation tissue containing lymphocytes, macrophages and multinucleated giant cells (Figs. 14.24, 14.25). The inflammatory changes eventually subside, and although the original vascular lumen has been obliterated there is often a surprising degree of recanalisation. The inflammation of the vessel wall also progresses to a chronic stage but without the degree of disruption which occurs in polyarteritis nodosa (see below). Fibrosis extends into the surrounding connective tissue, and the burned-out lesions thus consist of recanalised

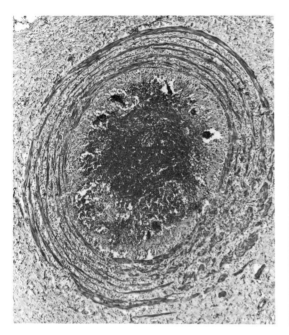 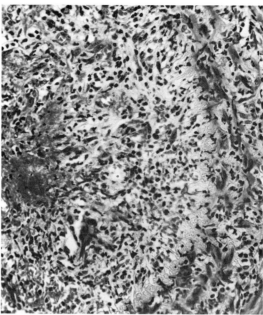

Fig. 14.25 Thrombophlebitis in Buerger's disease. *Left*, a superficial vein, showing inflammation of the wall, thrombosis and early organisation. Several multinucleated giant cells lie in and adjacent to the thrombus. × 60. *Right*, an older lesion with more advanced organisation of the thrombus: note the giant cell (*below centre*) and pleomorphic inflammatory infiltrate. × 250.

vessels with thickened fibrosed walls, enclosed in fibrous tissue which may envelop and compress adjacent nerves and vessels (Fig. 14.24).

The lesions affect short lengths of the small and medium-sized arteries and veins of the legs and feet, but seldom the larger vessels. Similarly, when the upper limbs are affected, the lesions are mainly in the vessels of the forearms and hands. The disease is chronic, acute lesions developing intermittently over a period of years. It may involve mainly either arteries or veins, but usually both. The changes of ischaemia, including gangrene of the extremities of the affected limbs, eventually result.

Aetiology. Features which distinguish Buerger's disease from atheroma with superadded thrombosis are its relatively early onset, inflammatory nature, predilection for smaller vessels, involvement of veins as well as arteries and of the upper limbs as well as the lower, and its rarity in women. It is a common misconception that the disease occurs especially in Jews, but a high incidence of HLA antigens A9 and B5 in sufferers has been reported, suggesting a genetic predisposing factor.

The inflammatory nature of the early lesions suggests a specific causal agent (as was postulated by Buerger) but none has been detected. The single known important predisposing factor is cigarette smoking. The disease is practically confined to heavy smokers, and there is a strong clinical impression that its progress is arrested or diminished by giving up smoking. Hypersensitivity to tobacco proteins has been suggested as a causal factor.

Clinical features. The symptoms are varied and depend on the degree of arterial obstruction. The earliest are pain, paraesthesia and circulatory disturbances e.g. local redness which disappears on elevating the limbs. On walking there is often cramp-like pain and inability to progress—'*intermittent claudication*'; this is a result of ischaemia of the calf muscles and occurs in other forms of arterial disease. Later, more severe trophic changes appear, including intractable ulceration, and gangrene which is apt to spread slowly; amputation, sometimes repeated, is often necessary but the need for surgery may be minimised by therapy which improves the collateral circulation. In view of the widespread involvement of the arteries, amputation, if required, should be performed at a high level. If the vessels of the arms are severely affected, the condition may simulate Raynaud's disease in the male.

Giant-cell or temporal arteritis. This is a fairly uncommon condition, occurring mostly in old people of both sexes. It affects mainly arteries of the head, but is sometimes much more widespread, and the aortic arch and its major branches are occasionally involved. Diagnosis is often based on clinical examination and biopsy of the temporal artery, which is conveniently superficial and often affected.

The lesion is an inflammation of the whole thickness and whole circumference of the affected arteries, affecting either a continuous length of the vessel or appearing as multiple focal lesions along it. The vessel wall is infiltrated with leucocytes (mainly polymorphs) in the early stages, but the subsequent reaction is granulomatous, with accumulation of lymphocytes, macrophages and multinuclear cells (of both Langhans' and 'foreign-body' types) which sometimes appear to develop in relation to fragments of the disrupted internal elastic lamina. Fibrous thickening of the intima, fibrous replacement of the media, and commonly thrombosis and organisation, result in a severely scarred vessel with a narrowed or obliterated lumen (Fig. 14.26).

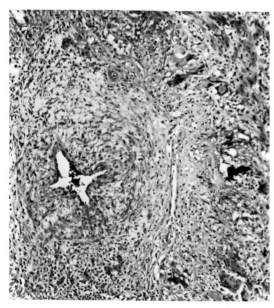

Fig. 14.26 Section of the temporal artery in giant-cell arteritis, showing multinucleated giant cells lying in relation to the internal elastic lamina (now disrupted and seen only as small fragments). There is gross intimal thickening and a very narrow lumen. × 120.

Clinically there may be localised reddening of the skin over an affected vessel, which is usually tender or painful and sometimes nodular. Depending on which arteries are involved, there may be headache, visual disturbances and even blindness (from involvement of the retinal arteries), facial pain, and sometimes cerebral infarction and other features resulting from more extensive arteritis. In some instances, the disease occurs in association with polymyalgia rheumatica. It is of entirely unknown aetiology and usually self-limiting.

Polyarteritis nodosa

The lesions of this disease consist of multiple foci of necrosis, inflammation and usually thrombosis, followed by healing, in the walls of medium-sized and small arteries and arterioles. Vessels in any part of the body may be affected, and there is involvement of many organs and tissues. The condition occurs over a wide age range, but mainly between 20 and 40 years and in men more often than women.

Pathological findings. The early lesion consists of a focus of fibrinoid necrosis of the media and intima of a small or medium-sized artery (up to about 3 mm diameter) or an arteriole. Necrosis is accompanied by acute inflammation with polymorph infiltration (often including eosinophils) of the whole thickness of the vessel wall and particularly intense in the adventitia and surrounding tissue (Fig. 14.27). Lesions affect the whole circumference of smaller arteries, but often only a segment of the wall of the larger vessels (Fig. 14.28). Occlusive thrombosis is common in the acute stage, but in some cases there is severe haemorrhage. The acute changes progress to more chronic inflammation, with replacement of the necrotic vessel wall by fibrous tissue infiltrated with lymphocytes, plasma cells and macrophages, and the thrombus undergoes organisation. The weakened wall may stretch to form an aneurysm (Fig. 14.29), but even without this the healed lesion may project as a nodular thickening of the vessel wall, and microscopy then shows a sharply-defined zone of fibrous replacement of the artery wall.

The lesions are multiple; they occur in almost any small or medium-sized artery or arteriole, but are commonest in those of the kidneys, heart, liver, pancreas, nervous system and skeletal muscles. Their effects, apart from haemorrhage, are due to acute or chronic ischaemia, and depend on the distribution of the lesions and arterial anastomoses in particular sites. Infarcts and patches of chronic ischaemic atrophy result in the heart, kidneys, etc.

The disease may be severe and progress rapidly to death, but more often the course extends over some years, with periods of quiescence alternating with the developing of new lesions. In most cases, death

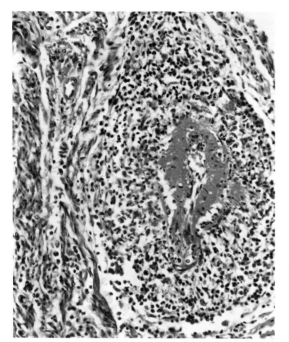

Fig. 14.27 An acute lesion of polyarteritis nodosa in a small artery in the kidney. There is fibrinoid necrosis and an intense inflammatory cellular infiltrate in and around the wall of the artery. × 100.

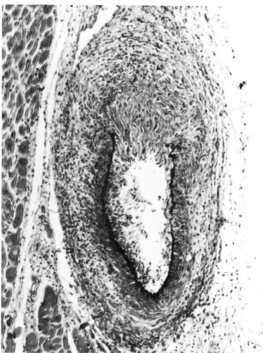

Fig. 14.28 Polyarteritis nodosa involving a coronary artery. The lesion is less acute than in the previous figure. Part of the circumference of the vessel wall (*above*) has been severely damaged, with interruption of the internal elastic lamina (stained black) and replacement of the inner part of the wall by fibrous tissue. There is more diffuse inflammatory cellular infiltrate. × 70. (The late Dr. Janet Niven.)

eventually results from lesions in the kidneys, heart or other vital organs.

Clinical features depend on the number and sites of lesions, and as these are widespread and vary greatly in their distribution, the clinical features also show great variation. In severe cases there is fever, prostration, neutrophil (and sometimes eosinophil) leucocytosis and a very high ESR. In less acute cases the disease fluctuates, with quiescent periods and exacerbations. Lesions in the small arteries of peripheral nerves result in paraesthesias, and symptoms may arise from ischaemia of virtually any tissue. Angina, cardiac failure, renal failure and hypertension are among the commoner clinical manifestations, but infarction of the gut, etc., can also cause death.

The diagnosis can be confirmed by skeletal muscle biopsy, particularly if tissue is removed from a tender spot in a muscle. Inflammatory changes are much more severe than in the necrotising arteriolar lesions of malignant hypertension.

Aetiology. The arterial lesions of experimentally induced acute immune-complex disease (p. 7.15) resemble those of polyarteritis nodosa. To explain the development of acute lesions over a prolonged period, as in polyarteritis nodosa, it is necessary to assume that fluctuations in the plasma levels of postulated antigen and antibody results, from time to time, in the formation of heavy concentrations of immune complexes in the circulation. In support of the disease being due to a hypersensitivity type 3 reaction, immunoglobulins and products of activation of complement have been demonstrated in the acute lesions, accompanied by hypocomplementaemia. The condition sometimes occurs in chronic carriers of hepatitis B virus with circulating HBsAg-Ab complexes, and also in patients with connective tissue diseases (see below). In most cases, however, the postulated antigen has not been identified, although there is often an association with various drugs, notably sulphonamides and penicillin.

Arteritis with lesions indistinguishable from polyarteritis nodosa occurs occasionally in patients suffering from the **connective tissue diseases**. It is usually associated with circulating immune complexes and is accompanied by a fall in serum complement levels. It occurs in patients with severe *rheumatoid arthritis* with high titres of rheumatoid factor and antinuclear antibodies, and in *systemic lupus erythematosus* it is usually associated with the presence of precipitating antibody to DNA. The immunological associations

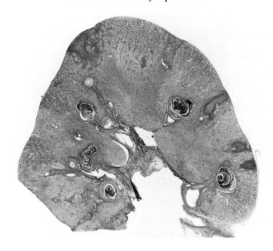

Fig. 14.29 Transverse section of the kidney of a patient who died of acute polyarteritis nodosa. In this instance, the necrotising lesions have resulted in aneurysmal dilatations, together with thrombosis. This has led to multiple infarcts. × 1·4.

of arteritis accompanying *progressive systemic sclerosis* and *dermatomyositis* are less clear.

Histological lesions identical with polyarteritis nodosa are occasionally found incidentally on histological examination of various organs, most commonly the appendix and gallbladder. Such localised arteritis has an excellent prognosis.

There are three conditions which are now considered to be distinct from polyarteritis nodosa. In **Wegener's granulomatosis** there is an arteritis and necrotising granulomatous inflammation in the tissues supplied by the affected arteries. The nasal passages, upper airways, lungs and kidneys tend to be involved. Men are affected twice as commonly as women. There is little evidence of hypersensitivity and serum complement levels are normal. There is a good clinical response to cytotoxic drugs. **Allergic granulomatosis and angiitis** (*Churg–Strauss syndrome* or *eosinophilic granulomatous vasculitis*) is a syndrome characterised by asthma, vasculitis of small arteries and veins and extravascular granulomatous inflammation with necrosis and intense eosinophil infiltration in the surrounding tissues. The lungs are most commonly affected although many other organs may be involved. The prognosis is better than in polyarteritis nodosa or Wegener's

granulomatosis. **Kawasaki disease** or *mucocutaneous lymph node syndrome* affects mainly children. It is a febrile illness characterised by skin rashes, inflammation of the conjunctival and buccal mucosae, generalised lymphadenopathy and sometimes arthritis. There is an arteritis resembling polyarteritis nodosa but, unlike infantile polyarteritis nodosa, spontaneous recovery usually occurs in 3–6 weeks.

Vasculitis of small vessels

In **anaphylactoid (Henoch–Schonlein) purpura** (p. 22.35) necrotising vasculitis of arterioles, capillaries and venules gives rise to small haemorrhages, especially in the skin and gut, and there may also be an associated glomerulonephritis. There is often clinical suspicion of hypersensitivity to microorganisms, for example some cases occur following streptococcal infections.

A **micro-angiopathic form of polyarteritis nodosa** is confined to small arteries, arterioles and capillaries and gives rise to a glomerulonephritis (p. 22.35). In some cases there is evidence of hypersensitivity with formation of immune complexes, for example deposits of HbsAg-Ab complexes (p. 20.11) have been detected in the serum and in the lesions, but in most cases the cause is unknown.

There are many other types of small vessel vasculitis, with or without necrosis, and often predominantly affecting the skin. Since hypersensitivity to drugs, micro-organisms and foodstuffs has been implicated in some cases the term *hypersensitivity vasculitis* is often used, but in most cases the aetiology remains obscure.

Other microangiopathies

As noted above, some generalised forms of vasculitis affect the glomeruli, giving rise to glomerulonephritis. In other instances, the glomeruli are the sole sites of lesions resulting from deposition of immune complexes and this accounts for most of the various types of glomerulonephritis (pp. 22.15–39).

In **diabetes mellitus** of all types there is very commonly a micro-angiopathy of unknown cause (p. 20.64), the most serious consequences of which result from lesions in the retina (p. 21.82) and in the glomeruli (p. 22.39).

Aneurysms

An aneurysm is a localised dilatation of an artery caused by stretching of the wall. Symmetrical stretching of the whole circumference produces a *fusiform* aneurysm, while stretching of part of the circumference causes a *saccular* aneurysm, which bulges from one side of the artery and may be connected to it by a quite small aperture These terms may not be applicable to advanced lesions, which are often very irregular in form.

The term *dissecting aneurysm* is used to describe a condition in which the wall of an artery (usually the aorta) splits, and blood tracks along the media, separating the inner from the outer layers. The lumen is not dilated and so the condition is not really an aneurysm. Some other lesions are loosely described as aneurysms (p. 14.34).

Pathogenesis. The force which expands an aneurysm is the blood pressure, but for an aneurysm to form there must be an arterial lesion which weakens the media locally. Stretching usually results in further weakening, so that once an aneurysm has started it tends to expand and commonly ruptures. Occasionally thrombus forms in thick layers which fill the whole sac.

Atheromatous aneurysm

In Europe and N. America, atheroma is now the most common cause of true aortic aneurysm, due to the early treatment of syphilis and the concurrent increase in atheroma. Atheromatous aneurysms occur usually after the age of 50, and much more commonly in men than women. They are usually fusiform (Fig. 14.30) and may rupture while still quite small. The aneurysm forms as a result of weakening of the media overlying atheromatous plaques or actual extension of the plaque into the media. The microscopic changes seen at the edges of the aneurysm are those of atheroma, sometimes with a marked leucocytic reaction around the fatty debris, and there may be some lymphocytic infiltration round the vasa vasorum in the adventitia and media. These aneurysms are usually a complication of *severe* atheroma and affect especially the abdominal aorta or a common iliac artery. They usually arise below the level of the renal arteries.

Effects. Large aneurysms are very liable to rupture with retroperitoneal or intraperitoneal haemorrhage, the clinical features being those of an acute surgical abdominal emergency. The aneurysmal sac is nearly always partly filled by thrombus which may cause ischaemia of the legs, either by occluding the iliac arteries or by embolism. Pressure effects are not conspicuous.

Syphilitic aneurysm

This occurs as a complication of syphilitic aortitis, usually above the age of 40. Large aortic aneurysms were previously due in most instances to syphilis, but are now very rare as a result of successful treatment in the primary and secondary stages of the disease. The commonest site is the aortic arch, because it is the part most frequently affected by syphilitic mesaortitis (p. 14.22), of which aneurysm is a complication. The focal loss of elastica and muscle in the media results in weakening of the wall, and there may be diffuse dilatation of the ascending aorta and arch: more localised stretching results in a fusiform or saccular aneurysm, which is often accompanied by smaller aneurysmal bulgings, along with the stellate scars and intimal thickening characteristic of syphilitic mesaortitis. If dilatation of the root of the aorta results in aortic valve incompetence, the forcible systolic thrust (p. 15.32) increases the likelihood of aneurysm formation. As an aneurysm forms, the elastic tissue and muscle of the artery wall soon degenerate and the sac comes to be composed of layers of fibrous tissue, on which laminated thrombus forms (Fig. 10.18, p. 10.15). Blood may infiltrate the wall of the aneurysm and ooze for some distance into the tissues around, obscuring its outer surface.

Effects. *Pressure* on surrounding structures leads to the syndrome of superior mediastinal compression; the great veins may be displaced and undergo thrombosis, resulting in congestion of the head and neck and enlargement of

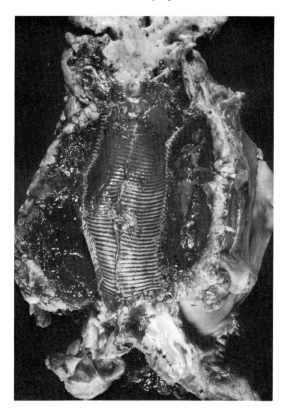

Fig. 14.30 Atheromatous aneurysm of the abdominal aorta arising below the origins of the renal arteries. The aneurysm, which is fusiform, has been repaired by a dacron tube, but death resulted from haemorrhage from rupture at the suture line.

collateral veins. Involvement of the oesophagus may cause dysphagia, while pressure on a major bronchus may cause a chronic cough and suppurating bronchopneumonia. Aneurysms of the transverse part of the aortic arch may compress and stretch the left recurrent laryngeal nerve and cause paralysis of the left vocal cord. Rigid structures such as the bodies of vertebrae may be eroded and incorporated into the wall of the sac; the intervertebral discs offer greater resistance to absorption and persist longer.

Rupture of an aneurysm results in massive haemorrhage into an adjacent body cavity or any hollow viscus to which the aneurysm has become adherent, and occasionally externally through the chest wall.

Embolism from thrombus formed within an aneurysm is surprisingly uncommon.

Cardiac hypertrophy and dilatation occur only when the syphilitic mesaortitis results in aortic valve incompetence. Otherwise aortic aneurysms, even very large ones, do not affect the heart as there is no interference with cardiac output.

Dissecting aortic aneurysm

Although not common, this is the least rare cause of rupture of the aorta. The initiating event is usually a tear in the inner part of the wall of the aorta, through which blood enters and tracks betweeen the inner two-thirds and outer third of the media, dissecting the wall into inner and outer layers. In most patients the blood bursts through the thinner outer layer of the wall, usually within the first few days, and without surgical treatment the condition is usually fatal from massive haemorrhage. The lumen of the aorta is not enlarged and the condition is therefore not a true aneurysm: *dissecting aortic haematoma* would be a better name.

The initial tear usually occurs transversely in the ascending aorta (Fig. 14.31). It is usually less than 3 cm in length but may involve almost the whole circumference. The extent of dissection varies greatly: in some patients the blood entering the media bursts out through the remainder of the wall almost immediately, with little dissection; occasionally the dissection remains localised and thrombosis and organisation of the blood in the media result in healing. In most cases, however, blood tracks proximally and distally in the media. Commonly it reaches the aortic ring and ruptures into the pericardial sac, causing death from cardiac tamponade. It may also track distally along the arch and abdominal aorta, and rupture may result in fatal haemorrhage into the mediastinum, pleura, retroperitoneal tissue or peritoneal cavity.

Depending on the extent of the dissection, the blood in the media can compress any of the vessels leaving the aorta and can track along them, causing acute ischaemia: the coronary arteries are most often affected in this way and myocardial infarction can result.

Occasionally a second tear occurs in the inner part of the aortic wall before the blood in the media has clotted. This sometimes happens in an atheromatous patch in the abdominal aorta and the blood can pass through the second tear

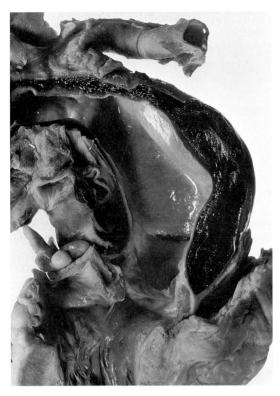

Fig. 14.31 Dissecting aneurysm of the aorta. There is a transverse tear of the inner part of the wall of the ascending aorta and blood has tracked proximally and distally within the media. Death was caused by haemopericardium. × 0·5.

and re-enter the lumen. If the patient survives, the second channel thus formed in the media becomes thickened by fibrous tissue formation and lined by endothelium, giving a 'double-barrelled' aorta (Fig. 14.32).

Clinically, dissecting aneurysm is usually accompanied by severe tearing pain in the chest; the patient becomes shocked and death may occur at any time from haemorrhage or from compression of the coronary or other aortic branches. Most cases are fatal within a few days, but early diagnosis and prompt surgical treatment to arrest the dissection by sutures have greatly improved the immediate prognosis.

Aetiology. The two important causal factors in dissecting haematoma of the aorta are the blood pressure and weakness of the media. It occurs most often during physical exertion and in hypertensives. Men are affected more often than women, in whom the condition tends to occur during or just after pregnancy. Weakness of the media is attributed to a change known as

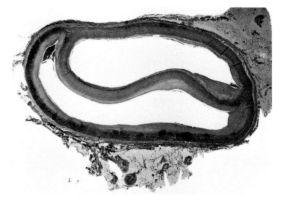

Fig. 14.32 Dissecting aneurysm of the aorta. In this case the blood burst back into the lumen through a second rupture, giving a 'double-barrelled' aorta, seen here in cross section. × 2·5.

Erdheim's medial degeneration, which consists of breaks in elastic fibres and patchy replacement of the musculo-elastic tissue of the media by amorphous metachromatic material resembling ground substance (Fig. 14.33). There may also be foci of necrosis, hence the alternative term *medionecrosis*, although this is rare. During ventricular systole the frictional force of the blood thrusts the intima in the direction of blood flow, and it seems likely that the patchy degeneration of the media allows irregular increase in this sliding movement of the inner part of the wall and that eventually this leads to the tear. Once this has happened the lesions in the media facilitate dissection by the escaping blood. This explanation is largely speculative. The medial degeneration is fairly common after middle age, particularly in hypertensives, and while it is often severe in patients with dissecting aneurysm, it is sometimes minimal. However, changes resembling Erdheim's degeneration are a feature of Marfan's syndrome (see below) in which it no doubt explains the high incidence of dissecting aneurysm.

Various other arteries may be affected apart from the aorta, usually following trauma or in relation to a pregnancy.

Disorders of connective tissue formation. Some of the inherited defects of formation of connective tissue result in formation of aneurysms, in dissecting aneurysm of the aorta, or in rupture of various arteries. The least rare example in **Marfan's syndrome**, which is inherited usually as an autosomal dominant, and characterised by laxity of ligaments, e.g. of

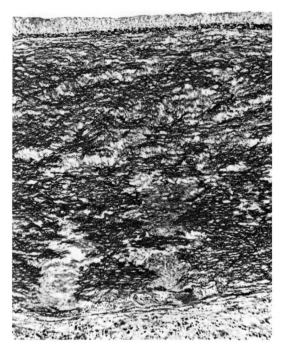

Fig. 14.33 Medial degeneration of the aorta. There are irregular gaps in the elastic tissue of the media, which is stained black. The patient was a woman of 24 who died of spontaneous rupture of the aorta. × 50.

joints and of the eye lens, inadequate elastic fibre formation in the aorta, tall slim build, long tapering fingers (*arachnodactyly*) and other skeletal abnormalities. Disturbances of vision result from subluxation of the lens, and there may also be deafness. The aortic media lacks elastic fibres, the appearances resembling those in Erdheim's medial degeneration. Fusiform aneurysm or dissecting aneurysm may result, and at necropsy there may be multiple healed aortic intimal tears.

Dissecting aortic aneurysms and rupture of various arteries occur also in some types of the Ehlers–Danlos syndrome.

Other causes of aortic rupture. Apart from aneurysm, rupture of the aorta may result from damage to its wall from outside, as by the perforation of an impacted fishbone or other sharp foreign body in the oesophagus; also from very severe injury such as crushing of the chest. In children traumatic rupture can occur without fracture of the ribs. Carcinoma of bronchus or oesophagus may invade the aortic wall and cause fatal haemorrhage.

Infective (mycotic) aneurysm

This may occur at the beginning of the aorta by direct extension of micro-organisms from vegetations in bacterial endocarditis, particularly *Staphylococcus aureus*. The organisms settle on the intima, an infective thrombus forms, invasion and weakening of the wall follow, and an *acute aneurysm* is produced, which may rupture.

Depending on the virulence of the micro-organisms, host resistance and antibiotic therapy, impaction of infected emboli in an artery or its vasa vasorum may be followed by elimination of the bacteria and organisation of the embolus or by suppurative destruction of the artery wall, rupture and severe haemorrhage. Between these two extremes, less severe inflammatory damage to the artery wall may result in a mycotic aneurysm. Multiple embolic arterial lesions are commonly seen in pyaemia, and are known as **pyaemic abscesses** (p. 9.8).

A mycotic aneurysm is sometimes seen in the wall of a tuberculous pulmonary cavity and may cause fatal haemoptysis. Usually, however, occlusion of the vessel by endarteritis obliterans or thrombosis prevents aneurysm formation.

Cerebral aneurysms

Aneurysms of the major cerebral arteries, commonly termed 'berry' aneurysms, occur in 1–2% of adults. Most of them are apparently symptomless and are found incidentally at autopsy, but they may rupture and bleed into the subarachnoid space or adjacent brain tissue and are responsible for about 4000 deaths annually in the UK. For their size, the cerebral arteries are thin-walled; the media is particularly thin, and the internal elastic lamina is often fragmented at the sites of arterial branching, which is where most of these aneurysms develop from adolescence onwards (the term *congenital aneurysm* is incorrect). Congenital gaps in the medial smooth muscle have been blamed, but such gaps are commonly present in the cerebral arteries of people who do not develop aneurysms. Deficient production of type III collagen, which is a major constituent of vascular walls, has been reported in a proportion of patients with ruptured cerebral aneurysms (Pope *et al.*, 1981),

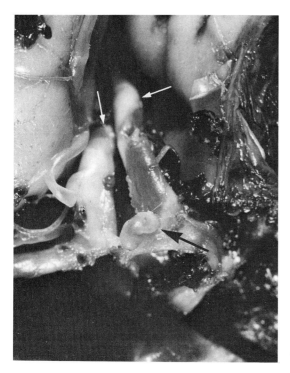

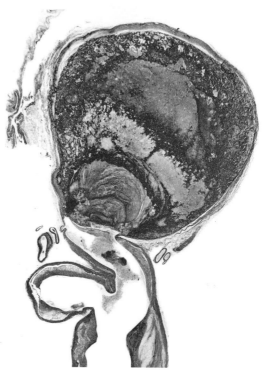

Fig. 14.34 Base of the brain showing subarachnoid haemorrhage which resulted from rupture of a berry aneurysm of the basilar artery (not shown). A second, intact aneurysm (*black arrow*) is seen on the anterior communicating artery. (The anterior cerebral arteries are marked by white arrows.)

Fig. 14.35 Aneurysm of circle of Willis, almost completely filled with thrombus. × 7·5.

and atheromatous thinning of the media (p. 14.7) may sometimes be involved. The discerning reader will have realised that the cause of these aneurysms is obscure. While rupture may occur in young or middle-aged adults, the peak incidence is between 40 and 50. Rupture often occurs during physical exertion, and systemic hypertension probably increases the risk of aneurysm formation and rupture.

A berry aneurysm is a small rounded sac projecting from the wall of an artery (Fig. 14.34): most are 2–6 mm in diameter, but an occasional aneurysm grows as large as 4 cm. The wall is thin, delicate and transparent and consists mainly of fibrous tissue lined by endothelium. It usually contains little or no trace of the internal elastic lamina or medial smooth muscle. As with aneurysms elsewhere, the sac may be partly or completely occluded by thrombus (Fig. 14.35).

The sites of occurrence and effects of rupture are described more fully on pp. 21.20–22.

Micro-aneurysms. The occurrence of multiple micro-aneurysms of the small cerebral arterial twigs in hypertensive subjects was described over a century ago, but they are difficult to find by routine autopsy methods. Using radiological techniques combined with histological examination, Ross Russell (1963) and Cole and Yates (1967) have confirmed the occurrence of multiple micro-aneurysms (usually 15–25) in the brain in over 50% of hypertensive subjects more than 50 years old, and only in occasional normotensives, usually over 65 years old. The aneurysms develop in arteries of 50–300 μm diameter and measure up to 900 μm; they are most numerous in and around the basal ganglia, where they arise at bifurcations of the smaller striate arterial branches. They are found also, although less frequently, in the cerebral subcortical white matter, midbrain and cerebellum.

The aneurysms may be saccular (Fig. 14.36) or fusiform, and the adjacent artery and wall of the sac show hyaline thickening of the intima, sometimes with fibrinoid change: the internal

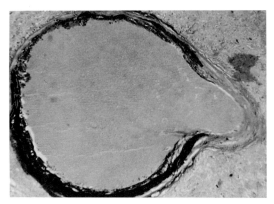

Fig. 14.36 A micro-aneurysm of a small cerebral artery. The wall of the sac is thinned and hyaline and is impregnated with fibrin (*stained black*). × 180 (By courtesy of Dr Ross Russell and the editor of *Brain*).

elastic lamina is usually absent from, or fragmented in, the wall of the sac, and muscle is usually absent. Thrombus, sometimes organised, may adhere to the wall or fill the sac, and there is often evidence of old or recent leakage of blood into the surrounding tissues.

Micro-aneurysms are detectable in most individuals dying from cerebral haemorrhage, and the above workers have provided evidence which suggests strongly that rupture of such aneurysms is the usual cause of cerebral haemorrhage in hypertensive subjects.

Other forms of aneurysm

Injury to the wall of an artery by a penetrating wound or blunt trauma may result in the development of a **traumatic aneurysm** due to stretching of the fibrous scar. Complete rupture of an artery may give rise to a **false aneurysm** in which the sac is formed by fibrous tissue.

Injury of an adjacent artery and vein may result in an arterio-venous fistula: in some instances the connection is by a channel with a fibrous wall, which may dilate to form an **arterio-venous aneurysm**.

A **cirsoid** or **racemose aneurysm** is a form of arterio-venous fistula which appears as a pulsatile swelling consisting of tortuous and dilated arteries and veins with multiple intercommunications. The commonest site is the scalp, and it may cause pressure atrophy of the underlying bone. The condition is sometimes congenital, but more often the result of a blow on the head; some of the allegedly congenital cases are probably the result of birth injury. Similarly a carotid-cavernous sinus aneurysm resulting from fracture of the skull base gives rise to great engorgement of the orbital veins and oedema of the orbit and conjunctiva.

Other arterial diseases

Raynaud's disease

Nomenclature. In 1862 Maurice Raynaud described a series of cases of intermittent impairment of the circulation through the extremeties, usually presenting as an abnormal response to exposure to cold. It has since become apparent that these effects can occur in subjects with or without organic vascular disease. There has been considerable confusion over nomenclature, but it is now customary to apply the term *primary Raynaud's disease* to cases apparently due wholly to abnormal angiospasm and to group together under the term *secondary Raynaud's disease* cases in which organic vascular changes play a major role.

Primary Raynaud's disease occurs mainly in women, usually starting in adolescence and often continuing indefinitely. It usually affects the fingers of both hands symetrically and occasionally the tip of the nose, ears and toes. On exposure to cold the fingers become cold, white or cyanotic and may be numb or extremely painful. The circulation is restored by warmth, but trophic changes may occur in the skin and whitlows are common: ulceration and gangrene seldom occur unless exposure to cold is prolonged.

Histological reports on the condition are few, because material is not usually excised unless gangrene develops. Thickening of the digital arteries has been reported, but these vessels are normally very thick walled, and reports of

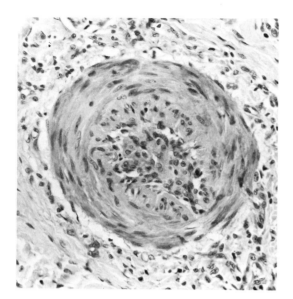

Fig. 14.37 Transverse section of a digital artery in Raynaud's disease. The lumen is obliterated by cellular fibrous tissue which has resulted from organisation of thrombus. × 250.

thickening have usually been erroneous. In cases where gangrene develops, however, there may be thrombosis and recanalised vessels may be found (Fig. 14.37).

The condition appears to be an exaggeration of the normal response to exposure to cold. Preganglionic sympathectomy is not curative.

Secondary Raynaud's disease. This consists of symptoms similar to those of Raynaud's disease, but attributable to organic vascular disease, including thromboangiitis obliterans, use of vibratory power tools, progressive systemic sclerosis and systemic lupus erythematosus. It can result also from vasoconstriction in response to cold superimposed on organic vascular disease, from arrest of the circulation in the extremities by cryoglobulins, and from agglutination of red cells in cold-antibody auto-immune haemolytic anaemia.

Involvement is not always symmetrical, and sympathectomy does not usually improve the condition. Both sexes are affected and, depending on the causal condition, gangrene may develop.

Calcification of the media (Mönckeberg's sclerosis)

Definition. This is a degenerative disease of unknown cause characterised by dystrophic calcification in the media, especially common in the major arteries of the lower limbs in elderly people. It may also affect the arteries of the upper limbs, and less commonly visceral arteries.

Naked-eye appearances. The affected vessels are generally dilated and show transverse bars of medial calcification due to deposition of calcium in the circular medial muscle layer (Fig. 14.38). At a later

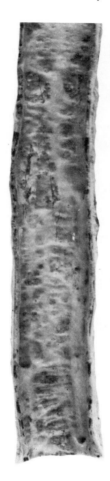

Fig. 14.38 Calcification of media of iliac artery, showing transverse markings caused by confluent calcification. × 0·8.

stage, lengths of the arteries may be converted into rigid tubes. There may be no noteworthy alteration of the intima though atheroma is sometimes present in addition.

Microscopy shows that the earliest change is hyaline degeneration of the muscle fibres and fibrous tissue, usually starting about the middle of the media. Calcium salts are deposited first as fine granules, and confluent calcification follows (Fig. 14.39). There may be little or no cellular reaction. Occasion-

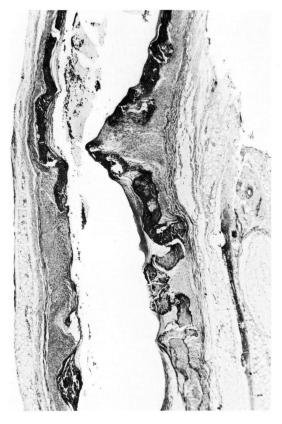

Fig. 14.39 Calcification of media. The calcified tissue is darkly stained. × 16.

ally true bone may be formed in an area of calcification, and may even contain red marrow.

Aetiology. This is generally regarded as an exaggeration of the normal increase of calcium salts in the arteries with age. It sometimes occurs earlier in arteriosclerotic vessels but in man is not intimately related to high blood pressure. A similar lesion has been produced in the aorta of rabbits by injections of adrenaline.

Effects. The radiological appearance is striking but the lumina of the arteries are seldom narrowed, and ischaemic effects, if present, are usually due to co-existing atheroma.

Fibromuscular dysplasia

This is a condition of unknown aetiology which affects medium and large arteries. There are various types but in all of them the structure of the artery wall is focally abnormal. Most often there is fibrous or fibromuscular thickening of the wall leading to stenosis. Sometimes alteration of the normal structure of the media gives rise to true aneurysms and occasionally to dissecting aneurysms. These conditions are rare and occur mainly in females. The renal arteries are most commonly affected, giving rise to renal hypertension (p. 14.15), but the carotid, vertebral and splanchnic arteries may also be involved.

Diseases of Veins

Compensatory enlargement of the veins takes place, as in the arterial system, when there is a sustained increase in blood flow, as in the uterine veins during pregnancy and in the collateral veins following obstruction of a major vein. As in the case of arteries, dilatation is followed by hypertrophy of the various elements in the wall of the vessels. Veins are, of course, not exposed to the marked variations of blood pressure which occur in arteries, but when they are subject to persistent over-distension, compensatory changes occur in their walls. There is little or no hyperplasia of the muscle, but the elastic tissue increases greatly and then undergoes degeneration; the fibrous tissue also increases and becomes hyaline (Fig. 14.40). Localised patches of thickening in the intima of veins are quite common and probably result from organisation of thrombus.

Acute thrombophlebitis

A distinction is sometimes made between *thrombophlebitis*, by which is meant a primary inflammatory condition of the vein, with secondary thrombosis, and *phlebothrombosis* (p. 10.15), in which a bland thrombosis of the vein occurs with, at most, mild preceding inflammatory change. In many instances the distinction is more theoretical than practical because

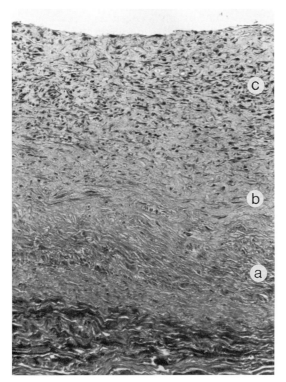

Fig. 14.40 Longitudinal section of the wall of a saphenous vein used to replace a length of an atheromatous coronary artery two years before death. The lumen is at the top and the dark fibres at the bottom are dense collagen fibres of the adventitia. The smooth muscle of the media has undergone atrophy and persists only as an ill-defined dark layer (a) near the periphery of the wall. Above this, the relatively acellular layer (b) represents fibrosed and thickened media and the more cellular (inner) layer (c) consists of greatly thickened intima which contains elastic fibres, collagen and large spindle cells. × 120.

the presence of thrombus in the lumen of the vein sets up reactive changes so that differentiation between mild thrombophlebitis and phlebothrombosis may no longer be possible. In **thromboangiitis obliterans**, however, veins are often affected and exhibit the same rather characteristic florid inflammatory lesions seen in arteries in this condition (Fig. 14.25, p. 14.25). The available evidence suggests that the inflammation is primary and the thrombosis a consequence of it.

Multiple venous thrombosis also occurs in **thrombophlebitis migrans** but without arterial involvement: it usually affects superficial veins, but sometimes also deeper ones, in any part of the body. In many cases the cause is not apparent, but in others it is associated with a carcinoma, most often of the pancreas but also of breast, stomach, bronchus, ovary, etc. The thrombotic episodes may be the first clinical manifestation of the cancer. In some cases, small vegetations form on the cardiac valves.

Outbreaks of a condition known as **tropical thrombophlebitis** have been reported in Africans: thrombosis is widespread and death may result from involvement of visceral veins. The cause is unknown.

Infective thrombophlebitis used to be seen commonly in the veins of the diploë and dural sinuses in middle-ear disease, in the uterine veins in puerperal sepsis, in the veins of the bone marrow in suppurative osteomyelitis, and occasionally in the pulmonary veins in cases of bronchiectasis. Veins involved in such lesions undergo thrombosis and the thrombus becomes invaded by bacteria, and then by polymorphs: fragments may break away and produce pyaemia.

In the rare condition known as *pylephlebitis suppurativa* (*portal pylephlebitis*) infection, e.g. from appendicitis, involves a small tributary of the portal vein and leads to progressive ascending thrombosis and suppuration, from which multiple abscesses in the liver may result.

Thrombophlebitis may also appear as a complication of conditions in which there is a bacteraemia, notably typhoid fever, and it is presumed that organisms circulating in the blood settle in the intima and produce an acute endophlebitis with secondary thrombosis.

Chronic phlebitis

Chronic inflammatory processes may spread to the walls of the veins and lead to reactive thickening; in fact, the smallest veins are affected in this way in all chronic inflammatory conditions. Chronic phlebitis of obscure origin is occasionally observed in the large vessels, for example in the portal vein, and may lead to thrombosis; cavernous tissue develops in the portal fissure and after some time it may be impossible to say whether the changes are congenital or secondary to the thrombosis.

Endophlebitis of the hepatic veins is the basis of the veno-occlusive disease of Jamaica and certain other tropical regions (see p. 20.5) and involvement of the hepatic ostia with thrombosis gives rise to the Budd–Chiari syndrome (p. 20.5). Hepatic endophlebitis also results from infestation with liver flukes and schistosomes.

Tuberculous invasion of veins most commonly results when a caseous lesion—usually in a pulmonary hilar lymph node—involves and destroys the wall of a vein: huge numbers of tubercle bacilli then enter the bloodstream and cause generalised miliary tuberculosis.

Veins are often invaded by **malignant tumours** which may then release cells singly or in groups, with the danger of metastatic growth in the lungs, etc. Cancer may also grow along the lumen of veins, an example being clear-cell carcinoma of the kidney, which commonly extends along the renal vein and even the inferior vena cava. Such invasion is usually accompanied by thrombosis.

Varicose veins

Dilatation and tortuosity of veins is termed *varicosity*. The changes may affect a group of veins diffusely or take the form of saccular dilatations. Varicosity of veins arises from chronic continuous or recurrent increase in the pressure of the blood within them, and this results mainly either from (*a*) the effects of gravity, e.g. in the leg veins, sometimes aggravated by compression proximally, or (*b*) obstruction of a major vein, leading to increased pressure in collateral veins.

'Gravitational' varicosity occurs in the saphenous system of the legs, notably the long saphenous vein. The condition is much commoner in women and there is a distinct *hereditary predisposition*. *Prolonged standing* upright without much muscular movement causes marked rise in pressure and distension of the long saphenous vein, for the valves can only play their part in breaking the venous pressure gradient between the heart and the foot if assisted by the pumping action of muscular activity of the lower limbs. Eventually the veins become permanently stretched, so that the valves are now incompetent, and even muscular activity does not protect the veins from increased pressure in the upright position; in consequence, stretching tends to progress and the

veins become visibly swollen and tortuous, i.e. varicose. Venous stasis occurs in the legs due to the pressure of the gravid uterus on the iliac veins and without doubt *pregnancy* is a predisposing cause of varicose veins; this probably accounts for the higher incidence in women, although *obesity* is also a predisposing factor. The venous valves and the muscle and elastic tissue of the vein walls atrophy somewhat irregularly so that thinning of the wall and pouch-like dilatations occur; finally the wall comes to be composed chiefly of fibrous tissue. The nutrition of the skin over varicose veins of the legs may be impaired. The skin becomes eczematous and pigmented, and chronic indolent 'varicose ulceration' often follows; dilated veins involved in such ulcers may bleed severely, but this is easily stopped by raising the leg with the patient lying flat. Thrombosis is also apt to follow. Organisation of the thrombus is generally imperfect and it may become calcified.

Varicocele is another common example of 'gravitational' varicosity, in the pampiniform plexus of veins around the spermatic cord: it is commoner on the left side than on the right and various ingenious explanations have been suggested for this. The distended veins feel like a bag of worms. It often depresses spermatogenesis and impairs fertility, particularly if bilateral. This may be a temperature effect.

Haemorrhoids consist of varicosities of the haemorrhoidal venous plexuses, projecting from the surface just above or below the anorectal junction. They are common in pregnancy, probably due to the pressure of the uterus on the pelvic veins, and also in people over 40 in whom constipation and straining at stool are causal factors. Portal hypertension, e.g. in cirrhosis, is also believed to be a predisposing factor.

Haemorrhoids may bleed and cause iron deficiency, or they may rupture into the perianal subcutaneous tissue, causing painful swellings. They may also become thrombosed or prolapse through the anal sphincter and become strangulated.

'Obstructive' varicosity. This is exemplified by chronic *obstruction to the portal venous blood flow* (due most commonly to cirrhosis or schistosomiasis of the liver), in which the vessels which form anastomoses between the portal and systemic venous systems become varicose (p. 20.34): the most important ones are those run-

ning longitudinally in the oesophageal and gas
tric submucosa (Fig. 19.18, p. 19.13), for they
may rupture and bleed profusely. *Obstruction
of the inferior vena cava* brings about dilatation
of the veins of the abdominal wall, establishing
a collateral circulation through veins in the
thoracic wall (Fig. 10.7, p. 10.6). *Obstruction
of the superior vena cava* may occur in cases of
bronchial carcinoma and other mediastinal
masses and leads to severe dusky cyanosis of
the head, neck and arms, sometimes accompanied by pitting oedema of the hands.

Tumours and Malformations of Blood Vessels

Angiomas

Haemangioma. A haemangioma consists of a
mass of blood vessels, atypical or irregular in
arrangement and size. A corresponding growth,
lymphangioma, is composed of lymphatic vessels similarly altered; but, as this is rarer, the
term angioma is often used as synonymous with
haemangioma.

The majority of the lesions called angiomas
are not true tumours, but hamartomas (p.
12.47). They are present at birth, even if not
always visible, and their enlargement ceases
with the growth of the patient. Most angiomas
are well-defined masses of vascular tissue which
resemble tumours sufficiently to justify their inclusion here. The two common varieties are as
follows.

(*a*) *Capillary angiomas* consist of dense
branching network of vessels of capillary size
(Fig. 14.41). They occur especially in the skin,
where they form one of the two common types
of **naevus** or birthmark, but are also seen in the
internal organs. Most are small, but larger
lesions occur, e.g. the 'port wine stains' of the
face, which consist of capillary-like vessels with
an abnormally large lumen. Capillary angiomas
are usually well defined, and deep red or purple.
The vessels have a more prominent endothelial
lining than normal capillaries and endothelial
cells may be seen scattered or in clusters without formation of a lumen (Fig. 14.41). The
stroma consists of well-formed collagen. There
is no capsule, and at the margin the capillaries
often give a false impression of invasion of the
adjacent tissues. The blood supply is usually
clearly separated from that of the surrounding
tissues, there being generally only one artery of
supply.

(*b*) *Cavernous angiomas* are found in the skin,
subcutaneous tissue, lips and tongue and also
in the liver. They consist of relatively large interconnecting sinus-like vascular spaces (Fig.
14.42). In the liver they form deep-purple well-
defined masses, usually polygonal rather than
round and not raised above the surface, signs
of their lack of expansile growth.

Angiomas are often multiple, and are also an
important component of several diseases with
a strong genetic predisposition, e.g. hereditary

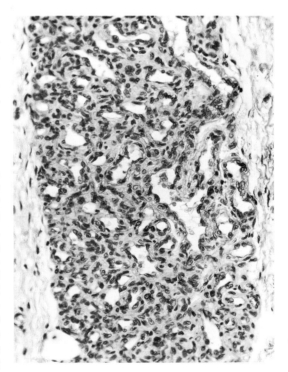

Fig. 14.41 Capillary angioma showing well-formed
capillaries with prominent endothelial cells. The solid
areas between capillaries include many cells which
appear to be endothelial cells not related to a lumen.
× 200.

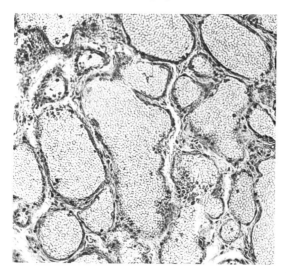

Fig. 14.42 Cavernous angioma of subcutaneous tissue, showing large intercommunicating spaces filled with blood. × 130.

haemorrhagic telangiectasia (multiple small angiomas in skin and mucosae with a strong tendency to haemorrhage—p. 17.64), Lindau's disease (cerebellar and retinal angiomas with cysts of liver and pancreas) and Sturge–Weber syndrome (facial and meningeal angiomas).

The nature of 'sclerosing angioma' (*histiocytoma* or *dermatofibroma*) of the skin is uncertain (p. 27.36).

Glomangioma (glomus tumour). This uncommon but interesting lesion apparently arises from the glomus bodies, small arteriovenous anastomoses with a coiled arteriole and abundant nerve supply, which control blood flow and temperature, particularly in the fingers and toes. In its most characteristic form, the glomangioma is a small bluish nodule, usually near the end of a finger, and extraordinarily tender to even light touch. On microscopic examination the tumour is found to consist of two kinds of tissue variously interblended (Fig. 14.43). The first is angiomatous, with spaces containing blood, lined by endothelium, and separated by connective tissue containing varying amounts of smooth muscle. The other is cellular, with rounded or cuboidal cells called 'myoid', as transitions to smooth muscle fibres can be found. The growth contains numerous myelinated and non-myelinated nerve fibres and the pain is apparently due to distensile pressures in the blood-containing spaces, though the painfulness is not in proportion to the neural content. Glomangiomas have been described in deeper tissues, including the gut, but the characteristic pain occurs only with those in the limbs.

Small dermal leiomyomas, apparently derived from vascular smooth muscle, are also sometimes painful and may be related to glomangioma.

Chemodectoma. This tumour arises from the glomus tissue derived from the branchial arches, viz. the carotid body, glomus jugulare and aortico-pulmonary bodies. Chemodectomas occur also in various other sites, including the organ of Zuckerkandl. They are sometimes (incorrectly) termed non-chromaffin paragangliomas, and do not appear to produce any

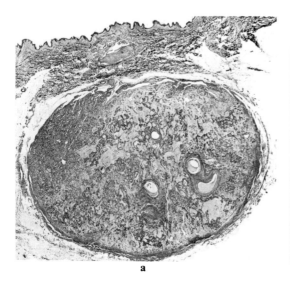

a

Fig. 14.43a Glomangioma. Small subcutaneous encapsulated growth showing the coiled arteriole. × 8.

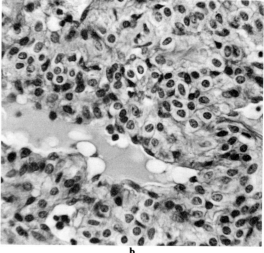

b

Fig. 14.43b The clear myoid cells surrounding a vascular space. × 350.

endocrine effect. They are nearly always benign but their anatomical site may render complete removal difficult. The least rare example occurs in the carotid body: it has an increased frequency in people living at high altitudes, for example in the High Andes (and also in their cattle) where hyperplasia due to hypoxaemia (p. 16.63) is a predisposing factor. Most carotid body tumours seen in clinical practice at sea level are not, however, associated with chronic hypoxia. These tumours may grow to several centimetres in diameter. They embrace and press on the bifurcation of the common carotid artery and torrential haemorrhage is a danger during surgical removal. Histologically, the tumour is composed of clusters of chief cells with clear cytoplasm and a round nucleus, the so-called 'zellenballen', enclosed in a box-like framework of fine fibrous tissue and with a rich sinusoidal blood supply (Fig. 14.44) The tumour cells are usually polygonal but may be spindle-shaped in places. Uncommonly there are aberrant cells with hyperchromatic nuclei, which are not an indication of malignancy, but rare tumours are malignant and metastasise to the regional lymph nodes.

Chemodectomas at other sites have the same general features as those of the carotid bodies. **Glomus jugulare** tumours present usually as recurrent bleeding aural polyps arising in the middle ear, but they may also present intracranially.

Structures resembling glomic tissue and of unknown function are seen occasionally around pulmonary venules. They resemble small chemodectomas or hyperplastic nodules of glomic tissue but on electron microscopy their cells are elongated and resemble sustentacular (type II) rather than chief (type I) cells.

Malignant vascular tumours

With the possible exception of Kaposi's sarcoma, which is relatively common in parts of Africa, true tumours of blood vessels are rare.

Occasionally a lesion with the histological features of haemangioma grows unusually rapidly and is classed by some as a *haemangio-endothelioma*. Very rarely an apparent capillary haemangioma gives rise to metastases and thus merits the term *haemangio-endotheliosarcoma*. This latter term is also applied to malignant tumours which show the cellular abnormalities characteristic of malignancy, but in which the neoplastic cells also show, in places, the structural arrangement of endothelial cells lining a lumen.

Rare tumours also arise from vascular pericytes (*haemangio-pericytoma*), the tumour cells being separated from vascular endothelium by basement-membrane material demonstrable by silver impregnation staining techniques. Some remain localised, but others metastasise.

Exposure to vinyl chloride monomer predisposes to the otherwise very rare *haemangiosarcoma of the liver* (p. 20.42), but it is not certain that this tumour arises from vascular endothelium.

Kaposi's Sarcoma

In 1872 Moricz Kaposi described five patients with an unusual vascular tumour of the skin. Similar cases were subsequently reported from many parts of Europe and North America, though it was an extremely rare malignancy except in southern Europe, being observed particularly in Italians and in Jews. In the United States the tumour occurred with equal frequency in black and white races.

This **sporadic form** of Kaposi's sarcoma usually occurs in elderly men and is characterised by the development of multiple haemorrhagic lesions of the skin, particularly on the hands and feet; these lesions are nodular or plaque-like and the disease often runs a benign course, though a few patients develop systemic spread.

Histologically, the tumour has a characteristic appearance. It consists of groups of spindle cells with slits between the cells giving a sieve-pattern (Fig. 14.45). Red cells are often seen in these slits, though the appearances are not those of endothelial-lined blood vessels: they may be present in the centre or periphery of the nodules of tumour. Kaposi's sarcoma appears to be derived from a primitive angioformative mesenchymal cell and can be differen-

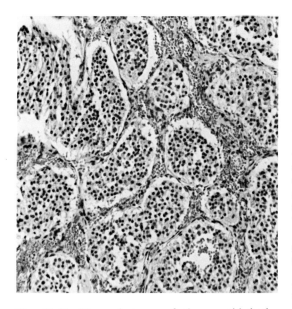

Fig. 14.44 Chemodectoma of the carotid body, showing the characteristic boxlike pattern and highly vascular stroma. × 160.

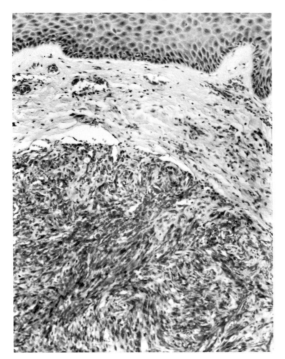

Fig. 14.45 Kaposi's sarcoma. The vascular spindle-celled tumour is separated from the epidermis by a layer of stretched dermis. × 130.

tiated from angiosarcomas, vascular leiomyomas and peritheliomas. Cellular variants without slits and anaplastic types are occasionally seen.

During the 1950s it became apparent that Kaposi's sarcoma was a much commoner tumour in the black populations of sub-Saharan Africa where, in many countries, it accounted for more than 4% of all malignancies: it is the fifth commonest malignancy in males in Zaire and Uganda. This **endemic form** of the tumour occurs in a younger age group than in Europe and some cases run a more aggressive course. The skin lesions in such patients are often florid and fungating and local lymph node metastasis may occur. Death is due to widespread systemic involvement, when nearly all organs may be affected. A par-

ticular feature of this aggressive form is the presence of multiple plaques or nodules in the mucosa of the gastro-intestinal tract. An unusual clinical variant is *lymphadenopathic Kaposi's sarcoma* which is characterised by massive and generalised tumour deposits in the lymph nodes of young children, usually without skin lesions. These patients have a very poor prognosis and die within a year of onset with multiple metastases. Unlike adult cases, the lymphadenopathic form does not show a marked male predominance.

In the 1970s, Kaposi's sarcoma was reported with unusual frequency in patients on prolonged immunosuppression, particularly in those with renal transplants. In 1981, several cases of Kaposi's sarcoma were described in the United States in young homosexual men who subsequently were shown to have AIDS (p. 25.5). In these **epidemic cases** the disease runs a very aggressive course and the early lesions, which consist of small patches, may not show the classical tumour histology but consist of rather bizarre vascular spaces in the dermis; spindle cell proliferation is usually found if carefully sought.

Recently, type III human T-cell leukaemia virus (p. 25.5) has been isolated from these cases and antibodies to this virus are present in most cases. This virus is the cause of AIDS, in which it destroys the T lymphocytes. Immunosuppressed patients with Kaposi's sarcoma also have a high frequency of infection by cytomegalovirus (CMV) and high titres of CMV antibody have also been found in African cases. CMV-related antigens have been demonstrated in tumour biopsies and CMV DNA and RNA in some tumours.

The role of genetic factors in Kaposi's sarcoma has been substantiated by the observation that HLA-DR5 occurs with undue frequency in both epidemic and sporadic cases. The male dominance in endemic cases in Africa and the unusual distribution of incidence in that continent remains unexplained. Some degree of immune depression is common in these populations as a result of their parasitic load in childhood and it is possible that, in such populations, infections with CMV and/or other viruses at an early age may be oncongenic.

Diseases of Lymphatic Vessels

The lymphatic vessels form a closed system separated by an endothelial layer from the tissue spaces. The walls of the small lymphatics are, however, extremely delicate, consisting mainly of a very thin endothelium and an in-

complete basement membrane. Moreover, the junctions between endothelial cells are readily separated (p. 4.24). In consequence organisms, leucocytes and tumour cells readily pass into the lymphatic vessels; also red cells which escape from the capillaries by diapedesis may be present in large numbers in the lymphatics draining an inflamed area. The lymphatic vessels thus afford an easy means of communication between the tissues and lymph nodes. Involvement of the lymph nodes in this way occurs in two main conditions, **infections** and **tumours**, especially carcinoma. In both, the extension may be due to transport of organisms or tumour cells by the lymph stream, i.e. metastasis in the strict sense. There may also be progressive involvement of the lymphatic vessels by the disease. Infections may cause either acute or chronic lymphangitis; in tumours, lymphatic permeation may occur, columns of cancer cells extending along the lymphatics (Figs. 12.33–35, p. 12.23).

Acute lymphangitis. This is seen in pyogenic infections, and is a feature of erysipelas and infections of the extremities, due to haemolytic streptococci. The spread of infection along the lymphatics is sometimes accompanied by visible reddening of the overlying skin, with pain and tenderness and often swelling. Spreading lymphangitis is an important feature in puerperal sepsis and septic abortion and may be followed by cellulitis of the loose connective tissue around the uterus. In other cases of bacterial infection, the organisms are carried by the lymphatic vessels and reach the lymph nodes without causing lymphangitis. A similar striking example is seen in bubonic plague, where even at the site of infection there is usually no inflammatory reaction, the first lesion appearing in the related lymph nodes.

Chronic lymphangitis occurs in various conditions; it may follow *repeated acute attacks of erysipelas*, and is an important feature in many types of *chronic inflammation*. In various chronic infections the spread of organisms by the lymphatics is of great importance. In *tuberculosis*, a disease which in the early stages may be regarded as essentially one of the lymphatic system, the organisms may be carried to lymph nodes without causing lesions on their way. They may, however, settle in the walls of the lymphatic vessels and give rise to tubercles which thus come to form rows along the vessels. In tuberculous ulceration of the intestine, small tubercles may be found along the lymphatics passing from the floor of the ulcer (Fig. 19.59, p. 19.47), and also in the mesenteric lymphatics. The thoracic duct may become involved by

spread of bacilli along the lymph stream and ulceration of these lesions may set free a large number of tubercle bacilli into the circulation to set up acute miliary tuberculosis (p. 9.21).

Lymphatic obstruction: lymphoedema. Chronic obstruction of lymphatics may give rise to interstitial accumulation of lymph (lymphoedema). When this is prolonged there is proliferation of connective tissue in the lymphoedematous area, resulting in a firm, non-pitting oedema. The most striking examples are seen in *filariasis*, in which obstruction of major lymphatics, together with recurrent inflammation in the affected region, may lead to gross thickening of the tissues known as **elephantiasis**: the lower limbs and sometimes the male external genitalia may be involved (p. 28.41). Genital elephantiasis may also occur in the sexually transmitted diseases *lymphogranuloma venereum* (p. 25.3) and *granuloma inguinale* (p. 25.3). In non-tropical countries, extensive carcinomatous permeation of lymphatics is a more common cause of lymphoedema, and also surgical removal of lymphatics or destruction of lymphatics by radiotherapy. This is sometimes seen following radical mastectomy and radiotherapy of the axilla for breast cancer, where the arm may be sufficiently deprived of its lymphatic drainage to develop gross lymphoedema without carcinomatous involvement of lymphatics. Occasionally a malignant tumour develops in the lymphoedematous arm, and has a poor prognosis. In some instances, it is not clear whether the tumour is a sarcoma or metastatic breast carcinoma the appearance of which is modified by the lymphoedematous environment.

Tumours and malformations of lymphatics

Lymphangioma. This may be composed of numerous lymphatic vessels—the *plexiform* lymphangioma—but more frequently it has a *cavernous* structure. Dilatation and diffuse growth of vessels may give rise to enlargement of a part, e.g. the tongue (*macroglossia*). In such lesions there is even less evidence of neoplastic growth than in haemangiomas, and the more diffuse lesions may be hard to distinguish from the effects of lymphatic obstruction, though in most cases it is clear from the anatomy that no such obstruction can be present, and that the lesion is a hamartoma (p. 12.47). It is becoming increasingly common to describe such lesions as *lymphangiectasia* rather than lymphangioma. Lesions, whether diffuse or compact, are commonest in the skin and subcutaneous tissue. Each forms a somewhat ill-defined, doughy or semi-fluctuant swelling, containing large, intercommunicating lymphatic spaces. They contain clear lymph with occasional lymphocytes. Sometimes bleeding into the spaces renders the diagnosis between haemangioma and lymphangioma difficult. Lymphangiomas occur occasionally also in mucous membranes in the wall of the bowel (Fig. 14.46), in the tissues of the orbit and mesentery, and elsewhere.

In rare cases lymphangiomas of neck, retroperitoneum or mesentery undergo great dilatation, forming a multilocular ramifying cystic mass which may become very large. Occasionally a single cyst is formed which may be distinguished from other cysts by its endothelial lining.

Lymphangio-endothelioma (lymphangiosarcoma) is a very doubtful entity, but has been described as arising in the lymphatics of the arm, following their obstruction by mastectomy and irradiation for mammary cancer (see above).

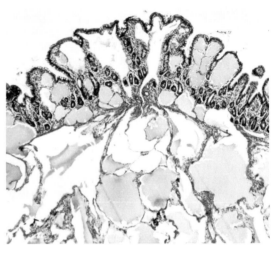

Fig. 14.46 Cavernous lymphangioma of small intestine. It is made up of large intercommunicating spaces filled with clear lymph (which has coagulated and then shrunk in processing the tissue). The lesion occupies both mucosa and submucosa, the mucosa being distorted but otherwise not much damaged.

References and Further Reading

Benditt, E. P. (1974). Evidence for a monoclonal origin of human atherosclerotic plaques and some implications. *Circulation*, **50**, 650-2.

Cardiovascular Pathology (1983). Ed. M. D. Silver, pp. 1407. Churchill Livingstone, Edinburgh, London, New York, etc.

Cole, F. M. and Yates, P. O. (1967). The occurrence and significance of intracerebral micro-aneurysms. *Journal of Pathology and Bacteriology* **93**, 393-411.

Duguid, J. B. (1946). Thrombosis as a factor in the pathogenesis of coronary atherosclerosis. *Journal of Pathology and Bacteriology*, **58**, 207-12.

Hjermann, I., Holme, I., Velve Byre, K. and Leren, P. (1981). Effect of diet and smoking intervention on the incidence of coronary heart disease. *Lancet*, **ii**, 1303-10.

Kannel, W. B., Castelli, W. P., Gordon, T. (1979). Cholesterol in the prediction of atherosclerotic disease. *Annals of Internal Medicine*, **90**, 85-91.

Keys, A. (1970). Coronary heart disease in seven countries. *Circulation* **41**, Supplement 1, pp. 1-211.

Keys, A. *et al.* (1981). The diet and all-causes death rate in the seven countries survey. *Lancet*, **ii**, 58-61.

Lancet (1982) Editorial. Coronary disease and multiple risk factor intervention **1**, 1395.

McGill, H. C. Jr. (1968). Fatty streaks in the coronary arteries and aorta. *Laboratory Investigation*, **18**, 560-4.

McGill, H. C. *et al.* (1968). International atherosclerosis project. The geographic pathology of atherosclerosis. *Laboratory Medicine*, **18**, 463-653. (A very large study involving over 20 000 autopsies in many countries).

Mitchison, M. J. (1984). The vasculitis syndromes, pp. 223-40 in *Recent Advances in Histopathology*, No. 12. Ed. P. P. Anthony and R. N. M. MacSween, pp. 293. Churchill Livingstone, Edinburgh, etc.

Niehaus, C.E., Wotton, R., Lewis, L., Nicoll, A., Williams, B., Coltart, D.J. and Lewis, B. (1977). Influence of lipid concentrations and age on transfer of plasma lipoprotein into human arterial intima. *Lancet*, **ii**, 469-71.

Orr, J. D., Sing, C. F. and Moll, P. P. (1981). Analysis of genetic and environmental sources of variation in serum cholesterol in Tecsumeh, Michigan—VI. A search for genotype by environmental interactions. *Journal of Chronic Diseases,* **34**, 545–59.

Pearson, T. A., Dillman, J., Solez, K. and Heptinstall, R. H. (1979). Monoclonal characteristics of organising arterial thrombi: significance of the origin and growth of human atherosclerotic plaques. *Lancet,* **i**, 7–11.

Pocock, S. J., Shaper, A. G., Cook, D. G., Packham, R. F., Lacey, R. F., Powell, P. and Rusell, P. F. (1980). British Regional Heart Study: geographic variations in cardiovascular mortality and the role of water quality. *British Medical Journal,* **280**, 1243–9.

Pooling Project Research Group. Final report (1978). Relationship of blood pressure, serum cholesterol, smoking habit, relative weight and ECG abnormalities to incidence of major coronary events. *Journal Chronic Diseases,* **31**, 201–306.

Pope, F. M., Narcisi, P., Neil-Dwyer, G., Nicholls, A. C., Bartlett, J. and Doshi, B. (1981). Some patients with cerebral aneurysms are deficient in type III collagen. *Lancet,* **i**, 973–5.

Prevention of coronary heart disease (1982). Technical Report Series No. 678. pp. 53. World Health Organisation, Geneva.

Ross, R. (1981). Smooth muscle cells and atherosclerosis, pp. 53–77. In *Vascular Injury and Atherosclerosis.* Ed. S. Moore, Vol. 9 in The Biochemistry of Disease, pp. 239. Dekker, New York, Basel.

Ross Russell, R. W. (1963). Observations on intracerebral aneurysms. *Brain,* **86**, 425–42.

Smith, J. P. (1956). Hyaline arteriosclerosis in spleen, pancreas and other viscera. *Journal of Pathology and Bacteriology,* **72**, 643–56.

Strong, J. P., Solberg, L. A. and Restrepo, C. (1968). Atherosclerosis in persons with coronary heart disease. *Laboratory Investigation,* **18**, 527–37.

Woolf, N. (1982). *Pathology of Atherosclerosis,* pp. 322. Butterworth Scientific, London, Boston, etc.

World Health Organisation European Collaboration Group (1982). Multifactorial trial in the prevention of coronary heart disease: 2. Risk factor changes at two and four years. *European Heart Journal,* **3**, 184–90.

Wright, H. P. (1971). Areas of mitoses in aortic endothelium of guinea-pigs. *Journal of Pathology,* **105**, 65–7.

15

The Heart

Heart disease is the commonest cause of death in most industrialised countries. It is responsible for more than one-third of deaths in the United Kingdom, and most other Western countries have similarly high rates. Most of these deaths are caused by ischaemic heart disease, which is nearly always due to atheroma, often with superadded thrombosis, of the coronary arteries. Other important causes of heart disease include systemic arterial hypertension and chronic diseases of the lungs which lead to hypoxia or pulmonary arterial hypertension. In most of the developing countries the incidence of ischaemic heart disease is relatively low, but rheumatic fever and malnutrition are still important causes of heart disease, while in Latin America Chagas' disease is a major cause. Bacterial infections, notably diphtheria, can cause serious toxic injury to the heart, and various virus infections are sometimes complicated by cardiac involvement. Finally, congenital abnormalities and acquired valvular lesions are increasing in medical importance because of the extending scope of cardiac surgery.

The work of the heart. Assuming a resting stroke volume of the heart is 66 ml and 72 beats per minute, the left ventricle has a minute volume of about 5 litres, and a daily output of 7200 litres (about $7\frac{1}{2}$ tons). The normal heart has great reserve power, and this can be substantially increased by physical training. During exertion, there is a greater venous return to the heart with consequent increase in diastolic filling and stretching of the muscle fibres; the response is a more vigorous contraction (Starling's law) and a greatly increased stroke volume. The heart rate also increases during exertion and these two factors together can raise the minute volume to about seven times that of the resting state.

This physiological performance can be maintained only if (1) the myocardium is intrinsically healthy, (2) the valves function efficiently, (3) the conducting system of the heart co-ordinates contraction of the chambers, and (4) peripheral resistance to blood flow is not grossly abnormal. Disturbance of any of these requirements can cause cardiac failure.

Cardiac Failure

Definition. Cardiac failure is that state in which the ventricular myocardium fails to maintain a circulation adequate for the needs of the body despite adequate venous filling pressure. Because the work of the heart falls mainly on the ventricles, heart failure is usually due to impaired function of one or both ventricles. Impaired atrial function may, however, affect ventricular function by interfering with ventricular filling, altering the rate of the heart or initiating arrhythmias.

Causes

Cardiac failure is due to weakness or inefficiency of myocardial contraction, to an abnormal increase of the work required of the myocardium, or to a combination of both. These two basic causes may be further classified as follows.

(1) Intrinsic pump failure. This is usually due to *weakness of the ventricular contraction*, the main cause of which is myocardial ischaemia resulting from coronary artery disease. Other causes of myocardial weakness include viral myocarditis, severe toxic bacterial infections and nutritional deficiencies, e.g. beriberi.

Expulsion of blood by the affected ventricle(s) is inadequate because the force of contraction is reduced, and during diastole the chamber dilates to contain both the residual blood and that entering from the atrium. Such dilatation places the failing ventricle(s) at a disadvantage, because the force required to provide a given pressure is greater in a large than in a small chamber. Consequently, unless the cause is reversible, dilatation and failure tend to be progressive. Moreover, left or right ventricular dilatation results in stretching and incompetence (secondary incompetence) of the mitral or tricuspid valve respectively, and this, as described below, increases the work of the dilated ventricle.

A less common cause of intrinsic pump failure is *impaired compliance of the myocardium* which in plain language means that the ventricles are too stiff to relax and fill properly during diastole, e.g. in hypertrophic and restrictive cardiomyopathies. The abnormal rigidity may also interfere with myocardial contraction. By restricting cardiac filling, pericardial haemorrhage or effusion and restrictive pericarditis can produce similar effects.

Disorders of cardiac rhythm, resulting from various conditions, are also included in this group. Although minor irregularities such as sinus arrhythmia and occasional extrasystoles do not significantly impair cardiac function, severe tachycardia so shortens the time for diastolic filling of the ventricles and diastolic flow in the coronary arteries that the efficiency of the heart is substantially decreased; this happens in atrial fibrillation and flutter and the paroxysmal tachycardias. The bradycardia of complete heart block (about 30 beats a minute) also causes a marked fall in cardiac output.

(2) Increased pressure load results from any condition which increases the resistance to expulsion of blood from the ventricles. The commonest causes affecting the left ventricle are systemic hypertension and aortic valve stenosis, while resistance to emptying of the right ventricle is usually due to pulmonary arterial hypertension resulting from left ventricular failure, various diseases of the lungs or mitral stenosis.

If the cause is chronic, the affected ventricle undergoes hypertrophy, but eventually dilatation and failure may develop.

(3) Increased volume load. This arises when a ventricle is required to expel more than the normal volume of blood. It occurs when, owing to incompetence of a heart valve, some of the blood leaks backwards (e.g. through the aortic valve during diastole), and also in conditions in which the general circulation is increased, e.g. anaemia, thyrotoxicosis, and hypoxia resulting from lung disease. Other causes include arterio-venous shunts between the left and right sides of the circulation.

(4) Multiple factors. Each of the above aetiological groups may independently produce cardiac failure, but various factors often operate simultaneously. For example, a patient with mitral stenosis may have only impaired exercise tolerance (i.e. diminished cardiac reserve), but atrial fibrillation commonly develops and may promote cardiac failure even at rest. An individual with systemic hypertension may develop cardiac failure as a result of occlusion of a minor coronary artery which would go virtually unnoticed but for the hypertension, or cardiac failure may be precipitated by an attack of pneumonia in a person with pulmonary hypertension due to chronic lung disease.

Manifestations of cardiac failure

In mild degrees of cardiac failure the heart is no longer able to increase its output sufficiently to fulfil extreme metabolic demands, as in strenuous physical activity, but is still able to meet lesser demands. With increase in severity the cardiac reserve is further diminished, with decreasing exercise tolerance until, in severe failure, the circulation is inadequate even at rest.

Failure may be **acute** or **chronic** depending on whether the causal factors—impaired myocardial efficiency or increased workload—develop rapidly or slowly. The causal factors may affect predominantly either ventricle, giving rise to **left** or **right ventricular failure**, or both may be affected, with consequent **total heart failure**.

Acute heart failure occurs when the causal factors develop rapidly or suddenly. Examples include myocardial infarction, gross pulmonary embolism, arrhythmias, viral myocarditis, acute bacterial toxaemias, rheumatic fever and rupture of a valve cusp.

In severe acute failure (most often due to myocardial infarction) the cardiac output falls drastically and a condition closely similar to hypovolaemic shock develops, with selective peripheral vasoconstriction due to increased sympathetic activity. The term **cardiogenic shock** (p. 10.41) is appropriate, but the central venous pressure is raised and the principles of treatment are quite different from those for hypovolaemic shock. The full picture of shock develops in only a small proportion of cases, but when it does the outlook is poor. Conversely, acute heart failure may supervene in hypovolaemic or septic shock (p. 10.40).

A sudden severe fall in cardiac output in acute heart failure may so diminish the blood supply to the brain that the patient loses consciousness and there is a danger of rapidly fatal cerebral hypoxia.

Chronic heart failure occurs when the causal factors develop slowly. The commonest causes are myocardial ischaemia due to gradual atheromatous narrowing of the lumen of the major coronary arteries, systemic arterial hypertension, chronic valvular lesions and chronic diseases of the lungs which cause hypoxia or pulmonary artery hypertension. Chronic failure usually develops insidiously, but acute failure may also progress into chronic failure. Regardless of whether either one or both ventricles are involved in chronic failure, cardiac output is diminished and tissue hypoxia results. This is not so dramatic as in acute failure, but sometimes causes mental confusion and is responsible for the profound muscular weakness of severe heart failure. A compensatory increase in red cells (erythrocytosis) may result from hypoxia.

As with acute failure, the clinical and pathological changes depend on the nature of the causal factors and whether they affect mainly the left, right or both ventricles.

Left ventricular failure (LVF). The common causes of cardiac failure usually affect the left ventricle more than the right, and most cases of cardiac failure therefore present initially as LVF. However, as explained in the next section, LVF usually leads to right ventricular failure so that, in the later stages, the picture is that of total, or congestive failure.

The commonest causes of LVF are chronic

systemic hypertension and ischaemic heart disease, particularly myocardial infarction. Other causes include aortic valve disease and mitral valve incompetence.

As failure develops, the left ventricle can no longer pass on all the blood it receives and so it contains an increasing volume of blood at the end of systole and this, together with the blood entering it during diastole, causes dilatation which further increases the inadequacy of contraction (Fig. 15.5, p. 15.9). Eventually the dilatation results in stretching of the mitral ring with consequent mitral valve incompetence. When this develops, some of the blood expelled during systole passes through the leaking mitral valve into the left atrium with consequent rise in pressure in the left atrium which in turn leads to *venous congestion and oedema of the lungs*. Retrograde loss of blood through the leaking mitral valve also reduces further the effective output of the left ventricle.

The main **clinical features** of left ventricular failure are dyspnoea and cough due to pulmonary congestion and oedema. In acute failure, e.g. due to myocardial infarction, death may occur rapidly from acute pulmonary oedema, but the picture is often complicated by cardiogenic shock (p. 10.41). In chronic failure, the left ventricle fails initially to meet increased circulatory demands so that undue dyspnoea and cough are brought on by physical activity. As failure increases, exercise tolerance diminishes until pulmonary congestion is present even at rest. Acute exacerbations of LVF commonly occur at night, sleep being disturbed by attacks of **paroxysmal nocturnal dyspnoea** in which severe respiratory distress and cough result from a sudden worsening of the pulmonary congestion and oedema. Respirations may be wheezy and the old name for the condition is '*cardiac asthma*'. Such attacks are apparently due to improved venous return from the lower limbs on lying down; there is a redistribution of fluid, with an increase in blood volume. They may be prevented by sleeping in an inclined or sitting position and are gradually relieved by sitting up. Diuretics and salt restriction are helpful in prevention and treatment.

The pulmonary congestion and oedema of LVF are most pronounced when there is severe imbalance between the functional capacities of the left and right ventricles. In chronic LVF the right ventricle eventually fails also (see below) and when this happens the functional imbalance is reduced: the mean left atrial pressure falls, the pulmonary congestion diminishes and there is less danger of the development of severe pulmonary oedema. Accordingly, in this stage of total failure the dyspnoea and cough improve and features of right ventricular failure, including systemic venous congestion and oedema, supervene.

In patients dying in LVF the findings depend on the causal factors, whether failure was acute or chronic, and whether death resulted from pulmonary oedema. The left ventricle and atrium are dilated and the mitral ring is enlarged. The lungs show the changes of acute or chronic congestion (p. 10.5) and contain various amounts of oedema fluid, while in chronic cases the changes of chronic right ventricular failure usually supervene.

Right ventricular failure (RVF) occurs most often as a consequence of pulmonary arterial hypertension, and in most industrialised countries the commonest cause of this is left ventricular failure due to ischaemic heart disease. When the left ventricle fails, the increased pressure in the left atrium and pulmonary veins induces pulmonary arteriolar vasoconstriction with a rise in pulmonary arterial pressure. The mechanism of this is not understood, but the raised pulmonary arterial pressure increases the workload on the right ventricle with consequent hypertrophy and, in some patients, eventual failure. The pulmonary hypertension is not the only factor involved, another being the hypertrophied and dilated left ventricle, which is likely to distort the right ventricle and interfere mechanically with its function. The raised left atrial pressure associated with mitral stenosis can also lead to RVF, although the hypertrophied right ventricle may maintain an adequate output for many years.

Many of the causal factors of heart failure, and notably myocardial ischaemia, usually affect the left ventricle more than the right, and *primary* RVF is relatively uncommon. It does, however, occur in patients with chronic pulmonary hypertension due to chronic destructive lung diseases such as chronic bronchitis and emphysema and extensive pulmonary fibrosis. RVF from other causes is unusual: tricuspid or pulmonary valve lesions are seldom responsible, but acute heart failure resulting from virus myocarditis and chronic failure in Chagas' disease are sometimes predominantly of right ventricular type.

The most acute form of RVF is seen in pulmonary embolism. A massive embolus is, of course, fatal within minutes, but multiple large emboli can cause acute RVF and multiple embolism over a long period occasionally causes chronic RVF.

When it fails, the right ventricle cannot pass on all of the blood reaching it and becomes dilated (Fig. 15.28, p. 15.28). Stretching of the tricuspid ring results in incompetence and blood accumulates in the right atrium and systemic and portal venous systems, with rise in central venous pressure and the changes of *systemic venous congestion* (p. 10.3) and 'cardiac' type of oedema (p. 10.32).

Total (congestive) heart failure combines the features of left and right ventricular failure. As noted above, it develops most often in cases of left ventricular failure, but both ventricles may fail simultaneously as a result of diffuse or extensive myocardial damage, e.g. extensive infarction, viral or severe toxic myocarditis (as in diphtheria), beriberi and congestive cardiomyopathy (Fig. 15.17, p. 15.17). Total failure can also result from conditions which increase the workload of both ventricles, for example chronic rheumatic lesions of the mitral and aortic valves and states in which there is a persistently raised cardiac output, such as thyrotoxicosis, anaemia and some congenital abnormalities of the heart and great vessels. In these latter states, failure is associated with the usual fall in cardiac output but the fall is relative to the previous abnormally high output and even in failure the absolute output may be normal or even increased. Accordingly, the term **'high output failure'** is applied. By contrast, failure developing in subjects with a previously normal cardiac output is associated with an abnormally low output and is sometimes termed **'low output failure'**.

Thrombo-embolic phenomena. Patients with cardiac failure are especially prone to develop deep venous thrombosis in the legs as a result of venous stagnation and muscular inactivity associated with lying in bed: in consequence, there is a serious risk of pulmonary embolism. The pulmonary circulation is already compromised by heart failure, and superadded embolism often results in infarction with pleural pain, bloodstained sputum and more severe heart failure. Thrombosis is also common in the atria and, in some forms of heart failure, in the ventricles: such cardiac thrombi, depending on their site, can give rise to pulmonary or systemic emboli. These complications are described in Chapter 10.

Compensatory enlargement of the heart

The compensatory changes which develop in the heart subjected to persistently increased workload often prevent heart failure or at least postpone its onset, sometimes for many years. **Compensatory myocardial hypertrophy** occurs in the walls of the affected chambers in response to increased pressure load. In conditions of increased volume load, due for example to valvular incompetence, **hypertrophy** of the affected ventricle(s) is accompanied by **passive dilatation** during diastole, thus compensating in some degree for the blood which, instead of passing onwards, is regurgitated through the leaking valve. This occurs before the supervention of heart failure, i.e. when ventricular systolic emptying is normal, and has been termed **compensatory dilatation**. This must be distinguished from the dilatation of ventricular failure, in which emptying is incomplete due to weakness of the myocardial contraction. Both hypertrophy and compensatory dilatation cause cardiac enlargement, which may be further increased by the dilatation of cardiac failure.

Because of the vascular arrangements of the coronary supply, ventricular hypertrophy renders the inner part of the myocardium particularly liable to ischaemia (p. 15.16).

The assessment of cardiac enlargement. In left ventricular hypertrophy, the weight of the heart is increased above the normal 300–350 g often to over 500 g. Because of its smaller mass, hypertrophy of the right ventricle is not usually sufficient to increase markedly the total heart weight. Although gross hypertrophy of either ventricle is usually obvious at autopsy from the increased thickness of its wall (Fig. 15.1), the degree of hypertrophy is not readily assessed without taking account of the volume of the chambers, i.e. the degree of dilatation. A more reliable method is to separate and weigh the individual ventricles, making allowance for

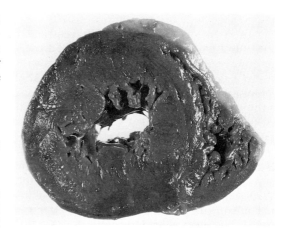

Fig. 15.1 Transverse section through the ventricles, showing left ventricular hypertrophy. From a patient with systemic arterial hypertension. (The dark area in the inferior wall of the left ventricle is a very recent infarct—see later).

epicardial fatty tissue and any gross fibrous scars, etc.

Increase in size of the hypertrophied heart is often not readily detected by clinical or radiological measurements unless there is also dilatation, in which case it is difficult to distinguish, from size alone, between the two processes.

Characteristic electrocardiographic changes accompany ventricular hypertrophy, especially when one ventricle is involved.

The **atria** also undergo compensatory changes when subjected to increased workload. Their capacity for hypertrophy is limited, but compensatory dilatation may be demonstrable radiologically.

Causes of compensatory changes

Compensatory changes in the ventricles result from increased workload which, if severe, may lead eventually to chronic cardiac failure. The causes therefore overlap with those of chronic cardiac failure. Examples have already been given, but fuller lists are provided below.

Left ventricular hypertrophy. The common causes of marked left ventricular hypertrophy are (1) systemic hypertension; (2) stenosis of the aortic valve; (3) aortic or mitral incompetence, in which hypertrophy is accompanied by compensatory dilatation; (4) coarctation of the aorta and some other congenital abnormalities; (5) persistently high cardiac output (thyrotoxicosis, anaemia, arterio-venous fistula and Paget's disease of bone). Mild left ventricular hypertrophy is found in the absence of hypertension or valvular lesions in some patients with healed myocardial infarcts, and is presumably compensatory for the loss of muscle. Various cardiomyopathies (p. 15.16) are a less usual cause of hypertrophy.

Right ventricular hypertrophy. Most examples of right ventricular hypertrophy are attributable to pulmonary arterial hypertension. The common causes are (1) left ventricular failure; (2) chronic lung disease, especially bronchitis and widespread pulmonary fibrosis; (3) stenosis and/or incompetence of the mitral valve; (4) congenital heart disease with large shunts of blood from one side of the heart to the other; (5) stenosis of the pulmonary valve (6) massive hypertrophy of the left ventricle, which is often accompanied by right ventricular hypertrophy

without any other obvious cause. Rarer causes of right ventricular hypertrophy include multiple small pulmonary emboli and other unusual causes of pulmonary hypertension (pp. 16.23–26).

Compensatory dilatation. Compensatory dilatation of the left ventricle results from incompetence of the mitral or aortic valve or of both, and right ventricular dilatation from incompetence of the tricuspid and/or pulmonary valves. Left/right shunts, as in ventricular septal defects, cause dilatation of both ventricles, and this occurs also, in lesser degree, in patients with persistently high cardiac output, e.g. in thyrotoxicosis or arterio-venous shunts.

Compensatory dilatation is accompanied by hypertrophy of the affected ventricle, the degree of which depends on the increase in its workload.

Ischaemic Heart Disease (IHD)

Death rates from ischaemia of the myocardium increased enormously in most industrialised countries during the first half of this century, and indeed it has become the leading cause of death, accounting for approximately one-third of all deaths in some countries. The rates increase with age and most deaths occur beyond the age of 40. By contrast, most of the developing countries have a low incidence of ischaemic heart disease (IHD) and it is not a major cause of death. There are also surprising differences in the death rates from IHD between industrialised countries. Among the highest are Finland, the British Isles, the USA, Australia, New Zealand and Canada. In most other European countries the rates are distinctly lower but nevertheless high, while in France, Italy and Switzerland the rates are less than half those in Finland and Britain. The outstanding exception to the relationship between industrialisation and IHD deaths is provided by Japan, in which the rate is less than 15% of that in the USA. In general, death rates are slightly higher for men than for women, but IHD affects men earlier and for age groups up to 65 the rates are much higher for men.

During the past 20 years, death rates for IHD have fallen in both men and women in the non-European industrialised countries mentioned above, including Japan. The fall has been greatest (about 30%) in the USA. Rates have fallen also in Finland, Belgium and Norway, but not in the other European countries, and indeed they have risen in France, Sweden, Denmark, Ireland and the Balkans. In Britain, overall rates have remained steady, although there has been a fall within the higher socio-economic classes, and particularly in doctors (a group who have reduced smoking more than most others). Scotland and Northern Ireland now appear to have the highest rates in the world (see Pisa and Uemura, 1982).

IHD is due almost always to narrowing of the lumen of one or more major coronary arteries by atheroma, often with complete occlusion by superadded thrombosis. It can present as (1) **angina pectoris**, severe chest pain brought on by factors which increase the work of the heart; (2) **myocardial infarction**, usually precipitated by coronary thrombosis; (3) **sudden death**, usually from ventricular fibrillation; (4) **cardiac failure**, and (5) **cardiac arrhythmias**.

Before describing these effects of IHD, the pathology of coronary artery disease merits a brief account.

Atheroma of the coronary arteries shows the

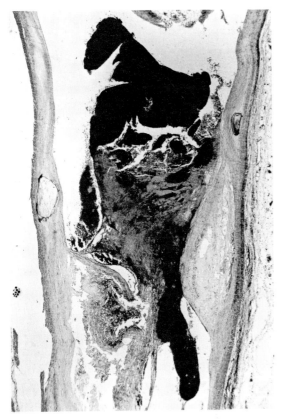

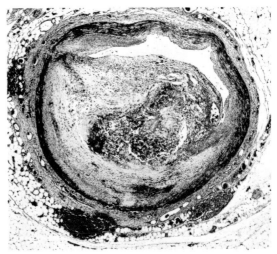

Fig. 15.3 Severe atheromatous narrowing of a coronary artery. The lumen has been further reduced by haemorrhage into the soft lipid-rich material, seen as the dark area in the atheromatous patch. × 20.

Fig. 15.2 Coronary artery in longitudinal section, showing an ulcerated atheromatous plaque (*left, lower*) with occlusion of lumen by thrombus. × 15.

general features of atheroma described on p. 14.3–8. It affects the major coronary arteries most severely, and may involve also the smaller branches in the epicardium, but branches that have penetrated the myocardium are usually unaffected.

The atheromatous plaques consist of patchy accumulations of lipid-rich debris deep in the intima with overlying fibrosis. As a plaque gradually enlarges, it encroaches progressively on the lumen and eventually may almost obliterate it. Rapid obliteration may result from superadded thrombosis (Fig. 14.9, p. 14.6) which in some cases follows ulceration or rupture of the plaque (Fig. 15.2). Haemorrhage into the soft lipid debris of the plaque (Fig. 15.3) may also greatly reduce or occlude the lumen.

In the atheroma-ridden industrialised countries the lesions are seen even in young adults, while men of over 40 years, dying from all causes, show degrees of coronary atheroma ranging from occasional isolated plaques to almost confluent involvement of the major arteries. The plaques are commonly heavily calcified and when numerous may convert the arteries into rigid tubes which are too hard to cut with a knife and can only be examined satisfactorily after decalcification.

Coronary artery atheroma tends to progress more slowly in women than in men until after the menopause. This accounts for the higher death rates for IHD in men up to the age of 65.

Other coronary artery lesions causing IHD are uncommon. They include the lesions of polyarteritis nodosa, embolism, and narrowing of the mouths of the coronary arteries by syphilitic aortitis.

Angina pectoris

This consists of attacks of sudden, severe, sometimes agonising chest pain caused by inadequate perfusion of a part of the myocardium relative to its metabolic needs. Attacks are brought on by factors which increase the work of the heart, notably physical exertion, and are relieved after a few minutes by rest.

Causal factors and pathological changes. Angina occurs in subjects in whom there is a precarious balance between perfusion of the myocardium and its metabolic needs. The attacks of pain occur when the balance is upset, usually by a sudden increase in myocardial workload. It is thus necessary to consider both the underlying predisposing factors and the causes of the individual attacks.

The most important underlying factor is impaired perfusion, due nearly always to coronary artery atheroma, and the incidence of angina therefore increases with age. There is usually severe atheromatous narrowing of one or more major coronary arteries, and often occlusion by old organised thrombus. Arteriograms also show some restoration of blood supply by enlarged anastomotic arteries which by-pass atheromatous constrictions or occlusions (Fig. 15.4). In most cases autopsy reveals myocardial scarring (Fig. 15.5) or more recent infarction, but myocardial lesions are not always present. Myocardial infarction may either promote angina by diminishing the blood supply to surviving myocardium around the infarct, or relieve it by eliminating an area of myocardium with a previously inadequate blood supply.

Anaemia also predisposes to angina, suggesting that oxygen supply to the myocardium is a critical factor. Other underlying factors increase the resting workload of the heart and thus the metabolic activity of the myocardium: examples include hypertension, valvular lesions which increase the pressure or volume load of the heart, impairment of efficiency of the heart by arrhythmias, cardiomyopathies, viral myocarditis and hyperthyroidism. In aortic valvular disease the left ventricular workload is increased and coronary perfusion is relatively or absolutely reduced (p. 15.32). In consequence, angina may occur without significant coronary artery disease, and this may happen also in gross ventricular hypertrophy from any cause.

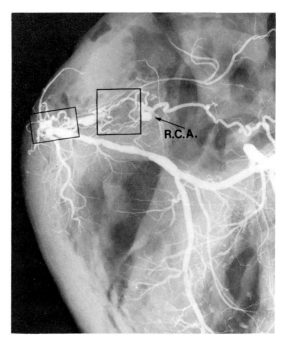

Fig. 15.4 Post-mortem radiograph of part of the right coronary artery in a case of angina. Shortly after its origin (*arrow*), a length of the artery is occluded (*square*) and adjacent vessels have enlarged to provide a collateral route, so that the artery is filled beyond the occlusion. A second occlusion (*oblong*) is present, but is partly obscured by the curving course of the artery. (Professor M. J. Davies.)

Factors which precipitate attacks include physical activity, exposure to cold, strong emotions, a heavy meal, serious injury and shock, all of which increase the workload of the heart. Coronary arterial spasm may also promote anginal attacks. Vasodilator drugs such as nitroglycerin are often effective in preventing and relieving attacks, presumably either by a direct effect on the coronary arterial tree or by reducing the resistance to cardiac output by causing more general peripheral vasodilation.

Clinical features and course. Anginal pain is often described as 'gripping' or 'crushing'. It is usually retrosternal and may radiate to the neck and jaw and ulnar side of the left arm. During an attack there is usually dyspnoea and tachycardia and there may be ECG changes suggestive of myocardial ischaemia. Angina is often stable and many sufferers live for over 30 years

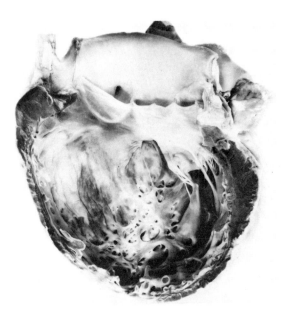

Fig. 15.5 Extensive fibrosis of the left ventricle secondary to coronary disease. The left ventricle also shows the marked dilatation of chronic failure. × 0·5.

with little change. Coronary artery atheroma does, however, tend to progress and the anginal patient may become increasingly prone to attacks until finally they occur even at rest. There is also an increased risk of myocardial infarction, heart failure, and sudden death from ventricular fibrillation. In general, the prognosis depends on the extent and degree of coronary artery atheroma and the presence of other underlying causal factors mentioned above.

Replacement of narrowed or occluded stretches of the coronary arteries by vein grafts is very often effective in patients for whom conservative treatment is unsatisfactory.

In **variant angina pectoris** (Prinzmetal's angina) the attacks of pain are not related to increases in workload of the heart and can occur at rest in bed. It has been shown conclusively that they are caused by spasm of the large and medium-sized coronary arteries, and in about 15% of cases the arteries appear otherwise normal.

Myocardial infarction (MI)

Myocardial infarction is the major cause of disability and death from coronary artery disease. In various industrialised countries it accounts for 10–25% of all deaths. In approximately 50% of patients the condition is fatal, and many of the remainder suffer from impaired cardiac function. Many patients die within a few hours of the onset, and advances in treatment have not improved the prognosis very much.

Myocardial infarcts affect mainly the ventricular myocardium. Over 90% of infarcts are **regional**, i.e. involve part of the myocardium lying within the region supplied by a major coronary artery. The supply artery is atheromatous and in most cases is occluded by thrombus. Less than 10% of MIs are **subendocardial**, affecting the inner part of the wall of the left ventricle throughout most or all of its circumference. In such cases the major coronary arteries are severely narrowed by atheroma but recent occlusion by thrombus is unusual. These two types of MI differ in their manifestations and causation, and are described separately below.

Regional MI

Structural changes

As indicated above, there is good correlation between thrombotic occlusion of a particular coronary artery and the site of associated MI. For reasons given below, regional infarcts vary greatly in size, but most are at least 2 cm across, and many are much larger. They may affect mainly the inner part of the myocardium, but most are **transmural**, i.e. affect the whole thickness of the muscle. In most cases, there is extensive and severe coronary artery atheroma but in some there are only one or two patches causing severe narrowing. The occluding thrombus typically forms on an atheromatous plaque but may then extend along a consider-

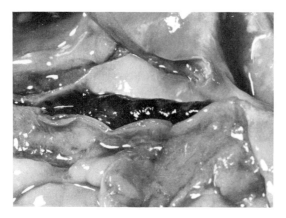

Fig. 15.6   Recent thrombotic occlusion of the right main coronary artery; death resulted 12 hours after the onset of symptoms. The artery has been opened longitudinally to reveal the thrombus. × 2·5.

able length of the vessel (Fig. 15.6). Initially, such propagated thrombus is mainly red, but subsequently it becomes pale and eventually organised, often with some recanalisation (Fig. 15.7).

Thrombotic occlusion occurs most often (about 40% of cases) in the *anterior descending artery* and the infarct is *anterior*, extending from the apex up the anterior wall of the left ventricle, often involving the anterior part of

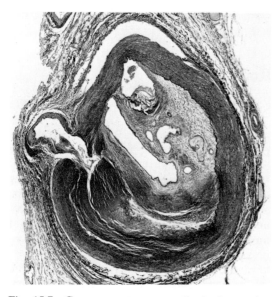

Fig. 15.7   Coronary artery recanalised after occlusion by thrombus. There was extensive healed myocardial infarction. × 25.

the interventricular septum and adjacent part of the anterior wall of the right ventricle (Fig. 15.8). Occlusion of the *right main artery* is almost as common and the infarct is then *inferior* (*posterior*), extending from the apex up the inferior wall of the left ventricle, often involving also the adjacent part of the interventricular septum and adjacent part of the inferior wall of the right ventricle. In about 15% of cases, the *left circumflex artery* is occluded, with infarction of the lateral margin of the left ventricle. Thrombosis of the left main artery or of two major arteries occurs much less commonly, and is associated with more extensive infarction.

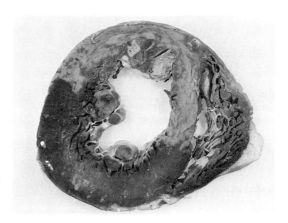

Fig. 15.8   Anterior myocardial infarction of several days duration, due to occlusive thrombosis of the anterior descending coronary artery. The infarct appears pale and involves the anterior parts of both ventricles and of the septum. The coronary arteries have been injected for radiography (Professor M. J. Davies). × 0·5.

The extent of infarction varies considerably, depending on the severity and distribution of atheroma throughout the coronary arteries and on the presence or absence of old thrombosis. There is considerable normal variation in the relative sizes of the left and right arteries, and gradual atheromatous narrowing of a major branch may result in enlargement of collateral vessels (Fig. 15.9) so that its final occlusion by thrombosis causes a lesser infarct or even none at all.

The detection of thrombotic coronary artery occlusion at autopsy is not always easy. If the arteries are opened lengthwise by scissors, a small thrombus may be dislodged or disrupted

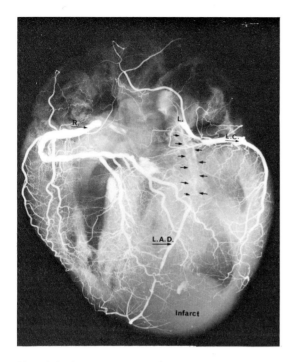

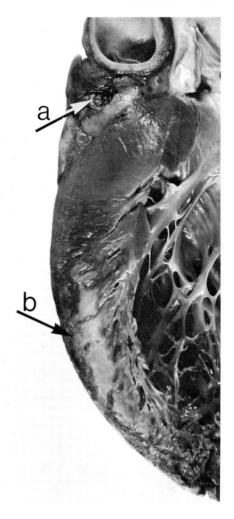

Fig. 15.9 Post-mortem angiogram in a case of recent myocardial infarction. The anterior descending artery (LAD) is occluded proximally (*arrows*), and although there was sufficient collateral supply to fill the artery distally, extensive infarction had occurred over the anterior wall and apical region. Note also the atheromatous narrowings of the right coronary artery. (Professor M. J. Davies.)

by the point of the blade and may escape notice. A more satisfactory method of examination is by transverse section of the arteries at intervals of not more than 2 mm. Extensively calcified arteries must be decalcified before they can be examined satisfactorily. Perfusion with radio-opaque material is of great help in assessing the state of the coronary arteries (Figs. 15.4, 15.9).

The infarct. Myocardial infarction can be induced experimentally by complete clamping of a major coronary artery for about fifteen minutes. Initially the dead muscle appears grossly and microscopically normal, morphological evidence of necrosis only becoming apparent after some hours. Similarly in man, myocardial necrosis cannot be recognised morphologically in patients dying less than 6–8 hours after the onset. Earlier changes can be detected by electron microscopy but cannot be

Fig. 15.10 Myocardial infarction of 11 days' duration. The anterior descending branch of the left coronary artery (**a**) is occluded by thrombus and there is extensive infarction of the wall of the left ventricle, seen as areas of pallor and surrounding congestion (**b**). Note also mural thrombus at the apex.

distinguished with certainty from post-mortem changes.

The sites of regional MI are described above: they depend on which coronary artery is occluded, but in nearly all cases the left ventricular myocardium is mainly affected, usually with involvement of the septum and often the adjacent part of the right ventricle. The first changes visible at autopsy are congestion (Fig. 15.1), or blotchy congestion and pallor, throughout the affected myocardium. During the next day or so the dead muscle is usually palpable as a patch of softening. The colour gradually pales to grey-brown and then to yellow-grey (Fig. 15.10), and there may be haemorrhages, particularly at the margin. After a few days the infarct becomes more sharply defined by development of a red zone of vascular granulation tissue along the margin, and removal of the dead myocardium by organisation proceeds gradually. There may be a fibrinous or haemorrhagic pericarditis localised to the area of infarction or more generalised. On the inner aspect of the infarct the endocardium and a thin layer of sub-endocardial myocardium remain alive, nourished by blood from the lumen, but in patients surviving for several days this does not prevent the formation of mural thrombus (see below). *Microscopically*, the infarcted muscle begins to show the changes of 'coagulative necrosis' (p. 3.32) after 8 or so hours: it is invaded by polymorphs and after a few days digestion by macrophages and organisation can be seen at the margins (Fig. 15.11). The dead muscle is replaced by fibrous tissue over the succeeding weeks or months, depending on the size of the infarct, and eventually the affected part of the ventricular wall is replaced by a thin layer of fibrous tissue (Fig. 15.12). In patients dying in the first few weeks it is not unusual to observe more recent infarction adjacent to the original infarct. This may be due to extension of thrombus along the affected coronary artery. It is also common to find old scars, suggestive

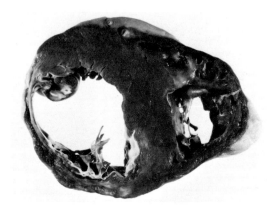

Fig. 15.12 Old infarct represented by replacement of the lateral and posterior wall of the left ventricle by a relatively thin fibrous scar.

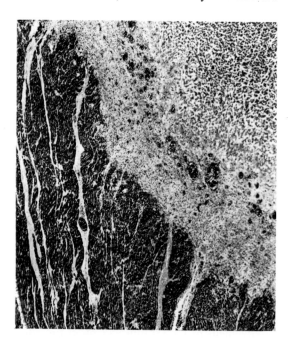

Fig. 15.11 Infarct of myocardium of 12 days' duration. The necrotic heart muscle (*upper right*) is separated from the surviving muscle by a zone of cellular and vascular granulation tissue. × 401

of previous infarcts, in patients dying from recent infarction. Regional scarring is suggestive of old infarction, particularly if accompanied by fibrous occlusion of a coronary artery resulting from organisation of an old thrombus. In some instances, however, myocardial fibrosis is more diffuse, and survival of some myocardial fibres throughout the fibrous tissue (Fig. 15.13) suggests chronic ischaemia with gradual loss of myocardial fibres and fibrous replacement.

Causal factors in regional MI

The important cause of regional myocardial infarction is occlusion of the lumen of a major coronary artery and in most cases this is caused by thrombosis superimposed on atheroma.

As it is frequently clinically silent unless complicated by superadded thrombosis, uncomplicated coronary atheroma is not readily studied epidemiologically. Factors carrying an increased risk of ischaemic heart disease, including MI, have been discussed on p. 14.8–14. They include raised levels of various plasma lipids associated with a lipid-rich diet, hypertension,

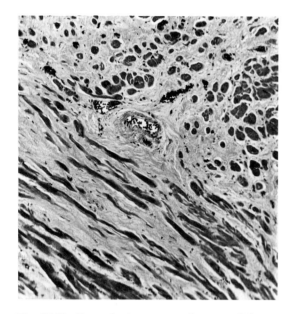

Fig. 15.13 Part of a large zone of myocardial scarring throughout which some myocardial fibres have survived.

cigarette smoking, a sedentary occupation, consumption of alcohol and genetic factors. These are all 'chronic' factors, and while they promote the development of atheroma they may also predispose to superadded thrombosis. Enhanced coagulability of the blood has been shown to be common in patients with ischaemic heart disease, and correlates partially with the levels of plasma lipids.

Patients with severe coronary atheroma are particularly liable to myocardial infarction following a severe injury or major surgical operation. This may occur during a period of shock, but the risk is high for some weeks following the injury, etc. The circulatory disturbances of shock, the effect of anaesthetic agents on the heart, and the increased coagulability of the blood in the weeks following injury are all probably of importance.

Role of coronary thrombosis. Over the past decade the causal role of coronary artery thrombosis has been questioned and it has been suggested that it is a secondary phenomenon, occurring after infarction has developed. This is based largely on the finding that the incidence of coronary thrombosis in fatal infarction depends on the length of time between the onset of symptoms and death. Thus in sudden cardiac deaths the incidence of coronary thrombosis is

only about 30%; in patients dying within 12 hours it is about 50%, and in those dying after 12 hours it is considerably higher. These findings are open to the following criticisms. (a) There is evidence that over 50% of sudden cardiac deaths are not related to myocardial infarction (p. 15.16). (b) In some series, the distinction has not been made between regional and subendocardial infarction: it is widely agreed that the latter usually occurs without coronary thrombosis. (c) Occlusive thrombosis over an atheromatous patch is often inconspicuous. During the next day or so propagation of the thrombus often renders it conspicuous (Fig. 15.6, p. 15.10), thus providing an explanation for the relationship between the incidence of thrombosis and the duration of survival. Some reports are unacceptable because the coronary arteries were not examined with sufficient care, and in particular the need for decalcification of extensively atheromatous and calcified arteries before they can be examined for thrombosis has not always been appreciated. Ideally, post-mortem angiography should first be performed to indicate the site of occlusion.

Evidence that coronary thrombosis *precedes* regional infarction is supported by the following points. (i) In animals, temporary clamping of a major coronary artery causes infarction, but such experimental infarction is not usually followed by occlusive thrombosis. (ii) Careful examination of the coronary arteries reveals coronary artery thrombosis in virtually all patients dying 12 or more hours after the onset of regional infarction (Davies, Woolf and Robertson, 1976): in patients dying earlier than this the diagnosis of infarction is often presumptive (p. 15.11). (iii) In a majority of patients dying of regional MI, coronary thrombosis has occurred over a *ruptured* atheromatous patch (Fig. 15.2, p. 15.7); this is strong evidence that the rupture has caused thrombosis, and it follows that, in such cases, MI is the *result* of the thrombosis and not its cause, for it is difficult to believe that MI predisposes to rupture of an atheromatous plaque. (iv) In his extensive studies on MI, Fulton has found no evidence against the orthodox view that coronary artery thrombosis precedes and causes regional infarction. In particular, when patients were injected intravenously with radio-labelled fibrinogen soon after the onset of MI, auto-radiography of slices of the thrombosed coronary arteries of those who subsequently died gave findings entirely consistent with thrombotic occlusion preceding infarction, with subsequent propagation of the thrombus. (Davies, Fulton and Robertson, 1979).

In conclusion, although it cannot be proved that thrombosis usually precedes and causes regional MI, the evidence in favour of this is strong, and the evidence against it rather weak. Vascular spasm can cause MI, but this is probably unusual.

Unusual causes. Occlusion of a coronary artery by an embolus, with consequent regional infarction, is much less common than thrombosis; the embolus usually originates from intracardiac thrombus, and particularly from thrombotic vegetations on the aortic valve in infective endocarditis. Rare causes include involvement of the coronary arteries in polyarteritis nodosa and in Buerger's disease, and occlusion of the ostia of the coronary arteries by dissecting aneurysm of the aorta or by syphilitic aortitis.

Clinical features and course

The dominant early symptom of MI is usually severe retrosternal pain. As in angina, it may radiate to the neck, jaw or left arm, but it is not relieved by rest or vasodilator drugs and persists for at least a few hours and usually 1–2 days. It is generally accompanied by nausea, vomiting, sweating, weakness and prostration. These early features are usually dramatic, but in some cases MI is remarkably silent, with little or no pain.

Within the first few hours there is usually mild fever and moderate neutrophil leucocytosis and characteristic electrocardiographic changes. Necrosis of myocardium is followed by release of cellular enzymes with consequent rise in the serum levels. Serum glutamic-oxalacetic aminotransferase rises in 6–8 hours, peaks at about 36 hours and returns to normal usually within a week. Lactic dehydrogenase (LDH) rises and peaks slightly later. These enzymes are released also by injury to other organs or skeletal muscle, but rise in serum LDH5, an LDH isoenzyme, is more specific, while serum CPK-MB, a creatine phosphokinase isoenzyme, rises in 2–3 hours, peaks at about 36 hours, and is virtually diagnostic of myocardial necrosis.

About 25% of patients with MI die from heart failure or ventricular fibrillation before reaching hospital. A further 25% die in the first year, following which the mortality gradually diminishes to about 5% annually. The most important single prognostic factor is the size of the infarct. In patients with a small uncomplicated MI the prognosis is good. The following complications occur more frequently with extensive infarction, and are responsible for most of the deaths.

(a) Arrhythmias. Ventricular fibrillation is the commonest cause of death in MI. It is especially liable to occur during the acute illness, after which the danger diminishes gradually. The occurrence of premature ventricular beats after the first month or so indicates a particular liability to ventricular fibrillation. Cigarette smoking greatly increases the incidence of sudden death following recovery from MI, and long-term administration of sulphinpyrazole greatly reduces the risk. By involving the conducting system, MI often causes various grades of heart block and other irregularities.

(b) Cardiac failure. Extensive infarction of left ventricular muscle can cause acute heart failure, and if severe this results in **cardiogenic shock**, the prognosis of which is poor. Loss of the infarcted muscle also predisposes to chronic heart failure, which may develop at any time after infarction.

(c) Mural thrombosis. Following acute myocardial infarction, release of tissue thromboplastin from the damaged muscle and localised eddying of blood may lead to mural thrombosis in the ventricles (Fig. 10.15, p. 10.14). This is seen at autopsy in about 30 per cent of cases; in patients who survive, the thrombus is eventually organised. *Systemic emboli* can result from mural thrombosis, but are not very common.

(d) Venous thrombosis. Systemic venous thrombosis is an important early complication of myocardial infarction and tends to occur especially in the veins of the legs (p. 10.16). Detachment of such thrombus is common and consequently pulmonary embolism is not infrequently a cause of death in myocardial infarction.

(e) Rupture of infarcted myocardium due to autolytic softening (**myomalacia cordis**) occurs in about 5% of cases, usually during the first few days. Most often the rupture occurs in the wall of the left ventricle and causes haemopericardium and sudden or rapid death from cardiac tamponade. The pressure of blood accumulating rapidly in the pericardial sac

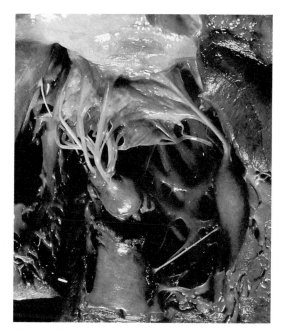

Fig. 15.14 Rupture of a necrotic papillary muscle in a patient with myocardial infarction.

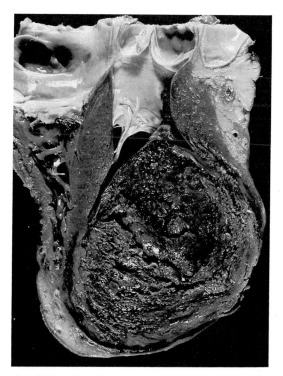

Fig. 15.15 Cardiac aneurysm following myocardial infarction. The wall of the left ventricle is stretched and thinned: thrombus has built up on it and now fills the aneurysm.

prevents diastolic filling of the cardiac chambers. Rupture of either the interventricular septum or of a mitral papillary muscle (Fig. 15.14) causes a sudden onset or worsening of acute heart failure accompanied by a loud cardiac murmur: these latter complications are usually rapidly fatal and may warrant surgical treatment.

(f) Cardiac aneurysm. Occasionally the fibrous scar of a healed infarct of the left ventricle may stretch to form a cardiac aneurysm. As with other aneurysms, laminated thrombus tends to form in the cavity (Fig. 15.15).

(g) Angina pectoris. Whenever myocardial infarction has occurred, the adjacent myocardium, although not infarcted, is likely to be ischaemic (and is presumably the source of the prolonged pain associated with infarction). As anastomotic channels dilate and enlarge, the blood supply to such areas of partial ischaemia will improve. However, in some patients angina pectoris dates from a myocardial infarction, and it is apparent that thrombosis of a major coronary vessel may render areas of myocardium chronically ischaemic. In some instances, angina is cured by myocardial infarction, presumably because an area of myocardium which was previously chronically ischaemic has been included in the infarct and destroyed.

(h) Recurrence of infarction. Because atheroma is generally extensive, individuals who have had a myocardial infarct are prone to recurrence. Cigarette smoking greatly increases the risk of this.

Diffuse subendocardial MI

Less than 10% of myocardial infarcts are subendocardial, affecting the inner part of the left ventricular myocardium throughout most or all of its circumference (Fig. 15.16). Necrosis is usually patchy, often with scattered haemorrhages, but may be confluent in patients surviving a week or more. All the major coronary arteries are usually severely narrowed by atheroma but in about two-thirds of cases there is no recent thrombotic occlusion, and the immediate cause of infarction is not usually apparent. In some patients, however, it develops during a period of shock. The left ventricle is usually hypertrophic and occasionally

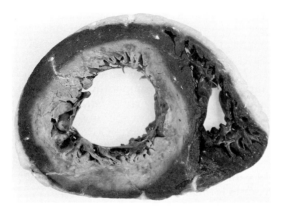

Fig. 15.16 Diffuse subendocardial myocardial infarction of several days duration. The infarcted myocardium is pale. Note also mural thrombi. The coronary arteries have been injected for radiography (Professor M. J. Davies).

subendocardial MI occurs in a hypertrophic right ventricle. It appears that the blood supply to the inner part of the ventricular myocardium is relatively precarious, and that the combination of ventricular hypertrophy and coronary atheroma predisposes to diffuse subendocardial infarction, often without superadded coronary thrombosis. In some instances, particularly when left ventricular hypertrophy is due to aortic valve disease, subendocardial MI occurs even without serious coronary artery disease.

Subendocardial MI is not complicated by pericarditis, nor by rupture of the ventricular wall or septum; otherwise its clinical features and complications resemble those of regional MI. In patients who recover, the dead muscle is gradually replaced by organisation leading to subendocardial scarring.

It is important to distinguish between subendocardial MI and small (sometimes microscopic) foci of myocardial necrosis which develop in dying patients with a failing circulation and which are of little significance.

Other effects of IHD

Ischaemic heart disease is the usual cause of **sudden cardiac death**. There may be a history of angina, previous infarction, evidence of chronic heart failure, or chest pain immediately before death, but sometimes there have been no warning symptoms. At autopsy there is usually severe coronary atheroma with or without old organised thrombotic occlusions. Recent occlusive coronary thrombosis is found in only about 30% of such cases, and the majority of patients resuscitated from what would undoubtedly have otherwise been sudden cardiac death do not develop regional MI (Cobb et al., 1975, Buja and Willertson, 1981). Accordingly, while coronary thrombosis is an important cause of sudden death, coronary artery atheroma without recent superadded thrombosis is even more important.

Ischaemic heart disease is also the commonest cause of various grades of **heart block** and other arrhythmias and of chronic heart failure (p. 15.3), whether or not there has been previous myocardial infarction.

The Cardiomyopathies

Patients with myocardial dysfunction, regardless of the underlying cause, usually present with chest pain and/or features of cardiac failure. Arrhythmias are common, and the heart is usually enlarged due to either myocardial hypertrophy or dilatation of one or more chambers, or to a combination of both. The commoner causes include ischaemia, systemic or pulmonary hypertension, valve lesions, rheumatic, viral or toxic myocarditis and congenital abnormalities. These conditions are described elsewhere in this chapter but there remains a heterogenous group of patients with chronic myocardial dysfunction of unknown cause. The term **cardiomyopathy** is most useful when applied to patients of this sort and its diagnosis must usually be based on exclusion of the commoner causes listed above, although endomyocardial biopsy is a very promising diagnostic procedure. Depending on the mechanical effects of the myocardial disorder, cardiomyopathy may be subdivided into the three types described below. There has been a tendency to include most or all myocardial disorders under the term cardiomyopathy, but this seems unnecessary and confusing.

1. Hypertrophic cardiomyopathy. In this condition there is asymmetrical hypertrophy of the left ventricle, and especially of the septum. Function is affected by (a) undue rigidity of the left ventricle, which interferes with diastolic filling; (b) the hypertrophied septum is widely assumed to obstruct the outflow from the left (less often the right) ventricle, but the frequency of this is now disputed; (c) mitral regurgitation is common, probably due to distortion of the ventricle by the asymmetrical hypertrophy.

The symptoms are those of atypical angina or of left and finally total heart failure but without dilatation of the left ventricle. Symptoms may occur at any age and sudden death is common. The condition is sometimes familial and has been detected (by echo cardiography) in some apparently healthy relatives. It appears to be inherited as a Mendelian dominant with a high degree of penetrance. The ventricular septum is grossly hypertrophied and there is also diffuse ventricular hypertrophy. Microscopy shows interstitial fibrosis, areas of disordered, whorled arrangement of muscle fibres and very marked thickening of the individual fibres, with enlarged, pleomorphic nuclei and increased glycogen content. These features are useful in diagnostic biopsy. The nature of the basic abnormality is unknown and current views are largely speculative.

The changes in the heart in Friedreich's ataxia are similar to those in HCM and 50% of patients die of heart failure.

2. Congestive cardiomyopathy (CCM). This presents as congestive heart failure in the absence of any of the usual causes, and is often accompanied by thrombo-embolic episodes. It is thus diagnosed by exclusion. At autopsy all the chambers are dilated, the myocardium is pale and unduly flabby, and there is often ventricular mural thrombus and endocardial thickening (Fig. 15.17). Microscopy may show gross hypertrophy of some myocardial fibres, with conspicuous nuclear enlargement, and atrophy of others. There may also be interstitial fibrosis. These changes are not diagnostic.

CCM sometimes shows a familial tendency, and may also be associated with alcoholism or follow childbirth, but the causation is entirely unknown and it occurs from childhood to old age. Conditions in which congestive failure arises from an unusual cause may be misdiagnosed as CCM unless the underlying cause is recognised, e.g. beriberi, haemochromatosis, transfusional haemosiderosis, acromegaly and Pompe's disease (in which glycogen storage accounts for the thickened myocardium and heart failure—p. 3.15).

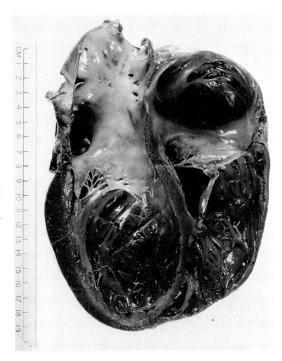

Fig. 15.17 Congestive cardiomyopathy. The anterior half of the heart is viewed from behind. The chambers are grossly dilated and there is some mural thrombus at the apex of the left ventricle.

3. Restrictive (obliterative) cardiomyopathy. In this disorder, abnormal rigidity of the affected chambers interferes with both filling and emptying and progressive heart failure results. The following two conditions are commonly included in this group, although in both of them the rigidity is due mainly to gross endocardial thickening, and not to myocardial disease.

Endomyocardial fibrosis (EMF). This condition is characterised by fibrosis of the endocardium and underlying myocardium of the inflow tracts of the ventricles. It may affect either or both ventricles. The fibrosis involves also the papillary muscles and chordae, causing incompetence of the mitral and/or tricuspid valve. The fibrous tissue restricts the ventricular muscle, impairing myocardial function. Ventricular dilatation or hypertrophy are not usually features though the atria are often grossly dilated. Mural thrombosis and embolic phenomena may occur.

EMF was first described by Loffler in 1936 and occurs sporadically throughout the world, usually associated with marked eosinophilia. However, the condition is endemic in tropical Africa, with a high incidence in Uganda and Nigeria, parts of southern India and, with a lower frequency, in Venezuela and Brazil. In all these regions EMF occurs in children and young adults and is a significant cause of cardiac morbidity and mortality. The geographical distribution of tropical EMF remains unexplained. However, there is evidence that the initial endocardial damage, in both sporadic and endemic forms of the disease, is related to eosinophilia and specifically to the effects on the heart of eosinophil leucocyte major basic proteins released following degranulation.

Endocardial fibroelastosis. This is an unusual cause of heart failure in infants and young children. A diffuse layer of dense white avascular tissue, composed largely of elastic fibres, develops in the mural endocardium, usually of the left atrium and ventricle. It obscures the trabecular pattern of the endocardial surface and affects also the papillary muscles and chordae and sometimes the cusps of the mitral and aortic valves, which become thickened, rigid and distorted. The mechanical effects of the thickened endocardium and valve lesions lead to fatal heart failure. The condition sometimes accompanies various congenital anomalies of the heart and is of unknown aetiology.

By increasing the rigidity of the myocardium, amyloid disease of the heart may simulate restrictive cardiomyopathy, while constrictive pericarditis (p. 15.43) produces the same picture of heart failure with small ventricles.

Inflammatory Lesions of the Heart

Myocarditis

Inflammatory lesions of the myocardium may be clinically silent or may give rise to fever, chest pain, tachycardia, heart block and other arrhythmias, heart failure and sudden death. A firm diagnosis of myocarditis is often difficult, for until recently there has been no widely applicable method of myocardial biopsy and histological investigation has been restricted largely to autopsy material.

The known causes of myocarditis include invasion of the myocardium by viruses, bacteria and parasites, bacterial toxins from infections of other tissues, hypersensitivity reactions and drugs. In addition, there are a number of ill-defined conditions of unknown cause.

In fatal cases of acute myocarditis the myocardium is flabby, usually pale, the ventricles are dilated and there may be mural thrombus.

Viral myocarditis. Coxsackie viruses, usually of Group B, and *Echovirus* type 8 give rise to acute myocarditis, usually accompanied by mild acute pericarditis. Individual cases occur in infants and outbreaks in nurseries, but young adults, particularly men, are more often affected. In fatal cases there is widespread interstitial oedema and infiltration of the myocardium by macrophages and lymphocytes (Fig. 15.18) and sometimes plasma cells and eosinophils: necrosis of scattered individual muscle fibres occurs, but is not conspicuous. The con-

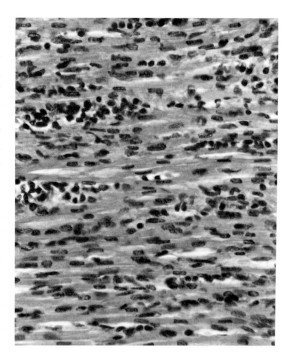

Fig. 15.18 Myocarditis due to Coxsackie B virus from a child of 11 months. The field illustrates the extensive focal infiltration with macrophages, lymphocytes, etc. × 320. (Dr J. F. Boyd.)

dition is usually mild and complete recovery is the rule. It may, however, be more severe, and is sometimes fatal.

Acute viral myocarditis with features similar to those described above occurs in some

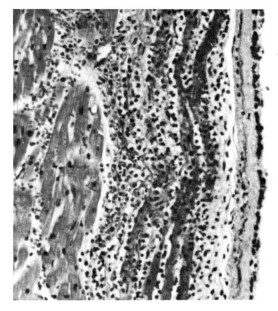

Fig. 15.19 Necrosis of the fibres of the left bundle branch, with an inflammatory reaction, in a fatal case of diphtheria. × 225. (Professor A. C. Lendrum.)

patients with poliomyelitis and as a complication of influenza. Rarely, it accompanies or follows chickenpox, measles, rubella or mumps, and it is a common feature of intra-uterine rubella infection.

Toxic myocarditis is a major feature of diphtheria. Similar appearances, presumed to be toxic in origin, may be seen in pneumococcal pneumonia, typhoid fever, septicaemia and other severe acute bacterial infections.

Morphological changes. The gross changes, mentioned above, are not diagnostic. Microscopically there are numerous small foci of coagulative necrosis in the muscle. The affected fibres appear swollen and glassy, with loss of striations and nuclei, and around them there is infiltration, mostly of macrophages and lymphocytes, but polymorphs also may be present. The necrotic fibres afterwards undergo absorption (Fig. 8.1, p. 8.5), fibroblasts proliferate, and small fibrous patches ultimately result. In some cases of toxic myocarditis due to diphtheria, the conducting system is severely affected (Fig. 15.9), with resultant heart block.

Clinically toxic myocarditis is recognised by the onset of cardiac arrhythmia or acute cardiac failure in a patient with diphtheria, pneumonia or other toxic infection. It may cause sudden death. Peripheral circulatory failure may also be present in severe cases.

Suppurative myocarditis caused by pyogenic bacteria, usually *Staph. aureus* or *Strep. pyogenes*, occurs in septicaemia and pyaemia, and also as a serious complication of acute infective endocarditis in which infection is by embolisation of the coronary arteries or direct spread from the valve lesions (p. 15.37). As in other tissues, *Staph. aureus* gives rise to localised abscesses while *Strep. pyogenes* causes a spreading infection with extensive necrosis and haemorrhage.

Chagas' disease. The chronic form of the disease is an extremely important cause of myocarditis in South America, for its affects up to 30% of the population in endemic areas and has a high mortality rate. The features are described on pp. 28.12–13.

Toxoplasmosis. Infection with *Toxoplasma gondii* is a cause of congestive heart failure of obscure aetiology, often associated with chest pain, atrial fibrillation and heart block.

Trichinosis. In *Trichinella spiralis* infection, some of the larvae invade individual myocardial fibres, and in heavy infection the myocarditis may be sufficiently severe to cause heart failure. (p. 28.46).

Hypersensitivity. Myocarditis is one of the most serious features of **rheumatic fever**, and is widely believed to result from a hypersensitivity reaction to antigens shared by the causal streptococcus and heart muscle (p. 15.24–25). Myocarditis may also complicate rheumatoid arthritis and systemic lupus erythematosus (p. 23.59), but is among the less common and less serious lesions of these conditions.

Administration of the cytotoxic drug daunorubicin and certain derivatives is sometimes associated with inflammatory myocardial injury which may cause congestive heart failure. The condition is dependent on dosage of the drug. The myocardium is a site of gumma formation in **syphilis**, but such lesions are now rare. The granulomatous lesions of **sarcoidosis** may occur in the myocardium, but seldom in sufficient numbers to interfere seriously with cardiac function.

Myocarditis of unknown cause. Acute or subacute myocarditis, unaccompanied by pericarditis or endocarditis and of unknown cause, is known as *iso-

lated myocarditis. The lesions sometimes resemble those of viral myocarditis, described above, while in other cases there is a focal granulomatous reaction resembling sarcoidosis.

This group of conditions includes also *Fiedler's* or *giant-cell myocarditis* in which the ventricles are dilated and hypertrophied and mural thrombi are common. The lesions may be just visible as yellow-white foci: there may be focal necrosis, interstitial infiltra-

tion with macrophages, lymphocytes, plasma cells and eosinophils, and a granulomatous reaction, sometimes with formation of multinucleated giant cells apparently derived from damaged muscle fibres. As with other forms of myocarditis, clinical features include chest pain and fever, embolic phenomena and arrhythmias. Sudden death or acute or chronic heart failure occur in some cases.

Rheumatic heart disease

Acute rheumatic fever

This is an acute febrile illness in which lesions occur in the heart, the joints and the subcutaneous tissue. It follows an attack of streptococcal pharyngitis and occurs mainly in children and young adults. Its incidence has fallen greatly in developed countries as a result of improved living conditions and use of antibiotics, but it is common in some parts of Africa, India, the Arab states and South America.

The most immediate hazard is diffuse myocardial injury during the acute illness: this is occasionally fatal, but otherwise myocardial function usually recovers completely. Subsequent disability is usually due to the effects of injury to the cardiac valves which results in their permanent distortion, often leading eventually to chronic heart failure. Rheumatic fever shows a marked tendency to recur after subsequent attacks of streptococcal pharyngitis, and each recurrence increases the risk of serious valvular disease.

Changes in the heart

Although all three layers of the heart are affected in acute rheumatic fever (pancarditis) the severity of their individual involvement varies greatly.

The **pericarditis** is exudative with effusion of serous fluid and deposition of fibrin on both pericardial surfaces, sometimes as a thick layer, giving them a rough, shaggy appearance (Fig. 4.22, p. 4.21) which has been compared with that observed when two generously buttered pieces of bread are pressed together and then

pulled apart. The fibrin may glue the pericardial surfaces together and is removed by the process of organisation which results in fibrous thickening and often permanent adhesion of the layers with partial or complete obliteration of the sac.

The development of pericarditis in the acute illness may precipitate or aggravate failure of the already weakened myocardium, particularly if there is much pericardial effusion.

In fatal acute cases, the **myocardium** is flabby and the ventricles, particularly the left, are dilated. Apart from this, there are no obvious naked-eye myocardial changes, but sometimes tiny pale foci may be just visible: these are the **Aschoff bodies** which are pathognomonic of rheumatic carditis. They are scattered throughout the myocardium (Fig. 15.20), being particularly numerous in the left atrium and ventricle. The Aschoff bodies develop in the fibrous tissue septa which run through the myocardium, and microscopy reveals a focus of eosinophilic hyaline material which contains fibrin and indicates exudation of plasma proteins from small vessels. This is surrounded by an aggregate of lymphocytes, macrophages, occasional polymorphs, and larger cells with two or three nuclei or a single convoluted nucleus (Fig. 15.21). The hyaline material is globular and appears to reflect necrosis of the infiltrating cells. In time, the Aschoff bodies subside and healing occurs with fibrosis, leaving minute focal scars in the connective tissue of the myocardium.

Although the function of the myocardium is seriously impaired in rheumatic fever, diffuse myocardial changes in fatal cases are neither

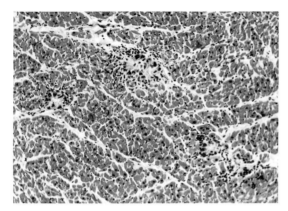

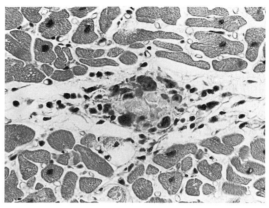

Fig. 15.21 Early Aschoff body in the myocardium of a child who died of heart failure during an attack of acute rheumatic fever. Central hyaline material is surrounded by macrophages, some with large or multiple nuclei, and by lymphocytes, etc. × 310.

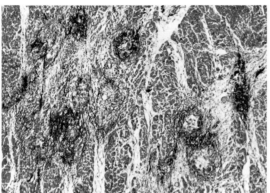

Fig. 15.20 Rheumatic myocarditis. *Above*, the acute stage, showing several Aschoff bodies. × 80. *Below*, later stage, showing fibrosis around the Aschoff bodies (Masson's trichome stain: collagen appears dark). × 48.

characteristic nor impressive. There is some inflammatory oedema and a light scattering of lymphocytes and occasional polymorphs. The functional disturbance appears to be due to an immunological reaction (see below).

The **endocardium** (like the myocardium) shows diffuse inflammatory oedema and light cellular infiltration. Aschoff bodies also develop in the endocardium and are particularly numerous in the posterior wall of the left atrium just above the insertion of the posterior mitral cusp; their healing may result in thickening and irregularity of the endocardium in

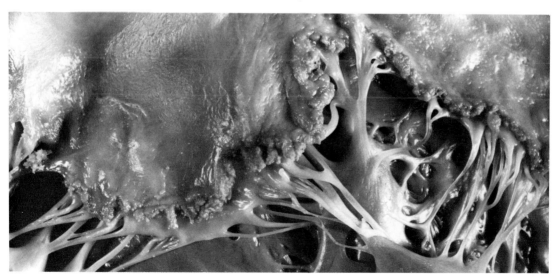

Fig. 15.22 Mitral valve in acute rheumatic endocarditis, showing the small vegetations which form along the line of apposition of the cusps. × 2.

this area. (McCallum's patch). In the acute fever, however, the most prominent endocardial lesion is seen on the heart valves and consists of small **thrombotic vegetations**, forming an interrupted or continuous line of fine grey-pink, firm nodular deposits on the surface of the valve cusps. They form mainly on that part of each valve cusp which comes into contact with the opposing cusp when the valves close, and are thus seen near the free margins of the cusps, on the atrial surface of the mitral (Fig. 15.22) and the ventricular surface of the aortic cusps. Vegetations develop most commonly on both these valves, but quite often on the mitral valve alone and occasionally on the aortic valve alone. The tricuspid also is occasionally affected, but vegetations are rarely seen on all four valves.

Microscopically, an important feature of the affected valves is the presence of blood vessels in the cusps (which are normally avascular). Capillaries grow into the cusps from their base early in the first acute attack of rheumatic fever and some of these subsequently enlarge and develop into arterioles and venules. Capillarisation is followed by acute inflammatory oedema, infiltration with polymorphs, macrophages, lymphocytes and plasma cells, and proliferation of fibroblasts. In some instances there are foci of fibrinoid necrosis in the valve cusps with surrounding aggregation of inflammatory cells, the appearances resembling Aschoff bodies, but cellular infiltration is usually more diffuse (Fig. 15.23). Superficial ulceration occurs at and around the parts of the valve cusps which are in contact during closure and is due to loss of endothelium resulting from the impact of valve closure on the inflamed oedematous cusps. Platelets and fibrin are deposited on the exposed fibrous tissue of the cusps and build up to form the vegetations, which appear eosinophilic and refractile (Figs 15.24 and 10.14, p. 10.13). Valvular function is not seriously impaired at this stage, although the vegetations tend to glue together the margins of adjacent cusps close to the commisures. Being composed largely of platelets, the vegetations are firmly adherent and do not give rise to emboli. Vegetations may also form on the chordae, which become matted together, and also on McCallum's patch in the left atrium. Bacteria cannot be detected in the heart in rheumatic fever.

The acute changes are followed by organisa-

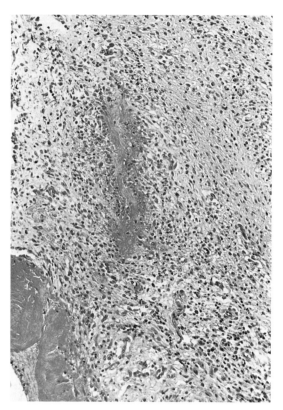

Fig. 15.23 A mitral valve cusp in acute rheumatic fever. Note the diffuse cellular infiltration and elongated patch of fibrinoid necrosis. Part of a surface vegetation is seen at bottom left. Capillaries can also be discerned in the cusp. × 130 (preparation kindly supplied by Professor A. C. Lendrum).

tion of the vegetations and more diffuse fibrous thickening of the cusps. Organisation of the vegetations on the cusps results in fibrous union between adjacent cusp margins and organisation of vegetations on the chordae lead to their becoming matted together as thick fibrous bands, particularly at their valvular ends: this has the effect of apparent shortening of the chordae and extension of the cusps. With recurrent attacks, the acute changes are superimposed on the valves and further fibrous thickening and deformity result.

In patients dying in the acute illness, all four valves are commonly inflamed, but residual effects with permanent distortion are usually confined to the mitral and aortic valves. These late effects are described on pp. 15.24, 15.26–32.

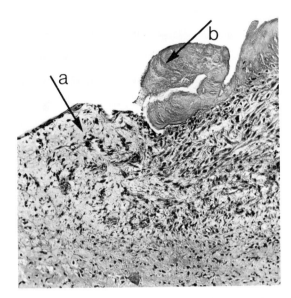

Fig. 15.24 Section of the mitral valve in acute rheumatic endocarditis. The cusp shows inflammatory oedema **(a)** and cellular infiltration, and appears to be vascularised. Where the cusps meet, the oedematous tissue has ulcerated and platelets have been deposited on the ulcerated surface to form the early vegetation **(b)**. × 80. (Professor A. C. Lendrum.)

Changes in other tissues

In patients dying of acute rheumatic fever, the **lungs** are congested, heavy, and feel firm and rubbery. Microscopy shows acute congestion, accumulation of oedema fluid containing some macrophages and desquamated pneumocytes, and lining of the alveolar ducts by a dense layer of fibrin ('hyaline-membrane disease', Fig. 15.25). These changes appear to result from fairly acute left ventricular failure and are sometimes seen when this occurs from causes other than rheumatic fever. The **joints** show mild inflammatory changes in the synovium with cellular infiltrates resembling Aschoff bodies but more diffuse; the tendons and their sheaths may show similar changes.

In some cases, **subcutaneous nodules** develop over bony prominences of the arms and legs, the commonest sites being the extensor surface of the elbow and overlying the ulna. The nodules are usually between 1 and 2 cm in diameter, painless, and consist of a patch of eosinophilic hyaline swelling of collagen surrounded by a granulomatous reaction in which the cells are mainly lymphocytes, plasma cells,

macrophages and fibroblasts. As in the Aschoff bodies, the hyaline change in collagen appears to be due to deposition of fibrin following permeation by plasma proteins exuded from the small vessels. Various erythematous skin rashes may occur, the commonest being *erythema marginatum*, and in some cases there may be a mild *encephalitis*, causing chorea (p. 15.24).

Clinical features

Rheumatic fever develops usually 2 to 4 weeks after a streptococcal sore throat. Symptoms may be mild, but there is usually fever, tachycardia, malaise and arthralgia flitting from joint to joint; the affected joints are sometimes swollen. The subsequent course depends on the degree of cardiac involvement: the most serious effect at this stage is on the myocardium, and various degrees of acute heart failure are observed. Signs of acute pericarditis usually appear later in the acute illness, and the valvular lesions are undetectable at this stage, although there may be

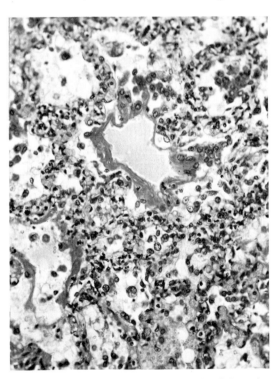

Fig. 15.25 The lung in a case of cardiac failure due to acute rheumatic myocarditis. The lung shows hyaline membranes lining alveolar ducts and mononuclear cells in the alveolar walls and lying free in the alveoli. × 220.

evidence of secondary mitral incompetence due to dilatation of the left ventricle, or valvular abnormalities resulting from previous attacks. Involuntary movements (*chorea*) attributable to involvement of the brain may occur during or apart from the acute illness, as may the skin rashes and subcutaneous nodules.

There is no specific test for rheumatic fever. A raised erythrocyte sedimentation rate, anaemia, slight leucocytosis and high titres of stretococcal antibodies are usually present. C-reactive protein, one of the so-called 'acute phase reactants', appears in the serum at an early stage but is found in many other acute illnesses.

Chronic rheumatic heart disease

Following recovery from rheumatic fever the function of the myocardium usually returns to normal, although minute fibrous scars mark the site of healed Aschoff bodies. Organisation of fibrinous pericarditis commonly results in fibrous pericardial adhesions or even obliteration of the sac, but the fibrous tissue is seldom thick or rigid enough to impair cardiac function. By contrast, *injury to the valves in rheumatic fever commonly causes permanent deformity resulting in stenosis or incompetence or a combination of both defects*. The acute changes leading to fibrous thickening and fusion of the cusps and to thickening and shortening of the chordae have been described above (p. 15.22). In about 30% of patients with rheumatic fever these valve lesions lead eventually to heart failure. The risk, however, depends on age, being higher following rheumatic fever in early childhood and in patients with repeated attacks. Sometimes the valvular changes progress rapidly and cause heart failure within weeks or months, but more often there is an interval of 5–30 years of apparent good health before the clinical features of valvular disease develop. Clearly, valve lesions can progress slowly and silently for many years after rheumatic fever. In patients treated surgically for post-rheumatic valvular disease, Aschoff bodies can often be detected in excised atrial tissue, particularly in patients under 50 years old. This suggests that rheumatic heart disease can smoulder on subclinically for many years, and this may possibly explain the slow progression of the valvular disease. However, distortion of a valve from any cause subjects it to increased mechanical injury

and stress with recurrent deposition of fibrin and platelets on the surface. Organisation of such deposits could account for the development of valvular disease many years after recovery from rheumatic fever.

In chronic post-rheumatic valvular disease, both the mitral and aortic valves are affected in about 50% of cases and the mitral valve alone in about 25%. The mitral, aortic and tricuspid valves are involved in about 15% of cases, while involvement of all four valves, or of the aortic valve alone, is rare. The susceptibility of the mitral and aortic valves to rheumatic injury is probably due to the relatively high pressure they must withstand. The valves on the right side of the heart are virtually never affected alone.

The chronic lesions of the individual valves and their effects are described on pp. 15.26–32.

Aetiology of rheumatic heart disease

Rheumatic fever (RF) occurs as a sequel to pharyngeal infection with *Streptococcus pyogenes*. It develops after an interval, usually 2–4 weeks, following an acute attack of streptococcal pharyngitis, including scarlet fever, and streptococci are not found in the heart in fatal cases of RF. Most individuals do not develop rheumatic fever after an attack of streptococcal pharyngitis, but those who do are very liable to have recurrent attacks of RF after subsequent attacks of pharyngitis whether due to the same or different serotypes of *Strep. pyogenes*. There is thus strong individual predisposition, and this appears to be genetically determined, for approximately 75% of RF patients have been shown to possess a B-cell allo-antigen, possibly of HLA-DR nature, which occurs in only 20% of the general population (Patorroyo *et al.*, 1979). There is also evidence that the serotypes of *Strep. pyogenes* are of importance, for some outbreaks of streptococcal pharyngitis are not associated with RF, even in subjects who have had previous attacks of RF.

Treatment for streptococcal pharyngitis with antibiotics does not abolish the risk of subsequent RF, but long-term administration of penicillin prevents further attacks of streptococcal pharyngitis and of RF.

It is unlikely that the acute carditis of RF is caused directly by streptococcal toxins, because it develops after recovery from the infection and is associated with unusually strong and persistent antibody responses to various streptococcal antigens. Indeed, a high titre of anti-streptolysin O (ASO) is widely used as a diagnostic aid. The association of RF with a strong immune response raises the possibility that it is caused by a hypersensitivity reaction and this received strong support from the work of Kaplan and Frangley (1969) who performed immunofluorescence tests on heart tissue from fatal cases of acute RF myocarditis: they demonstrated immunoglobulin and complement diffusely bound to the myocardial fibres and also, in some instances, to the tissue of the cardiac valves. The binding of antibody and complement to cardiac tissues, and particularly to myocardial sarcolemma, was subsequently confirmed. The next step was to determine the nature of the antigen(s) involved in this reaction. Was it streptococcal antigen which had bound to the heart during the acute infection, or was it a normal constituent of the heart muscle? The answer was provided by the demonstration that the serum of RF patients contains antibodies which react with normal myocardial sarcolemma and which can be absorbed by both normal myocardial and streptococcal antigens. It was subsequently shown that rabbit antisera to streptococcal antigen(s) react with human (and rabbit) sarcolemma. It is thus clear that *Strep. pyogenes and myocardium share common antigens.*

It is tempting to conclude that RF is due to a type 2 hypersensitivity reaction in which antibodies to streptococci react with the myocardial and endocardial tissues and, together with complement, cause the myocardial and endocardial injury. As usual, the story is more complex than this, for the heart-reactive autoantibodies induced in rabbits by streptococcal antigens, and also those in the serum in RF, react also with vascular smooth muscle and skeletal muscles. Nor are such antibodies found only in association with RF: they occur (although usually in lower titres) after uncomplicated streptococcal infections and in patients who develop post-streptococcal glomerulonephritis. Another difficulty is that, although rabbits immunised with streptococcal antigens develop antibodies reactive with autologous myocardium, these do not gain access to the rabbit's own myocardium, and it is necessary to postulate an initial myocardial vascular injury in RF which allows antibodies and complement to enter the tissue and bind to sarcolemma. In view of the delayed onset of RF, injury from streptococcal toxins is unlikely, and it may be that cell-mediated injury, i.e. a delayed hypersensitivity reaction, triggers off the cardiac lesion. In support of this possibility, it has been shown that immunisation of animals with streptococcal antigens results in production of lymphocytes which are cytotoxic to myocardial myocytes in tissue culture and less cytotoxic to skeletal muscle and other tissues. Investigations on cell-mediated immunity in RF have so far been inconclusive.

The streptococcal antigen(s) responsible for inducing antibody to myocardial sarcolemma has not been identified; it is of protein nature and is apparently associated with two distinct streptococcal components, M protein of the fimbriae, and the protoplast membrane. It is not known whether these contain the same or different cross-reacting antigens.

RF is also accompanied by the development of antibody to streptococcal cell-wall carbohydrate, and these persist for years in patients who develop rheumatic valvular disease. It has been reported that these antibodies react with human valvular tissue (and various other tissues, including joint synovia) and that experimentally-induced antibodies to valvular tissue can be absorbed by streptococcal carbohydrate. These findings have, however, been disputed and require further study.

It is not known why streptococcal infections of tissues other than the pharynx are not followed by RF, although pharyngeal infections invoke particularly strong antibody responses. Nor is the nature of the Aschoff bodies and rheumatic nodules understood: little or no immunoglobulin can be detected in these lesions.

In conclusion, RF is preceded and accompanied by the development of antibodies reactive with streptococcal components and with myocardium and heart valves. The streptococcal antigens involved are complex and have not been characterised. However, the binding of antibody and complement to myocardial sarcolemma and cardiac valves in acute RF suggests that these cross-reacting antibodies are of major pathogenic importance, in which case RF is an auto-immune disease.

Disorders of the heart valves

Normal cardiac function requires mechanical efficiency of the four cardiac valves. Deformity of a valve which results in serious reduction in the size of its aperture (**stenosis**) will increase the pressure load in the preceding chamber, while failure to close completely (**incompetence**) will result in regurgitation of blood and thus increase the volume load on the chambers on both sides of the valve. Either defect, if severe, is likely to result, sooner or later, in cardiac failure.

Abnormalities of the cardiac valves may be congenital or acquired. Congenital lesions are often associated with other malformations of the heart and great vessels: the more important lesions are described briefly on pp. 15.39–42. In many parts of Africa, Asia and South and Central America rheumatic fever is still common and is the major cause of acquired valvular disease at all ages. In most industrialised countries rheumatic fever has diminished greatly and chronic rheumatic valvular disease is now encountered mostly in middle and old age, while valve lesions from other causes have increased in relative importance.

The accurate diagnosis and assessment of valvular lesions by echocardiography, fluoroscopy and measurements of central pressures and blood flow have become more important in recent years because of the increasing availability of more effective treatment, e.g. by replacement of damaged valves by prostheses or tissue valve grafts.

Abnormalities of any of the cardiac valves increases the risk of infective endocarditis (p. 15.33).

The mitral valve

Normal functioning of the mitral valve depends on the mechanical efficiency of its cusps, chordae and papillary muscles, on the pliability and size of the fibrous valve ring 'or annulus, and on the adequacy of left ventricular contraction which normally halves the area of the orifice during systole. Because of the complex interaction of these components it is often difficult to assess the efficiency of the mitral valve at autopsy, and particularly to diagnose incompetence. As a rough guide, the circumference of the normal adult valve is approximately 8 cm and valves measuring less than 5 or more than 12 cm are likely to have been functionally defective.

Changes with age. In old people the mitral valve cusps are slightly thickened and appear relatively opaque, and there may also be a row of fine nodular thickenings along the line of contact of each cusp. Secondly, the posterior cusp often becomes stretched and bulges towards the atrium, apparently a minor degree of the 'floppy mitral valve' changes (p. 15.28). Lastly, calcification of the mitral ring is quite common in old age. These changes do not usually have serious effects on the functioning of the valve.

Mitral stenosis

Post-rheumatic. Rheumatic fever is still the major cause of mitral stenosis, even in the developed countries. Women are affected more often than men, and in approximately two-thirds of cases the aortic valve is also involved.

Each mitral cusp consists of a central fibrous plate (fibrosa) covered on either side by loose sub-endothelial connective tissue. The cusps are normally avascular except for a few small blood vessels at their bases. In chronic rheumatic disease, they are thickened and distorted, vascularised throughout, and consist of dense fibrous tissue which may be infiltrated with lymphocytes and plasma cells and in some cases irregularly calcified. The cusps are fused together along much of their free margins, thus forming a fibrous diaphragm with a central curved slit-shaped ('button hole') or oval orifice (Fig. 15.26), the area of which depends partly on the extent of fusion of the cusps and partly on their rigidity. Pure stenosis results when the diaphragm formed by the fused cusps is relatively thin and pliable. Greater thickening and rigidity usually results in a combination of stenosis and incompetence, particularly when the chordae become fused to form a rigid channel below the valve cusps, giving the valve a funnel-shape (Fig. 15.27).

Other causes. The changes described above

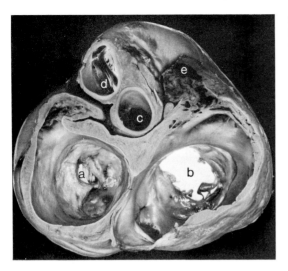

Fig. 15.26 Horizontal section through the atria in a case of mitral and tricuspid stenosis, as seen from above. **a,** mitral, valve, severely stenosed; **b,** tricuspid valve, moderately stenosed; **c,** aorta; **d,** pulmonary artery; **e,** right atrial appendage containing thrombus. × 0·6.

are the result of inflammatory valve damage. The rheumatic nature of the lesion must usually be based on a history of acute rheumatic fever or chorea, supported in some instances by involvement also of the aortic valve, McCallum's patch, and sometimes by the detection of Aschoff bodies (p. 15.20) in the myocardium or endocardium or the persistence of auto-antibody to myocardium (p. 15.25). Without such evidence, the possibility that mitral stenosis has resulted from a viral or other causal agent cannot be excluded.

In *rheumatoid arthritis* minor degrees of fibrous thickening and distortion of the mitral valve are common but seldom cause disability. Valve lesions resembling those following rheumatic fever are seen occasionally in patients with *systemic lupus erythematosus*.

Effects. The capacity of the left atrial myocardium to undergo hypertrophy is very limited and the obstruction to blood flow by a stenotic mitral valve soon results in a rise of pressure and accumulation of blood in the left atrium and pulmonary veins with gradual development of the changes of chronic pulmonary venous congestion (p. 10.5). Increased pulmonary venous pressure leads, by mechanisms which are not well understood, to pulmonary arterial hypertension and right ventricular hy-

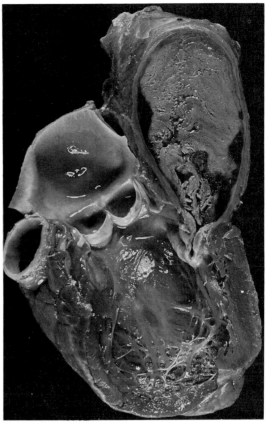

Fig. 15.27 Severe post-rheumatic mitral stenosis. The cusps are grossly thickened and the chordae are thickened and fused, forming a narrow channel below the cusps. The left atrium is grossly distended and almost filled with thrombus.

pertrophy, and eventually to structural changes in the pulmonary arterial tree (p. 16.25).

Initially the raised left atrial pressure is sufficient to drive the normal volume of blood into the left ventricle, but as mitral stenosis increases in severity the requirement for increased blood flow during physical exercise cannot be met and with severe stenosis even the resting blood flow is reduced. Dyspnoea and persistent cough result from pulmonary congestion and oedema and attacks of acute pulmonary oedema are brought on by exercise and occur also during the night as paroxysmal nocturnal dyspnoea (p. 15.3). Other effects of the pulmonary congestion include haemoptysis from the engorged capillaries and from broncho-pulmonary venous anastomoses, and recurrent pulmonary infections which may be promoted by pulmonary oedema.

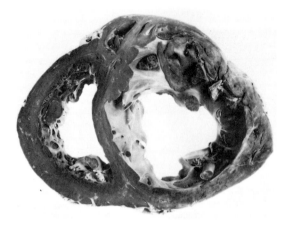

Fig. 15.28   Transverse section of the ventricles from a patient with mitral stenosis who died of right ventricular failure. The right ventricle (on the right) is hypertrophied and dilated, the left one relatively small. × 0·75.

Increased tone and hypertrophy of the pulmonary arterial tree tends to reduce the danger of pulmonary oedema, but restricts further the pulmonary blood flow and, by causing pulmonary hypertension, leads to right ventricular hypertrophy (Fig. 15.28) and eventual failure with generalised oedema, etc. (p. 15.4). In most cases the pulmonary hypertension is reversible and is relieved by surgical correction of the mitral stenosis.

Some degree of left atrial dilatation is usual in mitral stenosis (Fig. 15.27), although there are considerable variations which remain unexplained: in some patients the atrium is virtually normal in size, while at the other extreme its volume may exceed 400 ml. Gross dilatation is accompanied by atrophy of the left atrial myocardium, the wall becoming a thin layer of fibrous tissue. Atrial fibrillation is common and almost always accompanies gross atrial dilatation, but the cause/effect relationship is obscure.

Thrombus formation is common in the left atrium, particularly in its appendage, and is almost always present in patients with atrial fibrillation. In some cases the atrium may be almost filled with thrombus (Fig. 15.27) leaving a narrow irregular channel through which the blood flows. Systemic embolic phenomena often complicate the course of mitral stenosis, the commonest serious effect being cerebral infarction; they are more likely to occur when atrial fibrillation is present, and particularly when it alternates with periods of sinus rhythm.

Mitral incompetence

This may result from abnormalities of the valve cusps and their supporting chordae, from loss of function of papillary muscles, and from dilatation of the valve ring. The main causes are as follows.

(1) Lesions of the valve cusps and chordae. Injury to the mitral valve in *rheumatic fever* may be followed by reduction in the area of the cusps due to fibrosis and contraction, and by thickening and rigidity of the chordae which, if severe, may hold the cusps firmly in a partly open position. Increased rigidity of the cusps and fusion along part of their free margins often results in a combination of stenosis and incompetence and pure incompetence is unusual.

Another valve lesion termed the *floppy mitral valve* or *mitral valve prolapse syndrome* is becoming relatively important as a cause of mitral incompetence in developed countries as the incidence of rheumatic heart disease declines. The valve cusps and chordae become stretched and the latter may rupture. It is due to loss of collagen, and an increase in ground substance, in the cusps and chordae. During ventricular systole the slack is taken up and the chordae are jerked taut giving an audible systolic click. Part or all of one or both cusps bulge into the atrium (Fig. 15.29) and regurgitation may result, with a systolic murmur following the click.

Minor degrees of 'floppy valve' change occur in about 5% of people. The posterior cusp is usually more affected. Its segments or scallops become slightly thickened and at autopsy appear dome-shaped, bulging towards the atrium. The anterior cusp shows a single dome-shaped bulge. Incompetence is usually slight unless one or more of the chordae rupture. As in any abnormal valve, haemodynamic disturbance and mechanical trauma may lead to some thickening of the cusps and thickening and occasionally fusion of the chordae, the appearances sometimes being confused with rheumatic lesions. The changes of floppy mitral valve occur also in some cases of Marfan's syndrome, osteogenesis imperfecta and pseudoxanthoma elasticum.

Rapid or sudden mitral incompetence may develop in *infective endocarditis* as a result of

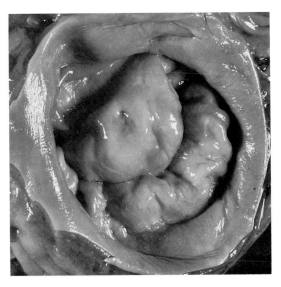

Fig. 15.29 Floppy mitral valve. The left atrium has been opened to show the thickened cusps bulging into it.

destruction of cusps and rupture of affected chordae.

(2) Papillary muscle ischaemia. Loss of contractility of a papillary muscle as a result of ischaemia may cause incompetence by allowing the related cusp to prolapse into the atrium. Accordingly, mitral incompetence is a common feature of myocardial infarction, particularly when the posterior wall of the left ventricle is infarcted. In some instances the papillary muscle is only partially ischaemic and recovers its function. In others, the muscle undergoes necrosis, followed by organisation and fibrosis, sometimes accompanied by stretching and various degrees of persistent regurgitation. Rupture of an infarcted papillary muscle causes sudden and severe regurgitation which usually results in rapidly fatal left ventricular failure.

(3) Dilatation of the mitral ring is rare as a primary event, but occurs in some cases of Marfan's syndrome, pseudoxanthoma and osteogenesis imperfecta. It is seen much more often as a consequence of the dilatation of a failing left ventricle, e.g. in ischaemic heart disease or systemic hypertension.

Effects. Incompetence of the mitral valve allows regurgitation of blood into the left atrium during ventricular systole. This additional volume of blood accumulating in the left atrium can pass freely into the left ventricle during ventricular diastole, and stretching of the left ventricle by the extra volume load results in more forcible contraction. When mitral incompetence develops gradually, there is time for the left ventricle to respond to the increased load by hypertrophy, and unless the leakage is very severe this enables it to eject the normal amount of blood into the aorta in spite of the mitral leak.

The left atrium becomes distended by the increased volume of blood entering it during ventricular systole, but as it empties during ventricular diastole the pressure within it falls to near normal, and so pulmonary venous congestion with consequent pulmonary arterial hypertension are not features of compensated mitral incompetence. Although atrial fibrillation commonly develops, left atrial thrombosis and embolic phenomena are observed less often than in mitral stenosis.

Although 'compensated', the left ventricle is handicapped by the mitral leak, and in all save the mildest cases its *maximal* effective stroke volume will be reduced. Accordingly, exercise tolerance is usually diminished and fatigue and weakness are often the presenting symptoms. Even during exercise, the pressure in the left atrium does not increase greatly during ventricular diastole, and attacks of acute pulmonary oedema with exertional and nocturnal dyspnoea are much less common than in mitral stenosis.

Eventually the increased volume load takes its toll and in some patients the left ventricle fails. As its contractions weaken and residual blood accumulates in it, the pressure in the left atrium rises also during ventricular diastole and pulmonary congestion and oedema develop. Death may result from left ventricular failure, but in some cases pulmonary congestion leads to pulmonary arterial hypertension and right ventricular failure may thus supervene.

In **sudden mitral incompetence**, as in rupture of a cusp in infective endocarditis or rupture of a papillary muscle in myocardial infarction, the left ventricle is unable to compensate and fails rapidly. The left atrium cannot dilate rapidly to accommodate the additional volume of blood entering it and so the left atrial pressure rises rapidly, leading to severe pulmonary congestion and oedema.

In cases of **combined mitral stenosis and incompetence**, pulmonary congestion and oedema lead to pulmonary arterial hypertension and right ventricular hypertrophy and eventual failure.

The aortic valve

The fibrosa of the aortic cusps is continuous with the valve sleeve which consists of fibrous and elastic tissue. Proximally the sleeve is attached to the muscular interventricular septum and to the fibrous base of the anterior mitral cusp. Distally it continues into the aortic media at the level of attachment of the aortic cusp commissures. The sleeve thus supports the valve cusps and forms the sinuses of Valsalva.

When the aortic valve closes, the areas of the cusps which are in mutual contact (the lunules) extend from the free margin to slight ridges passing obliquely across the cusps from the nodula Arantii towards the commissures.

With age, the cusps thicken slightly, but the lunules may be stretched, thinned and fenestrated, while the sinuses of Valsalva tend to bulge outwards. These changes are of no pathological significance. Calcification of the cusps is also common in old age and if extensive can cause aortic stenosis.

Aortic valve stenosis

In this country rheumatic endocarditis accounts for about 20% of cases of aortic stenosis, about 65% of cases are due to calcific aortic stenosis and 5% to congenital abnormalities. In the remaining 10% the cause is uncertain.

In *post-rheumatic aortic valve disease* the cusps are thickened, rigid and partly adherent and stenosis is usually combined with incompetence. In over 90% of cases the mitral valve is also affected. By contrast, *calcific aortic stenosis* is usually associated with a normal mitral valve and presents as stenosis, usually without serious incompetence: the changes are an exaggeration of those seen commonly in old age: the cusps become thickened by fibrosis and irregular nodules of dystrophic calcification develop, usually starting at the base of the cusps and extending towards the free margin. The irregular calcified nodules project from the aortic surface of the cusps, rigidity of which converts the orifice to a narrow slit. (Fig. 15.30). In con-

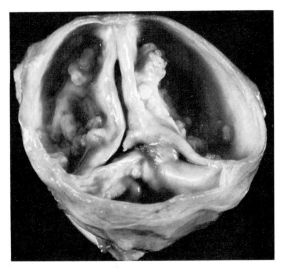

Fig. 15.30 'Senile' calcific stenosis in an aortic valve without obvious predisposing abnormality. × 2.

trast to rheumatic valvulitis, the cusps are not vascularised and usually there is no cusp fusion. In almost 80% of patients, calcific aortic stenosis develops in a *congenitally bicuspid aortic valve* (Fig. 15.31) and becomes apparent between 40 and 60 years of age. In the remaining 20% the lesion develops in an otherwise normal valve and causes symptoms after the age of 60.

In *congenital aortic valve stenosis* the cusps are usually fused to form a diaphragm with a central or eccentric orifice.

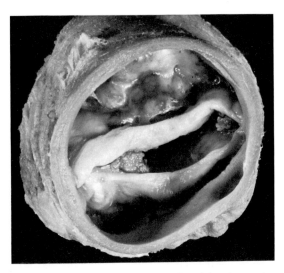

Fig. 15.31 Calcific aortic stenosis arising in a congenitally bicuspid valve. × 1·8.

Effects. Reduction of the area of the valve orifice by over 50% increases significantly the resistance to ejection of blood into the aorta and in consequence the left ventricle undergoes compensatory hypertrophy. In most patients this maintains adequate circulation for many years, during which there may be no symptoms. However, to achieve this compensated state, the left ventricle must generate a considerable pressure (sometimes over 250 mmHg) to overcome the resistance of the stenotic valve. Since the pressure in the aorta is not increased, and may fall below normal during ventricular diastole, the coronary perfusion pressure is diminished. These two factors—increased pressure load and diminished coronary circulation—predispose to angina pectoris, which is often the first symptom and sometimes occurs in the absence of coronary atheroma. Attacks of fainting are a common feature, perhaps due to transient arrhythmias triggered by the increased workload on the left ventricle. Indeed, approximately 15% of people with aortic stenosis die suddenly, presumably from ventricular fibrillation; nearly always there is a history of previous symptoms.

Eventually the left ventricle may fail and dilate, with consequent rise in left atrial pressure, pulmonary congestion and oedema. Death may result from left heart failure or pulmonary hypertension may lead also to right heart failure (p. 15.4).

Aortic valve incompetence

This increases the workload of the left ventricle, which, to maintain the circulation, must expel at each contraction both the normal stroke volume and the amount of blood regurgitated during ventricular diastole.

Causes. Incompetence may result from abnormalities of the cusps or from stretching or distortion of the root of the aorta. Fibrous thickening and contraction of the cusps in *rheumatic heart disease* is still an important cause of aortic incompetence, but this is usually combined with stenosis and in most cases the mitral valve is also affected. Incompetence may also be associated with *calcific aortic stenosis*, while some bicuspid valves, particularly those with grossly unequal cusps, are incompetent at birth or become so in youth.

In some cases of *infective endocarditis*, ero-

sion or rupture of a cusp causes acute or sudden aortic incompetence.

Dilatation of the aortic valve sleeve, with consequent aortic incompetence, may be inflammatory or non-inflammatory. Of the inflammatory lesions, syphilitic aortitis was formerly the usual cause, but it has become rare in most countries. A similar form of aortitis occurs occasionally in association with inflammatory joint disease, e.g. in ankylosing spondylitis and rarely in Reiter's syndrome and rheumatoid arthritis. More often, inflammatory dilatation of the aortic root is of unknown cause and occurs without associated disease.

Non-inflammatory stretching of the aortic valve sleeve is rare and usually of unknown cause. Various degrees of loss of medial elastic fibres and smooth muscle account for the weakness of the wall. Similar changes are seen in some of the genetic disorders of connective tissue, e.g. Marfan's syndrome.

In aortic incompetence due to dilatation of the aortic valve sleeve, the cusps become thickened, particularly along their free margins, and tend to sag downwards into the ventricle (Fig. 15.32). These changes, which may aggravate the

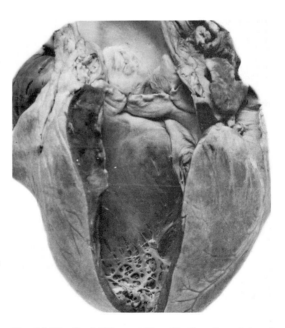

Fig. 15.32 Syphilitic aortitis, affecting the origin of the aorta. Stretching of the aortic ring has resulted in sagging and thickening of the cusps: dilatation and hypertrophy of the left ventricle are secondary to aortic incompetence. × 0·5.

incompetence, are well seen in syphilitic aortitis which is believed to cause medial damage by ischaemia and does not appear to attack the aortic cusps directly.

In *dissecting aneurysm of the aorta*, the lesion may extend down to involve the aortic valve sleeve and displace one or more aortic cusps, causing acute incompetence.

Effects. The increased volume of blood expelled by the left ventricle in aortic incompetence results in a raised systolic blood pressure, while during diastole the regurgitation of blood results in a rapid fall to abnormally low pressure. The pulse pressure is thus increased, giving a bounding or 'Corrigan' pulse. In response to the increased volume and pressure loads, the left ventricle hypertrophies and also dilates to accommodate more blood during diastole (Fig. 15.32), and a state of compensation usually lasts for many years. However, coronary blood flow, compromised by the reduced diastolic pressure, may not meet the demands of the hypertrophic left ventricle and so, as in aortic stenosis, angina pectoris is often a feature. Arrhythmias and sudden death are less common than in aortic stenosis. Eventually the left ventricle fails and this is usually fatal within three years unless the defective valve is replaced.

The tricuspid valve

In about 15% of cases of *post-rheumatic valvular disease* the mitral, aortic and tricuspid valves are affected. The changes in the tricuspid are similar to those in the mitral valve, but usually less severe (Fig. 15.26), and give rise to tricuspid stenosis or a combination of stenosis and incompetence. *The carcinoid syndrome* (p. 19.61) also causes tricuspid stenosis, either pure or combined with incompetence, and stenosis also results from *congenital malformations* of the valve. Pure incompetence due to dilatation of the valve ring is a feature of *right ventricular failure*.

Tricuspid stenosis or incompetence or a combination of the two all have similar effects. Pressure rises in the right atrium, which dilates, the central venous pressure increases and systemic venous congestion develops with 'cardiac' oedema. When associated with mitral stenosis or left ventricular failure these tricuspid lesions

tend to reduce the degree of pulmonary venous congestion and pulmonary arterial hypertension by limiting the volume of blood reaching the left side of the heart.

The pulmonary valve

Pulmonary stenosis is a feature of the carcinoid syndrome (p. 19.61) and occurs also as a congenital malformation (p. 15.40). It causes hypertrophy and eventual failure of the right ventricle.

Pulmonary incompetence may accompany stenosis in the carcinoid syndrome, but is more often secondary to pulmonary hypertension with dilatation of the pulmonary artery and valve ring. It occurs also as a congenital malformation and in infective endocarditis.

The mechanical effects are not serious unless there is pulmonary hypertension, and indeed the valve may be excised in patients with refractory infective endocarditis without greatly impairing cardiac function.

Infective endocarditis

When micro-organisms gain entrance to the bloodstream, they are usually rapidly eliminated. In circumstances favourable to them, however, they may succeed in gaining a foothold on the endocardial surface, usually of the valve cusps, and promote the formation of large infected thrombi. This condition—infective endocarditis—is characterised by fever, toxaemia, embolic phenomena, heart failure and sometimes glomerulonephritis. It is usually fatal unless the infection can be eliminated by antibiotic therapy, which has greatly reduced the mortality.

Traditionally, infective endocarditis is classified into **acute** and **subacute** types, the former being caused usually by bacteria of high virulence and the latter being a more prolonged illness due to less virulent organisms. Because of the differences in the clinical picture and pathological changes, the distinction between the two types is still valid but nowadays the disease is seen in patients treated by immunosuppressive therapy and commonly as an 'opportunistic' infection (p. 8.1) and often presents features intermediate between the two types. The causal agents include a wide range of bacteria and also fungi, *Coxiella burneti* and possibly viruses. Accordingly, while most cases are caused by bacteria, the generic term 'infective endocarditis' is preferable to the older 'bacterial endocarditis' which should be restricted to cases caused by bacteria.

Causal factors

The main factors which predispose to the development of infective endocarditis are (i) conditions which cause bacteraemia, septicaemia or pyaemia; (ii) abnormalities of the heart which favour the lodgement of micro-organisms on the endocardial surface, usually of the valves; (iii) depression of the defence mechanisms against micro-organisms.

Bacteraemia, septicaemia and pyaemia. It is probable that everyone develops transient and clinically silent bacteraemia from time to time. In many cases, however, infective endocarditis is preceded by a condition known to cause bacteraemia, and when the source of the bacteria can be traced, it is usually in the mouth, skin, genito-urinary or gastro-intestinal tracts.

Transient bacteraemia commonly follows tooth extractions, tonsillectomy and adenoidectomy, and even hard chewing or vigorous use of a toothbrush, particularly when there is periodontal infection, which is very common. Obvious infections, such as boils, carbuncles, bacterial pneumonias and infections of the urinary, gastro-intestinal and biliary tracts are associated with bacteraemia and, much less often, septicaemia and pyaemia.

Surgery on the gut, biliary or genito-urinary tracts, and even such minor procedures as urethral catheterisation, cystoscopy and sigmoidoscopy have been shown to be capable of causing transient bacteraemia, but such procedures do not carry a significant risk of infective endocarditis unless there is predisposing valvular disease or depression of defence mechanisms against infection.

Other causes include the use of intravenous injections by drug addicts and the introduction of micro-organisms during open heart surgery.

Predisposing cardiac lesions. Distortion of the heart valves predisposes to infective endocarditis, and in many cases there is evidence of preceding rheumatic or other valvular abnormalities. Despite the fall in incidence of rheumatic fever in many countries, chronic rheumatic valvular disease is still the most important underlying condition, but in developed countries other valve lesions, notably calcific aortic stenosis, floppy mitral valve and congenital abnormalities such as bicuspid aortic valve, have increased in relative importance. Even the minor changes which occur with age (pp. 15.26, 15.30) predispose to infective endocarditis, and help to explain its occurrence in middle-aged and old people without any other predisposing valve lesions.

Curiously, syphilitic aortic valve disease (now rare in most countries) was apparently seldom complicated by bacterial endocarditis.

It has been shown experimentally that when minor vascular lesions are caused by abrasion of the endothelium, intravenously injected bacteria adhere to and persist in small thrombi which form on such lesions. This helps to explain why congenital or acquired valve lesions predispose to infective endocarditis, for the uneven surfaces of distorted valve cusps are subjected to repeated trauma by forcible contact during closure and by unduly rapid and turbulent flow of blood through the deformed valve orifice. A fine layer of fibrin and platelets, to which micro-organisms can adhere, is frequently demonstrable on surgically-excised distorted valve cusps. Trauma and formation of fine mural thrombus occurs also at extra-valvular sites where rapid jets of blood passing through a distorted valve strike the endocardium, and this accounts for the development of infective endocarditis at such sites.

The mural thrombi which form at sites of endocardial injury, particularly on distorted valve cusps, are not usually visible macroscopically, but they provide shelter for entrapped micro-organisms and as these multiply they invade the underlying valve cusp and also promote the deposition of larger, readily visible thrombi which provide some protection from the host's defence mechanisms. The organisms embedded in thrombus may thus continue to multiply even when the level of antibodies in the plasma is sufficient to destroy any which are shed from the lesions into the bloodstream. The protection afforded by gross valvular abnormalities is a particularly important factor in the development of subacute infective endocarditis, which is usually caused by micro-organisms of low virulence. For bacteria of high virulence, such protection is less essential, and they frequently colonise valves with no gross preceding abnormalities. Valve prostheses and transplanted tissue valves and their supporting metal frame are also predisposed to deposition of thin layers of thrombus and over the years a significant proportion of patients with them develop infective endocarditis.

Impaired defence mechanisms. Depression of specific immunity, complement deficiencies and inadequate function of phagocytes, whether caused by cytotoxic therapy or by natural disease, predispose to infective endocarditis. This is partly because they increase the liability to infections, and thus to bacteraemia and septicaemia, and partly because they afford micro-organisms settling on the heart valves a better chance of survival and multiplication. Examples include the impaired specific immunity associated with lymphomas, and the deficiency of neutrophil polymorphs and monocytes in some forms of haemopoietic failure and leukaemia. Cytotoxic drugs used in the treatment of patients with various types of cancer, renal transplant recipients, etc., result in depression of immune responsiveness and of production of polymorphs and monocytes, and thus predispose to infections of various sorts. Such therapy increases the risk of infective endocarditis, and the range of micro-organisms responsible includes opportunistic pathogens which are normally of low virulence, as well as virulent bacteria.

Subacute infective endocarditis (SIE)

This is usually caused by bacteria of relatively low virulence, the most common being the 'viridans' group of α-haemolytic stretococci which form part of the normal flora of the mouth and pharynx and participate in periodontal infection, followed by *Streptococcus bovis*, which inhabits the gastro-intestinal tract, and *Staphylococcus epidermidis*, a skin commensal which inevitably infects indwelling venous catheters, exteriorised pacemaker wires, etc. Other skin and gastro-intestinal commensals, such as diphtheroids, coliform bacilli, bacteroides and mycoplasmas are responsible for occasional cases, while *Coxiella burnetii*, the cause of Q fever and subclinical infections, also accounts for about 3% of cases, occurring usually in

young and middle-aged adults. Fungal endocarditis occurs particularly in drug addicts from use of dirty syringes and solutions for intravenous injections, and also in immunosuppressed patients and following open heart surgery. The fungi most often involved are candida, aspergillus and, in some warm countries, histoplasma.

In most cases subacute infective endocarditis (SIE) develops on abnormal valves, and in countries where rheumatic fever is still rife it occurs most often in children and young adults with chronic rheumatic valvular disease. In the developed countries where rheumatic fever is now rare, chronic rheumatic valvular disease is seen mainly in middle and old age, and the age incidence of SIE has changed accordingly. Also, because of the decline in rheumatic fever, the other predisposing valve abnormalities noted below have increased in relative importance, and the overall incidence of infective endocarditis does not seem to have fallen significantly.

Changes in the heart. The mitral and aortic valves are most commonly affected, either separately or together. They may show evidence of previous rheumatic fever or the changes of 'floppy mitral valve', bicuspid aortic valve or calcific aortic stenosis. In some cases the valves show no evidence of previous abnormality or merely the minor changes which develop with age, and sometimes they are so altered by infective endocarditis that their previous state cannot be assessed.

The lesions consist of large friable soft shaggy thrombi, of various colours from yellowish-grey to reddish-brown, projecting from the surface of the valve cusps (Fig. 15.33). They usually develop on the contact surface of a cusp and spread along the lines of contact, where they may be patchy or continuous, and also to the contact surfaces of the adjacent cusp(s). The micro-organisms eventually invade the underlying cusp tissue and cause necrosis, which may result in aneurysm formation or rupture of the cusp, and they may also extend along, and cause rupture of, the chordae, although these destructive changes are more frequent and severe in acute bacterial endocarditis. The lesions may spread also from the mitral valve to McCallum's patch in the left atrium, and from the base of a valve cusp into the adjacent myocardium or into the root of the aorta. Spread from the aortic valve to the

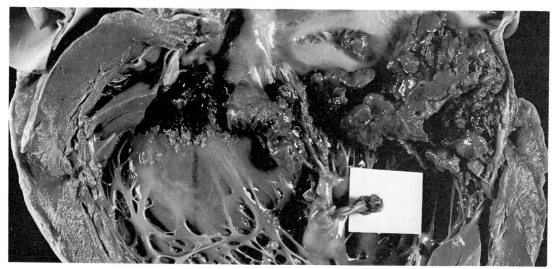

Fig. 15.33 Infective endocarditis of the mitral valve. The vegetations have covered the cusps and extended on to the posterior wall of the left atrium. A ruptured chorda is displayed.

anterior mitral cusp, and *vice versa*, is common.

The tricuspid valve is sometimes affected, particularly in drug addicts and as a complication of vascular catheterisation. Involvement of the pulmonary valve is rare. Other sites of infective endocarditis include the margins of ventricular septal defects and the sites where jets of blood from distorted valves strike the endocardium (p. 15.33), e.g. on the interventricular septum or anterior mitral cusp in aortic valve incompetence, and similar lesions (although not strictly endocarditis) sometimes develop in congenital vascular lesions, notably patent ductus arteriosus and coarctation of the aorta.

Microscopically, the vegetations are seen to consist mostly of fibrin and platelets and contain colonies of micro-organisms (Fig. 15.34). Polymorphs are usually scanty. The underlying cusp is vascularised, thickened and fibrosed. It is infiltrated with polymorphs and macrophages and may show invasion by bacteria and necrosis.

Eradication of the infection by antibiotic therapy is followed by gradual repair of the damaged cusps and slow organisation of the vegetations, resulting in gross and irregular scarring and distortion of the cusps and fibrous thickening and matting of the chordae. The end result may be indistinguishable from chronic rheumatic valvular disease, but usually the cusps are more irregularly thickened and calcified.

Embolic and other phenomena. Embolic phenomena result from detachment of fragments of the vegetations. Infarction of the brain, kidneys and spleen are common complications, and myocardial infarction, either gross or affecting multiple small areas, also occurs, particularly when the aortic valve is involved. The embolic

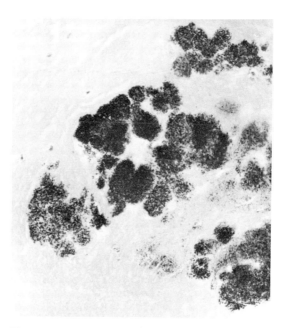

Fig. 15.34 Colonies of *Streptococcus viridans* in a section of a vegetation in subacute infective endocarditis. (Eosin, methylene blue.) × 320.

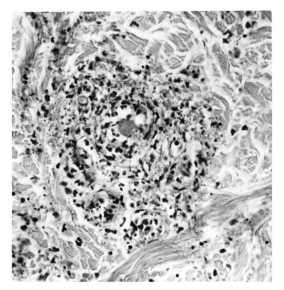

Fig. 15.35 Section through haemorrhagic spot in dermis in subacute infective endocarditis. Note small thrombosed and degenerate arteriole surrounded by leucocytes—the result of infective embolism. × 160.

lesions do not usually suppurate, perhaps because there are usually high plasma levels of antibodies to the causal micro-organisms. Unless the infection is cut short by early treatment, focal glomerulonephritis (p. 22.34) develops in about 30% of patients; diffuse glomerulonephritis is much less common. The spleen is moderately enlarged as a result of increase in mononuclear cells in the red pulp.

Clinical correlations and course. SIE often starts insidiously with irregular fever, malaise and mild anaemia. As it progresses, petechiae may appear, usually in small numbers, in the skin, mucous membranes and retina, and 'splinter' haemorrhages under the nails: these are probably embolic (Fig. 15.35). The spleen may become palpable and cardiac murmurs may be present from previous heart disease or may develop and change in quality as the infective lesions progress. Clinical features may arise from embolisation and infarction of the brain, myocardium, spleen, etc., and gross or microscopic haematuria due to renal infarction or glomerulonephritis. Heart failure eventually develops and is the commonest cause of death. It may be progressive and due mainly to increasing valvular damage, but it may come on or deteriorate suddenly from rupture of a valve cusp or chordae or from myocardial infarction. The other major causes of death are embolic phenomena and renal failure.

Without antimicrobial therapy, SIE is usually fatal within a few months. Early and adequate administration of an antibiotic to which the micro-organism is sensitive reduces the mortality to under 10%. Isolation of the micro-organism is thus urgent and sometimes requires repeated blood cultures. In about 20% of cases no causal organism can be found. In some instances this is due to recent administration of antibiotics, usually in amounts sufficient to sterilise the blood temporarily without eradicating the infection. In other instances, negative cultures occur because the micro-organisms do not grow in ordinary cultures, e.g. coxiella or mycoplasma. Occasionally an organism is cultured but is mistakenly regarded as a contaminant, e.g. diphtheroids or *Staph. epidermidis*. The prospect depends largely on the sensitivity of the micro-organisms to antibiotics, streptococcal cases, for example, having a good prognosis and those caused by fungi and *Coxiella burneti* a poor one. If blood cultures are negative, the decision on when to stop searching for micro-organisms and start therapy on suspicion is often very difficult.

Acute infective endocarditis

This is a much more severe infection than subacute infective endocarditis (SIE) and without effective treatment is fatal within a few weeks. It may arise as a complication of septicaemia or pyaemia or without obvious preceding infection. The commonest causal organism is *Staphylococcus aureus*, followed by *Streptococcus pyogenes* and *Enterococci*. In states of diminished resistance, however, less virulent bacteria, including those responsible for SIE, can cause acute endocarditis or conditions of intermediate severity.

Pathological features. The vegetations resemble in appearance those of SIE, but tend to be larger and more patchy and may be localised to one part of a valve (Fig. 15.36). They consist mainly of fibrin containing large clusters of bacteria surrounded by neutrophil polymorphs. The organisms rapidly invade the affected cusps, causing necrosis and suppuration, often with formation of cusp 'aneurysms' or complete rupture (Fig. 15.36). The vegetations commonly extend to the chordae, which may also rupture. Spread of infection from the aortic valve to the adjacent aorta may cause a mycotic aneurysm

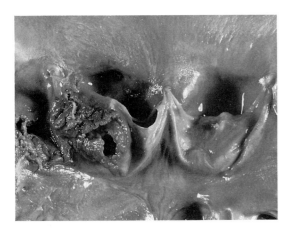

Fig. 15.36 Acute infective endocarditis of the aortic valve. The lesion has involved the adjacent parts of two cusps, one of which (left) is largely destroyed and the other (centre left) is perforated. There is an early vegetation on the remaining cusp.

or rupture and the organisms may also spread from the affected valve cusps into the adjacent myocardium where they cause necrosis and formation of abscesses.

When *Staph. aureus* is responsible the tricuspid valve is often affected, especially in drug addicts, but otherwise the mitral and aortic valves are more commonly involved and frequently there is no evidence of previous valvular abnormality. Rapidly fatal septicaemia may develop and fragments of the vegetations break away and produce septic infarcts in the brain, kidneys, lungs, etc.

The clinical features are those of a severe acute bacterial infection, usually accompanied by cardiac murmurs which may change rapidly as the valve cusps are destroyed. In the absence of previous antibiotic therapy, blood culture is nearly always positive. Various symptoms arise from septic infarction and in the absence of early and effective antibiotic therapy, the condition is fatal within days from overwhelming infection or within weeks from acute heart failure due to a combination of toxaemia, rapid destruction of the affected valves and septic infarcts. Even with intensive treatment the mortality is over 50%.

Other valvular lesions

Non-infective thrombotic endocarditis consists of the formation of sterile thrombotic vegetations on the heart valves, usually in a patchy fashion along the lines of closure of the cusps of the mitral and aortic valves. The vegetations are usually smaller than those in infective endocarditis and softer, larger, more friable and less regular than those in rheumatic endocarditis (Fig. 15.37). They are composed of mixed thrombus, fragments of which may break off and cause systemic embolism and infarction. In most instances, this condition is discovered at autopsy on patients who have died of cancer or other wasting diseases, and it is sometimes called *marantic* or *terminal endocarditis*. It may be associated with the venous thrombosis which occurs in some patients with carcinoma of the pancreas or of other internal organs (p. 10.17).

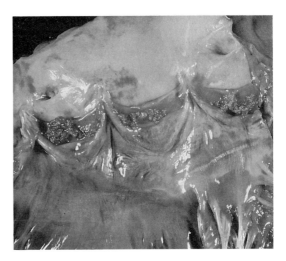

Fig. 15.37 'Terminal' thrombotic endocarditis of the aortic valve in a patient who died of cancer.

Libman–Sacks endocarditis occurs in many patients with systemic lupus erythematosus. The vegetations are sterile and are softer and more friable and usually larger than those of rheumatic endocarditis. They are also more widely dispersed on the cusps, usually affect the mitral and tricuspid valves, and may extend onto the adjacent mural endocardium or over the ventricular surface of the valve cusps (i.e. the surface away from the bloodstream).

Atheroma-like degeneration of mitral valve. Yellowish patches of thickening and degeneration similar in structure to atheroma are fairly common in the mitral valve and may be attended by fibrosis and calcification, especially at the base of the cusps. The chordae tendineae are not affected and there is seldom any effect on cardiac function.

Disorders of the conducting system

As indicated in preceding sections of this chapter, disturbances of cardiac rhythm commonly complicate various types of heart disease. Many of them, e.g. extrasystoles, paroxysmal tachycardia and atrial fibrillation, are not usually attributable to changes in the conducting system.

The most vulnerable part of the system is the A–V bundle and its right and left branches: injury may result from the various types of myocarditis (see Fig. 15.19, p. 15.19), chronic myocardial ischaemia or myocardial infarction, trauma during cardiac surgery, and invasion by metastatic tumour. Bundle branch fibrosis may also arise from unknown cause. The various grades of heart block can often be explained by such injuries (Figs. 15.38, 15.39), but in some instances lesions have been sought in vain, while in others the finding of lesions has been associated with normal ECG patterns during life. This lack of close correlation probably reflects the large amount of work involved in thorough histological examination of the conducting system and the difficulties which arise from various artefactual changes.

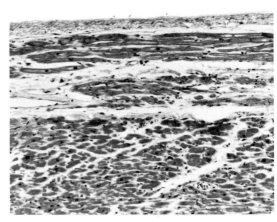

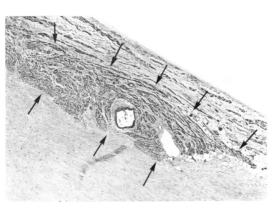

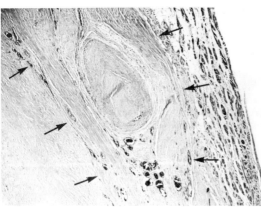

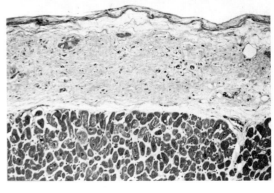

Fig. 15.38 Ischaemic fibrosis of A–V node. *Above*, normal A–V node (*outlined by arrows*), lying between the endocardium and central fibrous body. *Below*, ischaemic fibrosis of A–V node from a patient with heart block. (Professor M. J. Davies.)

Fig. 15.39 'Idiopathic' bundle branch fibrosis. *Above*, normal left bundle branch from the heart of a young man, consisting of groups of fibres lying between the ventricular myocardium and endocardium surface. *Below*, almost complete loss of left bundle branch in a case of heart block. (Some loss of fibres occurs as a normal feature of ageing). (Professor M. J. Davies.)

Congenital Abnormalities

Little is known of the causation of congenital abnormalities, but the part played by rubella infection of the mother in the first three months of pregnancy is well established. About 10–20% if the infants show serious abnormalities, of which heart disease constitutes about 50%.

Normal development

A high proportion of congenital abnormalities of the heart result from defects or variations in the formation of the septa in the primitive heart. For details the student must consult a work on embryology and the classical studies of Maude Abbott and Helen Taussig, but it may be recalled that the heart at an early stage of development consists of three chambers or parts, an atrial, a ventricular and the aortic bulb; division of each of these into two takes place separately. Of special importance in this connection is the relation of the ventricular septum to the division of the distal portion of the bulb into the beginning of the aorta and of the pulmonary artery. The ventricular septum grows upwards from the apex, with a curved margin resulting from the growing folds on the anterior and posterior walls, until ultimately there is a relatively small aperture at the base. The aortic bulb undergoes division into two nearly equal parts by the formation and fusion of two longitudinal folds in its wall, and the two vessels formed must rotate spirally in order to establish their normal continuity with the ventricles. The septum of the bulb ultimately fuses with the upgrowing ventricular septum, the last portion to close being represented by the membranous part of the septum. Important abnormalities occur in connection with the growth of these two septa. It is to be borne in mind that the positions of the semilunar valves do not correspond exactly with the junction of the primitive ventricle and the aortic bulb. This is especially the case on the right side, where the lower part of the bulb becomes the upper part of the right ventricle or conus, and, as we shall see, this part is sometimes abnormally narrow.

While some of the anomalies are incompatible with extra-uterine life, in many the circulatory dynamics are such that the patients may survive birth for varying periods of time. With the diagnostic methods of cardiac catheterisation and angiocardiography, successful surgical cure or alleviation of many of the conditions can be effected. It is convenient to divide the anomalies into those which produce *cyanosis* and those which do not. The cyanosis is produced by admixture of a relatively large amount of reduced haemoglobin from the systemic venous blood, with the oxygenated blood leaving the heart, i.e. a venous-arterial shunt exists. The resulting unsaturation of the arterial blood leaving the heart leads to compensatory rise in the red cell count, which makes cyanosis more prominent. Later, changes in the pulmonary vessels occur (pp. 16.23–25) and the heart begins to fail. Cyanosis may then increase owing to impaired oxygenation of the blood by the lungs.

Cyanotic group

Malformations of the aortic bulb—pulmonary and aortic stenosis. The commonest of these result from an unequal division of the bulb. Most frequently the septum is pushed to the right, so that the aorta is abnormally large and arises partly from the left and partly from the right ventricle, there being usually also a defect in the ventricular septum. The result is **pulmonary stenosis** or obstruction, but the site of the narrowing varies: sometimes the pulmonary artery is small, the division of the bulb being markedly unequal, and occasionally the small pulmonary artery is completely obliterated. In other cases the narrowing is mainly at the valve, the cusps sometimes being partly fused to form a thickened diaphragm with a reduced aperture. More rarely, there is a narrowing of the part of the right ventricle below the valve, that is, the part which is derived from the bulb. All these abnormalities interfere with the flow of blood into the pulmonary artery, and lead to a varying degree of hypertrophy of the right ventricle. Part of the blood from the right ventricle passes through the aperture in the interventricular septum and then into the aorta, and after birth the ductus arteriosus usually remains open and the lungs receive part of their blood supply through it. The foramen ovale also remains open and may be very large.

The commonest anomaly of this group and one which is amenable to surgery is the **tetrad of Fallot**. In this there is obstruction in the outflow tract of the right ventricle, usually from stenosis of the pulmonary valve, though the obstruction may be in the infundibular part of the right ventricle. This results in right ventricular hypertrophy and the pressure in this chamber is raised so that some of the reduced blood in the chamber is shunted through a high interventricular septal defect into the aorta, which, in addition to receiving the oxygenated blood from the left ventricle, partially overrides the septal defect and is thus in communication with the cavity of the right ventricle. All degrees of severity exist in the stenosis of the right ventricular outflow, the size of the septal defect and the dextraposition of the aortic root. In extreme cases the pulmonary orifice and artery may be atretic and blood reaches the lungs from the aorta through a patent ductus arteriosus.

In about 25% of cases of Fallot's tetrad, there is a right aortic arch.

Eisenmenger's complex. In this there is a strong resemblance in the gross morphology of the heart to that just described, but there is no obstruction to the outflow from the right ventricle. The pressure gradients across the high interventricular septal defect are such that little right-to-left shunting of blood, and hence little cyanosis, occurs at first. Later, with onset of pulmonary hypertension and changes in the pulmonary vessels, overt cyanosis occurs, partly from admixture cyanosis and partly from faulty oxygenation of the blood by the lungs.

Transposition of the great vessels. A curious anomaly results from failure of the proximal aorta and pulmonary artery, formed by division of the aorta bulb, to undergo the rotation necessary for the establishment of their correct relationships with the ventricles. In consequence, the aorta arises from the right ventricle and the pulmonary artery from the left. While such a condition alone is incompatible with extra-uterine life, it may sometimes be compensated, for a time, by persistence of the ductus arteriosus, patent foramen ovale, or a defect of the interatrial or interventricular septum; often these defects are present in combination. In this condition, the chief difficulty is not the volume

of blood reaching the lungs but the effectiveness of the mechanism allowing oxygenated blood to reach the systemic circulation. Hence the greater the volume of the shunt, the better the admixture of arterial blood to venous blood and the less marked is the cyanosis.

Truncus arteriosus. In this the arrangement of the heart and emergent arteries resembles that in elasmobranch fishes in which the aorta and the pulmonary arteries arise from a common stem vessel. The pulmonary arteries may be replaced by enlarged bronchial arteries. The truncus arises from both ventricles, overriding a ventricular septal defect. Sometimes the septum may be missing so that a single ventricular cavity exists. Defects of the interatrial septum are also common.

Single ventricle with a rudimentary outlet chamber. In this condition, a single ventricle provides blood to both the aorta and pulmonary artery, which may arise separately or from a rudimentary outlet chamber. The interatrial septum may or may not develop normally, resulting in cor binatrium triloculare or cor biloculare respectively.

Tricuspid atresia. This is associated with defective development of the right ventricle which in extreme cases is virtually absent. Blood passes from the right to the left atrium through a defect in the interatrial septum. The pulmonary artery is small, arising from the underdeveloped right ventricle. In some cases the vessel is atretic or occupies an abnormal position. Usually blood reaches the lungs from the aorta by a patent ductus arteriosus.

Aortic atresia. In this rare condition the aortic orifice is hypoplastic, the ascending aorta hypoplastic or atretic, and the left ventricle poorly developed or absent. Circulation of blood is maintained by shunting of oxygenated blood from the left atrium into the right atrium and thence to the right ventricle and pulmonary artery. From this, the aorta is filled via a patent ductus arteriosus.

Pure pulmonary stenosis. Here the course of the circulation is essentially normal but sometimes there is a patent interatrial septum. The lesion is a stenosis of either the pulmonary valve or the infundibulum of the right ventricle. The right ventricular myocardium is hypertrophied and able to force the blood to the lungs past the obstruction. If the interatrial septum is intact, cyanosis is not necessarily present; if there is interatrial communication a right-to-left shunt may be established with consequent cyanosis.

Anomalies of the venous return. These may involve the systemic or the pulmonary veins and vary greatly in detail. The superior and/or the inferior vena cava may open into the left atrium, thus shunting reduced systemic venous blood into the arterial side of the systemic circulation. In other cases, some of the pulmonary veins open into the right atrium: this results simply in an excessive amount of oxygenated blood being pumped around the pulmonary circulation and cyanosis will not occur.

Acyanotic group

Aortic valve stenosis and subaortic stenosis may each occur as an isolated abnormality as may also a **bicuspid aortic valve**. The incidence of the latter is approximately 2% and it is usually symptomless, but predisposes to the development of infective endocarditis or calcific aortic stenosis.

Patent ductus arteriosus. As indicated above, this may co-exist with many other anomalies, but it may be the only abnormality present, in which case closure by surgery restores the circulation to complete normality. Failure to close the ductus leads eventually to heart failure or the development of infective 'endocarditis' (endarteritis) of the ductus. In a few cases there is associated pulmonary hypertension and the direction of blood flow in the ductus may then be reversed so that unoxygenated blood passes from the pulmonary artery into the aorta via the ductus, usually immediately beyond the origin of the left subclavian artery. Such a patient may thus have a cyanotic tinge in the nailbeds of the toes but not in those of the hands.

Interatrial septal defect. This is one of the commonest congenital malformations of the heart. Even when the defect is large, it appears to have little effect on the circulation. Rarely a piece of detached thrombus, e.g. from the leg veins, passes from the right atrium through the defect to reach the left atrium and causes *crossed* or *paradoxical embolism*. While probe patency of the foramen ovale is very common in normal hearts (approx. 25%), the important malformations are of three main types: persis-tent ostium primum, ostium secundum and persistent atrio-ventricularis communis. In this last condition, there is often fusion of the tricuspid and mitral valves to form a common atrioventricular valve. Lutembacher's disease consists of an interatrial septal defect with mitral stenosis.

Interventricular septal defect. A high septal defect is frequently part of another congenital anomaly, e.g. tetrad of Fallot, but an isolated high interventricular septal defect is not uncommon. Maladie de Roger is the name sometimes applied to an isolated defect in the interventricular septum; the size and location of the aperture varies.

Anomalies of the aortic arch. As shown by Blalock, these are common in association with tetrad of Fallot (see above), but as isolated anomalies they rarely cause symptoms. When, however, a vascular ring is formed around the trachea and oesophagus by a right aortic arch and left descending aorta together with a persistent ductus arteriosus, ligamentum arteriosum or an anomalous left subclavian artery, pressure effects, mainly on the trachea, may result. A double aortic arch may give similar symptoms.

Coarctation (stenosis) of the aorta. Slight narrowing of the aorta between the left subclavian artery and the orifice of the ductus arteriosus, i.e. in the interval where the two main streams of the fetal circulation cross, is not very uncommon. The stenosis is rarely marked, but it may be severe and all degrees of narrowing up to complete atresia of the aorta at this point have been recorded. With major narrowing, an extensive collateral system from the carotids and subclavians links the aorta above and below the narrowed segment. The pulses in the lower limbs are poor as compared with those of the upper. Hypertension develops and death is likely to ensue from cardiac failure, cerebral haemorrhage or less commonly from local complications associated with the coarcted site, e.g. aneurysm or rupture of the aorta. Coarctation of the aorta may be associated with other congenital abnormalities, but frequently it is the only abnormality present and, moreover, it is one that can be cured by surgery. The condition is distinctly commoner in the male sex.

Ebstein's disease. In this condition there is downward displacement of the tricuspid valve so that the upper part of the right ventricle comes to be a functional part of the right atrium. The course of the circulation is normal.

Other abnormalities of the valves. Sometimes there is excess or deficiency in the number of the cusps of the semilunar valves; occasionally there are four cusps, usually somewhat unequal in size, but, as a rule, there is no interference with the efficiency of the valve. There may,

however, be only two cusps, usually in the aortic valve. One cusp is usually larger than the other and often shows evidence of fusion of two cusps. Such bicuspid valves tend to develop calcific aortic stenosis and also bacterial endocarditis. Very rarely cases have been recorded in which two mitral valves have been present.

Diseases of the Pericardium

Acute pericarditis

This illustrates the usual features of an acute inflammatory reaction of a serosal lining. Active hyperaemia, inflammatory oedema and emigration of leucocytes occur in the pericardial tissue, exudate accumulates in the pericardial sac and fibrin is deposited on its surfaces. Depending on the cause, these changes may be mild and brief, with accumulation of clear or slightly turbid fluid and dulling of the inflamed surfaces by a fine layer of fibrin, or they may be of greater severity, with turbid, bloodstained or purulent fluid and formation of a thick layer of fibrin on the surfaces. The volume of exudate in the pericardial sac and the amount of fibrin deposited on its surfaces are not closely related (p. 14.22), and a large amount of either can cause problems. The parietal pericardium can dilate to contain over a litre of fluid without rise in pressure, but only if the fluid accumulates slowly. If accumulation is rapid, even a small volume of fluid raises the pericardial pressure and may interfere with filling of the atria and thus with the general circulation (**cardiac tamponade**). A fine deposit of fibrin on the pericardial surfaces undergoes lysis, but a thicker layer is removed by organisation with consequent fibrous thickening of the two layers of the pericardium and formation of fibrous adhesions between them or even obliteration of the sac. If gross, fibrous thickening of the pericardium (*constrictive pericarditis*) can cause progressive heart failure (see below).

The clinical features of acute pericarditis include fever, tachycardia and usually chest pain, although the condition is sometimes clinically silent. If the volume of exudate in the sac is small, as in early or mild pericarditis, pain results from rubbing together of the inflamed, roughened pericardial surfaces; it is sharp

and 'stabbing', and accompanied by an audible friction rub synchronous with the heart beat. If fluid is more abundant, it separates the pericardial layers: the heart sounds are muffled and pain, if present, is usually dull and increased by movement. Cardiac tamponade is associated with dyspnoea, tachycardia, distension of the jugular veins and a low pulse pressure, particularly during inspiration (pulsus paradoxicus).

Causes. These include acute bacterial and viral infections, myocardial infarction, rheumatic fever, the connective tissue diseases and uraemia. Often, however, the cause is unknown.

Viral and 'idiopathic' pericarditis. This is a mild acute pericarditis which occurs most often in young adults, and is now commoner than bacterial pericarditis in most of the developed countries. It usually subsides within two weeks, but is sometimes more persistent and in some patients recurrent. Some pericardial thickening and adhesions may result from organisation of fibrin, but they are usually of no consequence.

Attempts to isolate a virus are successful in only a small minority of cases—most often Group B *Coxsackievirus* and occasionally *Echovirus* or the other viruses which can cause acute myocarditis (p. 15.18). Indeed, mild pericarditis and myocarditis are frequently associated, and in some instances accompanied by acute pleurisy.

Bacterial pericarditis may complicate septicaemia or pyaemia, bacterial pneumonia, empyema, an ulcerating carcinoma of the oesophagus or bronchus, etc. The causal organisms are most often pyogenic cocci, notably *Staphylococcus aureus. Streptococcus pyogenes* and *Streptococcus pneumoniae*, and systemic effects of a severe infection accompany the clinical features of pericarditis. In the early stages, the exudate may be clear or only slightly turbid, and fibrin deposition scanty, but unless treatment is early and effective the exudate become turbid or purulent and fibrin deposition increases, leading to formation of abundant granulation and eventually fibrous tissue, which in some cases results in constrictive pericarditis.

Tuberculous pericarditis is quite common in chronic pulmonary tuberculosis. The route of infection of the pericardium is usually not apparent, and is presumed to be by lymphatics or from an infected pleura. The pericarditis is exudative and may develop acutely. The exudate is slightly turbid or bloodstained and tubercles may be visible on the pericardial surfaces unless there is sufficient fibrin deposition to obscure them. The condition usually subsides, but in some instances becomes chronic with formation of a thick layer of fibrous tissue enclosing caseous foci and largely obliterating the sac. Calcification may be extensive and constrictive pericarditis may result.

Rheumatic pericarditis is part of the pancarditis of rheumatic fever (p. 15.20). It may persist for some weeks and a thick layer of fibrin may be deposited (Fig. 4.22, p. 4.21) with subsequent organisation and fibrous thickening and sometimes obliteration of the sac. It is presumably due to a hypersensitivity reaction, although it is even less understood than rheumatic myocarditis.

Myocardial infarction. Mild acute pericarditis usually develops during the first week in patients with a transmural myocardial infarct: it is localised to the area overlying the infarct, but in patients treated by anticoagulants may become diffuse and haemorrhagic. For some months after myocardial infarction there is a risk of the development of a mild acute diffuse pericarditis ('*post-infarction syndrome*') and this may occur also following cardiac surgery ('*post-cardiotomy syndrome*') or injury to the heart ('*post-traumatic syndrome*'). In all three conditions the detection of antibody reactive with extracts of myocardial tissue has been reported, suggesting an auto-immune hypersensitivity reaction triggered by injury to the heart. The presence of blood in the pericardial sac has been regarded as a predisposing cause, although the condition may follow non-cardiac thoracic surgery or injury.

Other causes. Acute pericarditis occurs in some cases of *systemic lupus erythematosus* and occasionally in *rheumatoid arthritis*, but is not usually severe. Fibrinous pericarditis is a feature of *uraemia* and is sometimes of importance when life is prolonged by haemodialysis. Finally, *carcinomatous infiltration* of the pericardium commonly induces a pericarditis of serofibrinous or haemorrhagic type. Small carcinomatous nodules and lymphatic permeation may be visible on the pericardial surfaces unless obscured by fibrin, and carcinoma cells may be detectable in the exudate.

Chronic pericarditis

Unless treated effectively, bacterial, and particularly tuberculous pericarditis may become chronic and viral or idiopathic pericarditis occasionally does so.

Constrictive pericarditis is a rare condition characterised by obliteration of the pericardial sac by a thick layer of dense fibrous tissue which sometimes becomes calcified. It can result from prolonged pyogenic or tuberculous pericarditis and also occurs as a complication of rheumatoid arthritis, but in many cases it develops without known cause.

By constricting the heart, the fibrous tissue interferes with the filling of the cardiac chambers and this may be aggravated by constriction of the lumen of the great veins as they enter the atria. The clinical picture is thus one of progressive congestive heart failure associated with a small heart and low stroke volume. If the heart can be freed by resection of the thickened pericardium the symptoms are relieved and for most patients the long-term outlook is good.

Hydropericardium

Accumulation of a transudate of clear fluid in the pericardium occurs in conditions of generalised oedema. In contrast to pericarditis with effusion, the pericardial surfaces retain their smooth shining appearance. Unless it collects rapidly or in large volume, the fluid does not seriously embarrass cardiac function.

Haemopericardium

Haemorrhage into the pericardial sac, giving rise to *haemopericardium*, may be due to rupture of the heart itself following infarction, to rupture of an aortic aneurysm, most often an acute dissecting aneurysm which strips open the aortic wall to the base of the heart (p. 14.30), or to a stab wound involving the heart or a large vessel. When the bleeding is rapid, the pressure of the blood in the pericardial sac interferes with the diastolic filling of the chambers (cardiac tamponade). The output of blood from the left ventricle is greatly diminished, the blood pressure rapidly falls and death results.

Multiple minute haemorrhages occur into the layers of the pericardium in the various purpuric conditions. They are sometimes a prominent feature also in cases of death by suffocation.

Tumours of the Heart and Pericardium

Primary tumours of the heart are rare. *Fibroma, myxoma, lipoma, haemangioma* and *lymphangioma* are occasionally encountered, especially in the left atrium, the least rare being a myxomatous mass of up to several centimetres in diameter, the so-called **cardiac myxoma**, projecting into the cavity from the margin of the foramen ovale: the commonly-associated mitral valve lesions may be due to haemodynamic or traumatic effects of the tumour. Cardiac myxoma sometimes has various unexplained effects, including weight loss, anaemia, a high ESR, serum protein disturbances, Raynaud's phenomenon and arthralgia. *Rhabdomyoma* of congenital origin occurs especially in the ventricles as multiple rounded nodules of pale and somewhat translucent tissue. It consists of large branching cells in which striped myofibrils are found; the cells have a somewhat vacuolated cytoplasm and contain much glycogen. In a number of cases, the tumour has been associated with multiple discrete gliomatous growths in the cerebral hemispheres—*tuberous sclerosis* (p. 21.48); in some cases there have also been malformations of the kidneys and liver, and adenoma sebaceum on the face (Bourneville's disease).

Metastatic tumours in the heart and pericardium are common, occurring in about 10% of all fatal malignancies. Bronchial carcinoma spreads to involve the heart more frequently than any other neoplasm (31% of cases); no doubt the proximity of the primary growth is a factor in this high incidence, as direct extension readily occurs to the base of the heart and pericardium. Melanoma metastasises surprisingly often to the heart.

As noted above, neoplastic invasion of the pericardium often causes a haemorrhagic inflammatory exudate. Spread of tumour into the wall of the right atrium is liable to cause arrhythmias.

References

Buja, L. M. and Willertson, J. T. (1981). Clinicopathological correlates of acute ischemic heart disease syndromes. *American Journal of Cardiology*, **47**, 343–56.

Cobb, L. A., Baum, R. S., Alvarez, H. and Schaffer, W. A. (1975). Resuscitation from out-of-hospital ventricular fibrillation: 4 years follow up. *Circulation*, Suppl. III, 223–40.

Davies, M. J., Fulton, W. F. and Robertson, W. B. (1979). The relation of coronary thrombosis to ischaemic myocardial necrosis. *Journal of Pathology*, **86**, 99–110.

Davies, M. J., Woolf, N. and Robertson, W. B. (1976). Pathology of acute myocardial infarction with particular reference to occlusive coronary thrombi. British Heart Journal, **38**, 658–64.

De Wood, M. A., Spores, J., Notske, R., Lowell, T., Mouser, L. T., Burroughs, R., Golden, M. S. and Lang, H. T. (1980). Prevalence of total coronary occlusion during the early hours of transmural myocardial infarction. New England Journal of Medicine, **303**, 897–902.

Kaplan, M. H. and Frangley, J. D. (1969). Autoimmunity to the heart in cardiac disease. Current concepts of the relation of autoimmunity in rheumatic fever, postcardiotomy and postinfarction syndromes and cardiomyopathies. *American Journal of Clinical Pathology*, **24**, 459.

Patarroyo, M. E., Winchester, R. J., Vejerano, A., Gibafsky, A., Chalem, F., Zabriskie, J. B. and Kunkel, H. G. (1979). Association of a B-cell alloantigen with susceptibility to rheumatic fever. Nature, **278**, 173-4.

Pisa, Z. and Uemura, K. (1982). Trends of mortality in ischemic heart disease in 27 countries, 1968-1977. *World Health Statistics Quarterly*, **35**, 11-47.

Further Reading

Abott, M. E. S. (1954). *Atlas of Congenital Cardiac Disease*, pp. 62. American Heart Association, New York.

Cardiovascular Pathology (1983). Ed. M. D. Silver, pp. 1407 Churchill Livingstone, Edinburgh, London, New York, etc.

Crawford, Sir Theo. (1977). *Pathology of Ischaemic Heart Disease*, pp. 170. Butterworth, London and Boston.

Davies, M. J. (1980). *Pathology of cardiac valves*, pp. 180. Butterworths, London and Boston.

Hudson, R. E. B. (1965-71). *Cardiovascular Pathology*, Vols. 1-3. Edward Arnold, London.

Paul Wood's Diseases of the Heart and Circulation (1968). Various Authors. 3rd edn, pp. 1164. Eyre and Spottiswoode, London.

Pomerance, Ariela and Davies, M. J. (Eds.) (1975). *The Pathology of the Heart*. Blackwell Scientific, Oxford and Melbourne.

Taussig, H. B. (1960). *Congenital Malformations of the Heart*. 3rd edn, pp. 204 and 1049. Harvard University Press, Cambridge, Mass.

16

Respiratory System

Introduction

The primary function of the respiratory system—oxygenation of the blood and removal of carbon dioxide—requires that air be brought into close approximation with blood. Accordingly, **the respiratory tract is particularly exposed to infection**, both by microbes in the inspired air and by spread downwards of the bacteria which commonly colonise the nose and throat. Another important hazard is presented by **inhalation of pollutants** contributed to the air we breathe in the form of dusts, smokes and fumes, a particularly important example being cigarette smoke. These pollutants are responsible for the high incidence of chronic bronchitis and chronic lung disease and also bronchial carcinoma in many parts of the world. Thirdly, the lungs are the only organs, apart from the heart, through which all the blood passes during each circulation: accordingly, cardiovascular diseases which disturb pulmonary haemodynamics are likely to have serious secondary effects on the lungs, such as pulmonary oedema, and conversely diseases of the lungs which interfere with pulmonary blood flow have important effects on the heart and systemic circulation. In short, *normal cardiac and pulmonary function are closely interdependent.*

Apart from infections, injury due to inhaled pollutants and the effects of cardiovascular disease, the respiratory tract is remarkably trouble-free, and most of this chapter will be devoted to the effects of these three hazards.

Although the respiratory tract, like other systems, is best considered on a regional basis, the continuity of the mucous membranes from nose to alveolus, and the microbial contamination of inspired air, allow ready spread of infection, and accordingly it seems appropriate to give a brief general account of the main factors concerned in respiratory tract infections before proceeding on a regional basis.

Respiratory infections

The defences of the respiratory tract against infection have been described in Chapter 8: they include (1) upward flow of the surface film of mucus which coats the air passages and is impelled by ciliated epithelium, (2) the cough reflex; (3) the secretion of IgA antibodies and (4) the phagocytic activity of alveolar macrophages.

Bacterial infections of the respiratory tract may be primary (i.e. occur in healthy individuals), or secondary to a large number of conditions which depress resistance. **Primary infections** have become much less common in many of the developed countries: they include laryngeal or nasal diphtheria, bacterial pneumonia due usually to *Streptococcus pneumoniae*, and pulmonary tuberculosis. Other examples include pneumonic plague and anthrax pneumonia. *Primary pneumonia due to various pyogenic bacteria is, however, relatively common in infants and old people.* **Secondary bacterial infections** occur especially when the local resistance of the respiratory mucosa is lowered by various virus infections, e.g. the common cold, influenza and measles; in these conditions, bacteria growing in the nose and throat extend downwards, usually giving a mixed infection, but in hospitals and other institutions, outbreaks of respiratory virus infections may be complicated by spread of virulent pathogenic bacteria from patient to patient. Chronic liability to bacterial infections also results from persistent abnormalities of the bronchi, especially chronic bronchitis and bronchiectasis, from various debilitating and wasting diseases, and from congenital and acquired immunodeficiencies.

Virus infections. *Most acute respiratory disease seen in general medical practice every winter is caused by viruses.* Over 150 different viruses have been isolated and antibody acquired against one virus rarely gives any cross-protec-

Table 16.1 The respiratory viruses

Virus group	No. of serotypes	Disease
Influenza viruses	3*	Influenza
Parainfluenza viruses	4	Croup, colds, lower respiratory infections in children
Respiratory syncytial virus	1	Bronchiolitis and pneumonia in infants, colds in older children
Rhinoviruses	>100	Colds
Adenoviruses	33	Pharyngitis, conjunctivitis
Coronaviruses	3	Colds
Coxsackieviruses	Types A21, B3	Colds
Echoviruses	Types 11, 20	Colds
'Virus pneumonia agents' (not true viruses)	A heterogeneous group	Atypical pneumonia

*There is considerable antigenic variation within the three major types (A, B and C) of influenza virus.

tion against any of the others. Acute viral pharyngitis (presenting as 'sore throat') and the common cold are frequent and comparatively trivial. Others, like bronchiolitis in infants due to respiratory syncytial virus, may be fatal.

Respiratory viruses fall into a few well-defined major groups (Table 16.1), most (but not all) of which replicate readily in tissue culture.

The clinical syndromes due to acute respiratory virus infections depend to some extent on the age of the patient and the depth to which the respiratory tract is invaded. These syndromes are not sharply defined and may be produced by many different viruses. Nevertheless, recognisable clinical syndromes produced by viruses in the respiratory tract are the common cold (coryza), viral sore-throat, influenza, infantile croup, infantile acute bronchiolitis and 'atypical pneumonia'.

The common cold occurs throughout the world, including tropical countries, and exposure to low temperature does not appear to be a predisposing factor. It is caused mainly by the *rhinoviruses* of which there are more than a hundred serologically distinct types. There is no cross immunity so that repeated infections are common. Rhinoviruses belong to the family of picornaviruses which also include enteroviruses. Other viruses which cause common colds are parainfluenza, respiratory syncytial, corona, and more rarely some coxsackie and echo viruses.

Adenoviruses are the main cause of 'viral sore-throat' in which the pharyngitis is some-times accompanied by conjunctivitis. They cause epidemics of acute respiratory disease as well as endemic pharyngitis and follicular conjunctivitis. There are about thirty serological types of these DNA viruses.

The *parainfluenza viruses* cause a respiratory infection intermediate in severity between the common cold and influenza. They are the major cause of acute laryngo-tracheobronchitis (succinctly termed 'croup') in young children. There are four serological types of these large RNA viruses.

Respiratory syncytial virus infection is common in young children, generally giving rise to trivial signs and symptoms. However, *it is highly virulent for children under one year of age and especially in infants less than six months old. It accounts for most of the young children admitted to hospital each winter with acute bronchiolitis or pneumonia.*

The most serious virus infection of the respiratory tract is **influenza**. This usually involves mainly the upper respiratory tract and is a febrile illness often followed by lassitude and depression. From time to time new antigenic strains arise and cause world-wide pandemics. Influenza virus is an RNA virus (Fig. 16.1) and three major antigenic types exist, A, B and C. Strains of the virus are further classified by two outer antigens—H antigen or haemagglutinin and N or neuraminidase antigen. However, these antigens are not stable because the virus undergoes considerable genetic reassortment (*antigenic shift*) and also minor but progressive

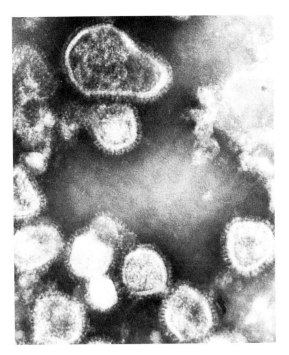

change (*antigenic drift*). When the H antigen undergoes shift, a new strain emerges to which there is no pre-existing immunity and a pandemic develops. This happened in 1918, 1957 (strain H2N2) and 1963 (strain H2N3). In such pandemics, rapidly fatal *influenza viral pneumonia* may occur in previously healthy young people. However, in most epidemics bacterial complications are the chief cause of pneumonia. During influenza epidemics it is important to protect those who are at special risk, such as chronic bronchitics. The pathology of influenza and viral pneumonias is considered on pp. 16.41–43. **Measles,** and in lesser degree the other viral exanthemata of childhood, may be followed by acute tracheobronchitis, which is commonly associated with bacterial infection sometimes progressing to pneumonia.

Fig. 16.1 Individual virus particles of the influenza H3N2 Hong Kong strain showing spikes of haemagglutinin by which the particle attaches itself to susceptible cells in the respiratory mucosa. Electron micrograph. × 128 000. (Dr D Hobson.)

Nose, Nasal Sinuses and Nasopharynx

Inflammatory conditions

Acute rhinitis is the common inflammatory disorder of the nasal mucosa. The familiar clinical form, **the common cold (acute coryza),** is usually caused by rhinoviruses and may be followed by secondary bacterial infection. The specific infectious fevers, such as measles, are often preceded by acute rhinitis. Nasal diphtheria is another cause but is now a rarity in many countries.

Another common clinical disorder is **hay fever,** or *acute allergic* or *atopic rhinitis*, which occurs as a result of sensitisation to certain pollens, such as that of Timothy grass, or to house dust, animal dandruff, feathers or other specific antigens (p. 7.6). Atopic hypersensitivity is also a factor in some cases of nasal polyps.

Acute sinusitis is generally a complication of acute infection of the nose, less commonly of dental sepsis. Gram + ve cocci such as *Streptococcus pyogenes*, *Streptococcus pneumoniae* or *Staphylococcus aureus* are the usual causal organisms.

Acute nasopharyngitis usually accompanies either acute rhinitis or acute tonsillitis in which *Streptococcus pyogenes* is the common pathogen.

The histopathology of acute inflammation of the nose, sinuses and nasopharynx is similar. There is hyperaemia and oedema of the mucosa, and the mucosal glands are hyperactive. In **virus infections,** neutrophil polymorphs are generally sparse in both the mucosa and the exudate until secondary bacterial infection supervenes, but thereafter increasing numbers of neutrophils migrate through the mucosa and the exudate becomes mucopurulent in charac-

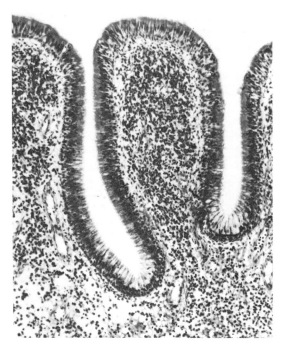

Fig. 16.2 Section through the surface of a nasal polyp, showing the respiratory epithelium and the loose oedematous stroma infiltrated with chronic inflammatory cells. × 100.

ter. There is a variable degree of loss of the superficial ciliated epithelium. In **atopic inflammation**, oedema of the submucosa is a prominent feature, giving rise to polypoid thickening of the mucosa. The mucosal glands are often enlarged and distended and the oedematous stroma is characteristically infiltrated by numerous eosinophil polymorphs.

Chronic rhinitis, sinusitis and nasopharyngitis may follow an acute inflammatory episode which has failed to resolve. Inadequate drainage of the sinuses, nasal obstruction due to polyps, or enlargement of the nasopharyngeal lymphoid tissue (adenoids), may be underlying factors.

Nasal polyps. Chronic inflammation of the nose may lead to polypoid thickening of the mucosa. Polyps are rounded or elongated masses commonly arising from the region of the middle turbinate. They are often bilateral, a point of distinction from nasal tumours. Nasal polypi are usually gelatinous in consistency with a smooth, shiny surface. Their microscopic structure consists of a core of loose oedematous connective tissue containing occa-

sional mucous glands and covered by normal ciliated respiratory type of epithelium (Fig. 16.2), but squamous metaplasia is common. Lymphocytes, plasma cells and eosinophils infiltrate the submucosa to a variable degree. Polyps in which eosinophils predominate are considered to have an atopic basis.

Chronic granulomatous rhinitis. In contrast to acute infection, specific forms of chronic infection of the nose are rare in most communities. Chronic granulomas may be due to tuberculosis, tertiary syphilis, leprosy, scleroma or fungal infections such as aspergillosis or rhinosporidiosis.

Two rare forms of necrotising granuloma of uncertain nature occur in the upper respiratory tract. In one form, **Wegener's granuloma**, (p. 14.28), a necrotising lesion with giant cells develops usually in the nose or the maxillary sinuses, followed by necrotic lesions in the lung and associated with disseminated lesions of polyarteritis (p. 14.26), particularly in the lungs and kidneys. The other, so-called **malignant granuloma of the nose**, presents as an ulcerated lesion which spreads progressively to erode the soft tissues and bones around the nose. Histologically the lesion consists of proliferating lymphocytes and macrophages: some authorities consider it to be a lymphoid neoplasm.

Tumours

Benign tumours. The common benign lesions of the nose are **haemangioma** of the septum and **squamous papilloma** of the vestibule. A much less common tumour is the **juvenile angiofibroma** which usually occurs in the nasopharynx. It appears in childhood, almost exclusively in boys, and tends to become quiescent by the end of the second decade. It is an enlarging vascular tumour which may cause bone erosion and destruction by pressure atrophy. Microscopically, it is seen to consist of small vascular spaces set in poorly cellular fibrous tissue. The histogenesis of the lesion is uncertain and, like haemangiomas, it may be a hamartoma of the nasal erectile tissue rather than a true neoplasm. Angioma may also occasionally present as a nasal polypoid lesion, but this form does not occur particularly in boys.

Malignant tumours. *Transitional-cell epithelial*

tumours are common in the nasal passages. Some of these do not recur, and may be termed *transitional cell papillomas*: some recur in the same form, and some show a rapid change to *squamous carcinoma*. Transitional cell tumours are found mainly in the nasal cavity itself, probably because most of those in the nasal sinuses remain undiscovered unless they become squamous-cell carcinomas. **Squamous-cell carcinomas** are common in the nose and nasal sinuses, but anaplastic carcinoma and adenocarcinoma also occur. The so-called lymphoepithelioma of the nasopharynx is now generally accepted as a highly anaplastic carcinoma invading the normal non-neoplastic lymphoid tissue of the region.

Nasopharyngeal carcinoma, usually squamous-cell, often poorly differentiated or of lympho-epitheliomatous (i.e. anaplastic) type, is particularly common in China, Malaysia, Indonesia and East Africa, where there is some evidence that the anaplastic forms of this tumour are associated with the same (EB) virus as Burkitt's lymphoma (p. 13.17). There is also an association with certain tissue antigens, e.g. (HLA-A2). *Adenocarcinoma of the nose and nasal sinuses*, especially in the ethmoid, has been found to be unduly frequent in woodworkers in the furniture industry in Southern England. It arises after a very long latent period, sometimes of forty years or more.

Larynx and Trachea

Inflammatory conditions

Acute inflammation

Mild *acute laryngitis and tracheitis* are commonplace in the conditions of modern urban life with its atmospheric pollution with cigarette smoke, car exhaust fumes, industrial and domestic smoke, etc. While these factors in themselves are rarely the cause of significant clinical laryngeal disease, they may be of importance in predisposing to viral and bacterial infections. The viruses concerned have been considered above. The bacteria commonly involved are *Streptococcus pneumoniae*, *Streptococcus pyogenes* and *Neisseria catarrhalis*. Once secondary bacterial invasion occurs it may progress to bronchitis. Acute laryngo-tracheitis commonly complicates acute febrile states such as measles, influenza and typhoid. It usually subsides but it may pass into the chronic stage.

Pseudomembranous inflammation may be due to diphtheria (see below) or may be associated with secondary infection by *Streptococcus pyogenes*, *Staphylococcus aureus* or *Streptococcus pneumoniae* following infection with parainfluenza virus. Frequently such infections spread to involve the bronchial tree as laryngo-tracheobronchitis. In this condition there is necrosis of epithelium and the formation of an extensive fibrinous membrane in the trachea and main bronchi. There may be pronounced oedema of the subglottic area, resulting in stridor. In a minority of cases *Haemophilus influenzae* is the secondary invader, with severe sore throat, fever, tender lymph nodes and swelling of the epiglottis. In laryngo-tracheobronchitis the danger of laryngeal obstruction is, in general, greater than that of toxaemia or lung infection but bronchopneumonia and lung abscess are recognised complications. Pseudomembranous inflammation may result also from the action of corrosive substances or from the inhalation of irritating gases, notably ammonia.

Diphtheria is an acute pseudomembranous inflammation which is now very rare in countries where prophylactic immunisation is carried out. It usually affects the fauces, soft palate and tonsils but may also involve the nose, larynx, trachea and bronchi. The local lesions are characterised by the formation on the affected surface of a false membrane composed of fibrin, neutrophil polymorphs and necrotic epithelium and containing clumps of *Corynebacterium diphtheriae*. In the lower larynx and trachea the epithelium is columnar and the coagulated exudate rests on the basement membrane from which it separates easily and is coughed up. Over the vocal cords, where the mucosa consists of squamous epithelium, the membrane is firmly adherent. When it is coughed up from the trachea, it may remain attached to the vocal cords and may then impact in the larynx and cause death from suffocation. In nasal diphtheria the infection is often unilateral and the child may appear to have a cold with discharge from one nostril. This type may be overlooked until the appearance of palatal paralysis, myocardial failure or other clinical manifestations of the serious toxic effects of diphtheria (pp. 3.10, 8.5).

Acute epiglottitis. This condition, which is caused by *Haemophilus influenzae* type b, is a disease of early childhood which may lead to death within a few hours of onset. Histological examination shows swelling of the tissues due to acute inflammatory oedema and infiltration by neutrophil polymorphs. There is no mucosal ulceration.

In typhoid fever there may be laryngitis and bronchitis. Typhoid bacilli may be recovered from such lesions but more commonly the inflammatory reaction is produced by infection by other bacteria. Occasionally ulceration involves the perichondrium of the laryngeal cartilage, sometimes followed by necrosis and suppuration.

Endotracheal intubation. Sore throat, hoarseness, subglottic oedema and non-specific arytenoid granuloma may follow brief endotracheal intubation during general anaesthesia for a surgical operation. Endotracheal intubation exceeding forty-eight hours, using a tube with an inflatable cuff, may lead to pressure injury and abrasion of the trachea with production of large ulcers which expose the underlying cartilaginous rings. Such ulcers, which may be oval or linear transverse lesions, are often located on the antero-lateral surface of the trachea: they may become infected by organisms such as *Pseudomonas aeruginosa* and *Candida albicans* and may be covered by a pseudomembrane. Occasionally, prolonged intubation is complicated by the development of tracheo-oesophageal fistula or tracheal stenosis.

Oedema of the glottis. This is an acute inflammatory oedema of the loose tissue of the upper part of the larynx and not of the vocal cords. The aryepiglottic folds and the tissues around the epiglottis become greatly swollen and tense. The false cords also are affected. This is an important lesion as *the swelling may lead to obstruction and death by suffocation.* It should be noted that after death the tissues become less swollen and tense than they were during life.

Oedema of the glottis may occur in cardiac and renal diseases but rarely to such an extent as to cause serious results. The severe type occurs as a complication of other lesions of the larynx such as diphtheria or the deep-seated ulceration and perichondritis seen in tuberculosis and syphilis and sometimes in typhoid. It may result also from erysipelas or from the spread of inflammation from tonsillitis and suppurative conditions in the neighbourhood, or from agranulocytic angina. Oedema of the glottis is also caused by the trauma following impaction of a foreign body in the larynx and may be produced by irritating gases or scalding fluids. It occurs in angio-oedema (p. 10.31) and in some cases this form has proved fatal.

Chronic laryngitis

Chronic catarrhal inflammation of the larynx and trachea is frequently associated with excessive smoking. The mucous glands are swollen and give the surface a granular aspect. Heavy smoking also leads to squamous metaplasia. The normal adult larynx is lined by squamous epithelium over the true cords, posterior glottis, a variable rim at the lateral margins and tip of the epiglottis on its posterior surface. Respiratory epithelium covers the central parts of the posterior surface of the epiglottis, the false cords, the ventricles and the subglottis. Squamous metaplasia is common among city dwellers, chronic bronchitics and smokers. Among heavy smokers, the entire larynx, including the subglottis and upper trachea, may become lined by squamous epithelium, thus interfering with clearance of mucus. Extensive squamous metaplasia is almost always present in patients who develop laryngeal carcinoma.

Tuberculous laryngitis occurs secondary to pulmonary tuberculosis, the tubercle bacilli being carried directly to the larynx in the sputum: they enter the mucosa and give rise to tubercles which caseate and form small ulcers with a tendency to spread. Any part of the larynx, or less commonly the trachea, may be affected but the disease usually starts first, and is most pronounced, in the arytenoid region and on the vocal cords. Occasionally small papillary outgrowths form at the margins of the tuberculous ulcers, and epithelial hyperplasia in biopsy material may be mistaken for carcinoma. Tuberculosis may spread deeply and involve the perichondrium of the arytenoid cartilages; there is chronic thickening, caseation and ulceration, and fragments of dead cartilage may be discharged. The lesion is often very painful; there may be considerable inflammatory swelling and oedema of the glottis may supervene.

Syphilis. In the secondary stage there may be a catarrhal laryngitis, white 'mucous' patches of hyperkeratinisation or 'snail-track' ulcers (p. 9.29). The most important effects, however, are in the tertiary stage: the lesions usually start in the submucosa of the larynx or trachea, or in the perichondrium as a diffuse but irregular thickening and stiffening which often leads to immobility of the cartilage. Gummatous change follows. The epiglottis and affected cartilages may be extensively ulcerated and the latter may become necrotic and separated. There is a pronounced tendency to extensive scarring. with stenosis and deformity of the larynx.

Tumours

Benign tumours. Small inflammatory polyps are common and may contain amyloid or show myxoid degeneration. They may simulate neoplasms. *Squamous papilloma* is the commonest benign tumour of the larynx. It occurs usually on the vocal cords and especially at the commissure. In adults it is generally single, and may recur after removal, but seldom becomes malignant. *Papillomas in children*, usually under the age of 5 years, are mostly of viral nature, multiple, occur anywhere in the larynx, and regress spontaneously at puberty, sometimes with great rapidity. The *laryngeal fibroma* is less common. It is usually small, rounded, and sometimes pedunculated. Like the papilloma, it occurs on the vocal cords, and both are apt to occur in singers and others who use their voices a lot. Angioma, myxoma and lipoma are all very rare.

Granular cell myoblastoma (p. 23.71) sometimes arises in the larynx.

Malignant tumours. *Carcinoma* is the commonest malignant tumour of the larynx: it is usually squamous, and occurs most often in

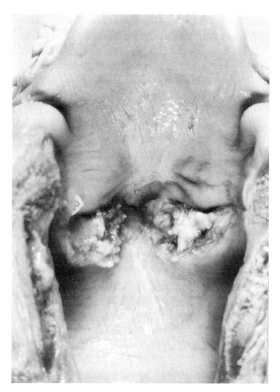

Fig. 16.3 Carcinoma of the larynx, causing extensive ulceration of the vocal cords. The false cords are intact. × 2. (Dr J. Watt.)

men over fifty years old. The incidence in Britain has declined steadily over the past twenty years and an association with pipe smoking has been postulated. When the tumour is on the true or false vocal cords, it is usually less invasive and has a better prognosis than when it arises in the upper part of the larynx or in the subglottic region. Carcinoma of a vocal cord appears first as a small indurated patch, sometimes with a papillary surface, and subsequently ulcerates (Fig. 16.3). In the latter case, diagnosis will be unsatisfactory if only a superficial part is removed for microscopic examination. A carcinoma of the larynx infiltrates and destroys the surrounding tissue; ulceration may be accompanied by septic infection from which the discharge passes down the bronchi into the lungs and causes aspiration pneumonia (p. 16.40).

In contrast to the larynx and bronchi, **the trachea** is a rare site of tumours.

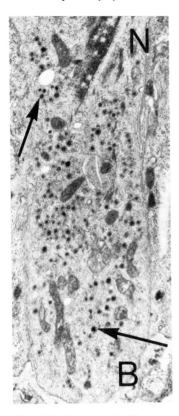

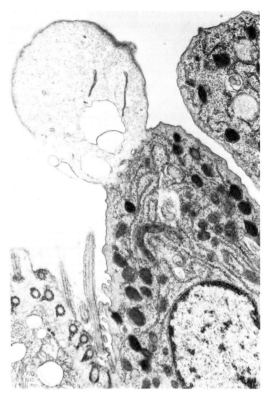

Fig. 16.4   Feyrter cell. Electron micrograph of bronchial epithelium from a neonatal rat showing the cell lying on a basement membrane (B). The cell contains characteristic round osmiophilic neurosecretory vesicles (arrows) and elongated mitochondria. Part of the nucleus (N) is shown in the figure. × 12 500.

Fig. 16.5   Clara cell. Electron micrograph of bronchiolar epithelium from a neonatal rat showing the apex of the cell caught in the process of extrusion into the bronchiolar lumen. It contains little smooth endoplasmic reticulum. The main body of the cell contains rough endoplasmic reticulum and mitochondria. × 12 500.

The Bronchi

The cells of the bronchial epithelium in health and disease

As explained in Chapter 8, the ciliated and mucus-secreting cells of the bronchial epithelium are intimately concerned in the defence of the airways and lungs against bacteria and foreign material. Certain viruses may damage the ciliary mechanism of the respiratory epithelium, thus facilitating invasion of the deeper parts of the bronchial tree and lung by bacteria. Chronic irritation of the bronchi by polluted air and particularly by cigarette smoke may lead to the hyperplasia and hypertrophy of goblet cells and mucous glands which is an important feature in chronic bronchitis.

Other, less familiar cells, whose functions are not yet well understood, are present in the bronchial epithelium. They include the argyrophilic **Feyrter cells** (Fig. 16.4) which contain neurosecretory vesicles and belong to the **apud** system of cells responsible for the secretion of polypeptide hormones (p. 12.43). On exposure to chronic hypoxia, the Feyrter cells respond (like the chief cells of the carotid body) by degranulation and microvacuolation of neurosecretory vesicles, suggesting that they may act as airway chemoreceptors, perhaps by secreting catecholamines. At birth they may play an important role in the adaptation of the pulmonary circulation to extrauterine life by dilating the muscular pulmonary vasculature of the fetus. The bronchial carcinoid tumour and small-cell bronchial carcinoma are both derived from Feyrter cells and their dense core vesicles reflect the abnormal secretion of hormones which is often a feature of these tumours.

Scattered among the ciliated respiratory epithelial cells in the bronchi and especially in the respiratory bronchioles are the non-ciliated **Clara cells** (Fig. 16.5). These have all the features of apocrine secretory cells; the secretory product accumulates within smooth cisternae at the apex of the cell, and the apical region is then extruded into the bronchiolar lumen. They are thought to secrete a surfactant-like substance.

Brush cells are also found in the epithelium of the conducting airways. Their most striking feature is the large regular microvilli which cover their relatively small free surface. Their function is as yet unknown but they may be some type of receptor because their fine structural features are similar to those of the chemoreceptor cell in taste buds.

Acute bronchitis

A distinction must be made between acute inflammation of the larger, extralobular bronchi (**acute bronchitis**) and of the small, intralobular bronchi and bronchioles (**acute bronchiolitis**). These different anatomical sites influence the likely consequences and hence seriousness of the inflammatory reaction. *The common acute bronchitis of the adult affects the large and medium-sized bronchi.* It is usually mild but may be the cause of much disability when it aggravates an established chronic bronchitis, especially in aged or debilitated subjects. *Except as a complication of influenza, acute bronchiolitis is rare in healthy adults,* because bacteria do not readily become established so far down the bronchial tree. It does, however, occur in children, old people and in states of debility: it is a serious condition owing to the liability of the organisms to spread to the adjacent acini and cause bronchopneumonia. Accordingly, acute bronchiolitis is dealt with in relation to pneumonia on p. 16.35 *et seq.*

The larger bronchi have mucous glands in their walls and their involvement in acute inflammation is characterised by excessive production of mucus. Acute bronchitis may be catarrhal, membranous or putrid.

Catarrhal bronchitis is characterised by exces-

sive secretion of mucus together with inflammatory exudation. If the inflammatory stimulus (usually bacterial infection) persists, neutrophil polymorphs appear and the sputum changes from a mucoid secretion to yellow muco-pus. In very severe cases the superficial part of the bronchial wall may be shed with exposure of deeper tissues—the so-called ulcerative bronchitis. *Much acute bronchitis is probably initiated by viruses or mycoplasma which impair local defence mechanisms and allow secondary bacterial invasion by the more pathogenic bacteria among those present in the upper respiratory tract at the time:* Haemophilus influenzae *and* Streptococcus pneumoniae *are the commonest, being found in the upper respiratory tract in half the adult population and in an even higher proportion of children.* Staphylococcus aureus *and* Streptococcus pyogenes *can produce a severe purulent bronchitis in infants.* Sometimes catarrhal bronchitis is an early symptom of typhoid fever. A much rarer cause of acute bronchitis is the inhalation of smoke or irritant gases such as sulphur dioxide or chlorine.

Pseudo-membranous bronchitis sometimes occurs in diphtheria (p. 16.5). Rarely it may be produced by severe infections due to *Staphylococcus aureus* and parainfluenza viruses.

Putrid bronchitis commonly occurs in dilated bronchi or bronchiectatic cavities as a result of decomposition of stagnating bronchial secretions by putrefactive bacteria, such as *Borrelia vincenti* and anaerobic streptococci. It is also associated with aspiration pneumonia following inhalation of infected fluids during narcosis or coma, and is a common result of ulceration of malignant tumours growing into the trachea or bronchi.

The bronchi become covered with necrotic debris consisting of fibrin, dead tissue and the various bacteria concerned, and the sputum is abundant and foul-smelling.

Chronic bronchitis

In spite of its name, *chronic bronchitis is not primarily an inflammatory disease but consists of metaplastic and other changes resulting from chronic irritation of the bronchial epithelium.* The two main irritants responsible are cigarette smoke and atmospheric pollution, aggravated by dampness and fog. Accordingly, it is exceptionally common in heavy smokers and in industrialised areas. It is especially prone to occur in middle-aged men and is a major cause of absenteeism from work, of great economic and sociological importance. Under certain atmospheric conditions, sulphur dioxide and other pollutants accumulate in the air and give rise to the lethal aerosol called smog which will kill sufferers from the disease. *One serious aspect of chronic bronchitis is that it is frequently associated with the condition of pulmonary emphysema, which is described later* (p. 16.29).

The chronic irritation of the bronchial epithelium leads to a pronounced hypertrophy and hyperplasia of mucous glands within the bronchial wall and an increase in the number and proportion of goblet cells, at the expense of ciliated cells, in the lining epithelium. Goblet cells appear also in the terminal bronchioles, where they are normally absent. These changes can be detected and assessed by quantitative histological techniques, such as point counting, or less accurately by comparing the thickness of the mucous gland layer, which is in fact very irregular, with that of the bronchial wall. The changes are persistent and lead to an excessive production of mucus, which is the hallmark of both the histological and the clinical pictures. In fact chronic bronchitis has been defined by the British Medical Research Council as a clinical entity characterised by a cough productive of sputum, in the absence of cardiac or other pulmonary disease: to fulfil the definition sputum must be produced on most days for a period of at least three months of the year, during at least two consecutive years. Areas of squamous metaplasia of the bronchial epithelium are common in chronic bronchitis, especially in heavy cigarette smokers.

Excessive production of mucus, combined with the loss of ciliated epithelium, results in accumulation of mucus which may cause obstruction of bronchi and penetrates even into the alveolar spaces. There is a tendency for colonisation of the retained secretion by bacteria, although they are of little importance in the primary causation of the disease. The bacteria usually found are *Haemophilus influenzae* and *Streptococcus pneumoniae*. Thus in chronic bronchitis the lower respiratory tract, which is normally sterile, is very liable to be infected, and an episode of virus infection or of irritation

by atmospheric pollution, fog or cigarette smoke could be sufficient to precipitate an acute exacerbation, with more extensive invasion by bacteria already present in the bronchial tree.

When such secondary pyogenic infection occurs, the sputum changes from a glairy mucus to a frankly yellow pus. Bouts of acute infection of this type may occur several times during the course of a year, especially during winter.

It is important to distinguish between chronic bronchitis, which is based on a chronic irritation of the bronchial tree, and emphysema, which is a destructive disease of the lung substance. The two conditions commonly exist together but they are quite distinct. Chronic bronchitis must also be distinguished from bronchial asthma. Clinicians and respiratory physiologists are inclined to refer to chronic bronchitis and emphysema together as '*chronic obstructive airways disease*' but this is not a pathological diagnosis. Organic obstruction to airways may, in fact, occur in cases of chronic bronchitis without emphysema. The episodes of mucopurulent inflammation may give rise to ulceration, scarring and destruction of the walls of bronchioles and this may lead to multiple stenoses and airway obstruction. This should be contrasted with the much rarer condition of *bronchiolitis obliterans* where the bronchiolar epithelium may be destroyed by irritant gases such as ammonia or by a severe infection, and replaced by polypoid masses of granulation tissue.

Bronchial asthma

In bronchial asthma there is widespread bronchial obstruction due to muscular spasm and plugging by thick mucus.

Aetiology and types. Bronchial asthma may be classified into extrinsic and intrinsic types. **Extrinsic asthma** usually starts in childhood or early adult life and may be preceded by infantile eczema or hypersensitivity to foodstuffs in childhood. It is due mainly to atopic (type I) hypersensitivity (p. 7.6) to one or more extrinsic antigenic substances ('allergens') and inhalation of the offending allergen brings on an attack within a few minutes. As already explained, such hypersensitivity occurs in individuals who have a genetically-determined predis-

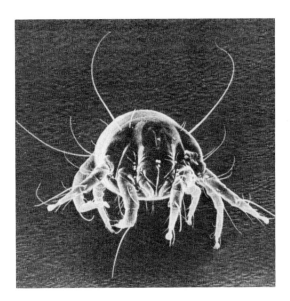

Fig. 16.6 The house-dust mite. *Dermatophagoides pteronyssinus.* × 300. (By courtesy of Bencard.)

position to develop reaginic antibodies of IgE class, and skin tests or provocative inhalation tests with the allergen(s) responsible typically produce an immediate (type I) reaction. The allergens commonly responsible include various pollens, animal dandruff, house dust and various fungi.

The most important allergen in house dust is provided by house-dust mites, notably *Dermatophagoides pteronyssinus* (Fig. 16.6) which infests mattresses and lives on human squames. This mite is commonly found in house dust, and inhaled excreta or fragments of the mite produce an asthmatic reaction in sensitised individuals. *The prognosis in extrinsic asthma is good, although deaths may result from over-medication or from sudden withdrawal of corticosteroids.*

Intrinsic asthma usually develops later in adult life in subjects without an individual or family history of atopic diseases. In contrast to extrinsic asthma, skin tests or provocative inhalation tests fail to reveal a responsible allergen. Nasal polypi are common, and microscopic examination of them shows infiltration with eosinophils. The prognosis is less good than in extrinsic asthma. Patients tend to develop drug hypersensitivities, particularly to aspirin and penicillin, and administration of these drugs may then be followed by a generalised atopic reaction which is sometimes fatal. *Intrin-*

sic asthma is commonly associated with chronic bronchitis, and atopic hypersensitivity to allergens provided by bacteria in the infected bronchi has been suggested, although this has seldom been established.

Psychological factors are of importance in asthma and in many patients the attacks are more likely to occur during periods of anxiety or emotional disturbance.

Clinical features. Asthmatic patients usually suffer from acute attacks characterised by a feeling of tightness in the chest, difficulty in breathing, and particularly in exhaling, which is accompanied by loud wheezing, and often coughing which, during the attack, tends to be non-productive. As the attack subsides, thick viscid sputum, which contains eosinophils, is coughed up. An attack may last from a few minutes to days and may vary in severity from mild dyspnoea to wheezing with severe respiratory distress. Attacks may occur almost continuously, so-called *status asthmaticus*. Some years ago there was a striking increase in mortality in Britain associated with the use of pressurised aerosols of sympathomimetic drugs. This declined following the issue of warnings against excessive use of such aerosols.

During attacks the lungs become overdistended with air, but such distension should not be confused with pulmonary emphysema (p. 16.29), which is only likely to complicate bronchial asthma when there is associated chronic bronchitis. *Right ventricular hypertrophy does not result from uncomplicated bronchial asthma.*

Pathology. When death has occurred during an acute attack, at autopsy the lungs appear overdistended with air and fail to collapse. Their cut surfaces show occlusion of many segmental bronchi by plugs of tough mucoid material (Fig. 16.7). Occasional areas of bronchiectasis (see below) may be present but chronic emphysema (p. 16.29) is slight or absent. The outstanding feature in sections of asthmatic lung during an attack is the plugging of bronchi by mucinous material containing eosinophils and normal or degenerate columnar respiratory epithelial cells. The cellular elements tend to form twisted strips, known as Curschmann's spirals, which may be found in asthmatic sputum. The bronchial epithelium is shed into the lumen, exposing the basal layer of cells overlying the basement membrane which shows a characteristic hyaline thickening. The submucosa shows vascular congestion, oedema and infiltration by eosinophils from which Char-

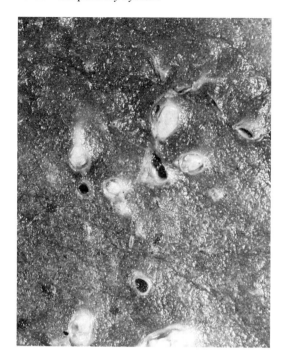

Fig. 16.7 The cut surface of a lung from a patient who died during an acute attack of bronchial asthma. The bronchi are distended by plugs of tough white mucoid material. × 2. (Dr P.S. Hasleton.)

cot's crystals are derived. There have been claims that the number of mast cells is increased. There is hypertrophy of the smooth muscle of the small bronchi and bronchioles, clearly associated with the repeated spasm of these airways (Fig. 16.8). Eventually the changes of chronic bronchitis may supervene (p. 16.10).

Bronchiectasis

Definition and classification. *Bronchiectasis means an abnormal and irreversible dilatation of the bronchi, which may be generalised or localised, and may result in the formation of multiple large spaces or cavities.* It is said to be *cylindrical* when the bronchi are affected over most of their length; this is most pronounced in the lower lobes. In the *saccular* form the dilatation is more localised and severe. *Congenital bronchiectasis* results from failure of development (agenesis) of pulmonary alveolar tissue or failure of large portions of a lobe or lobes to ex-

pand at birth (atelectasis): the affected lobe is small and shrunken and dilated bronchi form cyst-like spaces which extend almost to the pleural surface, there being virtually no trace of lung substance between them.

Structural changes. In chronic bronchitis the transverse markings of the bronchial lining are often increased and depressions are present between the ridges; from this condition all degrees of generalised dilatation are seen up to fully

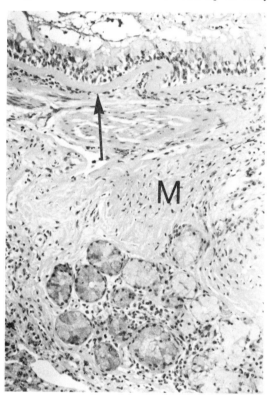

Fig. 16.8 Bronchial asthma. The bronchial lumen (top) contains mucinous material and is lined by intact respiratory epithelium. The basement membrane shows a characteristic hyaline thickening (arrow). The layer of bronchial smooth muscle (M) is hypertrophied and there is a proliferation of mucous glands (bottom). × 130.

established cylindrical bronchiectasis. Saccular bronchiectasis (Fig. 16.9) is usually due to fibrosis of the surrounding lung tissue with obliteration and destruction of the smaller bronchi and bronchioles. The dilated sacs so clearly displayed in a bronchogram appear to be the expanded terminations of the first few branches of the segmental bronchi (Fig. 16.10). The lin-

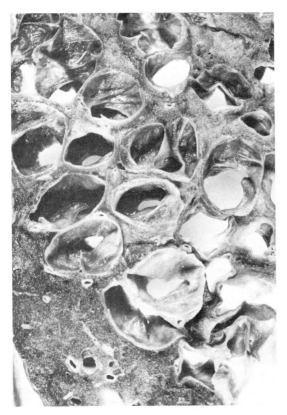

sometimes there is squamous metaplasia. In specimens removed surgically at an early stage, the walls of the larger affected bronchi often show surprisingly good preservation of their structural elements, the chief change being dilatation of the lumen, with collapse and obliteration of their terminal divisions and fibrosis of the lung tissue. In later stages the epithelium disappears, the surface being formed by a thinned basement membrane beneath which there is granulation tissue. Deeper ulceration also may be present. The muscle, elastic tissue and glands of the bronchial wall become atrophied and may eventually disappear.

Effects. Without effective treatment, bronchiectatic cavities eventually become persistently infected with putrifying micro-organisms: purulent fluid accumulates in them and is decomposed, causing foul-smelling breath and sputum. Organisms may spread from the bronchiectatic cavities to the alveolar tissue, either by the air passages or by direct ulceration, and cause pneumonia or a lung abscess. In such conditions the wall of a vein may become involved, with the formation of septic emboli and the development of secondary abscesses, partic-

Fig. 16.9 Bronchiectasis. There is pronounced dilatation of bronchi which appear crowded together with obliteration of intervening lung substance. The dilated bronchi have thick white fibrous walls and their lumina are tortuous and lined by congested mucosa.

ing of the bronchiectatic spaces resembles an irregularly swollen and vascular bronchial mucosa and is often congested. For a time the cavities are almost dry, but later secretion accumulates, becomes purulent, and ulceration of the wall occurs. Bilateral saccular bronchiectasis is seen in the upper lobes in the more fibrotic varieties of chronic tuberculosis, where the true nature of the lesion may be difficult to prove; such cases are now becoming rare in countries where tuberculosis has declined. Apart from tuberculous infection, saccular bronchiectasis is usually unilateral and is commonest in the lower lobes of the lung, especially in the left posterior basal segment.

Microscopic examination. The bronchiectatic cavities may be wholly or partly lined by epithelium, the cells being columnar, rounded or flattened and forming a single or several layers;

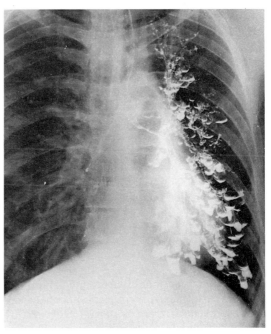

Fig. 16.10 Chest radiograph in which cystic bronchiectasis has been demonstrated in the left lung by the introduction of contrast medium. (Dr. R. Galloway.)

ularly in the brain. The abundant putrid secretion from the cavities may lead to infection of the nasal sinuses. Severe haemoptysis is another serious complication.

In chronic bronchiectasis pulmonary haemodynamic changes may result from such factors as alveolar hypoxia and fibrous obliteration of pulmonary arteries. There is usually considerable enlargement of the bronchial arteries with the development of bronchopulmonary anastomoses and substantial increase of the bronchial blood flow may contribute to the raised pulmonary arterial pressure and right ventricular hypertrophy that develops. Left ventricular hypertrophy may also occur.

Aetiology. Three main factors may be involved: (**a**) loss of aerated lung substance so that the force of inspiratory expansion of the chest falls, in the affected part of the lung, on the bronchial walls alone; (**b**) mechanical weakening of the supporting tissue of the bronchial wall caused by inflammatory changes, and (**c**) contraction of fibrous bands connecting the bronchial wall with the fibrosed and adherent pleura. In long-established cases these factors are variously combined and usually all three are present, but it is important to ascertain which is of primary pathogenic importance.

Bronchiectasis is usually a sequel of bronchiolitis and bronchopneumonia in childhood with partial collapse and imperfect resolution; it may also follow failure of a part of the lung to expand at birth (*atelectasis*). In children the bronchopneumonia may be primary or may complicate whooping cough or measles. In adults it is often secondary to influenza. Some cases of juvenile bronchiectasis were shown by Macfarlane and Somerville (1957) to be associated with adenovirus infection; the bronchi show pronounced irregularity and narrowing of the lumen by hyperplastic submucosal lymphoid tissue. The condition closely resembles that seen in certain virus infections of the lung in cattle ('cuffing pneumonia'), and is called *follicular bronchiectasis*.

There has been much uncertainty about the relative parts played by infection with consequent weakening of the bronchial walls and by collapse of lung tissue with subsequent fibrosis. Radiological investigations clearly indicate that any major degree of pulmonary collapse with negative intrapleural pressure is followed almost at once by dilatation of the bronchi

supplying the collapsed zone; this dilatation may subsequently disappear when the lung becomes re-expanded. Permanent collapse is, however, followed by fibrosis and the bronchi remain dilated. Radiographic examination indicates that this state is commoner than had been supposed and that it may exist for long periods without the clinical symptomatology associated with bronchiectasis. The dilated bronchi are relatively dry, and if lobectomy is performed at this stage, remarkably little structural change in the larger bronchial walls may be seen. Infection, with destruction of the specialised elements and consequent weakening of the wall cannot, therefore, be the primary change in these cases, and *it is probable that pulmonary collapse is the all-important initial causal lesion*. No doubt bronchial dilatation is hastened by the forced inspiration which follows the act of coughing. A vicious circle is thus set up, the effects of which become more severe when the accumulation of infected secretions has produced inflammatory damage to the bronchial walls with loss of the cartilage, muscle and elastic tissue.

Undoubtedly *the bronchopneumonias of childhood* are the most important antecedent to bronchiectasis, but any extensive pulmonary fibrosis may have this effect. In *chronic pulmonary tuberculosis* with fibrotic change, saccular bronchiectatic cavities are common in association with tuberculous cavities, and they also occur in silicosis and fibrotic conditions generally. In infants a few months old suffering from *fibrocystic disease* (*cystic fibrosis*) *of the pancreas*, the trachea and bronchi are lined by tough mucoid secretion which soon becomes purulent; bronchopneumonia follows and if the infant survives, bronchiectasis is a common sequel (p. 20.60).

Bronchial obstruction

Various degrees of obstruction may occur up to complete occlusion and either large or small bronchi may be affected, the causation being different in the two cases. Progressive obstruction of a **large bronchus** is most frequently produced by a primary carcinoma infiltrating the wall and growing into the lumen, less commonly by pressure of massively enlarged lymph nodes and rarely by pressure of an aneurysm of the aortic arch. Sudden obstruction may be produced by a foreign body lodging in a large bronchus. This may obstruct the bronchus completely, whereupon the air in the related part of the lung is absorbed rapidly and pulmonary collapse follows. Usually, however, obstruction is partial at first, resulting in the accumulation of oedema fluid and secretions with some degree of bronchial dilatation. Bacterial infection in the part beyond the obstruction follows, leading to a purulent bronchitis which by further extension may bring about suppurative bronchopneumonia. This is the usual sequence of events when a major bronchus is invaded by a neoplasm or is otherwise progressively obstructed. Occasionally, when infection is less severe, there may be considerable aggregation of lipid-rich macrophages—*endogenous lipid pneumonia* (p. 16.44).

Obstruction of individual **small bronchi** does not lead to collapse of the segment of lung supplied, because collateral ventilation from adjacent lobules through the pores of Kohn and canals of Lambert, connecting bronchioles to distal air passages, supplies enough air to expand the obstructed segment. In fact, it is more likely to become distended.

Obstruction of **bronchioles** is usually produced by purulent or fibrinous inflammatory exudate, notably in bronchopneumonia. In bronchial asthma the obstruction is due to the spasmodic contraction of the walls of the bronchioles, aided by the presence of tough secretion. If the obstruction is such that air can be sucked in and cannot be expelled, as may occur in bronchiolitis and in asthma, then hyperinflation may occur in the area supplied by the obstructed bronchioles. Such hyperinflation is at first reversible when the obstruction is removed. When the bronchiolitis is repeated, destruction of the wall of the respiratory bronchiole may occur, leading to centrilobular emphysema (p. 16.31).

The Lungs

Functions

The essential function of respiration is to provide oxygen to the cells of the body and to remove excess carbon dioxide from them. In large animals such as man, *respiration in its broader physiological context involves four processes*. The first act of respiration is **ventilation** which is the exchange of gases between the alveolar spaces and external atmosphere. Then in the lungs the blood gases exchange with alveolar air by **diffusion** across the alveolar walls. Finally the blood circulatory system is used to **transport** gases to and from the tissues, while **exchange** between blood and tissue cells occurs in the systemic capillaries. *Respiration in its clinical sense is generally restricted to those aspects which concern the major airways and lungs.* The primary function of the lungs is, therefore, to oxygenate mixed venous blood. This involves the controlled absorption of oxygen and the elimination of carbon dioxide so that the blood gas tensions are maintained within normal limits.

Although primarily involved in gas exchange, the lungs also have important non-respiratory functions: they act as a filter for the blood passing through them and are also concerned in the metabolism of certain vasoactive substances. Their anatomical situation is ideal for these roles for, apart from the heart, the lungs are the only organs through which all the blood passes in a single circulation. The pulmonary capillary bed is a huge network, the average diameter of the capillaries being about $8\,\mu m$. Particles ranging in diameter from 10 to $75\,\mu m$ tend to be delayed in passing through the pulmonary circulation. Small emboli such as fibrinous clots, bone marrow, fat, placental tissue and particulate matter contaminating intravenous infusions, are trapped in the lungs and may be cleared by the action of proteolytic enzymes and phagocytosis. The lung, therefore, plays an important role as a sieve in protecting organs such as the brain and kidney.

The lungs also have the ability to clear certain vasoactive substances from the blood and to synthesise or activate others. Thus significant proportions of the 5-hydroxytryptamine, bradykinin, prostaglandins and noradrenaline are removed from the blood during its passage through the lungs. The lung is probably the main site for the conversion of the relatively inactive decapeptide angiotensin I to the potent systemic vasoconstrictive octapeptide angiotensin II. The enzyme mechanisms responsible for the clearing and activation of these vasoactive substances are probably localised in the endothelium of the pulmonary arteries, capillaries and veins.

Respiratory failure

The primary function of the lungs is to maintain the blood gas tensions at normal levels. *Respiratory failure exists when a patient is unable to maintain blood gas tensions within normal limits* and is usually said to be present when the systemic arterial oxygen tension (Pa_{O_2}) falls below 60 mm Hg or when the carbon dioxide tension (Pa_{CO_2}) exceeds 50 mm Hg, while the patient is breathing air. Figures such as these imply that the patient's respiratory function is impaired, but it should be emphasised that many people are able to live comparatively unrestricted lives with blood gas tensions at least as abnormal as these.

The maintenance of normal gas tensions depends on the following factors.

1. Adequate ventilation of the alveolar spaces.
2. Unimpaired diffusion across the alveolar-capillary wall.
3. An even distribution of ventilation to the alveoli relative to the pulmonary capillary blood flow (perfusion).

The causes of respiratory failure may, therefore, be divided into three groups: *hypoventilation, impaired diffusion* and *uneven ventilation and perfusion.*

Hypoventilation

Ventilation of the lung is the volume of gas inspired in unit time and is 7 litres per minute in a normal adult breathing a tidal volume of 500 ml at a respiratory rate of 14 breaths per minute. This quantity of gas does not reach the alveoli because part of each breath merely fills the large conducting airways and takes no part in gaseous exchange. This is the *anatomical dead space* which amounts to about 150 ml. *Alveolar ventilation* in a normal adult, therefore, amounts to $(500 - 150) \times 14 = 4900$ ml per minute. Alveolar ventilation is achieved not only by the mass movement of gases caused by the rhythmic expansion and deflation of the lungs, but also by diffusion of gas molecules within the airways. The total cross sectional area of the airways at the level of alveolar ducts and spaces is many times greater than that at the levels of the bronchi and bronchioles. This means that the mass flow of gas in the relatively narrow bronchi and bronchioles suddenly drops to nearly zero as the airways abruptly widen into the alveolar ducts and spaces. Thus, transport of gas over the few millimetres between the respiratory bronchioles and alveolar-capillary wall is achieved by molecular diffusion. An important adverse effect of airways obstruction is to impede the mass transport of gases and consequently increase the distance over which molecular diffusion has to take place, so giving rise to a state of alveolar hypoventilation.

Causes of alveolar hypoventilation. In its broadest sense the term alveolar hypoventilation means that the volume of gas reaching the alveolar gas-exchanging interface is inadequate to maintain the normal systemic arterial tensions of oxygen and carbon dioxide. However, *alveolar hypoventilation in the clinical sense is usually applied to those patients with evidence of respiratory failure without underlying disease of the lungs.* Ventilation is a complex process which requires intact airways and involves the co-ordinated action of the respiratory centre, peripheral nerves, respiratory muscles and thoracic cage. Hypoventilation may, therefore, be caused by depression of the respiratory centre, neurological disease, muscular disorders and disorders of the chest wall and pleura.

Respiratory centre depression. Alveolar hypoventilation, leading to cyanosis and carbon dioxide retention, is a common complication of overdosage or poisoning with narcotic drugs such as the barbiturates and morphine. The action of the medullary respiratory centre may also be impaired by the direct or indirect effects of cerebral infarcts, cerebral haemorrhage and intracranial neoplasms.

Neurological disease. Conditions such as poliomyelitis, acute polyneuritis and spinal cord lesions at or above the origin of the phrenic nerve (C3, 4, 5) may cause hypoventilation due to paralysis of the respiratory muscles. Tetanus, botulism and neuromuscular block produced by curare or by ganglion-blocking agents may have a similar effect.

Muscular disorders. These include conditions such as myasthenia gravis, dermatomyositis and muscular dystrophy which may affect the intercostal muscles and diaphragm.

Chest wall disorders. Multiple fractures of the ribs produce a 'flail chest' in which the affected part of the chest wall collapses inwards on inspiration, so reducing effective ventilation of the alveoli. Severe kyphoscoliosis can interfere with the respiratory excursions of the thoracic cage and produce hypoventilation.

Pleural disease. Large pleural effusions and pneumothorax induce hypoventilation by causing compression collapse of the adjacent lung.

Excessive obesity (*Pickwickian syndrome*). Some excessively obese people develop hypoventilation although objective tests of pulmonary function are normal. They are liable to episodes of somnolence and develop cyanosis with secondary polycythaemia, hypercapnia and often pulmonary hypertension leading to right ventricular failure. Numerous factors have been suggested to account for the ventilatory disorders in these subjects, including mechanical impairment of respiration due to fatty infiltration of the respiratory muscles, excessive elevation of the diaphragm in the supine posture and decreased compliance of the thoracic cage.

Effects of hypoventilation. Alveolar gas differs from the inspired air because carbon dioxide is being continually added to it, and oxygen removed from it, by the blood perfusing the alveolar capillaries. Its composition depends on a balance between ventilation and blood flow. Hypoventilation causes a fall in alveolar oxygen tension and an increase in the carbon dioxide tension. This is accompanied by an elevation in the systemic arterial carbon dioxide tension (*hy-*

percapnia) and an arithmetically equivalent depression of the oxygen tension. *The main effects of hypoventilation are attributable to hypercapnia*: oxygen desaturation and cyanosis are late events. The symptoms and signs of hypercapnia are a rapid bounding pulse, moist warm hands, constricted pupils and elevation of the systemic blood pressure. Dyspnoea is often absent. Severe carbon dioxide retention leads to confusion, drowsiness, coarse tremors and eventual coma. The tendon reflexes are depressed and the plantar response is extensor. An important feature of hypoventilation as a cause of respiratory failure is that the lungs are normal and the prognosis is excellent if the precipitating cause can be removed.

Impaired diffusion

In the normal lung, alveolar gas is separated from capillary blood by the alveolar-capillary membrane which is $0.2\,\mu$m wide at its thinnest points and is composed of three distinct anatomical layers: *alveolar epithelium*, a narrow *interstitial zone*; and *capillary endothelium* (Fig. 16.11). The exchange of respiratory gases between the alveolar space and capillaries is by diffusion, the gases flowing from a region of high partial pressure to one of low partial pressure. Blood entering the alveolar capillaries is mixed venous blood with a relatively high carbon dioxide tension and a low oxygen tension. It gives off carbon dioxide and takes up oxygen from the alveolar gas. In a healthy individual at rest, equilibration between alveolar gas and capillary blood is virtually complete. Lung disease may impede the diffusion of gases if the thickness of the alveolar-capillary membrane is increased, or if there is a decrease of the anatomical surface area available for diffusion due to excision of lung tissue or its destruction by disease such as emphysema. The term *alveolar-capillary block* is sometimes applied to conditions in which thickening of the alveolar-capillary wall is accompanied by hypoxaemia. Examples include diffuse fibrosing alveolitis, pulmonary sarcoidosis, asbestosis, and alveolar-cell carcinoma. However, oxygen diffuses readily through the tissues and the degree of alveolar-capillary thickening in these conditions is usually not sufficient to impair

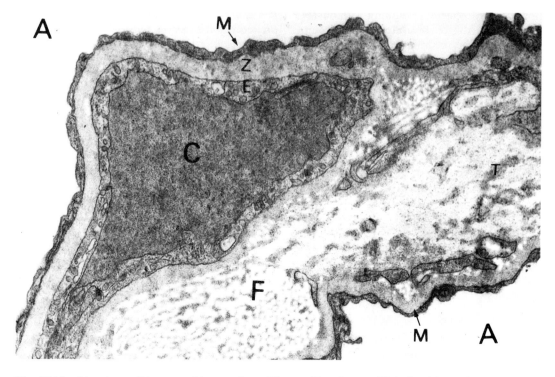

Fig. 16.11   Alveolar wall in normal human lung. The capillary lumen (C) is lined by endothelial cells (E). The alveolar spaces (A) are lined by membranous pneumocytes (M). In the thinnest portion of the blood-air pathway the endothelial cell is separated from the membranous pneumocyte by a granular amorphous zone (Z) consisting of their fused basement membranes. Elsewhere, the endothelial and epithelial cells are separated by an interstitial space containing collagen (F) and elastic fibres (T). Electron micrograph. × 25000.

oxygen diffusion seriously: the hypoxaemia is likely to be due mostly to a disturbed ratio of ventilation/perfusion (see below).

The functional effect of impaired alveolar-capillary gas exchange is interference with oxygen uptake and the development of systemic arterial desaturation. Patients with impaired diffusion are particularly liable to develop sudden systemic arterial desaturation with cyanosis on exercise or if alveolar hypoxia occurs. The effect of exercise is to reduce the time spent by the blood in the pulmonary capillaries and thus reduce the time available for diffusion and equilibration. In alveolar hypoxia the difference between the oxygen tension of alveolar gas and mixed venous blood is reduced, so decreasing the diffusion gradient across the alveolar-capillary wall and slowing the rate of diffusion of oxygen. Carbon dioxide is much more soluble than oxygen and diffuses twenty times more readily through the tissues, so that thickening

of the alveolar-capillary wall has no effect on the exchange of carbon dioxide between alveolar gas and capillary blood.

Uneven ventilation and perfusion

A factor of fundamental importance in gas exchange in the lungs is the distribution of alveolar ventilation relative to the pulmonary capillary blood flow. This is referred to as the ventilation/perfusion ratio. In the normal lung, total alveolar ventilation and pulmonary capillary blood flow both approximate to 5 litres per minute and the ratio is therefore near unity. Gravity affects the normal distribution of ventilation and perfusion throughout the lung so that the two are not closely matched in every alveolus. In a normal healthy individual who is upright, the alveoli at the apex of the lung have a very low blood flow and moderate ventilation, while at the base the blood flow is much larger but the ventilation only slightly increased. The result is that the ventilation/perfusion ratio decreases down the lung.

The anatomical organisation and physiological regulation of the lungs, which are composed of three hundred million functioning alveolar units, allow a large volume of gas and blood to be brought into close proximity over an enormous area (about 70 m^2). The efficiency of gas exchange is largely dependent upon the precision with which appropriate proportions of the total ventilation and total pulmonary blood flow are conveyed to each alveolus. *Abnormal distribution of ventilation and perfusion is the most common cause of respiratory failure.* It may arise either because ventilation is abnormally distributed, as in acute bronchial asthma, or because perfusion is abnormally distributed, as in multiple pulmonary emboli. More commonly, both ventilation and perfusion are abnormally distributed as in chronic bronchitis and diffuse fibrosing alveolitis.

Excessive ventilation of an alveolus cannot materially increase the oxygen tension of the blood perfusing it. Any ventilation which is superfluous to the respiratory capacity of the perfusing blood is wasted. The *physiological dead-space* is wasted alveolar ventilation added to the anatomical dead space. Mixed venous blood reaching a hypoventilated alveolus cannot be fully saturated with oxygen. Thus any alveolar capillary blood flow which is superfluous to the ventilatory capacity is wasted. Although the total blood flow and ventilation of a diseased lung may be the same as in a healthy lung, the effect of abnormally uneven distribution of ventilation and perfusion in numerous individual alveoli is to produce a decrease in the oxygen tension of arterial blood.

Although inequalities of both ventilation and perfusion commonly occur together in the same patient, it is easier to consider the pathological causes of each separately.

Uneven distribution of ventilation. This may be caused by widespread or focal narrowings or dilatations of airways, by variations in the distensibility of airways, and by the presence of oedema fluid and exudate.

Narrowing of airways. This occurs in acute bronchial asthma, chronic bronchitis and acute bronchiolitis.

Dilatation of terminal airways. If the finer airways are dilated, e.g. the respiratory bronchioles in bronchiolar emphysema, ventilation of the alveoli diminishes because part of every inspired breath is used to fill these abnormal airspaces. The distance over which gas molecules have to travel by diffusion to reach the alveolar wall is increased.

Variation in distensibility of different airways leads to uneven ventilation because those with stiff, inelastic walls expand less for a given intrathoracic pressure change than those which are compliant and easily distensible. This type of uneven ventilation is probably the major cause of impaired gaseous exchange in patients with diffuse pulmonary fibrosing diseases.

Alveolar exudates. In pneumonia, the alveolar capillaries are perfused but the alveolar spaces are filled with inflammatory exudate and so the affected lung tissue is not ventilated.

Uneven distribution of perfusion. This may be due to conditions leading to obstruction of the pulmonary vascular bed. Examples include multiple pulmonary emboli, fibrous obliteration secondary to pneumoconiosis or diffuse fibrosing alveolitis, the occlusive lesions of severe hypertensive pulmonary vascular disease, and pulmonary vasoconstriction resulting from hypoxia of lung tissue. This last mechanism may have a compensatory effect by reducing perfusion of poorly ventilated alveoli and thus improving the ventilation/perfusion ratio.

Pulmonary oedema

This condition may be defined as an excessive extravascular accumulation of fluid within the lung. It can result from (1) an *imbalance of hydrodynamic forces* across the alveolar-capillary wall which causes more fluid to leave the capillaries than can be removed from the tissues, and (2) *increased permeability* of the endothelial layer of the pulmonary capillaries (p. 4.8).

The fine structure of the alveolar septum is shown in Fig. 16.11. Capillary blood is separated from alveolar air by three distinct anatomical layers: capillary endothelium; a narrow interstitial zone; and alveolar epithelium. The alveolar capillaries are lined by the thin cytoplasmic extensions of endothelial cells which contain few organelles apart from numerous small pinocytotic vesicles. Normal alveolar capillary endothelial cells are not fenestrated. They are joined by 'tight junctions' containing narrow constrictions (p. 4.6). Sandwiched between the capillary endothelium and alveolar epithelium is an interstitial zone of variable width. Over the convexities of the capillaries protruding into the alveoli, there is no true interstitial space because the contact surface between the endothelium and epithelium is formed exclusively by the fused basement membranes of these two cell layers. In other regions, the epithelial and endothelial basement membranes are separated by an interstitial space containing fine elastic fibres, bundles of collagen fibrils, fibroblasts and macrophages. The alveolar septa are devoid of lymphatics, which first appear in the interstitial space surrounding terminal bronchioles, small arteries and veins. Over 95% of the area of the alveolar walls is lined by the thin, extensive membranous pneumocytes. The cytoplasm of these epithelial cells closely resembles that of the subjacent endothelial cells. The margins of adjacent membranous or granular pneumocytes (p. 16.51) abut bluntly or overlap with the formation of narrow clefts. However, unlike the endothelial cell junctions, which allow exchange of fluid between intravascular and extravascular spaces, the clefts between adjacent epithelial cells are actually obliterated by fusion of opposing cell membranes. Escape of fluid through the interendothelial junctions is dependent, as elsewhere, on capillary intraluminal pressure: a rise in intravascular pressure results in an increase in the amount of fluid entering the interstitial space of the alveolar septum.

Accumulation of fluid in the alveolar spaces is a late and not an inevitable manifestation of pulmonary oedema. It is preceded by a sequence of changes which is largely independent of the cause of the oedema. The pulmonary lymphatics have a considerable reserve capacity but when this is exceeded, fluid begins to accumulate in the lung. It first accumulates in the loose, readily distensible connective tissues around the bronchi and larger vessels and next distends the thick, collagen-containing portions of the alveolar wall. Fluid does not accumulate in the thinnest portions of the blood–air pathway, i.e. over the convexities of the alveolar capillaries, until a very late stage because, as mentioned above, the membranous pneumocytes and capillary endothelial cells in this zone share a common basement membrane, and relatively high pressure is necessary to separate them. The final stage of pulmonary oedema is accumulation of fluid within the alveolar spaces. The route whereby fluid escapes from the interstitial tissues to the alveolar spaces is uncertain, although it is usually assumed that it is related to the opening, perhaps temporarily, of some of the intercellular junctions between membranous pneumocytes.

A striking fine structural feature, not observed in systemic capillaries, may be seen in the alveolar capillaries in pulmonary oedema: the thin layer of endothelium lining the alveolar capillary may lift away from the underlying basement membrane to form a bleb or vesicle which protrudes into the lumen of the capillary (Fig. 16.12). It has been suggested that the thin endothelium is floated off its basement membrane by oedema fluid and projects into the lumen because of the low pressure within the capillaries. This hypothesis could account for the absence of endothelial vesicles in patients with pulmonary oedema due to pulmonary venous hypertension, where the capillary intraluminal blood pressure is increased. There is no evidence that the vesicles, although morphologically striking, have any significant effect upon the flow of blood through the affected capillaries.

Pulmonary oedema may occur in patients with *left ventricular failure* or *mitral stenosis* who develop elevation of the pulmonary venous pressure (pp. 15.3, 16.25). Pulmonary oedema which follows overloading of the circulation with *intravenous infusions* is probably also due to failure of the left ventricle. The acute pulmonary oedema which may follow *sudden withdrawal of a pleural effusion* is generally attributed to a sudden increase in the negative intrathoracic pressure. Pulmonary oedema may occasionally occur in patients with *raised intracranial pressure* resulting from head injuries, neurosurgical operations, intracerebral haemor-

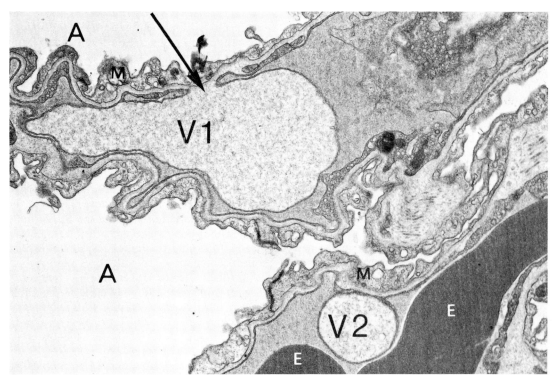

Fig. 16.12 Electron micrograph of two pulmonary capillaries from a rat showing the features of pulmonary oedema caused by acute exposure to simulated high altitude corresponding to the summit of Mount Everest (elevation 8850 metres; atmospheric pressure 250 torr.). The lower capillary contains two erythrocytes (E). Two endothelial vesicles, V1 and V2 are seen. The upper has been cut in longitudinal section and assumes the shape of the capillary into which it projects. Its pedicle is indicated by an arrow. The lower vesicle, V2, has been cut in transverse section and gives the spurious appearance of lying free in the capillary. The alveolar spaces (A) are lined by membranous pneumocytes (M). × 12 500.

rhage and neoplasms. The mechanism of production of this oedema is not clear. *High altitude pulmonary oedema* is an uncommon complication following ascent to altitudes over 3000 metres. It is unusual in that it occurs in otherwise healthy individuals, such as mountain climbers and military personnel. The mechanism of its production is unknown. Susceptibility to high altitude pulmonary oedema is not limited to men from low altitude, for if a high-altitude dweller spends a few weeks at sea level, he may develop pulmonary oedema soon after returning to his usual altitude of residence. *Toxic gases and fumes* such as nitrogen dioxide, chlorine and phosgene may damage the alveolar wall and produce pulmonary oedema.

Hyaline membrane disease. The respiratory distress syndrome is a serious disorder of newborn infants with a mortality rate of between 20 and 40%. It is most common in premature infants and 10–15% of those with a birth weight of 2500 g or less develop the syndrome. Infants born by Caesarian section and those born of mothers with diabetes mellitus are also particularly susceptible. The disorder is characterised by increasing respiratory difficulty which starts a few minutes to a few hours after birth. There is hypoxaemia and cyanosis despite high concentrations of inspired oxygen. Physiologically, the babies have large functional right-to-left shunts and very low lung compliance. At necropsy the lungs are collapsed, firm, and resemble liver in appearance and consistency. Microscopically, the alveoli are collapsed while the terminal and respiratory bronchioles are distended and lined by thick, eosinophilic 'hyaline membranes' of variable composition: they may contain fibrin, necrotic epithelial cell debris, and keratinised cells presumably derived from inhaled amniotic fluid. If the infants survive the first few days, they seem to recover completely, although pulmonary fibrosis may ensue in a small minority.

The aetiology of this disorder remains obscure. Important factors seem to be high pulmonary vascular resistance, impaired or deficient surfactant activity, increased permeability of the alveolar capillaries, and inhalation of amniotic fluid. The lungs of infants dying at the height of the disease invariably have a deficiency of pulmonary surfactant, which normally lowers the surface tension of the alveoli. Although this deficiency is regarded as a crucial factor by some workers, whether it is a cause or effect of the disease remain unsettled.

Massive pulmonary haemorrhage in the newborn. Sometimes infants thought clinically to have died from hyaline membrane disease are found at autopsy to have massive haemorrhage involving two or more lobes of the lungs. The condition may arise from about half-an-hour to two weeks after birth. Sometimes it becomes apparent in a baby already being treated for respiratory insufficiency in a respirator, when bloodstained fluid is discovered in the endotracheal tube. Evidence of disseminated intravascular coagulation (p. 17.68) has been found in some babies. Haemorrhage into the subarachnoid space or cerebral ventricles is sometimes also found at autopsy. At present, it is impossible to ascribe a single common cause for massive pulmonary haemorrhage. Some believe that it may be due to oxygen toxicity or to the insertion of a catheter too far down the endotracheal tubes.

Uraemic lung. This term is used to describe a chronic form of pulmonary oedema long known to radiologists on account of the butterfly-shaped shadow that extends outwards from the hilum of both lungs. At autopsy, the lungs are voluminous and rubbery and, on squeezing, a frothy fluid exudes from the cut surface. Microscopically the reluctance of the oedema fluid to drain out of the cut surface is seen to be due to a fine fibrin network in the alveoli, and hyaline membranes may be formed. In longstanding cases organisation of the exudate may take place in some areas.

Shock lung and adult respiratory distress syndrome. It has been known for some years that respiratory failure is the cause of death in many patients who have suffered major trauma, haemorrhage or other catastrophe causing shock. With improved techniques of resuscitation and blood transfusion, *the syndrome of post-traumatic pulmonary insufficiency or 'shock lung' has emerged as one of the most frequent and life-threatening complications to occur in both civilian and military casualties.* Shock lung occurs within one or two days of the traumatic episode, following the initial resuscitation procedures. The patient gradually becomes hypoxic with acidosis despite oxygen therapy, and mortality is high. Initially, the chest radiograph shows patchy opacities attributed to pulmonary oedema and collapse, which progress to almost totally opaque lung fields in the severely affected patient. At autopsy, the lungs are heavy, beefy and oedematous. Microscopically, in early cases there is intra-alveolar oedema with extravasation of erythrocytes. Fibrinous exudate and hyaline membranes which line the alveolar walls develop later. In long-standing cases, pulmonary fibrosis ensues, and the alveolar walls become lined by metaplastic cuboidal epithelium.

There are many possible explanations for shock lung, including fat embolism, over-transfusion, pulmonary oedema, aspiration of gastric contents, oxygen toxicity and pulmonary micro-embolism. It is probably not a single entity, but has several causes. It has been suggested that micro-emboli originating in damaged tissue, in transfused whole blood or reconstituted dried plasma, may be responsible for the pulmonary changes. Disseminated intravascular coagulation and endotoxaemia have been recognised in some cases.

Pulmonary vascular disease

Diseases of the heart affect the lungs and diseases of the lungs affect the heart. The anatomical basis of this interrelationship is the pulmonary vasculature. Normally the blood

Table 16.2 The causes of pulmonary arterial hypertension and hypertensive pulmonary vascular disease

Disease group	Examples
Pre-tricuspid congenital cardiac septal shunts.	Atrial septal defect.
Post-tricuspid congenital cardiac septal shunts.	Ventricular septal defect. Patent ductus arteriosus.
Elevation of left atrial pressure.	Mitral stenosis. Chronic left ventricular failure. Left atrial myxoma.
Massive pulmonary fibrosis.	Silicosis.
Fibrosing alveolitis.	Rheumatoid disease. Progressive systemic sclerosis. Berylliosis.
Chronic hypoxia.	Normal subjects living at high altitude. Chronic bronchitis and emphysema. Kyphoscoliosis. Pickwickian syndrome.
Liver disease.	Cirrhosis. Portal vein thrombosis.
Pulmonary thrombo-embolism.	Secondary to thrombosis in deep veins of limbs.
Primary pulmonary hypertension.	Classical variety. Pulmonary veno-occlusive disease.
Diet.	Crotalaria alkaloids. Some anorexigens suspected. Toxic oil syndrome in Spain (adulterated rape-seed oil).

pressure in the pulmonary arterial tree is only one-sixth of that in the systemic. This is reflected in the fact that the right ventricle is thinner than the left. The pulmonary arteries are also thinner than the systemic, and consist of a layer of circularly orientated smooth muscle sandwiched between well-formed elastic laminae. The pulmonary arterioles, unlike the systemic ones, do not have a muscular media, their walls consisting mainly of a single elastic lamina. Normal pulmonary arterioles are thus incapable of exerting significant resistance to the flow of blood through the lungs. The main way in which diseases of the heart and lung affect each other is through the production of pulmonary arterial hypertension and associated hypertensive pulmonary vascular disease.

Pulmonary hypertension

There are many diseases which will cause pulmonary arterial hypertension and associated pulmonary vascular disease (Table 16.2). Pulmonary hypertension may be arbitrarily defined as a systolic blood pressure in the pulmonary circulation exceeding 30 mmHg. There are various forms of hypertensive pulmonary vascular disease, and one cannot predict what vascular lesions are present from a knowledge of the level of the pulmonary arterial pressure. Rather the form of the hypertensive pulmonary vascular disease depends upon the nature of the underlying disease process. This is of considerable practical importance, since the different forms of pulmonary vascular disease are reflected in different levels of pressure, flow and resistance in the pulmonary circulation, which, in turn, have an important effect on the clinical picture and course. The causes of pulmonary hypertension and the various forms of hypertensive pulmonary vascular disease that they are associated with are as follows:

Congenital cardiac shunts. A large congenital cardiac defect between the right and left ventricles or between the aorta and the pulmonary trunk will lead to pulmonary arterial hypertension from birth, due to direct transmission of systemic arterial pressure and flow into the pulmonary circulation. Examples of such **post-tricuspid shunts** are ventricular septal defect, patent ductus arteriosus, persistent truncus arter-

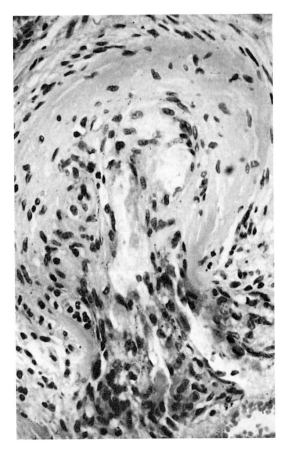

Fig. 16.13 Plexiform lesion from a girl of 12 years with a large ventricular septal defect. The parent muscular pulmonary artery shows fibrinoid necrosis. Its dilated sac contains a proliferation of myofibroblasts and fibrillary cells. × 150.

iosus and aorto-pulmonary septal defect. **Pre-tricuspid shunts**, such as atrial septal defects, produce pulmonary hypertension in adolescence or adult life as a result of the effect of a prolonged excessive blood flow on the pulmonary vasculature.

Provided the defect is large enough, a characteristic form of pulmonary vascular disease occurs in association with the raised pulmonary arterial pressure. The form of disease produced by pre- and post-tricuspid congenital cardiac shunts is identical. Initially there is increased thickness of the medial coat of the small pulmonary arteries, while pulmonary arterioles develop a distinct muscular media and resemble systemic arterioles. This is followed by intimal thickening of the pulmonary arteries and arter-

ioles, at first cellular, then fibrous, and finally fibro-elastic. *These intimal changes lead to organic occlusion of pulmonary arteries.* This is followed by dilatation of the pulmonary vasculature which may be generalised or localised. Localised 'dilatation lesions' develop. These are clusters of thin-walled branches of small pulmonary arteries arising proximal to the sites of occlusion. They form a collateral circulation to maintain a flow of blood to the pulmonary capillary bed, and are termed **'angiomatoid lesions'**. Sometimes a characteristic proliferation of myofibroblasts and fibrillary cells* takes place within them in a plexiform pattern to give the structure its name of **'plexiform lesion'** (Fig. 16.13). These thin-walled branches rupture to give rise to **pulmonary haemosiderosis**. Finally, **fibrinoid necrosis** of the small pulmonary arteries may occur if the pulmonary arterial pressure rises rapidly or severely.

This form of pulmonary vascular disease offers a good example of how pathological changes in the pulmonary circulation may exert a profound effect on the clinical picture and course. It illustrates too how these effects may change with progression of the pulmonary vascular disease. Thus the early stages of medial hypertrophy and intimal fibrosis are associated with pulmonary arterial hypertension with a high pulmonary flow, and a moderate increase in pulmonary vascular resistance which is largely reversible. The later dilatation lesions and necrotising arteritis are associated with severe pulmonary hypertension, a reduced pulmonary blood flow, and a severely and irreversibly increased pulmonary vascular resistance. Hence, *the early phase of the clinical picture of a large congenital cardiac shunt is dominated by signs of left ventricular hypertrophy, increased pulmonary blood flow, and left-to-right shunting of blood with no cyanosis. The later phase, however, is dominated by clinical signs of right ventricular hypertrophy, diminished pulmonary blood flow, and right-to-left shunting of blood with cyanosis.* In the early stages of hypertensive pulmonary vascular disease, surgical correction of septal defects is usually followed by the reversal of the associated pulmonary hypertension. In the later stages, however,

---

*Fibrillary cells are primitive vasoformative reserve cells which contain within their cytoplasm whorls of intermediate filaments.

the pulmonary hypertension is irreversible and this contra-indicates attempts at corrective surgical treatment.

This florid form of hypertensive pulmonary vascular disease, designated **plexogenic pulmonary arteriopathy**, is characteristic of *congenital cardiac septal defects* but is not exclusively produced by them. It can also complicate an *acquired ventricular septal defect* such us septal rupture following infarction, or the rare cases of cirrhosis of the liver associated with pulmonary hypertension. It is also found in *primary pulmonary hypertension* which is a rare disease occurring largely in young women with no underlying disease of the heart or lungs.

Hypoxia. *Any state of chronic hypoxia will induce pulmonary arterial hypertension and associated changes in the pulmonary arteries.* Thus pulmonary hypertension occurs in anyone living at high altitude and is consistent with a healthy and active life. It also complicates chronic bronchitis and emphysema when there is associated chronic hypoxia. Kyphoscoliosis, Monge's disease (so-called 'chronic mountain sickness') and the Pickwickian syndrome are all likely to become complicated by hypoxic hypertensive pulmonary vascular disease, which also occurs occasionally in individuals with enlarged adenoids.

The hallmark of this variety is muscularisation of the terminal portions of the pulmonary vascular tree, which increases pulmonary vascular resistance. There is insignificant intimal fibrosis and the important functional implication of this is that *the pulmonary hypertension and associated pulmonary vascular disease of chronic hypoxia are largely and rapidly reversible.* Another effect of hypoxia is the development of longitudinal muscle in the intima of pulmonary arteries and arterioles.

Another feature of chronic hypoxia, **hyperplasia of the carotid bodies** is discussed on p. 16.63.

Elevation of left atrial pressure. *Any disease that brings about a sustained significant elevation of blood pressure in the left atrium is complicated by pulmonary venous and arterial hypertension and associated hypertensive pulmonary vascular disease.* This is characterised in its early stages by medial hypertrophy and intimal fibrosis of pulmonary arteries and muscularisation of pulmonary arterioles. Rarely in the later stages there is fibrinoid necrosis of pulmonary arteries.

Plexiform and other dilatation lesions do not occur in this group. The pulmonary hypertension associated with the early vascular changes is reversible whereas that associated with fibrinoid necrosis is not. Conditions which lead to chronic left atrial hypertension include chronic left ventricular failure from any cause (p. 15.3), mitral stenosis or incompetence (acquired or congenital), and the rare myxoma of the left atrium. The interesting association of pulmonary capillary hypertension and normal left atrial blood pressure occurs in pulmonary veno-occlusive disease which is a rare form of primary pulmonary hypertension.

The direct effects of pulmonary *venous* hypertension are grouped together under the term *chronic venous congestion* and are described in outline on p. 10.5. The congestion may cause pulmonary oedema in which fluid accumulates not only in the alveolar spaces but also in the interlobular septa and in distended perivascular lymphatics; this is sometimes seen radiographically as *basal horizontal lines* (Kerley B lines), which indicate that the pulmonary venous blood pressure exceeds a mean level of 25 mmHg.

Persistent pulmonary congestion and oedema are associated with a hyperplasia of granular pneumocytes (p. 16.51) and the development of interstitial fibrosis of the lung. Red blood cells may be extruded from the distended pulmonary capillaries into the alveolar walls and spaces (Fig. 16.14). Their phagocytosis and destruction in macrophages results in collections of haemosiderin-laden macrophages within the alveoli—*pulmonary haemosiderosis* (Fig. 11.10, p. 11.12) which may present radiologically as a 'snow storm effect'. The liberated ferric iron salts may also be deposited on reticulin and elastic fibres in the walls of alveoli and in pulmonary arteries and veins where it may provoke a giant cell reaction. The combination of rusty discoloration of the lung due to this deposition of ferric salts, and firmness of the pulmonary parenchyma due to increase in fibrous tissue in the alveolar walls, accounts for the classical term of *brown induration*.

Other mineral deposits which may occur in chronic pulmonary venous hypertension include nodules of osseous metaplasia which present a characteristic radiological picture. A much rarer manifestation is the deposition in the alveolar spaces of myriads of microliths composed of laminated concretions of

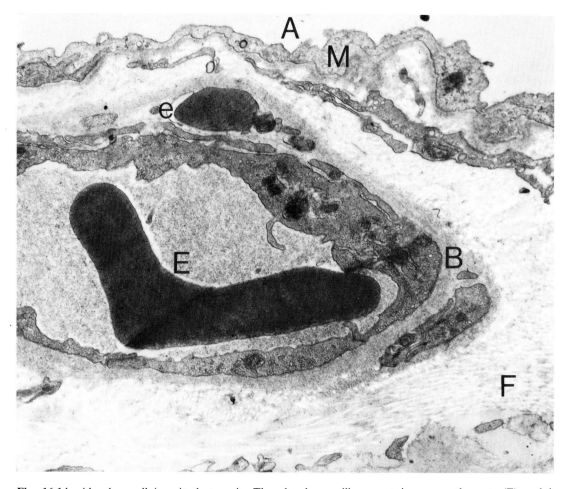

Fig. 16.14 Alveolar wall in mitral stenosis. The alveolar capillary contains an erythrocyte (E) and is surrounded by dense fibrous tissue (F) which displaces it inwards from its normal superficial position beneath the membranous pneumocyte (M) lining the alveolar space (A). The capillary basement membrane (B) is thickened and contains a disintegrating extravasated erythrocyte (e). Electron micrograph. × 16 500.

calcium phosphate bound within an organic envelope containing ferric salts. This condition, which may transform the lung into a rock-hard mass that may require sawing for dissection, is called *microlithiasis*.

The pulmonary veins themselves show the effects of increased venous pressure by the formation of a distinct muscular media so that they may resemble small muscular pulmonary arteries. They also show intimal fibrosis.

Pulmonary fibrosis. Both massive and interstitial pulmonary fibrosis may become complicated by pulmonary hypertension and pulmonary vascular changes which are initially muscular in type and reversible. Later there is obliterative fibrosis of pulmonary arteries and arterioles with an irreversible increase in pulmonary vascular resistance.

'Cor pulmonale.' The term 'cor pulmonale' has been used in a general sense to mean involvement of the heart secondary to lung disease. Unfortunately it is used equally to describe either hypertrophy or failure of the right ventricle, brought about by involvement of the pulmonary circulation by lung disease. Since this term has no precise meaning its use is best avoided.

Pulmonary hypotension

Diminished pulmonary arterial pressure due to pulmonary stenosis is commonly associated with redirection of pulmonary blood flow when there is an associated congenital cardiac septal defect such as a ventricular septal defect. This occurs in Fallot's tetrad where a reversed flow (from right to left) causes pronounced cyanosis and leads to compensatory erythrocytosis. The net result is the circulation of viscous blood at diminished pressure and flow through the pulmonary vessels. This leads to atrophy of the media of the pulmonary arteries with thrombosis, subsequent organisation, and recanalisation of these vessels. The media of the pulmonary trunk shows atrophy with clumping of its elastic tissue. This is in contrast to states of pulmonary arterial hypertension where there is thickening of the media even to the extent of the pulmonary trunk becoming as thick as the aorta. In states of pulmonary hypotension with an inadequate flow of blood to the pulmonary capillary bed, there is compensatory enlargement of the bronchial arteries.

Pulmonary embolism

Thrombo-embolism

By far the commonest sites of origin of thrombi leading to pulmonary embolism are the deep veins of the legs, especially in the calf. Pulmonary thrombo-embolism is very rare in children but opinion is divided as to whether age or sex affects its incidence in adults. Predisposing factors are described on p. 10.16.

There is no doubt that pulmonary thrombo-embolism is very common indeed. In one study, carried out in hospitals in Oxford, its incidence, as determined by examination of the left lung in a routine autopsy service, was 12%. A detailed histological examination of the right lung from the same cases revealed an incidence of 52%. Morrell and Dunnill (1968) believe that pulmonary thrombo-embolism is even commoner than indicated by their results and that it is almost ubiquitous in hospital patients coming to autopsy.

The lungs have an astonishing capacity to dispose of thrombo-emboli. Even large fresh thrombi are absorbed by the lungs in dogs in six weeks and small ones much more rapidly. Two main groups of processess are involved, chemical and cellular. Chemical disposal is by *fibrinolysis* and predominates in the disposal of small thrombi. Lung tissue has a high content of fibrinolysins, which have been shown to be present in the intima of both pulmonary and systemic arteries. Cellular processes of *organisation* and *recanalisation* seem to be more important in the disposal of larger thromboemboli. In a few days fibroblasts and capillaries grow into the emboli, which are gradually reduced to patches of intimal fibrosis.

The clinical effects of pulmonary thromboemboli depend upon the size of the pulmonary artery involved and on the speed with which the occlusion occurs. Sudden blocking of the pulmonary trunk or a large pulmonary artery may be rapidly fatal owing to the inability of the right ventricle to maintain the circulation. Under certain conditions, blockage of smaller pulmonary arteries will give rise to pulmonary infarction. In the third and rarest groups of patients, multiple small thrombo-emboli lodge in the smaller branches of the pulmonary arterial tree over a period of time and give rise to severe pulmonary hypertension.

Massive pulmonary thrombo-embolism. Massive pulmonary embolism is a classical clinical emergency brought about by sudden occlusion of the pulmonary trunk (Fig. 10.24, p. 10.20) or one of its main branches by a large embolus (Fig. 16.15). In the normal human lung, rather more than half the pulmonary arterial bed must be occluded before the clinical syndrome of acute massive embolism will appear. In the presence of pre-existing pulmonary hypertension, however, occlusion of one primary branch of the pulmonary trunk has important haemodynamic effects. The increased pulmonary vascular resistance which occurs in pulmonary embolism in man is more likely a mechanical effect of blockage of pulmonary arteries rather than due to the effect of serotonin liberated from pulmonary emboli: the latter has a greater effect on the pulmonary circulation of dogs and cats than on that of man.

Pulmonary infarction. Pulmonary arterial occlusion alone commonly fails to produce infarction of the lung and an additional important requirement appears to be an increased pulmonary venous pressure. Infarction is, there-

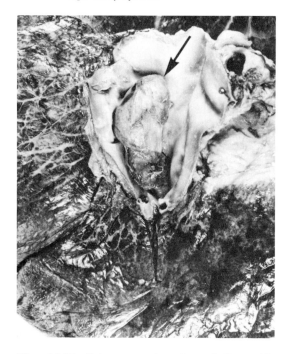

Fig. 16.15 Pulmonary thrombo-embolism. The main pulmonary artery at the hilum of the lung has been opened to reveal a pale thrombo-embolus (arrow) lying free in its lumen.

fore, common in patients with mitral stenosis. In experimental studies, the presence or absence of the bronchial arterial supply seems to make no difference to the development of infarction. Pulmonary infarction occurs more often in the lower lobes, where the pulmonary venous pressure is likely to be higher. In addition, the lung bases are more prone to be affected by bronchial occlusion, pleural effusion and infection, all factors shown experimentally to favour infarction. The appearances of pulmonary infarcts are described on p. 10.25.

Recurrent pulmonary embolism. In this condition there is a gradual occlusion of the pulmonary arterial bed over a period of time which may extend to several years. Infarction is not a feature but *there is a progressive increase in the pulmonary vascular resistance, leading to severe pulmonary hypertension, right ventricular hypertrophy and failure.* The muscular pulmonary arteries show medial hypertrophy and excentric nodular fibro-elastic thickening of the intima due to organisation of the thrombo-emboli. The larger elastic pulmonary arteries may show lattices, due to recanalisation of thrombo-

emboli. Smooth muscle develops in the walls of pulmonary arterioles.

In many patients with recurrent pulmonary thrombo-embolism the source of venous thrombi is not found. As already explained, the recurrent impaction of small thrombo-emboli in the pulmonary circulation is a normal phenomenon. Hence it may well be that chronic pulmonary thrombo-embolism is not caused by the production of an excessive number of thrombo-emboli, but by the intrinsic inability of the pulmonary circulation to deal with them. So far, no evidence has been found of inadequate fibrinolytic activity in the blood of these patients. The abnormality may lie in the pulmonary vascular endothelium.

Non-thrombotic pulmonary embolism

The pulmonary capillary bed is a most effective filter of particulate matter in the blood and all manner of fragments may be found impacted in it. The commonest and most important clinical form is pulmonary thrombo-embolism, but fragments of various materials other than thrombus can cause pulmonary embolism, as described below.

Bone marrow embolism may follow accidents with bone fractures, thoracic operations involving cleavage of the sternum, rib fractures due to external cardiac massage, or spontaneous fracture due to tumour metastases in bones. Masses of megakaryocytes may be found impacted in the pulmonary capillaries, especially after surgical operations and in cases of pulmonary thrombo-embolism. **Fat embolism** (p. 10.20) commonly occurs after accidents involving fractures of bones or contusion of adipose tissue . It is detected as oily patches in the blood and can be readily demonstrated by the usual stains for fat. Fat embolism in the lungs is very common: it rarely causes significant symptoms, unless very extensive, when it can even be fatal. **Amniotic fluid embolism** to the lung, which may occur in women during or shortly after childbirth, may be fatal: it is also a possible cause of primary pulmonary hypertension. By contrast, small fragments of trophoblast are frequently found in the lungs of pregnant women dying from various causes, but rarely give rise to symptoms. **Cancer cells** are trapped in the pulmonary capillary bed like other particulate matter: they may degenerate or grow to form metastases. Recurrent emboli from the right atrium in cases of cardiac myxoma may lead to pulmonary hypertension. **Air embolism** (p. 10.21) may arise from many causes, including various surgical and diagnostic procedures such as intravenous infusions, abortions, and the induction of a pneumothorax. If the volume of air is large, it may cause death by arresting the pulmonary circulation. At autopsy, the pulmonary trunk must be opened under water to reveal air embolism. Other materials entering the pulmonary circulation include cotton-wool fibres and materials injected by drug addicts.

Pulmonary emphysema

Pulmonary emphysema is a permanent enlargement of the respiratory passages or air spaces distal to the terminal bronchiole. The definition of emphysema must include the concept of *permanent* enlargement of air spaces, implying destructive changes, in contrast with their temporary over-inflation as, for example, in bronchial asthma. It must be admitted, however, that the mechanisms of destruction are usually not understood. For this reason the term 'distensive emphysema' should be avoided. Under certain circumstances, air may escape into the interstitial connective tisues of the lung. This quite different condition is called *interstitial emphysema* and should not be confused with pulmonary emphysema as defined above. It will be considered briefly later.

Bronchi and bronchioles. To understand emphysema it is necessary to be familiar with the micro-anatomy of the terminal air passages. Large bronchi have complete rings of cartilage in their walls. They divide into small bronchi with cartilage in the form of plates which do not completely surround the lumen of the bronchus. With further division, the airways increase in number and decrease in size, and the point at which the cartilage disappears is taken as the dividing line between the small bronchus and the bronchiole. Small bronchi still have a few mucous glands left in their wall, whereas in the bronchioles the only mucin-secreting cells are goblet cells in the lining epithelium. The terminal bronchiole is the last small air passage not to bear alveoli and the respiratory bronchiole is the first in which they appear.

The cut surface of distended lung shows hexagonal areas of parenchyma, some 1 or 2cm across, delineated by fibrous septa (Fig. 16.16). Each hexagonal area is a section of a **secondary lung lobule**; it contains the lung tissue supplied

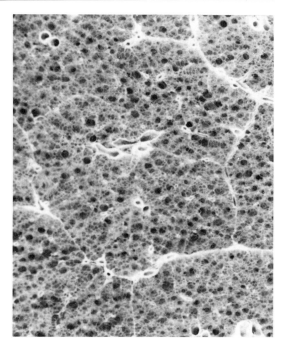

Fig. 16.16 Normal adult lung. Note the hexagonal lobule in the centre of the field with the terminal bronchioles in its centre. (Barium sulphate inpregnation.) × 4. (Professor W.R. Lee.)

by the three to five terminal bronchioles, which radiate from the centre, accompanied by muscular pulmonary arteries. This is the unit referred to subsequently in this account as 'the lobule'.

The respiratory acinus. The structure of the respiratory acinus is central to our understanding of the pathology of pulmonary emphysema. The acinus (previously termed a 'primary lobule') is that portion of lung tissue formed by the branching from a single terminal bronchiole (Fig. 16.17a). Hence one lung lobule (see above)

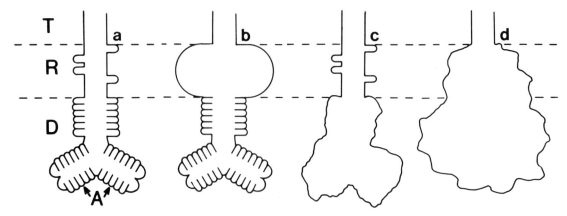

Fig. 16.17   Models of the normal respiratory acinus and the changes of emphysema. The normal acinus **(a)** consists of a terminal bronchiole (T), leading into respiratory bronchioles (R) and alveolar ducts (D) from both of which alveoli (A) arise. (For clarity, only one respiratory bronchiole is shown arising from the terminal bronchiole.) Dilatation of air spaces is confined initially to the respiratory bronchioles in centrilobular and focal duct emphysema **(b)**, and to the alveolar ducts and spaces in alveolar duct emphysema **(c)**. In panacinar emphysema **(d)** dilatation of the alveolar ducts and spaces extends to the respiratory bronchioles.

consists of three to five respiratory acini. The respiratory bronchioles may branch from three to five times. The first order of respiratory bronchioles have only a few alveoli but they increase in number with each division. The walls of the alveolar ducts are lined entirely by alveoli, the dividing walls between the spaces ending in small knots of smooth muscle.

The varieties of pulmonary emphysema

There are complicated and detailed classifications of all the possible localised and generalised forms of pulmonary emphysema but a simple classification of the **generalised form**, which may cause death from respiratory or cardiac failure, follows from the micro-anatomy of the lung that we have just considered. The respiratory acinus consists of respiratory bronchioles, alveolar ducts and alveoli (Fig. 16.17a). *There are two main forms of pulmonary emphysema. One is characterised by permanant dilatation of the respiratory bronchioles, the other by permanent dilatation of the alveolar ducts and alveoli.*

   Bronchiolar emphysema. In this type, the enlarged terminal air spaces are respiratory bronchioles (Fig. 16.17b). In the early stages of the disease the alveolar ducts and alveoli distal to the dilated bronchioles are normal. The disease is readily recognised by naked-eye examination of slices of fixed distended or inflated lungs, as the enlarged air spaces are seen in clusters, at

the centres of the seconary lung lobules, surrounded by normal lung tissue (Fig. 16.18). In histological sections, the emphysematous spaces

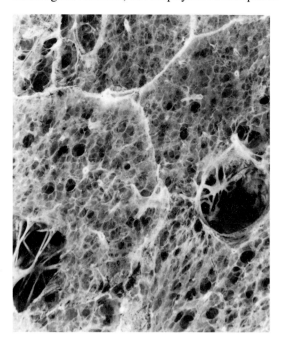

Fig. 16.18   Section of lung impregnated with barium sulphate, showing centrilobular emphysema. Note the punched out centrilobular spaces containing fibrous strands and blood vessels and the relatively normal parenchyma at the periphery of the lobules. × 7. (Professor W. R. Lee.)

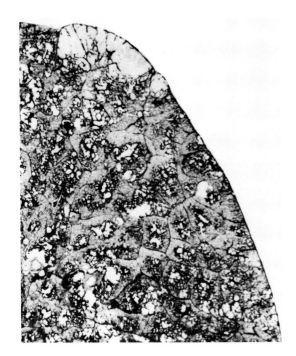

Fig. 16.19 Focus dust emphysema in coal-workers' pneumoconiosis. × 1.

appear to be derived from respiratory bronchioles, but it may be difficult to be certain of this unless many lesions or serial sections of a single lesion are examined. There is a great contrast between the greatly enlarged respiratory bronchioles and the normal alveolar ducts and alveoli distal to the emphysematous spaces. There are two varieties of bronchiolar emphysema. The first is **focal dust emphysema** which occurs with varying degrees of severity in all those exposed to carbon dust inhalation such as coal workers, coal trimmers in docks, and in graphite and foundry workers (Fig. 16.19). A minor form has even been reported in the general population of urban areas and has been termed '*soot emphysema*'. The second, more serious and commoner form is found in the general population and is called **centrilobular emphysema** (Fig. 16.18). As there are two to five respiratory bronchioles in each secondary lung lobule the dilated spaces are not strictly in the centres of lobules in either centrilobular or focal dust emphysema. However, in both conditions the emphysema is centriacinar.

The distinction between focal dust emphysema and centrilobular emphysema depends to some extent on the occupational history but there are also micro-anatomical differences. In the focal variety, there is a fusiform dilatation of all orders of respiratory bronchioles and they are surrounded by coal dust. In centrilobular emphysema, the distal orders of respiratory bronchioles are first affected and there is little surrounding dust but evidence of chronic bronchiolitis. *Right ventricular failure is common in centrilobular but not in focal dust emphysema,* which is discussed in the later section on pneumoconioses (p. 16.57).

Alveolar emphysema. In this type, there is permanent enlargement initially of alveolar ducts and alveoli and subsequently of respiratory bronchioles. The first stage is called **alveolar duct emphysema** (Fig. 16.17), although it has also been called the *vesicular* variety. In slices of distended or inflated lung it may be recognised as diffuse areas of abnormally large air spaces. Histological sections show enlarged alveolar ducts and alveoli, the latter becoming wider at their mouths and shallower in depth. The respiratory bronchioles are normal. In the second stage of alveolar emphysema, the enlargement of air spaces extends from the alveolar ducts proximally in the respiratory acinus to involve the respiratory bronchioles and so the entire acinus (Fig. 16.17). This is called **panacinar emphysema**: in lung slices it is readily recognised by areas of grossly abnormal air spaces (Fig. 16.20) scattered irregularly throughout the lung: macroscopically the lungs appear voluminous, the anterior surface of the heart is covered and the diaphragm pressed downwards. The edges of the emphysematous lung are raised above the surface, rounding off the sharp edges. The emphysematous tissue is paler than the rest of the lung as less carbon pigment is present: it contains little blood and pits on pressure owing to lack of elasticity. Emphysema is most pronounced at the apices of the lungs and along the margins, especially the anterior borders, but in extreme cases practically the whole of the lung substance may be affected, although the condition is usually slight on the posterior aspect. In severe panacinar emphysema, the involved areas frequently merge with one another so that there is little or no intervening normal lung tissue. Some of the enlarged abnormal air spaces in the lung may become cystic and project from the pleural surface; these are called *bullae*. In histological sections the alveoli are few and greatly

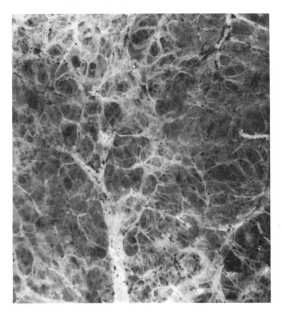

Fig. 16.20 Severe panacinar emphysema. Parts of two secondary lobules are shown, with a thickened interlobular septum (lower central). The alveolar walls throughout the lobules have been largely destroyed, with formation of emphysematous spaces. Atrophic lung tissue and some surviving small vessels are seen as fine strands. Barium sulphate preparation. × 8. (Professor W.R. Lee.)

enlarged. In some cases of centrilobular emphysema the dilatation of the respiratory bronchioles may be so pronounced that it becomes impossible to distinguish them from cases of panacinar emphysema.

The demonstration of emphysema at autopsy

Adequate fixation is very important for the demonstration of emphysema. The usual practice of cutting lungs at autopsy results in collapse and could hardly be better designed to obscure the appearances of the air spaces. Careful examination or 'point-counting', as described below, requires that the whole lungs should be distended with formol-saline until the pleural surfaces are smooth and then left for two to three days before cutting. Impregnation of slices of fixed lung with barium sulphate will allow the relationship of the abnormal air spaces and their connections to be assessed in three dimensions with the dissecting microscope (Figs. 16.18 and 16.20). Sections of an adequately fixed lung can be used for 'point-

counting' to estimate the distribution and severity of emphysema. This may be carried out by placing over the slice of lung a perspex sheet divided into equilateral triangles with 1 cm sides, at the corners of which are small punched-out points. This enables one to determine the percentage of emphysema present by counting the number of points lying over air spaces. Such quantitative studies have not revealed any simple relation between the amount of lung destroyed by pulmonary emphysema and the weight of the right ventricle (see below). Another technique for the demonstration of emphysema is the preparation of sections, approximately 300 μm thick, of gelatin-embedded lungs (Fig. 16.19). Such sections may be mounted on paper and preserved as dry specimens. If morphometric studies on histological sections are to be carried out, the lung should be inflated with formalin vapour in a vacuum chamber.

Clinicopathological correlations. There are two main clinical syndromes associated with what physicians call '**chronic obstructive airways disease**', the pathology of which is chronic bronchitis and emphysema. The 'type A' patient is characterised by obvious radiological evidence of emphysema, reduced diffusing capacity; Pa_{O_2} and Pa_{CO_2} are both normal at rest, and there is little tendency to develop systemic oedema. This patient is the 'pink puffer' and his main disability is breathlessness. He has emphysema without significant hypoxia and the emphysema is commonly but not invariably of the panacinar type. The 'type B' patient does not have much radiological evidence of emphysema; diffusing capacity is normal; at rest, Pa_{O_2} is low and Pa_{CO_2} raised. This is the 'blue bloater' who has significant hypoxia and is likely to develop systemic oedema and eventually right ventricular failure. The emphysema is commonly of centrilobular type. Chronic hypoxia causes pulmonary hypertension and the hypoxic form of pulmonary hypertensive vascular disease (p. 16.24) (Fig. 16.21).

Morphometry in emphysema. Quantitative methods have proved useful in the study of pulmonary emphysema. It is quite inadequate now to talk of 'severe' or 'moderately severe' emphysema. The application of histological morphometric techniques derived from principles used by geologists for a century in the study of rocks enables one to establish fairly easily the

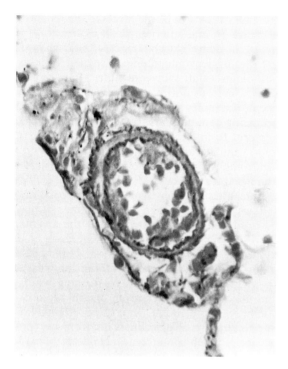

Fig. 16.21 Transverse section of muscularised pulmonary arteriole from a man with centrilobular emphysema and right ventricular hypertrophy. The vessel has been converted into something akin to a systemic arteriole which offers resistance to pulmonary blood flow. (Elastic tissue appears dark). × 150

internal surface area of the lung and the number of surviving alveolar spaces. In one study the normal internal surface area of both lungs together was 70 m². The corresponding area in centrilobular emphysema was reduced to 61 m² and in alveolar emphysema to 46 m². The total number of alveolar spaces in the normal left and right lungs together was 273 × 10⁶, while in centrilobular emphysema it was 215 × 10⁶, and in panacinar emphysema 63 × 10⁶. *There is no relation between the reduction in internal surface area in pulmonary emphysema and the weight of the right ventricle, suggesting that the classical concept that right ventricular hypertrophy in emphysema is due to loss of pulmonary capillary bed is incorrect.* In fact, right ventricular hypertrophy appears to be commoner in centrilobular emphysema in which the reduction in internal surface area, and so presumably in capillary bed, is smaller.

The pathogenesis of emphysema

There is evidence to suggest that certain proteolytic enzymes can cause emphysema. It can be induced in animals by aerosols of papain, a proteolytic enzyme which selectively attacks the amorphous component of elastic fibres leaving the microfibrils intact. Emphysema can also be produced in dogs by aerosol homogenates of human leucocytes which contain an elastase apparently capable of damaging the lung. Alpha₁-antitrypsin, which is an inhibitor of such enzymes, is synthesised in the liver and is a normal constituent of the α_1-globulin fraction of the plasma proteins. Some people have an inherited deficiency of this inhibitor in their blood. In the rare homozygous state, the deficiency is severe and there is a high frequency of panacinar emphysema. It is not generally accepted that heterozygotes are more prone to emphysema but deterioration in lung function in cigarette smokers (which is usually due to centrilobular emphysema), and the loss of elastic recoil with increasing age, proceed more rapidly in heterozygotes than in the normal population. It is now possible to measure the serum trypsin inhibitory capacity. The panacinar emphysema associated with homozygous α_1-antitrypsin deficiency in man develops before the age of 40 years, and is mainly basal in situation.

By contrast, *the known air-borne factors predisposing to emphysema, including cigarette smoke and coal dust, tend to induce either centrilobular or focal dust emphysema*, most severe in the apices of the lung. Dunnill (1982) believes that the effects of cigarette smoke are greater in the upper lobes due to its high temperature (and so low density). The smoke appears to act initially by stimulating a mild inflammatory reaction, with aggregation of macrophages and neutrophil polymorphs, around the first-order respiratory bronchioles. This is an important transition zone in the lung where the respiratory acinus begins and beyond which the mass movement of air is replaced increasingly by diffusion. The pulmonary macrophages of smokers contain a pigment in which refractile crystalloid inclusions, abnormally high concentrations of acid hydroxylases, and some aluminium silicate, may be detected. The macrophages aggregated around the respiratory bronchioles appear to be damaged by a toxic component of smoke thought by some to be cadmium. This renders the lysosomes of macrophages and polymorphs more labile, releasing their proteolytic enzymes. Centrilobular emphysema thus appears to result from an imbalance between elastase and anti-elastase activity, with enzyme release from macrophages and neutrophils in the region of respiratory bronchioles initiating tissue destruction. There seems no doubt that the smoking of tobacco is of considerable importance in the pathogenesis of centrilobular emphysema, which is rare below the age of 40 years and increases rapidly with continuation of the habit.

Once the initial damage to the lung tissue had occurred, the force which expands the damaged portions into emphysematous spaces is the atmospheric pressure of the inspired air. The force required to distend an elastic sphere is inversely related to the radius and therefore becomes progressively less as the sphere enlarges. A vicious circle is initiated as soon as a weakness develops in the air passages, and continuing dilatation and destruction is inevitable, particularly if the emphysematous lung is subject to the powerful inspiratory effort of the coughing which is associated with chronic bronchitis.

Other types of emphysema

'**Compensatory emphysema**' is a term sometimes used to describe the overdistension of alveoli which may occur around areas of collapsed lung tissue and during acute attacks of bronchial asthma.

With increasing age there is a concomitant increase in the size of the alveolar spaces and a decrease in the internal surface area of the lungs. In some elderly subjects these changes are of sufficient magnitude to suggest to some pathologists that they constitute '**senile emphysema**'. Various forms of **localised emphysema** occur. Examples are paracicatricial emphysema occurring around scars, paraseptal emphysema adjacent to interlobular septa or to the pleura, and unilateral emphysema (MacLeod's syndrome) in which radiography demonstrates abnormal translucency of only one lung.

'**Interstitial emphysema.**' This condition follows laceration of the lung substance. It may be produced by overdistension of the alveolar spaces as may occur with severe coughing or in dyspnoea with forced inspiration. It may also follow traumatic laceration of the lung tissue by a fractured rib or by a perforating wound and may occur in divers from unduly rapid decompression (p.10.22). Interstitial emphysema due to rupture of alveolar walls from overdistension is much commoner in children than adults and occurs in such conditions as whooping cough, bronchiolitis, and in diphtheria of the larynx and trachea. The alveolar walls rupture as the result of over-expansion during forced inspiration, and air, in the form of small bead-like collections or blebs, extends along the lines of junction of the interlobular septa with the pleura, thus producing a reticulated appearance on the pleural surface. When the air is abundant, it passes by the lymphatics to the rest of the lungs, and in some cases it extends to the tissues at the root of the neck and gives rise to subcutaneous emphysema.

Collapse of lung tissue

Atelectasis and collapse. The term *atelectasis* is derived from the Greek for 'imperfect expansion' and it should be restricted to denote failure of the lungs to expand properly at birth and distinguished from acquired *collapse* of a previously expanded lung. A lung may collapse because something presses on it from without— *pressure collapse*, or because there is obstruction of a bronchus with resulting absorption of air in the corresponding area of lung tissue— *absorption collapse*.

Pressure collapse. The lung may be compressed from without by a pleural effusion, haemothorax, empyema or pneumothorax. The absence of bronchial obstruction leaves the secretions from lung and bronchi free to drain up the bronchial tree and the collapsed lung tissue does not usually become seriously infected. The changes in it result from the haemodynamic alterations and associated vascular changes. Collapse due to pyothorax (empyema) may be considerable so that the lung becomes very small and lies posteriorly against the side of the vertebral column. When the exudate on the visceral pleural surface becomes organised, pleural thickening results and prevents re-expansion of the lung even when the infection is overcome. Accordingly it is important to drain the pleural cavity and obtain re-expansion of the lung before this happens.

Absorption collapse. This is a commoner condition than pressure collapse and follows *acute and complete obstruction* of a large bronchus. Following such obstruction, collateral air ventilation may for a time keep the obstructed segment of lung filled with air provided the surrounding lung is free from pulmonary oedema, haemorrhage or pneumonia. However, as the air gradually disappears it is largely replaced by secretion and oedema fluid so that the lung does not change very much in size. Acute absorption collapse follows inhaled foreign bodies and collections of mucus occurring in terminal illnesses, after tracheostomy, during and after anaesthetics or in lung infections. *Chronic bronchial obstruction* may be caused by tumours growing in the wall of the affected bronchus or pressing on it from without. Other lesions which may press on bronchi and obstruct them are aneurysms and enlarged lymph nodes. In absorption collapse, bronchial secretions beyond the obstruction are very likely to become infected and suppuration may extend through the collapsed segment of lung tissue.

In collapse of the lung the pleural surfaces are wrinkled and the cut surface is airless. Portions of the collapsed tissue sink in water. The reduction in volume is often much greater in pressure than in absorption collapse. There is no respiratory movement of air in the collapsed area of lung so that the haemoglobin in its alveolar capillaries is in a reduced state, and the affected lung appears purple. When the collapse has lasted for some time, there is a progressive pulmonary fibrosis which permanently prevents re-expansion and a return to normal. In the early stages there is a constriction of the pulmonary arteries but later they show intimal fibroelastosis.

Atelectasis. Incomplete expansion of the neonatal lung may be caused by failure of the respiratory centre or, in premature infants, because the lung is insufficiently developed. It may follow hyaline membrane disease (p. 16.21), or may result from laryngeal dysfunction and obstruction of the air passages. These causes are, however, responsible for only a small proportion of atelectatic neonatal lungs. In many infants with severe atelectasis, no cause can be demonstrated at autopsy.

Acute pulmonary infections

Bacterial pneumonias

The most common acute inflammatory disorders of the lung are the various types of **pneumonia**, which is defined as an inflammatory condition of the lung characterised by consolidation due to the presence of exudate in the alveolar spaces. The pneumonias may be classified anatomically into **bronchopneumonia** and **lobar pneumonia.**

Bronchopneumonia is an inflammatory condition of the lung that occurs when microorganisms colonise the bronchioles and extend into the surrounding alveoli, leading to numerous discrete foci of consolidation (Fig. 16.22). The many causal bacteria include *Streptococcus pneumoniae, Staphylococcus aureus, Streptococcus pyogenes, Klebsiella* and *Haemophilus influenzae.* It occurs most commonly in infancy, in old age, and in patients with some debilitating condition such as cancer, uraemia or a stroke. Acute respiratory virus infections, and chronic diseases such as chronic bronchitis, bronchiectasis and cystic fibrosis predispose to bronchopneumonia. It may develop in patients with congestive cardiac failure and after surgical operations under general anaesthesia, due to the adverse effect of narcotic drugs on respiration and ciliary activity. Bronchopneumonia occurs most often in the lower lobes of the lungs and at autopsy is seen as focal dark red or grey areas of about 1 cm diameter, which are firmer than the surrounding lung; each appears to be centred around a bronchiole from which a bead of pale yellow pus can be expressed. If progressive, the focal areas

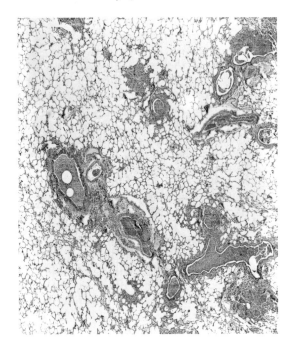

Fig. 16.22 Acute bronchiolitis and early broncho-pneumonia. The bronchioles are filled with exudate which is extending into the associated respiratory acini and peribronchiolar alveoli. × 10.

of consolidation become larger and eventually coalesce to simulate lobar pneumonia. The microscopic lesions of bronchopneumonia are an acute bronchiolitis with filling of the surrounding peribronchiolar alveoli with inflammatory exudate rich in neutrophil polymorphs. Complete resolution is uncommon, except in mild cases, because there is usually a variable amount of damage to, and destruction of, the walls of bronchioles. In consequence, the lesions usually result in the development of small foci of fibrosis. If fibrosis of the lung is extensive, bronchiectasis may develop.

Lobar pneumonia. In this condition infection leads to a watery inflammatory exudate in the alveoli. This flows directly into bronchioles and related alveoli, filling them and spilling over into adjacent lobules and segments of the lung. Damage to the bronchiolar walls, although present, is relatively unimportant. The exudate and bacteria spread through the lumens rather than the walls of the terminal airways. The consolidation is sharply confined to the affected lobe, which is diffusely affected.

The anatomical type of pneumonia (lobar or bronchopneumonia) and the subsequent liability to develop complications depend on the aetiological agent responsible. Hence the older anatomical classification has been superseded by a classification based on the causative agent.

Pneumococcal lobar pneumonia

Since the widespread use of antibiotics the fully-developed picture of classical lobar pneumonia is not often seen in Britain. However, fatal untreated cases may still be encountered in those who lie neglected at home or who decline medical aid, in vagrants and in alcoholics who become exposed to cold. Classical lobar pneumonia is still a common disease in many areas of the world where medical services are poorly developed. The disease predominates in males and occurs at all ages, although it is uncommon below the age of one year. It is still most often seen in healthy adults between the ages of 30 and 50 years.

The causative agent is *Streptococcus pneumoniae*, a Gram +ve diplococcus which can be serologically typed according to the antigenic properties of its polysaccharide capsule. The capsule prevents effective phagocytosis by polymorphs and macrophages unless type-specific antibody is present. About 80% of cases are caused by the following types in descending order of frequency: I, III, II, V, VII, VIII and IV. The first three types are responsible for 40% of cases. Types I and II cause pneumonia mainly in younger persons who were previously healthy, and type III mainly in patients over the age of fifty suffering from some other form of chronic disease. Type III has always been known as a particularly lethal strain and it is likely to cause high mortality in spite of the use of antibiotics and modern supportive measures.

Structural changes. Infection is acquired by inhalation of pneumococci. If the organisms are virulent and the resistance of the patient low, a disease process commences which, if untreated, runs a fairly well-defined course, usually terminating in resolution. It has been customary to recognise the following four stages in the progress of untreated pneumococcal lobar pneumonia: acute congestion; red hepatisation; grey hepatisation; and resolution. It must be emphasised that these stages occur in untreated cases in adults. The use of sulphonamides and

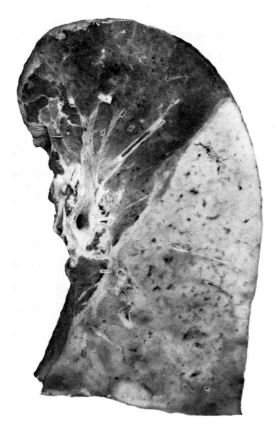

Fig. 16.23 Acute lobar pneumonia with grey hepatisation in lower lobe and red hepatisation in part of upper lobe. × ⅓.

antibiotics profoundly alters the classical clinical and pathological picture.

Acute congestion. This initial phase, which lasts for one or two days, is one of acute congestion and oedema. Macroscopically the affected lobe is heavy, dark red and firm: abundant frothy red fluid can be squeezed from it. Large numbers of pneumococci are seen in stained smears prepared from the cut surface. Microscopically, the alveolar capillaries are engorged with erythrocytes. The alveolar spaces are filled with eosinophilic oedema fluid containing many Gram +ve diplococci and neutrophil polymorphs, which also show margination of the venules.

Red hepatisation. This phase lasts from the second to the fourth days of the disease. The pleural surface of the affected lobe is covered by greyish-white friable tags of fibrin. The cut surface appears dry, firm, red and granular and feels like liver. Affected lung tissue is airless and

sinks in water. Microscopically, the capillary engorgement persists, but the exudate occupying the alveolar spaces now contains a fine network of fibrin (Figs. 16.24 and 4.2, p. 4.4), large numbers of extravasated red cells and increasing numbers of emigrated neutrophil polymorphs.

Grey hepatisation. In this stage of late consolidation (4 to 8 days) the affected lung may weight up to 1500 g. Fibrinous pleurisy is present and the cut surface is dry, granular and grey (Fig. 16.23). The affected lobe still feels like liver and slices of it retain straight, sharp edges. Microscopically, the alveolar spaces are distended and consolidated by a denser network of inspissated fibrin containing neutrophil polymorphs, many of which are dead and disintegrating (Fig. 16.24) and occasional degenerating erythrocytes. During this stage, antibodies to pneumococci appear in the blood, pneumococci are rapidly eliminated, and the fever subsides by crisis.

Resolution begins on the eighth day with the migration of macrophages from the alveolar septa into the exudate, which is gradually liquefied by fibrinolytic enzymes and absorbed or

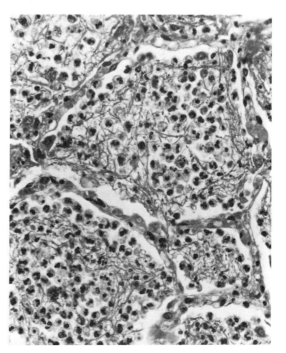

Fig. 16.24 Lobar pneumonia. The alveolar spaces are filled with exudate containing a fibrin network and many neutrophil polymorphs. × 235.

coughed up. The cut surface of the affected lung is at first friable and mottled red and grey in colour. Complete resolution and re-aeration take from one to three weeks. Since there is virtually no tissue destruction in lobar pneumonia, the lung parenchyma returns to normal, but the pleural exudate is commonly organised with the formation of fibrous adhesions between the two surfaces.

The above account refers to cases not receiving antibacterial therapy. Sulphonamides or antibiotics rapidly abort the infections and resolution follows.

Clinical features. The onset is sudden and the patient has a fever with rigors and sharp pleuritic pain on respiration. When a lower lobe is involved, diaphragmatic pleural pain may be referred to the tip of the shoulder. Partly because of the pain, breathing is shallow and rapid, and there is usually a cough productive of brown or bloodstained sputum. There is a well-marked neutrophil polymorphonuclear leucocytosis from an early stage. Bacteraemia may occur, blood cultures being positive in about

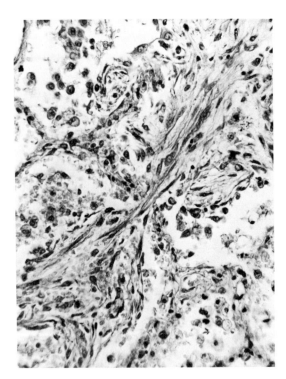

Fig. 16.25 Organisation of alveolar exudate in the lung. The inflammatory exudate has been replaced by cellular fibrous tissue which can be seen passing from one alveolus to another through the pore of Kohn in the centre of the picture. × 390.

30% of cases. The systemic arterial oxygen saturation is usually only slightly reduced.

Complications. The principal complications of pneumococcal lobar pneumonia are as follows:

Organisation of exudate. In about 3% of cases resolution does not occur and the fibrinous exudate occupying the alveoli becomes organised (Fig. 16.25). The fibrin is slowly digested by macrophages, while fibroblasts grow in from the alveolar septa, and the tissue becomes fibrosed, tough, airless, leathery and grey.

Pleural effusion occurs in about 5% of treated cases.

Empyema occurs in less than 1% of treated cases.

Lung abscess is a complication which has practically disappeared since the introduction of antibiotics.

Cardiac complications include suppurative pericarditis, acute bacterial endocarditis and various degrees of acute failure from toxic myocarditis.

Bacteraemic complications include bacterial endocarditis, suppurative meningitis, acute otitis media and arthritis.

Staphylococcal pneumonia

Staphylococcus aureus rarely causes pneumonia as a primary event; it is usually encountered as a secondary infection in patients debilitated by chronic lung disease, such as cystic fibrosis, where antibiotics have been used for long periods. Its incidence rises sharply during epidemics of influenza, measles and pertussis, when it may be responsible for an acute, short-lived, lethal haemorrhagic bronchopneumonia in affected children and adults. In this severe form, staphylococci invade the lungs about 36 hours after the onset of influenza. At autopsy, the lungs appear purple and are heavy due to haemorrhagic pulmonary oedema. The bronchi are filled with blood-stained fluid which drains away to reveal an inflamed mucosa, sometimes covered by a grey membrane of fibrin. There is no pleural reaction. Microscopically there is an acute ulcerative bronchitis and bronchiolitis: the alveolar spaces are filled with oedema fluid containing fibrin coagulum, much extravasated blood, scanty neutrophil polymorphs and abundant clusters of Gram +ve cocci.

In patients who survive this acute phase, multiple foci of greyish-white bronchopneumonic consolidation develop and suppurate, forming abscess cavities containing sticky yellow pus. There is much lung destruction and the pleura at this stage is thickly coated with fibrinous or fibrino-purulent exudate. Empyema and pneumothorax may occur from rupture of pulmonary abscesses into the pleural cavity. In children, a valvular obstruction may occur at the junction of an abscess cavity and bronchus to produce a rapidly-expanding air-filled *tension cyst* or *pneumatocele*. The cyst, which can be several centimetres in diameter, may rupture into the pleural cavity to produce a *tension pneumothorax*. Usually the air is absorbed after the infection is overcome.

Occasionally staphylococcal pneumonia may be lobar in type and produce clinical and radiological signs which may mimic classical pneumococcal lobar pneumonia.

Haemophilus pneumonia

Haemophilus influenzae has a polysaccharide capsule which interferes with phagocytosis in the absence of specific antibody. Haemophilus pneumonia is most often seen in children less than 10 years old. Viral infection is a common precursor, but it also occurs sporadically in adults whose pulmonary defence mechanisms are impaired by chronic bronchitis and emphysema. The consolidation may be lobar or bronchopneumonic in type. Examination of the sputum may be valuable in provisional diagnosis, since it may contain abundant small Gram − ve bacilli.

Klebsiellar pneumonia

Klebsiella pneumoniae (Friedlander's bacillus) is a Gram − ve bacillus with a very thick mucoid capsule that inhibits phagocytosis. It is an infrequent cause of pneumonia but important because the infection is destructive, with a high mortality rate and a high incidence of complications. The organism is a commensal in the upper respiratory tract in about 5% of normal individuals, but more frequently in people with advanced dental caries and periodontal disease. Klebsiellar pneumonia tends to occur especially in men over the age of fifty who are chronic alcoholics, diabetics, or have oral sepsis. Most

infections commence in the right lung, usually in the posterior segment of the upper lobe. Clinically, the onset is acute with severe prostration and a cough with bloodstained gelatinous sputum resembling red currant jelly. Pathologically, red-grey areas of consolidation become confluent, leading to involvement of the entire right upper lobe. The cut surface of the affected lung is mucoid. Destruction of lung tissue often leads to the formation of a large apical abscess which may be mistakenly diagnosed as tuberculosis. The infection may become chronic with severe progressive destruction of lung tissue so that the patient becomes a permanent respiratory cripple.

Steptococcal pneumonia

Pneumonia due to *Streptococcus pyogenes* is rare and usually secondary to influenza or measles. In severe cases death occurs within 36 to 72 hours and the lungs appear purple with a fibrinous pleurisy. In cases dying after a week, yellow areas of consolidation are present in the lungs. These consolidated foci may cavitate, with the formation of abscesses leading to empyema and bronchopleural fistulas.

Pseudomonas pneumonia

Following the introduction and combined use of antibiotic and corticosteroid drugs, Gram − ve organisms in general, and *Pseudomonas aeruginosa* in particular, have become of greater importance as causes of bacterial pneumonia. Another factor is the increased use of tracheostomy and mechanical ventilation. Both the tracheostomy wounds and ventilation apparatus commonly become colonised by *Pseudomonas aeruginosa*, which spreads rapidly to infect neighbouring patients. It is most important to sterilise respiratory equipment properly after use to prevent the spread of infection. Unfortunately, *Pseudomonas aeruginosa* may survive and proliferate in water, soap solution, stored blood, infusion fluids, and in some antiseptics. In pseudomonas pneumonia, the air spaces in the affected lung are filled with blood, oedema fluid, scanty neutrophil polymorphs and innumerable causative organisms which can be demonstrated by appropriate staining methods. A characteristic feature of pseudomonas pneumonia is bacterial invasion of pulmonary arteries, leading to necrosis of the vessel with subsequent haemorrhage or thrombosis and then pulmonary infarction.

Legionnaires' disease

An outbreak of severe pneumonia affected 180 of about 4400 persons attending the Annual Convention of American Legionnaires in Philadelphia, USA, during July 1976, causing twenty-nine deaths. Investigation revealed that the pneumonia was caused by a hitherto unknown Gram −ve coccobacillus which has been named *Legionella pneumophila*. One proved source of infection is the water in air-conditioning systems. Pathological examination of the lungs shows either a lobar or a bronchopneumonia (Fig. 16.26). The intra-alveolar exudate contains abundant fibrin and variable numbers of macrophages and neutrophil polymorphs. Unlike many bacterial pneumonias, macrophages may predominate. Acute vasculitis and focal necrosis of alveolar septa occur in

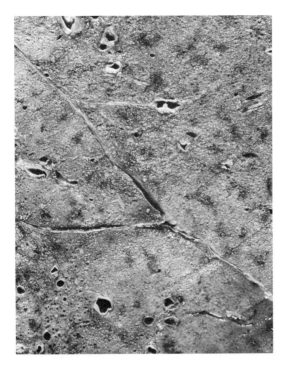

Fig. 16.26 The cut surface of the right lung in legionnaire's disease, showing the adjacent parts of upper, middle and lower lobes, all of which are diffusely consolidated by inflammatory exudate. × 0·7 (Dr J.F. Boyd.)

about one-third of cases. *Legionella pneumophila* can be demonstrated histologically using the Dieterle's silver staining method and also by immunofluorescence microscopy. Culture is extremely difficult. Since the original description of the disease, numerous cases have been reported in North America and Europe and several other species of *Legionella* are now known to cause pneumonia (Blackmon *et al.*, 1981).

Aspiration pneumonia

This results from the inhalation of food, gastric contents, or infected material from the oropharyngeal region. It may follow anaesthesia administered on a full stomach for an obstetric or other emergency. It may complicate pyloric stenosis, hiatus hernia, oesophageal obstruction and any condition associated with persistent vomiting. The likelihood of food or gastric contents being inhaled is increased in unconscious patients, drunkenness, epilepsy and neurological disorders affecting swallowing.

Massive inhalation of gastric contents may lead to rapid death from asphyxia. The aspiration of smaller amounts of sterile acid gastric contents produces pulmonary oedema due to chemical irritation of the alveolar walls: a few hours after aspiration the patient dramatically develops cyanosis, dyspnoea and shock, and cough with bloodstained sputum. If the acute episode is survived, secondary bacterial infection is likely to follow. Non-sterile aspirate rapidly causes widespread bronchopneumonia, which becomes confluent with multiple areas of necrosis. The microscopic picture is of a suppurative bronchopneumonia with destruction of alveolar walls. A granulomatous reaction with foreign-body giant cells may be seen surrounding vegetable matter from food.

Aspiration pneumonia with suppuration may also result from partial drowning, particularly in dirty water. There is development of rapidly progressive multiple abscesses in which anaerobic organisms e.g. bacterioides, streptococci, clostridia and fusiform bacteria and also aerobic organisms, play an active role. The lesions are rapidly enlarging, irregular abscess cavities containing foul-smelling pus surrounded by soft, friable, moist, green or black necrotic tissue. The necrosis and putrefactive infection warrant the term gangrene or gangrenous bronchopneumonia.

Hypostatic pneumonia

In severely debilitated bedridden patients, some oedema fluid and secretion tends to accumulate in the dependent parts of the lungs. This may become infected by bacteria from the upper respiratory tract, and the resultant pneumonia, termed hypostatic pneumonia, is likely to be fatal unless treated by antibiotics. Hypostatic pneumonia is a common terminal event in patients with cancer, in comatose states, e.g. due to a stroke, and in the old and feeble: it used to be known as the old peoples' friend.

Lung abscess

Lung abscess presents clinical and radiological features which must be distinguished from those of necrosis in a malignant tumour or cavitation due to tuberculosis; these two diagnoses must be considered automatically whenever there is a clinical suspicion of lung abscess.

Causes. The commonest cause of a lung abscess is *inhalation of infected material* during unconsciousness and sleep, for example, gastric contents, decaying teeth or necrotic tissue derived from lesions in the mouth, upper respiratory tract or nasopharynx. An abscess may form beyond an *obstructed bronchus* and this may be the first sign of a bronchial carcinoma or impacted foreign body. Pyogenic infection of *bronchiectatic* or *tuberculous cavities* results in abscess formation, and another important group of lung abscesses may complicate pneumonia caused by type III *Streptococcus pneumoniae, Klebsiella pneumoniae, Staphylococcus aureus* or *Streptococcus pyogenes*. Less common causes of lung abscess include infection of a pulmonary infarct, septic emboli in the lung as in pyaemia due to acute osteomyelitis or acute infective endocarditis, amoebic 'abscesses' due to *Entamoeba histolytica*, trauma to the lung, or direct extension from a suppurating focus in the oesophagus, mediastinum, subphrenic area or vertebral column.

Localisation. Abscesses due to inhalation of infected foreign material are likely to be located in the lower part of the right upper lobe or at the apex of the right lower lobe. The right bronchus is more in line with the trachea than the left and is thus more likely to receive aspirated foreign material. An abscess resulting from inhalation of a large foreign body will develop beyond its site of impaction. Small foreign particles are able to travel further into the lung and may produce an abscess just beneath the pleura. An abscess arising as a result of bronchiectasis tends to be centred around the affected bronchus, while an abscess complicating pneumonia has no primary relationship to a major bronchus. Pyaemic abscesses, which are usually staphylococcal or streptococcal, are scattered widely throughout the lungs, although they are likely to be small and mainly subpleural.

Complications. It is possible for a small lung abscess to heal completely, leaving a fibrous scar with a small central sterile cavity. An abscess near the pleura induces a fibrinous or purulent pleurisy which may progress to *empyema*. An abscess communicating with a bronchus may rupture into the pleural cavity to give a *bronchopleural fistula* and *pyopneumothorax*. Serious *haemorrhage* may occur if an abscess erodes a pulmonary or bronchial artery. Abscess formation in staphylococcal pneumonia may result in *tension cysts* or *pneumatoceles* (p. 16.39).

In 5–10% of patients with lung abscess, *meningitis* or *cerebral abscess*, develop from bloodstream spread of the infection.

Virus pneumonia

In viral respiratory infections there may be proliferation of bronchial, bronchiolar and alveolar epithelium, sometimes with formation of multinucleated giant cells, followed by necrosis. The bronchial, bronchiolar and alveolar walls are infiltrated by lymphocytes and mononuclear cells. Neutrophil polymorphs are few or absent in the inflammatory cell infiltrate, which is mainly interstitial except in influenza. Inclusion bodies may be demonstrated in lung tissue and secretions in infections with *Chlamydia trachomatis* or cytomegalovirus but otherwise the viral nature of a pneumonia can often only be inferred from the above histological features. Moreover, as noted earlier, *viral infections of the lung, and especially influenza, predispose the respiratory tissues to secondary bacterial invasion and when this occurs the distinctive histological appearances of viral pneumonia are often obscured.*

The nature of a viral pneumonia can be confirmed by isolation of the virus or by demonstrating a rising or high titre of specific antibodies in the patient's serum. In spite of their varied pathogenesis, viral pneumonias mostly present a broadly similar clinical picture which is commonly referred to as **atypical pneumonia**.

Influenza

Influenza occurs endemically in most countries, but about every three years it causes an epidemic. Every forty years or so a major epidemic or worldwide pandemic appears, as in 1918 when a large percentage of the world's population was affected. Infection is spread by inhalation of droplets of infected secretions.

Influenza virus colonises and causes necrosis of the columnar epithelium of the respiratory tract. At this stage the tracheobronchial mucosa is lined by basal or reserve cells and the submucosa is acutely inflamed but infiltrated mainly with lymphocytes. In mild cases these changes are probably restricted to the trachea and larger bronchi, but in severe cases they extend down to involve the terminal bronchioles or even the alveoli, causing *primary influenzal pneumonia*. In patients who recover from the initial infection, the epithelium regenerates: at first it is of simple squamous type and devoid of cilia. During this phase the lung defence mechanisms are impaired and there is a considerable risk of invasion by *Staphylococcus aureus*, *Haemophilus influenzae* and *Streptococcus pneumoniae*, any of which may give rise to secondary bacterial pneumonia (Fig. 16.27). Differentiation to pseudostratified ciliated columnar epithelium occurs in about three weeks.

In **primary influenzal pneumonia**, which is almost always fatal, the alveoli are filled with a mixture of oedema fluid, fibrin, red blood cells and mononuclear cells (lymphocytes and macrophages). These changes are accompanied by an interstitial mononuclear cell infiltrate in half the cases. In the most severely affected parts of the lung there may be focal necrosis of the alveolar walls, which are lined by hyaline membranes. In fatal cases, the lungs are heavy, bulky and purple-red. The cut surfaces exude bloodstained frothy fluid from the bronchi and lung parenchyma; the latter shows focal dark areas of collapse, particularly in the lower lobes, and possibly due to loss of surfactant resulting from viral destruction of granular pneumocytes.

Recent pandemics have all been caused by type A virus and the subtypes causing successive pandemics have differed markedly in their important outer (H and N) antigens. Pandemics are thus caused by apparently 'new' strains of virus, possibly resulting from recombination between 'human' and 'animal' strains.

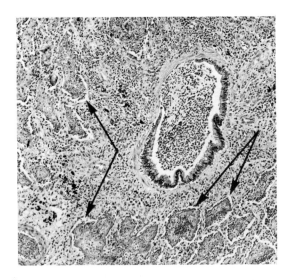

Fig. 16.27 Influenza with secondary bacterial bronchopneumonia. There is acute inflammatory exudate in the bronchiole and in the surrounding alveolar spaces (arrows): the exudate in the alveoli is rich in fibrin and appears dark. × 60.

Other viral pneumonias

Cytomegalovirus lung disease. Cytomegalovirus causes opportunistic infections in man, notably in the fetus, in premature infants, and in subjects with immunodeficiency diseases or whose immunity is depressed by corticosteroid therapy, immunosuppressive drugs, irradiation or cytotoxic drugs. Patients treated by bone marrow transplantation are particularly susceptible to pulmonary cytomegalovirus infection. In the adult form of disease, the lungs may be involved as part of a serious widespread infection, the salivary glands and kidney being affected more frequently than the lungs. The changes occur in both bronchiolar and alveolar epithelium. Cells enlarge so that they are five to six times the size of their uninvolved neighbours

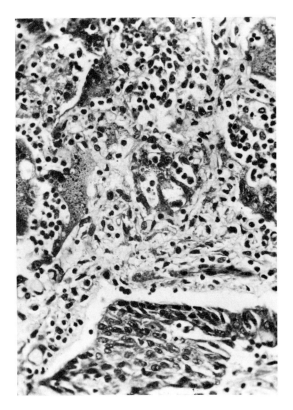

Fig. 16.28 Giant-cell pneumonia in measles. There is hyperplasia of the bronchiolar epithelium and numerous giant cells in the alveolar spaces. × 240.

(Fig. 13.10, p. 13.16). *Pneumocystis carinii* is often present in addition (see below).

Giant-cell pneumonia. In patients with measles dying early in the disease, notably in children with a deficiency in cell-mediated immunity, the epithelium of the bronchioles may be hyperplastic (Fig. 16.28). Numerous giant cells may develop by fusion of alveolar lining epithelial cells and may contain inclusion bodies. This form of giant-cell pneumonia is due to measles virus and represents a deficient immune response to the virus. In patients developing a secondary bacterial pneumonia the characteristic changes are obscured.

Other types of pneumonia

Psittacosis (ornithosis). Infection with various species of *Chlamydiae* (p. 9.34) is very common in birds. Infection in man is acquired by inhalation of elementary bodies derived from the excreta of infected birds. Cross infection from human patients to healthy attendants may occur by droplet spread. The infection should be suspected in any patient who presents with atypical pneumonia where there is a history of contact with birds, especially parrots, budgerigars and pigeons. Infection produces a broncho-pneumonia in which the alveoli are filled with exudate containing mainly macrophages, fibrin and often red cells. Very few polymorphs are present. The disease is occasionally fatal.

Q fever. This condition is caused by *Coxiella burneti* which primarily infects cattle, sheep and goats. Man is usually infected by handling carcasses of infected cattle and sheep, by inhaling dust from infected barns and straw, or by drinking raw milk containing the organisms. Stockyard workers, farmers, shepherds and medical laboratory staff may be exposed to infection during the course of their work. The disease most commonly presents as an atypical pneumonia, with headache and muscle pains as prominent symptoms. The course of the illness is usually short (up to eight days) and benign, but chronic infection can occur. Endocarditis is a rare complication and is frequently fatal.

Mycoplasmal pneumonia. This is caused by *Mycoplasma pneumoniae* (p. 9.34). It causes a low-grade bronchopneumonia in which the walls of the bronchioles are thickened by interstitial mononuclear cell infiltration, while the lumina contain mucopurulent material. In some alveoli there is fibrinous exudate tending to undergo organisation, in others oedema and haemorrhage. The onset is usually gradual and the mortality is low but resolution is often somewhat delayed.

Pneumocystis pneumonia is caused by opportunistic infection with *Pneumocystis carinii* (p. 28.20).

Unusual causes of pulmonary consolidation

Lymphoid interstitial pneumonia is characterised by a chronic cough, dyspnoea and pyrexia, together with enlargement of the spleen and liver. Many patients have hypergammaglobulinaemia. The disease, which is of unknown cause, affects persons of all ages, including infants. It is a slowly progressive condition and the diagnosis is usually made following lung biopsy. Histologically, the alveolar septa are distended with masses of mature lymphocytes intermingled with large pale macrophages and plasma cells. Large lymphoid follicles may be present. Differentiation from a malignant lymphoma may be difficult.

Eosinophilic pneumonia. This may occur in acute and chronic forms, both of which may be accompanied by peripheral blood eosinophilia. Acute eosinophilic pneumonia is a brief, mild, self-limiting illness commonly referred to as *Löffler's syndrome*. In chronic eosinophilic pneumonia, which may last for several months or years, the alveolar spaces contain proteinaceous exudate mixed with eosinophils and mononuclear cells. The alveolar septa and pulmonary interstitial tissues are heavily infiltrated with plasma cells, lymphocytes, eosinophils and macrophages. Most cases of eosinophilic pneumonia are of unknown cause but some are related to adverse drug reactions, or infection by helminths, *Aspergillus*, *Filaria* and *Dirofilaria*.

Pulmonary alveolar proteinosis. This is a rare chronic disease of unknown cause, which can affect persons of all ages from infancy to old age. It is manifested clinically by dyspnoea, a cough often productive of yellow sputum, increasing fatigue and loss of weight. Some patients recover spontaneously but the disease is fatal in about one-third of cases. At autopsy, confluent grey areas of consolidation are found in the lungs. A little milky or pale yellow fluid may be squeezed from the cut surface. Histologically, the alveolar spaces are distended by granular eosinophilic material, and lined by prominent granular pneumocytes. The granular eosinophilic intra-alveolar material contains lipid and protein and is apparently derived from the cytoplasm of granular pneumocytes which have degenerated, become necrotic and detached from the alveolar walls. The alveolar septa are devoid of inflammatory cells and fibrosis is usually absent. The nature of pulmonary alveolar proteinosis is obscure. It may represent a stereotyped reaction of the lung to different types of injury, rather than being a single disease entity.

Pulmonary granulomatosis. The lungs are sometimes the principal site of involvement by a number of distinctive types of focal destructive and infiltrative vascular disease and granulomatosis not produced by known infectious agents, nor associated with rheumatoid arthritis. By granulomatosis is meant necrosis of tissue with a peripheral, chronic, cellular inflammatory reaction, not ascribable to occlusive lesions of the blood vessels. The necrotic lesions are surrounded by granulation tissue rich in plasma cells, lymphocytes, large macrophages and multinuclear giant cells. Several forms of granulomatosis have been identified and classified by Liebow (1973) according to their histological picture, location within the lung and behaviour. They include Wegener's granulomatosis (p. 16.4), lymphomatoid granulomatosis, bronchocentric granulomatosis and necrotising sarcoid granulomatosis (Churg, 1983).

Lipid pneumonia. The inhalation of oily material into the lungs may cause **exogenous lipid pneumonia**. This is associated with the long-term use of oily drops or sprays taken for rhinitis. Mineral oil (liquid paraffin) taken regularly at bedtime is readily aspirated during sleep in small amounts which fail to excite the cough reflex. There is a danger of aspiration when oily vitamin preparations are given to reluctant young children or debilitated elderly persons. **Exogenous lipid pneumonia** tends to be symptomless and is usually revealed by chance during radiographic examination or at necropsy. The lesions are commonly located in the middle or lower lobes of the right lung or in the left lower lobe. There may be diffuse fibrosis of the affected lung or the formation of a well-circumscribed *oleogranuloma*. This latter firm tumour-like mass may be mistakenly diagnosed as carcinoma in a chest radiograph or during thoracotomy. Microscopically the oil may be seen lying free or in foamy macrophages, and there are multinucleate giant cells with accompanying lymphocytic infiltration and fibrosis.

Exogenous lipid pneumonia must be distinguished from the more common **endogenous lipid pneumonia** that is occasionally seen distal to obstruction of a major airway. Macrophages with foamy cytoplasm accumulate within alveolar spaces. They may degenerate with the liberation of cholesterol and other lipids and the formation of cholesterol clefts. Foreign body giant cells surrounding large lipid droplets are not seen.

Chronic bacterial infections

Pulmonary tuberculosis

A general account of tuberculosis is provided on pp. 9.15–22, and the basic information contained in it is essential to the understanding of this account of pulmonary tuberculosis.

Tuberculosis affects the lungs more often than any other organ, partly because inhalation is now the commonest mode of infection, but also because lung tissue provides a favourable environment for the growth of the organism. Certain diseases and occupations predispose to the development of pulmonary tuberculosis. Thus it occurs with increased frequency in chronic alcoholics and in workers with silicosis. It is an occupational hazard for all hospital personnel, particularly those who work in pathology laboratories and autopsy rooms. Corticosteroid therapy, diabetes mellitus and partial gastrectomy are associated with an increased liability to develop the disease. The pattern of tuberculosis varies greatly in different populations. In those with a high prevalence of the infection, there is a high rate of primary infection in young childhood, and survivors may remain free of further clinical evidence of infection or may subsequently develop secondary (chronic or re-activation) pulmonary tuberculosis. This is the traditional pattern which was also seen in this country and elsewhere following the industrial revolution and gave rise to the terms 'childhood' (i.e. primary) and 'adult' (i.e. secondary) tuberculosis. The pattern has, however, changed in many of the developed countries where a combination of high nutritional and housing standards, population screening, immunisation and effective drug therapy has very greatly reduced the prevalence of all forms of tuberculosis. The result is that tuberculosis in childhood has become increasingly rare; primary tuberculosis is seldom seen because of a high level of immunisation and most 'new' cases are now in the middle-aged or elderly and represent recrudescence from a healed primary or secondary lesion which has remained latent for many years. Such old latent lesions are liable to be activated by any chronic debilitating disease, notably by corticosteroid or other immunosuppressive therapy, by chronic alcoholism, the development of diabetes mellitus, etc.

Primary pulmonary tuberculosis

In patients who have not previously had tuberculosis, inhalation of tubercle bacilli and subsequent infection gives rise to a **primary lesion** (p. 9.20), also termed the *Ghon focus*. This is usually single, 1 to 2 cm in diameter, and situated just beneath the pleura, usually in the mid-zone of either lung. Microscopic examination of the early Ghon focus shows central caseation and peripheral tubercles; the lesion enlarges by spread of mycobacteria, which are taken up and carried by macrophages, so that tubercles form in the adjacent lung tissue, replacing alveolar walls and filling air spaces, and as they enlarge these peripheral tubercles become incorporated in the central caseous area.

Lymphatic spread of *Mycobacterium tuberculosis* occurs in the primary infection; tubercles are often seen along the line of the lymphatics between the Ghon focus and the hilar lymph nodes, and both the tracheobronchial and adjacent mediastinal nodes often become extensively involved, greatly enlarged and caseous (Fig. 16.29). The combination of the Ghon

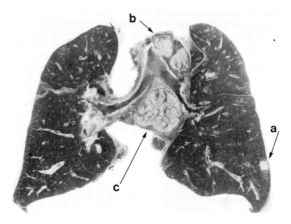

Fig. 16.29 Primary pulmonary tuberculous complex. Lung of child with primary lesion (a) in right lower lobe and enlarged tracheobronchial lymph nodes (b and c).

focus and tuberculous lymphadenitis is termed the **primary complex**. In children, the affected hilar and tracheobronchial lymph nodes form a caseous mass which is much larger than the peripheral Ghon focus. In some adults with a primary infection, the reverse is the case.

In most instances, the Ghon focus undergoes healing: if small, by fibrous tissue; if larger, the caseous centre usually persists and is converted into a hard calcified nodule, often partly ossified and enclosed in fibrous tissue. Such a healed lesion is readily visible in chest radiographs. The affected hilar and tracheobronchial lymph nodes usually heal and may become heavily calcified.

Spread from the primary complex. The primary complex is often symptomless, but the pleura may be infected directly from the Ghon focus, causing a *pleural effusion* or rarely *tuberculous empyema*. (Unless there is superadded pyogenic bacterial infection, tuberculous lesions do not usually suppurate, but tuberculous lesions of the kidney, bones and pleura sometimes do so.) In some cases the Ghon focus or hilar lymph nodes may involve and ulcerate into a bronchus, with consequent *tuberculous bronchopneumonia* (see below) or dissemination may occur by the bloodstream resulting in either *generalised miliary tuberculosis* (p. 16.48) or one or more metastatic lesions, e.g. in the kidneys or joints. These serious complications are particularly liable to develop in very young, malnourished or debilitated children.

Acute tuberculous bronchopneumonia can develop from the primary infection by aspiration of infected caseous material throughout the bronchial tree, either from the Ghon focus or, more commonly, from caseous lymph nodes at the hilum. In the former case, the Ghon focus continues to enlarge until eventually it incorporates a bronchus in the caseous process. Caseous material is then discharged into the lumen, from where it may be aspirated through adjacent and more distant parts of the bronchial tree. Bronchial dissemination results similarly when a caseating hilar lymph node ulcerates into a major bronchus. The resulting tuberculous bronchopneumonia is relatively acute, and usually affects both lungs, although one is often involved more extensively than the other. The lung tissue is studded with numerous small pneumonic patches (Fig. 9.17, p. 9.19), which are arranged in groups or clusters around the terminal bronchi. The microscopic features (p. 9.19) are quite atypical for tuberculosis. The lesions spread rapidly and are exudative, with accumulation of macrophages and lymphocytes in the alveolar spaces, followed by necrosis.

They may become confluent in the lower parts of the lungs, where they are most numerous. The enlarging necrotic patches may discharge into bronchi, with further dissemination throughout the lungs. The cavities resulting from discharge of caseous material have ragged caseating walls and, unlike chronic tuberculous cavities, no surrounding fibrosis. Tuberculous pleurisy usually develops and a small cavity opening into a bronchus may rupture also into the pleura, resulting in pneumothorax. Extensive tuberculous bronchopneumonia is associated with fever, severe debility and rapid weight loss and was formerly known as 'galloping consumption'. Unless treated early and effectively it is rapidly fatal. As stated below, acute tuberculous bronchopneumonia can

occur also in patients with reactivation pulmonary tuberculosis.

Secondary (re-activation or chronic) pulmonary tuberculosis

During the primary tuberculous infection, or following BCG immunisation, the patient develops cell-mediated immunity to antigens of the tubercle bacillus; this is demonstrable by a positive tuberculin skin test (a delayed hypersensitivity reaction to tuberculoprotein) which is associated with increased resistance to subsequent infection.

Post-primary infection can be endogenous, resulting from reactivation of a dormant primary or post-primary lesion, or it may be exogenous, i.e. caused by organisms in inhaled dust, etc. The causes of re-activation of a dormant primary lesion include malnutrition, the development of other severe illness, intercurrent lung infection, and systemic immunosuppressive therapy, but in many instances, none of these factors is responsible.

The common sites for post-primary pulmonary tuberculosis are the posterior segment of the upper lobe and the apical segment of the lower lobe. The anatomical location of the lesion is attributed to the good ventilation but relatively low blood flow in these areas. The re-infection lesion results from proliferation of *Mycobacterium tuberculosis* in the wall of a bronchiole or alveolus. The usual reaction takes place, with formation of tubercle follicles, and the lesion enlarges by formation of new tubercles at the margin and in the adjacent lung tissue. The infection spreads by the lymphatics, but, because of the immune state, it induces a delayed hypersensitivity reaction from the onset, lymphatic spread is strictly localised, and the hilar lymph nodes are not usually affected. The early re-activation lesion thus comes to consist of a cluster of follicles which, as they enlarge and caseate, become confluent, producing one or more larger lesions. Because of the partial state of immunity which exists, progress of the lesions is slow, the tubercles are well developed and there is conspicuous formation of fibrous tissue at their periphery. The caseous material is yellowish or sometimes greyish due to inclusion of carbon pigment, which is often abundant in the fibrous tissue. If healing does not now occur, some of the nodules will spread to involve the wall of a bronchus in caseous necrosis and blockage of the lumen follows. The lesion may become encapsulated by fibrous tissue or the caseous material may be gradually discharged along the bronchus leaving a small cavity. Bronchial spread to the upper parts of other lobes and to the other lung may occur, and chronic pulmonary tuberculosis is frequently bilateral.

The cavities may coalesce and can become very large (Fig. 16.30). Even with cavitation,

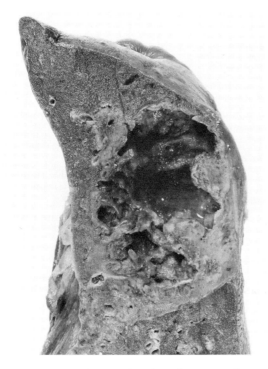

Fig. 16.30 Cavitating chronic pulmonary tuberculosis. Much of the upper lobe is occupied by a large irregular cavity with a necrotic lining and a fibrous wall in which paler caseous patches are seen. Fibrosis is most extensive below and lateral to the cavity, where it extends to the pleura. Irregularity of the cavity is due to persistence of fibrosed remnants of bronchi and blood vessels involved in the lesion.

enlargement of the tuberculous lesions is usually slow: there is considerable overgrowth of fibrous tissue, not only around the cavities, but also in a diffusely spreading manner. In this way the lung shrinks and bronchiectasis may be superadded. Ultimately a cavity may become

very large and occupy a considerable portion of the upper lobe. The walls of the chronic cavities are somewhat irregular and contain raised bands, which represent obliterated blood vessels and other structures with more resistance than the rest of the tissue. The surface is usually lined by caseous material or by pus and debris sometimes mixed with blood; if the disease becomes inactive, the lining of the cavities becomes smooth. The contents of the cavities do not usually have a putrid odour, and the organisms present along with the tubercle bacilli are chiefly pyogenic cocci. Pulmonary and bronchial blood vessels involved in the wall of a cavity usually become occluded by endarteritis obliterans (p. 14.2). Sometimes, however, the wall of an artery may be weakened and rupture; this may be preceded by aneurysm formation. Serious and sometimes fatal haemorrhage results. This is to be distinguished from the coughing up of bloodstained sputum, or the slight bleeding which commonly occurs from small vessels in the wall of a cavity.

If at any time there should occur a rapid diffusion of large numbers of bacilli by the air passages, as may happen when a caseous focus suddenly discharges into a bronchus, the patient's resistance may be overcome and acute *rapidly spreading tuberculous bronchopneumonia* supervenes. It is not uncommon to find the latter in the lower parts of the lungs, while chronic cavity formation is present in the upper lobes (Fig. 9.18, p. 9.20). This is likely to occur if the patient is debilitated by intercurrent disease such as influenza or diabetes, or by overwork, malnutrition and unfavourable environmental conditions.

In patients dying from chronic pulmonary tuberculosis, and particularly when there has been breakdown of resistance and extensive bronchopneumonia, blood dissemination with *acute miliary tuberculosis* may occur, but this is much less common than in primary tuberculosis in young children.

Tuberculous ulcers may develop in the intestine from infection by bacilli in swallowed sputum (p. 19.46). *Tuberculosis of the larynx* (p. 16.6), likewise produced by direct infection from the sputum, is a serious complication.

Secondary amyloidosis is a common complication of chronic tuberculosis.

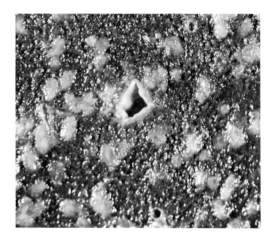

Fig. 16.31 Acute miliary tuberculosis. The cut surface of the lung shows numerous discrete grey tubercles. × 5.

Generalised miliary tuberculosis

The pulmonary lesions in this condition are part of an acute generalised tuberculosis, which occurs when a large number of mycobacteria gain entrance to the bloodstream. The ways by which this is brought about have already been considered (p. 9.21). In miliary tuberculosis, lesions are usually more numerous in the lungs than in any other organ. They consist of grey tubercles which may be too small to be visible by the naked eye or up to 3 mm in diameter (Fig. 16.31). Commonly, they are more numerous and rather larger in the upper lobes than in the lower.

Microscopically the early tubercles are seen to be in the peribronchial connective tissue, fibrous septa, and in the alveolar walls but they enlarge by extension to the surrounding alveoli. Necrosis then occurs in the centre of the tubercle. In very acute cases the tubercle follicles are poorly formed and giant cells are virtually absent. The miliary lesions do not cavitate and *Mycobacterium tuberculosis* is rarely found in the sputum.

The pleura in pulmonary tuberculosis

At a very early stage of localised lung disease, tubercles may form in the visceral pleura, and this may be followed by an extensive effusion into the affected pleural sac. Tuberculosis is a frequent cause of apparently idiopathic pleurisy. The fluid is usually clear and the cells in it are scanty and mainly lymphocytes: desquamated serosal cells are seldom conspicuous and tubercle bacilli often cannot be found. Sometimes the exudate is serofibrinous or blood-stained. The lesion usually resolves and the fluid is absorbed, leaving only scanty adhesions to mark its previous existence. In chronic pulmonary tuberculosis the underlying visceral pleura is thickened and rupture of a cavity into the pleural sac is usually prevented by fibrous adhesion between the two layers of pleura. As mentioned on p. 16.45, pulmonary tuberculosis sometimes causes empyema, and secondary pyogenic infection cannot always be incriminated.

The effects of specific chemotherapy

The above account refers essentially to the disease unmodified by chemotherapy. The general changes produced in tuberculous lesions by a combination of drugs, usually rifampicin, ethambutol and isoniazid have been discussed on p. 9.22. In pulmonary tuberculosis, combined therapy is imperative in order to render the patient non-infective and to reduce the risk of producing antibiotic-resistant strains. If adequately carried out in the early stages of the apical lesion, chemotherapy leads to rapid healing with minimal fibrosis. In excavated lesions, whether chronic or bronchopneumonic, the caseous lining disappears and is replaced by a layer of vascular granulation tissue which, in turn, is converted to a thin smooth fibrous layer, over which an epithelial lining may eventually grow, leaving a persistent cavity which may or may not communicate with a bronchus.

Provided it is not too advanced, pulmonary tuberculosis of both major types can be arrested by drugs, although excision may still be required in some cases to avoid other infections of 'healed' cavities.

Sarcoidosis

Sarcoidosis is a systemic disease of unknown aetiology in which non-caseating epithelioid cell follicles are scattered throughout several organs. The general features of the condition are described on pp. 9.26–27.

The lungs are involved more frequently than

any other organ. In Europe and North America the commonest presentation of the disease is an abnormal routine chest radiograph. The four following patterns of radiological abnormality can be distinguished. (1) Hilar node enlargement with normal lung fields (38%). (2) Hilar node enlargement with pulmonary infiltration (50%). (3) Pulmonary infiltration without hilar node enlargement (7%). (4) Pulmonary fibrosis with honeycomb lung (5%). In active sarcoidosis the activity of angiotensin-converting enzyme in the serum may be increased, as may the number of lymphocytes in fluid obtained by broncho-alveolar lavage. These features may aid in diagnosis and in the assessment of response to therapy.

Most patients have no physical disability and the radiological changes regress within two to three years. About 13% of patients develop chronic progressive pulmonary sarcoidosis, which is frequently associated with crippling dyspnoea, respiratory failure and pulmonary hypertension. Right ventricular failure may also ensue. About half the patients with chronic progressive pulmonary sarcoidosis die within ten to fifteen years of the disease being recognised.

Pathological examination of the lungs at an early stage of the disease reveals typical non-caseating epithelioid-cell granulomas in the alveolar walls and fibrous septa; they usually heal with minimal fibrosis. In chronic progressive sarcoidosis with extensive involvement of the lung, an interstitial fibrosis develops which leads eventually to honeycomb change (p. 16.53): in this late stage, no trace of the original sarcoid granulomas can usually be found.

Syphilis

Pulmonary syphilis occurs in congenital and acquired forms, both of which are extremely rare in most medically advanced countries. The majority of infants with *congenital* pulmonary syphilitic lesions are stillborn. The lungs are enlarged, pale and firm due to diffuse fibrosis of the alveolar septa and peribronchial and perivascular tissue. The interstitial fibrous tissue is diffusely infiltrated by lymphocytes and plasma cells and contains abundant *Treponema pallidum*. In *acquired* syphilis, gummas may rarely develop in the lung.

Actinomycosis and nocardiosis

Actinomycosis is caused by *Actinomyces israeli* (p. 9.32) which produces a chronic granulomatous reaction with pus formation. About 20% of actinomycotic infections involve the lungs and thorax. Pulmonary actinomycosis may be primary or secondary, the latter usually resulting from the spread of disease from below the diaphragm, particularly from the liver. About 75% of pulmonary cases are primary and the disease commonly occurs in the lower lobes, where it forms a dense fibrotic lesion honeycombed with small abscess cavities. The pus contains 'sulphur granules' which are colonies of *Actinomyces israeli*.

Nocardia asteroides is an aerobic, branching filamentous organism similar in some respects to *Actinomyces*. The lungs are involved in about 60% of cases of nocardiosis. The incidence of infection appears to be increasing, and to be associated with diseases or therapy that impair the patient's immune mechanisms. At autopsy the lungs show a suppurative pneumonia that may be lobular in distribution. The organism does not form colonies, but occurs as branching filaments which are not stained with haematoxylin and eosin. It is Gram +ve and appears black using the silver methenamine stain.

Fungal infections (Mycoses)

Most pulmonary fungal infections are *opportunistic*, arising as a result of breakdown in cellular and humoral defence mechanisms (p. 7.32), and from the sustained use of antibiotics, which may so alter the normal human bacterial flora that fungi which are normally non-pathogenic may grow and invade the tissues. Until recent years, many of the pulmonary fungal diseases (mycoses) were little known and constituted an unimportant group of conditions. However, *since the introduction of the therapeutic immunosuppressive agents and antibiotics, the importance of fungal diseases has changed dramatically.*

The pulmonary mycoses usually encountered in Britain are aspergillosis, candidiasis and cryptococcosis, but increasing foreign travel has also brought occasional cases of histoplasmosis (p. 9.36), coccidiomycosis and blastomycosis from overseas.

Aspergillosis. This is the commonest pulmonary mycosis in the British Isles and it is usually due to infection by *Aspergillus fumigatus*. The hyphae are 3–4 μm in diameter, show frequent

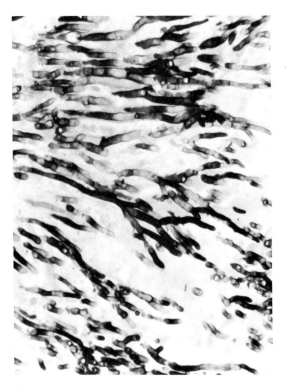

Fig. 16.32 Invasive pulmonary aspergillosis. The hyphae of *Aspergillus fumigatus* show frequent transverse septa and exhibit dichotomous branching at acute angles. From a patient who received cytotoxic therapy for Hodgkin's disease. Methenamine silver stain. × 375.

transverse septa, and exhibit dichotomous branching at acute angles (Fig. 16.32). It may give rise to four types of lung disease in man. Firstly, atopic subjects may develop reaginic antibodies to antigenic constituents of *Aspergillus*, and as a result suffer from attacks of **bronchial asthma** following heavy exposure to the spores. Secondly, some patients develop precipitating antibodies, and on further exposure to the spores may have attacks of **extrinsic allergic alveolitis** (p. 16.61). Thirdly, *Aspergillus* can colonise tuberculous or bronchiectatic cavities in the lung producing a rounded mass of fungus (**mycetoma**) with a characteristic radiographic appearance. The chest radiograph shows an opaque spherical mass which almost completely fills the cavity, leaving a crescentic 'halo' of air between the mycelial mass and the cavity wall. Fourthly, in immunosuppressed patients, and in patients with Hodgkin's disease or leukaemia, aspergillus infection may produce nodules of **haemorrhagic consolidation and necrosis** scattered throughout the lungs. Such consolidated areas contain ramifying hyphae of *Aspergillus fumigatus* which may invade pulmonary arteries and veins leading to thrombosis and metastatic foci in other organs.

Candidiasis. *Candida albicans* (p. 9.35) is a normal commensal in the pharynx, where it can give rise to the lesion of **thrush.** Bronchopulmonary infection with *Candida* is rare, occurring as a result of severe underlying disease, immunological deficiency, or because of long-term treatment with antibiotic or corticosteroid drugs. Sometimes the trachea and bronchi are lined by a mass of fungus and sections show hyphae growing down through the mucosa. The lungs may show pneumonic consolidation with areas of necrosis and infiltration by neutrophil polymorphs.

Cryptococcosis (torulosis). *Crytococcus neoformans* (p. 9.37) tends to cause disease in patients whose resistance to infection is diminished by leukaemia or Hodgkin's disease or by systemic corticosteroid therapy. Although rare, the incidence of infection is increasing. The most usual presentation is a meningoencephalitis, but respiratory tract infection can occur with the production of an atypical pneumonia. At autopsy, the lungs contain firm rubbery areas of consolidation which are devoid of necrosis but show a mucoid cut surface.

Pulmonary fibrosis

Pulmonary fibrosis is a result or complication of many of the diseases described in this chapter. Localised fibrosis, for example, may result from organisation of acute pneumonias and pulmonary infarcts or from tuberculosis. Chronic diffuse pulmonary fibrosis may be caused by inhalation of toxic dusts or fumes, certain connective tissue diseases, ionising radiation, sarcoidosis and as an adverse reaction to certain drugs. There is also an uncommon condition, cryptogenic fibrosing alveolitis (Hamman-Rich syndrome), the cause of which remains unknown.

We shall consider first the cells lining the alveolar walls and their reaction to injury.

Alveolar lining cells (pneumocytes). The alveolar walls consist of a meshwork of capillaries,

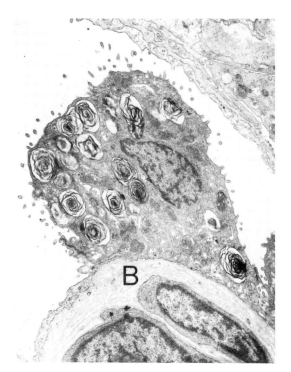

Fig. 16.33 Granular pneumocyte. The cell rests on the basement membrane (B) and projects into the alveolar space. Its surface is covered by microvilli and within its cytoplasm are lamellar bodies, considered by many to be the source of pulmonary surfactant. Electron micrograph. × 7500.

supported by scanty connective tissue, and covered largely by the ultrathin cytoplasmic extensions of **membranous (type I) pneumocytes**. These extensions have a large area but possess few organelles and are probably metabolically dependent upon the central perinuclear portion of the cells, which lie in the corners and angles of alveoli. This dependence may explain why membranous pneumocytes are vulnerable to a variety of injuries.

The **granular (type II) pneumocytes** are interposed between the membranous pneumocytes and unlike them do not have flat cytoplasmic extensions. The basal portion of the cell is attached to the underlying basement membrane; its free convex surface projects into the alveolar space (Fig. 16.33) and is covered by short, straight and fairly regular microvilli. Within the abundant cytoplasm are prominent lamellar bodies thought to be the source of pulmonary surfactant (Fig. 16.33). Granular pneumocytes have a much greater capacity for division and a shorter turnover time than membranous pneumocytes and probably represent the reserve (stem) cells of the alveolar lining epithelium. They proliferate and replace membranous pneumocytes when the latter are destroyed. Thus, proliferation of granular pneumocytes can occur in a wide variety of circumstances and appears to be a non-specific reaction to injury.

Fibrosing alveolitis and interstitial pneumonia

The term **fibrosing alveolitis** was suggested by Scadding for a disease process characterised by inflammatory changes in the lung beyond the terminal bronchiole and having as its essential features cellular thickening of the alveolar walls with a tendency to fibrosis and the presence of mononuclear cells within the alveolar spaces. Since the inflammatory reaction takes place predominantly in the supporting structures of the lung, rather than the alveolar spaces, the term **interstitial pneumonia** is preferred by some. In most cases there is patchy involvement of the lungs, and in the lesions the alveolar walls are thickened due to a combination of fibrosis and infiltration by lymphocytes and plasma cells with smaller numbers of eosinophils and

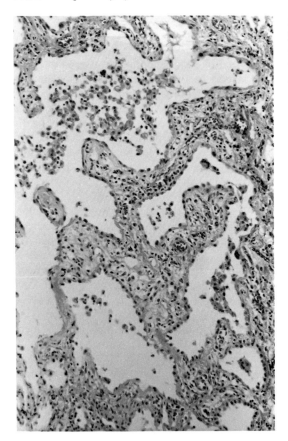

Fig. 16.34 Usual interstitial pneumonia. The alveolar walls are thickened due to a combination of fibrosis and infiltration by lymphocytes and plasma cells with smaller numbers of eosinophils and neutrophil polymorphs. Many of the alveolar walls are lined by cuboidal epithelial cells. Scanty mononuclear cells are present in the alveolar spaces. × 120.

neutrophil polymorphs. Many of the alveolar walls are lined by cuboidal or columnar granular pneumocytes which have proliferated and replaced necrotic membranous pneumocytes. Some of the alveolar spaces contain small clusters of macrophages, sometimes accompanied by scanty proteinaceous exudate. This histological picture is sometimes referred to as **usual interstitial pneumonia** (Fig. 16.34). Less commonly the lesion is more diffuse and the alveoli are filled with macrophages: the alveolar walls show minimal fibrous thickening, only a scanty infiltrate of lymphocytes, plasma cells and occasional eosinophils, and are lined by prominent, proliferated granular pneumocytes. This second histological picture is sometimes

referred to as **desquamative interstitial pneumonia** (Fig. 16.35) because it was believed originally that the intra-alveolar macrophages were desquamated granular pneumocytes. Desquamative interstitial pneumonia has a better response to steroids and has a better prognosis than usual interstitial pneumonia. However, both are probably non-specific reactions of the lung to diverse forms of injury rather than distinct pathological entities.

Fibrosing alveolitis may be associated with the connective tissue diseases, usually rheumatoid arthritis or progressive systemic sclerosis. It may also occur as an adverse reaction to drugs, especially chemotherapeutic agents like busulphan and bleomycin, to pulmonary infection by viruses, chlamydiae and mycoplasmas, or to the inhalation of toxic gases and dusts, especially asbestos. In most cases, however, no cause can be found and the condition is then called cryptogenic fibrosing alveolitis.

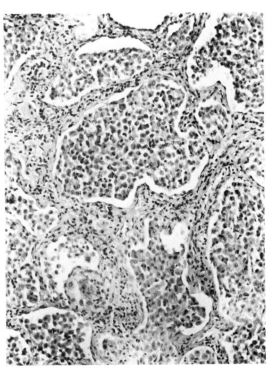

Fig. 16.35 Desquamative interstitial pneumonia. The alveolar spaces are filled with macrophages. There is only slight fibrous thickening of the alveolar walls. × 130. (Section donated by Professor D.B. Brewer.)

Cryptogenic fibrosing alveolitis. This condition, also known as *idiopathic diffuse interstitial pulmonary fibrosis* or the *Hamman-Rich syndrome*, is an uncommon disease that affects middle-aged and elderly people of both sexes, although occasionally it occurs in young people. It is characterised clinically by the insidious onset of dyspnoea, and usually pursues a chronic and progressive downhill course with death from respiratory failure or right ventricular failure, often precipitated by a superimposed respiratory tract infection. The mean survival time from the onset of the first symptom until death is 4 years, but may range from a few months to 20 years.

Although the pathogenesis is unknown, about one-third of patients have antinuclear antibodies in the serum and about one-third have rheumatoid factor, although only a few have both and the titres are usually low. Several investigators have demonstrated circulating immune complexes and/or deposition of immunoglobulin and complement within the alveolar walls and capillaries of patients with active disease, and it has been suggested that the deposition of complexes is responsible for the inflammatory changes, as in other immune-complex diseases (p. 7.16).

Broncho-alveolar lavage. Cells and proteins recovered from the alveolar surface by lavage through a fibre-optic bronchoscope wedged in a subsegmental bronchus may give an indication of the inflammatory cells and their related proteins in the alveolar walls. Lavage fluid from normal non-smoking subjects yields a differential count of approximately 93% macrophages, 6% lymphocytes and 1% neutrophil polymorphs. In smokers, the number of neutrophils is slightly increased. In active fibrosing alveolitis and asbestosis there is a raised neutrophil count with a normal lymphocyte count, while in sarcoidosis and chronic extrinsic allergic alveolitis there is a high lymphocyte count with a normal neutrophil count in the lavage fluid. This technique may aid in the resolution of the differential diagnosis in a patient with diffuse interstitial lung disease. Serial broncho-alveolar lavage may also be used to assess the activity of the disease and response to therapy in patients with fibrosing alveolitis and sarcoidosis (Hunninghake *et al.*, 1979).

Honeycomb lung

Honeycomb lung describes the naked-eye appearance of an acquired condition in which a large number of small cystic spaces develop in fibrotic lungs. Honeycomb lung is the non-specific final end-stage of many disease processes of diverse aetiology including asbestosis and beryllium intoxication, extrinsic allergic al-veolitis, cryptogenic diffuse fibrosing alveolitis, sarcoidosis, rheumatoid disease, progressive systemic sclerosis and histiocytosis X. The cysts are up to 1 or 2 cm in diameter, have smooth grey-white walls, and the surrounding lung is pale, firm and fibrous (Fig. 16.36). The presence of cysts beneath the visceral pleura gives the external surface of the lungs a nodular appearance which simulates that of the liver in macronodular cirrhosis. The essential change in honeycomb lung is obliteration by fibrosis or granuloma of some of the bronchioles and alveolar spaces with compensatory dilatation of unaffected neighbouring bronchioles. Thus the cysts are lined by columnar or cuboidal epithelium which may be ciliated or mucin-secreting. The interstitial and pericystic tissue is composed of young fibroblasts and collagen infiltrated by scanty lymphocytes, plasma cells and macrophages. There may be an interstitial hyperplasia of smooth muscle cells probably derived from obliterated bronchioles and pul-

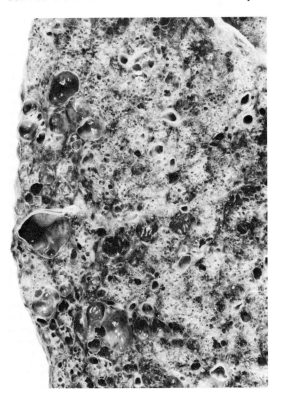

Fig. 16.36 Slice of lung showing a subpleural band of honeycomb change brought about by dilatation of terminal bronchioles. The condition is quite distinct from pulmonary emphysema.

monary blood vessels. Right ventricular hypertrophy is present in more than half the cases at autopsy. Pulmonary hypertension in honeycomb lung is attributed to a combination of chronic hypoxia, fibrous obliteration of the pulmonary vascular bed, and the development of bronchopulmonary anastomoses.

The effects of drugs and toxic compounds on the lung

A wide range of drugs and toxic compounds may give rise to clinical signs and symptoms which may resemble those of naturally occurring disease. Thus bronchial asthma may result from hypersensitivity to a wide variety of drugs, including aspirin. Some drugs, herbal substances and poisons, however, may give rise to other organic diseases in the lungs and we shall consider a few examples.

Paraquat. This is the widely used weed-killer, 1,1-dimethyl-4, 4-bipyridylium chloride. When ingested, it may produce ulceration of the mouth within two days. Acute renal failure may result from tubular epithelial injury, but renal function usually returns, sometimes with the help of haemodialysis. The most serious effect of paraquat, however, is on the lung. Within hours of ingestion there is an initial destructive effect on the alveolar epithelium. The membranous pneumocytes become swollen and vacuolated and project into the alveolar spaces. The granular pneumocytes also show vacuolation of their lamellar bodies and disruption of their endoplasmic reticulum. Two days after administration of paraquat, many alveolar walls are denuded of their epithelial lining and there is commonly pulmonary oedema and the formation of hyaline membranes. This destructive phase is followed by a proliferative phase.

Three days after a single injection of paraquat into rats, mononuclear cells are found in the alveolar spaces. They resemble macrophages, but mature into fibroblasts (Fig. 16.37) and accordingly may be termed profibroblasts. They form collagen in the alveolar spaces and thus paraquat produces intra-alveolar rather than interstitial fibrosis. There may be some associated dilatation of respiratory bronchioles. Paraquat appears to kill plants by entering the chloroplasts and then taking part in an oxidation-reduction cycle in which hydrogen peroxide is liberated. A similar type of catalytic activity may occur in animal tissue, in which a small concentration of paraquat can lead to the synthesis of a high concentration of toxic by-products such as

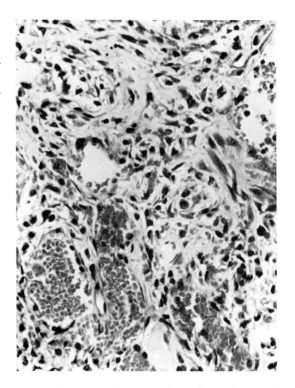

Fig. 16.37   Lung of a rat ten days after an intraperitoneal injection of paraquat. The lung architecture is obliterated by a dense mass of fibroblasts and small quantities of collagen. × 330.

hydrogen peroxide and the superoxide and peroxide free radicals which damage lipid membranes.

Busulphan. This drug is widely used in the treatment of chronic myeloid leukaemia. In a minority of patients heavy and prolonged dosage of the drug may induce interstitial pulmonary fibrosis which impairs oxygen diffusion and causes dyspnoea. Chest radiographs show perihilar infiltrates and subsequently diffuse mottling throughout both lungs. Lung functions tests often show considerable impairment of oxygen diffusion. A striking proliferation of granular pneumocytes, many of which disintegrate to produce intra-alveolar debris, precedes the fibrosis of the alveolar walls. Pulmonary fibrosis may also occur as a result of administration of bleomycin, salazopyrin, hexamethonium and methotrexate.

Pyrrolizidine alkaloids and anorexigens. Addition of the seeds or foliage of certain plant species of *Crotalaria* or *Senecio* to the diet of rats causes pulmonary hypertension and associated vascular disease of the lungs, with death from right ventricular failure in one or two months. The plants in question are *Crotalaria spectabilis*, a cover crop grown in the United States, *Crotalaria fulva*, used to prepare bush-tea in Jamaica and a cause of veno-occlusive disease of the liver, and *Senecio jacobaea*, the common 'ragwort' of British hedgerows. The effects of these plants are due to the pyrrolizidine alkaloids they contain.

An epidemic of primary pulmonary hypertension in Germany, Switzerland and Austria has been ascribed to the anorexigen, aminorex fumarate. There is as yet no proof of the association, and hypertensive pulmonary vascular disease has not been produced in laboratory animals fed on the drug.

Amiodarone. This is an iodinated benzofuran de-

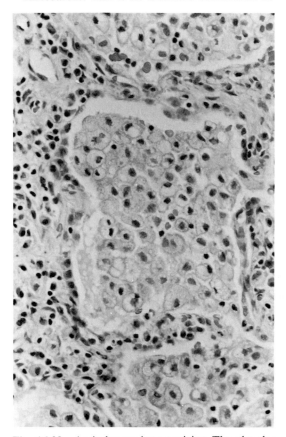

Fig. 16.38 Amiodarone lung toxicity. The alveolar spaces contain large macrophages with abundant pale foamy cytoplasm. The alveolar walls are thickened and infiltrated by plasma cells, lymphocytes and scanty neutrophils. There is patchy cuboidal cell metaplasia of the alveolar epithelium. × 300.

rivative and is used to suppress supra-ventricular and ventricular cardiac arrhythmias. In one study, 6% of patients receiving amiodarone developed serious pulmonary lesions in which large intra-alveolar macrophages with abundant pale foamy cytoplasm (Fig. 16.38) aggregate in the alveoli. Electron microscopy reveals laminated intracytoplasmic inclusions in interstitial cells, capillary endothelial cells, granular pneumocytes, bronchiolar epithelial cells, alveolar macrophages and leucocytes. The alveolar macrophages resemble those observed in rats after administration of chlorphentermine or iprindole, drugs which appear to interfere with lipid metabolism leading to the accumulation of various lipids within lysosomes. Experimental studies have shown that drug-induced phospholipidoses are reversible, suggesting that the prognosis of amiodarone pulmonary toxicity may be good providing the condition is recognized early and the drug is discontinued.

Pulmonary oxygen toxicity. One of the commonest therapeutic agents used in intensive treatment units is oxygen. The prolonged use of high concentrations of inspired oxygen can cause lung damage which may be irreversible and is potentially fatal. The free radical theory of oxygen toxicity attributes the damaging effects of hyperoxia to the intracellular production of oxygen radicals or other chemically active oxygen metabolites which inactivate enzymes, damage DNA and destroy lipid membranes. The initial damage in pulmonary oxygen poisoning seems to cause increased permeability, followed by disintegration, of capillary endothelial cells and alveolar epithelium. The alveoli become filled with oedema fluid, fibrinous exudate and extravasated blood. Hyaline membranes (p. 15.23) line the alveolar walls. If the patient survives, there may be replacement of the intra-alveolar exudate by cellular fibrous tissue which becomes incorporated into the alveolar walls. The thickened alveolar walls become lined by proliferated granular pneumocytes. It is of interest to note that some of the changes induced in the lung by oxygen toxicity are similar to those produced by the weedkiller, paraquat.

Pneumoconiosis and industrial lung diseases

Pneumoconiosis is a comprehensive term covering a group of lung diseases resulting from the inhalation of dust. This group of conditions grows continuously as fresh industrial hazards are created. The type of lung disease varies according to the nature of the inhaled dust. Some dusts are apparently inert and cause little or no damage, whereas others may cause widespread lung destruction and fibrosis. Certain dusts are antigenic and cause damage through immunological reactions, while others may predispose to tuberculosis or to neoplasia. The factors which determine the extent of damage caused by an inhaled dust include its physical state, its chemical composition, its concentration, the duration of exposure, and the co-existence of other lung diseases.

The size of the inhaled dust particles is of great importance as it is this factor which largely determines whether particles will reach the alveoli and whether they will adhere to the alveolar wall. Particle size is also important in determining whether dust will penetrate the thin alveolar epithelium or remain within the alveolar lumen. Practically all inhaled non-filamentous particles of more than $10\,\mu$m diameter are trapped in the nasopharynx, trachea and major bronchi, from where they are swept upwards, entangled in mucus, by the action of cilia. Many inhaled particles of $5\,\mu$m diameter or less gain access to the alveolar spaces, where they tend to collect in the lower halves of the upper lobes, the upper halves of the lower lobes, and the right middle lobe.

When particles measuring from 0.5 to $5\,\mu$m reach the alveolar walls, they adhere to the surface film of fluid and within minutes are ingested by macrophages. Ultra-fine particles, less than $0.02\,\mu$m in diameter, rapidly penetrate the alveolar epithelium. Coarse filamentous particles 30–$60\,\mu$m in length, such as asbestos fibres, can reach the alveoli, but they tend to slip down and lodge in the bronchi and the resulting lesions are found mainly in the lower lobes of the lungs.

The pneumoconioses may be classified according to whether the dusts inhaled are inorganic or organic.

Mineral dusts

The principal varieties are anthracosis, coal workers' pneumoconiosis, silicosis and asbestosis.

Anthracosis

This is caused by the inhalation of atmospheric soot particles; it is found in some degree in all adults, and is more marked in those who live in the highly polluted atmosphere of industrial areas. Most of the inhaled particles are removed by the normal mechanisms (pp. 8.2–4), but some are engulfed by macrophages and retained within the relatively immobile alveoli adjacent to bronchioles, blood vessels and fibrous septa, beneath the pleura and at the edges of lung scars. Some soot particles reach the lymphatic channels of the lung and are carried to the hilar lymph nodes. Anthracosis is the innocuous, well-known blackening seen in virtually every adult lung at autopsy. It may cause a minor degree of focal dust emphysema termed 'soot emphysema', but this is without clinical effect.

Coal-workers' pneumoconiosis

This is due to the inhalation of coal dust particles of less than $5\,\mu$m diameter and occurs in persons who handle soft bituminous coal with a low silica content, either in mines or by shovelling it in large quantities, as in the holds of ships. It occurs in two stages: (1) **Simple coal-workers' pneumoconiosis**, in which the lungs become impregnated with dust, leading to a minor degree of fibrosis and sometimes focal dust emphysema, which cause few if any symptoms and (2) **progressive massive fibrosis (complicated pneumoconiosis)** which develops in a small proportion of patients with simple pneumoconiosis.

Simple pneumoconiosis of coal workers. Coal dust particles reaching the alveoli are fairly evenly distributed within the lungs but maximal changes occur in the upper two-thirds of each lung. The particles are ingested by macrophages and, like soot particles (see above), are retained in relatively immobile alveoli, including those adjacent to the respiratory bronchioles in the centres of the lobules. Thus the respiratory bronchioles become surrounded by a sleeve of alveoli which are consolidated due to the accumulation of dust-laden phagocytes. The dust-laden macrophages eventually die and a network of fine collagen fibres develops in between the liberated dust particles; the aggregates also become covered by alveolar epithelial cells and thus incorporated into the alveolar walls. The upper two thirds of an affected lung contain numerous black, firm, spidery nodules and streaks measuring a few millimetres in diameter which produce a radiographic appearance known as **dust reticulation**. After several years there is fibrous obliteration of the peribronchiolar alveoli and atrophy of bronchiolar smooth muscle. The collagenous tissue then shrinks but the lung as a whole is not reduced in size, because the respiratory bronchioles dilate to produce **focal dust emphysema**, characterised by abnormal clusters of dust-blackened

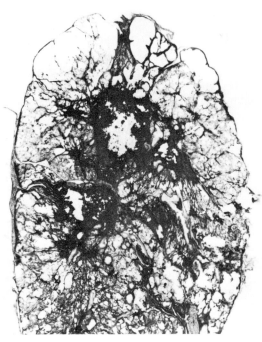

Fig. 16.40   Thick section of the lung of a coalminer, showing very severe emphysema and two foci of progressive massive fibrosis, seen as solid black areas with, in this instance, central cavitation. × 0·5.

centrilobular air spaces (Figs. 16.39, 16.19, p. 16.31). The respiratory bronchioles thus dilate and came to fill the space vacated by destruction of the adjacent alveoli.

Simple pneumoconiosis may be seen in the chest radiographs of coal workers who are free from symptoms. It appears to have no adverse effect on pulmonary function and does not significantly alter life expectancy. Coincidental chronic bronchitis in such patients may, however, cause great concern in men who are aware that their chest radiograph is abnormal.

Progressive massive fibrosis. After ten to twenty years at the coal face a small proportion of workers with simple pneumoconiosis develop massive confluent areas of fibrosis in one or both upper lobes, which may ultimately involve an entire lobe. Irregular masses of jet-black rubbery fibrous tissue with well-defined margins are present in the affected lobe, which is commonly adherent to the chest wall (Fig. 16.40). Sometimes the fibrous masses break down centrally, forming cavities filled with black fluid resembling India ink. These cavities result either from tuberculous infection or ischaemic

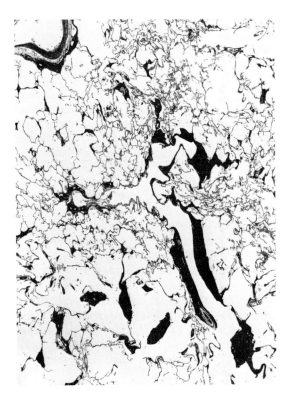

Fig. 16.39 Simple coal-workers' pneumoconiosis with focal dust emphysema, showing localisation of dust accumulation in the walls of the second order of respiratory bronchioles. × 7.

necrosis consequent upon fibrous obliteration of branches of the pulmonary artery in the affected lobe. Histological examination shows that the fibrous lesions are composed almost entirely of dense collagenous tissue arranged in bundles. Between the bundles are collections of coal dust and scattered lymphocytes. There has been considerable debate about the nature of progressive massive fibrosis and the factors which promote its development in a small proportion of cases of simple pneumoconiosis. Concomitant silicosis does not appear to be a factor. Careful examination of the lungs at autopsy, including culture and guinea-pig inoculation, yields evidence of tuberculous infection in up to 40% of cases, and some people accept that concomitant tuberculosis leads to the development of massive fibrosis in workers with simple pneumoconiosis. There is, however, a higher incidence of rheumatoid and antinuclear factors in the serum of workers with progressive massive fibrosis than in those with simple coal-workers' pneumoconiosis and the significance of immunological factors requires further study. Progressive massive fibrosis is a serious and incapacitating disease. It may develop years after exposure to coal dust has ended: eventually death results from respiratory failure, tuberculosis, or from right ventricular failure secondary to pulmonary hypertension due to a combination of chronic hypoxia from loss of lung tissue, and obliteration of major blood vessels incorporated into the fibrous masses.

Caplan's syndrome

This is characterised by rounded nodules, up to 5 cm in diameter, scattered fairly evenly throughout the lungs of workers who are exposed to inhaled dusts, including coal dust, silica and asbestos. *Rheumatoid arthritis* is usually present but occasionally the nodules develop several years before the arthritic manifestations. Rheumatoid factor is present in the blood. Cavitation and calcification of the nodules is common and clinically they may be mistaken for tuberculosis, bronchial carcinoma and secondary carcinoma. Not all patients with rheumatoid disease and pneumoconiosis develop Caplan's syndrome. The central parts of the nodules show concentric black and pale yellow rings, the pale zones frequently being liquefied.

Histologically, the lesions are modified rheumatoid nodules with a central zone of dust-laden fibrinoid necrosis, separated by a cleft from an outer layer of palisaded fibroblasts and mononuclear cells.

Silicosis

The changes of silicosis are seen in the lungs of workers who inhale fine particles of silica (SiO_2) for many years. Silica and silicosis have a world-wide distribution. Wherever rock is cut, as in granite, sandstone and slate quarries or in the mining of coal, gold, tin or copper, silica dust is likely to fill the air. In the case of coal, it is the hard anthracite variety which is accompanied by significant quantities of silica. Other workers also face the hazard, particularly stonemasons, sandblasters, boiler scalers and those involved in glass and pottery manufacture. Inhaled particles of less than $5 \, \mu m$ in diameter are liable to cause silicosis: they reach the alveoli, and, like other ducts, are phagocytosed by macrophages which tend to congregate in the relatively immobile alveolar spaces adjacent to respiratory bronchioles, blood vessels, fibrous interlobular septa, and beneath the pleura. The characteristic lesions therefore develop in these sites. Silica differs from coal dust, soot, etc., in stimulating an intense desmoplastic reaction with formation of relatively acellular collagenous fibrous tissue which is often hyaline and arranged in a concentric laminated fashion (Fig. 16.41). These silicotic nodules measure up to 5 mm in diameter and are pathognomonic of the disease. The fine silica particles are birefringent and are readily detected within the fibrous nodules by polarising microscopy. The fibrosis obliterates the lumen of bronchioles and pulmonary blood vessels. As nodules increase in size beneath the pleura, adhesions form and the pleural cavity may eventually be obliterated. At autopsy the pleura is thickened and adherent and the lungs feel gritty on cutting and palpation, due to the presence of multiple discrete fibrous nodules, some of which may coalesce to form large confluent masses of fibrous tissue. In a severe case the lungs may be largely solid. The silicotic nodules are well circumscribed and greyish-black. Some silica dust is carried to the hilar lymph nodes, which become enlarged and fibrous.

The cause of pulmonary fibrosis in silicosis is

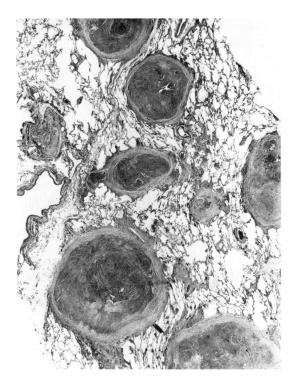

Fig. 16.41 Silicosis. The lung contains multiple nodules consisting of laminated fibrous tissue. There is no inflammatory cellular infiltrate. × 7.

uncertain. The solubility theory postulated that silica particles slowly dissolve to form silicic acid, which stimulates fibrogenesis: this is unacceptable because there is no relation between the severity of fibrosis and the solubility of different forms of silica. Two alternative but unproven biological theories are that silica is antigenic and provokes fibrosis through an immunological mechanism, and that collagen formation is stimulated by the release of lysosomal enzymes by macrophages which have ingested silica particles (p. 3.14).

Silicosis leads to progressive respiratory impairment, although twenty years' exposure may have occurred before symptoms appear. Death may be due to *respiratory failure*. Progressive fibrous obliteration of the pulmonary vasculature, together with chronic hypoxia, may induce *pulmonary hypertension* with the development of right ventricular hypertrophy and eventual failure. Silica increases susceptibility to tuberculosis, which has been observed in 10–75% of patients with silicosis and is of florid type, usually progressing rapidly to extensive tuberculous bronchopneumonia and sometimes to generalised miliary tuberculosis.

The effects of asbestos

Asbestos is a general term embracing a number of complicated fibrous silicates of magnesium of differing chemical composition and morphology. It is imported into Britain mainly from mines in South Africa and Canada. The three types of asbestos which are most important commercially are *chrysotile* (white asbestos), *crocidolite* (blue asbestos) and *amosite* (brown asbestos) which is rich in iron. Chrysotile consists of soft, curly pliable fibres which tend to split progressively into finer fibrils. Amosite and crocidolite fibres are in general rigid and harsh even when fine. The physical properties of the fibres determine the industrial use of various types of asbestos, and also influence the depth to which they travel along the airways during inspiration and thus their differing pathological effects. The behaviour of inhaled particles is determined by their aerodynamic properties as well as their size. Chrysotile fibres are apparently more likely to be retained higher up the small airways, particularly at bifurcations, while the rigid fibres of crocidolite and amosite travel readily in the air-stream and so reach the periphery of the lung. These properties may explain why chrysotile causes lesions in the lungs but rarely pleural mesothelioma (see below). All forms of asbestos are fire-resistant and are good acoustic and thermal insulators. Chrysotile can be spun into yarn and incorporated into textiles. Crocidolite and amosite are noted for their resistance to acids and alkalis. Large amounts of asbestos (mostly chrysotile) are used in asbestos-cement products for corrugated roofing, pipes, gutters, chimneys and tiles. Chrysotile is also used in the manufacture of floor tiles, brake linings, clutch facings, plastics, paint, and in asbestos-paper products including engine gaskets, roofing felts and wall coverings. Both crocidolite and chrysotile have been used for pipe and boiler lagging and as a spray with synthetic resins for thermal and acoustic insulation of buildings and ships.

Occupational exposure to asbestos occurs to a small extent in asbestos miners but more in the crushing and extraction processes which follow. Bagging of the fibre used to be a dusty

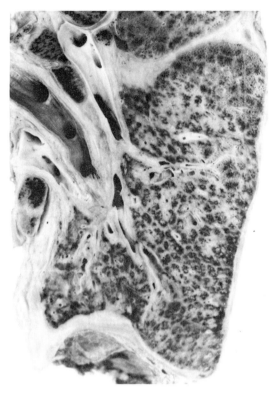

Fig. 16.42 Pulmonary asbestosis showing pronounced fibrosis and shrinkage of the lower lobe and gross pleural thickening. $\times \frac{3}{4}$.

process and before the introduction of modern methods and leakproof bags, dockers and warehouse personnel were exposed to hazard. The asbestos textile and insulation industries have produced the highest incidence of asbestosis. There is little risk associated with cutting, sawing and trimming asbestos-cement products because the fibres are trapped within the cement matrix. In Britain, rigorous standards came into force in May 1970. The most stringent rules apply to crocidolite because of its association with mesothelioma; the use of this fibre has latterly been discouraged and much reduced in many countries.

Exposure to asbestos dust may be associated with the development of *pleural fibrous plaques*, *pulmonary asbestosis* and *mesothelioma of the pleura or peritoneum*. Mesothelioma is considered on p. 16.72.

Pleural fibrous plaques. These are located in the parietal pleura on the postero-lateral aspects of the lower chest wall, mainly over the ribs, and on the diaphragm. They are bilateral,

well-circumscribed, irregularly-shaped white raised patches of hyaline fibrosis. The surface may be nodular, or smooth and polished resembling articular cartilage. Histologically the plaques consist of hyaline acellular collagenous lamellae. Extensive foci of calcification may be present. Asbestos bodies (see below) are not found in the plaques but may be detected in the lungs. Calcified parietal pleural plaques may be visible in chest radiographs but they do not produce symptoms and are free from complications. At present there is no evidence that pleural plaques are a precursor of malignant mesothelioma.

Asbestosis. This term means fibrosis of the lungs due to inhaled asbestos dust (Fig. 16.42). Chrysotile, crocidolite and amosite can all produce it, though in differing degrees of severity, probably due to differences in their penetration and retention in the lungs dependent on their aerodynamic and physical properties. The most important factors in the development of asbestosis is the amount of dust inhaled. Heavy exposure for a few years or exposure to fairly low concentrations over many years are equally likely to result in asbestosis.

Inhaled asbestos fibres ($50\,\mu$m long and $0.5\,\mu$m in diameter) are mostly retained in the respiratory bronchioles of the lower lobes. In time a number of them pass into the alveolar ducts and spaces. Experimental evidence suggests that short fibres or fragments less than $10\,\mu$m long are engulfed by macrophages, whereas larger fibres cannot be properly ingested but become surrounded by macrophages. In time, the asbestos fibres become coated with endogenous iron and protein to produce the characteristic **asbestos body** (Fig. 16.43). When well formed, these are long ($50\,\mu$m), golden-yellow or brown structures consisting of an asbestos fibre coated with layers of iron-containing protein which gives the prussian blue reaction for ferric iron (p. 11.15). The protein coat is usually segmented along the length of the fibre and bulbous at its ends, producing a 'dumbbell' or 'drumstick' appearance. It should be emphasised that *the finding of asbestos bodies in the sputum or lung is only an indication of past exposure to asbestos and is* not *proof of the presence of disease due to asbestos.* Asbestos bodies have been found at autopsy in the lungs of 20 to 60% of otherwise normal urban dwellers with no known industrial exposure to asbestos.

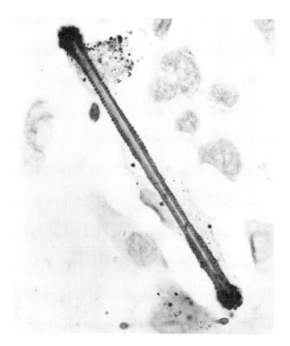

Fig. 16.43 An asbestos body in the lung. The needle-like asbestos fibre is enclosed in a crenellated protein-deposit with club-shaped ends. The body is partly enveloped by two macrophages (which also contain dust pigment), and a smaller asbestos body (below) is almost completely engulfed within a macrophage. × 900.

There is a tendency for these bodies to fragment. The mechanism by which asbestos causes pulmonary fibrosis is not understood. It has been suggested that, like silica (p. 16.59), asbestos stimulates macrophages to secrete fibrogenic lysosomal enzymes. Immunological factors may play a part: this is suggested by the finding of a high prevalence of circulating antinuclear antibody (25%) and rheumatoid factor (23%) in cases of asbestosis. Fibrosis is first evident around respiratory bronchioles and then spreads to involve alveolar ducts, atria and alveolar walls. There is progressive obliteration of alveolar spaces with compensatory dilatation of unaffected bronchioles which may progress to honeycomb lung. Asbestos bodies are found free in alveolar spaces and also enmeshed in fibrous tissue. The disease commences in the sub-pleural region of the lower lobes and causes fibrous thickening of the visceral pleura, which is quite distinct from the pleural fibrous plaques described above. Fibrosis then progresses inwards and upwards so that eventually the middle lobe and lower parts of the upper lobes may be affected.

Asbestosis causes *respiratory failure* due to destruction of lung tissue. The chief symptom is dyspnoea on effort, developing usually after 10–40 years exposure. Respiratory failure may be accompanied by *pulmonary hypertension*, which may in turn lead to right ventricular hypertrophy and failure.

Asbestosis does not predispose to pulmonary tuberculosis, but it is the only form of pneumoconiosis with a high risk of bronchial carcinoma. Approximately half of British male asbestos workers with asbestosis die of bronchial carcinoma, which arises in the vicinity of the fibrosis and is, therefore, most commonly found in the lower lobe. The neoplasm may be of any cell type but it is usually an adenocarcinoma. Surveys of the smoking habits of asbestos workers have shown only a slight increase in the prevalence of lung cancer among non-smokers. However, heavy smokers (more than 20 cigarettes a day) have an 80 to 90-fold greater predisposition to lung cancer. The combined effects of asbestos and smoking therefore appear to be synergistic rather than additive.

Other inorganic dust diseases

Pulmonary siderosis occurs in silver polishers (who use rouge containing iron oxide), arc-welders and haematite miners. Iron oxide itself appears to be almost innocuous, but often in haematite miners it is accompanied by silica and a modified form of silicosis may result: the lung becomes rusty-brown and extensively fibrosed. Microscopically, free haematite is brownish-yellow and prussian-blue negative, but after ingestion by macrophages it reacts positively. Inhalation of **beryllium compounds** induces sarcoid-like granulomas in the lung and sometimes in the liver and other organs; fibrosis and honeycomb lung may result. **Cadmium fumes** cause an acute pneumonitis with formation of hyaline membranes and fibrosis of the alveolar walls: this also may progress to honeycomb lung.

Biological dusts

Inhaled organic dusts may affect the bronchi, as in the case of byssinosis, or may produce an *extrinsic allergic alveolitis* (p. 7.14)

Extrinsic allergic alveolitis. In addition to

Table 16.3 Examples of extrinsic allergic alveolitis

Disease	Occupation	Dust Exposure	Circulating Precipitating Antibodies Against
Farmer's lung	Dairy farmers, cattle breeders	Mouldy hay	Thermophilic actinomycetes, usually *Micropolyspora faeni*
Bagassosis	Manufacture of paper and cardboard from sugar-cane bagasse	Mouldy sugar-cane bagasse	Thermophilic actinomycetes, usually *Micropolyspora faeni*
Mushroom worker's lung	Cultivation of mushrooms	Mushroom compost dust	Mushroom spores and/or *Micropolyspora faeni*
Maple-bark stripper's disease	Maple-bark stripping	Mouldy maple bark	*Cryptostroma corticale*
Suberosis	Cork workers	Mouldy oak-bark and cork dust	Mouldy cork dust
Malt worker's lung	Distillery or brewery workers	Mouldy barley, malt dust	*Aspergillus fumigatus*
Bird fancier's lung	Pigeon breeders, parrot and budgerigar fanciers, chicken farmers	Pigeon, parrot, budgerigar and hen droppings	Serum proteins and droppings
Pituitary snuff-taker's lung	Patients with diabetes insipidus	Porcine and bovine pituitary powder	Serum proteins and pituitary antigens

their causal role in asthma, inhaled organic dusts can induce in the alveoli an Arthus (type III) reaction (p. 7.13) in which circulating precipitating antibodies react with inhaled antigen. The clinical syndromes produced by this latter reaction are known collectively as *extrinsic allergic alveolitis*. Their symptoms and pathological manifestations are similar but their origins diverse. The individual diseases are generally recognised by names descriptive of their occupation or nature of the antigenic dust (Table 16.3). The clinical features consist of acute episodes of fever, headache and malaise with cough, dyspnoea and basal pulmonary crepitations, arising four or five hours after exposure to dust and persisting for twenty-four hours. There is seldom opportunity to examine the lung tissue during the acute stage of the Arthus reaction, with polymorphonuclear infiltration, acute exudation, etc. Subsequently, the alveolar walls are thickened by an infiltrate of lymphocytes, plasma cells and mononuclear cells and by sarcoid-like granulomas. Repeated exposure, as commonly occurs with bird fanciers, is associated with chronic ill health, weight loss, etc, rather than acute episodes, and leads to the development of a diffuse interstitial fibrosis which may progress to honeycomb lung. Of all the forms of extrinsic allergic alveolitis so far known, the most acute and severe is **farmer's lung** (which also occurs in cows). However, new sources of environmental contamination are constantly being found, and consequently new types of the disease emerge every year.

Byssinosis is an occupational disease which develops after many years of exposure to dust in the cotton, flax and hemp industries. The early stage presents as the syndrome of 'Monday fever': following the weekend break, the worker returns to the dusty atmosphere and after a few hours develops a characteristic tightness of the chest with a cough and scanty sputum. The symptoms persist during the day but regress for the remainder of the week. As time goes by, the symptoms persist for longer and finally progress to permanent dyspnoea with cough and sputum, and there may be severe disability. The disease is thought to be due to broncho-constriction induced by cotton dust or associated bacteria from the cotton bales. The pathological changes are indistinguishable from those of chronic bronchitis.

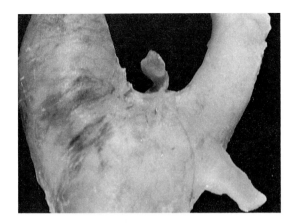

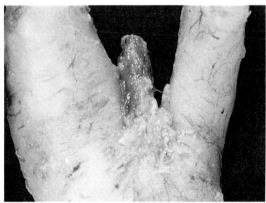

Fig. 16.44 The carotid body. *Upper*, the normal appearance (weight 10 mg). *Lower*, hyperplastic (weight 35 mg), from a 74-year-old man who died from chronic bronchitis and panacinar emphysema. Both × 3.

A note on the carotid bodies

These are ovoid bodies, a few millimetres across, lying in the bifurcation of the common carotid artery (Fig. 16.44), which is the usual source of their blood supply by glomic arteries. They are not invariably bilateral and rarely a carotid body may be double or bi-lobed. They have long been known to be chemoreceptor organs, monitoring the partial pressure of oxygen in arterial plasma and being capable of secreting catecholamines.

Hyperplasia of the carotid bodies occurs in conditions which cause chronic hypoxaemia. For example it has been observed in the dwellers in the High Andes, and also in such conditions as pulmonary emphysema (Fig. 16.44), kyphoscoliosis and the Pickwickian syndrome (obesity accompanied by narcolepsy, so-named

from the fat boy in Dickens' 'Pickwick Papers'). Perhaps more surprisingly, hyperplasia occurs also in people with systemic hypertension, and is observed in the Okamoto strain of rats which develop spontaneous systemic hypertension.

The histological features of hyperplasia of the carotid bodies are the same in hypoxaemia and hypertension. There is a striking proliferation of elongated cells between the clusters of so-called chief (type I) cells which contain neurosecretory vesicles and are regarded by many as the cells directly responsible for chemoreception (Fig. 16.45). The proliferating, elongated cells consist of sustentacular (type II) cells and Schwann cells. Both are closely associated with nerve axons, the sustentacular cells with small myelinated axons in and at the edges of clusters of chief cells, and the Schwann cells with larger myelinated axons in the interlobular connective tissue. Some fibroblasts and pericytes are associated with the proliferating sustentacular cells. There is some evidence that after prolonged exposure to chronic hypoxaemia or systemic hypertension there is focal proliferation of the dark cell variant of the chief cells.

Chemodectoma of the carotid bodies is described on p. 14.40.

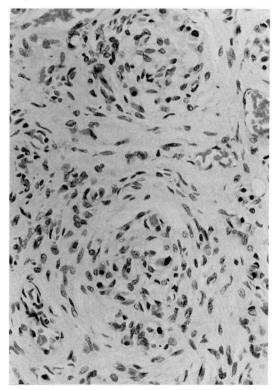

Fig. 16.45 Carotid body hyperplasia, showing proliferation of type II (sustentacular) cells. From a 69-year-old man with essential hypertension. × 270.

The Pleura

Pleural effusions

The passage of fluid in and out of capillaries is mainly dependent upon a balance between the colloid osmotic pressure exerted by the plasma proteins and the hydrostatic pressure within the capillary lumen (p. 4.7). In the systemic circulation the averages of these two forces in capillaries and venules are normally approximately equal. However, in the pulmonary circulation, which includes the vessels in the visceral pleura, the intracapillary hydrostatic pressure is only about one-third of that in the systemic capillaries, so that it is normally exceeded by the colloid osmotic pressure. In consequence the visceral pleura normally exerts a net absorptive force of about 13 mmHg on fluid accumulating in the pleural cavity.

Causes. Pleural effusions can be caused by diseases which interfere with the mechanisms that maintain the normal balance of entry and removal of water, electrolytes and protein into and out of the pleural cavity. The following are the more important causes.

Increased intracapillary pressure may cause a pleural effusion in patients with either left or right ventricular heart failure or an increased blood volume.

Increased capillary permeability is responsible for effusions complicating pleural inflammation which may be due to pneumonia, pulmonary tuberculosis, pulmonary infarction, connective tissue diseases, bronchial carcinoma, mesothelioma, subphrenic abscess and acute pancreatitis. The cells in the pleural fluid are mostly leucocytes, the numbers and types depending on the cause of the inflammation.

Hypoproteinaemia may cause pleural effusions in patients with the nephrotic syndrome or cirrhosis of the liver.

Impaired lymphatic drainage of the lung may occur in carcinomatous permeation of lymphatics and in neoplasms involving the hilum of the lung.

As with oedema fluid in general, pleural effusions may be rich in plasma proteins when they are due to increased capillary permeability, i.e. **inflammatory exudates**, or of low protein content when due to haemodynamic or osmotic disturbances or lymphatic obstruction, i.e. **trans-**udates. As elsewhere, inflammatory exudates may be serous, serofibrinous, purulent or haemorrhagic. A haemorrhagic exudate should always raise the suspicion of tuberculosis, neoplastic infiltration or pulmonary infarction.

Empyema or pyothorax is a collection of purulent exudate or pus in a pleural cavity. It may be due to infection of the pleura from the lung or occasionally from penetrating injuries of the chest wall. Less commonly infection of the pleura may arise from the bloodstream or through the diaphragm from abdominal disease such as a subphrenic abscess. In lung abscess, bronchiectasis and bronchial cancer, infection of the lung may extend into the pleural cavity and cause empyema. A post-pneumonic lung abscess may discharge both into a bronchus and into the pleural cavity, resulting in a **bronchopleural fistula** and **pyopneumothorax**. Empyema may also result from perforation of the oesophagus and mediastinitis, and as a complication of thoracic surgery. A large empyema compresses the lung, which becomes collapsed against the side of the vertebral column: a layer of granulation tissue then forms on the pleural surfaces and matures to dense fibrous tissue. This is followed by fibrosis in the collapsed lung. These changes prevent the proper expansion of the lung and hence *it is of great importance that pus in the pleural cavity should be evacuated without undue delay*. If the empyema is small, its contents may be absorbed or changed into inspissated material. Great pleural thickening, sometimes followed by calcification, is apt to occur.

Haemothorax is a collection of blood in a pleural cavity. It may be due to trauma to the chest wall and lung, or result from rupture of an aortic aneurysm. The pleural cavity may be distended with fluid and clotted blood, with associated compression-collapse of the lung on that side.

Chylothorax is the accumulation of an opalescent creamy fluid in the pleural cavity due to obstruction of, or injury to, the thoracic duct. Obstruction is commonly due to pressure exerted by enlarged mediastinal lymph nodes, while trauma may be accidental or a complication of thoracic surgery. The fluid is an emulsion of fat globules which may separate into an upper fatty layer on standing. It is odourless and alkaline, can be cleared by adding fat solvents, and stained with dyes such as Sudan III.

Pleural fibrosis

This condition, often with pleural adhesions, and sometimes with obliteration of the cavity, may follow acute pleurisy, e.g. in various pneumonias, or may be the result of chronic pulmonary lesions such as silicosis and tuberculosis, as already described. The presence of some pleural adhesions is common after middle adult life. Hyaline fibrous plaques may develop on the diaphragmatic and posterior costal portions of the parietal pleura in people exposed to asbestos.

Pneumothorax

Pneumothorax is the presence of air in a pleural cavity. It causes the lung on that side to collapse to an extent depending on the volume of air admitted. Pneumothorax may be therapeutic or traumatic, or it may arise spontaneously due to the escape of air from the lung through a hole in the visceral pleura. Traumatic pneumothorax may be due to a penetrating injury of the chest wall or it may occur accidentally during the withdrawal of pleural fluid.

Primary spontaneous pneumothorax occurs in the absence of any clinical evidence of underlying disease, most commonly in young males between the ages of 20 and 40 years. In some cases it is recurrent and rarely bilateral. Occasionally thoracotomy has revealed a tear in the visceral pleura at the site of attachment of a fibrous adhesion. The association of spontaneous pneumothorax with the Ehlers-Danlos syndrome and Marfan's syndrome (p. 14.31) is attributed to the rupture of gas-filled cystic spaces beneath the visceral pleura, formed as a result of the inherited defect of connective tissue.

Secondary spontaneous pneumothorax occurs in patients who have evidence of underlying lung disease—most commonly emphysema or active pulmonary tuberculosis. Other causes include sarcoidosis, honeycomb lung, pneumoconiosis, bronchial asthma, lung abscess, bronchiectasis, bronchial carcinoma, histiocytosis X and lymphangiomyomatosis.

Once rupture of the lung surface has occurred, air continues to escape into the pleural cavity until the pressure gradient reaches zero or until the aperture is sealed by collapsing lung tissue. Occasionally, a valve-like mechanism occurs so that air enters the pleural cavity during inspiration but cannot escape during expiration: the pressure within the affected pleural cavity then steadily increases to produce a **tension pneumothorax** leading to mediastinal shift and compression also of the opposite lung. In uncomplicated cases the hole in the pleura is sealed spontaneously and the air in the pleural cavity is gradually absorbed in a few weeks. Complications include pleural effusion, haemorrhage and infection.

Tumours of the Bronchi, Lungs and Pleura

Benign tumours. The so-called *chondroma* or *adenochondroma* of the lung forms an ovoid, largely cartilaginous mass. It usually presents as a chance finding on radiological examination as a discrete rounded shadow which requires surgical intervention to exclude a bronchial carcinoma. These tumours consist entirely of mature cartilage with clefts lined by flattened or respiratory type epithelium and with collections of adipose and fibrous tissue (Fig. 16.46). They are best regarded as hamartomas. The so-called *bronchial adenomas* are low-grade malignant tumours (see below). *Fibromas and lipomas* are very rare.

Malignant tumours

Bronchial carcinoma

This is the commonest primary tumour of the lung. At the turn of the century it was infre-

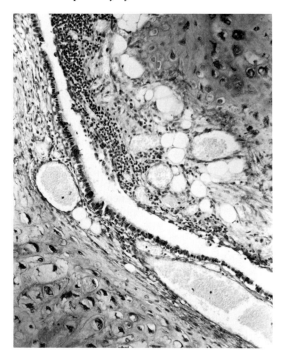

Fig. 16.46 Section of a cartilaginous hamartoma ('adenochondroma') of lung. This field shows an epithelial-lined space with cartilage on either side, some adipose tissue and blood vessels. × 50.

quent, but it has since become the commonest fatal cancer in men in many countries (Table 12.3, p. 12.16), and in women is second only to cancer of the breast. In England and Wales the annual number of deaths from cancer of the lung has risen from 6500 in 1944 to over 30 000 in 1982. Like other carcinomas, the incidence increases with age, but it is now not exceptional in young men in their thirties.

Aetiology. The most important factor in the dramatic rise in the incidence of bronchial carcinoma is the habit of **smoking, particularly cigarettes**. There is good statistical evidence that the risk increases proportionately to the consumption of cigarettes and inversely to the length of the cigarette stub left. The smoking of cigars appears to be safer and the smoking of pipes safer still. The risks have been clearly indicated by retrospective statistical studies and confirmed in a prospective study of the causes of death of medical practitioners. In the UK, the habitual smoking of twenty-five cigarettes or more a day has been shown to be associated with a 12% risk of dying from bronchial carci-

noma. *In ex-cigarette smokers the risk gradually diminishes and after ten years of abstinence it is not much greater than in non-smokers.* The mode of action of cigarette smoke is uncertain. Analysis of the 'tar' from cigarette smoke reveals at least 18 hydrocarbons, 10 of which can induce carcinomas when applied to the shaven skin of small experimental animals. There is as yet no clear relationship between atmospheric pollution and the development of bronchial carcinoma, although the incidence is higher in non-smokers who live in cities, in which the atmosphere is polluted by carcinogens, than in those living in rural areas. Recent reports also suggest that the incidence is also increased in the non-smoking spouses of cigarette smokers.

There are much rarer but established causes of bronchial carcinoma. Thus workers in the chromate industry have an abnormally high death rate from bronchial carcinoma. Other industrial workers at risk are those engaged in nickel refining, workers with asbestos and haematite miners. A much quoted example of industrial lung cancer, now of little practical importance, is that of the workers in the Schneeberg cobalt mines in Saxony. It is almost certain that radioactive substances were concerned.

Naked-eye appearances. Bronchial carcinoma presents a variety of appearances depending upon the site of origin, the extent of local spread, and the degree of bronchial obstruction produced.

Hilar type. Usually the tumour forms a mass surrounding the main bronchus to the lung or to one lobe (Fig. 16.47). The bronchial mucosa may be ulcerated or may be merely roughened and nodular. Lymphatic spread often produces further nodules in the mucosa towards the bifurcation of the trachea. The carcinoma narrows the lumen of the affected bronchus, causing obstruction. Retention of secretions then occurs and is followed by infection with consequent bronchopneumonia and abscess formation. The tumour soon spreads by the lymphatics, giving rise to massive metastases in the mediastinal nodes, which are often enveloped in the tumour mass and cannot easily be distinguished. Extension upwards into the lymph nodes of the neck is often seen. Retrograde spread also occurs along the peribronchial and perivascular lymphatics so that even the smaller bronchi and vessels may be ensheathed by

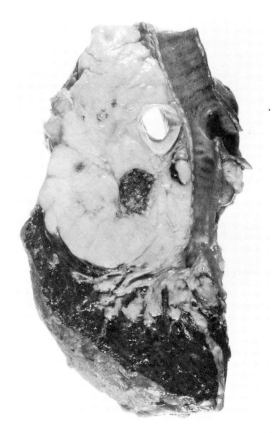

tain. Bronchiolo-alveolar carcinomas is a type of mucus-secreting adenocarcinoma which uses the alveolar walls as a stroma (Fig. 16.48). Such neoplasms may produce consolidation of large areas of the lung resembling pneumonia, the cut surface presenting a greyish, mucoid appearance.

The spread of lung cancer. The early and widespread invasion of the lymphatics has been emphasised and this may involve the pleura, forming a thick ensheathment of the surfaces or as multiple discrete nodules. Pleurisy with effusion, often haemorrhagic in character, is common. When the tumour is at the apex of the lung, extension to the adjacent thoracic cage may involve the lower cords of the brachial plexus and the sympathetic chain, so that pain and sensory disturbances occur ('*Pancoast's syndrome*'). Owing to the peripheral situation of the tumour, symptoms and signs referable to the lung may appear only late in the disease.

Metastases. Metastases are widespread and may involve virtually any organ in the body. Spread may occur to the lymph nodes of the

Fig. 16.47 Bronchial carcinoma. The main mass of tumour is at the hilum and has compressed and displaced the lung tissue. An enlarged lymph node, showing dust pigmentation and white flecks of tumour, lies within the mass. The major bronchi and pulmonary vessels are extensively infiltrated by tumour and appear thickened. The point of origin cannot be determined at this age.

whitish collars of tumour. Permeation of lymphatics just beneath the visceral pleura produces a delicate white lacework pattern, visible on the external surface of the lung. Invasion of the pericardial sac occurs by direct extension along the lymphatics around the walls of the pulmonary veins and the carcinoma may compress and occlude the superior vena cava, causing marked cyanosis. Infiltration of the heart is sometimes obvious on gross examination, and on careful histological examination of necropsy material it is found to be frequent.

Peripheral type. Less frequently the tumour originates from a peripheral bronchus and sometimes apparently arises in such a small bronchus that the exact site of origin is uncer-

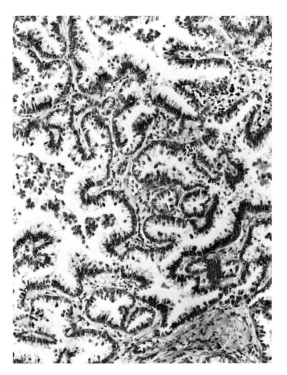

Fig. 16.48 Bronchiolo-alveolar carcinoma. The alveolar walls are lined by tall columnar neoplastic cells. × 125. (Section loaned by Dr F. Whitwell.)

neck, axilla or groin, before the primary tumour presents localising signs. Ipsilateral spread to the adrenals is common and this favours the lymphatics rather than the blood-stream as the route of spread. The kidneys, with a much larger arterial supply, are less often involved by metastases. Ipsilateral spread also tends to predominate in the liver and kidneys.

There is a special tendency to the formation of secondary tumours in the brain, which may overshadow the primary bronchial tumour clinically. Surgical exploration for a cerebral neoplasm should always be preceded by a careful survey of the lungs to exclude primary bronchial carcinoma. Metastases in the bones are common, the thoracic vertebrae being especially frequently involved, possibly by the retrograde venous route (p. 12.27). It should be kept in mind that *widespread metastasis may occur from a small and clinical silent bronchial carcinoma. Even at autopsy the primary tumour may be very difficult to find.*

Associated phenomena. Bronchial carcinoma is sometimes associated with neuropathy and myopathy mediated by humoral factors of the tumour. Cushing's syndrome with adrenal cortical hyperplasia is due to secretion of ACTH by the tumour, which is almost always of small-cell type. Other rare systemic effects of bronchial carcinoma are the carcinoid syndrome, hypercalcaemia, hyponatraemia, encephalopathies, neuropathies, hypertrophic osteoarthropathy and gynaecomastia. Migrating phlebitis and gross lymphoedema may also occur and may cause the initial symptoms.

Histological types. Lung tumours are usually classified according to the criteria recommended by the World Health Organisation (1982). There are four major histological types: *squamous-cell carcinoma, small-cell carcinoma, adenocarcinoma* and *large-cell carcinoma.* Sometimes a tumour may have a mixed histological pattern as in the so-called adenosquamous carcinoma. Precise histological classification is important because it has prognostic and therapeutic implications. In a recent large series of lung cancers the mean doubling times were estimated to be 187 days for adenocarcinoma, 100 days for squamous-cell carcinoma and large-cell carcinoma; and 33 days for small-cell carcinoma. Squamous-cell carcinomas, adenocarcinomas and large-cell carcinomas are treated by surgical resection whenever there is

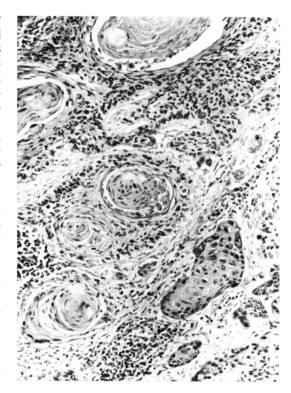

Fig. 16.49 Keratinising squamous-cell carcinoma of bronchus with well-developed cell nests. × 130. (From a section kindly loaned by Dr F. Whitwell.)

a reasonable chance of complete removal; small-cell carcinomas are treated by radiotherapy and chemotherapy because metastases are almost always present by the time the diagnosis is made.

Squamous-cell carcinoma (Fig. 16.49) usually arises in a large bronchus near the hilum. These tumours are prone to massive necrosis and cavitation, especially after radiotherapy, and cause severe or fatal haemorrhage more frequently than any other lung cancer. They probably arise from bronchial epithelium which has undergone squamous metaplasia, areas of which are frequently seen in the bronchial mucosa of cigarette smokers and patients with chronic bronchitis. In about two-thirds of cases exfoliated malignant squamous cells can be identified in the sputum.

Small-cell carcinoma also commonly arises from a main bronchus in the hilum and malignant cells can be identified in the sputum in about two-thirds of cases. Three varieties of small-cell carcinoma are recognised but their

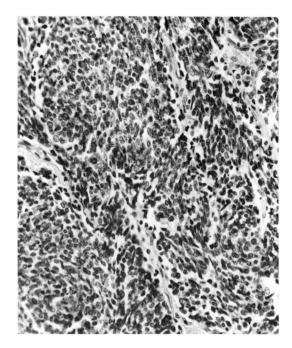

Fig. 16.50 Oat-cell carcinoma of bronchus. This neoplasm is composed of small, uniform, darkly-staining ovoid cells, with scanty supporting stroma. ×115.

biological behaviour and response to therapy are the same. All three types are highly cellular and stroma is usually scanty. The *oat-cell carcinoma* is composed of uniform small cells, generally larger than lymphocytes, with dense round or oval nuclei, diffuse chromatin, inconspicuous nucleoli, and very sparse cytoplasm (Fig. 16.50). The tumour cells appear to be separate or only loosely connected, but some are more adhesive and may palisade around small blood vessels. In some necrotic tumours, haematoxylinophilic material, consisting largely of nucleic acids, impregnates vessel walls. *Small-cell carcinoma, intermediate cell type* is composed of small cells with nuclear characteristics similar to the oat cell but with more abundant cytoplasm. The cells are less regular in size and shape than those of oat-cell carcinoma. *Combined oat-cell carcinoma* is a tumour in which there is a definite component of oat-cell carcinoma with squamous cell and/or adenocarcinoma. Small-cell carcinomas are believed to be derived from Feyrter cells in the bronchial mucosa (p. 16.8), which may explain the endocrine syndromes commonly associated with them (p. 12.43).

Adenocarcinoma. More than half of these tumours arise at peripheral sites within the lung, and malignant cells are detectable in the sputum in only about half the cases. They may be subclassified into *acinar adenocarcinoma* (Fig. 16.51), *papillary adenocarcinoma, bronchiolo-alveolar carcinoma* and *solid carcinoma with mucus formation.* Bronchiolo-alveolar carcinoma is a type of mucus-secreting tumour in which cylindrical tumour cells grow upon the walls of pre-existing alveoli (Fig. 16.48). Solid carcinoma is a poorly differentiated adenocarcinoma lacking structural differentiation, but with mucin-containing vacuoles in many of the cells. Histochemical and ultrastructural studies of pulmonary adenocarcinomas have suggested that they differentiate towards goblet cells, mucous cells of the bronchial glands, Clara cells and cells resembling granular pneumocytes. In reaching a diagnosis, special care must be taken to exclude metastasis from an adenocarcinoma in the gastrointestinal tract, pancreas or ovaries.

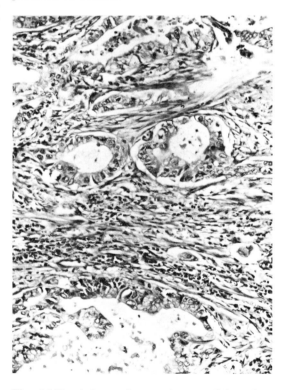

Fig. 16.51 Acinar adenocarcinoma of bronchus. The neoplasm is composed of columnar cells which form acini situated in a dense fibrous stroma. ×130. (From a section kindly loaned by Dr F. Whitwell.)

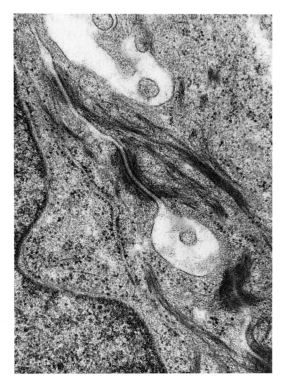

Fig. 16.52 Squamous-cell carcinoma of bronchus. Prominent desmosomes link two adjacent tumour cells. Dark bundles of tonofilaments run through the cytoplasm. Part of a nucleus at the left lower corners. × 30 500. (Dr W. Mooi.)

Large-cell carcinoma. This neoplasm is composed of cells with large nuclei, prominent nucleoli, abundant cytoplasm and usually well defined cell borders, without the characteristic features of squamous-cell, small-cell or adenocarcinomas. When large-cell carcinomas are examined with the electron microscope, they turn out to be poorly differentiated variants of squamous and adenocarcinoma.

Electron microscopy. The ultrastructural examination of bronchial carcinomas is helpful in their precise categorization, particularly in those cases in which light microscopy shows an undifferentiated type.

In squamous-cell carcinoma, the tumour cells possess prominent tonofibrils and desmosomes, but few other cytoplasmic organelles (Fig. 16.52). Adenocarcinoma cells show inter- and intra-cellular lumina lined by microvilli, and usually prominent secretory organelles (Fig. 16.53). Small-cell carcinomas show tumour cells with small dense-core neuroendocrine granules

within the sparse cytoplasm (Fig. 16.54), presumably reflecting their origin from apud cells. It is of interest that tumours which are undifferentiated on light microscopy generally show some features of differentiation, as outlined above, at the electron-microscopic level. Mixed forms of differentiation are more often detected ultrastructurally than on light microscopy alone, but their clinical significance is not yet known.

'Bronchial adenoma'

This term should mean a benign glandular tumour of bronchial epithelium. However, in practice it is used to designate a group of slowly growing malignant tumours which not uncommonly metastasise to regional lymph nodes and other organs such as the liver. A disturbing feature is that it is not possible to predict their prognosis on the basis of their histological

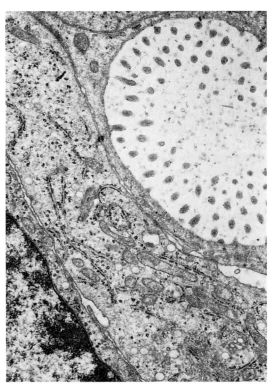

Fig. 16.53 Adenocarcinoma of bronchus. A small lumen lined by microvilli mostly transversely cut is seen at the right upper corner. The cytoplasm is rich in organelles. Part of a nucleus at the left lower corner.   × 12 500. (Dr W. Mooi.)

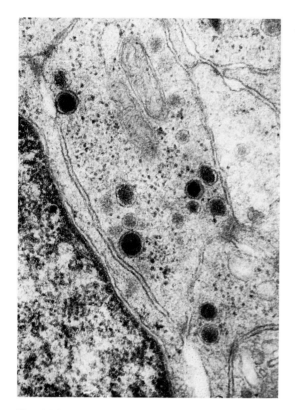

Fig. 16.54 Small-cell carcinoma of bronchus. Small dense-core (neuroendocrine) granules within the cytoplasm. × 39 000. (Dr W. Mooi.)

appearance. 'Bronchial adenomas' comprise about 1% of tumours of the lung and they occur most commonly in people under the age of 40 years and with equal frequency in the sexes. Macroscopically the tumour forms a 'dumb-bell' lesion, intraluminal growth being connected by a relatively narrow neck to invasive growth in the adjacent lung tissue. Endoscopic resection is therefore not practicable. The tumour sometimes causes haemoptysis and usually partial bronchial obstruction, with bronchiectasis beyond. Histologically, most 'bronchial adenomas' resemble the carcinoid tumours of the alimentary canal. About 50% show the argyrophil reaction (p. 19.60) and 20% show the argentaffin reaction. They occasionally give rise to the carcinoid syndrome (p. 19.60). On electron microscopy, they show characteristic intracytoplasmic secretory vesicles (Fig. 16.55). The remaining adenomas show a glandular histological pattern rather like tumours of the salivary glands: this sug-

gests that they arise from the bronchial sub-mucosal glands. These glandular variants are designated cribriform (adenoid cystic) and muco-epidermoid carcinomas.

Secondary tumours in the lung

The lung is the great filter of the bloodstream so it is not surprising that a wide variety of tumours may give rise to pulmonary metastases. Sarcomas of all types commonly metastasise to the lung by the bloodstream. Spread of carcinoma to the lungs is also common both by the lymphatics and by the bloodstream. **Spread by lymphatics** is common in *breast carcinoma*, the tumour cells of which may spread to the pleural lymphatics and thence to the lungs. *Abdominal carcinomas* may spread to hilar lymph nodes and thus extend into the lung (Fig. 12.33, p. 12.23). When the lymphatics of the lung are involved, extensive cuffing of blood vessels and bronchi may result—*lymphangitic carcinomatosis*. *Malignant lymphomas* may involve the hilar lymph nodes, and show a tendency to extend along peribronchial lymphatics, forming an encasing sheath to the bronchi. Some **blood-borne metastases** may be very large.

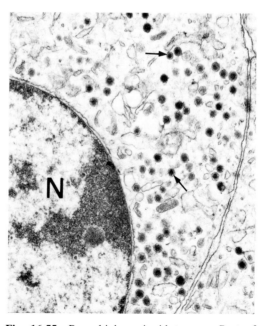

Fig. 16.55 Bronchial carcinoid tumour. Part of a neoplastic cell containing a nucleus (N) and numerous small electron-dense neurosecretory granules (arrows). × 18 750. (Dr W. Taylor.)

Such is the case with the 'cannon-ball' metastases which may originate from a renal carcinoma or from testicular tumours.

Pleural mesothelioma

Until recently this neoplasm was considered to be very rare. In 1960 a relation was noted between mesothelioma and occupational and environmental exposure to asbestos in South Africa. Since then the number of recorded pleural and peritoneal mesotheliomas has been steadily increasing in many countries. Only about 10 to 15% of the cases recorded in the UK appear to be unrelated to asbestos. On the other hand the incidence of the tumour in people with industrial exposure to asbestos is very low. In cases of pleural mesothelioma, the duration of exposure to asbestos varies from as little as three months to sixty years. The degree of exposure is, however, likely to have been intense for at least part of the time. The latent period which elapses between exposure to asbestos and the development of mesothelioma is very long, usually more than twenty years and sometimes more than forty. Because of this long delay an increasing number of mesotheliomas can be expected to occur until well into the twenty-first century. The fibre type which

has been most associated with mesothelioma is **crocidolite**. The source of exposure has usually been occupational but cases have occurred in people exposed to air pollution in the vicinity of asbestos mines and factories. The tumour affects both the visceral and parietal layers of the pleura, leading to the formation of a layer of grey-white tissue 0·5 to 3 cm in thickness, which obliterates the pleural cavity, ensheaths and compresses the lung, and extends into the interlobar fissures. Areas of necrosis within the tumour give rise to large cystic spaces containing mucinous fluid. The histological picture presents a variable pattern with either carcinomatous or sarcomatous features or a mixture of the two. The carcinomatous pattern usually consists of tubular and papillary structures in a loose stroma. The sarcomatous pattern consists of spindle cells. Asbestos bodies are seen in the lungs but not in the tumour, which is thought to be derived from the mesothelial lining of the pleura. Metastasis to hilar and abdominal lymph nodes is fairly common. A few years ago it was believed that distant metastasis did not occur: recent studies have, however, shown that secondary deposits can arise in the other lung, the liver, thyroid, adrenals, bone, skeletal muscle and brain.

Congenital anomalies

Unilateral agenesis of a lung does not in itself endanger life but other serious malformations often accompany it. Sometimes one lobe or an entire lung may be **hypoplastic**. It is not uncommon to find an excessive or diminished number of lobes in a lung and this rarely has an effect on pulmonary function. A **sequestered pulmonary segment** is one which is totally or partially separated from the normal lung. It is usually intralobar but an extralobar variety also occurs. Intralobar sequestration is observed in young adults in whom a large mass is found, usually in the lower lobe of the left lung. The sequestrated segment does not communicate with the bronchial tree and is supplied with blood from an artery which arises from the aorta above or below the diaphragm. In extralobar sequestration, which is usually encountered in infancy, the lesion is usually basal and on the left side either in the pleural cavity or within the substance of the diaphragm. It is covered by its own pleura and does not communicate with the bronchial

tree. Its arterial blood supply is derived from the aorta and its veins drain into the azygos system. Rarely, a sequestration of either variety is served by a bronchus growing directly out of the oesophagus or gastric fundus.

Congenital cysts occur and may or may not communicate with the bronchial tree. In older children and adults, congenital *pulmonary cysts* may be so altered by inflammation and fibrosis that distinction from acquired bronchiectasis and honeycomb lung may be difficult. Cysts arising near the hilum of the lung may be bronchial or derived from the foregut. *Bronchial cysts* are lined by bronchial epithelium and their walls contain cartilage, smooth muscle and bronchial glands. Some bronchial cysts may arise near to or within the wall of the oesophagus. *Enterogenous cysts* derived from the foregut are lined by gastric or intestinal epithelium. Multiple small cysts in the periphery of the lung may be congenital anomalies of the distal bronchi or may be derivatives of the visceral pleura. Multiple lung cysts may be present in patients with Marfan's syndrome.

Congenital cystic adenomatoid malformation is a rare form of diffuse hamartoma usually found in the lungs of premature or stillborn infants. The lesion is generally confined to one lobe which is greatly enlarged to form a firm, white fibrous mass containing small cysts. There is commonly mediastinal displacement to the opposite side and compression of normal lung. Microsopically, the hamartoma consists of an inter-communicating mass of tubules and spaces resembling fetal bronchioles and alveoli. Mucous glands and cartilage may be present.

References and Further Reading

Blackmon, J.A., Chandler, F.W., Cherry, W.B., England, A.C., Feeley, J.C., Hicklin, M.D., McKinney, R.M. and Wilkinson, H.W. (1981). Legionellosis. *American Journal of Pathology* **103**, 429–465.

Churg, A. (1983). Pulmonary angiitis and granulomatosis revisited. *Human Pathology* **14**, 868–83.

Dunnill, M.S. (1982). *Pulmonary Pathology*, pp. 496. Churchill Livingstone, Edinburgh.

Harris, P. and Heath, D. (1985). *The Human Pulmonary Circulation*, 3rd edn. Churchill Livingstone, Edinburgh.

Heath, D. and Williams, D.R. (1981). *Man at high altitude*, 2nd edn., pp. 368. Churchill Livingstone, Edinburgh.

Hunninghake, G.W., Gadek, J.E., Kawanami, O., Ferrans, V.J. and Crystal, R.G. (1979). Inflammatory and immune processes in the human lung in health and disease: evaluation by bronchoalveolar lavage. *American Journal of Pathology* **97**, 149–206.

Katzenstein, A-L.A. and Askin, F.B. (1982). *Surgical Pathology of Non-Neoplastic Lung Disease*, pp. 430. W.B. Saunders Company, London.

Liebow, A.A. (1973). Pulmonary angiitis and granulomatosis. *American Review of Respiratory Disease* **108**, 1–18.

Macfarlane, P.S. and Somerville, R.C. (1957). Non-tuberculous juvenile bronchiectasis: a virus disease? *Lancet* **i**, 770–71.

Morrell, M.T. and Dunnill, M.S. (1968). The postmortem incidence of pulmonary embolism in a hospital population. *British Journal of Surgery* **55**, 347–52.

Spencer, H. (1984). *Pathology of the lung*, 4th edn., pp. 1200. Pergamon Press, Oxford.

Wagenvoort, C.A. and Wagenvoort, N. (1977). *Pathology of Pulmonary Hypertension*, pp. 345. John Wiley & Sons, London.

World Health Organization Histological Typing of Lung Tumors. 2nd ed. (1982). *American Journal of Clinical Pathology* **77**, 123–136.

17

The Blood and Bone Marrow

Introduction

This chapter is devoted to abnormalities of (1) the red cells, leucocytes, and platelets of the blood, (2) disorders of the production of these elements of the blood in the haemopoietic marrow, and (3) disturbances of clotting and fibrinolysis, i.e. the haemostatic system. Lymphocytes and their disorders are considered mainly in Chapters 6 and 7 and in the following chapter on the lympho-reticular tissues. Lymphoid leukaemias are, however, included with other forms of leukaemia in this chapter.

With the exception of most of the lymphocytes, all the cells of the blood are produced in the haemopoietic bone marrow, which is also the site of platelet production, and changes in peripheral blood commonly reflect abnormalities of haemopoiesis in the bone marrow. Primary haematological diseases are less common than haematological abnormalities resulting from disease in other systems, an obvious example being the leucocytosis accompanying pyogenic infection. The connection between the primary disease and changes in the peripheral blood may, however, be obscure and the haematological abnormality may be mistakenly regarded as indicative of the primary pathology. For example, severe anaemia is a common complication of renal failure, metastatic carcinoma, or a lesion causing blood loss, while an increase in red cells may result from chronic pulmonary disease, congenital heart disease or a renal tumour.

Physical features of blood

Blood volume. The volume of circulating blood in a normal adult male is about 5 litres in men and slightly less in women. Blood volume is related to body weight, but more closely to lean body mass; it can be estimated approximately from a height/body weight nomogram. Centrifuging a column of venous blood in a glass tube shows that about 44% by volume consists of cells (*packed cell volume* or *haematocrit value*), and the remaining 56% of plasma; this procedure gives a rough estimate of the proportion of cells to plasma in the blood as a whole. A rise in the haematocrit value results either from an increase in red cell mass (*erythrocytosis*) or a decrease in plasma volume (*haemoconcentration*). Conversely, a fall in the haematocrit value may result from a reduction in red cell mass (*anaemia*) or a rise in plasma volume (*haemo dilution*). Other haematological measurements dependent on concentration (e.g. red cell count and haemoglobin level) vary in a similar way.

Blood viscosity. Specific gravity and viscosity of the blood are dependent largely on the concentration of red cells and the protein content of the plasma. Important increases in specific gravity and viscosity may thus occur in erythrocytosis and in conditions such as myeloma where there is a high concentration of globulin in the plasma; similar increases may be associated with very high leucocyte counts in leukaemia. This increased viscosity may slow the circulation and contribute to the vascular occlusive episodes sometimes found in these conditions.

Erythrocyte sedimentation rate (ESR). This is determined by placing blood, to which anticoagulant has been added, in an upright calibrated tube and observing the rate of sedimentation of the red cells, as indicated by the length of the column of plasma after a given period of time. The range of normality depends on the details of technique, and is greater for women than for men. Abnormal variations are chiefly in the direction of increased rapidity of sedimentation and are associated with increased concentration of fibrinogen or various globulins in the plasma. The test has no specific value but has been found useful as an aid to detection of organic disease in the absence of physical signs, and notably as a prognostic aid in particular conditions e.g. in tuberculosis or rheumatoid arthritis where return of the rate to normal is taken as a favourable sign. The finding of a normal ESR does not exclude the existence of serious disease.

Development of the blood cells

Sites of blood cell formation. During the first few weeks of gestation the embryonic yolk sac is the main site of haemopoiesis. At six weeks the liver becomes a haemopoietic organ and by the twelfth week is the major organ of haemopoiesis. The spleen is a minor haemopoietic organ during the hepatic phase of blood formation. Haemopoiesis commences in the bone marrow at the twentieth week of gestation and by the twenty-eighth week has become the major source of blood cells. *During childhood and adult life the bone marrow is normally the only source of new blood cells.* In infancy all marrow is haemopoietic (red marrow), but during childhood progressive replacement by fatty or yellow marrow commences in the limb bones so that by early adult life haemopoietic marrow is confined to the proximal ends of long bones, the skull, vertebrae, pelvis, ribs and sternum. In old age, even these sites become increasingly replaced by fatty marrow. In persisting haemopoietic areas about 50% of the marrow volume consists of fat cells (Fig. 8.6, p. 8.17). These changes in distribution of haemopoietic tissue determine the sites which are suitable for aspiration or trephine biopsy of the bone marrow for morphological examination. Whereas the tibial tubercle is the site of choice in infants, in older children and in adults the sternum, iliac crest and tips of the vertebral spines are the only suitable sites. Haemopoietic activity in these sites is variable and the appearance in a single sample does not necessarily represent the overall pattern. Fatty marrow is capable of reversion to haemopoiesis in certain pathological states, for example in compensatory erythroid hyperplasia in chronic haemolytic anaemias, in which there is premature destruction of red cells. Also, the liver and spleen may revert to their fetal haemopoietic function, a process known as **extramedullary haemopoiesis.** This is also seen, for example, in chronic haemolytic anaemias.

Release of cells from bone marrow. The marrow cavity is partially compartmentalised by bony trabeculae protruding into the cavity from the cortex. Haemopoietic marrow within this space is a gelatinous tissue rich in fat. The exchange vessels in the marrow are interconnecting thin-walled sinusoids. Electron microscopy has confirmed that haemopoiesis occurs in extravascular spaces between the sinusoids. Whether permanent fenestrations exist or gaps develop transiently to permit transendothelial passage of cells into the vascular system is not clear, nor are the mechanisms for control of cell release fully elucidated. Granulocytes are motile and can migrate towards the adjacent sinusoid. Megakaryocytes (which provide the platelets) usually lie close to the sinusoidal membrane and the platelets may be released from cytoplasmic processes projecting between the endothelial cells. The mechanism permitting release of the non-motile red cell is not known but cell deformability appears to be an important factor. Increased release of neutrophils in infection, or platelets in auto-immune thrombocytopenia, can occur as isolated events, whereas increased release of red cells, for example after acute haemorrhage, is usually accompanied by increased release of leucocytes and platelets. Such observations suggest that specific humoral release factors exist for platelets and neutrophils but red cell release may depend more on mechanical factors. The destruction of the sinusoidal architecture in myelofibrosis (p. 17.57), or following invasion of bone marrow by disseminated carcinoma, may explain the frequent occurrence of immature cells in the circulating blood in these diseases, although it is also a feaure of the extramedullary haemopoiesis which occurs in these conditions.

Haemopoietic stem cells. Proliferation of stem cells in haemopoietic tissue not only maintains the stem-cell pool but also provides the precursors of the red cells, granulocytes, monocytes, B Lymphocytes and platelets. Some of the stem cells enter the blood and settle in the thymus, where they are the source of T lymphocytes (Fig. 6.13, p. 6.14).

The pluripotential nature of the haemopoietic stem cell was first demonstrated convincingly by experiments involving intravenous injection of marrow cells from a normal mouse into a mouse whose own haemopoietic cells had been destroyed by wholebody x-irradiation. The injected cells were found to produce colonies of cells in the bone marrow and spleen and each colony was further shown to arise from a single stem cell. Such colonies show restricted differentiation: in the spleen over 60% differentiate into erythroid cells and these, together with megakaryocytic colonies, develop superficially in the spleen whereas mixed granulocytic/monocytic colonies develop more deeply in the organ. If the cells of a single colony are injected into a second irradiated mouse, they produce colonies of all three types. These findings have been interpreted as indicating (1) that the mouse haemopoietic stem cell is pluripotent, and (2) that the micro-environment promotes differentiation of the stem cell into a restricted precursor or progenitor cell. This technique also provided a method of assay of pluripotential stem cells, expressed as CFU-S (colony forming units—spleen).

Haemopoietic stem cells have been described as small mononuclear cells resembling lymphocytes, but they cannot yet be identified from their morphology and the numbers of human stem cells can only be estimated either (1) by studying the cytokinetics of haemopoiesis, i.e. the numbers of mitoses which occur between the stem cell and the mature red cell, megakaryocyte, granulocyte or monocyte and calculating the numbers of stem cells from the numbers of mature cells produced; or (2) by culture of bone marrow cells in a suitable gelatinous medium: this technique does not support the proliferation of stem cells, but of committed progenitor cells (Fig. 6.13, p. 6.14), each of which is capable of producing a colony of differentiating cells. In the steady state i.e. when the haemopoietic activity is constant, the numbers of progenitor cells forming colonies of monocytes and granulocytes (CFU-C), erythrocytes (CFU-E) and megakaryocytes (CFU-Mk) reflect the number of stem cells, although it is likely that some progenitor cells fail to form colonies *in vitro*. Like stem cells, committed progenitor cells cannot be identified morphologically in bone marrow.

The control of haemopoiesis

This is by no means fully understood. In the normal individual, haemopoietic activity is fairly constant and produces sufficient cells and platelets to maintain the blood levels of these elements. Excessive loss or destruction of cells or platelets is followed by a compensatory hyperplasia in the marrow with increased production until the blood levels are restored. It is thus apparent that haemopoietic activity is controlled by feedback mechanisms which depend on the composition of the blood, but the nature of these mechanisms is mostly obscure. Clearly there must be a mechanism for controlling stem-cell proliferation and the size of the stem cell pool. From the experiments outlined above, it is apparent that the micro-environment of the haemopoietic tissue plays a major role in setting the direction of differentiation of individual stem cells into committed progenitor cells. The micro-environment of the marrow and humoral stimulatory and inhibitory factors are believed to play complementary roles in the level of production of each type of blood cell.

The haemopoietic micro-environment provides factors essential for haemopoiesis, although very little is known about these. As mentioned earlier, haemo-poiesis begins in the embryonic yolk-sac, and then proceeds in the liver and spleen, followed by the bone marrow, which is the only normal site in childhood and adult life. In various pathological conditions, however, extramedullary haemopoiesis can recommence in the liver and spleen and foci of haemopoiesis can develop in the kidney, lymph nodes and peritoneum: this requires the development of a haemopoietic stroma and the ratio of erythropoiesis to granulopoiesis varies from one potential haemopoietic tissue to another. This provides confirmation that the haemopoietic stroma can direct the transformation of a stem cell into a particular type of committed progenitor cell.

Humoral haemopoietic factors. Proliferation of committed progenitor cells into clones of cells which differentiate into red cells, leucocytes or megakaryocytes is known from cell-culture studies (see above) to be influenced by humoral factors. The first of these to be recognised was the granulocyte/monocyte stimulating factor (GM-CSF or CSA—colony stimulating activity) which is produced by various human cells (p. 8.18), the richest known source being lymphocytes. Subsequently, factors have been detected which stimulate specifically the development of erythroid or megakaryocytic clones. There is also evidence of specific inhibitory factors, for example lactoferrin, the iron-binding glycoprotein present in the granules of mature granulocytes, inhibits the production and release of GM-CSF by monocytes, and various prostaglandins may have a stimulatory or inhibitory effect on proliferation of granulocyte or monocyte precursors. Humoral factors influencing red-cell production are described later.

Assessment of haemopoiesis

In many disorders of the blood, accurate diagnosis depends on estimations of the production of cells and platelets in the marrow. The traditional method is by morphological study of sections and smears of haemopoietic marrow obtained by aspiration or trephine. This provides an indication of total marrow cellularity and of the proportions of precursors of each blood cell type. The proportion of granulocyte/erythrocyte precursors is normally about 3 to 1 and variations in the ratio reflect changes in production of granulocytes or red cells. An increase in the proportion of primitive precursors ('shift to the left') of a particular cell line suggests increased proliferation or a failure of maturation. The proportion of cells in mitosis, or mitotic index, normally about 1–2%, also provides an indication of haemopoietic activity. The kinetics of haemopoiesis may also be studied by means of tritium-labelled thymidine which is incorporated as thymine into DNA and thus provides a measure of DNA synthesis. This is difficult to apply *in vivo*, but it can be used *in vitro* to measure the labelling index of cells in culture, i.e. the duration of the S phase of the cell cycle divided by the duration of the whole cycle (see Fig. 5.15, p. 5.11). The kinetics of red cell production are now well defined and are described below. The kinetics of production of leucocytes and platelets is at an earlier stage of investigation.

Erythrocyte production (Erythropoiesis)

The developing erythrocyte passes through successive changes which involve (1) progressive diminution in cell size, (2) progressive reduction of nuclear size with condensation of chromatin, pyknosis and eventual extrusion from the cell and (3) progressive loss of cytoplasmic RNA and concurrent production of haemoglobin (a unique property of erythroid cells). The earliest morphologically recognisable erythroid precursor is the **pro-erythroblast (pronormoblast)**. Between this cell and the late normoblast there exists a period of maturation and division associated with synthesis of a variety of constituents including haemoglobin, carbohydrate and various enzymes. Although this process occurs in a continuum, it is convenient to define cells at various stages of maturation as in Fig. 17.1. Three mitotic divisions occur during evolution of proerythroblast to *late normoblast* with intermitotic intervals of 16 hours, the entire process taking 48 hours in the normal subject. A number of kinetic variations occur in diseases which produce abnormal circulating red cells. A shortening of the intermitotic interval with a normal maturation time results in the formation of an increased number of cells in a given time and this is the usual response to anaemia caused by acute haemolysis or haemorrhage. When severe anaemia exists there may also be shortening of the maturation time with release of immature cells into the circulation. The number of mitoses may be reduced, notably in *megaloblastic haemopoiesis* which results from deficiency of vitamin B_{12} or folic acid. Both of these factors are necessary for synthesis of DNA in the S phase of the cell cycle (p. 17.36), and their deficiency results in accumulation in the marrow of abnormal large

erythroblasts termed *megaloblasts*: the nucleus is large with a finely reticulated chromatin pattern and abundant cytoplasm which becomes haemoglobinised as usual (Fig. 17.2). Red cell production is diminished and the cells are unduly large (*macrocytes*). These changes are described in detail on pp. 17.35–38. By contrast, in iron deficiency additional mitoses occur with production of unduly small red cells (*microcytes*).

The **reticulocyte** is the young red cell remaining after ejection of the nucleus from the late normoblast. Maturation of the reticulocyte to the mature **erythrocytes** takes 48 to 72 hours, of which the last 24 hours are spent in the circulation. Reticulocytes contain both polyribosomes and mitochondria and are thus still capable of synthesising both globin and haem. In a Romanowsky-stained peripheral blood smear the reticulocyte is larger than the mature erythrocyte and possesses a distinctive diffuse basophilia described by the term polychromasia. To count reticulocytes accurately, supravital staining is necessary using either brilliant cresyl blue or New methylene blue. *The reticulocyte count in the peripheral blood is the most commonly used clinical measurement of erythropoietic activity* and is usually expressed as a percentage of the erythrocyte count. More accurate measurements are provided by (a) the absolute reticulocyte count ($\times 10^9/1$) or (b) the reticulocyte index, which corrects the reticulocyte percentage for haematocrit level assuming the normal haematocrit to be $0.45 \, 1/1$ (45%).

Mediators of erythropoiesis. In order to maintain haemopoietic populations in their normal steady state or to adapt to stress or environmental change, a series of regulatory mechanisms must exist at each developmental stage. It is now recognised that control of haemopoietic cell proliferation is effected by a series of integrated inhibitor/stimulator feedback loops. The proliferation and progressive differentiation during erythropoiesis is under the control of **erythropoietin**, a hormone derived from a plasma α_2-globulin (probably produced in the liver) by the action of **erythrogenin** which is produced in the kidney. Tissue hypoxia resulting, for example, from a reduced total red cell mass in anaemia or following haemorrhage triggers increased erythropoietin production, which in turn stimulates erythropoiesis. As the red cell mass returns to normal, erythropoietin

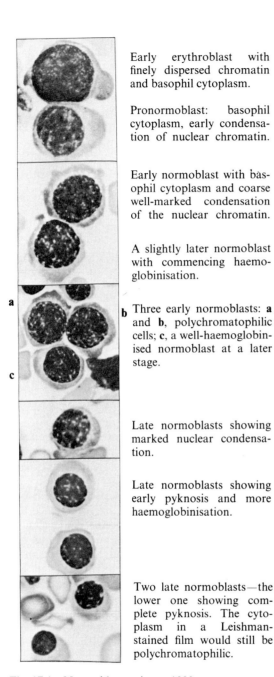

Early erythroblast with finely dispersed chromatin and basophil cytoplasm.

Pronormoblast: basophil cytoplasm, early condensation of nuclear chromatin.

Early normoblast with basophil cytoplasm and coarse well-marked condensation of the nuclear chromatin.

A slightly later normoblast with commencing haemoglobinisation.

Three early normoblasts: **a** and **b**, polychromatophilic cells; **c**, a well-haemoglobinised normoblast at a later stage.

Late normoblasts showing marked nuclear condensation.

Late normoblasts showing early pyknosis and more haemoglobinisation.

Two late normoblasts—the lower one showing complete pyknosis. The cytoplasm in a Leishman-stained film would still be polychromatophilic.

Fig. 17.1 Normoblast series. × 1000.

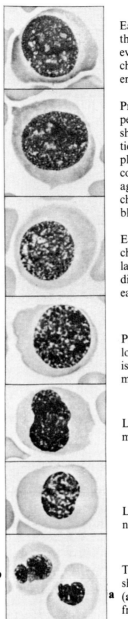

Early erythroblast: note the basophil cytoplasm and evenly dispersed nuclear chromatin containing several nucleoli.

Promegaloblast: nucleoli persist, nuclear chromatin shows commencing fine reticular condensation, cytoplasm basophilic. Note contrast to the coarse aggregation of nuclear chromatin in the normoblast series.

Early megaloblast: nuclear chromatin is finely reticulate, cytoplasm shows diminished basophilia and early haemoglobinisation.

Polychromatophilic megaloblast with haemoglobinisation in advance of nuclear maturation.

Later polychromatophilic megaloblast.

Late megaloblast with some nuclear condensation.

Two late megaloblasts, one showing nuclear pyknosis **(a)** and the other nuclear fragmentation **(b)**.

Fig. 17.2 Megaloblast series. × 1000.

production is reduced. Primarily, erythropoietin controls the rate at which the committed erythroid progenitor (CFU-E) gives rise to pronormoblasts, but it also influences the rate of maturation, synthesis of haemoglobin and release of red cells from the marrow into the circulation. Erythropoietin may be detected in both plasma and urine and a number of assays exist for its measurement, but none is yet suitable for routine use.

'End-product feedback' is yet another mechanism for regulation of erythropoiesis and implies that products released by red cell destruction may influence the rate of red cell production. Thyroxine, growth hormones and androgens stimulate erythropoiesis by increasing erythropoietin production. Helper T cells also influence erythropoiesis but only in the presence of erythropoietin.

Measurement of erythropoiesis. Assessment of the extent, rate and effectiveness of erythropoiesis frequently provides important clinical information. The reticulocyte level in peripheral blood is the most frequently used index of erythropoietic activity and is raised in proportion to the degree of anaemia when erythropoiesis is effective (see below). Elevation of the reticulocyte count occurs following haemorrhage or haemolysis, and during the treatment of deficiency states by specific haematinics (vitamin B_{12}, iron, etc.). Conversely, the reticulocyte count is low when erythropoiesis is ineffective (i.e. is not progressing normally to the stage of red cell production, as occurs, for example, in untreated megaloblastic anaemia). Assessment of overall marrow cellularity and estimations of the myeloid:erythroid (M:E) ratio provide simple tests of total erythropoiesis. The normal M:E ratio ranges from 2·5:1 to 12:1. This does not, however, provide a test of the effectiveness of marrow function. For the latter, ferrokinetic studies must be performed which analyse the fate of an injected dose of radioactive iron. A variety of measurements may be made. From the plasma iron clearance, i.e. the rate of clearance of transferrin-bound iron from the plasma and the plasma iron content, it is possible to calculate the plasma iron turnover (normally 72–144 μmol/1/day). Most iron leaving the plasma is taken up by erythroblasts and reticulocytes and the iron turnover is therefore related to the total amount of erythropoietic tissue, both effective and ineffective. Plasma iron turnover rises or falls in proportion to erythropoietic activity. Reappearance of radioactive iron in circulating red cells provides an indication of effective erythropoiesis. Normally, 70–80% of the administered iron is so utilised and can be detected 7–9 days after injection. Finally, sites of erythropoiesis may be demonstrated by *surface counting* radioactivity over various parts of the body e.g. spleen, liver and sacrum. Using these tests, functional diagnoses of a variety of important haematological diseases may be made.

Granulopoiesis

The development of granulocytes in the bone marrow is described on p. 8.16 in relation to leucocytosis.

Platelet production

Platelets are produced by mature megakaryocytes in the bone marrow (Fig. 17.3) and released into the blood. The megakaryocyte arises from the haemopoietic stem cell by an unknown number of cell divisions, followed by repeated divisions of its nucleus in a common cytoplasm (endomitotic replication). The cytoplasm of mature megakaryocytes differentiates into platelets. There is approximately one megakaryocyte per 500 nucleated red cells in the bone marrow. It is probable that platelet production is regulated by a humoral factor, corresponding to the regulation of erythropoiesis by erythropoietin.

The red cell

Primary red cell measurements. The conventional basic red cell measurements include the red blood cell count, the packed cell volume, and the haemoglobin concentration. *The red cell count* (RBC) is of diagnostic value in only a minority of blood diseases, but, since the advent of electronic cell counters, it can be performed as quickly and accurately as the measurement of the haemoglobin concentration. Direct measurement of the **packed cell volume (PCV or haematocrit)** is determined by centrifuging whole blood in a capillary tube at 12 000 g for 3–5 minutes. During this procedure a certain amount of plasma remains trapped in the red cell column, variously estimated at 1·5–3·0% for normal individuals, but considerably more in certain disease states in which the red cells are distorted, including spherocytosis (p. 17.22), iron deficiency, thalassaemia (p. 17.27) and sickle cell disease (p. 17.26). Electronic cell counters use indirect methods for calculation of the PCV which exclude trapped plasma and therefore give lower PCV values. This is of importance in the interpretation of absolute values calculated from RBC, PCV and Hb concentration (see below). **The haemoglobin con-**

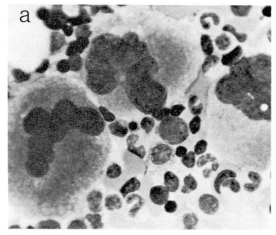

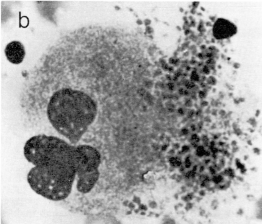

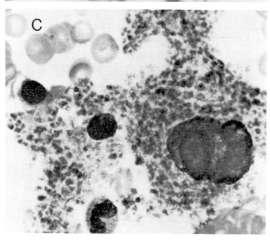

Fig. 17.3 Megakaryocytes and platelets. **a**, Young megakaryocytes with commencing granulation. × 900. **b**, More advanced cell showing partial conversion of the cytoplasm to platelets. × 600. **c**, Mature megakaryocyte with platelet formation throughout the cytoplasm. × 600.

centration (Hb) in g/dl* is measured photometrically following red cell lysis and conversion of haemoglobin to cyanmethaemoglobin. The range of normal values for all three basic measurements is wide (Table 17.1) and for any

Table 17.1 Normal adult values expressed as mean ± 2 SD.

	RBC ($\times 10^{12}/1$)	PCV (1/1)	Hb (g/dl)
Male	5.5 ± 1.0	0.47 ± 0.07	15.5 ± 2.5
Female	4.8 ± 1.0	0.42 ± 0.05	14.0 ± 2.5

given individual, significant fluctuations can occur within the accepted range. The normal range varies with age, sex and elevation above sea level

Absolute values. Anaemias can be classified on a morphological basis by microscopic examination of stained peripheral blood smears to assess the *size of blood cells* and their *degree of haemoglobinisation*. A similar but quantitative assessment can be made using the basic red cell measurement of RBC, PCV and Hb, to obtain estimates of average volume of red cells, the average amount of haemoglobin in each cell, and the concentration of haemoglobin in the red cells. The **mean cell volume (MCV)** is calculated by dividing the PCV (1/1) by the RBC ($\times 10^{12}/1$), the resultant volume being expressed in femtolitres (fl). The **mean cell haemoglobin (MCH)** expresses the average amount of haemoglobin per red cell and is derived by dividing the haemoglobin concentration in g/l by the red cell count ($\times 10^{12}/1$), the result being expressed in picograms (pg). The **mean cell haemoglobin concentration (MCHC)** measures the concentration of haemoglobin in g/dl of red cells and is obtained by dividing the haemoglobin concentration of whole blood (g/dl) by the PCV (1/1). Normal ranges for MCV, MCH and MCHC are shown in Table 17.2. *The absolute values are uninfluenced by age, sex and altitude.* Obviously, these values will be influenced by any inherent errors in the individual measurements on which they are based. Using manual methods, the MCHC was the most accurate absolute value because, being calculated from the Hb and PCV only, the major errors

*The World Health Organisation has recommended a change in the unit of measurement for Hb from g/dl to g/l.

Table 17.2   Normal ranges of red cell absolute values

Mean cell volume (MCV)	80 – 100 fl
Mean cell haemoglobin (MCH)	27 – 32 pg
Mean cell haemoglobin concentration (MCHC)	30 – 36 g/dl

associated with manual red cell counting were avoided. Using such techniques the MCHC could range from as low as 26 g/dl in iron deficiency anaemia to 40 g/dl in hereditary spherocytosis (p. 17.22). On the introduction of electronic cell counters the range has contracted to 30–36 g/dl and study of this phenomenon revealed that the previous wide range was a measure of variation in plasma trapping (see above). The degree of accuracy of red cell counting now achieved by automated counters has made the MCV and MCH prime diagnostic measurements (Table 17.3). Less use is now made of the MCHC, although it provides an important quality control measurement for automated counters.

The red cells of an individual are never totally uniform in volume, but exhibit a range of volumes. In traditional clinical practice the average or mean cell volume is widely used. The automated determination of 'average' volumes gives useful information in cases of marked abnormality, but it suffers from two inherent weaknesses: (a) it is insensitive to minor but significant variations at extremes of the volume distributions and will, therefore, miss some abnormalities and (b) it is incapable of detecting the presence of more than one population of red cells. Accordingly, the manufacturers of automated cell counters have concentrated, in recent years, on the analysis of cell volume distributions. These may be displayed graphically (Figure 17.4) or they may be analysed mathematically to provide a quantitative measure of the dispersion by volume of red cells in a given patient (expressed as standard deviation of coefficient of variation of the population distri-

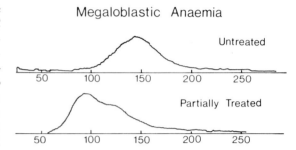

Megaloblastic Anaemia

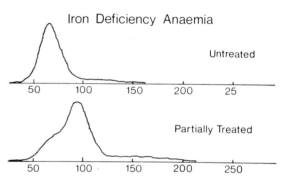

Iron Deficiency Anaemia

Fig. 17.4   Red cell volume distributions in untreated and partly treated megaloblastic anaemia (above) and untreated and partly treated iron-deficiency anaemia (below).

bution under study). Modern automated cell counters routinely provide information on red cell volume distribution both in graphical and numerical form, the dispersion measurement used being called the **red distribution width** (**RDW**). The RDW thus indicates the amount of variation in cell volumes and is a measure of anisocytosis (*see below*): it is increased in iron deficiency and in megaloblastic anaemias.

Table 17.3   Morphological classification of anaemias

	Absolute values	
Type of Anaemia	MCV	MCH
Normocytic, normochromic	normal	normal
Microcytic, hypochromic	low	low
Macrocytic, normochromic	high	normal

Examples of multiple red cell populations are shown in Fig. 17.4.

Erythrocytosis. Chronic hypoxia from any cause, e.g. chronic respiratory or heart failure, congenital heart disease or living at high altitude, stimulates erythropoietin production with consequent increase in erythropoiesis and the red cell count may be above the normal range (*erythrocytosis*). This condition is sometimes termed secondary polycythaemia, which is inappropriate because it implies increase also in granulocytes and platelets, as in primary polycythaemia (*polycythaemia rubra vera*), a neoplasm of haemopoietic tissue. Only the red cells are increased in erythrocytosis and when due to hypoxia it can be regarded as a compensatory effect. *Rarely*, erythrocytosis results from increased formation of erythropoietin due to secretion of erythrogenin by certain tumours—most commonly renal carcinoma—or by cystic lesions or ischaemia of the kidney.

Morphological changes in red cells

Red blood cells vary little in size and shape in healthy individuals. The majority of red cells are biconcave discs, smooth in contour, and of average diameter $7.0\,\mu m$ (range $6.0-8.5\,\mu m$). The diameter of the nucleus of the small lymphocyte is also $7\,\mu m$ and serves as a useful gauge. In a normal blood film up to 10% of red cells may appear oval rather than round and a very small number of irregularly contracted cells and red cell fragments may be observed (less than 0.1% in adults and children but rather more in neonates). Because the red cell is a biconcave disc, staining is heavier around the periphery of the cell, the central area being pale. This area of central pallor should not normally exceed one-third of the total surface of the cell (**normochromia**).

Changes in size and shape. Anaemia is frequently associated with abnormal variation in erythrocyte size (**anisocytosis**) and irregularities in shape (**poikilocytosis**). Abnormally large cells, macrocytes, are numerous in megaloblastic anaemias, aplastic anaemia and liver disease. Although red cell fragments are also frequently present in megaloblastic anaemia (Fig. 17.5), the average size (MCV) of the red cells is usually greater than normal and the anaemia is described as **macrocytic**. Abnormally small cells or **microcytes** occur in all forms of anaemia, but

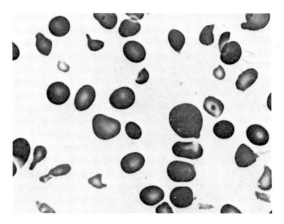

Fig. 17.5 Red cells in pernicious anaemia, prepared from below the buffy coat, showing gross anisopoikilocytosis. × 650.

in certain types they predominate so that the average size of cells is diminished. Iron-deficiency anaemia and thalassaemia are typical causes of **microcytic anaemia**.

Small poikilocytes may occur in any severe anaemia (Fig. 17.5). While their presence is of no absolute diagnostic importance, they are usually prominent in megaloblastic anaemia (p. 17.35) and may appear even before the anaemia is pronounced. Mechanical injury of red cells by intravascular fibrin in micro-angiopathic haemolytic anaemia (p. 17.32), may result in the appearance of numerous triangular, helmet-shaped cells in the circulation (Fig. 17.6), often along with obvious red cell fragments (**schistocytes**).

The term **spherocytosis** is applied to red cells which have assumed a globular shape and so are reduced in diameter and appear uniformly densely stained. Spherocytosis is associated with abnormalities of the red cell membrane and a reduced red cell lifespan. Other morphological changes are associated with genetic errors of haemoglobin structure e.g. a sickle shape assumed by de-oxygenated cells containing HbS (p. 17.26) and the abnormally thin cells which sometimes have a central area of thickening (**target cells**) found in thalassaemia and other haemoglobinopathies. In hereditary **elliptocytosis** the majority of the erythrocytes are oval but in most instances this is a harmless trait.

Variations in haemoglobin content. Reduction in the amount of circulating haemoglobin may be the result of diminution in the

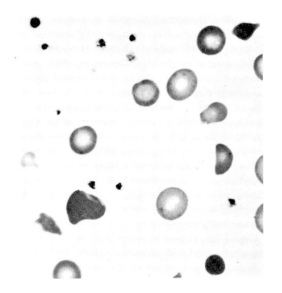

Fig. 17.6   Fragmentation of red cells in microangio-pathic haemolytic anaemia. × 1000.

numbers of circulating red cells, in the *size* of the red cells, their *concentration of haemoglobin*, or any combination of these. For example, in megaloblastic anaemia, reduction in the number of red cells is the cause of the anaemia; the increase in size of the individual cells does not compensate for this. By contrast, the anaemia of iron-deficiency states is due initially to a reduction in red cell size (MCV) and also in MCH but a reduction in cell numbers eventually contributes to the anaemia. In established iron deficiency, the cells show staining only at the periphery (**hypochromia** or '*ring-staining*'—Fig. 17.29). Iron deficiency is the most common but not the only cause of hypochromia, which occurs also in sideroblastic anaemia, the anaemia of chronic infection (defective haem synthesis) and in thalassaemia (defective globin synthesis). The term **anisochromia** describes a mixture of normochromic and hypochromic red cells and is seen in iron-deficiency anaemia responding to treatment, following transfusion of normal cells to a patient with a hypochromic anaemia, and in sideroblastic anaemia.

Polychromasia and reticulocytosis. If a film of normal blood is stained by a Romanowsky method, practically all the erythrocytes are purely eosinophilic. In some conditions, however, a proportion of the erythrocytes show a superimposed slight bluish-violet tinge and the term

polychromasia is applied to this double staining. These are young cells which have recently lost their nuclei but still retain ribosomal RNA to give a basophilic tinge to the otherwise eosinophilic haemoglobin-rich cytoplasm. As these young cells mature in the circulation, the polychromasia gradually disappears and they become normochromic. The young erythrocytes tend also to be slightly larger than older ones. By supravital staining with certain dyes, e.g. brilliant cresyl blue, any RNA remaining in the erythrocytes is precipitated or condensed within the cells as a sharply-stained skein or reticulum and such young cells are therefore called **reticulocytes** (Fig. 17.7). They are normally present in a proportion of less than 1% in males but may rise to 2% in females after menstrual loss. It is preferable to report the reticulocyte count in absolute numbers (normal range $10-100 \times 10^9/l$) rather than as a percentage of the total red cell count (range $0.2-2.0\%$) (see p. 17.4).

Red cell inclusions. Various inclusions may be present in erythrocytes; some are vestiges of cell elements lost during maturation, while others are due to pathological changes in the cells. A normal function of the spleen is to remove such inclusions from erythrocytes without destroying the cells themselves; this is achieved in the red pulp and is known as the 'pitting' function of the spleen. If the spleen has been

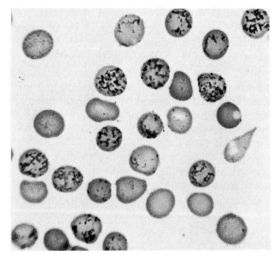

Fig. 17.7 Blood smear in haemolytic anaemia, showing numerous reticulocytes containing various amounts of reticulum. Supravital staining with cresyl blue. × 100.

removed, is atrophied or is congenitally absent, cells with such inclusions may be present in large numbers in the circulation without necessarily indicating any blood disorder.

Pappenheimer bodies are small, deeply basophilic granules, usually solitary and less than 1 μm in diameter, which give a positive prussian blue reaction for ferric iron. Red cells containing them are abundant in the blood of adults after splenectomy and are present in some erythroblasts in normal marrow (sideroblasts).

Howell-Jolly bodies are granules of nuclear chromatin, 1–2 μm or more in diameter (Fig. 17.25, p. 17.36). If very small they resemble Pappenheimer bodies but they are iron-negative. They are most common in the red cells in macrocytic anaemias, but are also found in various other blood disorders or following splenectomy, even in haematologically normal individuals.

Heinz bodies are not visible in Romanowsky-stained films but they are readily demonstrated in supravital methyl violet preparations (Fig. 17.18, p. 17.25) or when stained by brilliant cresyl blue. They consist of granules of denatured globin, and are numerous in many forms of chemically-induced haemolytic anaemia, especially those caused by oxidant drugs (*see below*). Evidence of oxidative change of the iron in the haem moiety (producing methaemoglobin) often co-exists. Heinz bodies are seen when the blood of patients with unstable haemoglobin disease (p. 17.27) is incubated. A few Heinz bodies are seen following splenectomy.

In *punctate basophilia* some of the red cells contain clumps of RNA seen as minute blue granules in smears stained with Romanowsky dyes (Fig. 17.8). This is observed mainly in infections, intoxications such as chronic lead poisoning and in red cell injury by haemolytic chemicals, but can also occur in other types of anaemia.

Presence of erythroblasts. The term **erythroblast** is used throughout to mean nucleated red cells at all stages of maturity; normally in the adult they are present only in the marrow but they appear in the blood in various conditions.

Normoblasts are late erythroblasts, about the size of an ordinary red cell or a little larger, and have a single spherical nucleus which is condensed and thus stains very deeply. The chromatin appears as a course network, or may

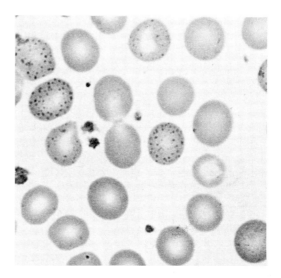

Fig. 17.8 Blood smear showing punctate basophilia. × 1250.

be very dense and practically homogenous in the pyknotic nuclei of the more mature normoblasts (Fig. 17.1). The presence of normoblasts in the blood is a characteristic feature in extramedullary haemopoiesis, but may develop suddenly, together with reticulocytosis, in acute anoxic states e.g. in acute cardio-respiratory failure, or during an active marrow response to haemorrhage or haemolysis.

When megaloblastic change (p. 17.4) takes place in the marrow, megaloblasts may appear in the blood and are most easily found in buffy coat smears (a smear of the top layer of cells including most of the leucocytes, in a centrifuged preparation of blood).

Leucocytes

The three classes of leucocytes in the blood, granulocytes (polymorphs), monocytes and lymphocytes, differ in their precursor cells, their morphology and their functions. The three types of **granulocytes**—neutrophil, eosinophil, and basophil—originate in the bone marrow (p. 8.16). The neutrophil granulocytes, as already explained in Chapter 4, are concerned in inflammatory reactions and their chief function is the phagocytosis and digestion of micro-organisms and other foreign materials, damaged tissue elements, dead cells and immune complexes. The eosinophil granulocytes increase in the blood and appear in the lesions of patients with atopic hypersensitivity (p. 7.9) and in parasitic infestations, in which they play a defensive role. The **monocytes** of the blood are also phagocytic; they belong to the mononuclear phagocyte system (p. 4.33) and provide most of the macrophages in inflammatory lesions. Disturbance of the functions of neutrophil granulocytes and monocytes, with consequent tissue injury, is a feature of certain types of hypersensitivity reaction (Chapter 7). The origins of **lymphocytes**, and their essential function in immune responses and reactions have been considered in Chapters 6 and 7.

Increase or decrease of the leucocytes in disease can affect any or all of the different types. In practice, increase in the total number above $11 \times 10^9/1$ is termed **leucocytosis** while diminution below $4 \times 10^9/1$ is termed **leucopenia**; to determine the absolute numbers of different types of leucocytes, it is necessary to determine the total number and also the proportion of different types by performing a *differential leucocyte count* on a stained film. The normal range of numbers of the leucocytes in adults is shown in Table 17.4. The advantage of determining the absolute numbers for each class, rather than percentages, must be stressed.

Table 17.4 The normal numbers of leucocytes

	No. $\times 10^9/1$	No. per μl blood
Granulocytes		
neutrophil	2·0 — 7·5	2000 — 7500
eosinophil	0·04 — 0·4	40 — 400
basophil	0 — 0·1	0 — 100
Lymphocytes	1·5 — 4·0	1500 — 4000
Monocytes	0·2 — 0·8	200 — 800
Total WBC	4·0 — 11·0	4000 — 11 000

Neutrophil granulocytes

An account of the production of neutrophil granulocytes and of **neutrophil leucocytosis,** with its accompanying myeloid hyperplasia of the haemopoietic marrow, is given on pp. 8.15–19). The commonest cause is *bacterial infection* which should always be suspected, particularly in the range $15-25 \times 10^9/1$, and occasionally causes counts up to $50 \times 10^9/1$. Moderate rises may accompany *tissue necrosis* without infec-

tion in such diverse conditions as myocardial infarction, burns, crush injuries and rapidly growing *cancers* which tend to outgrow the blood supply and become necrotic; leucocytosis also develops within a few hours after a large *haemorrhage*, passing off after a day or so; *acute haemolysis* (abnormal destruction of red cells) is also accompanied by a neutrophil leucocytosis, and *drug reactions* e.g. to steroids, sometimes promote a leucocytosis. In any active neutrophil leucocytosis, the proportion of young neutrophils in the blood increases (Fig. 17.9)

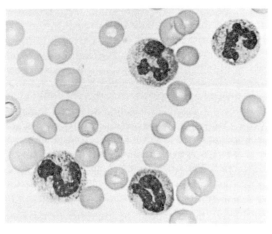

Fig. 17.9 Blood smear in neutrophil leucocytosis. $\times 850$. (Dr. I. Evans.)

and myelocytes or metamyelocytes may also be found ('shift to the left'). Another change is a moderate increase in neutrophil alkaline phosphatase. In severe infections and toxic states the neutrophil granulocytes may show morphological evidence of damage; their cytoplasm contains deeply-staining granules showing abnormal variations in size (*toxic granulation*) and their nuclei fail to undergo the normal degree of segmentation. More severe toxic injury results in failure of production of granulocytes and leucopenia is thus a grave sign when associated with severe infection by pyogenic bacteria. Reactive neutrophil leucocytosis as described above may be regarded as a physiological reaction on the part of the granulopoietic marrow. By contrast, the neutrophil leucocytosis which occurs in chronic granulocytic leukaemia is not a controlled response to a known stimulus but is of neoplastic nature.

Leukaemoid reaction. This consists of a

reactive outpouring of leucocytes with the appearance of immature forms including myelocytes, promyelocytes and even myeloblasts and requires to be distinguished from chronic granulocytic leukaemia. The phenomenon is seen in severe and chronic infections (notably haematogenous tuberculosis), in severe haemolysis and occasionally with some solid cancers e.g. of the breast, kidney, lung and metastatic tumour: the precise mechanism is unknown. The total leucocyte count may be as high as 50–$100 \times 10^9/1$. The cells show toxic granulation and the neutrophil alkaline phosphatase score is high (c.f. chronic granulocytic leukaemia). Occasionally a lymphocytic leukaemoid reaction may occur.

Leuco-erythroblastic reaction. This term denotes the presence in the circulation of immature granulocytes accompanied by substantial numbers of nucleated red cells. Although not uncommonly seen in patients with massive haemorrhage, severe haemolysis, acute hypoxia or severe infection e.g. miliary tuberculosis, the most common causes are invasion of the bone marrow by metastatic cancer and lymphomas, leukaemia and myelofibrosis.

Neutrophil leucopenia (Neutropenia) occurs both as an isolated haematological feature and also as part of a reduction of all cell types in the blood (**pancytopenia**). Neutropenia can result either from failure of the marrow to produce adequate numbers of neutrophils or from excessive peripheral destruction or consumption of these cells. Examples of the former include bone marrow aplasia (p. 17.43) bone marrow replacement with secondary tumour, leukaemia, myeloma or severe megaloblastic anaemia (p. 17.35). Toxic chemicals (e.g. benzene), ionising radiation and the cytotoxic drugs used in the treatment of malignant disease cause predictable depression of the bone marrow. Marrow production may also be severely depressed in overwhelming infections such as septicaemias and disseminated tuberculosis, and neutropenia in such conditions is a bad prognostic sign. Many acute virus infections cause a temporary neutropenia but the mechanism is uncertain. A large number of different drugs can cause neutropenia, the most important being phenylbutazone, chlorpromazine and other phenothiazines, sulphonamides and related compounds e.g. cotrimoxazole and sulphasalazine, frusemide and antithyroid

drugs. In large doses many compounds may depress the marrow but neutropenia more often results from the development of an idiosyncrasy towards a particular compound, subsequent administration of even a small dose being capable of inducing the condition. Such idiosyncrasy is usually unpredictable, although the risk is probably greater in people prone to hypersensitivity reactions. *In every case of severe neutropenia the possibility that it is drug induced must be thoroughly investigated.*

The term **agranulocytosis** is now commonly reserved for a well-defined syndrome consisting of marked neutropenia and severe infection of drug-induced origin. It is thought that the mechanism of neutropenia is immunological, circulating neutrophils, coated by a drug-antibody complex, being preferentially removed by the mononuclear phagocyte system. Alternatively a drug which does not bind to the leucocyte surface may act as a hapten to form an antigen and the resulting antigen-antibody complexes are apparently capable of binding to and damaging the circulating leucocytes and their late-stage precursors in the marrow. (Red cells and platelets may also be destroyed by such mechanisms). With so many new synthetic drugs being introduced, the dangers of sensitisation of this kind must always be kept in mind, because the haemopoietic system, and in particular its granulocytic component, is often the first to exhibit signs of unwelcome side effects.

Immunological reactions may also be involved in the neutropenia of mycoplasmal pneumonia, infectious mononucleosis, disseminated lupus erythematosus (p. 26.30), cyclical neutropenia and the recently-described autoimmune neutropenia. In anaphylactic shock (p. 7.6), marked leucopenia results apparently from aggregation of leucocytes in the capillaries of the lungs and other internal organs. This occurs also in endotoxin shock (p. 10.42). The syndrome of *hypersplenism* (p. 17.32), in which leucocytes, erythrocytes and platelets each or all are sequestered in an enlarged spleen, is another example of neutropenia due to 'peripheral' mechanisms.

Severe neutropenia has a high mortality, especially when the absolute neutrophil count falls below $0.5 \times 10^9/1$. There is an increased likelihood of major infection by pathogenic organisms while opportunistic infection with organisms normally of commensal type, e.g.

gut coliforms and fungi, may become a major factor.

Defects of neutrophil function. An abnormal susceptibility to infection can be produced not only by a reduction in circulating neutrophils but also by defective neutrophil function even when their number is normal. The capacity of the neutrophil to combat infection by pathogenic micro-organisms is dependent upon its ability to respond to chemotactic stimuli, to phagocytose the offending micro-organisms and to bring about their subsequent destruction intracellularly (p. 8.9). Intrinsic defects in all three of these components of neutrophil function have been described and must be distinguished from impaired leucocyte function due to defects of the complement system or of antibody production. The type of disorder can often be inferred from the history and diagnosed from (a) measurement of serum immunoglobulin and complement levels, (b) tests of neutrophil migration and phagocytic capacity and (c) tests of neutrophil oxygen metabolism.

Disorders of chemotaxis and opsonisation. Patients with *antibody deficiency syndromes* and *complement disorders* often have recurrent bacteraemias, meningitis and pulmonary infections. Normal synergistic activity of antibody and complement components leads to the formation of chemotactic factors and opsonisation of bacteria (p. 8.11): absence of these serum proteins leads to recurrent infection, usually with streptococci, pneumococci, *Neisseria*, *Haemophilus influenzae* and *Pseudomonas*. Such diseases include congenital and acquired agammaglobulinaemia, the latter often in association with multiple myeloma or lymphoproliferative disease; congenital or acquired deficiency of C3 (the latter occurring in advanced liver disease, systemic lupus erythematosus and immune-complex disease).

Disorders of locomotion and ingestion. The defect of neutrophil function associated with *glucocorticoid therapy* falls into this category: neutrophils are unable to migrate to inflammatory lesions and to phagocytose, and monocytes and macrophages are similarly affected. In the *lazy leucocyte syndrome* there also exists a defect in neutrophil motility. The *Chediak-Higashi syndrome* is a rare congenital disorder transmitted as an autosomal recessive character: it is charaterised by defective chemotaxis, neutropenia, and by the presence in neutrophils and other cells of giant lysosomes which fail to disrupt following phagocytosis of bacteria. In consequence there is a failure to destroy bacteria intracellularly. Other variable features include defective skin pigmentation and neuropathies, and most patients die soon after

entering an accelerated phase characterised by lymph node enlargement and massive hepatosplenomegaly.

Disorders of bactericidal activity. Perhaps the most important example of this group is **chronic granulomatous disease of childhood** in which the neutrophils and monocytes do not metabolise oxygen to superoxide or hydrogen peroxide (p. 8.10), and as a result lack the capacity to kill some species of bacteria, especially staphylococci, Gram −ve bacteria and certain fungi. The disease is transmitted by a gene defect in the X chromosome and so, like haemophilia, affects males. Female carriers have a mixture of normal and defective neutrophils in their blood, and this supports the Lyon hypothesis, which postulates that the inactive X chromosome represented by the sex chromatin of females' cells (p. 25.20) can be either of the X chromosomes, selection being random in early embryonic cells. From early childhood, affected males suffer from recurrent and protracted infections with extensive suppuration and granulation tissue formation, particularly in the skin, bones and viscera, even from bacteria of low pathogenicity. The enzyme defect can be demonstrated *in vitro* by the failure of neutrophils and monocytes to reduce the yellow dye, nitroblue tetrazolium (NBT) to an insoluble precipitate of blue-black formazan.

Patients with **myeloperoxidase deficiency** demonstrate a bactericidal defect but this is less severe than in chronic granulomatous disease and in most cases there is no undue susceptibility to infection.

Abnormalities of granulocyte morphology. A number of hereditary and acquired defects of granulocyte morphology occur. *Döhle bodies* are intracytoplasmic inclusions seen in mature neutrophils and are thought to be ribosome-containing remnants of promyelocyte cytoplasm. They have been observed in pregnancy and in a variety of acquired states e.g. severe infection, burns and cancer, but they also occur in a rare autosomal dominant trait called the *May-Hegglin anomaly*. This condition, characterised by giant platelets and Döhle bodies in granulocytes is usually benign but some patients develop a bleeding tendency associated with thrombocytopenia or a qualitative platelet defect. *Hypersegmented neutrophils* (macropolycytes) are characteristically found in megaloblastic anaemia but also in uraemia. These cells have more than 5 lobes to their nuclei.

The Pelger-Huet anomaly is a rare hereditary abnormality characterised by failure of nuclear segmentation. It is transmitted as a simple autosomal dominant trait and is clinically silent. In the typical heterozygous individual, the majority of mature neutrophils possess bilobed nuclei: in the homozygous state the nucleus is unsegmented. Rather more common is an acquired disorder known as *pseudo-Pelger change* occurring in the course of myeloproliferative syndromes and various infections.

Eosinophil granulocytes

These differ from neutrophil granulocytes in possessing large brightly eosinophilic granules, which often appear closely packed. In addition, the nucleus usually has only two lobes (Fig. 17.10). Eosinophil granules are rich in a distinctive type of peroxidase and on electron microscopy they display a crystalloid core containing the *major basic protein (MBP)* of eosinophils, a functionally important protein. Eosinophils have the ability to inhibit degranulation of mast cells and can thus modulate atopic reactions (p. 7.9). In addition, they exert some control over metazoan parasitic infestations (p. 28.21).

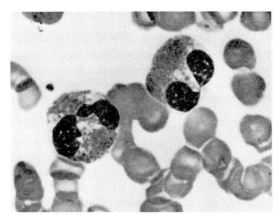

Fig. 17.10 Blood smear showing two eosinophil granulocytes. × 1250. (Dr. J. Browning.)

Eosinophil leucocytosis (eosinophilia) occurs in the following conditions:

(*a*) *Parasitic infections* by amoebae, hookworms, tape worms, ascaris, filariae and trichinella. The eosinophil level sometimes exceeds $3 \times 10^9/1$ and may represent an atopic reaction.

(*b*) *Hypersensitivity reactions:* In atopic hypersensitivity reactions such as asthma and hay fever, eosinophilia is usually present and is related to the local migration of eosinophils into the affected tissues. Eosinophilia may also be found in angio-oedema, food sensitivity, and in hypersensitivity reactions to certain drugs, e.g. penicillin. An increase in eosinophils may also occur in polyarteritis nodosa and other so-called hypereosinophilic syndromes including eosinophil granuloma of bone, Loeffler's syndrome, etc.

(*c*) *Chronic skin diseases* such as dermatitis herpetiformis, psoriasis, etc. In some generalised skin conditions, a hypersensitivity mechanism may be present, e.g. in eczema or urticaria. Eosinophilia also occurs early in scarlet fever.

(*d*) *Malignant tumours* The eosinophil count rises in some patients with cancer involving the bone marrow. In chronic granulocytic leukaemia, eosinophils may be increased along with the other granulocyte cells. In certain forms of Hodgkin's disease the lymph nodes are infiltrated with eosinophils and about 10% of cases show eosinophila in the blood.

Eosinophil leucopenia is a practically constant response to increased secretion or therapeutic administration of glucocorticoids or adrenocorticotrophic hormone.

Basophil granulocytes

These constitute a small fraction of the total blood granulocyte pool and contain heparin, hyaluronic acid, serotonin and histamine. Basophils resemble, but present certain differences from, the tissue mast cells, and have been shown to be involved in hypersensitivity reactions, at least in animal studies. In chronic granulocytic leukaemia and the chronic myeloproliferative syndromes they sometimes contribute to the leucocytosis and basophil myelocytes also may appear in the blood. As an isolated finding, basophil increase is observed in myxoedema and less frequently in chickenpox, chronic ulcerative colitis, and (formerly) in smallpox.

Lymphocytes

Recent advances in understanding of the life cycle and immunological functions of the lymphocytes have been described in chapters 6 and 7. Like many other cells, they are known to be capable of producing interferon (p. 9.2).

Lymphocytosis. Normally, lymphocytes account for a higher proportion of total leucocytes in the child than in the adult. The number is highest after birth, probably because of the build-up of antigenic experience at this time, and gradually falls in subsequent years. The presence of lymphocytosis is a useful diagnostic feature in whooping cough, in which it occasionally rises to $100 \times 10^9/1$. Lymphocytosis also occurs in virus infections and particularly in infectious mononucleosis (p. 18.10), in which the cells are large and of abnormal appearance. Other infections in which lymphocytosis may be seen include typhoid and paratyphoid fevers, brucellosis, influenza, secondary syphilis, toxoplasmosis and cytomegalovirus infections. High lymphocyte counts are also seen in the acute infective lymphocytosis of young children. The outstanding cause of gross lymphocytosis is, however, chronic lymphocytic leukaemia (p. 17.49) and an increased proportion of lymphocytes may sometimes be observed (by a differential count) to precede the actual rise in total leucocyte count.

Lymphopenia is found commonly in the elderly and in any stressful situation and is therefore of limited diagnostic value. In infancy, it is a cardinal feature of some rare immunological deficiency syndromes (p. 7.32), and has also been reported in intestinal lymphangiectasia (p. 14.44) and in coeliac disease, especially when there is splenic atrophy (p. 19.53). Severe lymphopenia results also from irradiation and the use of cytotoxic drugs, including glucocorticoids, for immunosuppressive therapy or treatment of neoplasia.

Monocytes

Monocytes (Fig. 17.11) are circulating cells of the mononuclear-phagocyte system (p. 4.33). When stimulated, they enlarge and increase in motility and metabolic activity, becoming macrophages. Their role in the immune response is described in Chapter 6, and the release of lymphokines which influence monocytes and macrophages in delayed hypersensitivity reactions is discussed on p. 7.20.

Like the neutrophil granulocytes, monocytes migrate into inflammatory foci and phagocytose bacteria, damaged tissue elements, dead cells, etc., but they leave the circulating blood later than the neutrophils and are seen in increasing numbers in the late stages of pyogenic infections, in the outer part of the wall of persistent abscesses, and in chronic inflammations of various types and causes.

Monocytosis is commonly present in subacute infective endocarditis and in brucellosis. Macrophages constitute an important component of the local cellular reaction to tuberculosis and a circulating monocytosis may also occur in this condition. They are also increased in typhus and some other rickettsial diseases, and in certain protozoal infections, e.g. malaria, trypanosomiasis and kala-azar, in which diseases there is no increase of the neutrophils. In chronic malaria, monocytosis is often a striking feature and some of them may contain small granules of pigment (Fig. 17.12). Monocytosis is not uncommon in Hodgkin's disease and in patients with carcinoma. The possibility of monocytic and myelomonocytic leukaemia must always be considered in patients with monocytosis. Some of the functional defects of neutrophil granulocytes e.g. chronic granulomatous disease of childhood, are shared by

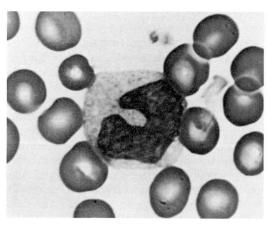

Fig. 17.11 Monocyte in a blood smear. × 1250. (Dr I. Evans.)

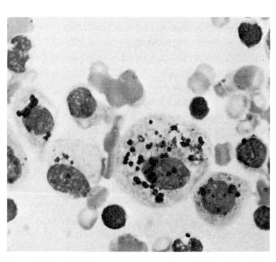

Fig. 17.12 Buffy coat preparation of the blood in malaria, showing monocytes containing pigment. × 680.

monocytes; the latter are also functionally impaired in carcinomatosis and some other conditions.

Blood platelets

Platelets are anucleate fragments of megakaryocyte cytoplasm and although not cells in the true sense, they possess a complex structure of organelles and tubular systems. Platelets are capable of adhering to the walls of damaged blood vessels and to each other forming aggregates or haemostatic complexes (p. 10.7). In addition, they secrete a number of important biological mediators and are weakly phagocytic. Platelets can, therefore, perform a number of important functions: (1) they help maintain the integrity of the vascular endothelium; (2) they form a primary haemostatic plug following vessel injury; (3) they are capable of activating the blood coagulation system, and (4) they produce mediators involved in vessel wall repair, in regulation of vascular tonicity and in inflammatory reactions. Accordingly, diminution in the number of circulating platelets or disorders of platelet function can result in a state of purpura in which spontaneous haemorrhages occur.

The number of platelets in blood is normally between $150-400 \times 10^9/1$. The newer automated haematological instruments, in addition to performing platelet counts, measure platelet size, expressing this as a mean platelet volume, or MPV (cf MCV of red cells). An interesting and diagnostically useful inverse but non-linear relationship exists between platelet count and mean platelet volume, i.e. the lower the platelet count, the greater is the MPV and *vice versa*. So long as this relationship is preserved it can be inferred that megakaryocytes are continuing to produce platelets, a low platelet count with increased MPV indicating peripheral destruction or consumption of platelets as a cause of the thrombocytopenia. When thrombocytopenia is accompanied by a low MPV, myelosuppression is the cause of thrombocytopenia.

Platelet disorders may be grouped into three categories: (1) an increase in platelet count which may be reactive (*thrombocytosis*) or neoplastic (*thrombocythaemia*); (2) a reduction in platelet count (*thrombocytopenia*), and (3) a normal platelet count but platelets which are functionally defective (*qualitative platelet disorders*). These disorders are described in the section on abnormal haemorrhagic states (p. 17.62 *et seq.*).

Anaemia

Definition and types of anaemia

Anaemia is defined as a *reduction in the concentration of haemoglobin in the blood below the normal range* and is usually but not invariably accompanied by reduction in the number of red cells. Anaemia develops when the rate of red cell production by the bone marrow fails to keep pace with the destruction of red cells or with any losses from haemorrhage. Accordingly, the anaemias can be classified simply as follows:

(1) **Excessive loss or destruction of red cells**
   (a) loss—*post haemorrhagic anaemia*
   (b) destruction—*haemolytic anaemias*
(2) **Failure of production of red cells**
   (a) diminished production with marrow hyperplasia—*dyserythropoietic anaemias*

(b) diminished production with marrow hypoplasia—*hypoplastic* or *aplastic anaemias*

Although such a classification is essential for accurate diagnosis and rational treatment, in most examples of anaemia more than one of the above mechanisms is involved, e.g. in megaloblastic anaemias there is not only insufficient output of red cells by the marrow, but those cells which are produced wear out too quickly, i.e. there is also excessive destruction.

Effects of anaemia

The main effect of anaemia is a reduction in the oxygen-carrying capacity of the blood with resulting **tissue hypoxia.** The patient may complain of tiredness, dizziness, paraesthesias of the extremities, anginal chest pain and breathlessness on effort.

Certain **compensatory adjustments** of the circulation occur in anaemia. There is a reduction in arteriolar tone, while the stoke volume and to a lesser extent the heart rate increase. Cardiac output thus rises, circulation time falls and tissue perfusion is increased. These changes may be reflected clinically in a bounding pulse with a high pulse pressure, palpitations, cardiac enlargement and haemic murmurs; if the condition continues or the anaemia worsens, *cardiac failure* is a serious risk, especially if the load on the heart is increased by injudicious blood transfusion. These effects do not depend only on the severity of the anaemia; if it develops rapidly the symptoms are correspondingly severe, whereas remarkable tolerance is often seen when the haemoglobin level has fallen slowly. Co-existing atheroma, so common in the elderly, also enhances the effects of anaemia. Pallor, mild pyrexia and slight splenomegaly may be attributed to anaemia *per se*.

Tissue hypoxia resulting from anaemia stimulates the production of erythropoietin (p. 17.4), which in turn leads to *erythroid hyperplasia*; the yellow fatty marrow of the long bones becomes progressively replaced by dark red cellular marrow and in extreme cases resorption of bone trabeculae may occur. In haemolytic and post-haemorrhagic anaemias, this leads to a useful output of new red cells from the marrow (*effective erythropoiesis*); in the dyshaemopoietic states, however, although marrow hyperplasia occurs, cell maturation is slow and some red-cell precursors are destroyed, so that red cell production is not correspondingly increased (*ineffective erythropoiesis*). In aplastic or hypoplastic anaemias, compensatory hyperplasia cannot occur despite stimulation by erythropoietin.

Fatty change, especially in the liver (p. 20.7) and heart, is the most constant pathological change in patients dying with severe anaemia.

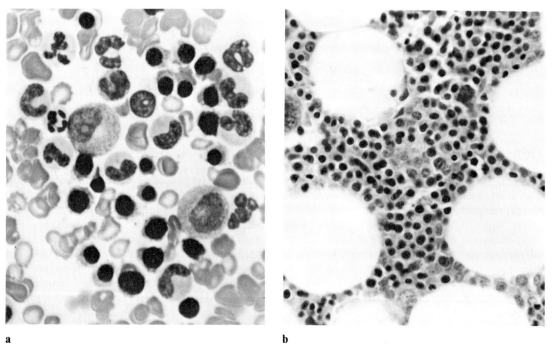

a   b

Fig. 17.13   The haemopoietic marrow, showing an erythroblastic reaction following haemorrhage. **a** Marrow smear: there is an increased proportion of normoblasts, at various stages of maturity, as compared with myelocytes. × 850. **b** Marrow section: the cellular haemopoietic tissue has increased at the expense of the fat cells. × 500.

Post haemorrhagic anaemia

The restoration of the plasma volume after *acute haemorrhage* causes a temporary dilution of the blood with accompanying fall in red cell count. The first evidence of regeneration of red cells after a large haemorrhage is a progressive increase in the number of reticulocytes in the blood and the degree of increase is an indication of haemopoietic activity. Occasionally normoblasts may also be seen, and after repeated haemorrhage they may be numerous. As regeneration becomes complete the reticulocytes gradually return to their normal level and normoblasts disappear. These changes are the result of erythroblast proliferation in the bone marrow, in which they form a larger proportion of the cells than normally (Fig. 17.13). A neutrophil leucocytosis and thrombocytosis, both of moderate degree, appear within a few hours after haemorrhage; they pass off in two or three days unless the haemorrhage is repeated.

Chronic loss of small amounts of blood does not necessarily produce anaemia because the number lost is rapidly replaced. *Iron-deficiency anaemia* (p. 17.40) may, however, develop, chronic haemorrhage being its most important cause.

Haemolytic anaemias

General features

The haemolytic disorders comprise a group of conditions characterised by an increased rate of red cell destruction with a shortening of mean red cell lifespan. There is a compensatory increase in the rate of red cell production, and anaemia will develop only when the rate of destruction exceeds that of production. The absence of anaemia, therefore, does not exclude the existence of haemolytic disease. In all haemolytic disorders, irrespective of cause, there is evidence of increased rates of haemoglobin catabolism and erythropoiesis, and this combination provides the laboratory basis for the diagnosis in this group of disorders.

In most haemolytic conditions, red cell destruction occurs in macrophages, mainly in the spleen, liver and bone marrow (**extravascular haemolysis**). As much as 20% of the total red cell mass may be destroyed daily in this way. Mildly or moderately damaged red cells are phagocytosed mainly in the spleen whereas more severely damaged cells undergo phagocytosis in all tissues containing vascular channels lined by macrophages (notably the liver, spleen and bone marrow). **Intravascular lysis**, i.e. escape of haemoglobin from red cells in the circulation, is due mainly to severe red cell membrane damage by antibody and complement, toxic chemicals or mechanical trauma.

The 'ghosts' or lysed red cells are phagocytosed by macrophages as described above.

Changes resulting from increased destruction of red cells. Following *phagocytosis of red cells by macrophages*, haemoglobin is degraded to haem and globin. Haem iron is released and transported to the marrow and the residual porphyrin rings are broken down to bilirubin; the peptide chains of the globin moiety are hydrolysed to their constituent amino acids and re-enter the general metabolic pool (p. 11.11). In haemolytic disorders, the production of bilirubin may exceed the capacity of the liver to remove it, and plasma levels rise; clinical jaundice results when the level exceeds $50\,\mu$mol/l (3 mg/dl). *The bilirubin is unconjugated but bound to albumin and therefore does not pass into the urine* (**acholuric jaundice**). The increased excretion of *conjugated* bilirubin by the liver leads to excessive formation of stercobilinogen in the gut, so that the faeces are dark. There is increased absorption of stercobilinogen from the gut which often cannot all be dealt with by the liver and so appears in the urine as urobilinogen. While the finding of increased urinary urobilinogen is a useful qualitative screening test for increased red cell destruction, measurement of urobilinogen or stercobilinogen in faeces is not useful in the diagnosis of haemolytic anaemia because of the wide normal range and technical difficulties both in sample collection and in estimation. The high bilirubin content of the bile may predispose to the formation of pigment gallstones, which are seen most often in chronic haemolytic anaemias of the inherited type, and the high levels of plasma bilirubin found in haemolytic disease of the newborn may cause toxic damage to the brain—kernicterus (p. 21.44).

Intravascular lysis leads to the appearance of free haemoglobin in the plasma (normally less than 1 mg/d1); a proportion of this is bound at once to plasma *haptoglobin* to form a haemoglobin/haptoglobin complex of molecular weight 150 000 and therefore too large to pass into the urine. This complex is removed by the hepatocytes and, if intravascular haemolysis is severe, haptoglobins disappear from the plasma. Some reduction in the levels of haptoglobins is also observed when the haemolytic mechanism is predominantly extravascular. The estimation of plasma haptoglobulins as a test for haemolysis is of limited value, because haptoglobin levels are increased in a variety of inflammatory states. In intravascular lysis, haemoglobin in excess of the haptoglobin-binding capacity circulates as the free protein. Unless performed under very carefully standardised conditions, the result of plasma haemoglobin estimations can be most misleading. Some of the free haemoglobin is removed by hepatic cells but two other pathways also exist for its removal: it may dissociate into half-molecules ($\alpha\beta$ dimers of mol. wt. 32 000 which pass into the glomerular filtrate), or it may be oxidised to *methaemoglobin* from which the haem is then dissociated and either (a) complexes with *haemopexin* and passes to the hepatocytes, or (b) combines first with albumin to form *methaemalbumin* which subsequently transfers the haem to haemopexin as the latter becomes available. Measurement of plasma methaemalbumin has long been used in the diagnosis of intravascular haemolysis (**Schumm's test**). Haemosiderin granules in exfoliated epithelial cells in the urine are also a sensitive indicator of intravascular lysis.

Measurement of red cell lifespan. A sample of the patient's red cells can be labelled *in vitro* with radiochromium and returned to the circulation where their fate can be closely followed. The rate of disappearance of radioactivity from the circulation can be estimated by serial blood samples and is proportional to the rate of red cell destruction. It is customary to calculate the time taken for the concentration of ^{51}Cr to decay to 50% of its initial value. Provided haemorrhage can be excluded, the red cell lifespan can be estimated from these data. In addition, by placing an external scintillation counter over the liver, spleen and bone marrow, the sites of red cell sequestration and destruction can be ascertained. Such information may help to predict the potential benefits of splenectomy on red cell survival.

Changes associated with compensatory erythropoiesis. In haemolytic states, erythropoietin stimulation of the marrow induces compensatory hyperplasia of red cell precursors. Kinetic studies show that the marrow is capable of increasing red cell production to a maximum of six times the normal. There is thus an increased number of young red cells in the blood; in a Romanowsky-stained blood film many of the erythrocytes show polychromasia and there may be both early and late normoblasts. Reticulocytes are always increased, often exceeding 20% (Fig. 17.7). In any untreated case of anaemia such a reticulocytosis is strong evidence of a haemolytic process provided blood loss can be excluded. It is usually assumed that the magnitude of reticulocytosis reflects the degree of shortening of red cell lifespan, but the relationship is inexact. When erythropoietic activity is increased, the reticulocytes may be released prematurely from the bone marrow ('shift reticulocytes') and survive longer in the circulation. Such early reticulocytes are larger than those normally released and contain inclusions such as basophilic stippling and Howell-Jolly bodies. The anaemia in haemolytic disease is usually normocytic but may be mildly macrocytic (see below). The marrow shows erythroblastic hyperplasia (Fig. 17.14) and the fat cells are partly or even completely replaced by haemopoietic tissue which may also extend down the shafts of the long bones. Eventually the medullary cavity may become widened with loss of bony trabeculae and thinning of cortical bone. The greatly increased erythropoiesis may result in enlargement of erythroblasts (*macronormoblasts*) with dyserythropoietic features (p. 17.34) and the production of *macrocytic red cells*. Megaloblastic change due to folic acid deficiency may also develop (p. 17.40). In severe

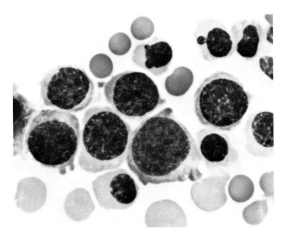

Fig. 17.14 Marrow smear in haemolytic anaemia due to hereditary spherocytosis, illustrating normoblastic hyperplasia: the cluster of erythroblasts includes all stages from early basophilic cells to late normoblasts. × 1100.

chronic cases, extramedullary haemopoiesis occurs in the spleen and other sites (p. 17.2).

Classification of haemolytic disorders

Shortening of the red cell survival time is the essential diagnostic feature of haemolytic disease. The pathogenesis of the different types of haemolytic disease is not fully understood and no single classification is entirely satisfactory. Important points in producing a classification of the haemolytic disorders include (1) site of haemolysis (extravascular or intravascular); (2) intrinsic defect of the red cells ('intracorpuscular defect') or the action of an extrinsic agent on normal red cells ('extracorpuscular defect'); (3) hereditary or acquired disorders (see Table 17.5).

A1. Hereditary red cell membrane defects

The red cell membrane, as in nucleated cells, consists of a lipid bilayer. Recent studies have suggested that the physical properties of the membrane are largely due to a sub-membrane protein meshwork which functions as a

membrane skeleton. Included in the latter are the proteins spectrin and actin. *Spectrin* is an important major membrane protein possessing contractile properties which may alter the shape of the red cell; mice with hereditary spectrin deficiency have extremely fragile cells which spontaneously lose fragments of membrane with resultant marked spherocytosis and severe haemolysis, and there is evidence that a similar

Table 17.5 Classification of haemolytic anaemia

A. Hereditary
1. Red cell membrane defects
   (a) hereditary spherocytosis
   (b) hereditary elliptocytosis
2. Red cell enzyme defects
   (a) Embden-Meyerhof pathway defects
   (b) hexose monophosphate shunt defects
3. Haemoglobinopathies
   (a) synthesis of abnormal globin chains—haemoglobin variants
   (b) defective globin chain synthesis—thalassaemia syndromes

B. Acquired
1. Auto-immune haemolytic anaemia
   a) warm antibody type
   b) cold antibody type
2. Iso-immune haemolytic anaemia
   a) haemolytic transfusion reaction
   b) haemolytic disease of the newborn
3. Drug-induced immune haemolytic anaemia
4. Haemolysis due to toxins and chemicals
5. Red cell fragmentation syndromes
      (mechanical damage to red cells)
   (a) march haemoglobinuria
   (b) micro-angiopathic haemolytic anaemia
6. Hypersplenism
7. Paroxysmal nocturnal haemoglobinuria
8. Parasitic invasion of red cells

mechanism may be operative in human hereditary spherocytosis. Since red cell *membrane lipids* are in equilibrium with the plasma lipids they may be altered by diet or disease, and the ratio of cholesterol to phospholipid influences the deformability of the red cell membrane, increase in cholesterol tending to make the cell less deformable.

Like all cells, the red cell regulates its volume and water content primarily through control of sodium and potassium ions (pp. 3.1–5), maintenance of the cytosol concentrations of which depends on an intact cell membrane and a supply of energy in the form of ATP (p. 3.5).

The surface-to-volume ratio of red cells varies considerably in some disease states. Red cells become spherocytic as surface-to-volume ratios decline and this can arise because of loss of membrane surface (**microspherocytes**) or by gain in red cell volume (**macrospherocytes**). The red cell becomes less deformable as spheroidicity increases. Correspondingly, an increase in the surface-to-volume ratio may be due either to an increase in membrane surface area or to a decrease in cell volume, either change resulting in the appearance of target cells in peripheral blood smears. **The osmotic fragility test** is a useful indirect measurement of the surface-to-volume ratio. When red cells are placed in a hypotonic salt solution they swell and rupture and the haemoglobin diffuses out. With normal red cells, the first trace of lysis is usually seen in 0·42% saline; initial lysis occurring below 0·4% or above 0·5% is abnormal, indicating diminished or increased fragility respectively.

(a) Hereditary spherocytosis (HS). This common type of chronic haemolytic anaemia occurs in most parts of the world; it is caused by a red-cell membrane defect probably involving spectrin (see above), and is inherited as an autosomal dominant trait with incomplete penetrance. In about 25% of patients, however, there is no family history, and the defect presumably arises as a spontaneous genetic mutation. The membrane defect results in excessive permeability to sodium ions, and red cell integrity can only be maintained by increased glycolytic activity which provides the ATP, and thus the energy, required to 'pump' sodium ions out of the cell. This metabolic activity is associated with an increased turnover and loss of membrane lipid, resulting in the development of **microspherocytes,** a process which is greatly accelerated in the red pulp of the spleen where the availability of glucose is diminished. Microspherocytic red cells are trapped in the red pulp, and subsequently destroyed, because they lack the deformability necessary to enable them to pass through the clefts between the endothelial cells in the venous sinusoids and return to the circulation. The spleen itself occupies a critical role in the disease process and *following splenectomy the survival of red cells returns to normal*. Transfused cells survive normally in HS. Clinically, the disease is characterised by acholuric jaundice, often mild and fluctuating and usually dating from early childhood. Anaemia may be mild or even absent although acute episodes of severe anaemia (crises) are sometimes experienced. These crises may result from either (1) an increase in red cell destruction (*haemolytic crises*), sometimes related to infection or pregnancy and associated with deepening jaundice, fever and leucocytosis or (2) reduction in erythropoietic activity in the marrow, when increased anaemia is accompanied by a fall in reticulocyte count ('*hypoplastic crisis*'). *Splenomegaly* is invariable in HS and some patients develop *chronic leg ulceration*. Most untreated patients develop *pigment gallstones*. The diagnosis is proven when signs of haemolysis, such as persistent reticulocytosis and urobilinogenuria, are associated with the presence in the peripheral blood of numerous *microspherocytes*, seen in blood films as small, intensely stained spheroidal red cells (Fig. 17.15). Demonstration of **increased osmotic fragility** of the red cells helps to confirm the diagnosis. If the HS cell is deprived of its source of energy, namely glucose, the sodium leak can no longer be balanced and intravascular lysis occurs. This observation forms the basis of the *incubated osmotic fragility test*, which is useful for diagnosing patients with a mild form of the disorder. A rather more sophisticated test is the **autohaemolysis test** which again involves incubation

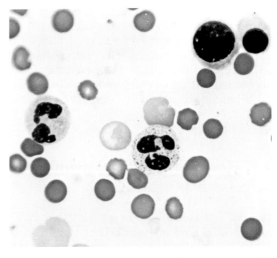

Fig. 17.15 Blood film in hereditary spherocytosis. Note the small, densely staining spherocytes. ×780.

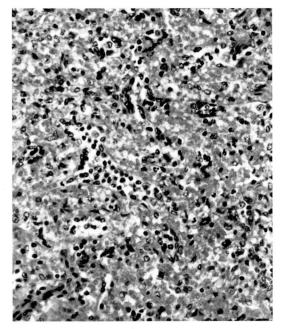

Fig. 17.16 Spleen in hereditary spherocytosis. The pulp is intensely congested and the sinuses are inconspicuous. × 230.

and lysis of red cells with and without added glucose. Cells from HS show a type I reaction in the auto-haemolysis test, lysis occurring in the absence of glucose and being prevented by addition of glucose. (The type II reaction is seen when utilisation of glucose via the glycolytic pathway is impaired as in pyruvate kinase deficiency. In this case the increased rate of auto-haemolysis is not reduced by glucose.)

The spleen usually weighs 500 g or more. Histologically the red pulp is distended with red cells, and the venous sinusoids are compressed (Fig. 17.16). Although splenectomy relieves the haemolysis, microspherocytosis and increased osmotic fragility of the red cells persist.

(b) Hereditary elliptocytosis. This diagnosis probably includes several inherited disorders characterised by the presence of elongated red cells in the peripheral blood. At least two variants have been recognised by genetic studies: both have an autosomal dominant inheritance, but in one form the abnormal gene is linked to the Rh blood-group genes on the same chromosome, while the other shows no such linkage.

This disorder occurs more frequently than hereditary spherocytosis and is probably also due to abnormalities in the spectrin molecule (p. 17.21). Clinically, red cell production keeps pace with destruction in about 90% of cases, and anaemia is minimal. In the remaining 10%, anaemia is overt: the latter patients have osmotically fragile red cells and respond to splenectomy.

A2. Hereditary red cell enzyme defects

Normal red cell survival is dependent upon the integrity of the two enzyme systems concerned in glucose metabolism, (a) the Embden-Meyerhof anaerobic glycolytic pathway supplemented by (b) the hexose monophosphate shunt to provide additional reducing power (Fig. 17.17). Conversion of glucose to pyruvate in the **Embden-Meyerhof pathway** results in the production of two moles of adenosine triphosphate

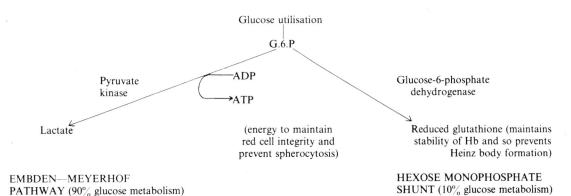

Glucose utilisation

G.6.P

Pyruvate kinase   ADP → ATP   Glucose-6-phosphate dehydrogenase

Lactate   (energy to maintain red cell integrity and prevent spherocytosis)   Reduced glutathione (maintains stability of Hb and so prevents Heinz body formation)

EMBDEN—MEYERHOF PATHWAY (90% glucose metabolism)   HEXOSE MONOPHOSPHATE SHUNT (10% glucose metabolism)

Fig. 17.17 Two enzyme systems of importance in determining the lifespan of the red cells.

(ATP) for each mole of glucose catabolised. In addition, NAD is reduced to NADH. ATP maintains the internal environment of the red cell by regulation of the membrane cation pump and also preserves membrane flexibility and red cell shape. Lack of ATP leads to shortening of red cell survival and extravascular haemolysis, although there is marked variation in severity of haemolysis due to defects in different glycolytic enzymes. The NADH produced by this pathway is necessary to maintain the iron of haem in the ferrous state, i.e. to reduce methaemoglobin (see below) to haemoglobin. The **hexose monophosphate shunt** produces reducing power in the form of NADPH; this additional reducing power is required in circumstances of oxidative stress which would otherwise lead to oxidation of membrane components, causing both membrane rigidity and increased 'leakiness' of cations. Oxidation of the haemoglobin to (non-functional) methaemoglobin, with precipitation of globin chains as Heinz bodies, occurs in infections (due to production of oxidants by macrophages), following absorption of oxidising agents from the gut, and after administration of certain drugs. Red cells contain a relatively high concentration of reduced glutathione (GSH), an intracellular buffer with protective effects against these exogenous and endogenous oxidants, which convert it to GSSG. The maintenance of GSH levels is accomplished by glutathione reductase which catalyses NADPH-mediated reduction of GSSG to GSH. Although deficiencies of most enzymes involved in these pathways have been described, only a few are of clinical importance. The deficiency may be severe so that enzyme activity is insufficient under physiological conditions, or it may be inadequate only under conditions of increased oxidant activity. Deficiency may occur either because of failure to synthesise an enzyme, or because a functionally abnormal molecule is produced. For each category of enzyme deficiency there are certain general characteristics which point to the pathway involved. For example microspherocytosis is not a feature of some enzyme defects, and these cause the *hereditary non-microspherocytic haemolytic anaemias*.

(a) **Defects of the Embden-Meyerhof pathway.** The least rare abnormality of this system involves **deficiency of pyruvate kinase (PK).** This disorder is inherited as an autosomal recessive trait and haemo-lysis is seen only in the homozygous state. The anaemia, which may be moderate to severe, causes relatively mild symptoms because of a shift to the right in the oxygen dissociation curve (due to a rise in intracellular 2, 3-diphosphoglycerate which enhances oxygen release from haemoglobin). PK deficiency presents in childhood with mild jaundice and slight to moderate splenomegaly. The red cells show only minimal morphological abnormality, despite the paradoxically high reticulocyte counts sometimes observed. Osmotic fragility of non-incubated blood is decreased due to the large numbers of osmotically resistant reticulocytes. Diagnosis may be difficult unless careful enzyme studies are performed *in vitro*. Trapping of red cells in the spleen is not a prominent feature and splenectomy affords only minimal benefit except in those patients requiring repeated blood transfusions. Many other defects of the Embden-Meyerhof enzymes are reported, but they are very rare.

(b) **Defects in the hexose monophosphate shunt** only produce haemolysis under the stimulus of oxidative stress, and with the exception of **glucose-6-phosphate dehydrogenase (G-6-PD) deficiency,** are very rare. G-6-PD deficiency is, however, one of the most common of all genetic defects, affecting up to 40% of individuals of Mediterranean, South East Asian and Negro ancestry. By contrast, the incidence is low in Europeans and Japanese. The deficiency is most common in areas where malaria is endemic and this probably reflects the protection which the deficient cells appear to afford against falciparum malaria. More than 150 G-6-PD variants are recognised but only a few are clinically important. Inheritance of the defect is sex-linked, affecting males and carried by females, who have approximately half of the normal G-6-PD values. *The principal effect of the deficiency is a decrease in reduced glutathione; in consequence, oxidants are free to damage cellular constituents and haemoglobin is readily oxidised to methaemoglobin, intracellular precipitation of which is seen as Heinz bodies* (Fig. 17.18).

G-6-PD deficiency may present clinically in four ways, the occurrence of which varies, for reasons unexplained, in affected individuals of different ethnic groups. (1) Most often haemolysis is precipitated by bacterial infections: this applies everywhere. (2) The second commonest precipitating factor is ingestion of compounds with oxidative potential. In Mediterranean peoples, it may be induced even by the mild oxidant in fava beans (favism). The list of oxidant drugs is long and includes antimalarials, sulphonamides and other antibacterial compounds (nitrofurantoin, penicillin and anti-tuberculous drugs), phenacetin, anti-helminthics and many others. (3) Chronic low-grade haemolytic anaemia is being recognised increasingly in northern Europeans with G-6-PD deficiency, and is exacerbated by infec-

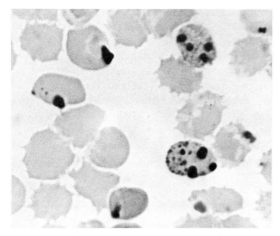

Fig. 17.18 Blood film in sodium chlorate poisoning, stained with methyl violet to show Heinz bodies. × 1400.

tion or oxidant drugs but, surprisingly, not by eating fava beans. The most dramatic clinical presentation is severe acute intravascular haemolysis accompanied by pains in the abdomen or back; apart from this, haemolysis is usually mild and may readily be overlooked. (4) Spontaneous haemolysis occurs in about 5% of affected neonates in the Mediterranean countries, Nigeria, Thailand and China, but not in other parts of the world: the main danger is brain damage by bilirubin (*kernicterus*—p. 21.44) and if this can be prevented the prognosis is good, haemolysis ceasing spontaneously after 2–3 months.

The diagnosis of G-6-PD deficiency is suggested by the presence of contracted and fragmented cells in the peripheral blood film and by the demonstration of cells containing Heinz bodies, together with the features of intravascular haemolysis. Reticulocytes have a higher level of G-6-PD than older cells and enzyme assays may therefore give false normal results during an exacerbation. Subsequent assay at a later stage may reveal the deficiency. A number of screening tests are available of widely varying sensitivity.

A3. Haemoglobinopathies

Haemoglobin is a globular protein of molecular weight 64000 consisting of two pairs of coiled polypeptide chains and four prosthetic haem groups, one being attached to each of the four chains. The role of these haem groups is to transport oxygen and it is the function of the surrounding globin to provide a suitable environment for this to be achieved. The type of haemoglobin is determined by the amino-acid sequence in polypeptide chains. Four different chains occur normally in adults, termed α, β, γ and δ. The normal haemoglobin consists of a pair of α chains and another pair of β, γ or δ chains (Fig. 17.19). Alpha chains contain 141 amino acids and the others each contain 146. Each globin chain has a spiral configuration and the constituent amino acids are located both internally (non-polar, non-charged radicals) and externally (polar, charged radicals). The internal polypeptide amino acids are vital for the structure and function of the chain, forming an internal scaffold which preserves the rigidity and stability of the tertiary configuration. Haemoglobins differ in their electrophoretic mobility (Fig. 17.20), solubility and resistance to denaturation by alkalis; these features, together with chromatography, are used for their identification. Replacement of 'fetal' haemoglobin (HbF) by HbA starts before birth and HbA and HbA_2 account for over 99% of the haemoglobin normally present by one year of age. In the adult less than 2% is HbF. Haemoglobinopathies result from abnormalities arising in the synthesis of the globin fraction from gene mutation, deletion, etc., the haem groups being normal. Mutations are of two main varieties, resulting in the *haemoglobin variants* and the *thalassaemia syndromes*.

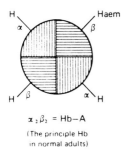

$\alpha_2\beta_2$ = Hb–A

(The principle Hb in normal adults)

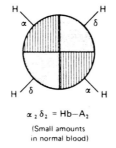

$\alpha_2\delta_2$ = Hb–A$_2$

(Small amounts in normal blood)

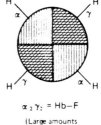

$\alpha_2\gamma_2$ = Hb–F

(Large amounts in fetal and neonatal blood)

Fig. 17.19 The structure of the normal haemoglobins.

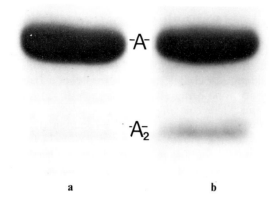

Fig. 17.20 Starch-gel electrophoresis of haemoglobins. **a** Normal. **b** Thalassaemia minor, showing increase in HbA$_2$.

The effect of a haemoglobinopathy, however caused, is to impair Hb synthesis and so red cell production, with resulting anaemia: the red cells also have a reduced survival time in the circulation, and the anaemia is therefore partly dyserythropoiesic, partly haemolytic.

Haemoglobin variants

These are haemoglobins with abnormalities in the amino-acid sequence of the globin chains, most often substitution of a single amino acid. Over 300 such haemoglobin variants have been recognised but only a few of these result in disease, the best known being S, C, D and E haemoglobins, in each of which the β chains contain an abnormal amino-acid sequence. The inheritance of such haemoglobin variants follows a simple Mendelian pattern, being heterozygous or homozygous for the structural variant. Of greater importance, however, in terms of the severity of the clinical disorder, is the polarity of the substituted amino acid. Haemoglobin variants resulting from substitution of external (polar) amino acids only produce clinical disease in the homozygous state, whereas the internal (non-polar) amino-acid variants produce disease in heterozygotes, and homozygotes are non-viable.

Haemoglobin variants due to substitution of external amino acids. The commonest and most important condition of this type is **sickle-cell** or **HbS disease.** Individuals who are homozygous for HbS (HbS/S) always have the clinical manifestations of *sickle-cell disease.* Heterozygotes develop symptoms only under certain circumstances and are said to have the *sickle-cell trait* (see below). The abnormal gene occurs among Negroes and those with Negro ancestry. **Sickle-cell disease** is often fatal in childhood. It has a geographical distribution similar to falciparum malaria and patients who carry the gene are protected from malaria. HbS ($\alpha_2\beta_2^{6\,val}$) differs chemically from HbA in the substitution of valine for glutamic acid in the sixth position of the amino-acid sequence of the β chain. When the α chains move apart to give up oxygen, the amino-acid substitution results in locking of the adjacent ends of the α chains with the abnormal β chains, and the haemoglobin molecules become stacked in rows. This causes distortion of the red cells to a sickle shape in deoxygenated blood, and sickling is demonstrable *in vitro* by adding a reducing agent to the blood (Fig. 17.22). Clinically, there is a chronic haemolytic anaemia, painful sickling crises, leg ulceration, recurrent respiratory infection and myocardial insufficiency. The crises affect especially the abdomen, bones and joints; they are due to blocking of small vessels by sickled cells and infarcts of the spleen, bones, etc. commonly result. The severity of haemolysis and anaemia is modified by elevation in the HbF concentration. In the Middle East, sickle-cell disease is often a benign disorder due to the presence of up to 30% of HbF; this reflects a high incidence of genes determining persistence of HbF production.

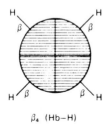

β_4 (Hb–H)

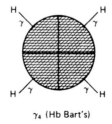

γ_4 (Hb Bart's)

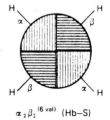

$\alpha_2\beta_2^{(6\,val)}$ (Hb–S)

Fig. 17.21 The structure of some abnormal haemoglobins.

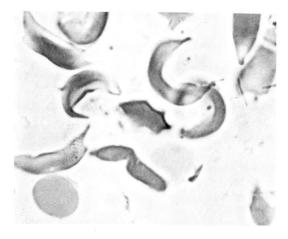

Fig. 17.22 Blood from a subject with sickle-cell trait showing the characteristic distorted shapes assumed when the red cells are subjected to a low oxygen tension. × 1000.

The sickle-cell trait, due to the heterozygous state (HbA/S), occurs in 12–20% of Negroes. Symptoms are usually absent or mild but sickling is demonstrable *in vitro*. It is, however, important to establish the diagnosis because sickling can occur if such individuals are subjected to severe and prolonged hypoxia. All patients of Negro ancestry should be screened for HbS on admission to hospital.

Combinations of HbS with other variants are not uncommon. The most frequent, HbS/C, results in features very similar to sickle-cell disease in HbS/S individuals. Pregnancy occurring in individuals with HbS/S and HbS/C leads to a worsening of the clinical disorder: crises are more frequent and both morbidity and mortality are increased. Suppression of the haemoglobin variant by repeated transfusion gives temporary improvement. The existence of HbS/S should not pose an anaesthetic risk provided anaesthesia is rapidly induced and prolonged hypoxia avoided. The combination of HbS/thalassaemia is described on p. 17.28.

Haemoglobin variants due to substitution of internal amino acids. Three categories of abnormality occur in this group, all representing heterozygous expression. **HbM variants** produce one variety of *congenital methaemoglobinaemia* characterised clinically by cyanosis due to the failure of methaemoglobin to bind oxygen. Haemolytic anaemia is not usually evident but there may be mild reticulocytosis. **Altered affinity haemoglobins** constitute the second group and most bind oxygen strongly, with consequent tissue hypoxia and erythrocytosis. The third and largest group comprises **the unstable haemoglobin variants** producing clinical conditions called *congenital Heinz-body hae-*

molytic anaemias. These haemoglobin variants are highly unstable because the causative amino-acid substitutions affect the attachment site of haem. Even individuals heterozygous for such abnormal haemoglobins, of which **Hb Köln** is the commonest, suffer from a spontaneous *hereditary non-spherocytic haemolytic anaemia*. Since unstable haemoglobins readily become denatured, Heinz body formation is a typical feature and this can readily be demonstrated when the cells are incubated *in vitro* (Fig. 17.18). Heinz bodies are not, however, observed *in vivo* unless splenectomy has been carried out, because the spleen is capable of removing them from circulating red cells.

The thalassaemia syndromes

This second main group of haemoglobinopathies are caused by genetic defects which result in diminished production of one of the normal globin chains, most often the α or β chain. Reduced α-chain synthesis (α *thalassaemia*) leads, in fetal life, to a compensatory excess of γ chains which tend to form tetrameric (γ_4) haemoglobin molecules (Hb Barts), and in adults to an excess of β chains which combine to form the unstable β_4 tetramer, HbH (Fig. 17.21). Deficient production of β chains (β *thalassaemia*) does not result in formation of abnormal haemoglobins because although α chains are produced in excess, they are incapable of forming tetramers.

The thalassaemia syndromes comprise a complex group of heterogeneous disorders in which the red cells are deficient in haemoglobin and are hypochromic and microcytic. New types of thalassaemia are still being described and advances in cytogenetics and molecular biological techniques, particularly restriction enzyme analysis, have revealed a molecular complexity comparable to the diversity of clinical types.

Some of the thalassaemias arise from gene deletion; in others the genes are present but transcription defects result in diminished synthesis of mRNA, while in a third group mRNA is produced but translation defects prevent production of normal gobin chains. To complicate matters still further, each disorder may occur in a homozygous or heterozygous form.

Alpha thalassaemia. There are two pairs of genes responsible for α-chain production and accordingly there are four forms of thalassaemia, depending respectively on deletion or defective expression of 1 to

4 genes. They are as follows: (1) *Silent α thalassaemia*, in which the blood picture is normal; (2) *α-thalassaemia trait*—mild anaemia and hypochromia; (3) *HbH disease*, in which the Hb is typically 7–9 g/dl, the red cells are severely hypochromic, and aggregates of β-chain tetramers precipitate as HbH inclusions. In a variant of HbH disease occurring in SE Asia there is deletion of only two of the genes but, because of a translocation, a third gene is abnormal and codes for Hb Constant Spring; (4) *Hb Barts*, in which there is complete absence of α chains and no production of HbF or HbA. The haemoglobin consists mainly of γ tetramers (*Hb Barts*). Anaemia is severe and causes death *in utero* from hydrops fetalis (p. 17.30).

The β thalassaemia syndromes are no less complex. They result from defective synthesis of the β and sometimes also the γ chains. In *β° thalassaemia* the β-globin genes are intact but there is failure to synthesise β chains, in some instances because mRNA is not produced, in others because mRNA is structurally abnormal or there is an error in its translation to β chains. In *β⁺ thalassaemia*, β-globin mRNA synthesis is reduced, but some β chains are formed.

The effects of these defects in β-chain production are, of course, more severe in homozygotes than in heterozygotes. *Homozygous β° thalassaemia* results in absence of HbA and the haemoglobin consists of HbF (98%) and HbA₂. Such patients are severely anaemic and dependent on blood transfusions and so are thus classed as suffering from *thalassaemia major*.

Heterozygous β° thalassaemia causes mild or moderate anaemia, hypochromic and microcytic red cells and elevated HbA₂ (5%) but only slight rise of HbF level; it is graded as *thalassaemia minor*. *Homozygous β⁺ thalassaemia* presents a range of severity and is graded as either *thalassaemia major* or *intermedia*: in contrast to homozygous β° thalassaemia, HbA, HbA₂ and HbF are all detectable. *Heterozygous β⁺ thalassaemia* causes mild or moderate anaemia, elevation of HbA₂ and in some forms also elevation of HbF; it is graded as *thalassaemia minor*. The δβ thalassaemias are rare and arise because of deficient production of both δ and β chains. The most common form is represented by Hb Lepore.

The traditional clinical grading of thalassaemia into major, intermedia and minor types is useful clinically. In *thalassaemia major*, severe anaemia develops within a few weeks of birth and splenomegaly becomes prominent. The peripheral blood (Fig. 17.23) shows reticulocytosis, many nucleated red cells, and target cells (p. 17.9) with high osmotic resistance. Many patients die in infancy or childhood, while those surviving longer develop widespread haemo-

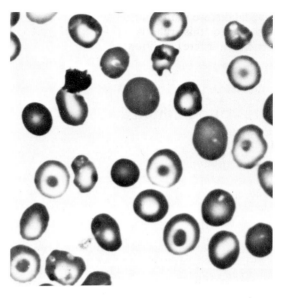

Fig. 17.23   Target cells in a case of thalassaemia. × 1000.

siderosis with consequent hepatic cirrhosis and cardiac failure. Prolonged marrow hyperplasia causes bone changes e.g. thickening of the calvarium, giving a mongoloid appearance. *Thalassaemia intermedia* is less severe whereas in *thalassaemia minor* the effects are much less serious, the condition usually presenting in adult life as mild hypochromic microcytic anaemia which is often symptomless. The diagnosis rests initially on the discovery of abnormal absolute values, hypochromia, microcytosis and target cells (p. 17.9) in the peripheral blood film and changes in the proportions of HbF and HbA₂ (Fig. 17.19). Confirmation of the diagnosis is by measurement of α and β globin chain synthesis ratios (normally 1:1).

The thalassaemias are world-wide and occur in nearly all ethnic groups, but they are particularly prevalent in the Mediterranean region, the Indian subcontinent and South East Asia. The combination of haemoglobin variants with thalassaemia occurs in areas where both groups of gene defects have a high frequency. The finding of HbS/β thalassaemia is not uncommon and produces a wide spectrum of clinical severity ranging from a disorder indistinguishable from severe sickle-cell disease to a clinically benign condition. Likewise, β thalassaemia in association with other haemoglobinopathies, e.g. HbC and HbD, usually presents with mild clinical disease not requiring treatment. The exception to this rule is HbE/β thalassaemia which is a severe condition.

B1. Auto-immune haemolytic anaemias

One of the commonest causes of acquired haemolytic anaemia is the development of an auto-antibody capable of binding to and damaging the red cells. By far the most useful test for detecting such antigen-antibody interaction is the antiglobulin (Coombs') test (p. 6.11). The mechanism of auto-antibody formation is uncertain, but in most instances it seems likely that suppressor T-lymphocyte function is defective, allowing the development of reactive clones of lymphocytes. In other cases, exogenous agents such as drugs or micro-organisms may stimulate the formation of antibodies which cross-react with red cell surface antigens.

Auto-immune haemolytic anaemia occurs in two major forms which differ in the thermal range of reactivity of the antibody and are termed *warm* and *cold antibody types.*

(a) Warm antibody type. This is usually due to IgG class auto-antibody which binds strongly to the red cells at 37°C. The antibody is sometimes specific for one of the Rh antigens of the red cells and, like Rh iso-antibodies, is 'incomplete', i.e. it does not cause agglutination of red cells suspended in saline (p. 6.10). *In vivo,* the red cells usually become microspherocytic and undergo phagocytic destruction in spleen, liver, marrow, etc., i.e. extravascular haemolysis (p. 17.19).

This type of haemolytic anaemia can occur at any age and in both sexes, but is commonest in women over 40. Most cases are chronic, almost half occurring without other associated disease and the remainder complicating systemic lupus erythematosus, less often rheumatoid arthritis, other putative auto-immune disorders and malignant lymphomas, including chronic lymphocytic leukaemia. Acute but self-limiting forms are seen in children following various infections, and some cases are caused by drug therapy, most often with α-methyldopa (p. 7.12). In the chronic disease, the clinical picture is one of fluctuating haemolytic anaemia with mainly extravascular haemolysis and usually splenomegaly. Microspherocytosis and increased osmotic fragility are usual, particularly during exacerbations (in which there may also be intravascular haemolysis). Antibody bound to the red cells is detectable by the direct antiglobulin test with anti-IgG; antibody can be eluted from the red cells and is sometimes detectable in low titre in the serum.

(b) Cold-antibody type. This is usually caused by IgM class auto-antibody which binds to the red cells at temperatures below 37°C and most strongly at about 4°C. The antibody produces effects in two ways—by causing auto-agglutination of the red cells and by sensitising them to complement activation with consequent intravascular haemolysis (p. 17.20). Either effect may predominate, causing respectively *cold agglutinin disease* and *paroxysmal cold haemoglobinuria.*

Cold agglutinin disease is a chronic condition of middle or old age. Anaemia is usually moderate to mild but may become severe in cold weather. It is sometimes idiopathic (*chronic cold agglutinin syndrome*) but more commonly secondary to other diseases, especially lymphoma, adenocarcinoma and the connective tissue diseases. An acute self-limiting form follows certain infections, especially pneumonia due to infection by *Mycoplasma pneumoniae*: it is usually mild and subsides within a few months. Acrocyanosis is a prominent feature and must be distinguished from primary Raynaud's disease. The antibody is of the IgM class and commonly reacts with the antigen I, which is present on the red cells of nearly all individuals. In the chronic disease, the antibody is monoclonal and there may be sufficient in the serum to give a monoclonal band on electrophoresis (p 17.60). The thermal amplitude of antibodies of this type varies and the disease occurs only in those subjects with antibody reacting at temperatures up to about 30°C. The direct antiglobulin test is usually positive using antibody to complement components, e.g. anti-C3, but negative with class-specific anti-IgG. The haemagglutinin titre of the serum is usually 2000 to 64000 when tested at 4°C. In all forms of cold agglutinin disease, marked red-cell agglutination is seen in peripheral blood films and when blood counts are performed on automated equipment such agglutination may produce erroneous values with falsely reduced PCV and falsely elevated MCV.

Paroxysmal cold haemoglobinuria. The classical chronic form of this condition occurred in association with congenital syphilis and is now rare. It is seen occasionally as an acute, usually transient complication of virus infections (where it is often accompanied by a false-positive Wassermann reaction) or as an apparently primary auto-immune disorder in adults. Unlike most cold antibodies, the antibody is of IgG class; it reacts with antigens of the P system present on the red cells of nearly all individuals, is capable of strong complement fixation, and causes intravascular haemolysis on exposure to cold. The mechanism of haemolysis was elucidated by Donath and Landsteiner who demonstrated haemolysis *in vitro* by first chilling the blood to allow the cold antibody to react with the red cells, followed by warming to allow complement activity. This was the first demonstration of an auto-immune disease mechanism and the test is still used.

B2. Iso-immune haemolytic anaemias

(a) Haemolytic disease of the newborn (HDN). Fetal red cells commonly enter the maternal circulation shortly before or during labour, in the course of obstetric manipulations and during abortion. They may provoke formation of maternal antibodies to blood-group antigens foreign to the mother; such immune iso-antibodies are often mostly of IgG class, and are thus capable of crossing the placental barrier in subsequent pregnancies, when they may cause haemolytic anaemia of the fetus (Fig. 7.5, p. 7.12). Since there are at least 20 common blood group systems, some degree of fetal/maternal incompatibility is inevitable, but in practice the Rh system (p. 10.45) and particularly the antigen D, is responsible for most of the severe cases of HDN. The disease occurs in only a small proportion of those pregnancies at risk (i.e. of those with an Rh−ve mother and an Rh+ve father). This is because: (a) the first-born child is not affected unless the mother has been previously immunised by blood transfusion or abortion; (b) the father is sometimes heterozygous (Dd), in which case the fetus has a 50% chance of being Rh−ve; (c) ABO incompatibility between mother and fetus often prevents immunisation of the mother by fetal (e.g. D) antigen: incompatible fetal red cells (say Group A) entering the maternal circulation are destroyed by maternal natural (anti-A) iso-antibody before they can stimulate production of Rh antibodies. ABO incompatibility itself rarely causes severe HDN because the antibodies are usually of the IgM class and incapable of crossing the placenta, although occasionally IgG antibody is present and causes a relatively mild form of the disease.

HDN varies considerably in severity. In mild forms there may be merely transient jaundice and anaemia—*congenital haemolytic anaemia*, and treatment is often unnecessary or simple blood transfusion alone is sufficient. The more dangerous form, known as **icterus gravis neonatorum,** is of extreme importance, for urgent treatment is required and is often successful. In this condition, jaundice develops shortly after birth and if the level of unconjugated serum bilirubin is allowed to exceed 15 mg/dl (250 μmol/l) there is a serious danger of permanent brain damage—**kernicterus** (p. 21.44). The infant is usually moderately anaemic, with reticulocytosis and many nucleated red cells in the blood. Marked hepatosplenomegaly is usual and in fatal cases there is widespread liver cell necrosis together with extensive extramedullary haemopoiesis in the spleen, liver, kidneys and adrenals. The only effective treatment of this condition is exchange transfusion in which the red cells of the fetus are replaced by compatible red cells (i.e. lacking D antigen). Very severe anaemia causes intrauterine or neonatal death due to marked anaemia and congestive cardiac failure—**hydrops fetalis.** The possibility of HDN should become known from parental blood grouping early in pregnancy, and where there is incompatibility, the mother's serum should be examined during pregnancy for Rh and other antibodies. Confirmation of HDN can be obtained by detecting a raised level of bilirubin in samples of aspirated amniotic fluid. Early delivery may save some infants, but with others intra-uterine fetal transfusion with Rh−ve blood is indicated. Once the infant is born, the diagnosis and treatment are based on the detection of IgG antibody on its red cells by the direct antiglobulin test and assessment of the blood changes and clinical features outlined above. Iso-immunisation of an Rh−ve woman by red cells entering the maternal circulation from the fetus may be prevented by intravenous injection of anti-D within three days of delivery. The anti-D coats the fetal (Rh+ve) cells and causes their rapid clearance from the circulation before an immune response can be initiated. Prophylaxis is also appropriate for all Rh−ve women with Rh+ve husbands following abortion, amniocentesis or other obstetric manipulation. It is, of course, most important to avoid transfusing Rh−ve girls and women with Rh+ve blood. Incompatibilities in other blood group systems, e.g. Kell and Duffy, also occasionally cause HDN.

(b) Transfusion reactions. When incompatible blood is transfused into a recipient who has already developed the corresponding antibodies, a haemolytic transfusion reaction results and the transfused cells are rapidly destroyed. The results of an incompatible transfusion depend to some extent on the speed of destruction of the transfused red cells and this is likely to be greater when abundant iso-antibody is present, e.g. in ABO incompatibility, and especially when group A blood is given to a Group O recipient or Rh+ve blood to a Rh−ve iso-immunised recipient. These are not the only incompatibilities encountered but are so much the most common that stringent precautions must be taken to avoid them. The patient is likely to suffer a rigor, pain in the back and pyrexia. Shortly thereafter, haemoglobinuria appears, followed by jaundice. In a severe reaction, death from shock may occur within a few minutes. If the patient survives, DIC and haemostatic failure (p. 17.67) may develop or acute renal failure may ensue (p. 22.8). Similar clinical effects may result from the transfusion of blood which is time-expired or contaminated by Gram−ve bacteria, some of which are cryophilic and grow freely in stored blood at refrigerator temperature.

B3. Drug-induced immune haemolysis

Various drugs are capable of inducing an immune reaction which results in the destruction of red cells. Two types of reaction are recognised: (1) where the antibody is directed against the drug or a drug-plasma protein complex, and (2) where the drug induces formation of an antibody which cross-reacts with a normal red cell antigen.

Antibody directed against drugs. Two subdivisions of this mechanism occur. First, the drug may bind very firmly to the red-cell membrane and antibody may then be formed against the drug/red cell complex. The antibody is usually IgG; haemolysis is not often severe and ceases promptly on discontinuing the drug. This is the mechanism of haemolysis in some patients receiving high doses of penicillin or cephalosporin. A second mechanism exists when an antibody is formed against a drug-plasma protein complex which binds to red cells; the reaction of antibody and complement with the bound complex results in red cell destruction. Moderate to severe haemolytic anaemia develops, accompanied by haemoglobinuria. Drugs which can cause this type of reaction include quinidine, phenacetin, digoxin, sulphonamides and chlorpropamide.

Antibody directed against normal red cells. In this variety, the drug appears to induce autoantibody formation against normal red cells by a mechanism which is not fully understood. The most common cause is the drug α-methyldopa. The Coombs' test becomes positive in some 10% of patients on long-term treatment with methyldopa (usually for hypertension) some months after starting therapy, but only a small proportion develop a frank haemolytic anaemia. In most patients, the antibody possesses a specificity within the Rh system. It has been suggested that methyldopa in some way alters the antigen and thus stimulates the formation of antibody capable of cross-reacting with the normal antigen. The Coombs' test may remain positive for many months after discontinuing therapy.

B4. Haemolytic toxins and chemicals

Extensive infections with bacteria which secrete haemolytic toxins (e.g. phospholipases) can result in acute haemolysis. Examples include *Clostridium welchii* and *Streptococcus pyogenes*. The cells become spherocytic and massive intravascular haemolysis may occur. Haemolytic chemicals are numerous and include such substances as phenylhydrazine, compounds of lead, arsenic and copper, saponin and potassium chlorate. In chronic lead poisoning the red cell membrane is rendered brittle, with increased mechanical but diminished osmotic fragility; such cells are short-lived, and mild anaemia results. Lead also interferes with haemoglobin synthesis, particularly iron utilisation, and in consequence sideroblasts are seen in the marrow and the mature red cells tend to become microcytic although the patient is not iron-deficient. Lead also precipitates the RNA of reticulocytes, producing punctate basophilia (Fig. 17.8). Early and reliable diagnosis is provided by detecting a raised level of lead in the blood. The disorder of haemoglobin synthesis induced by lead is reflected in the high levels of erythrocyte protoporphyrin, urinary coproporphyrin and δ-aminolaevulinic acid. Vegetable compounds may also be responsible (p. 17.24). A number of spider and snake venoms have been shown to produce haemolysis, presumably by enzyme-mediated red-cell damage.

B5. Mechanical damage to red cells (red cell fragmentation syndromes)

(a) **March haemoglobinuria** consists of acute haemoglobinuria, usually mild, resulting from long marches or marathon running. The haemolysis is now believed to be due to mechanical injury to the red cells sustained in the circulation through the soft tissues of the plantar aspect of the feet and brought on by the prolonged mild trauma of long walks, particularly on hard surfaces and carrying heavy loads. Haemoglobinuria has also been reported from mechanical trauma of red cells in the soft tissues of the hands in over-enthusiastic exponents of karate.

(b) **Micro-angiopathic haemolytic anaemia** is a haemolytic state of varying severity, associated with red-cell fragmentation (Fig. 17.6, p. 17.10) and thrombocytopenia: it is observed in various clinical situations, including obstetric complications such as ante-partum haemorrhage and pre-eclampsia, in malignant hypertension, thrombotic thrombocytopenic purpura (Moschowitz syndrome), the 'haemolytic-uraemic' syndrome of childhood (p. 22.45), car-

cinomatosis, especially if the tumour is of mucin-secreting type, and septic shock (p. 10.42). A common factor in all these conditions is the presence of widespread fibrin deposition in small blood vessels due either to vascular damage (microangiopathy) or to intravascular activation of the clotting mechanism (p. 17.67). It is thought that the red cells are fragmented when they become enmeshed in fibrin strands or adhere to damaged endothelium. A similar form of red-cell fragmentation has also been observed in patients with prosthetic heart valves, which invariably produce some degree of red-cell damage and occasionally result in overt intravascular haemolysis with haemosiderinuria and even iron deficiency.

B6. Hypersplenism

Healthy blood cells traverse the normal spleen readily, whereas abnormal cells which have lost their ability to deform may be trapped and destroyed in the normal spleen. When the spleen becomes enlarged, the circulation through it becomes more circuitous and as a result red cells, leucocytes and platelets are retained for longer periods in the splenic cords; because of this delay, destruction of abnormal cells is increased, but in addition normal cells may also be destroyed. In most conditions characterised by splenomegaly, clinically-evident haemolysis does not occur although some shortening of red cell survival can be demonstrated. When anaemia occurs, it is usually due to impairment of the bone marrow compensatory response by the underlying disease process. Additional mechanisms which may be involved include expansion of the plasma volume with consequent dilution of the red cell mass: this dilution effect is not confined to splenomegaly of any particular cause and is cured by splenectomy. These phenomena are described as *the hypersplenism syndrome*, the components of which include: (1) splenic enlargement; (2) reduction in one or more of the cell types in peripheral blood; (3) normal or hyperplastic haemopoietic marrow with at least normal representation of the cells deficient in the peripheral blood; (4) correction of the cell deficit(s) by splenectomy. By convention, the syndrome does not include conditions in which splenomegaly *results from* haemolytic anaemia, thrombocytopenia, etc., for example hereditary spherocytosis or auto-immune thrombocytopenia.

The principal disorders leading to hypersplenism include congestive splenomegaly (see p. 18.5); various malignant neoplasias including leukaemias and lymphomas; chronic myeloproliferative disorders (see p. 17.56); acute and chronic infections including tuberculosis, brucellosis, malaria and kala-azar; auto-immune, inflammatory and granulomatous diseases including sarcoidosis; Felty's syndrome and systemic lupus erythematosus; lipoid storage disorders. As noted above, hypersplenism is often occult, the increased destruction of formed elements being masked by compensatory hyperplasia of the marrow, a state which becomes recognisable only when the patient is exposed to a myelodepressant factor such as intercurrent infection.

B7. Paroxysmal nocturnal haemoglobinuria (PNH)

PNH is an uncommon chronic disease characterised by intravascular haemolysis, usually with paroxysmal acute exacerbations, repeated thrombotic episodes and increased liability to infections. It affects mainly young adults but can develop at any age.

PNH is caused by the clonal development of abnormal populations of haemopoietic stem cells, the end products of which (red cells, leucocytes and platelets) are abnormally susceptible to the action of complement. The disease is not inherited and the nature of the acquired stem-cell abnormality is unknown but the disorder can arise from other primary dysplastic disorders of haemopoietic marrow, such as aplastic anaemia, sideroblastic anaemia and myelofibrosis. It may also evolve into acute leukaemia.

A major feature of PNH is intravascular haemolysis due to the unusual sensitivity of the red cell membrane to the lytic action of complement (p. 7.11). Normal red cells possess membrane proteins which regulate the activity of cell-bound C3b, and it has recently been reported that PNH red cells lack this membrane regulatory activity. Activation of complement by the classical or the alternative pathways results in the deposition of more C3 on PNH cells than on normal cells. C3 conversion to active C3b is also markedly increased on PNH cells, resulting in enhanced activation of the subsequent complement components C5–C9, and lysis of PNH red cells. Because of these abnormalities, even the

normal low-grade continuous activity of the complement system is sufficient to damage PNH cells, and increase in complement activity, e.g. by infections, results in acute exacerbations. The increased sensitivity of red cells to complement-mediated lysis has long provided the basis for diagnosis. In *Ham's acidified serum test*, the increased complement activity of acidified serum (pH 6·4) is sufficient to lyse PNH red cells but not normal cells. Intravascular haemolysis in PNH is worse at night because of the slight fall of plasma pH during sleep. In the sucrose haemolysis test, red cells absorb complement components from serum at low ionic concentrations and PNH cells undergo lysis because of their enhanced sensitivity to complement. The most sensitive test for PNH cells is provided by determining their sensitivity to complement lysis following sensitisation with an antibody. Haemosiderin granules are usually detectable in the urine, but in mild cases haemoglobinuria may occur only during exacerbations.

Because PNH is due to a stem-cell abnormality, both platelets and leucocytes are also abnormally sensitive to complement-mediated lysis and this may be a factor in the pathogenesis of the venous throm-

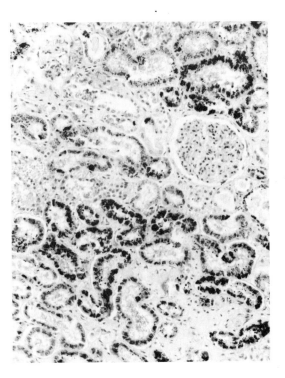

Fig. 17.24 The kidney in paroxysmal nocturnal haemoglobinuria, stained by the prussian blue reaction, showing accumulation of haemosiderin in the convoluted tubules due to prolonged haemoglobinuria. × 100.

bosis and liability to infections respectively which occur in this disorder.

The severity of haemolysis depends on the severity of the red-cell membrane abnormality and also on the proportion of circulating abnormal cells. The latter appears to vary from time to time, accounting partly for the characteristic exacerbations and remissions. Patients are commonly iron-deficient due to the high urinary iron loss during intravascular haemolysis. Abdominal, back and musculoskeletal pain may be due either to an episode of intravascular haemolysis or may be ischaemic in nature, secondary to venous thrombosis. Thromboses of portal, splenic, hepatic and cerebral veins are common causes of death. Repeated haemolytic crises cause marked anaemia with reticulocytosis, marrow hyperplasia and marked accumulation of haemosiderin in the kidneys (Fig. 17.24).

Blood transfusion is dangerous unless washed or reconstituted frozen cells are used, because transfusion of even small volumes of plasma produces haemolysis due to the presence of activated complement components. Iron therapy to the patient with PNH who is both anaemic and iron-deficient results in the rapid production of abnormal red cells with the consequent risk of severe haemolytic episodes. The course of PNH is highly variable. A number of patients may experience progressive diminution of the number of abnormal cells present and apparent spontaneous remission may occur, but the 10-year mortality is probably about 50%.

B8. Haemolytic disease caused by parasitic invasion of red cells

This occurs in malaria and oroya fever. Malaria is described on pp. 28.3-9: haemolysis is both intravascular and extravascular (in the spleen) but, unlike most haemolytic anaemias, splenectomy aggravates the haemolysis by impairing host defences against the parasite. The most serious haematological complication is **blackwater fever,** a severe acute attack of intravascular lysis. It occurred mainly in Europeans with falciparum malaria and was often fatal. It has, however, became rare since the replacement of quinine by modern anti-malarial drugs.

Dyserythropoietic anaemias

In these conditions the marrow is of normal or increased cellularity, but red-cell production is diminished (**dyserythropoiesis** or **ineffective erythropoiesis**) and anaemia results. Of the various types (Table 17.6) the most important are the megaloblastic and iron deficiency anaemias.

Congenital dyserythropoietic anaemia (CDA). In this group of rare congenital conditions with recessive inheritance, varying degrees of anaemia are associated with ineffective erythropoiesis and morphological abnormalities in red-cell precursors unrelated to B_{12} or folate deficiency. Three different types have been described, the least rare being characterised by *hereditary erythroblastic multinuclearity* together with a positive acid serum test for haemolysis (p. 17.33), hence the name HEMPAS. In other types, 'megaloblastoid' and giant erythroblasts have been described.

The megaloblastic anaemias

This form of anaemia is characterised by the presence in the bone marrow of a distinct abnor-mality of haemopoiesis known as megaloblastic change (Fig. 17.2, p. 17.5). This affects production of granulocytes and platelets as well as red

Table 17.6   Causes of dyserythropoietic anaemia

Primary
Congenital—Congenital dyserythropoietic anaemia
Acquired—The dysmyelopoietic syndromes (p. 17.58)
Secondary
Impaired DNA synthesis
      Vitamin B_{12} deficiency $\left.\begin{array}{l}\\\\\end{array}\right\}$ The megaloblastic
      Folic acid deficiency   anaemias
Impaired haem synthesis
      Iron deficiency—Iron deficiency anaemias
      Impaired iron utilisation—Sideroblastic anaemia
      Impaired globin synthesis—The haemoglobinopathies*

*The haemoglobinopathies are described with the haemolytic anaemias on pp. 17.25-9 because the lifespan of the red cells is shortened, but dyserythropoiesis is also an important feature and accordingly they are included in this table.

cells, but the abnormality of erythropoiesis is most conspicuous. *By far the commonest cause of megaloblastic haemopoiesis is deficiency of either vitamin B_{12} or folic acid;* less often similar changes occur (a) following therapy with cytotoxic drugs which inhibit DNA synthesis (e.g. cytosine arabinoside, hydroxyurea, 6-mercaptopurine and methotrexate), (b) in rare inherited enzyme defects such as methylmalonic aciduria, and (c) in erythroleukaemia (p. 17.49). In the peripheral blood, megaloblastic anaemia is characterised by an increase in the mean cell volume (MCV) of the red cells and is one of the commonest causes of *macrocytic anaemia*. It must be emphasised, however, that other forms of anaemia can be macrocytic in the absence of megaloblastic marrow change. This is especially true of the anaemia of alcoholic liver disease but anaemia following severe haemorrhage or haemolysis, or anaemia with extramedullary haemopoiesis, is occasionally macrocytic, presumably because of a high reticulocyte count, but some forms of aplastic or refractory anaemia with a low reticulocyte count also show this change.

The physiological actions of B_{12} and folic acid. These two substances are important for normal cell function, and in particular for normal cell division. Their activities are clearly interrelated, although the nature of this relationship has yet to be fully clarified. Certainly both act as co-enzymes in a number of biochemical reactions. The main co-enzyme function of folic acid is the transfer of single carbon units in such reactions as the breakdown of histidine, the synthesis of methionine and, of particular relevance to the pathogenesis of megaloblastic haemopoiesis, the synthesis of DNA and RNA. It now seems likely that only the polyglutamate form of folic acid is active biologically and that B_{12} is required for the intracellular conversion of the transport form of folic acid, 5-methyltetrahydrofolate, to the polyglutamate form. This would explain why B_{12} deficiency leads to megaloblastic haemopoiesis, which is largely due to a failure of DNA synthesis, and to neurological disturbance, apparently due to impaired RNA synthesis in nerve cells (Chanarin, 1979). It would also account for the observation that biochemical tests of folic-acid deficiency, such as the urinary excretion of formimino-glutamic acid (FIGLU) following a loading oral dose of histidine, are often positive in B_{12} deficiency. B_{12} has, however, other co-enzymic functions, including a critical action in the catabolism of methyl-malonic acid, an intermediate product of valine and propionic acid metabolism: B_{12} deficiency thus leads to appearance of this metabolite in the urine following a loading dose of valine, a test of possible diagnostic value.

Although existing in several forms, B_{12} **(cyancobalamin)** is made up of two major compounds; a planar group consisting of a corrin ring and a nucleotide group consisting of a base and phosphorylated sugar.

The effects of vitamin B_{12} and folic-acid deficiencies

These deficiencies affect all tissues with a high rate of cell turnover (p. 5.1). This explains the predominant involvement of the haemopoietic system, in which *the haemopoietic changes are identical in vitamin B_{12} and folic acid deficiency.* In some other tissues, however, the effects differ, for example, nervous system changes occur mainly in B_{12} deficiency.

Blood picture. In fully developed cases, the red cells, granulocytes and platelets are all reduced in number, i.e. there is **pancytopenia.** The red cells usually show an increase in MCV and this may precede the anaemia. As anaemia develops, however, the red cells show increasing variation in size (*anisocytosis*) with many small cells or red cell fragments as well as *macrocytes* over 10 µm in diameter, producing an increase in the red distribution width (p. 17.8) Red cells of grossly abnormal shape **(poikilocytes)** are also conspicuous in advanced cases (Fig. 17.5, p. 17.9). Nucleated red cells, often with megaloblastic features (Fig. 17.25), can almost always be detected in severe cases, especially in smears prepared from the buffy coat of centrifuged whole blood (p. 17.11). This technique may be diagnostically useful should marrow examination prove to be impracticable. The reticulocyte count is usually low although sometimes there is a slight increase in serum bilirubin resulting from shortened lifespan of macrocytes and breakdown of red-cell precursors in the marrow. There is usually significant *neutropenia* associated with the presence of large hypersegmented neutrophils with six or more lobes **(macropolycytes)** often detectable at an early stage of the disease, and occasional myelocytes

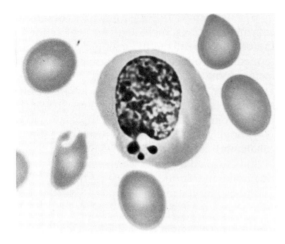

Fig. 17.25   Blood in pernicious anaemia showing a megaloblast with Howell–Jolly bodies. × 1300.

are seen in severe cases. Platelets are moderately reduced but occasionally there is severe thrombocytopenia resulting in purpura (p. 17.62).

Bone marrow. Diagnostic changes are observed in smears or sections of marrow aspirates. The cellularity in such sections is maximal, with complete loss of fat spaces (Fig. 17.26), even when anaemia is still minimal. Autopsy studies reveal also a marked expansion of haemopoietic tissue, which ultimately ex-

tends throughout the entire length of long bones (Fig. 17.27). Cytologically, all the haemopoietic elements are affected in some degree. Erythropoiesis undergoes a profound alteration described as **megaloblastic change**, *the essential feature of which is a delay in nuclear maturation with the accumulation of many cells in an early stage of development. Not only is there maturation arrest but many of the immature cells die in the marrow.* Nuclear immaturity is expressed by increased nuclear size with a delicately stippled chromatin pattern. A variety of other dyserythropoietic abnormalities occur, including nuclear polyploidy and fragmentation with formation of Howell-Jolly bodies (Fig. 17.25). Haemoglobinisation of the cytoplasm of developing erythroblasts is much less seriously affected and the asynchrony between nuclear and cytoplasmic maturation leads to the appearance of the most distinctive manifestation of megaloblastic erythropoiesis in the mar-

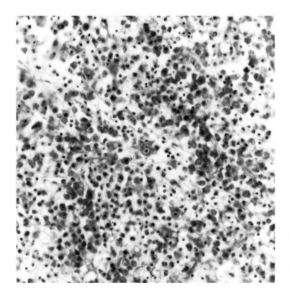

Fig. 17.26   Bone marrow from femoral shaft in pernicious anaemia, showing an extreme degree of megaloblastic hyperplasia with complete loss of fat and absorption of the bony trabeculae. × 250.

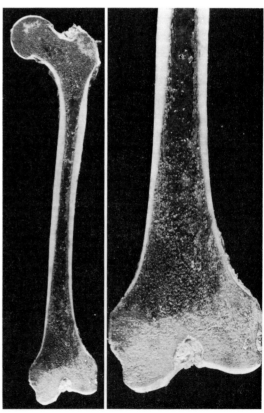

Fig. 17.27   Section of femur in pernicious anaemia, showing the dark red marrow throughout the shaft. *Left*, × 0·3. *Right*, lower end, × 0·7.

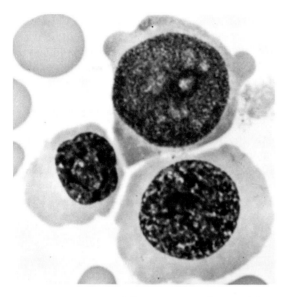

Fig. 17.28 Smear of bone marrow in pernicious anaemia, showing a promegaloblast (*above*) and two typical haemoglobinised megaloblasts. × 1700.

row (Fig. 17.28). The various stages of normoblastic and megaloblastic erythropoiesis are compared in Figs. 17.1 and 17.2 (p. 17.5). Interference with granulocyte development is most readily identified by the presence of abnormal metamyelocytes, which are greatly enlarged and possess a large horse-shoe shaped unsegmented nucleus. Megakaryocytes are often difficult to find, possibly as a result of a defect in the maturation of their precursors.

Neurological changes. *These are only conspicuous in B_{12} deficiency and they may develop before anaemia becomes apparent.* The principal lesion is referred to as **subacute combined degeneration,** characterised by a discontinuous demyelination of the long pyramidal tracts and posterior columns of the mid-thoracic region of the spinal cord. There may also be patchy demyelination of fibres of the large peripheral nerves and sometimes foci of demyelination are sometimes found in the cerebral hemispheres. Early clinical recognition of subacute combined degeneration is extremely important because, although it can be arrested by treatment, it is disabling and not completely reversible. Further, *the administration of folic acid alone can exacerbate the condition. Should urgent treatment of a megaloblastic anaemia be required before the cause can be established, it is advisable* to give both B_{12} and folic acid. Psychiatric disturbances are not uncommon in B_{12} deficiency ('*megaloblastic madness*').

Effects on other tissues. Epithelial changes can be detected in both B_{12} and folic-acid deficiencies. Atrophy and 'megalocytosis' of the epithelium of the tongue, sometimes associated with glossitis and oral ulceration, is a common feature of B_{12} deficiency and 'megalocytic' epithelial cells have also been detected in smears from the cervix uteri. In both B_{12} and folic-acid deficiency, mild villous atrophy (p. 19.51) may be found in the small intestine and 'megaloblastic' nuclear changes have been observed in cells of the crypts of Lieberkuhn. Sterility, presumably due to disturbed maturation of germ cells in the gonads, has been described in both sexes in B_{12} deficiency and can be reversed by specific therapy. Marked haemosiderin deposition in the renal tubules is observed in untreated cases of megaloblastic anaemia, probably as a result of the haemolytic element mentioned above. Slight to moderate splenic enlargement, due to increased red-cell destruction or to extramedullary haemopoiesis, is often present.

Causes of B_{12} deficiency

Vitamin B_{12} is synthesised only by micro-organisms and the sole source for humans is food of animal origin, notably liver and kidney but also meat, fish, chicken, eggs and dairy produce. The minimal daily requirement is approximately 1 μg. *Normally the liver stores sufficient vitamin to provide the total needs for 3–5 years.* Absorption from the gut is dependent on the binding of dietary B_{12} to gastric *intrinsic factor* (IF), a mucoprotein produced by the parietal cells. The B_{12}–IF complex thus formed passes to the terminal ileum where it attaches to specific receptor sites. The B_{12} enters the surface epithelial cells of the ileum, but the fate of the intrinsic factor is unknown. The vitamin B_{12} transport proteins in the plasma are *transcobalamin I* (TCI), its iso-enzyme transcobalamin III (TCIII), which bind B_{12} tightly and do not readily give it up to the tissues, and *transcobalamin II (TCII)* which is the major B_{12} transport protein. Congenital absence of TCII results in megaloblastic anaemia with normal plasma B_{12} and folate levels, developing a few weeks after birth. Congenital TCI deficiency is not associated with clinical abnormality, but the plasma B_{12} level is low. Elevated TCI levels in association with increased B_{12} levels have been observed in chronic myeloproliferative states and in a variety of tumours e.g. carcinoma of the breast and hepatoma.

Dietary deficiency of B_{12} is largely restricted to underdeveloped parts of the world, where it is quite common. Strict vegetarians can theoretically be expected to develop B_{12} deficiency but this is observed only occasionally because their diets are seldom totally lacking in B_{12}.

Malabsorption of B_{12}. This may be caused by deficient production of IF in the stomach or by intestinal disorders which interfere with absorption of B_{12} complexed to IF. By far the commonest cause of deficient IF production is severe **chronic gastritis** of the body of the stomach (p. 19.20). This is the underlying cause of pernicious anaemia, which was first described by Addison in 1853 and is a major type of megaloblastic anaemia. This form of gastritis is a good example of an organ-specific auto-immune disease, and it is a curious coincidence that both of 'Addison's diseases' should turn out to belong to this group. *Total gastrectomy* also eliminates IF secretion but overt signs of B_{12} deficiency may be delayed for as long as 10 years if the liver stores are normal. A proportion of patients also develop B_{12} deficiency following partial gastrectomy, usually due to chronic gastritis in the remaining portion of the stomach. Rarely impaired B_{12} absorption is *congenital*, IF being absent or of abnormal structure and functionally defective, although the gastric mucosa is morphologically normal. **Intestinal disorders** causing malabsorption of B_{12} include intestinal stasis, fish tape-worm infestation and disease or resection of the ileum. Various other disorders lead to mild malabsorption of B_{12} without the manifestations of severe clinical deficiency; they include severe chronic pancreatitis and the Zollinger–Ellison syndrome (p. 20.65).

In *intestinal stasis*, uptake of B_{12}-IF complex by bacteria proliferating abnormally in the more proximal parts of the small bowel may cause B_{12} deficiency. Almost any form of intestinal stasis, if sufficiently prolonged, can promote such colonisation, although surgical blind loops, jejunal diverticula and chronic obstruction are most often responsible, and co-existent malabsorption of fat can usually be demonstrated. Stasis in the afferent jejunal loop may

be involved in some cases following partial gastrectomy of the Polya type. *Infestation with Diphyllobothrium latum* (p. 28.32), which absorbs B_{12} (free and bound to IF) rendering it unavailable for absorption, is a common cause of megaloblastic anaemia in Finland, and is acquired by eating raw or partially cooked fish. *Extensive disease of the distal ileum* interferes with the final stage of B_{12} absorption. This occurs invariably in tropical sprue but in only 30% of cases of adult coeliac disease (p. 19.53), in which the mucosal lesions tend to be mild or even absent in the distal ileum. In Crohn's disease (p. 19.33), in which the terminal ileum is frequently involved, B_{12} deficiency is a recognised complication and surgical resection of the ileum inevitably abolishes B_{12} absorption.

In a rare congenital condition, Imerslund's syndrome, there is an isolated defect of B_{12} absorption in the ileum, associated with proteinuria.

Pernicious anaemia (PA)

This disease was the first cause of B_{12} deficiency to be described and remains one of the most important. It is particularly prevalent in individuals of North European stock and is predominantly a disease of the elderly. There is a strong familial tendency, relatives of patients being at much greater risk of developing it than the general population. Both patients and their relatives also have a high incidence of auto-immune thyroiditis and there is convincing evidence that the chronic gastritis of PA belongs to the group of organ-specific auto-immune disturbances (p. 7.24). Antibodies to parietal cells are found in the serum of 90% of patients and in 60% antibodies to IF can also be demonstrated. More significantly, IF antibodies are present in the gastric juice in about 50% of patients and in most of these the antibody reacts with and blocks the B_{12}-binding site of IF, thus inactivating what little IF is secreted by the atrophic gastric mucosa. Appearance of antibody to IF in the gastric juice is often the final event precipitating overt B_{12} deficiency. In the few young patients with PA, IF antibody is more often present and the chronic gastritis is frequently accompanied by other organ-specific auto-immune disorders, notably adrenal insufficiency and hypoparathyroidism and also by malabsorption. The role of auto-immunity in the atrophic gastritis responsible for PA is discussed on pp. 7.26 and 19.20. The changes in the blood and bone marrow are those of megaloblastic anaemia (pp. 17.35-6). Symptoms due directly to the gastritis are seldom evident and the effects of B_{12} deficiency, especially anaemia and neurological disturbances, dominate the clinical picture. There is, however, an increased risk of gastric carcinoma in patients with pernicious anaemia. The anaemia is usually insidious and many patients are severely anaemic before they seek medical advice.

Diagnosis of vitamin B_{12}-deficiency states

Once evidence of megaloblastic anaemia has been obtained, usually by marrow examination, it is necessary to establish whether B_{12} or folic acid deficiency exists. B_{12} deficiency is usually established by the demonstration of a reduced level of the vitamin in the serum, which is assayed by radio-immunoassay (p. 6.11) or by a microbiological technique. Having diagnosed B_{12} deficiency, the cause can usually be determined by the Schilling test for intestinal absorption: a small dose of B_{12} labelled with ^{58}Co is administered orally, followed by a parenteral 'loading dose' of $1000\,\mu g$ of unlabelled B_{12} (to minimise utilisation of the labelled B_{12} absorbed from the gut). The degree of absorption is assessed by measuring either the urinary excretion of labelled vitamin over a 24-hour period, or the serum level after 36 hours. If dietary deficiency is responsible, absorption is normal, whereas if IF is deficient, as in pernicious anaemia, absorption is subnormal but labelled B_{12} given orally together with IF is absorbed normally. In the blind-loop syndrome (in which the B_{12} is used up by the intestinal bacteria) IF does not improve absorption of B_{12} although broad-spectrum antibiotics usually do so. More specific therapy is, however, required to improve B_{12} absorption in malabsorptive states, e.g. a gluten-free diet in coeliac disease (p. 19.53). Although the demonstration of IF deficiency is necessary for certain diagnosis of pernicious anaemia, the demonstration either of histamine fast achlorhydria or of IF antibody in a patient with megaloblastic anaemia establishes the diagnosis beyond reasonable doubt. Antibody to parietal cells is not so helpful because it is common in people with less severe gastritis without pernicious

anaemia (p. 19.20). *The marrow reverts to normoblastic erythropoiesis within 24 hours following parenteral administration of B_{12} and confirmation of the diagnosis is provided by a reticulocytosis in the blood within 10 days.*

Causes of folic-acid deficiency

Folic acid (pteroyl-glutamic acid) consists of pteridine and para-aminobenzoic acid coupled to glutamic acid. The main dietary sources are fresh green vegetables, e.g. spinach and lettuce; cereals, meat, fish and eggs. The average Western diet contains about $650\,\mu g$ of folic acid daily, but up to 90% of this may be destroyed by cooking. The estimated minimum daily requirement is $50\,\mu g$, but more is needed in pregnancy and in some pathological states (see below). The storage capacity of the body is sufficient for about 80-100 days, i.e. about 10 mg, the principal storage site being the liver. Absorption of folic acid takes place predominantly in the upper small bowel. The causes of folic acid deficiency are as follows.

Dietary deficiency. This is a common contributory factor in many folic-acid deficiency states, and is of particular importance in elderly people on a poor diet and in infancy if weaning is delayed; dried milk is also a poor source of folic acid. Any condition in which there is anorexia and poor dietary intake, e.g. alcoholism or chronic gastro-intestinal disease, predisposes to folic acid deficiency. Nutritional folate deficiency also occurs in kwashiorkor, scurvy, and in infants with repeated infections or those fed solely on goat's milk, which has a very low folate content.

Malabsorption. Only two conditions are known with certainty to cause malabsorption of folic acid, namely **coeliac disease** (p. 19.53) in which folic-acid deficiency is invariable, and **tropical sprue** (p. 19.53). In both these diseases there are extensive pathological changes in the upper small bowel. Few other intestinal diseases produce such extensive chronic lesions and folic-acid deficiency arising in conditions such as Crohn's disease (p. 19.33) or following partial gastrectomy are more likely to be due to impaired dietary intake. There is, however, a very rare condition known as *congenital malabsorption of folate*, which is thought to be due to an inherited defect in the intestinal mucosal transport of folic acid.

Increased requirements. The most important condition in which the requirement for folic acid is increased is pregnancy, the haematological complications of which are discussed later. Premature babies are liable to develop folate-deficiency megaloblastosis, especially those who have feeding difficulties, suffer from infections, or who have received multiple exchange transfusions. Diseases in which there is greatly increased haemopoietic activity, such as chronic haemolytic states, leukaemia or the myeloproliferative disorders (p. 17.56), or rapid proliferation (usually neoplastic) of other tissues, can similarly predispose to folic-acid deficiency.

Drugs. It cannot be over-emphasised that *therapeutic agents can produce an astonishing variety of haematological disturbances*, and one of the most notable examples of this is the megaloblastic anaemia associated with *anticonvulsant drugs* such as phenytoin. The mechanism involved is uncertain, but these drugs probably interfere with folic-acid absorption. It is also suspected that oral contraceptives can produce folate deficiency. Some drugs are *folic-acid antagonists* and are given deliberately to induce folate deficiency in proliferating tumour cells (e.g. methotrexate, cytosine arabinoside) or to combat infection (e.g. cotrimoxazole, nitrofurantoin): inevitably, they cause some degree of megaloblastic change in the marrow.

The diagnosis of folic-acid deficiency

Anaemia with megaloblastic haemopoiesis in the absence of B_{12} deficiency strongly suggests deficiency of folic acid. Serum folate level may be measured microbiologically, using *Lactobacillus casei*, or by radioimmunoassay. Most laboratories quote the normal range as 3–15 µg/l. All folate-deficient patients show a low serum folate level but the serum folate is very sensitive to immediate dietary deficiency, so that *low serum levels may occur in the absence of genuine deficiency*. Most folate in the blood is located in the red cells and the red cell folate level, which can be measured by the same techniques used for serum assay, is a valuable test of body folate stores: the normal adult range is 160–640 µg/l of packed red cells. However, *the haematological response to folic acid remains the most convincing evidence of deficiency*.

Iron deficiency anaemia

There is no regulatory mechanism for iron excretion, and body iron content is controlled entirely by absorption from the gut. The mechanism of control of absorption and the distribution and forms of storage iron are discussed on page 11.13 *et seq.*

In children and adult males, less than 1 mg of iron is lost passively from the body every day and this is easily replaced by absorption of a similar amount of iron from a balanced diet. In females, however, the average daily loss is increased by menstruation to about 1·6 mg daily, and in the second and third trimesters of pregnancy the loss includes fetal requirements and is about 3·0 mg daily; *iron balance is thus more precarious in women of reproductive age and iron deficiency anaemia is common in them*.

Negative iron balance results from excessive losses of iron from the body or from impaired intake or absorption of iron relative to physiological requirements. In some patients both factors are involved. Negative iron balance is compensated, for a time, by mobilisation of the iron stores and by enhanced absorption from the gut, but eventually the stores may become depleted and the characteristic changes of iron deficiency begin to appear in the blood.

Causes of iron deficiency anaemia

Low dietary intake of iron is an important factor in iron deficiency, especially in developing countries and in infants before weaning. Dietary deficiency of iron is, however, often not the sole cause of anaemia.

Chronic blood loss. *This is the only way by which large amounts of iron can be lost from the body.* A litre of blood contains approximately 500 mg of iron and a loss of 10–15 ml blood daily (5–7 mg iron) is equivalent to the maximum amount of iron that can be absorbed from a normal diet. Heavy menstrual bleeding is important, but any source of chronic or recurrent blood loss has the same effect. Occult bleeding from unsuspected lesions of the gastro-intestinal tract, especially peptic ulceration or ulcerated carcinoma of the stomach, caecum or colon, is of diagnostic importance because iron deficiency anaemia may be the presenting feature of such underlying conditions. Infestation with hookworm (*ankylostomiasis*—p. 28.37), which causes considerable gastro-intestinal bleeding, is probably the most common cause of iron deficiency worldwide and an important cause of chronic morbidity in the tropics.

Malabsorption of iron. Iron is absorbed mainly in the duodenum and disease affecting it may cause iron deficiency, e.g. coeliac disease. Normal gastric acid secretion is also important for iron absorption and gastrectomy or achlorhydria predispose to iron deficiency.

Physiological increase in iron requirements. Infants, children and adolescents have increased requirements for iron because of the expansion of blood volume which accompanies growth. As noted above, menstrual loss of blood and fetal requirements also increase iron demands in women.

Changes in the blood

The laboratory findings in iron deficiency depend on its degree. When body iron stores are entirely depleted, no stainable iron is observed in biopsies of the bone marrow, transferrin saturation is less than 15% (normal 30%) and the serum ferritin level is less than 14 µg/l (normal range 20–100 µg/l—p. 11.15). The blood picture may still be normal (*latent iron de-*

ficiency), but any increase in the deficiency will result in anaemia with a fall in MCV and MCH and a rise in red distribution width (p. 17.8). As the deficiency progresses the red cells become obviously microcytic and hypochromic and poikilocytosis is evident (Fig. 17.29). The total iron binding capacity (TIBC) rises as a result of increased hepatic apotransferrin synthesis and the serum iron level falls, resulting in a decreased saturation of TIBC to less than 10%. The fall in the number of red cells is usually slight or moderate and erythroblasts are not seen in the peripheral blood. The leucocyte count is usually normal. The platelet count is also normal but in longstanding cases it may be increased. If blood loss is an important factor, there may be a reticulocytosis.

Bone marrow

In addition to absence of stainable iron, the marrow is hyperplastic due to erythropoietin stimulation but, because of lack of iron, pro-

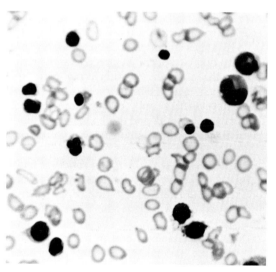

Fig. 17.30 Sternal marrow in severe microcytic anaemia, illustrating the increased proportion of erythroblasts, many of which are poorly haemoglobinised normoblasts. × 1000.

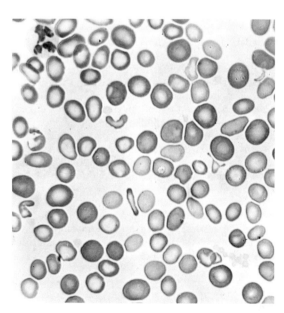

Fig. 17.29 Blood smear in iron-deficiency anaemia, showing some variation in the size of red cells and some rod cells: note also ring-staining which is, however, not diagnostic. × 800.

duction of haemoglobin, and therefore of red cells, is inadequate. Cytologically there is an increased number of both early erythroblasts and small, poorly haemoglobinised pyknotic normoblasts (Fig. 17.30).

Associated changes

In severe iron deficiency, the haematological effects are the most obvious, but other signs of tissue iron depletion may be found. The nails become striated and brittle and may eventually become spoon-shaped (*koilonychia*). Atrophic glossitis and *angular cheilosis*, with fissuring of the angles of the mouth, may also occur. A minority of patients suffer from *dysphagia* (difficulty in swallowing), which may be purely functional but is sometimes related to a folding of lax mucosa in the upper oesophagus. Such an 'oesophageal web' may disappear with successful treatment of the anaemia. The association of anaemia, glossitis and dysphagia is known as the *Plummer-Vinson syndrome*; it may predispose to the later development of post-cricoid carcinoma of the oesophagus. A high proportion of iron-deficient patients have achlorhydria and there may be various degrees of mucosal change in the body of the stomach, ranging from superficial gastritis to atrophic gastritis or gastric atrophy as severe as that found in pernicious anaemia. In most patients, however, it is likely that the achlorhydria is the *result* of iron deficiency, analogous to the other tissue changes mentioned above: only in a minority does it appear to precede and predispose to the anaemia by interfering with iron absorption. Once achlorhydria has developed, it will nevertheless tend to aggravate the iron deficiency. The oral and nail changes usually respond to iron, but achlorhydria may be permanent.

Iron deficiency is much the commonest cause of hypochromic microcytic anaemia, but any condition characterised by failure of haemoglobin synthesis will have the same effect. In some patients the fault may lie in globin chain synthesis (thalassaemia) and in others a failure to synthesise adequate amounts of haem (*sideroblastic anaemias*—see below).

Anaemias due to disorders of iron metabolism

While iron deficiency is a major cause of anaemia, abnormalities of iron metabolism also cause anaemia. Iron derived from haemoglobin catabolism by macrophages is mainly bound to plasma apotransferrin to form transferrin (p. 11.14) and returned to the bone marrow for haemoglobin synthesis; transferrin iron is donated to the developing normoblasts and is later inserted into protoporphyrin to form haem. This pathway may be compromised in two situations.

(a) The anaemia of chronic disease. In chronic infections, rheumatoid disease, systemic lupus erythematosus, renal failure with uraemia, disseminated carcinoma and other wasting diseases, there is often a mild microcytic anaemia due in part to a block in release of iron by macrophages: the plasma iron level is low but the total iron-binding capacity (TIBC), reflecting mainly the apotransferrin level, is also reduced so that the percentage saturation is not as low as in iron deficiency. The reduced level of plasma transferrin results in inadequate supply of iron to the marrow and maturation of erythroblasts is therefore delayed. The serum ferritin level is normal or raised. In addition to these effects, there is a quantitative depression of erythropoiesis and often a mild reduction in red cell lifespan. So long as the causal condition persists, treatment by oral iron therapy is ineffective.

(b) Sideroblastic anaemia. This is a heterogeneous group of disorders which have in common the presence of prussian-blue positive granules in the normoblasts, usually arranged around the nucleus in a ring fashion (*ring sideroblasts*) and representing mitochondria laden with ferric iron. This appearance results from impairment of iron utilisation in the cell; since iron is not being inserted into the porphyrin precursors, haem cannot be formed and there is thus poor haemoglobinisation of the red cells. The rare *primary congenital form* of this disorder is sex-linked, occurring in males in childhood or adolescence. The more common form, *primary acquired sideroblastic anaemia*, occurs in middle-aged and elderly subjects who usually present with symptoms of mild anaemia. Such patients may eventually develop acute myeloblastic leukaemia. *Secondary sideroblastic anaemia* may be due to specific toxins such as alcohol, anti-tuberculous drugs, chloramphenicol and lead, or may be associated with primary myeloproliferative disorders, various leukaemias, carcinomatosis and erythropoietic porphyria.

Anaemias of pregnancy

It is well recognised that the haemoglobin level tends to fall during normal pregnancy. This so-called 'physiological anaemia' is probably due to an expansion of the plasma volume rather than to any fall in the total haemoglobin content of the blood. Nevertheless, true anaemia is common, mainly because of the demands of the developing fetus on iron and folic acid, particularly during the later months of pregnancy. An adequate diet will normally meet the increasing requirements, but haematinic deficiency is especially liable to develop when a woman is in negative haematinic balance at the onset of pregnancy. **Iron deficiency** is common in non-pregnant women of reproductive age (p. 11.13) and not surprisingly is the commonest cause of anaemia during pregnancy; although debilitating, it is seldom severe. **Megaloblastic anaemia,** often severe, is not uncommon in the third trimester of pregnancy. It is due to deficiency of folic acid and so the traditional term 'pernicious anaemia of pregnancy' is inappropriate and should be discarded. Since it is potentially dangerous for a woman to begin labour in an anaemic state, supplementation of the diet with both iron and folic acid is now a routine part of ante-natal care, and it is recommended that the daily intake of folic acid should not be less than 200 µg during pregnancy. Occasionally almost any other form of anaemia may fortuitously complicate pregnancy.

Hypoplastic and aplastic anaemias

Anaemia due to diminution in the total cell mass of the haemopoietic marrow is termed aplastic when little or no cellular marrow exists, and hypoplastic when the marrow is merely of reduced cellularity, as is more commonly the case. Aplasia restricted to red-cell precursors **(pure red cell aplasia)** may be *congenital* (*Blackfan-Diamond anaemia or erythrogenesis imperfecta*) or *acquired*, usually in adults and often associated with thymic tumours. It is more usual for all the haemopoietic cell lines to be affected, resulting in reduced numbers of all the cellular elements in the peripheral blood **(pancytopenia).** This may also be *congenital* (*Fanconi anaemia*, usually associated with other mesenchymal, e.g. skeletal, abnormalities) or *acquired.*

These conditions are all rare apart from acquired aplastic anaemia.

Acquired aplastic anaemia with pancytopenia

The characteristic **changes in the blood** are normochromic normocytic anaemia, granulocytopenia and thrombocytopenia; these result respectively in anaemic manifestations which may be severe, increased liability to infection which is often fatal, and thrombocytopenic bleeding which increases the pancytopenia. The **bone marrow** is hypocellular and fatty (Fig. 17.31) and most of the few cells present are lymphocytes or plasma cells. There may be small haemopoietic foci or, in cases of very rapid onset, patches of cell debris lying between the fat cells.

Causes of aplastic anaemia include (1) damage to the haemopoietic stem cell by drugs, chemicals and x-rays, (2) an immune reaction against the stem cell or its progeny, and (3) marrow micro-environmental damage.

Drugs, chemicals and x-rays. *Cytotoxic drugs or x-rays used in the treatment of malignant disease regularly produce marrow depression in proportion to the dosage.* It is usually possible to avoid severe damage by careful monitoring of the blood and adjustment of dosage. In some patients, marrow aplasia results from an *idiosyncratic reaction to certain drugs*, particularly

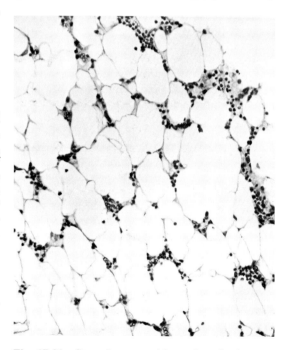

Fig. 17.31 Sternal marrow biopsy in aplastic anaemia due to chloramphenicol. There is great reduction in the numbers of all cell types. × 250.

chloramphenicol, sulphonamides, phenylbuta-zone and other anti-rheumatic agents and anti-thyroid drugs. Such drug reactions are now a major problem and are not infrequently fatal, but in some cases the condition is reversible on stopping the drug. Some hair dyes and many industrial organic chemicals, e.g. benzene, can also cause aplastic anaemia. When (as is usual) there is pancytopenia, the causal agent prob-ably affects the haemopoietic stem cells and there may also be lymphopenia. In other in-stances, however, the effect is mainly on com-mitted progenitor cells (p. 8.16) and there may then be red cell aplasia, agranulocytosis, or thrombocytopenia in any combination. In some cases there appears to be an inborn defect of haemopoietic cells which renders them sucepti-ble to injury by the drug. In others, immuno-logical reactions may be involved.

About 50% of cases of aplastic anaemia are 'idiopathic' and a virus aetiology has been sus-pected, but the only virus infections so far in-criminated are type A virus hepatitis and infec-tious mononucleosis. In these conditions, aplastic anaemia is a rare complication, usually severe and often fatal; it appears within 10 weeks of an (often mild) attack of hepatitis.

It is important to distinguish pancytopenia attributable to aplastic anaemia from other pancytopenias, e.g. in marrow replacement, leukaemia, megaloblastic anaemia or hyper-splenism.

Agranulocytosis and thrombocytopenia, due to failure of marrow production, may each occur in pure form and are considered respec-tively on pp. 17.13 and 17.62.

Neoplasia of the Haemopoietic Tissues

Precursor cells of the erythroid, myeloid, lym-phoid and megakaryocyte series may undergo physiological proliferation in response to appropriate stimuli. Each cell line may also undergo purposeless proliferation in the bone marrow, giving rise to conditions which must be regarded as neoplastic, although in some features they differ from typical tumours of other tissues. By far the commonest and most important are the **leukaemias** which are neopla-sias of leucocyte, usually myeloid (granulocytic) or lymphoid, precursors and in which the neo-plastic cells, like their normal counterparts, enter and circulate in the blood. There is also a group termed the **dysmyelopoietic syndromes** which, although not initially neoplastic, often progress to leukaemia and include many of the disorders classified as *pre-leukaemias*. The **myeloproliferative disorders** form another large group of not uncommon conditions exemplified by (a) *polycythaemia rubra vera*, a proliferation mainly of the erythroid series, (b) *myelofibrosis*, a related condition in which there is also fibro-sis of the marrow, and (c) *essential thrombo-cythaemia*, in which megakaryocytic prolifer-ation predominates. These three apparently neoplastic conditions have overlapping features and transitional or intermediate forms are sometimes observed, presumably reflecting an origin from pluripotent haemopoietic stem cells.

Neoplasias of lymphoid cells pose a problem in classification, for they include the **lymphoid leukaemias** and the **plasma-cell tumours,** most of which originate in the marrow, and also the **solid lymphomas** of the lymphoid and other tissues. Lymphoid leukaemias and plasma-cell tumours are included in this account but the solid lymphomas are described in Chapter 18.

General features. Although, as indicated above, haemopoietic neoplasia is classified by cell type, there may be proliferation of two or more lines. For example, megakaryocytic pro-liferation and thrombocytosis are common features of chronic granulocytic leukaemia while erythroid, myeloid and megakaryocytic cells all proliferate in polycythaemia rubra vera. There is, moreover, a tendency for one condi-tion to transform into another during the course of the disease.

Most forms of haemopoietic neoplasia differ from carcinomas and sarcomas in that they usually infiltrate the marrow, and sometimes other tissues, diffusely rather than forming dis-tinct tumour masses. They suppress and replace the normal haemopoietic elements, often with consequent reduction in the production of red and white cells and platelets. As with other neoplasias, a high degree of cell differentiation is usually associated with a relatively chronic course, and poor differentiation with more ag-gressive behaviour, *but virtually all forms of haemopoietic neoplasia are malignant and are likely to be fatal in the untreated patient.*

The leukaemias

The leukaemias are neoplastic proliferations of leucocyte precursors in the bone marrow. Like normal leucocytes, such neoplastic cells escape into the blood where they may be present in large numbers (hence 'leukaemia'). Leukaemic proliferation overwhelms normal haemopoiesis in the marrow and the leukaemic cells infiltrate many other organs. Traditionally, leukaemias are divided into two main classes, **acute** and **chronic**. Two decades ago, the patient with acute leukaemia followed a rapid, relentless, downhill course to death within a matter of weeks, whereas the patient with chronic leukae-mia survived for very much longer. Since the advent of more effective therapy this position has changed radically: prolonged remission can be achieved in over 50% of children with acute lymphoblastic leukaemia and many of these may be cured: the outlook is much better than in patients with chronic granulocytic leukae-mia. However, it is essential to retain the acute and chronic classification because this serves to highlight important differences in aetiology, pathogenesis, cell kinetics, diagnostic proce-dures, clinical features and treatment.

Leukaemias are further sub-divided into lym-phoid, myeloid (granulocytic) and (uncommon) monocytic types: the two main groups of acute leukaemias are **acute lymphoblastic (ALL)** and **acute non-lymphoblastic (ANLL)**: the latter includes also unusual types in which the leuk-aemic cells show features of monocytic or ery-throid precursors. The two main chronic types are **chronic lymphocytic leukaemia (CLL)** and **chronic granulocytic leukaemia (CGL)**. During the past decade, an increasing number of sub-sets of leucocytes and their precursors have been identified and application of marker tests and cytogenetic studies have resulted in further subdivisions; such studies are proving of prog-nostic and therapeutic relevance and are dis-cussed in the following account.

The acute leukaemias

It is now customary to divide acute leukaemias by age incidence into those occurring in child-hood, 80% of which are ALL (see above), and adult acute leukaemias (>15 years), 85% of which are ANLL. The predominant neoplastic cell in acute leukaemia is a poorly differentiated or immature cell, all types of which are widely termed 'blast' cells (the term is applied also to primitive non-neoplastic cells). The develop-ment of suitable cell culture techniques has re-sulted in some progress towards revealing the pathogenesis of acute leukaemia and it is now clear that, as in many other cancers, failure of cells to differentiate is a classical feature, the degree of which varies, giving different types of acute leukaemia. There is evidence that acute leukaemia cells in tissue culture can be induced to differentiate by addition of certain biological agents, including corticosteroids, physiological regulators of haemopoiesis (e.g. colony stimu-lating factor—p. 17.3) and some chemicals. However, therapeutic induction of remission of acute leukaemia depends on destruction of the leukaemic cells rather than correction of their behaviour.

As in other malignant neoplasias, many of the acute leukaemic cells are in a resting (non-dividing) state: the proportion of dividing cells varies, but is often relatively low before treat-ment and high during relapse. Many anti-leukaemic drugs have been introduced because of their known cytotoxic effects on actively proliferating cells and schedules of treatment are now designed to synchronise cell division and bring resting cells into a susceptible state of active proliferation.

Clinical picture. The clinical features of acute leukaemia are attributable mainly to rapidly developing failure of normal haemopoiesis. This results in the classical triad of pallor, fatigue and weakness due to anaemia, recurrent infections due to reduction of normal (non-leukaemic) leucocytes, and bleeding due to thrombocytopenia. The disease appears abruptly with fever, weakness, pallor, bleeding from the gums and petechial haemorrhages in the skin. Intercurrent infections are very common and without treatment the whole course from onset to death may be only a few weeks. In adults, the disease may be more insidious, but the clinical features are similar.

Blood picture. The leucocyte count is usually raised, often to $100 \times 10^9/l$ ($100\,000/\mu l$). Most of these cells are large primitive blasts, with nucleoli and a high nuclear/cytoplasmic ratio (Fig. 17.32). In over a third of cases, however, the total white cell count is normal or even reduced—so-called 'aleukaemic leukaemia—although primitive leukaemic cells can almost always be demonstrated.

Bone marrow. In smears of marrow aspirates, a marked increase in cellularity is usual and most of the cells are primitive 'blasts' (Fig. 17.33). Sections of the marrow show replacement of the fat spaces by the primitive leukaemic cells. Normal haemopoietic elements, especially neutrophils and megakaryocytes, are

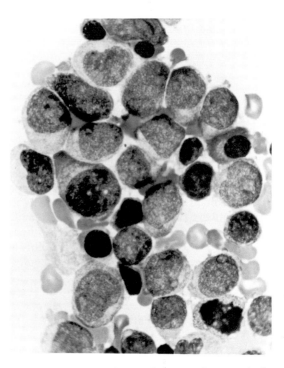

Fig. 17.33 Smear of sternal marrow in acute leukaemia. Nearly all the cells are primitive 'blasts', with a large nucleus containing one or more nucleoli, and with scanty basophilic cytoplasm. ×750. (Dr Annette Mallinson.)

sparse. At autopsy, in untreated cases there is a variable degree of extension of cellular leukaemic marrow along the shafts of the long bones, replacing the fatty tissue: it often has a reddish-grey or green hue and a firm consistency.

Other tissues. *Splenic enlargement* is common but seldom gross. *Lymph node enlargement* is unusual in ANLL but frequently occurs in ALL. In some instances of ALL a *thymic lymphoid tumour* (*Sternberg's tumour*) precedes the onset of ALL in childhood (p. 18.25). Rarely ANLL, especially in children, is preceded by the discovery of a tumour of ANLL cells, usually arising under the periosteum of the facial bones and termed a *granulocytic sarcoma* or *chloroma*, since it has a curious green colour which fades rapidly on exposure to air.

More extensive diffuse tissue infiltration occurs during the course of acute leukaemia, and almost any organ can be affected.

Leukaemic cells proliferating in the *subarachnoid space* often escape destruction during

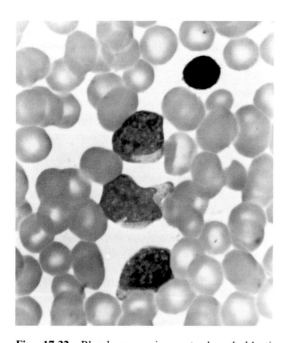

Fig. 17.32 Blood smear in acute lymphoblastic leukaemia, showing three large, primitive leukaemic cells with dispersed chromatin and basophilic cytoplasm. The cell at upper right is a mature lymphocyte. ×1000.

treatment because, with the exception of methotrexate in high dosage, most cytotoxic drugs do not reach an effective concentration in the cerebrospinal fluid. Such cells provided a nidus from which dissemination and relapse may occur. Similarly, leukaemic cells which have infiltrated *the gonads*, especially the testis, may escape destruction and be a source of relapse. Radiotherapy is also of value in eliminating leukaemic cells in these protected sites.

Diagnosis and types of acute leukaemia. The diagnosis of acute leukaemia is based on the clinical features, the blood picture, and the morphology of the bone marrow (see above). To assess the prognosis and select the most appropriate form of treatment it is necessary to distinguish between ANLL and ALL and to further identify the sub-types of leukaemia in each of these two major groups. Such detailed classification is not always easy and is best achieved by a combination of the morphological, cell-marker and cytogenetic studies described briefly below.

The distinction between ANLL and ALL can sometimes be made morphologically, lymphoblasts having a higher nuclear-cytoplasmic ratio, a denser nuclear membrane, coarser clumping of chromatin and fewer nucleoli than myeloblasts. The distinction is also aided by cytochemical tests; the most useful are the peroxidase and Sudan black B tests which demonstrate myeloperoxidase in the primary (azurophil) granules of granulocyte precursors. Cells of the monocyte line posess granules which stain with α-naphthyl acetate esterase.

Demonstration of large cytoplasmic granules ('blocks') of glycogen by the periodic acid-Schiff (PAS) stain in leukaemic blasts is indicative of ALL, although not all cases present this feature. The detection of deoxynucleotidyl transferase (TdT—a DNA polymerase) is also helpful, for it is present in over 95% of cases of childhood ALL (all except B-cell ALL) and negative in ANLL.

The further diagnosis of subtypes of ALL and ANLL is based on the widely-used classification devised by a collaborative group of French, American and British workers—**the FAB classification** (Bennett *et al.*, 1976, 1981). This provides a means of distinguishing between three types of ALL and six types of ANLL (Table 17.7) by the morphology of the leukaemic cells using Romanowsky stains and simple cytochemical tests. Additional cytochemical tests, use of monoclonal antibodies and other techniques to detect cell markers, and cytogenetic studies to detect chromosomal abnormalities, are all valuable adjuncts in the diagnosis of acute leukaemias. They augment morphological classification, demonstrate greater heterogeneity in both ALL and ANLL, and are of prognostic and therapeutic significance.

Acute lymphoblastic leukaemia (ALL) of childhood

This is classified in the FAB system into three types. L1 includes 85% of all childhood ALL:

Table 17.7 The French–American–British (FAB) morphological classification of the acute leukaemias

FAB Morphological classification	Type Name
Acute lymphoblastic leukaemia (ALL)	
L1: Small, uniform cell type	Common ALL (cALL)
	T-ALL
L2: Large, pleomorphic cell type	Null-ALL
L3: Vacuolated cytoplasm	B-ALL
Acute non-lymphoblastic leukaemia (ANLL)	
M1: Myeloblastic, no differentiation	AML without differentiation
M2: Myeloblastic, some differentiation, Auer rods	AML with differentiation
M3: Promyelocytic	Acute promyelocytic
M4: Granulocytic and monocytic differentiation	Myelomonocytic
M5: Monoblastic	Monoblastic
M6: Erythroblastic and myeloblastic	Erythroleukaemia

the leukaemic cells are mostly small blasts of uniform appearance with a large rounded nucleus, scanty cytoplasm and inconspicuous nucleoli. In L2 (14% of childhood ALL), the cells are heterogeneous in size, nuclear shape and chromatin pattern: the nuclear/cytoplasmic ratio is about 5:1 (in smear preparations) and some cells have large nucleoli. L3 is rare (1%); the cells are large with abundant basophilic, often vacuolated cytoplasm.

Membrane and immunological markers. T lymphocytes are identified by their ability to bind sheep erythrocytes, forming 'E' rosettes' (p. 6.33) and also by means of a series of monoclonal antibodies which react with T cells and with various functional subsets of T cells. B cells are identified by detecting their surface immunoglobulin (SIg): cytoplasmic μ heavy chain (Cμ) is formed in a stage of primitive, pre-B cells which lack SIg (p. 6.14). More recently a surface antigen has been identified, by means of a monoclonal antibody, on the surface of lymphoblasts of most children with ALL; it is called **the common ALL antigen (c ALLA)**.

Application of such markers in childhood ALL has shown that about 15% have T-cell markers (**T-ALL**) and 1–2% have B-cell markers (**B-ALL**). Over 80% have neither T nor B markers and are classified as **non-B, non-T ALL**, but they are a heterogeneous group, about 85% being cALLA +ve (**cALL**) and the remaining 15% are termed **null-ALL**. About one-third of the cALLA +ve non-B, non-T cases have demonstrable Cμ and are thus really pre-B ALL, and many of the rest have arrangements of the Ig genes which suggest that they too are committed to B-cell lineage. B-ALL cells (but not T-ALL cells) are also cALLA +ve.

The rather complex classification based on the above markers is of clinical significance. For example, **non-B, non-T cALL** (85% including pre-B ALL) is usually of L1 morphology, often PAS +ve, and occurs more commonly in girls than boys with a peak incidence between 3 and 7 years of age. The WBC is usually between $5-15 \times 10^9/1$ ($5-15\,000/\mu$l) and the response to treatment and prognosis are usually good.

Null ALL (10%) also usually presents L1 morphology, but has a worse prognosis than cALL. In **T-ALL** (15%) the morphology may be either L1 or L2: it tends to occur in older children, particularly boys, and is characterised by a high WBC (about $40 \times 10^9/1$) and a mediastinal mass (Sternberg's tumour—p. 18.25). Response to treatment is poor and relapse from surviving cells in the meninges (p. 17.46) is common. Accordingly, the prognosis is bad.

In the rare **B-ALL** (1–2%) the morphology is L3 with characteristic vacuolated blast cells. This type has the worst prognosis.

Cytogenetic changes. Chromosome analysis, including modern banding techniques (p. 2.4) has revealed abnormalities in the chromosomes of the blast cells in more than two-thirds of untreated patients with ALL, and it is likely that, as techniques continue to advance, they will be found in virtually all cases. Many of the chromosomal changes are non-random and they are of aetiological, therapeutic and prognostic importance.

About 5% of cases of **cALL** have a translocation t (9;22)—the 'Philadelphia chromosome' (Ph^1), which is a major feature of chronic granulocytic leukaemia (p. 17.52): occasionally t (4;11) is found in cALL and this is present in most cases of **null-ALL**. In **T-ALL**, t (9;22) or t (4;1) are occasionally present and t (8;14) is usually present in **B-ALL**. Other abnormalities include gain of a chromosome, usually 21, 14 or 13; a modal number of over 50 chromosomes is found in 30% of cases of **non-B, non-T ALL** and appears to carry a good prognosis. Apart from this, chromosomal anomalies usually worsen the prognosis and persistence of the abnormal clone after treatment is a grave prognostic sign.

Adult ALL

This differs clinically from childhood ALL in often having a more gradual onset. The proportion of cases with L1 morphology (FAB classification—p. 17.47 is lower (about 36%) and more cases are L2 (about 56%) or L3 (8%). Virtually all the L3 cases are of B-cell type.

About 70% of cases are non-B, non-T, but a smaller proportion (about 30%) of these are cALLA-positive and a higher proportion (about 20%) have the Ph^1 chromosome abnormality. The prognosis is, in general, worse than in children, but remission lasting 5 years or more is now being achieved by chemotherapy in about 25% of patients.

A rare form of aggressive T-cell lymphoma/leukaemia of adults occurs endemically in Japan and some other countries; it is of intense interest because of the recent discovery of an associated oncogenic virus and is described on p. 18.28.

The occurrence of a blast cell crisis resembling ALL in chronic granulocytic leukaemia is described on pp. 17.51, 17.53.

Acute non-lymphoblastic leukaemias (ANLL)

These include the six types (M1–6) of acute leukaemia listed in Table 17.7 (p. 17.47) and division into further sub-types has resulted from cell-marker and cytogenetic studies, which correlate only partially with the FAB classification. Types M1–3 are all leukaemias of the granulocyte series and differ in the degree of differentiation of the leukaemic cells. In **M1**, less than 10% of the cells differentiate sufficiently to develop a few azurophil granules and give a positive peroxidase or Sudan black B reaction. Most cells have large rounded nuclei and up to four prominent nucleoli. In **M2** the cells have bilobed or reniform nuclei, usually an Auer rod, azurophil granules, and are peroxidase and Sudan black B positive; variable numbers of cells differentiate into abnormal promyelocytes, myelocytes and even granulocytes. In **M3,** most of the cells are rich in peroxidase-positive azurophil granules, some contain bundles of Auer rods and resemble promyelocytes. Two populations of cells are present in **M4**, myeloblasts and monoblasts: they may be distinguished by non-specific esterase activity which is demonstrated by the splitting of a naphthol ester substrate (the NASDA reaction). Both cell types are positive but pre-treatment with sodium fluoride inhibits the reaction in monoblasts whereas myeloblasts are resistant. In **M5**, most of the leukaemic cells are monoblasts, less than 20% being myeloblastic. **M6** is characterised by the presence of both myeloblasts and abnormal primitive erythroblasts, some of which have abnormal multiple or lobed nuclei: the erythroblasts account for over 30% of nucleated cells in the marrow.

Over 50% of ANLL cases are M1 or M2, about 30% are M4, while M3, 5 and 6 are uncommon. With intensive chemotherapy, M3 cases have the longest survival while M6 has a very poor prognosis. The remaining types show considerable individual variation in the response to treatment.

Cytogenetics. About 50% of patients with AMLL show no cytogenetic abnormalities, although there is recent evidence of subtle chromosomal changes in many of these. The remaining 50% show a variety of abnormalities which mostly differ from those found in ALL and correlate only partially with M1–6 morphology. Examples include an extra chromosome 8, loss of a chromosome 7, t (8;21) which is seen only in some M2 patients and t (17;15), seen in most M3 cases only. About 2% of cases show the Philadelphia chromosome.

The chronic leukaemias

The two main types are **chronic lymphocytic leukaemia (CLL)** and **chronic granulocytic leukaemia (CGL)**. CLL is rare below 40 years of age, the median age of onset being 50–60 years, and it accounts for almost 50% of leukaemias occurring after the sixth decade of life. The median

age of onset of CGL is 30–40 years, but it occurs over a wide age range and is seen in children. In both diseases, large numbers of leucocytes circulate in the blood and eventually infiltrate various tissues. In most cases, the initial leukaemic proliferation is readily controlled by drugs, but many patients with CLL remain well without treatment and may never require specific anti-leukaemic therapy. By contrast, the prognosis is poor in CGL because the chronic phase is superseded sooner or later by an acute phase characterised by decreasing cell maturity and greater resistance to therapy.

Chronic lymphocytic leukaemia

Blood picture. The outstanding feature is a marked increase in leucocytes, commonly to around $100 \times 10^9/1$ ($100\,000/\mu l$): nearly all are lymphoid cells and most are mature small lymphocytes (Fig. 17.34), with only a small proportion of larger, more primitive cells. Although the disease usually appears to originate in the bone marrow, anaemia, granulocyto-

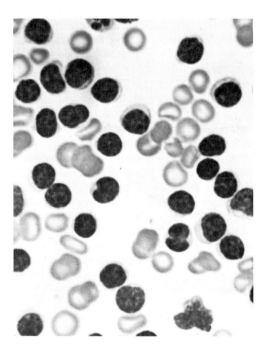

Fig. 17.34 Blood smear in chronic lymphocytic leukaemia. Most of the leukaemic cells have the appearances of normal small lymphocytes, a narrow ring of pale cytoplasm enclosing a round, dense nucleus of about the diameter of a red cell. × 750.

penia and thrombocytopenia due to marrow replacement are late features. Auto-immune haemolytic anaemia and mild thrombocytopenia,
possibly also of auto-immune nature, are complications which may occur quite early in the
course of the disease.

There is often a reduction in the normal
plasma immunoglobulin levels, decreased resistance to bacterial infection, and sometimes a
monoclonal gammopathy (p. 17.60) develops
due to secretion of Ig by the leukaemic cells. In
about 95% of cases the leukaemic lymphocytes
possess surface immunoglobulin (SIg) and
other markers characteristic of B cells. About
5% of cases are of T-cell origin, but the percentage is significantly higher in the Eastern
hemisphere.

Bone marrow. From an early stage the bone
marrow shows an excess of lymphocytes which
may initially be focal but later becomes diffuse
and gradually replaces the normal haemopoietic cells. Eventually the fatty marrow is also
replaced and the shafts of the long bones
become filled with pale leukaemic marrow
resembling that seen in CGL.

Other tissues. Generalised enlargement of the
lymph nodes is a conspicuous feature and commonly the presenting sign of the disease. The
nodes are soft and rubbery and appear homogeneous and pinkish-grey on cutting. Large
nodes may cause clinical effects by compressing
important structures such as the common bile
duct. Microscopically, the nodal architecture is
lost and replaced by massive diffuse lymphocytic infiltration, the appearances being those of
lymphocytic lymphoma (p. 18.22). The **spleen** is
enlarged but seldom as massive as in CGL. It
usually weighs between 1 and 2 kg and microscopy shows extensive infiltration by mature
lymphocytes which fill the red pulp and obscure
the Malpighian bodies.

Involvement of other organs is usually extensive, although it tends to be patchy. The **liver** is
usually enlarged due to infiltration of the portal
and periportal areas by leukaemic cells (Fig.
17.35). The **kidneys** are also usually enlarged,
either diffusely or with nodules of leukaemic
infiltration. As with CGL, the extent of infiltration of the various organs varies greatly. The
risk of secondary gout and renal damage by
urate crystals is not as great as in CGL.

Other features include fatty change due to
the anaemia, which develops late in the disease,

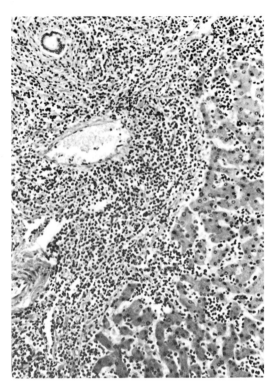

Fig. 17.35 Section of liver in chronic lymphocytic
leukaemia, showing infiltration of lymphocytes
around the portal tracts. × 60.

and bacterial infection, especially bronchopneumonia, which is often the immediate
cause of death.

Diagnosis and course. The minimum diagnostic criteria for CLL are: (a) persistent lymphocytosis of more than $5 \times 10^9/1$ (5000/μl), of
mature small lymphocytes and (b) a bone marrow lymphocytosis in excess of 30%, CLL is an
extremely variable disease. The course may be
rapidly progressive with a fatal outcome in 1–2
years or it may be static over several decades.
The overwhelming majority of cases are of B-
cell lineage (B–CLL); monoclonal SmIg at low
density and receptors for mouse erythrocytes
are detectable on a high proportion of cells.
T-CLL has a similarly variable course; it can
occur at a much earlier age and may show the
morphological and immunological features and
antigenic markers of suppressor/cytotoxic T
lymphocytes (see pp. 6.20 *et seq*).

Staging of CLL, based on physical examination and the blood picture, is designed to assess
the extent of the disease and to indicate the

likely prognosis. Two staging systems in common use are shown in Table 17.8. They are both of prognostic value and are also likely to be of help in assessing the effectiveness of various therapeutic regimes. The most important prognostic factor in CLL, however, is the rate of progression of the disease, and while a patient diagnosed at an early stage is more likely to progress slowly or remain static than a patient with advanced disease, this is not always the case.

Leukaemic states resembling CLL. The term **pro-lymphocytic leukaemia** is applied to leukaemia of either B (80%) or T (20%) lymphocyte lineage in which the tumour cells resemble small lymphocytes but have prominent nucleoli and conspicuously more cytoplasm. Typically the white cell count is very high. Splenomegaly is more pronounced and the disease progresses more rapidly than classical CLL. In **hairy cell leukaemia (leukaemic reticuloendotheliosis)** splenic enlargement is also marked and there is evidence of hypersplenism (p. 17.32). The leukaemic cells, which may be sparse in the blood, show prominent cytoplasmic projections (hence the name) and ovoid nuclei with finely dispersed chromatin. Nearly all cases are of B cell lineage. In the *Sezary syndrome* and *mycosis fungoides* (p. 22.37) there is neoplastic lymphocytic infiltration of the skin and the tumour cells, which are of T-cell origin, appear also in the blood. *Adult T-cell leukaemia/lymphoma,* as the name implies, may present as a solid lymphoma or as leukaemia: it is of great interest because of recent virological findings and is described on p. 13.7. The unfortunate term *lymphosarcoma-cell leukaemia* is sometimes used when cells from a solid lymphoma (especially follicular lymphoma, p. 18.23) enter and accumulate in the blood, giving a leukaemic picture. These cells may exhibit the 'cleaved' or irregular nuclear outline characteristic of centrocytes of the lymph-node follicles.

Chronic granulocytic leukaemic (CGL)

While commonest in adults, with a median age of 30–40, this disease can occur at any age from birth onwards. The clinical picture tends to be dominated initially by gross hepatic and splenic enlargement. Signs of impaired marrow function, such as anaemia and thrombocytopenia, are usually inconspicuous until late in the course of the disease. After a variable period, usually of some years, acute non-lymphoblastic leukaemia (ANLL) or common lymphoblastic leukaemia (cALL) supervenes (*blast transformation*). It is generally accepted that CGL arises as a result of a mutation or series of mutations in a single pluripotential haemopoietic stem cell. Evidence of this comes from studies of CGL patients heterozygous for the glucose-6-phosphate dehydrogenase (G-6-PD) isoenzymes (p. 2.11), which have demonstrated that all the leukaemic cells express the same iso-enzyme. Further support for the monoclonal original of CGL in a stem cell comes from the distribution of the Philadelphia (Ph[1]) chromosome in haemopoietic precursors of CGL patients: it is found in cells of granulocytic, erythroid, megakaryocytic and even B-lymphoid origin. As noted above, acute transformation in CGL may be along myeloid, lymphoid or even mixed cell lines.

Table 17.8 Methods of staging chronic lymphocytic leukaemia (CLL)

Rai *et al.* (1975)

Stage O	Lymphocytosis of blood and marrow only
Stage I	Lymphocytosis and enlarged lymph nodes
Stage II	Lymphocytosis and enlarged liver or spleen or both, with or without enlarged nodes
Stage III	As with O–II but Hb < 11 g/dl
Stage IV	As with O–III but with platelet count < 100 × 10⁹/1

Binet *et al.* (1981)

Group A (good prognosis):	$Hb > 10\,g/dl$: platelet count $> 100 \times 10^9/1$; fewer than three sites of palpable organ involvement
Group B (intermediate prognosis)	Hb and platelet count as for A but with 3 or more sites of palpable organ involvement
Group C (poor prognosis)	$Hb < 10\,g/dl$ and/or platelet count $< 100 \times 10^9/1$

The Philadelphia (Ph¹) chromosome was initially described in 1960 and was considered to be an anomaly of chromosome 21. This classical abnormality has since been shown to be a reciprocal translocation of parts of the long arms of chromosomes 9 and 22 (Fig. 17.36). Approximately 90% of patients with CGL are Ph¹+ve in most or all analysable marrow cell metaphases and have a median sur-

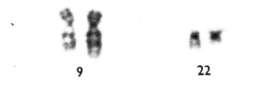

9   **22**

Fig. 17.36 The Philadelphia chromosome anomaly. This shows the classical anomaly, in which there is reciprocal translocation between chromosomes 9 and 22, with breakpoints in the long arms of the chromosomes: the right chromosome of each pair is the anomalous one. (Professor M.A. Ferguson Smith.)

vival of some 42 months whereas the remaining 10% are pH¹−ve and have only a 15-month median survival. In occasional patients the Ph¹+ve stem cells do not dominate haemopoiesis completely and both Ph¹+ve and Ph¹−ve metaphases continue to be detectable in marrow cells: this appears to be associated with a relatively long survival. The development of additional chromosomal changes during the chronic phase of CGL is, however, a grave prognostic sign and often indicates incipient blast transformation. About 80% of patients in the acute terminal phase show additional chromosome abnormalities superimposed on the Ph¹+ve cell line. A few cases of *de-novo* acute leukaemia, both ALL and ANLL, are Ph¹+ve (pp. 17.48, 17.49).

Blood picture. The outstanding feature is the huge number of circulating leucocytes, sometimes exceeding $300 \times 10^9/1$ (300 000/μl). Most of them are mature neutrophil granulocytes (Fig. 17.37), although metamyelocytes and myelocytes are almost always present and in more rapidly progressing cases myelocytes may

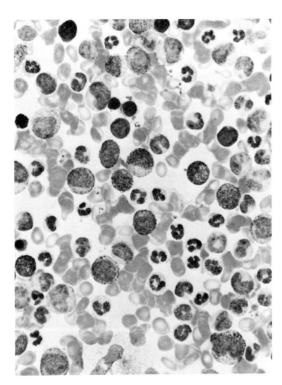

Fig. 17.37 Blood in chronic granulocytic leukaemia, showing myelocytes, neutrophil granulocytes and intermediate forms; two erythroblasts are seen above centre of field. × 500.

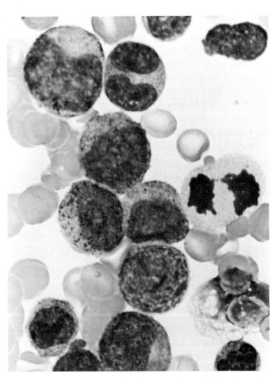

Fig. 17.38 Blood in chronic granulocytic leukaemia, showing finely granular myelocytes and neutrophil granulocytes. One cell is in mitosis. × 1000.

predominate (Fig. 17.38). Occasionally eosinophils are numerous and a significant increase in basophils is a useful diagnostic feature in the blood film. Anaemia is only moderate and indeed a polycythaemic state is observed initially in some cases.

Transformation to the aggressive, acute phase mentioned above is indicated by increasing anaemia and other features of marrow failure, as in acute leukaemia *de novo*. In about 75% of patients, the transformation is myeloblastic and accompanied by a rise in myeloblasts and promyelocytes in the blood. In the remaining 25%, transformation is lymphoblastic, usually of cALL type (p. 17.48), and accompanied by appearance of lymphoblasts and a high level of TdT (p. 17.47) in the blood. Occasionally the blast cells are of more than one lineage, e.g. myeloblasts and lymphoblasts. Most patients with a blast-cell crisis die within six months in spite of treatment.

Diagnosis is usually easy, but rarely a pronounced reactive leucocytosis (p. 17.12) can produce a blood picture closely resembling that of CGL, myelocytes and even less mature cells being observed. Features which help to confirm the diagnosis of CGL include (1) an unusually high proportion of myelocytes, (2) an absolute increase of basophils, (3) the presence of the Ph[1] chromosome in proliferating marrow cells in 90% of cases (see above), (4) the markedly reduced level of alkaline phosphatase in leukaemic neutrophils in contrast to the elevated levels observed in reactive leucocytosis, and (5) elevation of the serum vitamin B_{12}, probably due to an increase in plasma B_{12} binding protein.

Bone marrow. The red marrow is replaced by soft pale pink or greenish tissue, which usually also replaces the fatty marrow throughout the length of the long bones (Fig. 17.39). The marrow cavities are also expanded by reabsorption of bone trabeculae, and at autopsy the expanded marrow can be cut out in large pieces, although it is sometimes almost fluid from autolysis and may even resemble pus. Microscopy shows a massive increase in the marrow cells; granulocyte precursors predominate, myelocytes being most numerous except in the acute terminal stage. In some cases, megakaryocytes are also conspicuous, while in others there may be a pronounced increase in red cell precursors, the appearances resembling those of polycythaemia rubra vera (p. 17.56).

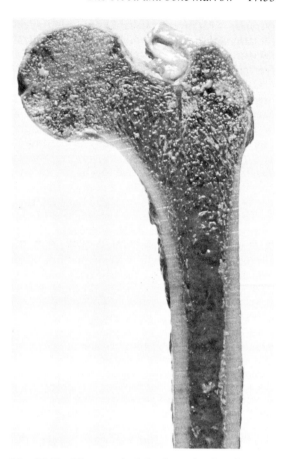

Fig. 17.39 Upper end of the femur in chronic granulocytic leukaemia. Pale cellular marrow occupied the whole shaft. The marrow cavity is also widened by resorption of bone trabeculae.

Other organs. There is usually massive enlargement of the **spleen**, which may exceed 3 kg, and often causes great discomfort. It is moderately firm and the cut surface has a pale red mottled appearance with paler patches of infarction. Microscopically, the red pulp is packed with leukaemic cells, but also shows non-leukaemic extramedullary haemopoiesis, erythroid precursors and megakaryocytes usually being conspicuous. The Malpighian bodies are largely obscured by massive cellular infiltration of the red pulp. In cases in which the disease progresses rapidly, splenic enlargement is usually not so great. The **lymph nodes** are not usually infiltrated until a late-stage of the disease, when they may be moderately enlarged. The **liver** is usually markedly enlarged and microscopy shows extensive sinusoidal infiltration with myeloid cells. Diffuse infiltration of any other organ, including the central nervous system, may occur, and accounts for the varied symptomatology.

Other features include fatty change of the organs due to anaemia, widespread petechial haemorrhages due mainly to thrombocytopenia or defective platelet function, occasionally more extensive haemorrhage, especially in the brain, and haemorrhagic infarcts in various organs due to diffuse microvascular occlusion by aggregates of leukaemic cells. There is usually a rise in the level of serum uric acid derived from the breakdown of nucleic acids from large numbers of leukaemic cells, especially during cytotoxic drug therapy. Unless prevented by appropriate treatment, e.g. with xanthine-oxidase inhibitors, the large uric acid load may lead to secondary gout (p. 23.51) and to formation of urate crystals in the renal tubules, with impairment of renal function.

Variants of CGL. It has become apparent from recent advances in the characterisation of leukaemic cells that CGL comprises a number of different but incompletely defined entities which differ in age incidence, clinical and haematological features, cytogenetics and response to treatment. The major categories of $Ph^1 + ve$ and $Ph^1 - ve$ CGL have already been described, leaving such entities as *juvenile CGL* and *chronic myelomonocytic leukaemia (CMML)*; the latter is more appropriately described under the dysmyelopoietic syndromes (p. 17.58). *Juvenile CGL* is a rare disorder occurring under the age of 5 years and with a very characteristic clinical and haematological picture. The leukaemia cells are $Ph^1 - ve$ and originate from a fetal stem cell; a high level of HbF is found in the red cells. Response to treatment is poor.

Aetiology of the leukaemias

The cellular changes involved in carcinogenesis and the various factors which induce such changes are discussed in Chapter 13. This should be read before the following account, which is restricted to leukaemogenesis but assumes a knowledge of carcinogenesis in general.

Hereditary factors. There is no strong evidence that heredity plays an important role in most cases of leukaemia. A very high incidence of CLL has been reported in some families, e.g. four of five siblings, and the concordance rate of ALL in monozygotic twins has been esti-mated to be over 20%, but there appears to be no strong relationship to particular HLA antigens and it is difficult to exclude environmental factors.

Ionising radiation. The leukaemogenic effect of radiation has been established by the detection of an incidence of leukaemia at least ten times as high as expected in the following three groups: (a) patients treated for ankylosing spondylitis by x-irradiation of the spine (AML and CGL), (b) radiologists practising in the 1930–40s (usually CGL), and (c) survivors of the atom bomb explosions in Japan in 1945 (mostly ALL in children and CGL in adults; less often AML). In each group, the incidence of leukaemia has peaked between 4 and 8 years after exposure. The clinical and pathological features (including age-groups of the various types) of post-irradiation leukaemias are the same as those of 'spontaneous' leukaemias. The incidence of leukaemia bears a close (but not linear) relationship to the dose of irradiation. There is less certainty about the possible leukaemogenic effects of exposure of the fetus to diagnostic x-ray examination in pregnancy or of treatment of patients with polycythaemia rubra vera with radioactive phosphorus.

Chemicals and drugs. The only industrial chemical known with certainty to be leukaemogenic is benzene, prolonged exposure to which increases the risk of developing ANLL and possibly CGL and CLL. The leukaemia is characteristically preceded by marrow hypoplasia, sometimes for several years. There is also firm evidence that cytotoxic and immunosuppressant drugs, and particularly alkylating agents, used to treat various neoplastic conditions (e.g. Hodgkin's disease and ovarian cancer) and non-neoplastic diseases (e.g. rheumatoid arthritis), increase the risk of ANLL. Leukaemia develops most often a few years after the start of treatment and is preceded by a variable period of dyserythropoiesis (p. 17.34). A number of other drugs are suspect, notably phenylbutazone, which is known to cause marrow aplasia and may be leukaemogenic.

Chromosomal abnormalities. As noted earlier, loss or gain of whole chromosomes or parts of chromosomes or translocation of part of one chromosome to another are detectable in at least 50% of all types of leukaemia, and there is recent evidence that such changes are present in most if not all cases of leukaemia. The causal role of such abnormalities is strongly suggested by (1) the association of particular chromosomal changes with particular types of leukaemia, e.g. the Ph[1] chromosome in CGL, trisomy 12 in CLL and specific abnormalities associated with the sub-types of ANLL (p. 17.48); (2) the increased incidence of leukaemia in individuals with certain syndromes attributable to congenital chromosomal abnormalities, e.g. the high incidence ($\times 20$) of ALL or ANLL in trisomy 21 (Down's syndrome) and of ALL in 47, XXY (Klinefelter's syndrome), and (3) the fact that radiation and most leukaemogenic drugs cause chromosomal abnormalities. The evidence that chromosomal abnormalities play a causal role in leukaemia, quite apart from chromosomal changes which occur as a secondary effect in genetically unstable leukaemic cells, is thus very strong.

Leukaemogenic viruses. The role of oncogenic retroviruses in animal species is discussed on pp. 13.6–7. The implication of oncogenic retroviruses in leukoses of domestic fowls and in a whole range of leukaemias and lymphomas in cats, rodents, cattle and non-human primates, has led to intensive search for leukaemogenic viruses in man. Many workers have reported the detection of retrovirus-like particles in human leukaemias, and viruses resembling the retroviruses of non-human primates have been isolated from a wide range of human leukaemias and lymphomas, but a causal relationship has not been established. There is, however, convincing evidence that a retrovirus termed the human T-cell leukaemia virus (HTLV) is responsible for a form of adult T-cell leukaemia/lymphoma which is endogenous in parts of Japan and some other parts of the world. This condition, which may present as a leukaemia or a solid lymphoma, is described on p. 18.28 and the evidence for its viral aetiology is reviewed on p. 13.7.

A unifying concept of leukaemogenesis. Most of the evidence on leukaemogenesis indicates the importance of chromosomal abnormalities, whether occurring 'spontaneously' (i.e. of unknown cause) or induced by irradiation, chemicals, or by integration of a retrovirus. Some of the ways in which chromosomal re-arrangements may effect transformation to a neoplastic cell are well illustrated by the leukaemias. In particular, it is noteworthy that many of the translocations observed in leukaemia affect regions rich in cellular oncogenes and sites of immunoglobulin genes. For example, some of the translocations observed in various leukaemias involve chromosomes carrying the genes for immunoglobulins (2, 22 and 14) and may activate cellular oncogenes (c-*oncs*) by bringing them into proximity with Ig promoter genes: this applies to the reciprocal Philadelphia chromosome changes in which c-*alb* in the translocated part of chromosome 9 is brought into proximity with the promoter genes for λ light chains in chromosome 22. Similarly, the translocations most often related to B-cell ALL are t (8;14), t (2;8) and t (8;22), each of which may transfer the cellular oncogene c-*myc* in chromosome 8 to the vicinity of Ig genes and their promoters. It is also of interest that the part of chromosome 22 transferred to chromosome 9 in Ph[1]+ve CGL contains c-*sis*, which may be a structural gene for the platelet-derived growth factor and has mitogenic activity.

The latent period of some years between exposure to radiation or leukaemogenic chemicals indicates that, like carcinogenesis in general, the development of leukaemia is a multi-step process. Chromosome abnormalities increase the chances of the development of further cellular genetic abnormalities by rendering the affected cells genetically unstable or conferring on them a growth advantage with increased mitotic activity. This is seen in individuals with Ph[1]+ve CGL in whom Ph[1]+ve stem cells gradually dominate haemopoiesis: the blast-cell crisis is attributable to an additional chromosomal abnormality which may occur in either a stem cell of the CGL clone or in a pluripotent Ph[1]+ve stem cell which is not yet neoplastic, converting it to a malignant cell whose progeny may be of any haemopoietic lineage, thus accounting for development of a blast-cell crisis of ALL or ANLL type. The development of resistance to cytotoxic drugs in leukaemia is also explicable by an additional chromosomal abnormality in a leukaemic stem cell, conferring on it resistance to the therapeutic agents being applied, and thus the ability to proliferate in spite of treatment.

Activation of cellular oncogenes by integrated proviruses of leukaemogenic retroviruses, which do not themselves possess a viral oncogene, has been discussed on p. 13.16. It depends on chance insertion of the provirus at a particular site in the cellular DNA. Apart from Burkitt's lymphoma (p. 18.13), there is no strong evidence that DNA viruses are involved in human leukaemias or lymphomas.

Finally, two further aspects of leukaemogenesis deserve comment. One is the suppressive effect of leukaemic proliferation on the haemopoietic activity of normal stem cells. This occurs in most forms of leukaemia. It may result from insensitivity of leukaemic cells to a factor termed **leukaemia-associated inhibitory activity (LIA)** which is an acidic iso-ferritin produced by monocytes and macrophages. LIA inhibits normal cells in the S phase of mitosis but fails to inhibit proliferation of leukaemic cells. The second aspect is the possible role of **immunosuppression** in leukaemogenesis. Radiation and leukaemogenic drugs are immunosuppressant and so are the leukaemogenic retroviruses of animals. There is, moreover, an increased incidence of leukaemia in several of the congenital immunodeficiency diseases.

The myeloproliferative disorders

This term was originally proposed by Dameshek in 1951 to describe a group of disorders characterised by abnormal, excessive and sustained proliferation of erythropoietic, granulopoietic and megakaryocytic components of the bone marrow, often accompanied by fibrosis (myelofibrosis) and myeloid metaplasia (extramedullary haemopoiesis—formation of haemopoietic foci in other tissues). Of the original group proposed by Dameshek, only three diseases are now classified under the heading of myeloproliferative disorders—*polycythaemia rubra vera, myelofibrosis* and *essential thrombocythaemia*. Grouping together of these three conditions is based on (1) the occurrence of cases with intermediate features, (2) the frequent evolution of one disease into another within the group e.g. polycythaemia rubra vera into myelofibrosis, and (3) the invariable involvement of more than one haemopoietic cell line in the neoplastic process: for example, red cell production is most conspicuously increased in polycythaemia, but also granulocyte and platelet production, reflecting abnormal proliferation of all three cell lines in the marrow. The leukaemias are classified separately, and the

rare erythroleukaemia, originally on the list, is now more appropriately classified as M6 subtype of ANLL (p. 17.49).

The above features suggest that the abnormal haemopoietic proliferation of the myeloproliferative disorders originates from a stem-cell abnormality. The neoplastic nature of the proliferation is suggested by the apparent absence of excess of any of the known physiological stimulating factors and by the demonstration of G-6-PD iso-enzyme homogeneity (p. 2.11) in the haemopoietic cells of heterozygotes with these diseases. This latter finding suggests a monoclonal proliferation from a single abnormal stem cell. Although chromosomal abnormalities occur in this group of diseases, they are neither consistent nor specific. Many of the morphological features are common to the group as a whole, and differ only in degree, particularly those in the bone marrow: they include (1) marked haemopoietic hyperplasia with extension into long bones, (2) an increase in reticulin or in some cases collagen deposition in the marrow spaces, (3) an increase of morphologically abnormal megakaryocytes often present in clusters and (4) the presence of myeloid metaplasia.

Polycythaemia rubra vera (Primary polycythaemia) is characterised by proliferation in the marrow, predominantly of red cell precursors but also of myeloid cells and megakaryocytes. It occurs in 1 per 100 000 of the population, nearly always after 40 years of age, and with a male preponderance. The clinical features are caused by an increase of red cell mass (see below) and consequently of blood volume and viscosity, and by the hypermetabolism associated with the myeloproliferation. Patients may complain of various non-specific symptoms of which headaches, blurring of vision and generalised pruritus, particularly after a hot bath, are especially common. The hypervolaemia results in engorgement of the microcirculation which, together with erythrocytosis, produces a florid appearance, particularly of the face. The elevated blood viscosity may lead to hypertension and a tendency to thrombosis, notably in the cerebral vessels. The platelets may be functionally deficient and, in spite of their increased number, spontaneous haemorrhage may occur, particularly into the gastro-intestinal tract. There is also an increased incidence of peptic ulceration. The spleen is usually palpably enlarged and firm. Increased cell turnover may be reflected by elevation of uric acid levels with secondary gout and renal impairment (p. 23.51). The outstanding feature is a marked increase in red cell mass; the red cell count usually exceeds

$7 \times 10^{12}/1$, and the haemoglobin concentration 18·0 g/dl. A packed cell volume of 0·6 1/1 (60%) at sea level is virtually diagnostic, but the total red cell volume should be estimated, both to confirm the diagnosis and to ascertain the severity of the disease, particularly as peripheral blood cell values do not correlate closely with the red cell volume. The increase in total red cell volume may exhaust iron stores and this, combined with the frequent occurrence of haemorrhages, may result in the association of a florid appearance and iron deficiency. About 50% of patients show elevation of the total white cell count and two-thirds have an elevated platelet count. The neutrophil alkaline phosphatase score is usually increased, often to very high levels. In addition, serum vitamin B_{12} and B_{12}-binding capacity are high.

The distinction between polycythaemia rubra vera and other causes of erythrocytosis is discussed on p. 17.9. Treatment is directed mainly at reducing the red cell mass and thus the blood viscosity; this may be achieved by repeated venesection or by administration of radioactive phosphorus or myelosuppressive drugs.

The disease is often advanced when first detected but may run a prolonged course. Death may result from the effects of hypertension or from thrombotic episodes, but with improved control and longer survival many patients eventually develop either myelofibrosis or acute myelomonocytic or lymphoblastic leukaemia.

Myelofibrosis. The essential feature of this condition, which occurs in elderly persons, is increased fibroblastic activity in the *haemopoietic marrow*, resulting in a great increase in reticulin fibres and sometimes coarser fibrosis with thicker collagen strands (Fig. 17.40). The increase in fibroblasts appears to be reactive rather than another aspect of the neoplastic haemopoietic process, for G-6-PD iso-enzyme studies indicate that it is not due to a monoclonal proliferation.

The onset of the disease is usually insidious, symptoms being due to either anaemia or splenomegaly. The *spleen* is greatly enlarged and often enormous, and this may cause abdominal discomfort, particularly after food. Abdominal pain due to splenic infarction may be the presenting symptom. The *liver* may also be enlarged and both organs are the site of extensive myeloid metaplasia, the microscopic appearances of which resemble those in the haemopoietic marrow, including the increase in reticulin or fibrous tissue. Needle aspiration of the marrow is often unsuccessful ('dry tap') and trephine or open biopsy may be necessary for diagnosis. In some cases there is an increase in the bony trabeculae (*osteosclerosis*). The haemopoietic elements in the marrow may be diffusely or focally increased or diminished, and abnormal megakaryocytes are seen.

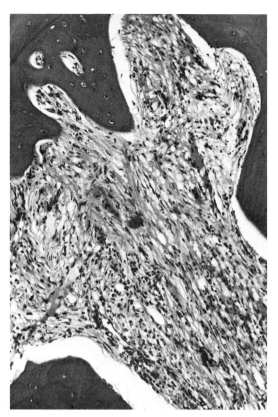

Fig. 17.40 Myelofibrosis. Section of bone showing replacement of the haemopoietic marrow by fibrous tissue.

The blood picture shows anaemia, marked polychromasia, anisocytosis, and poikilocytosis with 'tear-drop' red cells. A proportion of patients become folate-deficient, with a raised MCV and macrocytes (which may be oval). Nucleated red cells are regularly present and typically associated with immature cells of the granulocyte series **(leuco-erythroblastic reaction)**. The number of granulocytes may be low, normal or increased and the platelet count is usually increased at the time of diagnosis. As the disease progresses, all formed elements tend to decrease due to impaired haemopoiesis and sometimes also to hypersplenism. As in polycythaemia rubra vera, the neutrophil alkaline phosphatase score is very high, and the serum uric acid is raised. The median survival from the time of diagnosis is about 3 years. Most patients die from myocardial infarction or cerebro-vascular accidents, but some from bone marrow failure with severe haemorrhage or infection and about 10% develop acute myeloblastic leukaemia.

Essential thrombocythaemia. In this condition, megakaryocytic hyperplasia and excessive production of platelets predominate. The platelet count usually exceeds $1000 \times 10^9/l$ ($10^6/\mu l$) but many of the platelets are functionally defective and haemorrhage from the gastrointestinal tract is common, with consequent iron-deficiency anaemia. There may be a moderate neutrophil leucocytosis. Thrombotic episodes with infarction of internal organs are also common, particularly in the spleen, which is usually enlarged initially but may subsequently become atrophic from repeated infarction.

Although there is a high mortality from the effects of haemorrhage and/or thrombosis, a proportion of patients progress to myelofibrosis or acute myeloblastic leukaemia. The length of survival is very variable.

Bone marrow replacement syndrome

Extensive replacement of the bone marrow by other (usually neoplastic) tissue is accompanied by extramedullary haemopoiesis, notably in the spleen but sometimes in lymph nodes, liver etc. Immature cells of the granulocyte series and nucleated red cells escape from the abnormal marrow and from the extramedullary sites of haemopoiesis and appear in the blood (**leuco-erythroblastic reaction**). The spleen is enlarged and sometimes massive and eventually inadequate production of blood cells leads to normocytic normochromic anaemia, thrombocytopenia and diminution of mature granulocytes in the blood. The leukaemias are, by convention, excluded from this group of conditions and the most important causes are invasion of the marrow by metastatic carcinoma or (non-leukaemic) lymphomas and myelofibrosis (p. 17.57).

Carcinomatosis of the marrow. The bone marrow is a common site of metastases from various malignant tumours. In malignant melanoma and carcinoma of certain organs, especially the breast, bronchus, prostate and thyroid, the nodules may be very numerous and widespread in the marrow. They occur especially in the red marrow and are sometimes detectable in histological sections of marrow aspirates (Fig. 17.41) or by bone scanning. When the marrow of the short bones is extensively invaded, there is often a compensatory hyperplasia of red marrow in the long bones. *Leuco-erythroblastic anaemia* (see above) may result, particularly when metastases are

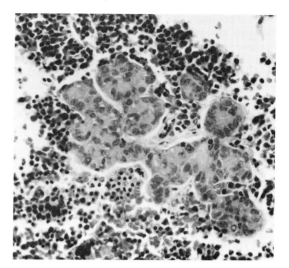

Fig. 17.41 Section of sternal marrow aspirate showing metastatic breast carcinoma. × 250.

numerous and widespread, or when they stimulate an osteosclerotic reaction, a common feature of metastases from prostatic cancer.

Dysmyelopoietic syndromes

The disorders in this group all arise from acquired stem-cell defects. They occur mostly in old people presenting with anaemia which is refractory to haematinic therapy and is associated with persistent neutropenia and/or thrombocytopenia, i.e. the features of bone marrow failure. In addition, there are qualitative defects in the erythrocytes and/or granulocytes and platelets. From the earliest stage, the marrow is hypercellular and some patients progress to acute non-lymphoblastic leukaemia (ANLL). In addition to detection of the peripheral blood and bone marrow abnormalities, precise diagnosis may require kinetic, cytogenetic and bone-marrow culture studies. The following four clinical entities are widely classified as dysmyelopoietic syndromes.

1. Primary acquired sideroblastic anaemia
2. Refractory anaemia and/or cytopenia
3. Refractory anaemia with excess of blast cells (RAEB)
4. Chronic myelomonocytic syndrome

Primary acquired sideroblastic anaemia has already been described (p. 17.42). About 10% of these patients develop ANLL. *Refractory anaemia and/or cytopenia* occurs in people less than 50 years old. A characteristic feature is the presence of micromegakaryocytes in the bone marrow, reflecting a failure of endomitotic replication (p. 17.6). Myeloblasts and promyelocytes together constitute less than 15% of marrow cells. Although the karyotype is normal, a proportion of patients ultimately transform to ANLL. *Refractory anaemia with excess of blasts* (RAEB) affects people of over 50 and shows an equal sex incidence. Neither ring sideroblasts nor micromegakaryocytes are found in the marrow. The aggregate proportion of myeloblasts and promyelocytes is between 15% and 30% and about 30% of patients develop ANLL. *The chronic myelomonocytic syndrome* (CMMS—sometimes called *chronic myelomonocytic leukaemia*) affects patients over 50 years of age and the clinical and haematological manifestations are essentially as for RAEB, but patients with CMMS have an absolute peripheral monocytosis greater than 2×10^9/l, often with abnormal monocytes. The bone marrow is hypercellular and the appearances are similar to RAEB but with rather more promyelocytes. ANLL develops in 40-50% of patients.

Prediction of transformation to ANLL within the group of dysmyelopoietic syndromes is difficult but the detection of cells with ANLL karyotype abnormalities (p. 17.49) indicates a high risk of this.

Plasma cell tumours

General features. Plasma cells are derived from B lymphocytes (p. 6.5) and are responsible for the synthesis and secretion of antibodies. Plasma cell neoplasias arise from neoplastic proliferation of a B cell, and there is good evidence for their monoclonal origin, for many of these tumours produce immunoglobulin (Ig) and the cells of any one such tumour cell produce molecules of Ig which are identical with one another, i.e. they have the same class of heavy chains (γ, α, μ, δ or ε), the same type of light chains (κ or λ), and identical sequences of amino acids in the variable regions of each chain (p. 6.15). These 'monoclonal' proteins are called *myeloma* or M *proteins*, and their investigation has contributed significantly to the understanding of both antibody production and neoplasia.

The most important and best defined of the plasma cell neoplasms is *multiple myeloma*, which differs from other lymphomas in affecting predominantly the bone marrow. Other members of the group are rare and include *Waldenstrom's macroglobulinaemia* and *heavy chain disease*, the morphological and other features of which are intermediate between multiple myeloma and other lymphomas.

Multiple myeloma (Myelomatosis; Myeloma)

Multiple myeloma (MM) is an uncommon disease characterised by neoplastic proliferation of plasma cells or their precursors, usually confined to the bone marrow and occurring in elderly subjects. It is rare before the age of 40 years. The disease varies greatly in aggressiveness; some patients with indolent forms live for many years while the most rapidly progressive form is fatal in 2-3 months. Untreated patients have an average life expectancy of less than a year, but this is increased by chemotherapy to 2-3 years, and with improvements in treatment an increasing number of patients now survive for 5 years or more. Death usually results from anaemia, infection, renal failure or the effects of skeletal lesions.

Diagnosis if MM is usually not difficult and depends on demonstration of the monoclonal protein in the serum, the typical cellular changes in the marrow, and osteolytic lesions on x-ray.

Pathological changes. The neoplastic tissue occurs usually in the form of numerous reddish nodules throughout the bone marrow (Fig. 17.42). The nodules are osteolytic so that absorption and rarefaction of the affected bones take place and *spontaneous fractures* are common, especially in the ribs. The lesions may be seen radiologically as sharply punched-out defects in the bone, for example in the skull. More often, widespread plasma cell proliferation in the marrow products a *diffuse osteoporosis*, sometimes without the formation of discrete defects, and *vertebral collapse* may occur. Rarely a solitary plasmacytoma may develop; usually in a long bone, but in most cases multiple myeloma develops sooner or later, and excision is unlikely to effect cure, though a few successful cases have been reported. A solitary plasmacytoma may occur in various other tissues, e.g. the nasopharynx, or stomach, and its relation to multiple myeloma is uncertain.

Microscopic appearances. The nodules and widespread infiltrates of myelomatosis are highly cellular and vascular. The appearance of

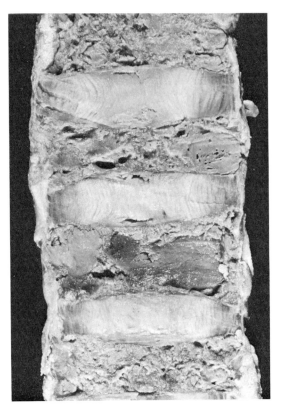

Fig. 17.42 Multiple nodules of myeloma in vertebral column. The vertebral bodies show compression collapse.

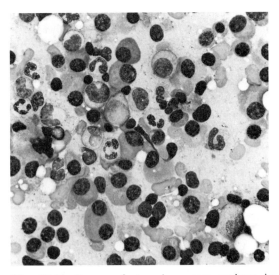

Fig. 17.43 Smear of sternal marrow aspirate in multiple myeloma, showing large numbers of plasma cells. ×600. (Dr. Annette Mallinson.)

the cells is variable, but most commonly many of them are recognisable as plasma cells (Fig. 17.43), having the typical eccentric cartwheel nucleus and cytoplasm of various grades of basophilia and pyroninophilia due to a high content of RNA. As in normal plasma cells, the Golgi zone may be seen as a crescent of pale-staining cytoplasm beside the nucleus, and bi- and tri-nucleate cells are often seen. More primitive cells—plasmablasts—are also present in varying proportions. Cells of intermediate appearance between small lymphocytes and plasma cells may occasionally predominate. There is usually little or no fibrous stroma. Plasma cells are present in the normal marrow and their number is increased in chronic infections, etc., but seldom to more than 10% of all nucleated cells.

Plasma proteins. In most (but not all) cases the myeloma cells synthesise and secrete immunoglobulin (Ig) and the level of serum Ig is usually raised, sometimes exceeding 100 g/l. This is composed almost exclusively of the monoclonal Ig and the normal polyclonal Ig is frequently reduced. The class of immunoglobulin secreted by myelomas is most often IgG, followed by IgA. Myelomas secreting IgM, IgD or IgE are rare. Many myelomas produce a relative excess of light chains and some product mainly light chains (light-chain myeloma). The homogeneity of the monoclonal Ig in MM is reflected in its appearance as a dense narrow band is serum electrophoresis (Fig. 17.44). This is termed an M or 'myeloma' band and its demonstration is important in diagnosis.

In about 50% of cases, light chains in the form of monomers and dimers, of molecular weights 22 000 and 44 000 Daltons respectively, are demonstrable in the urine where they are known as **Bence-Jones proteins**. Adjustment of the urine pH to 4–6 and heating results in precipitation of these light chain molecules at about 50°C and they redissolve at about 80°C, but this test has now been largely superseded by immunoassay. In any particular case, the light chains are all of one type (κ or λ).

Treatment and assessment of the prognosis of patients with MM have been improved by use of a clinical staging system based on indirect estimation of total myeloma tumour cell mass and on the presenting clinical features.

Associated changes. As noted above, electrophoresis of serum demonstrates the monoclonal

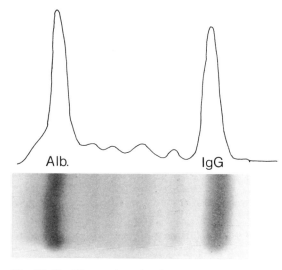

Fig. 17.44 Electrophoresis of the serum in a case of multiple myeloma (origin on right). The IgG (myeloma protein) forms a discrete dense band close to the origin. The other dense band (on the left) is the normal albumin. The scan (above) indicates the large amount of protein in these two zones. The levels of normal immunoglobulins are diminished. (Prof. I.W. Percy-Robb)

Ig in most cases. MM causes pronounced **bone resorption** with focal or generalised osteoporosis, hypercalcaemia and increased excretion of calcium and phosphorus in the urine. Serum alkaline phosphatase is usually not raised. These changes are brought about by an *osteoclast-activating factor* which is produced by myeloma cells.

The **hyperglobulinaemia** results in marked rouleaux formation, sludging of red cells and a high ESR. It also accounts for the increased background staining observed in blood films. Patients with light-chain or non-secretory MM often have a normal ESR. **Anaemia** results from extensive infiltration of the marrow by myeloma cells, and is usually of normochromic normocytic type, although blood loss from haemorrhage may bring about an iron-deficiency anaemia. There is often a tendency to *haemorrhage*, which may be due to formation of complexes between myeloma immunoglobulin and several of the clotting factors, but there may also be thrombocytopenia. Another feature is **increased viscosity of the blood** due to hyperglobulinaemia and sludging of red cells: this may cause secondary Raynaud's disease (p. 14.35) and occasionally gangrene of the extremi-

ties, particularly in patients with an M protein which gels on cooling (*cryoglobulin*). Rarely, the neoplastic plasma cells appear in the blood in numbers which warrant the term *plasma cell leukaemia*.

Infiltration of various organs occurs in occasional patients. **Renal changes** are common, and result from precipitation of Bence-Jones protein (light chains) in the lumen of the renal tubules to form dense hyaline casts. These cause tubular obstruction and also stimulate a foreign-body giant-cell reaction, and consequent tubular destruction may bring about renal failure. Nephrocalcinosis resulting from hypercalciuria may also be a contributory factor. **Immunodeficiency** results from the reduction of normal immunoglobulins mentioned above. This is due partly to an increased rate of catabolism of immunoglobulins, but there is also evidence that myeloma cells secrete a non-immunoglobulin factor which suppresses antibody production. Susceptibility to infections is increased and death often results from bronchopneumonia. **Amyloid deposition** is a common complication of MM, and usually presents the pattern of 'primary' amyloidosis: it occurs particularly in the light-chain and IgA myelomas and only rarely in IgG myeloma.

Waldenstrom's macroglobulinaemia is an uncommon and eventually fatal condition. It develops after the age of 50, in men more often than in women, and is a B-cell neoplasm involving the marrow, lymph nodes, spleen and liver. The tumour cells secrete IgM, thus accounting for the macroglobulinaemia. The serum IgM is usually between 25 and 80 g/dl and shows up as an M band (p. 17.60) on serum electrophoresis: it is insoluble in water and precipitates on diluting the serum with water (*Sia test*).

The high level of IgM increases the blood viscosity and so impedes the circulation through capillary beds: this is aggravated by red-cell aggregation and sludging of the blood and, in consequence, some patients have neural symptoms (dizziness, pareses, blurring of vision, etc.). In about 10% of patients the IgM behaves as a cryoglobulin (gels on cooling) and causes secondary Raynaud's disease and even gangrene of the extremities. Haemorrhages may occur into the respiratory, alimentary and urinary tracts and also in the periphery of the retina: they may be due to the impaired blood flow but the IgM also binds to platelets and interferes with both platelet function and coagulation.

The bone marrow, liver, spleen and lymph nodes are diffusely infiltrated with small lymphocytes and cells of intermediate appearance between lymphocytes and plasma cells ('plasmacytoid lymphocytes'), which may contain PAS + ve nuclear inclusions. Red cell aggregation occurs also *in vitro*, making cell counting difficult. There is usually a pancytopenia (but sometimes a lymphocytosis) and the anaemia, together with impaired circulation, causes weakness and tiredness.

The patient's condition is relieved briefly by plasmapheresis and in most cases chemotherapy induces a temporary remission. The condition is usually fatal in 3 years or so, although some patients live much longer.

Heavy-chain disease comprises a group of rare neoplastic conditions in which infiltration of the tissues by lymphoid cells is associated with the presence in the serum of a protein identifiable as the Fc fragment of Ig heavy chain. **Alpha-chain disease** is the least rare example: it is a follicle-centre-cell lymphoma which arises in the wall of the small intestine. When the normal lymphoid tissue of the gut responds to an antigen, many of the B cells produced pass into the blood and settle in the lamina propria of gut, where they differentiate into plasma cells and secrete IgA antibody. It is of particular interest that the neoplastic cells in α-chain disease behave similarly but produce α chains rather than whole IgA molecules: the disease occurs particularly in communities with a high incidence of intestinal parasites.

Haemorrhagic disorders

These fall into three major categories—disorders of platelets, of blood vessels, and of coagulation and fibrinolysis. They may also be classified as genetically determined or acquired. In coagulation defects, haemorrhage is usually initiated by trauma and is characterised by its persistence rather than its severity. In disorders of platelets and blood vessels, spontaneous bleeding (purpura) occurs into the skin and into, or from the surface of, mucous membranes. Before reading the following account of haemorrhagic disorders it is essential to have a basic understanding of the physiological principles involved in the process of coagulation of the blood and haemostasis (p. 10.7-11).

Platelet Disorders

Thrombocytopenia

Thrombocytopenia exists when the platelet count is less than $150 \times 10^9/1$ $(150\,000/\mu l)$. Bleeding is, however, unusual when the count is greater than $50 \times 10^9/1$ and spontaneous haemorrhage does not usually occur above $20 \times 10^9/1$ unless infection is also present.

Hereditary thrombocytopenias are rare. They include the *Bernard-Soulier syndrome* (large platelets), *May-Hegglin anomaly* (large platelets associated with Döhle bodies in granulocytes), and *Wiskott-Aldrich syndrome* (small platelets, progressive pyogenic infections and eczema).

Acquired thrombocytopenias

These are much more common. Some result from **depressed platelet production**, and are readily identified by a paucity of megakaryocytes in the marrow and by the small mean size of the circulating platelets (detected by determining the mean platelet volume—MPV). Other cell lines are often affected as well, and anaemia and/or leucopenia may be present. Causes include aplastic anaemia, megaloblastic anaemia (due either to Vitamin B_{12} deficiency or folate deficiency), bone marrow infiltration by neoplasm and administration of cytotoxic drugs or ionising radiation, which cause predictable dose-related thrombocytopenia. A number of drugs cause thrombocytopenia in occasional recipients; they include cotrimoxazole, phenylbutazone and gold compounds. Reduction in platelet count also occurs after drinking large amounts of alcohol and is due to defective production and reduced lifespan of platelets: it can occur independently of both folate deficiency and cirrhosis, both of which are common in chronic alcoholics.

Acquired thrombocytopenia may also result from **increased destruction of platelets**; normal or increased numbers of megakaryocytes are present in the bone marrow (Fig. 17.45) and the circulating platelets appear larger than normal and have a raised MPV. This type of thrombocytopenia usually results from immune mechanisms of platelet destruction and is

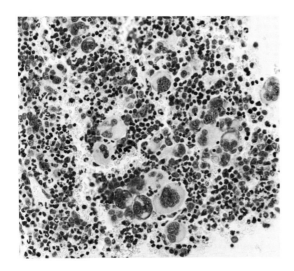

Fig. 17.45 Marrow biopsy in idiopathic thrombocytopenic purpura, showing increased numbers of megakaryocytes, many of which are immature. ×205.

caused either by hypersensitivity to drugs or the development of auto-antibodies to platelets. When caused by **hypersensitivity to drugs**, the thrombocytopenia develops suddenly following a single dose of a drug which the patient has received previously, or during the course of protracted treatment by the offending drug. There is evidence that the drug or one of its metabolites acts as a hapten, forming an antigenic complex by binding to a plasma protein, and that antibody (usually IgG) is formed against this complex. The resulting antigen-antibody complexes then bind to the platelets (which have surface receptors for reacted Fc of IgG) and bring about their destruction by phagocytosis. If this is the whole explanation, however, it is difficult to understand why thrombocytopenia is not a more prominent feature of serum sickness (p. 7.16) and other forms of immune-complex disease. The most notable drugs causing this type of thrombocytopenia are chlorothiazides, digitoxin, methyldopa, para-aminosalicylic acid, paracetamol, quinine, quinidine and sulphonamides.

In **auto-immune thrombocytopenia**, auto-antibodies, usually of IgG class, bind to platelets and bring about their destruction by complement activation and phagocytosis. Tests are available to detect IgG and complement bound to platelets but they are technically difficult and do not distinguish auto-antibodies from bound immune complexes; tests for platelet antibody in serum are not very satisfactory. Auto-immune thrombocytopenia may occur as an isolated disorder (*idiopathic thrombocytopenic purpura*—see below) or in association with other auto-immune disorders, e.g. systemic lupus erythematosus or myasthenia gravis, and rarely accompanies auto-immune haemolytic anaemia (Evans' syndrome). It may also complicate various lymphomas, including chronic lymphocytic leukaemia, although thrombocytopenia may also be due to marrow replacement in these conditions.

Post-transfusion purpura is a rare condition in which severe, sometimes fatal, thrombocytopenia develops acutely about 10 days after blood transfusion, usually in women. In some cases the patient lacks the almost universal platelet iso-antigen Pl^{A1} and apparently this antigen stimulates an immune response to the donor (Pl^{A1} +ve) platelets with production of antibodies not only to Pl^{A1} but also to antigens common to both donor and recipient platelets, resulting in auto-immune thrombocytopenia.

Bacterial and viral infections may also be followed by thrombocytopenia due sometimes to the binding of immune complexes as in some drug reactions (see above). In bacterial infections, platelet loss may also be caused by disseminated intravascular coagulation, another cause of thrombocytopenia, while viruses may stimulate the development of platelet auto-antibodies (see below).

Increased destruction of platelets also occurs in hypersplenism (p. 17.32) but if thrombocytopenia is severe, an additional cause should be suspected.

Detection of the cause of increased platelet destruction is often difficult, but the above underlying causes should be sought and eliminated before assuming that the patient has idiopathic thrombocytic purpura.

Idiopathic (Auto-immune) thrombocytopenic purpura

This disorder occurs chiefly in children and young adults. **In children** the onset is acute and is often preceded by a viral respiratory infection. In most cases the disorder is self-limiting, lasting only 2–4 weeks, and platelet destruction appears to be caused by auto-antibodies to platelets or virus-associated immune complexes. **The adult type**, occurring mainly in females aged 20–40 years, develops insidiously and usually persists for months or years. It is auto-immune in nature, the offending antibody usually belonging to subclass 3 of IgG. The clinical pattern of bleeding may vary from mild cutaneous purpura to gross uterine or gastro-intestinal haemorrhage. In severe cases, intra-cerebral bleeding is a particular danger. Many patients respond to immunosuppressive drugs, failing which splenectomy may be beneficial; this operation does not appear to affect the degree of platelet sensitisation by antibody but simply removes the site of their destruction. Following splenectomy there may be a remark-able transient overswing in the platelet count, which can exceed $1000 \times 10^9/l$. There is evidence that platelets which are very heavily coated by antibody are removed mainly by the Kupffer cells of the liver and that patients with such strong sensitisation are unlikely to benefit from splenectomy.

Qualitative platelet defects

A variety of haemorrhagic defects, both hered-itary and acquired, are recognised and are characterised by a normal platelet count but abnormal platelet function. Defects are recog-nised in all steps leading to formation of the haemostatic platelet plug (p. 10.7), including adhesion, release reaction and aggregation of platelets.

With the exception of von Willebrand's disease (p. 17.66), **hereditary disorders** are rare. Those due to defects of adhesion of platelets include *Bernard-Soulier syndrome* (p. 17.62) in which there is a platelet membrane abnormality and *Ehlers–Danlos syndrome* in which there is an abnormality in the collagen to which platelets usually adhere. Hereditary defects of the platelet release reaction include the various stor-age pool (dense body) deficiency syndromes, α-gran-ule deficiency and defects of thromboxane synthesis. Of the hereditary defects of platelet aggregation, the best recognised is *Glanzmann's disease* (*thrombas-thenia*), an autosomal recessive disorder resulting in a lifelong haemorrhagic tendency with multiple superficial bruises, epistaxis and menorrhagia. The clinical severity tends to lessen with age.

Acquired disorders of platelet function are more common, occurring in renal failure, the myeloproliferative syndromes and hyperglobu-linaemic states. Many drugs can interfere with platelet function, including aspirin-type anti-inflammatory drugs, dextran, dipyridamole, sulfinpyrazone and carbenicillin.

Disorders of blood vessels

Congenital vascular disorders. The least rare is *here-ditary haemorrhagic telangiectasia*, which is trans-mitted as a simple autosomal dominant trait. Haemorrhagic symptoms vary in severity and time of onset, but epistaxis is usually a prominent feat-ure. Multiple telangiectatic spots, which consist of arteriolar-venular anastomoses, occur in the skin and the mucous membranes: they cause recurrent haemorrhage and severe iron-deficiency anaemia may result. Similar lesions in the lungs may cause profuse haemoptysis. Vascular purpura due to defec-tive capillary support occurs in patients with Ehlers–Danlos syndrome, Marfan's syndrome, osteogenesis imperfecta or pseudoxanthoma elasticum.

Acquired vascular defects are much com-moner. Purpura is often due to a mechanical effect following sudden transient rise in capil-lary pressure with resultant leakage of red cells, e.g. in whooping cough, after prolonged vom-iting, and in epileptic fits. *Purpura simplex* or 'devil's pinches', the easy bruising seen parti-cularly in women, is also common. *Senile or cachectic purpura* on the backs of the hands and arms is probably attributable to poor capillary support from collagen, as is the purpura asso-ciated with *steroid therapy* or *Cushing's syndrome*. Ascorbic acid, together with the phosphatase of fibroblasts, is involved in the polymerisation of mucopolysaccharides neces-sary for collagen synthesis, and ascorbic acid may also have a role in the formation of inter-cellular cement substances. Haemorrhage from capillaries, most characteristically from the around carious teeth, subperiosteally, into muscles and also in various other sites, is seen in *scurvy*. The anaemia of scurvy usually results from haemorrhage but has a mild hae-molytic component. Ascorbic acid is concerned also in the conversion of folic acid to folinic acid, and megaloblastic anaemia may occur in scurvy.

The various types of *arteritis* and *vasculitis* (pp. 14.21–8) may also cause purpura, e.g. anaphylactoid (Henoch–Schonlein) purpura, or haemorrhage from larger vessels, e.g. in polyarteritis nodosa.

Finally, purpura from damage to capillaries may occur in severe acute bacterial infections e.g. acute meningococcal septicaemia (Fig. 9.10, p. 9.10) or subacute bacterial endocarditis; they are caused by microemboli or by toxae-mia.

Disorders of coagulation

Inherited disorders of coagulation

The coagulation cascade (p. 10.10) is composed of a series of limited proteolytic reactions ultimately leading to the generation of thrombin which then mediates the conversion of fibrinogen to fibrin. At each stage in the cascade, a parent zymogen is activated and catalyses a subsequent reaction. Many of the coagulation factors are simple peptides, the products of single structural genes (factors II, VII, IX, X, XI, XII and XIII belong to this group). Some, however, are more complex and products of more than one structural gene: fibrinogen, factor V and factor VIII belong to this category, at least two genes being responsible for factor V and from 3–5 genes for factor VIII. The precise roles of factors V and VIII in the coagulation system are not yet fully understood but, unlike the simple peptide factors, neither acts as an enzyme. As with other gene products, deletion can result in absence of a clotting factor, reduced expression can result in inadequate production, and a point mutation can result in adequate production, but of a non-functioning polypeptide. Such ineffective molecules are well recognised in Christmas disease (haemophilia B; factor IX deficiency), von Willebrand's disease and classical haemophilia (haemophilia A; factor VIII deficiency). Inherited coagulation defects usually occur singly, but occasionally combined defects occur, the most common being factors V/VIII deficiency.

The importance of factor VIII is obvious from the clinical features of the factor VIII deficiency diseases, haemophilia A and von Willebrand's disease. These disorders are the two most common inherited defects of coagulation and some knowledge of the structure and function of factor VIII is necessary to understand the molecular defects which cause them. Plasma factor VIII is now considered to be a complex of two components. The larger of the two, factor VIII/von Willebrand factor (VIII R:WF), is coded by autosomal genes (see below) and is deficient or defective in von Willebrand's disease. It promotes primary haemostasis by interacting with platelets and also appears to function as a carrier for the smaller component, factor VIII coagulant (VIII C), which is coded by an X-chromosome gene. VIII C participates directly in the cascade clotting reaction and is deficient in classical haemophilia. When assayed immunologically, these two components are expressed as antigen (Ag), i.e. VIII R:Ag and VIII C:Ag respectively. Such assays, supplemented if necessary by functional assays, are essential in distinguishing between haemophilia and von Willebrand's disease.

Haemophilia A (Classic haemophilia) Haemophilia A is the most common of this group of diseases; it has an incidence of 1 in 10 000 of the population and occurs in all ethnic groups. Transmission is by an X-linked recessive pattern and thus haemophilia A is a disorder of males (Figs. 17.46 and 3.9, p. 3.7). All the daughters of a haemophiliac will be carriers but all the sons will be normal and will not transmit the disease. Fifty per cent of the daughters of carrier mothers will be carriers and 50% of their sons will be haemophiliacs. By chance, several generations of an affected family may elapse without a haemophilic son being born, and this probably explains many of the 30% or so of cases apparently arising *de novo* with no affected relatives. However, some cases are attributable to spontaneous mutations.

The clinical features of haemophilia are virtually indistinguishable from those of other inherited defects of coagulation factors. Although the defect is present at birth, bleeding manifestations are uncommon during the neonatal period and usually appear only when the child begins to crawl. In severely affected patients the most common presenting features are haemarthroses, particularly of weight-bearing joints, bleeding into the muscles of the calf, thigh or forearm or within the iliopsoas sheath, and microscopic haematuria. The risk of intracranial

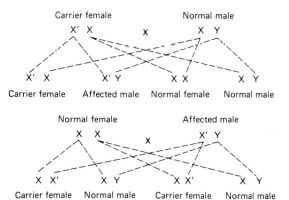

Fig. 17.46 The genetic transmission of the abnormal X chromosome (X′) responsible for haemophilia.

bleeding is low. These features are less common in moderate cases which, together with mild cases, may first present as prolonged bleeding after injury, tooth extraction or surgery. The severity of haemophilia is graded according to the level of VIIIC, measured as clotting activity, into (i) severe—VIIIC < 1% of normal; (ii) moderate—2–5% and (iii) mild—5–20% of normal. Clinical features correlate well with this grading, but the genetic basis of differences in severity is still obscure. The diagnosis of haemophilia A is confirmed by finding a low VIIIC activity, low VIIIC:Ag and normal VIIIR:Ag assays. The skin bleeding time, which depends on vasoconstriction. and formation of a platelet plug (p. 10.7), is normal Carrier detection is usually possible by the above factor VIII assays and is important for the purposes of genetic counselling; early prenatal diagnosis of haemophilia is also possible.

The increasing use of plasma products in the management of haemophiliacs has undoubtedly improved their quality of life, but there is increasing concern over the high prevalence of abnormal liver function tests in the multi-transfused haemophiliac, some of whom eventually progress to chronic active hepatitis. Occasional haemophiliacs have developed the acquired immune deficiency syndrome (AIDS—p. 25.5) following treatment with plasma products, and approximately 15% of haemophiliacs develop antibodies to human factor VIII:C, which can cause difficulties in the treatment of bleeding episodes.

Von Willebrand's disease. This is an inherited haemorrhagic disorder in which the skin bleeding time is prolonged in association with a quantitative or qualitative abnormality of the von Willebrand (VIIIR) factor (see above). This factor appears to have two roles: first, it is a 'co-factor' for platelet adhesion to vascular subendothelium (VIIIR:WF activity) and secondly, it seems to be the carrier protein for factor VIIIC, the coagulation protein absent or inactive in haemoglobin A. Von Willebrand factor is synthesised by vascular endothelium and also by megakaryocytes and is not a single substance but a complex of homologous oligomers, which are products of autosomal genes. Abnormalities include (a) reduced synthesis of all the oligomers, (b) reduced synthesis of some oligomers, and (c) an amino-acid defect which prevents formation of the complex. Accordingly, there is considerable heterogeneity of disease expression and in the results of laboratory tests, which may render diagnosis difficult. For reasons unknown, the classic form of the disease occurs more often in females than in males; the bleeding time is prolonged, low levels of both VIIIC and VIIIR:Ag occur, there is defective platelet adhesion to glass beads and platelets do not aggregate normally on exposure to ristocetin. In practice, any combination or permutation of these test results may be found.

In its rare homozygous form von Willebrand's disease usually presents in early childhood with spontaneous bruising and bleeding from mucous membranes, particularly epistaxis and melaena. The more usual heterologous form is less severe: excessive bleeding follows dental extraction and surgery, and in the adult female, menorrhagia is common but postpartum haemorrhage is unusual.

Factor IX deficiency (Haemophilia B or Christmas disease). This inherited disorder shows the same pattern of inheritance as haemophilia A and has an almost identical clinical presentation. Incidence, however, is only about one-fifth that of haemophilia A. Antibodies to factor IX result from treatment in 1–2% of patients.

Acquired disorders of coagulation

These arise in individuals without previous history of bleeding as the result of an inherent disease process which leads to defective synthesis or increased loss (usually consumption) of coagulation factors, or to the presence of interfering substances. Acquired coagulation-factor disturbances are usually part of a generalised failure of haemostasis.

Acquired inhibitors of coagulation include **auto-antibodies to clotting factors**, most often to factor VIII. Inhibitors to factor VIIIR result clinically in an acquired form of von Willebrand's disease; they occur mainly in patients with auto-immune disease, hypergammaglobulinaemia or lymphoproliferative disorders. 'Lupus anticoagulant' is an inhibitor found in 5–10% of all SLE patients and in a number of patients with haematological malignancies. Its precise mode of action is not known.

Coagulation defects result also from **deficiency of vitamin K**, which is necessary for the γ-carboxylation of precursors of factor II (prothrombin) and some other coagulation factors. It is a fat-soluble vitamin present in leaf vegetables and is also synthesised by the normal intestinal flora. Dietary deficiency of sufficient severity to produce bleeding is well recognised in neonates (haemorrhagic disease of the newborn), in whom the normal bacterial flora is not yet established. In children and adults, deficiency occurs in the grossly malnourished, particularly those receiving antibiotic therapy, and also in patients on parenteral nutrition if vitamin K supplements are not given. Absorption of vitamin K is impaired in biliary obstruction, coeliac disease and pancreatic insufficiency.

Liver disease is a common cause of complex haemostatic abnormalities associated with clinically significant haemorrhage. Since the liver is responsible for the synthesis of most coagulation factors, severe impairment of liver function can result in *combined factor deficiency*, particularly of factors II, VII, IX, X and I (fibrinogen). In addition, severe liver disease can result in the production of structurally abnormal clotting factors, disseminated intravascular coagulation (DIC), thrombocytopenia and failure of hepatic clearance of plasminogen activators, resulting in increased fibrinolytic activity. Similarly, in acute and chronic **renal disease**, there may be a bleeding tendency due to multiple haemostatic abnormalities, including thrombocytopenia, platelet function disorders, coagulation factor deficiency (mainly factors II, VII, IX, X and XIII), DIC and abnormal fibrinolysis. Fibrinogen and factor VIII are often increased.

Cardiac surgery with cardiopulmonary bypass is sometimes associated with severe bleeding, most frequently due to thrombocytopenia and functional platelet disorders, heparin-induced defects, coagulation-factor deficiencies and sometimes DIC. A dilutional coagulopathy may follow **massive blood transfusion** because stored blood is deficient in clotting factors (particularly V and VIII), and contains a reduced number of poorly functioning platelets, an excess of citrate ions and no ionised calcium.

Disseminated intravascular coagulation (DIC)

This term describes the virtual breakdown of haemostasis involving all its components and can complicate a wide variety of diseases. The basic defect, described on p. 10.11, is activation of the clotting system resulting in the deposition of fibrin in the small vessels of many organs causing tissue necrosis and multiple organ dysfunction, and a subsequent bleeding state due to consumption of platelets and clotting factors and secondary enhancement of fibrinolytic activity. Micro-angiopathic haemolytic anaemia is a common accompaniment. While a variety of trigger mechanisms can produce DIC, the end result is the same, namely the widespread intravascular deposition of fibrin and a consumption

coagulopathy. Damage to red cells, platelets, leucocytes and to vascular endothelium are all capable of initiating DIC. The conditions most often responsible are extensive burns, septicaemia, shock, liver disease and complications of labour (retroplacental haemorrhage and amniotic fluid embolism), but it may occur in many other conditions.

DIC may present as a catastrophic acquired haemorrhagic tendency, or as a more chronic bleeding disorder, or thrombotic features may predominate. Transition from the low grade or chronic forms to the acute disorder is quite common. The clinical management of the condition is difficult, and it should not be forgotten that *DIC is always secondary to a pre-existing disease or injury and treatment must be directed at correcting this where possible.* Therapeutic efforts to restore haemostasis, prevent further microthrombosis and to digest thrombi are difficult to control.

Hypercoagulable states

This term is widely but imprecisely applied to changes in the blood which predispose to thrombosis. It does not include changes in the blood flow or in vessel walls which also promote thrombosis (pp. 10.12 *et seq*), although two or even all three factors are sometimes involved.

Hypercoagulable states result from increased activity of factors which promote thrombosis—platelets and clotting factors, and/or decreased activity of factors which maintain the fluidity of the blood—the fibrinolytic or plasmin system and various clotting-inhibitory factors. Such changes occur in various physiological and pathological conditions, but are only occasionally severe enough to cause overt thrombosis.

Physiological conditions. In *stress* or *strenuous exercise* there is a rise in the plasma levels of both factor VIII and plasminogen activator, but the latter rapidly subsides, leaving an unbalanced increase in factor VIII level which can predispose to thrombosis. On *exposure to cold* there is a fall in the plasma level of antithrombin III which may contribute to the higher death rate from myocardial and cerebral infarction observed during cold weather. With *advancing age*, there is in both sexes a gradual increase in the levels of several clotting factors, including fibrinogen and factors V, VII, VIII and IX. In men, but not in women, there is also a decrease in fibrinolytic activity, and a reduction in antithrombin III levels. *In pregnancy* there is a progressive rise in the levels of coagulation factors, including fibrinogen, which becomes evident at 4 months and is particularly marked during the third stage of labour. Fibrinolytic activity decreases during this time except during parturition, when activation occurs: it returns to normal within 15 minutes of delivery of the placenta whereas the fibrinogen level does not fall to normal for a further 6 weeks; these changes may contribute to the recognised thrombotic complications occurring both during pregnancy and following childbirth.

The use of *oral contraceptives*, particularly those with high oestrogen content, has long been associated with an increased risk of thrombotic episodes: this tendency increases mainly during the first year of use and thereafter further progression does not occur. Most of the clotting factors are increased. Fibrinolytic activity is also increased although apparently not in smokers. These changes are influenced by age, ethnic origin and ABO blood group.

Hypercoagulability in various diseases. Increases in the levels of clotting factors occur in many and varied disease states. For example, the levels of fibrinogen and factor VIII are increased in acute pancreatitis, congestive heart failure, diabetes mellitus, widespread cancer, renal failure and many others. There is a known tendency to thrombosis in these conditions, but it is noteworthy that other factors, e.g. the reduced blood flow in congestive failure and both atheroma and micro-angiopathy in diabetes (in which thrombosis is often arterial), are likely to be involved. Following major surgery or trauma there is a rise in the levels of various clotting factors and an increase in both the number and adhesiveness of the platelets. As explained on p. 10.16, however, other factors are also involved in the common occurrence of deep leg vein thrombosis in these patients.

There is also a large group of conditions which predispose to DIC (see above), and while in some of these the clotting system is triggered by endothelial injury, in others it results from damage to red cells or platelets or to activation of Hageman factor, e.g. by endotoxin, and falls within the definition of hypercoagulability.

Most primary abnormalities of the clotting factors predispose to bleeding rather than thrombosis, e.g. haemophilia and von Willebrand's disease, but there are some rare inherited disorders which predispose to thrombosis, for example congenital deficiency of antithrombin III which is inherited as an autosomal dominant factor and causes repeated venous thrombosis and embolic phenomena, usually starting in adolescence. Some inherited abnormalities of fibrinogen also promote thrombosis.

References and Further Reading

Bennett, J.M., Catovsky, D., Daniel, M-T., Flandrin, G., Galton, D.A.G., Gralnick, H.R. and Sultan, C. (1976). Proposals for the classification of the acute leukaemias. *British Journal of Haematology*, **33**, 451–85.

Idem (1981) The morphological classification of acute lymphoblastic leukaemia: concordance among observers and clinical correlations. *British Journal of Haematology*, **47**, 553–61.

Binet, J.L. *et al.* (1981). A new prognostic classification of chronic lymphocytic leukaemia derived from a multivariate survival analysis. *Cancer*, **48**, 198–206.

Chanarin, I. (1979). *The Megaloblastic Anaemias*, 2nd edn., pp. 800. Blackwell Scientific Publications, Oxford, London and New York.

Clinics in Haematology. Saunders, Philadelphia, London and Toronto. (An excellent series of reviews on haematological topics, from 1972 onwards.)

Dacie, J.V. and Lewis, S.M. (1984) *Practical Haematology*, 6th edn., pp. 512. Churchill Livingstone, Edinburgh, London and New York.

Goldman, J.M. and Priester, H.D. (Eds) (1984). *Leukaemias* pp. 372. Butterworths, London, etc.

Hardisty, R.M. and Weatherall, D.J. (1982). *Blood and its disorders.*, 2nd edn., Blackwell Scientific Publications, Oxford, etc.

Hoffbrand, A.V. and Lewis, S.M. (1981) *Postgraduate Haematology* pp. 774. William Heinemann Medical Books Ltd., London.

McDonald, G.A., Dodds, T.C. and Cruikshank, Bruce. (1981). *Atlas of Haematology*, 4th edn. (reprint). Churchill Livingstone, Edinburgh, London and New York.

Rai, K.R., Sawitsky, A., Cronkite, E.P., Charona, A.D., Levy, R.N. and Pasternak, B.S. (1975). Clinical staging of chronic lymphocytic leukaemia and its relationship to survival. *Blood*, **46**, 219–34.

18

The Lympho Reticular Tissues

The lymphoid tissues subserve two major functions. First, they are responsible for specific immune responses to antigenic stimulation: this function has been described in Chapter 6 and its harmful and protective effects in the two subsequent chapters. Second, the **lymph nodes** and **spleen** also monitor the tissue fluid and blood respectively for abnormal constituents. To perform this second function they contain abundant macrophages capable of phagocytosis and digestion of micro-organisms, effete and abnormal cells, tissue and cell fragments and fibrin. These cells of the mononuclear phagocyte system occupy the sponge-like *reticular tissue* and *sinuses* of the spleen and lymphoid tissue and are also present in the lining of the sinusoids of various non-lymphoid tissues, e.g. in the liver (Kupffer cells), haemopoietic marrow, etc. Traditionally, all these tissue elements rich in macrophages are termed collectively the *reticulo-endothelial system* (p. 4.33). Specialised cells, now believed to be members of the mononuclear-phagocyte series, are also present in the epidermis (*Langerhans cells*), the B-cell zones (*dendritic reticulum cells*) and the T-cell zones (*interdigitating reticulum cells*) of the secondary lymphoid tissues including the lymph nodes, gut-associated lymphoid tissues and the spleen. These cells collaborate with lymphocytes in the immune response. The lymph nodes and spleen are thus subject to abnormalities of the lymphoid cells proper and also of macrophages and cells associated with them in the reticular tissue and sinuses. They are also involved in various 'storage diseases' in which enzyme defects result in failure to digest various metabolites and these accumulate in macrophages. **The thymus** differs from other mammalian lymphoid tissues in being a 'primary' lymphoid organ, concerned with antigen-independent lymphopoiesis (p. 6.19), and it lacks the filtering tissue of the lymph nodes and spleen. The **tonsils** and **Peyer's patches,** etc., are not sites of filtration of body fluids but are strategically placed in the wall of the alimentary tract to encounter micro-organisms or their products which penetrate the epithelium (p. 6.37) or are transported across it by phagocytes, and to mount the appropriate immune responses.

The Spleen

Functions

As indicated above, the spleen is a composite organ consisting of: (*a*) units of **lymphoid tissue** termed *lymphoid follicles* or *Malpighian bodies* or collectively the *white pulp*, and (*b*) the vascular network and sinuses termed the **red pulp,** which makes up most of the organ.

The spleen is not an essential organ, but its removal, especially in childhood, greatly increases the risk of septicaemia and meningitis by pneumococci and other pyogenic bacteria (Chilcote *et al.*, 1976). This is probably attributable in part to the capacity of the spleen to phagocytose micro-organisms in the blood before there has been time for the development of a specific immune response with production of protective antibody. Splenectomised animals, e.g. sheep, are abnormally susceptible to various parasitic infections. In both animals and man, the spleen is an important site of formation of antibodies in response to *intravascular* injection of antigens, and considerably less antibody is produced by splenectomised individuals. It is of less importance than the lymph nodes in the response to antigens injected into the tissues. The venous drainage of the spleen into the portal system allows antibodies produced in the spleen to encounter antigenic material absorbed from the gut, and this may facilitate phagocytosis of such material by the Kupffer cells.

The spleen plays an important physiological role in the removal from the blood of old or injured red cells, which are phagocytosed and digested by macrophages in the cords of the red pulp. The bilirubin formed from the breakdown of haemoglobin is secreted into the blood, to be extracted, conjugated and excreted by the liver cells, while the iron is re-utilised in haemoglobin synthesis in the marrow. The average life of the red cells and the number in the blood are not increased following splenectomy, and it is apparent that the phagocytic cells in the liver, marrow and other tissues also destroy old red cells. However, the macrophages in the red pulp of the spleen have a special function in extracting from the red cells various cytoplasmic inclusions, and also in removing the nuclei of any normoblasts which have gained entrance to the circulation, the cells then being returned to the blood. Loss of this function, which is known as 'pitting', is observed following splenectomy, when normoblasts and red cells containing Howell-Jolly bodies and siderotic granules, etc., may be found in blood films (p. 17.11).

It is less certain that the spleen is an important site of physiological destruction of leucocytes and platelets, but splenectomy is commonly followed by a polymorphonuclear leucocytosis of up to $30 \times 10^9/1$ (30 000 per μ1), a monocytosis, and a thrombocytosis of up to 10^{12} per litre ($10^6/\mu$l). The polymorphs reach a peak level during the few days following splenectomy, the platelets 2–3 weeks later. The levels decline thereafter, but monocytes and platelets may remain above the normal ranges for months or even years.

Structure

The vascular arrangements of the spleen are of particular importance in relation to its two major functions. The larger arteries branch within the trabeculae, and give off arterioles which leave the trabecula and become ensheathed in a cuff of lymphoid tissue—the *Malpighian bodies* or *white pulp*—to which they supply capillaries. The inner part of the lymphoid tissue (immediately around the arteriole) is occupied mainly by T lymphocytes, around which is a B-cell zone containing a lymphoid follicle. At the periphery of the lymphoid tissue, each central arteriole divides into several penicillar arterioles, which enter the red pulp. They show a fusiform swelling of the wall, termed an *ellipsoid*; this consists of an inner layer of prominent endothelium surrounded by layers of large pale cells and a basement membrane. The red pulp consists of a spongework of vascular channels rich in macrophages and plasma cells and termed the *splenic cords*. Lying within the red pulp are larger vascular channels which are known as *sinuses* and represent the radicles of the splenic vein. The sinuses are lined by elongated endothelial cells between which are fenestrations about 3μm in diameter. The endothelial cells are supported by reticulin fibres like the hoops of a wooden barrel. Some of the blood from the penicillar arterioles may pass directly into the sinuses (the 'closed' circulation), but mostly it enters the splenic cords of the red pulp (the 'open' circulation) and in order to reach the venous system the blood cells must pass between the endothelial cells lining the sinuses. The red cells must therefore retain elasticity or deformability and cells lacking these properties, e.g. spherocytes, are trapped in the cords and undergo premature destruction (pp. 17.22–23). The process of 'pitting', by which rigid inclusions are removed from the red cells (see above), also takes place as the red cells pass between the endothelial cells of the sinuses, the inclusions being extracted by macrophages in the adjacent red pulp. The 'open' circulation through the splenic cords clearly provides opportunity for phagocytic removal of abnormal materials or cells from the blood, whereas the 'closed' circuit is a more direct route. In man, the spleen normally contains only 20–30 ml of blood although it becomes enlarged and engorged with blood in various diseases.

Shrinkage of the spleen

Atrophy of the spleen occurs in old age, affecting both red and white pulp, and sometimes is seen in wasting diseases. Hyaline thickening of the walls of the small arteries and arterioles of the spleen is a normal feature of ageing. The resulting ischaemia brings about splenic atrophy with some increase in reticulin. Splenic ischaemia is also a feature of *sickle-cell disease* (p. 17.27) and is due to blockage of sinuses by hypoxic sickle-shaped red cells: infarcts and atrophy result, and eventually the spleen may be converted into a small fibrous remnant, often heavily pigmented by haemosiderin derived from phagocytosed red cells. Loss of splenic function may explain the predisposition to bacterial infections in sickle-cell disease. Severe splenic atrophy is also a feature of some cases of *coeliac disease* (p. 19.53), the mechanism being obscure.

Splenic infarcts

Infarcts in an otherwise normal spleen are a common result of emboli and are usually secondary to intracardiac thrombosis, e.g. in infective endocarditis. Less often they result from atheroma and thrombosis of the splenic artery. Unless extensive or multiple, as in sickle-cell disease (see above), they are of little importance. Infarction is very common in splenomegaly, particularly when the spleen is very large, e.g. in chronic granulocytic leukaemia, and often the immediate cause is not apparent. Clinically, infarction may be symptomless, or fibrin deposition on the overlying serosal surface may result in local or referred pain. The appearances of infarcts are described on p. 10.25.

Splenomegaly

As already stated, the two known major functions of the spleen are the production of specific immune responses and phagocytosis of abnormal materials in the blood. Accordingly, increased functional activity of the spleen, with hyperplasia of the lymphoid cells or macrophages, or of both, commonly results from antigenic stimulation or the presence of abnormal materials, for example micro-organisms, toxins or abnormal cells, in the blood. Splenomegaly is therefore a very common secondary phenomenon in a great many diseases. Conditions which involve the lympho-reticular tissues commonly result in enlargement of both the spleen and lymph nodes. However, in some conditions splenomegaly is an outstanding feature, while others present clinically as enlargement of the nodes. Accordingly, it is helpful to give separate consideration to the causes of splenomegaly and those of lymphadenopathy.

Participation of the spleen in immune responses involves hyperplasia of the Malpighian bodies, often with formation of germinal centres and also accumulation of plasma cells throughout the red pulp. These changes alone are, however, seldom sufficient to cause significant splenic enlargement and, apart from the lymphoid neoplasias, splenomegaly is usually due to enlargement of the red pulp. The major categories of splenomegaly are as follows.

(1) Infections and granulomatous conditions.
(2) Congestive splenomegaly.
(3) Diseases of the blood and bone marrow.
(4) Lipid storage diseases.
(5) Amyloid disease.
(6) The lymphomas.

Infections

Because of its vascular nature and phagocytic role, the spleen is exposed to *blood-borne infection*: it has, however, strong defences against pyogenic bacteria, and abscess formation is uncommon except for septic infarcts in pyaemia. However, bacteria are commonly arrested in the spleen and may be recovered from it in non-pyogenic generalised infections, as in typhoid fever, brucellosis and generalised tuberculosis. Significant splenomegaly is not usual in acute viral infections, but an exception is infectious mononucleosis, in which it is often palpable. Colonisation of the spleen with enlargement is brought about also by trypanosomes, and by micro-organisms which are capable of survival and multiplication within macrophages, as in leishmaniasis, histoplasmosis and brucellosis. The spleen is also enlarged in malaria, in which it is an important site of destruction of the infected red cells.

Acute pyogenic infections

The earliest change in the spleen is congestion of the cords of the red pulp. As the number of circulating polymorphs increases, they accumulate progressively in the red pulp of the spleen, and in septicaemia, or severe localised pyogenic infections with a high leucocytosis, they may be present in the spleen in huge numbers. At autopsy the spleen is slightly enlarged (200–300 g), acutely congested, and the splenic tissue may be so softened that it looks and feels almost like a bag of fluid; the cut surface is pinkish or deep red, and the tissue is semi-fluid. These changes, sometimes termed '*septic spleen*', are due to congestion, accumulation of polymorphs and marked terminal and post-mortem autolysis by the digestive enzymes released from degenerate polymorphs.

In fatal septicaemia, the bacteria can often be recovered from the spleen, as from other organs, unless they have been destroyed by antibiotics administered shortly before death. Microscopic examination of the septic spleen is seldom satisfactory owing to severe autolytic changes.

Non-pyogenic bacterial infections

Moderate degrees of splenic enlargement commonly accompany generalised non-pyogenic bacterial infections, and are due to hyperplasia of both the lymphoid tissue and red pulp of the organ, together with granulomatous lesions brought about by arrest and proliferation of bacteria in the red pulp. As enlargement is due mainly to accumulation and local proliferation of macrophages, lymphocytes and plasma cells, together with increase in reticulin, the spleen is usually firm, and post-mortem autolysis is not nearly so marked as in pyogenic infections. Some examples are given below.

In **typhoid fever**, splenic enlargement is an important feature, the weight sometimes reaching 500 g; the spleen is deep red from congestion and firm: as elsewhere in typhoid, there is a virtual absence of polymorphs and accumulation of macrophages (many of which contain ingested red cells), lymphocytes and plasma cells. Typhoid bacilli usually occur in clumps in the red pulp. There may be no sign of damage in their neighbourhood, but sometimes there is necrosis around them.

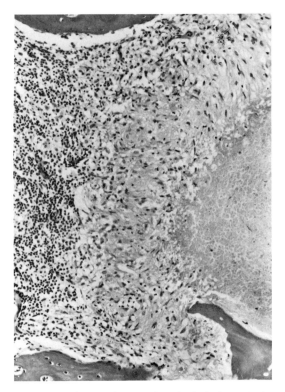

Fig. 18.1 Biopsy of a vertebral body in brucellosis. The lesion consists of an epithelioid macrophage granuloma with central necrosis (*right*) and peripheral aggregation of lymphocytes and plasma cells (*left*). × 130.

Undulant fever is due to infection with small Gram-ve bacilli, the *Brucellae*. There are three important species, *Brucella abortus*, *Br. melitensis* and *Br. suis*, which commonly infect cows, goats and pigs respectively. Traditionally, infection in man results from drinking the milk of infected cattle or goats. A combination of pasteurisation and elimination of infection from dairy herds has considerably reduced the incidence in many countries. In this country, infection with *Br. abortus* still occurs and is an occupational hazard of those who handle infected cattle, particularly in the veterinary profession: infection is also occasionally acquired in medical bacteriology laboratories.

The organisms, which are not easy to isolate in culture, colonise the macrophage system and cause lesions closely resembling tubercle follicles, sometimes with central necrosis (Fig. 18.1): these occur in the lymph nodes, spleen and liver, all of which may be enlarged, although the spleen becomes palpable in only a small proportion of cases. Other organs may be affected, and in some cases there is a transient polyarthropathy. The clinical features vary greatly; there is usually fever, either acute or low grade, with vague symptoms, malaise and weight loss. Bacteraemia is commonly intermittent and multiple blood cultures may be negative. Without treatment the condition usually subsides spontaneously but it may continue for months or even years. Diagnosis is dependent usually on either positive blood culture or demonstrating a high or rising titre of antibodies in the serum. Individuals with occupational exposure to brucellae frequently have antibodies but no symptoms, and diagnosis, particularly of chronic brucellosis, is accordingly difficult.

Tuberculosis. In acute miliary tuberculosis the tubercles are specially numerous in the spleen. They generally appear as minute grey points about the size of Malpighian bodies, from which they may be distinguished by appearing to project slightly from the cut surface when viewed by oblique lighting. In less acute generalised tuberculosis in children, the spleen is occasionally studded with yellowish caseous patches of 3–5 mm diameter. In chronic pulmonary and other forms of tuberculosis, a few tubercles of various sizes, and occasionally larger nodules, may be present in the spleen.

Sarcoidosis. The spleen is commonly involved in sarcoidosis, although it is not usually enlarged, and frequently the lesions are not visible macroscopically; their histological features are the same as in sarcoidosis elsewhere in the body (Fig. 18.8 and p. 9.26), i.e. epithelioid-cell granulomas resembling those of tuberculosis, but showing little or no necrosis, and with multinucleate giant cells which often contain curious stellate and laminated inclusions. In some cases the spleen is extensively affected and moderately enlarged; the coalescent lesions are then visible macroscopically. Hypersplenism may complicate the condition (p. 17.33).

Protozoal infections

In **malaria** (p. 28.3), the spleen swells acutely during each attack of pyrexia, due to the accumulation of red cells containing the parasites. After repeated attacks, thickening of the stroma with induration may ultimately occur and in chronic cases the organ becomes firm, brownish-grey owing to accumulation of malarial pigment, and may weigh 1–1·5 kg. The spleen is greatly enlarged in the *tropical splenomegaly syndrome* (p. 28.5) which appears to be caused mainly by chronic falciparum malaria.

Kala-azar is the generalised (visceral) type of leishmaniasis, in which there is widespread colonisation of macrophages by the leishmanial form of the protozoon, *Leishmania donovani* (p. 28.9). The spleen is greatly enlarged, often exceeding 1·5 kg.

Splenomegaly occurs also in early *trypanosomiasis* and in disseminated *histoplasmosis*, but is not an important feature of these conditions.

Congestive splenomegaly

This results from a persistent rise in pressure in the splenic vein. The most important causes are *systemic venous congestion* in right heart failure and *portal hypertension* most commonly due to hepatic cirrhosis or the 'pipestem' hepatic fibrosis of schistosomiasis (p. 28.25). Less commonly it results from occlusion of the hepatic or portal veins by thrombosis, tumour, etc.

In systemic venous congestion, the spleen is usually only slightly or moderately enlarged (up to 250 g), while in portal hypertension it usually weighs about 500 kg and sometimes exceeds 1 kg. Initially the splenic sinuses are distended with blood, the splenic cords are inconspicuous (Fig. 10.4, p. 10.4) and there is moderate increase in reticulin fibres throughout the red pulp. At this stage the spleen is dark red and blood may ooze from the cut surface. Later there is hyperplasia of macrophages and fibroblasts in the splenic cords and walls of the sinuses and an increase in fibrous tissue of the capsule and red pulp. At this stage the spleen is firm, the cut surface is grey-red and the sinuses are compressed. Organisation of haemorrhages may result in yellow or brown patches of fibrous tissue containing deposits of haemosiderin (*Gandy-Gamna bodies*).

Congestive splenomegaly in portal hypertension is the commonest cause of hypersplenism (see below).

Haematological disorders

The normal function of the spleen in destroying effete red cells, and probably also polymorphs and platelets, has been described on p. 18.2. Numerous abnormalities of the red cells, as for example in various types of *haemolytic* and *macrocytic anaemias*, are accompanied by an increased rate of their destruction in the spleen, and as a consequence there is a great increase in the number of macrophages in the red pulp. The degree of splenomegaly depends on the severity and duration of the process, and is due mainly to engorgement of the red pulp with red cells. Similarly, in idiopathic thrombocytopenic purpura there is increased splenic destruction of the antibody-coated platelets, although splenomegaly is usually absent or slight.

The spleen may become greatly enlarged in conditions in which the bone marrow is extensively replaced, e.g. in myelofibrosis (p. 17.57) or secondary carcinoma (particularly of the prostate): the enlargement is due to **extramedullary haemopoiesis** and the spleen is firm and red or pink, sometimes with deeper red patches, up to 1 cm across, in which the haemopoietic tissue is more abundant. All haemopoietic cell lines are present and sometimes megakaryocytes are very numerous. The haemopoietic activity may contribute significantly to the supply of blood cells, but in some cases hypersplenism is apparent (see below).

As usual with extramedullary haemopoiesis, the blood picture shows the features of leuco-erythroblastic anaemia (p. 17.58).

Splenomegaly is a feature of **leukaemia**. Great enlargement occurs in chronic granulocytic and sometimes in chronic lymphocytic leukaemia. In acute leukaemia, enlargement is usually moderate.

In summary, the haematological disorders accompanied by **great splenomegaly,** i.e. to about 2 kg, are chronic myeloid leukaemia, myelofibrosis and sometimes chronic lymphocytic leukaemia. **Moderate splenomegaly,** up to about 1 kg, occurs in acute leukaemia, various haemolytic anaemias and polycythaemia rubra vera. The changes in the spleen in these conditions have been described in the previous chapter.

Hypersplenism. Moderate or great enlargement of the spleen from any cause may be accompanied by destruction of normal red cells, leucocytes and platelets. This phenomenon is termed *hypersplenism* and contributes to the anaemia (*'splenic anaemia'*), leucopenia and thrombocytopenia observed in some patients with splenomegaly, although defective haemopoiesis and increased plasma volume are also contributory factors (p. 17.33).

Disorders involving lipid storage

Storage of lipids in macrophages occurs in human disease in two groups of conditions.

(a) The hyperlipidaemias include the familial forms of hyperchylomicronaemia, alpha-lipoprotein deficiency (pp. 3.11, 3.13), in which unstable beta-lipoproteins are formed in excess, and hyperbetalipoproteinaemia (pp. 3.15–16). In these conditions and also in poorly controlled diabetes, hypothyroidism, prolonged obstructive jaundice and dietary hypercholesterolaemia, various grades of accumulation of cholesterol or its esters occur in macrophages (Fig. 18.2), not only in the spleen, lymph nodes, liver, bone marrow, etc., but also in the form of xanthomas in the skin and elsewhere. The increased incidence and severity of atheroma in

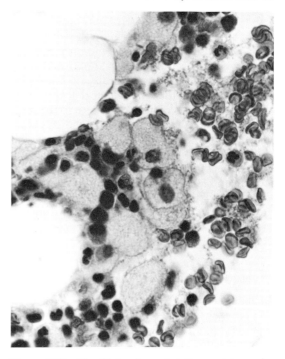

Fig.   18.2 Familial   hyperbetalipoproteinaemia. Bone marrow biopsy showing foamy cells. × 540.

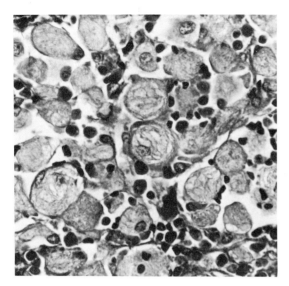

Fig. 18.3 Section of spleen in Gaucher's disease, showing the characteristic large cells with striated and vacuolated cytoplasm. × 440.

these conditions is discussed on p. 14.9. Accumulation of sufficient lipid to cause splenic enlargement occurs only occasionally. Macrophages in the red pulp increase in number and in size and excess lipid is present either as cytoplasmic globules which react variously with fat stains, or in a masked state apparently combined with protein. For example, cholesterol may be present in the spleen in increased amount without birefringent esters being detectable in the cells. Although deposition occurs secondarily to hypercholesterolaemia, it is not known what other factors determine the extent of deposition.

(b) Various rare hereditary lipid storage diseases, such as Gaucher's disease and Niemann-Pick disease, in which the lipid storage becomes excessive in various tissues and the enlargement of the spleen is very great. These conditions result from inborn abnormalities of lipid metabolism (p. 3.14). The composition of the lipids varies in different types.

Gaucher's disease. This uncommon condition was described by Gaucher in 1882. In its least rare form it becomes apparent in adult life, usually as slowly increasing and eventually extreme enlargement of the spleen and liver. This is due to accumulation of glucocerebrosides in macrophages which increase in number and size in the affected organs. The spleen may exceed 5 kg and microscopy shows huge numbers of macrophages termed **Gaucher cells:** they mostly have a single nucleus (but occasional cells

have two or three) and abundant cytoplasm which shows a characteristic streaky or irregularly vacuolated appearance (Fig. 18.3). Stains for fat are only weakly positive but the Gaucher cells are rich in acid phosphatase, the level of which may be raised in the plasma. The liver also is much enlarged by aggregation of Gaucher cells in the sinusoids. Involvement of the haemopoietic marrow may result in resorption of bone with widening of the marrow cavity, thinning of the cortex, and a tendency to pathological fractures. Anaemia, leucopenia and thrombocytopenia in any combination occur in most cases and are due to replacement of haemopoietic marrow by Gaucher cells and sometimes also to hypersplenism. Enlargement of lymph nodes, especially in the abdomen and mediastinum, is usual. In late cases, Gaucher cells may form aggregates in the skin and also in the conjunctiva where they may be seen as wedge-shaped yellow-brown patches, termed *pingueculae.*

The adult form of Gaucher's disease described above is due to a deficiency of a β-glucosidase resulting in accumulation of glucocerebroside derived from normal breakdown of red cells. The defect is consistent with long life, and death may eventually result from the effects of marrow replacement.

A second type of Gaucher's disease exists and becomes apparent in infancy: glucocerebrosides accumulate not only in macrophages but also in neurons and death occurs in infancy from the effects on the central nervous system. A third type develops in childhood: the features are intermediate between the infant and adult types and death results in a few years.

All three types are inherited as Mendelian recessive diseases and are caused by inheritance of a double dose of abnormal genes coding for a β-glucosidase. The different types are determined by inheritance of particular abnormal alleles. Diagnosis of the disease and the carrier (heterozygote) state can be made by assay of the β-glucosidase enzymes in leucocytes or cultured skin fibroblasts and diagnosis of the condition in the fetus can be made on cultured amniotic cells.

Niemann–Pick disease. This condition is an example of abnormal storage, chiefly of the phospholipid sphingomyelin, but also of cholesterol and other lipids. It is a very rare condition of early childhood which causes mental deficiency and is usually rapidly fatal. The storage of the lipid is very extensive, occurring in the specialised cells in the brain, intestinal mucosa, adrenals, lungs, pancreas, etc., as well as in macrophages in the spleen, liver, lymph nodes, bone marrow, etc. The accumulation of lipid enlarges the cells and gives their cytoplasm a foamy appearance. The lipid stains more readily with fat stains than in Gaucher's disease. The biochemical defect is probably an autosomal recessive trait and in some cases appears to be a deficiency of an enzyme involved in the breakdown of myelin. Occasionally similar lipid-storage diseases occur in which a different phosphatide accumulates, e.g. a cephalin, and it seems likely they are all founded on defects in the enzyme systems controlling lipid metabolism. As in Gaucher's disease, diagnosis in fetal life can be made on amniotic cell cultures.

Amyloid disease

The spleen is commonly involved in generalised amyloidosis. Deposition may be mainly in the Malpighian bodies, which are changed to translucent rounded patches (Fig. 11.5, p. 11.3)— *sago spleen*—or there may be diffuse involvement of the red pulp, in which case the spleen is most often enlarged, sometimes to over 1 kg. The occurrence of the two forms is unexplained, but diffuse involvement is said to be a feature of amyloidosis complicating syphilis.

Tumours

Malignant lymphomas. As in the lymph nodes, the commonest forms of primary neo-plasia in the spleen are the various malignant lymphomas (p. 18.16). It is often not possible to determine the site of origin of these tumours, for many lymph nodes and sometimes the spleen, bone marrow, etc., are commonly involved when the patient is first seen. Occasional less widespread tumours do seem, however, to have originated in the spleen.

Metastatic tumours. Splenic metastases occur more frequently in sarcoma than in carcinoma, but even in the former they are not common. The spleen contrasts with the bone marrow and lymph nodes in its low frequency of secondary carcinoma, and in some cases of widespread carcinoma, microscopic haematogenous foci of cancer cells undergoing degenerative change have been observed in the spleen. Direct invasion may, however, occur from cancer of the pancreas, etc.

Benign tumours of the spleen, including fibroma, myoma, haemangioma and lymphangioma have been described, but all are rarities. **Cysts** of the spleen are occasionally seen. They are usually small and multiple, though one may reach a large size and form a fluctuant swelling on the surface. They contain a clear serous fluid, but there may be an admixture of altered blood. They are regarded as usually of lymphangiomatous origin.

Lymph Nodes

A brief description of the structure of the lymph nodes has been given in Chapter 6. They consist essentially of two parts. First, the lymphoid tissue proper with its follicles and deep cortex (paracortex), which are responsible for mounting immune responses (pp. 6.36-7). Second, the lymph sinuses and medullary cords which not only house antibody-producing plasma cells, but are also involved in the phagocytosis and destruction of organisms or damaged cells carried from the tissues in the lymph. In fact, the lymph node medulla and sinuses have much the same relation to the lymph as the splenic red pulp has to the blood. The macrophages in both react similarly. In addition to being active phagocytes for particulate material, they exhibit a great capacity for uptake and storage of various substances present in solution.

These two functions of lymph nodes are interdependent, for the antigenic constituents of bacteria etc. phagocytosed by macrophages are presented in highly immunogenic form to responsive lymphocytes (p. 6.26), and antibodies released locally by plasma cells in the medullary cords of lymph nodes opsonise bacteria etc., thus promoting their phagocytosis and destruction.

Acute bacterial infections

Experimental studies have shown that in normal circumstances lymph nodes are not very efficient in removing particulate elements from the lymph passing through them: for example, bacteria and similar-sized inert particles have been shown to pass rapidly from the peripheral lymphatics, through the regional nodes, and to reach the blood stream. However, within less than an hour of the establishment of an acute infection, the sinuses of the draining lymph nodes are dilated by the increased flow of lymph, the node becomes acutely inflamed (see below), and neutrophil polymorphs migrate into the sinuses from the adjacent small blood vessels and aggregate particularly in the medulla where they provide a filter by actively phagocytosing bacteria in the draining lymph: the efficiency of the nodes in preventing spread of infection to the bloodstream is thus greatly increased. Unless the infection is overcome quickly, the numbers of macrophages in the sinuses and medulla increase and they also participate in the phagocytosis of bacteria, degenerate polymorphs, cell fragments, etc., in the lymph.

In addition to the migration of polymorphs and monocytes, the lymph nodes draining a focus of acute infection show the other features of acute inflammation, including dilatation of the small blood vessels and inflammatory oedema: these changes are due to the local effects of bacteria or their toxins, and various endogenous mediators, carried in the lymph from the focus of infection. Polymorphs are also carried in the lymph, and supplement those which have accumulated in the nodes by local migration. These inflammatory changes occur in the regional lymph nodes in various pyogenic infections, particularly those caused by *Streptococccus pyogenes* and *Staphylococcus aureus*: the nodes become swollen, tender and sometimes painful. Common examples include the axillary nodes draining a whitlow and the cervical nodes in streptococcal pharyngitis.

Organisms that have invaded a lymph node are often destroyed by the leucocytes and the inflammation then resolves. They may, however, continue to multiply, with consequent suppuration which may spread to the surrounding tissues and, if superficial, discharge on the skin surface.

The changes associated with immune responses (pp. 6.36–7) are also seen in the lymph nodes in the late stages of acute infections.

In **bubonic plague**, the causal organism, *Yersinia pestis*, usually gains entry by the bite of an infected black-rat flea. It is carried to the draining lymph nodes where it causes a painful swelling termed a *bubo*: the infected nodes become swollen with haemorrhage, oedema and suppuration and the surrounding tissues are

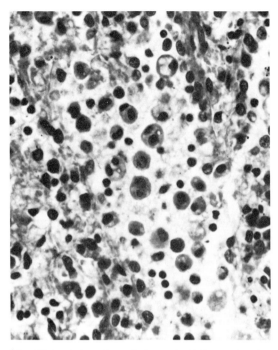

Fig. 18.4 A lymph node in typhoid fever, showing numerous macrophages in a sinus. Some of the macrophages contain ingested erythrocytes. × 520.

grossly oedematous (traditionally described as gelatinous). The bacteria usually cause a septicaemia with haemorrhagic, necrotic lesions in many tissues and a high mortality. Diagnosis is usually easy during an outbreak: the bacteria are present in large numbers in aspirates of the bubo and can also be cultured from the blood. In **anthrax** the lesion is mainly an inflammatory oedema with a varying amount of haemorrhage and necrosis (Fig. 9.12, p. 9.14).

In **typhoid fever,** large numbers of macrophages accumulate in the sinuses and medullary cords of the lymph nodes draining the intestinal lesions (Fig. 18.4). The macrophages contain ingested cell debris and often erythrocytes. Plasma cells are also numerous. Haemorrhage, necrosis and autolytic softening may follow (Fig. 19.55, p. 19.44) but, as in other typhoid lesions, neutrophil polymorphs are few or absent.

Acute suppurative granulomatous infections

A miscellaneous group of acute infections is characterised by lymphadenopathy in which epithelioid-cell granulomas undergo central suppuration. This occurs in **lymphogranuloma** venereum (p. 25.3), a venereal disease caused by *Chlamydia trachomatis*. In men, the inguinal nodes are involved and in women the inguinal, pelvic or para-rectal nodes. Microscopically, the lesions consist of stellate abscesses enclosed in a palisade of epithelioid cells. The pus eventually becomes inspissated and enclosed in dense fibrous tissue. Similar suppurating granulomas are seen in the mesenteric nodes in **yersinial infections** of the appendix or ileum (p. 19.50), in the axillary, cervical or inguinal nodes in **cat scratch disease** (which is of unknown cause and occurs in the nodes draining the site of a cat scratch within the preceding few weeks) and in the generalised lymphadenopathy of **tularaemia,** an infection with *Francisella tularensis* seen mostly in parts of the Americas and Asia.

Viral infections

Lymph node enlargement occurs in many acute viral infections but is usually overshadowed by other features and in most instances biopsy is neither necessary nor helpful in diagnosis. Occasionally, however, lymph node biopsy is performed particularly in infectious mononucleosis and acquired cytomegalovirus disease. The features of early measles are sometimes encountered incidentally in lymph nodes, tonsils or appendix excised for other reasons.

Infectious mononucleosis (IM). This is a viral infection which occurs sporadically and in small epidemics, mostly in adolescents and young adults. It is characterised by swelling and tenderness of cervical lymph nodes, fever lasting a week or two (it is also called **glandular fever),** and atypical lymphoid cells in the blood. The posterior cervical nodes are usually affected first, but other groups may be involved.

Splenomegaly is not uncommon and rupture, sometimes fatal, may follow a trivial injury. Apart from this, the disease is rarely fatal, and recovery usually occurs after 1 to 3 weeks. Sore throat is often a prominent clinical feature: it is due to a viral pharyngitis with mixed secondary infection, often including candida, and sometimes progressing to necrosis and ulceration of the mucosa. There may also be severe headache and a skin rash. After an initial neutrophil leucocytosis, the characteristic blood picture appears—a leucocyte count usually of $10–20 \times$

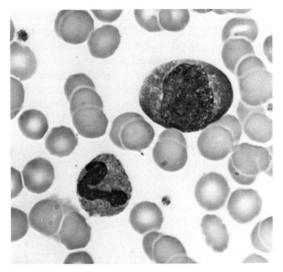

Fig. 18.5   Blood smear in infectious mononucleosis, showing an atypical lymphoid cell with enlarged irregular nucleus and abundant basophilic cytoplasm. It has the features of a lymphoblast, and is much larger than the adjacent polymorph. Leishman's stain. × 1400.

$10^9/1$ (10–20 000/μl), of which 50% or more are enlarged atypical lymphoid cells with a large irregular, sometimes convoluted nucleus and an increased amount of basophilic cytoplasm (Fig. 18.5). The lymph nodes show early prominence of the germinal centres, but soon the most striking change is accumulation of huge numbers of lymphoblasts in the paracortex and sinuses. Mitoses are frequent and the appearances are highly suggestive of a malignant lymphoma (Fig. 18.6), particularly as the blast cells may infiltrate the perinodal tissue. Cells indistinguishable from the Reed–Sternberg cells of Hodgkin's disease are sometimes present but the large numbers of lymphoblasts are not seen in Hodgkin's disease (p. 18.18). Also the nodal architecture is preserved in IM. Another feature is the formation of new blood vessels in the paracortex: they are lined by flat endothelial cells and are distended with blood. The most conspicuous microscopic change in the spleen is proliferation of lymphoblasts in the splenic cords and Malpighian bodies. Some patients develop *acute hepatitis*, the pathogenesis of which is obscure: liver biopsy shows changes resembling those of infectious hepatitis together with aggregates of lymphoblasts in the portal areas and sinusoids.

Aetiology. IM is caused by infection with

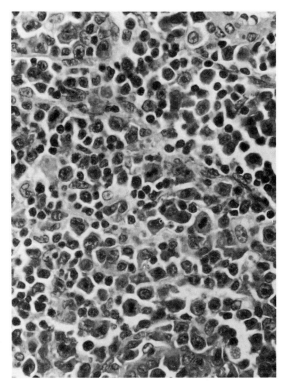

Fig. 18.6 Lymph node in infectious mononucleosis, showing large numbers of lymphoblasts in the paracortex. Mitoses are conspicuous and a sinus (upper right) also contains blast cells. × 520 (Slide provided by Dr G.B.S. Roberts).

Epstein–Barr virus (EBV), a member of the herpes group. Throughout the world, most people are infected sooner or later, and infection results in life-long immunity. Infection in childhood rarely results in clinical illness, but if the virus is first encountered in adolescence or adult life the development of immunity is accompanied in up to 50% of individuals by an attack of IM. Accordingly, the clinical illness is seen more often in the higher socio-economic communities in which infection is more likely to be delayed until adolescence or early adult life. Spread of infection is by close contact: the virus colonises the pharyngeal epithelium and is present in the throat washings and saliva shortly after infection. It is thought to be transmitted by kissing.

Following invasion of the pharynx, the virus infects B lymphocytes which have specific EBV receptors, and the viral genome becomes integrated into the lymphocyte DNA. It behaves like an oncogenic DNA virus (p. 13.6), transforming the lymphocytes into blast cells which proliferate rapidly and continue to do so in cell cultures. *In vivo*, the transformed B cells induce a remarkably intense cell-mediated immune response which accounts for the paracortical T-cell hyperplasia and the appearance of atypical mononuclear cells in the blood. Except in the early stages, most of the atypical cells are T immunoblasts, including cytotoxic cells which react with and kill most of the infected, transformed B cells and bring the illness to an end. Although the virus integrates into B-cell nuclei, in a small proportion of cells it replicates. In spite of the intense T-cell response, some infected B cells persist and infection is probably life-long, thus accounting for the permanent immunity to re-infection.

Infectious mononucleosis is of particular interest because in some ways it resembles a virus-induced B-cell lymphoma and yet is eliminated by a vigorous T-cell response to the transformed cells. EBV is also associated with Burkitt's lymphoma (p. 18.26) and with anaplastic nasopharyngeal carcinoma. There is, however, no evidence of an increased risk of these tumours following IM.

Serology. By the time symptoms develop, the patient has already developed a high titre of antibody to viral capsid antigen (VCA) and this persists for many years. Antibody to viral 'early antigen' (p. 13.13) develops during the illness and the titre falls in a few months. Antibody to a viral 'nuclear' antigen (EBNA) appears later in the illness and persists for many years. These antibodies can be detected by immunofluorescence, using EBV-infected B lymphoblasts in culture.

Heterophil antibody agglutinates sheep red cells, and appears in the serum in about 75% of patients in the early stages of IM. It is detected by the **Paul-Bunnell test** and is absorbed by bovine red cells but not by guinea-pig kidney, which distinguishes it from heterophil antibody in some healthy individuals and in some other diseases. The antibody disappears after several months.

Diagnosis can usually be made on the clinical features and a positive Paul-Bunnell test. If the test is negative, antibody to viral antigens, e.g. VCA, can be sought. Demonstration of IgM class antibody is particularly helpful, indicating recent infection.

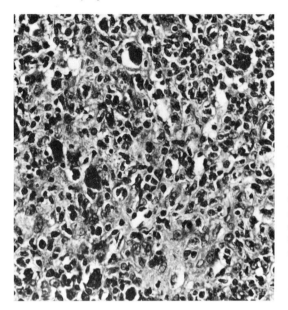

Fig. 18.7 Lymph node in the prodromal stage of measles, showing part of a germinal centre containing Warthin-Finkeldey giant cells. × 320.

Other viral infections

Various other acute viral diseases, including **varicella**, **rubella** and **herpes simplex** produce changes in the lymphoid tissues resembling those of infectious mononucleosis, but the T-cell proliferation is usually much less intense and more patchy and the number of lymphoblasts in the blood is correspondingly small.

Cytomegalovirus (CMV) infection. In the fetus, this virus (one of the herpes group) can cause fatal infection or a severe encephalomyelitis resulting in mental retardation (p. 21.33). In postnatal life, infection is usually subclinical but sometimes causes an illness closely resembling infectious mononucleosis: it is not, however, accompanied by a pharyngitis and the Paul–Bunnell test is negative. Antibodies to EBV do not develop during the illness although they may, of course, already be present in the serum. The virus also causes lesions in immunosuppressed patients, e.g. following renal transplantation, and is a common feature of the acquired immune deficiency syndrome (p. 25.5).

Measles. In measles, the lymph nodes show formation of multinucleated giant cells, termed Warthin-Finkeldey cells (Fig. 18.7). They are sometimes observed in an appendix or tonsils which happen to have been removed during the incubation period of measles, and it is important not to mistake the changes for anything more sinister. Multinucleated giant cells are formed by fusion of alveolar epithelial cells in the lesions of giant-cell pneumonia which sometimes complicates measles (Fig. 16.28, p. 16.43).

Chronic lymph node enlargement

This occurs in a very large number of conditions and is, of course, a most important clinical sign. The main causes may be classified as follows.

    (a) Chronic granulomatous lymphadenitis
    (b) Hyperplastic lymphadenopathies
    (c) Neoplastic conditions

Chronic granulomatous lymphadenitis

Granulomatous inflammation is a common cause of lymph node enlargement and diagnosis often depends on histological and microbiological examination of an excised node. Some diseases give rise to epithelioid-cell granulomas, while others have less characteristic appearances. The features of most of the conditions are described in detail elsewhere, and the present account merely summarises the histological changes in the nodes. Acute infections in which a granulomatous reaction is accompanied by suppuration are described on pp. 18.9–10.

Tuberculosis. Enlarged caseating lymph nodes are the major feature of the primary complex of tuberculosis (p. 9.20). Depending on the site of infection, the cervical, pulmonary hilar or mesenteric nodes may be affected. Occasionally tuberculosis is responsible for enlargement of one or more cervical nodes in an adult, due to recrudescence of old dormant tuberculosis: histological examination of an excised node shows the typical epithelioid- and

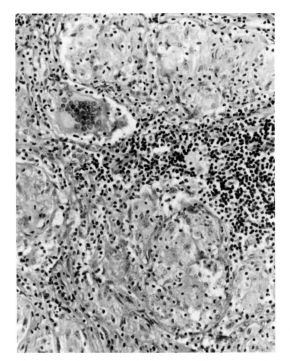

Fig. 18.8 Lymph node in sarcoidosis, showing tubercle-like epithelioid-cell granulomas and giant cells but without caseation. × 75.

giant-cell granulomas which tend to coalesce and usually (but not always) show central necrosis. In most cases the tubercle bacillus can be detected microscopically or by culture.

Sarcoidosis. This is a granulomatous condition of unknown aetiology (p. 9.26) in which lymph node enlargement is the commonest feature. The pulmonary hilar nodes are usually affected, although other deep and superficial nodes are commonly involved, and also the spleen, lungs and various other organs. The condition may be clinically silent and is often detected by the incidental finding of hilar lymph node enlargement in a young adult by routine chest x-ray. In other cases, fever or a persistent cough are the presenting symptoms. The affected nodes may be greatly enlarged, greyish or pinkish, and the condition may readily be mistaken clinically for Hodgkin's disease. The histological features of an excised node (described more fully on p. 9.27) consist of multiple epithelioid-cell granulomas which do not tend to coalesce and usually show little or no central necrosis (Fig. 18.8). Multinucleated giant cells may be present, and sometimes they contain curious stellate or conchoid bodies, which may

be calcified. The tuberculin test is usually negative in cases of sarcoidosis, and there is evidence that this is due to depression of cell-mediated immunity: delayed hypersensitivity to other antigens, e.g. mumps virus, is also depressed, although the serum contains the usual blood-group and other antibodies, and there may be a raised level of serum IgG. In some cases, delayed hypersensitivity to tuberculin has been observed to diminish or disappear following the onset of sarcoidosis, and to re-appear following remission. The Kveim test, a granulomatous sarcoid reaction at the site of intradermal injection of a sterilised extract of sarcoidosis lesions, is useful in diagnosis.

Non-caseating epithelioid-cell granulomas occur in the lymph nodes and spleen in some patients with **Hodgkin's disease** and are liable to be mistaken for sarcoidosis unless the biopsy material contains also Hodgkin's lesions. In some cases of **Crohn's disease** (p. 19.33) epithelioid-cell granulomas develop in the mesenteric lymph nodes, although enlargement is usually slight. In **syphilis,** the lymph nodes draining the primary sore become enlarged and indurated (p. 9.29), and the skin rashes of the secondary stage are usually accompanied by moderate or slight general enlargement of lymph nodes. In both stages, the enlarged nodes show follicular hyperplasia and plasma cells are numerous. There may also be epithelioid and multinucleated giant cells, singly and in small groups, in the paracortex, and sometimes formation of larger, tubercle like epithelioid-cell granulomas, together with endarteritis and periarteritis of small vessels. In the tertiary stage, gummas occur comparatively rarely in the lymph nodes.

There may be local or widespread enlargement of the lymph nodes in **chronic granulomatous disease of childhood** (p. 17.14) and in some cases the enlarged nodes contain epithelioid-cell granulomas closely resembling those of tuberculosis. In addition, there may be smaller groups of foamy macrophages, sometimes containing lipofuscin.

Histoplasmosis most commonly causes a localised respiratory infection with eventual healing and calcification (p. 9.36). It may, however, cause a generalised infection in which the macrophages in the spleen, lymph nodes, bone marrow, liver and elsewhere are colonised by huge numbers of *Histoplasma capsulatum*. These organs are enlarged and the masses of colonised macrophages may show foci of necrosis similar to tuberculous caseation. A positive skin test, indicating cell-mediated immunity, is of little value in inhabitants of endemic areas where most individuals are positive, and in generalised infection the test may become negative.

Toxoplasmosis. Infection with the protozoon *Toxoplasma gondii* is described on p. 28.17. Apart from the congenital form, it is usually symptomless but may cause lymph node enlargement, either localised or generalised, usually including the upper cervical nodes. There may be no other symptoms or a febrile illness, and a wide variety of symptoms may also result from involvement of one or more organs, including the lungs, heart and skeletal muscles. It may occur at any age, but is seen most often in young adults.

Hyperplastic lymphadenopathies

A number of miscellaneous, apparently non-infective conditions are characterised by lymph node enlargement due to hyperplasia of lymphoid cells or macrophages and related cells, or of more than one cell type. The hyperplasia may assume a lymphoid follicular pattern or the cells may occupy mainly the sinuses or the paracortex.

(a) Follicular hyperplasia

An exaggerated form of the physiological follicular hyperplasia of the humoral immune response (p. 6.37) is a common feature of **rheumatoid arthritis,** and the lymph nodes may be sufficiently enlarged to raise clinical suspicion of a lymphoma. Histologically, the nodes contain numerous enlarged follicles, usually with prominent germinal centres (Fig. 18.9). The appearances probably reflect production of rheumatoid factors, antinuclear antibodies, etc., but they may be difficult to distinguish from follicular lymphoma (p. 18.23). This form of lymphadenopathy is particularly common in Felty's syndrome (rheumatoid arthritis, splenomegaly and leucopenia) and in patients with the extra-articular lesions of rheumatoid arthritis.

In the rare condition of **angiofollicular hyperplasia** there is great lymph node enlargement, usually of the

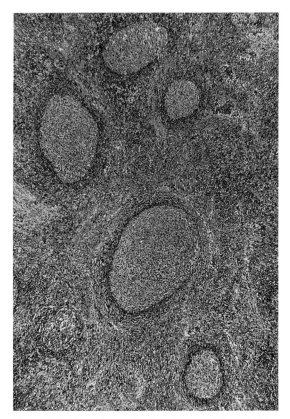

Fig. 18.9 Lymph node in rheumatoid arthritis, showing follicular hyperplasia with conspicuous germinal centres. × 50.

mediastinal nodes. The affected nodes consist mainly of large follicles composed of concentrically-arranged small lymphocytes but with a central small group of centrocytes enveloping a small blood vessel which may show hyaline change. The cause of the condition is unknown: it may occur at any age and the enlarged lymph nodes are sometimes detected incidentally on chest x-ray.

(b) Sinus hyperplasia

Sinus hyperplasia is a common cause of enlargement of the regional lymph nodes draining sites of chronic or repeated infection or tissue destruction. Histologically the sinuses, particularly those of the medulla, are distended by large numbers of macrophages (Fig. 18.10). Sinus hyperplasia commonly causes enlargement of the axillary nodes in carcinoma of the breast and may be mistaken clinically for metastasis. It is also very common in the inguinal nodes, presumably because of the frequency of mild injuries and infections of the feet: eventually the affected nodes become fibrosed, accounting for the firm, usually palpable nodes in the groin.

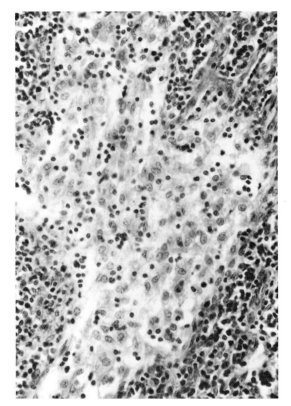

Fig. 18.10 Lymph node showing reactive sinus hyperplasia: an enlarged sinus containing increased numbers of macrophages. × 120.

Lymphangiopathic histiocytosis, also called *sinus histiocytosis with massive lymphadenopathy,* is an uncommon, chronic disease of unknown cause, occurring mainly in children and young adults, more often in boys than in girls: it may subside or cause death. Fever, neutrophil leucocytosis and hypergammaglobulinaemia suggest an infection, but no causal organism has been discovered. There is a marked lymphadenopathy, often noticed first in the cervical nodes, caused by distension of the sinuses with macrophages which show the usual cell markers (p. 4.36), and some of which contain ingested lymphocytes and occasional polymorphs and red cells. There may also be occasional multinuclear giant cells. The medullary cords are enlarged by increased numbers of plasma cells, lymphocytes and macrophages, together with polymorphs.

Histiocytosis X. This term is applied to local or widespread proliferation of Langerhans cells of the monocyte-macrophage system (p. 4.33). The proliferated cells appear uniform and mitoses are not seen. They have a folded or deeply indented nucleus, well seen in imprint preparations, and abundant slightly eosinophilic cytoplasm which may be vacuolated.

Their nature can be confirmed by demonstrating the markers of Langerhans cells (e.g. S-100 protein, strong staining for ATPase, Birbeck granules—p. 4.37). The lesions are commonly infiltrated also by ordinary macrophages and giant cells (both of which may contain phagocytosed material) by eosinophil polymorphs (aggregates of which may undergo necrosis) and by plasma cells and fibroblasts.

Histiocytosis X occurs predominantly in the first two decades. In infants, the lesions tend to be widespread, causing generalised lymphadenopathy, hepatosplenomegaly, skin rashes, often osteolytic lesions in the bones and infiltration of various other organs. In the affected lymph nodes the Langerhans and other cells are confined to the sinuses, which become grossly distended. This generalised form is known as **Letterer-Siwe** disease: it is accompanied by fever, loss of weight and anaemia, and is usually fatal within a few months, although glucocorticoids and cytotoxic drugs may prolong life.

In children, the lesions progress more slowly and the Langerhans cells may accumulate cholesterol esters and other lipids. The lesions occur particularly in the bones, skin, lymph nodes, spleen and lungs. Exophthalmos or diabetes insipidus may result from lesions of the skull involving the orbit or hypothalamus respectively. This more chronic form of histiocytosis X is called **Hand-Schuller-Christian disease.** It can occur at all ages, and may continue for years, particularly *in older children and adults,* the lesions, which may be multifocal rather than diffuse, eventually undergoing fibrosis. Although in some instances this condition runs a benign course, in other cases it assumes the more aggressive features of Letterer-Siwe disease.

The third member of the group is termed **eosinophil granuloma of bone:** it is usually a solitary lesion with a benign course, and occurs most often *in adolescents or young adults.* It is described with other bone lesions on p. 23.24.

The above three conditions illustrate the wide spectrum of behaviour of histiocytosis X—from the diffuse, often rapidly fatal condition in infants to the solitary benign lesion of adults. There are, however, instances in which one condition has transformed into another. The aetiology of histiocytosis X is unknown. Because of the associated inflammatory cells, low mitotic activity and lack of cellular atypia, it is widely regarded as non-neoplastic, although Letterer-Siwe disease behaves very much like a malignant tumour.

(c) Other patterns of hyperplasia

Dermatopathic lymphadenopathy is a cause of regional or generalised enlargement of lymph nodes draining chronic inflammatory or destructive lesions of the skin. Histology shows hyperplasia of inter-

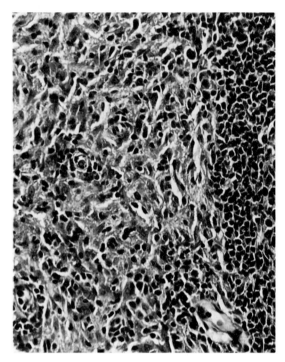

Fig. 18.11 Dermatopathic lymphadenopathy. Para-cortical tissue occupies most of the field, with a strip of cortex on the right. The paracortex is occupied by large, irregularly arranged elongated cells which can only be identified as interdigitating reticulum and Langerhans cells by marker studies or electron microscopy. × 300 (Dr A. McQueen)

digitated reticulum cells and accumulation of Langerhans cells in the paracortex (Fig. 18.11). The cells may be recognised by cell-marker studies and by electron microscopy (p. 4.37): some of them contain lipid and granules of melanin and haemosiderin, giving the alternative name of *lipomelanic reticulosis*. When accompanying T-cell lymphomas or other neoplastic conditions of the skin, the enlarged nodes may be mistaken clinically for metastatic spread.

Angio-immunoblastic lymphadenopathy or *immunoblastic lymphadenopathy* is an uncommon cause of generalised lymph node enlargement, occurring usually in old people, and accompanied by hepato-splenomegaly, cutaneous rashes, polyclonal hyper-gammaglobulinaemia and sometimes auto-immune haemolytic anaemia. Clinically, it develops rapidly and there may be fever, anorexia and weight loss which, together with the lymphadenopathy, may raise the suspicion of Hodgkin's disease. The lymph-nodes are greatly enlarged with a pale uniform cut surface. The nodal architecture is largely replaced by arborising small blood vessels with a prominent endothelium: the vessels lie in a mixed cell infiltrate, including lymphocytes, plasma cells, lymphoblasts and macrophages and sometimes eosinophils and groups of epithelioid cells. The nature of this condition is unknown, but death often results from aplastic anaemia with pancytopenia or from development of a lymphoma.

The lymphomas

The term 'lymphoma' is now widely used to describe a diverse group of tumours arising most often in the lymphoid tissues. Some would (with justification) restrict the term to those tumours which can be shown conclusively to derive from lymphocytes in their various functional phases. It is convenient, however, to include also within this general term tumours arising from cells of the mononuclear phagocyte system ('histiocytic lymphomas') which are intimately associated with lymphocytes in the development of the immune response (p. 6.26). Such histiocytic tumours, moreover, often exhibit characteristics similar to those of lymphocytic neoplasms.

All of the known lymphomas are malignant and without treatment they usually limit the lifespan of their victims. They vary considerably, however, in their degree of aggressiveness, some leading to death in a few weeks, others only after many years. Their natural course is modified by treatment and in some instances cure is possible.

Most lymphomas, whether of lymphocytic or histiocytic derivation, arise in lymph nodes or in other tissues rich in lymphoid tissue such as the spleen, bone marrow, pharynx and gastrointestinal tract. Lymphocytes and histiocytes are, however, ubiquitous cells and lymphomas may arise in almost any tissue, including the skin and CNS. While some lymphomas resemble other malignant neoplasms in forming distinct tumour masses, others, and in particular those of bone marrow derivation, present as forms of leukaemia (p. 17.46) and also produce tumour masses or organomegaly as a secondary phenomenon, and it is difficult to draw a sharp distinction between 'solid' and leukaemic variants of the lymphomas.

Classification

As with other tumours, the main purpose in classifying lymphomas is to provide an indication of how a particular example will behave and what form of therapy is likely to be most effective. Rapid progress has been made in relating the cells of most lymphomas to the types and stages of lymphoid cells found in normal lymphoid tissues, and this forms the basis of modern classifications. However, before considering the individual tumours and their classification, it is convenient to deal with *Hodgkin's disease*, which is quite distinct from the other lymphomas—now referred to as the *non-Hodgkin's lymphomas* (p. 18.21).

Hodgkin's disease

General features. Although this is the commonest form of lymphoma, the nature of the neoplastic cells (Reed–Sternberg and Hodgkin cells—see below) is uncertain. Recent cell-marker studies using a monoclonal antibody (Stein *et al.*, 1982) suggest that they are derived from a small population of lymphocyte-like cells widely distributed in the lympho-reticular tissues, but it is also possible that they are related to macrophages.

The disease can develop at almost any age, although there is a peak incidence in early adult life and a second peak in the older age groups. The usual presenting feature is progressive and usually painless enlargement of lymph nodes, most often those of the cervical, inguinal or axillary groups. Early involvement of the abdominal or mediastinal nodes, the pharyngeal lymphoid tissue or the spleen is, however, not uncommon. It is unusual for extranodal sites to be primarily affected, although almost any tissue may be implicated by metastatic spread of the tumour. Constitutional symptoms are sometimes conspicuous, especially in advanced

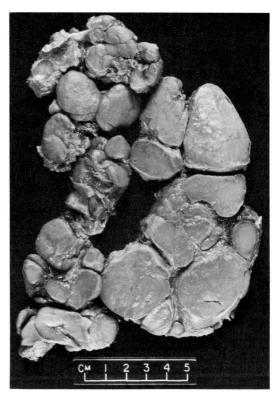

Fig. 18.12 A group of enlarged cervical lymph nodes in Hodgkin's disease. The largest nodes are becoming matted together.

cases; they include an irregular low-grade pyrexia which occasionally assumes a periodic pattern (Pel-Ebstein fever), and an anaemia usually of normochromic normocytic type, sometimes accompanied by a neutrophil—less commonly an eosinophil—leucocytosis. An important feature is an early depression of T-lymphocyte function with impairment of cell-mediated immunity. In consequence, patients are unusually prone to develop various infections, especially tuberculosis and herpes zoster (p. 7.36), but also fungal and other 'opportunistic' infections by organisms of relatively low pathogenicity.

Hodgkin's disease is classified on a histological basis into four types, which differ in their course from death in a few months to survival and good health for many years, even without treatment. *The histological pattern and the extent of the disease at the time of diagnosis have considerable prognostic significance.*

Macroscopic changes. Initially the enlarged **lymph nodes** are discrete (Fig. 18.12), soft and rubbery, with a greyish-pink cut surface. In

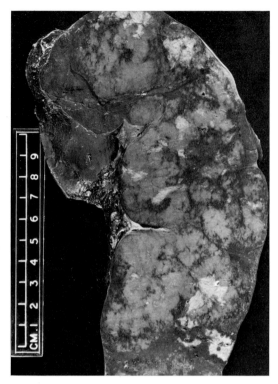

Fig. 18.13 Advanced involvement of the spleen in Hodgkin's disease. The neoplastic tissue is seen as pale, irregular patches on the cut surface. The whitish areas are foci of necrotic neoplastic tissue.

some forms of the disease, however, fibrosis is present from the outset. As they become larger, the nodes tend to become firmer and bound together by the spreading lesions, and they may produce serious pressure effects, for example on the trachea or mediastinal blood vessels. Foci of non-suppurative necrosis are also commonly observed in the lesions. **The spleen** is frequently involved and enlarged: the lesions develop in the Malpighian bodies, which become expanded and eventually confluent. This process ultimately produces the characteristic German sausage appearance of the cut surface, the pale neoplastic patches resembling flecks of suet (Fig. 18.13). Staging procedures in which splenectomy is carried out (see below) have shown, however, that the spleen may be involved without obvious enlargement, and also that splenomegaly may occur in the absence of tumour involvement, due to diffuse hyperplasia of the red pulp. Although the disease is often restricted at first to the lymphoid organs, almost any tissue may be affected at a later stage, the

lesions appearing as pale patches of neoplastic infiltration or replacement of the normal tissue. Lesions occur especially in the **liver, kidneys** and **bone marrow:** involvement of the **vertebrae** may lead to pressure on the spinal cord with paraplegia: focal or diffuse lesions in the **lungs** are not uncommon (Fig. 18.14), especially if the mediastinal nodes are affected, and ulcerating tumour masses occur in the **gastro-intestinal tract.**

Microscopic appearances. The diagnosis is usually made by biopsy of an enlarged lymph node. The tissue of the node is partly or completely replaced. The essential feature, without which the diagnosis cannot be made, is the presence of typical **Reed–Sternberg (RS) cells.** This cell measures 40 μm or more in diameter, and has an intricate double or bi-lobed nucleus, each component of which has a vesicular appearance due to condensation of chromatin peripherally, and a large central eosinophilic nucleolus (Fig. 18.15). The cytoplasm is abundant and amphophilic (i.e. purple with haematoxylin-eosin stain). Similar cells occur in some reactive lymph nodes and in some other lymphomas, so that the presence of RS cells is not alone diagnostic of Hodgkin's disease. Variants of these typical giant cells are common and may help in subclassifying Hodgkin's dis-

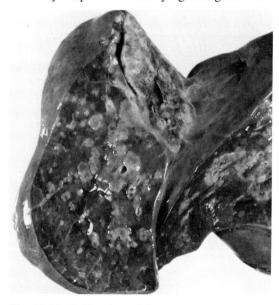

Fig. 18.14 Infiltration of the lung in Hodgkin's disease. In this instance the neoplastic tissue is seen as discrete pale patches: in some cases it is more diffuse. × 0·3.

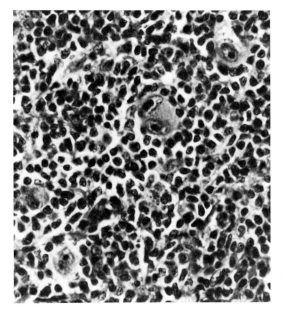

Fig. 18.15 Hodgkin's disease of lymphocyte-predominant type, Field chosen to show Reed–Sternberg cells, one of which shows the characteristic 'mirror-image' nuclei with large nucleoli. × 520.

ease (see below). Likewise, the Hodgkin cells, which have a single ovoid nucleus but are otherwise similar to RS cells, are not diagnostic except in the recognition of metastatic lesions. In the more aggressive forms of Hodgkin's disease (see below), aberrant neoplastic cells much larger than typical RS cells and with multiple or grossly irregular nuclei (Fig. 18.16), are commonly present. The neoplastic cells of Hodgkin's disease lie in a variable reactive cellular infiltrate which includes lymphocytes and sometimes plasma cells, macrophages, fibroblasts, neutrophil and eosinophil leucocytes: the proportions of these cells vary greatly from case to case. There is always some increase in reticulin fibres, particularly in the late stages, and abundant collagen is formed in some variants of the disease.

In some cases, sarcoid-like epithelioid-cell granulomas are found in the lymph nodes, spleen, etc.; they may be present in tissue unaffected by Hodgkin's disease and do not affect the prognosis.

Classification of Hodgkin's disease

For prognostic purposes, Hodgkin's disease has been subdivided, in the internationally agreed Rye classification, into four major types as follows.

(1) Lymphocyte-predominant (15% of cases). The important feature of this type is that *typical* RS cells are sparse and difficult to find. More numerous, and peculiar to the type, are variants of the RS cell with complex twisted nuclei and indistinct nucleoli. The infiltrate is mainly lymphocytic (Fig. 18.15) but there may be small aggregates of macrophages and sometimes sarcoid-like follicles. Eosinophils and other reactive cells are scanty or absent and capsular thickening and reticulin deposition are minimal, although sometimes a nodular pattern develops (see below).

(2) Nodular sclerosing type (40% of cases). In this type, the lymph node capsule is thickened and fine or coarse bands of collagen subdivide the node into nodules of various sizes (Fig. 18.17). Within the nodules, the neoplasm may show a mixed cellular reaction (see above) but lymphocytes are usually predominant. In addition to typical RS cells, a variant showing

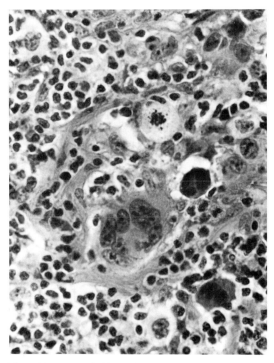

Fig. 18.16 Hodgkin's disease showing numerous neoplastic reticulum cells, including a multinucleated Reed–Sternberg cell. There was a mixed cell infiltrate in this case. × 450.

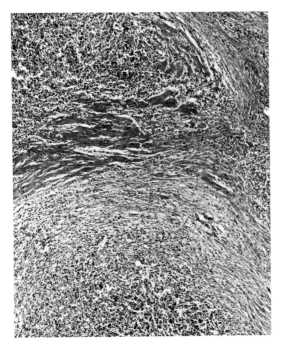

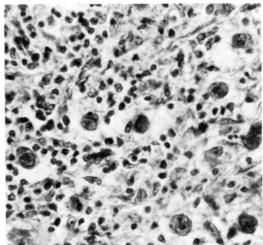

Fig. 18.18 Nodular sclerosing Hodgkin's disease in a lymph node, showing lacunar cells with vacuolated cytoplasm. × 375.

tissue varies greatly in amount, but in some cases is very abundant and diffuse.

Stage, histological type and prognosis

Hodgkin's disease often appears to start in a single lymph node or group of nodes, and may spread either by lymphatics or by the blood-

Fig. 18.17 Nodular sclerosing Hodgkin's disease in a lymph node. In this instance, the collagen dividing the 'Hodgkin's tissue' into nodules is abundant and the diagnosis is obvious. × 50.

pronounced vacuolation of the peripheral cytoplasm (the *'lacunar' cell*—Fig. 18.18) is regarded as characteristic of this type, which is often confined to the lower cervical lymph nodes, mediastinum and sometimes upper abdominal nodes. In some instances the thymus appears to be involved first and the condition has been misnamed *granulomatous thymoma*.

(3) Mixed-cellularity type (30% of cases). In this type, typical RS and Hodgkin cells, commonly showing mitotic activity, are numerous, and lie in a mixed cellular infiltrate of neutrophils, eosinophils, macrophages, plasma cells and lymphocytes (Fig. 18.16). Reticulin fibres are sometimes abundant, with early collagen formation, but this is diffuse and does not result in nodularity.

(4) Lymphocyte-depleted type (15% of cases) includes cases previously classed as *Hodgkin's sarcoma*. The histological picture in such cases is dominated by RS and Hodgkin cells (Fig. 18.19) and many larger pleomorphic neoplastic giant cells may also be present. Lymphocytes are sparse and other reactive cells, including eosinophils, are variable in number. Fibrous

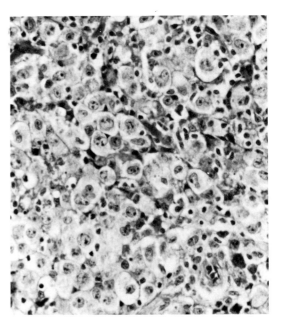

Fig. 18.19 Lymphocyte-depleted Hodgkin's disease. Most of the cells are neoplastic reticulum cells and lymphocytes are few. × 520.

stream to adjacent or distant tissues, both lymphoid and non-lymphoid. When limited to one area of the body, local ablation, e.g. by radiotherapy, is effective and sometimes apparently curative. Once the lesions are widely disseminated, systemic chemotherapy provides the only hope of controlling its otherwise relentless progress. *The extent of the disease is thus critical in determining the prognosis and in planning therapy.* To assess this accurately, clinical examination must be supplemented by at least bone marrow biopsy and abdominal lymphangiography, and many now advocate laparotomy with splenectomy and liver biopsy to detect and determine the extent of abdominal involvement. By these methods the disease can be subdivided into four **stages** (Table 18.1).

Table 18.1 Staging of Hodgkin's disease, based on the Ann Arbor system

STAGE I	Confined to a single lymph node or group of nodes.
STAGE II	Confined to upper or lower part of body, i.e. all lesions *either* above *or* below the diaphragm.
STAGE III	Involving lymph nodes above *and* below the diaphragm, with or without lesions in other tissues.
STAGE IV	Widespread involvement of one or more non-lymphoid tissues, with or without lymph node involvement.

The more extensive the disease, the worse, in general, is the prognosis, and most patients surviving for ten years or more were initially diagnosed in stage I. The prognosis can also be correlated with the **histological type.** In general, the outlook is most favourable when lymphocytes are abundant and RS and Hodgkin cells sparse. Thus the lymphocyte-predominant type is associated with a much longer survival than the lymphocyte-depleted type, while the mixed-cellularity type has an intermediate prognosis.

The histological type also correlates quite well with the clinical stage, most cases of lymphocyte-predominant Hodgkin's disease presenting in stage I. The great importance of staging, however, is best illustrated by the nodular sclerosing type. This shows no tendency to undergo transitions to other forms of the disease, and provided it is in stage I the outlook is good: indeed, most of the patients surviving

for many years belong to this group. In stages II and III, however, this variant has a prognosis scarcely better than the mixed-cellularity type. Apart from the nodular sclerosing type, Hodgkin's disease is unfortunately prone to progress to a worse type, i.e. from lymphocyte-predominant to mixed-cellularity and to lymphocyte-depleted.

Non-Hodgkin's lymphomas (NHL)

Apart from Hodgkin's disease, in which the nature of the malignant cell is uncertain, nearly all the lymphomas arise from cells of the lymphocyte series. Malignant tumours do, however, originate from cells of the monocyte-macrophage lineage; they are termed *malignant histiocytomas* but are usually included in the NHL group of lymphomas.

The recent advances in the recognition of sub-types of lymphocytes and the use of cell markers to relate the neoplastic lymphoid cells with their normal counterparts have revolutionised the classification of the NHL and have led to improvements in treatment of individual patients. These advances are still continuing and classification must be to some extent provisional. At present, the two most widely used are the Lukes–Collins classification (Lukes and Collins 1977) and the Kiel classification (see Lennert 1978, 1981). They have much in common and the classification used here (Table 18.2) is a simplification of the Kiel classification, in which a broad distinction is made between NHL of *low-grade* and of *high-grade malignancy.* The recognition of the cell type of the tumours in each group is based mainly on morphological study of histological sections and impression preparations, but this is being increasingly supplemented by more sophisticated immunological and histochemical methods of detecting cell markers and by cytogenetic and ultrastructural techniques.

It is now established that most lymphomas, and particularly those within the low-grade group, are derived from B lymphoid cells and that their morphological features are related to the stages in the normal life cycle of the lymphocyte sub-population to which they belong. Immunological marker studies on fresh cell suspensions or frozen sections from lymphoid

Table 18.2 Classification of the non-Hodgkin's lymphomas

Low-grade malignancy	Cell type
Lymphocytic (including CLL)	B or T
Lymphoplasmacytic	B
Plasmacytic	B
Follicle-centre-cell tumours	B
(predominantly centrocytic)	
Follicular	
Diffuse	
High-grade malignancy	
Lymphoblastic	B or T
Large cell	
Immunoblastic	B or T
Centroblastic	B
Histiocytic	Macrophage

Note. This classification corresponds closely to the Kiel classification of Lennert (1978) but rare types are ommitted. It includes also histiocytic tumours, which do not find a place in the Kiel classification.

tumours have shown, however, that T-cell tumours are by no means rare in Western countries and in Japan they are almost as common as B-cell tumours. T-cell lymphomas do not always fit readily even into the broad categories listed in Table 18.2 and some of the more recently described types are discussed separately (pp. 18.27–28).

While all lymphomas are to be regarded as malignant, they exhibit great variation in natural behaviour. The low-grade types of NHL, which occur almost exclusively in adults, are often widely disseminated within the lympho-reticular tissues by the time they cause symptoms, and frequently become leukaemic. In spite of this, they very often respond well to chemotherapy and the patient usually survives for years rather than months, although in some instances the tumour evolves into a highly malignant form. By contrast, the high-grade malignancy types of NHL quite often arise in childhood or adolescence and while they may also be widely disseminated at presentation, some, like carcinomas, are initially localised and only later become disseminated. Staging procedures like those used in Hodgkin's disease are therefore more important in the highly malignant types of NHL: in most instances, however, these tumours are fatal within a year or so.

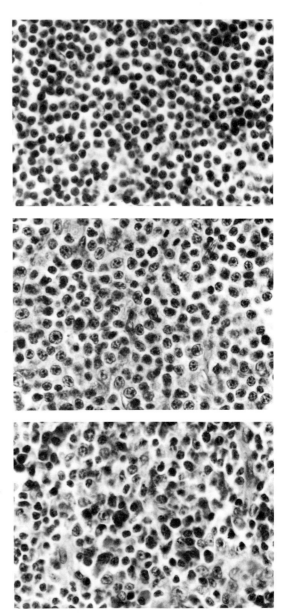

Fig. 18.20 Lymph nodes showing examples of diffuse lymphoma of low-grade malignancy. *Top,* lymphocytic type (from a case of chronic lymphocytic leukaemia). *Middle,* centrocytic type (also from a case of lymphoid 'leukaemia'). *Bottom,* lymphoplasmacytic type (Waldenström's macroglobulinaemia). × 520.

Non-Hodgkin's lymphomas of low-grade malignancy

(a) Lymphocytic lymphoma. The commonest form of this tumour is typical chronic lymphocytic leukaemia (CLL), originating in the bone marrow, usually after the age of 40, and progressing slowly (p. 17.49). There is often generalised lymphadenopathy with hepatosplenomegaly: in some instances this dominates the clinical picture and leukaemia does not develop. Histologically there is a diffuse monotonous infiltration of neoplastic small lymphocytes (Fig. 18.20, *upper*). In lymph nodes this results in loss of the normal architectural features, accompanied in B-cell types (i.e. in most cases) by nucleolated pro-lymphocytes and even blast cells lying singly or in groups ('proliferation centres'). Rarely blast cells come to dominate the neoplastic process and the disease becomes highly aggressive (*Richter syndrome*). Only a small proportion of tumours are of T-cell type. '*Hairy cell*' leukaemia (B cell), *pro-lymphocytic leukaemia* (B or T), *mycosis fungoides* (p. 27.37) and the *Sézary syndrome* (both T cell) are all considered to be variants of lymphocytic lymphoma.

(b) Lymphoplasmacytic lymphoma. These tumours show considerable variation in cell morphology and clinical expression. The neoplastic infiltrate, which is diffuse, differs from lymphocytic lymphoma in consisting not only of small lymphocytes but also of plasma cells and cells with intermediate features (plasmacytoid lymphocytes—Fig. 18.20, *lower*); immunoblasts and even germinal centre cells may, however, be found in some cases so that a wide spectrum of cells within the B lymphoid range is represented. The clinical features usually include diffuse lymph node enlargement with CLL, but the condition can present as a localised lymph node tumour and may also arise in an extranodal site such as the spleen or orbit. In all cases, monoclonal immunoglobulin can be demonstrated in those tumour cells showing plasmacytoid differentiation (Fig. 18.21), and a striking feature in some cases is the secretion of large amounts of immunoglobulin by the tumour cells: usually this is of the IgM class and is associated with the clinical syndrome of *Waldenström's macroglobulinaemia* (p. 17.61). In general, the tumours in this group progress slowly but occasionally they evolve into highly malignant lymphomas.

(c) Plasmacytic. Apart from multiple myeloma, which is a primary bone marrow neoplasm (p. 17.59), tumours consisting exclusively of plasma cells are uncommon. Such extra-

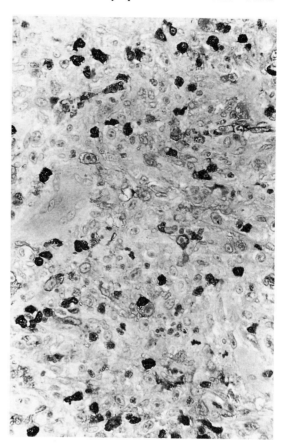

Fig. 18.21 Lymphoplasmacytic lymphoma. The section is stained for kappa light chains of Ig by the immunoperoxidase technique, and shows heavy staining of the cytoplasm of many of the tumour cells. × 300.

medullary tumours are most often found in relationship to the upper respiratory tract or oral cavity, and only rarely in lymph nodes or other sites. Unless they become disseminated (or are unusually large) a monoclonal immunoglobulin (p. 17.60) is not found in the serum. Microscopically, these tumours show the same features as multiple myeloma.

(d) Follicle-centre-cell tumours. The most important member of this group is widely known as **follicular lymphoma (FL),** which is one of the most common types of NHL: it is essentially a tumour of late adult life and rarely occurs before the age of 30. The neoplastic cells have the features of the B cells normally found in germinal centres. Follicular lymphoma usually arises in a lymph node, less often in some

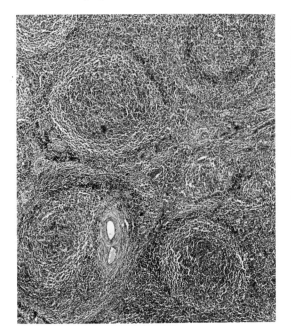

Fig. 18.22   Follicular lymphoma involving a lymph node. There are numerous follicles of roughly equal size. × 35.

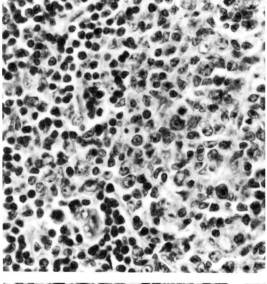

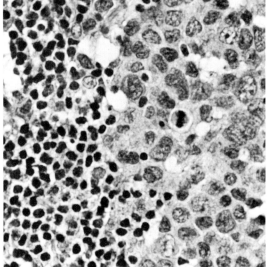

Fig. 18.23   *Above,* follicular lymphoma of predominantly small cleaved cell (centrocyte) type. *Below,* follicular lymphoma of large-cell (centroblast) type. Each photograph shows the edge of a follicular lesion, the lymphoma cells being on the right, and adjacent lymphoid tissue, containing small lymphocytes, on the left. × 520.

extranodal site such as skin or intestinal tract. While it may remain localised for some time, in most cases it is widely disseminated, with generalised lymphadenopathy and splenomegaly, when the patient is first seen. The bone marrow is often involved and tumour cells are found in the blood in about 10% of cases. Follicular lymphoma is perhaps the least malignant of the lymphomas but it has a tendency to change, sooner or later, into a highly malignant phase which is rapidly fatal and is often accompanied by a blood picture resembling acute lymphoblastic leukaemia (ALL) of B cell type (p. 17.48). It has been shown recently that in many cases of FL there is a translocation between chromosomes 18 and 14: the latter contains the genes coding for the synthesis of immunoglobulin heavy chains (Yunis *et al.,* 1982) .

Histologically, the characteristic feature of the tumour is the formation of follicular structures (Fig. 18.22) which mostly consist of an admixture of two types of lymphoid cell in variable proportion. The first of these, known as the **cleaved follicle centre cell** or **centrocyte,** is variable in size but relatively small and has an irregularly-shaped or indented nucleus and indistinct cytoplasm (Fig. 18.23, *upper*); while the

other cell, the **non-cleaved follicle centre cell** or **centroblast,** is generally larger and has a round nucleus with two or more distinct nucleoli, often peripherally placed (Fig. 18.23, *lower*). In an affected lymph node the neoplastic follicles resemble reactive germinal centres but usually have a more monotonous appearance due to a

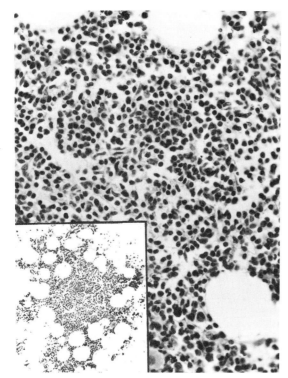

Fig. 18.24 Follicular lymphoma of small-cell type in a needle biopsy of the bone marrow. *Inset,* at low magnification, showing the follicular pattern.

predominance of small centrocytes, and lack the macrophages containing nuclear debris seen in reactive follicles. The neoplastic follicles also tend to have less well defined margins and to compress the interfollicular tissue, and the neoplastic infiltrate invariably extends beyond the sub-capsular sinus. In some cases, the follicular structure is lost and there is extensive and profuse proliferation of follicle centre cells: this may be accompanied by the formation of collagen bands, which is associated with a relatively good prognosis. Conversely, a predominance of centroblasts and prominent mitotic activity (Fig 18.23, *lower*) implies a more aggressive course and possibly indicates transformation into a highly malignant phase.

Neoplastic follicles can often be readily demonstrated in the bone marrow (Fig. 18.24). They usually consist of aggregates of centrocytes which may also appear in the peripheral blood.

Some follicle-centre-cell tumours are **diffuse** (i.e. non-follicular) from the outset (Fig. 18.20, *middle*); the neoplastic centrocytic cells may be

relatively large, and they tend to behave in a slightly more aggressive fashion than FL. They may, however, show the same admixture of centrocytes and centroblasts histologically—hence the old term '*mixed-cell lymphoma*'.

There are also tumours in this category which seem to consist exclusively of small cleaved cells **(centrocytic lymphoma).** This too tends to be more aggressive than FL and is often widely disseminated in the lymphoid system. Leukaemic changes are by no means unusual (20%). A particular variant of this tumour originates in the gut and produces the condition called **'lymphomatous polyposis'** (p. 19.61)

Non-Hodgkin's lymphomas of high-grade malignancy

(a) Lymphoblastic lymphoma. By definition, tumours in this group consist of lymphoid 'blast' cells with a high nuclear-cytoplasmic ratio and nuclei mostly smaller than those of normal macrophages. In fact, the nature of cells with this morphology is uncertain, but some at least appear to be lymphocyte precursors. Not surprisingly, it may not always be possible to determine the lymphocyte subpopulation to which they belong. It is also notable that tumours of these cells often arise in the primary lymphoid organs, i.e. bone marrow and thymus, and that many arise during childhood and adolescence. The pathological features of these highly malignant lymphoblastic tumours is variable. Some are leukaemic from the outset, the best example of this being the common type of ALL of childhood (cALL) which is a marrow-derived lymphoblastic neoplasia of 'non-B non-T' cell type (p. 17.48). Others become leukaemic after a variable phase of solid growth, often developing in the mediastinum and probably originating in the thymus. Tumours of this kind are generally of T-cell origin and predominantly affect males in late childhood or adolescence **(Sternberg tumour).** The blast cells may have a distinctive convoluted nuclear morphology. In a third form of lymphoblastic tumour, solid tissue growth is the dominant feature and leukaemia, if it develops at all, is a late event. Some tumours in this category are known to be of B cell origin and some of these may be of germinal centre derivation, Burkitt's tumour (see below) being the classic example. Many other solid lymphoblastic tumours arising both in childhood and in adult life are difficult to classify: these may arise in many different sites such as pharyngeal lymphoid tissue, the gut-associated lymphoid tissue, the skin and lymph nodes. Cytogenetic studies have shown that in tumours of this kind there may be translocation between chromosomes 8 and 14 (c.f. follicular lymphoma, p. 18.23) and less often between 8 and 2 or 22. The latter two chromosomes contain the genes coding for the light chains of immunoglobulin. Some of the B-immunoblast tumours (see below) may show similar translocations (Yunis *et al.*, 1982).

Burkitt's lymphoma. Between 1958 and 1962 an unusual variant of malignant lymphoma was described in children in sub-Saharan Africa. Over half these patients presented with jaw tumours, affecting one or more segments of the mandible or maxilla, but it was soon realised that other organs were often involved and that the initial manifestations were variable. Intra-abdominal masses due either to enlarged retroperitoneal lymph nodes or, in girls, to bilateral, often massive ovarian tumours, are commonly seen. Paraplegia may be a presenting feature and is caused by cord involvement by retroperitoneal tumour. The skin, bones, thyroid and testis are occasionally involved. Untreated cases run a rapid downhill course and die with widespread metastases to the liver, kidneys and other organs.

Burkitt's lymphoma is a tumour of B lymphoblasts. In impression preparations the tumour cells have a large rounded or indented nucleus and three or four nucleoli, and a thin layer of basophilic cytoplasm. In sections, macrophages with abundant pale, sometimes foamy cytoplasm and containing nuclear debris are seen scattered among the tumour cells and give the 'starry sky' appearance which is also observed in some other rapidly growing lymphomas.

Burkitt's lymphoma is endemic in many regions of sub-Saharan Africa but its occurrence is affected by altitude, temperature and rainfall. In Uganda it occurs everywhere in the country except in the mountainous southwest where it is extremely rare. The tumour is also endemic in Papua New Guinea where it occurs in the coastal regions. This geographical distribution corresponds very closely with the presence of endemic *P. falciparum* malaria. It is known that repeated attacks of malaria in early childhood give rise to depression of cellular immunity and this may play a role in the development of the tumour.

In 1964 Epstein and his colleagues isolated the virus now known as EB virus from a tissue culture of Burkitt's lymphoma tumour cells. Subsequently it was shown that all cases in Africa had antibodies to this virus and that the mean titres were higher than in controls. A study in the West Nile region of Uganda showed that EB infection precedes the development of the tumour and that in individuals who were later to develop Burkitt's lymphoma the antibodies to EB were often very high. Further evidence that EB virus is directly implicated in the development of the tumour is the finding of viral antigens in tumour cells and of EBV genomes in nuclear DNA. The epidemiological and laboratory findings suggest that the combination of recurrent malaria and EB infection very early in childhood may lead to the development of the tumour (see also p. 13.17).

(b) Large-cell lymphoma. Formerly included within the term *reticulum cell sarcoma*, it is now recognised that these highly malignant tumours constitute a heterogeneous group; most seem to arise from transformed lymphocytes but others are derived from large germinal-centre cells or possibly from cells of the mononuclear phagocyte system (see below). A feature of all these tumours is that the nuclei of the neoplastic cells are as large or larger than those of normal macrophages. Exact identification of the cell of origin is often difficult if not impossible, but the effort is worthwhile since the prognosis is better in some types than in others. The stage of the disease at the time of diagnosis is also critically important; only when it is localised is there any hope of controlling the disease, even for a short time. Probably the most common member of this group is the **tumour of B immunoblasts** which tends to arise in individuals whose immunity system is defective in some way, e.g. in congenital or acquired immunodeficiency disease, prolonged immunosuppression by drugs, or simply old age. It may arise either in lymph nodes or in an extranodal site and characteristically the tumour cells have vesicular nuclei with large central nucleoli and dense, sharply defined pyroninophilic cytoplasm (Fig. 18.25, *upper*). **Tumours consisting exclusively of centroblasts** (p. 18.24) may arise de novo or evolve from a pre-existing follicular lymphoma (p. 18.24). In the former case their behaviour is somewhat less aggressive than that of immunoblastic tumours, so it is worthwhile attempting to make the distinction. **Tumours of large centrocytes** (p. 18.25) also appear to be less malignant and are worth distinguishing from other tumours in the group. **Tumours of** T

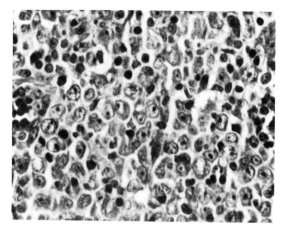

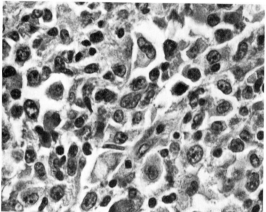

Fig. 18.25 Lymph nodes showing examples of highly malignant lymphomas. Both would formerly have been called 'reticulum-cell sarcoma'. Electron microscopy and immunohistology showed the lymphoma above to be of B immunoblastic type, and the lower to be a 'histiocytic lymphoma'. × 520.

immunoblasts have recently been identified and are highly aggressive: histologically, the tumour cells may be indistinguishable from those of B immunoblasts, but on occasion they show marked irregularity of nuclear shape and abundant clear cytoplasm.

(c) **Histiocytic lymphoma.** Some lymph node tumours within the so-called large cell group (Fig. 18.25, *lower*), are of histiocytic (macrophage) origin as revealed by their ultra-structural features, their possession of certain cytoplasmic enzymes (e.g. α_1 antitrypsin, muramidase) and their phagocytic activity. These tumours vary in behaviour but may be highly aggressive. The term **histiocytic medullary reticulosis** is applied to a rapidly advancing

form of histiocytic neoplasia which is usually widely disseminated within the lymphoreticular tissues by the time symptoms develop. The condition is characterised by hepatosplenomegaly, lymphadenopathy, and pancytopenia caused by phagocytosis of the formed elements of the blood by the neoplastic cells. Most cases have been encountered in East Africa and the Far East but the condition is world-wide. A variant of this condition, known as **malignant histiocytosis of the intestine,** is now recognised as the most common neoplastic complication of coeliac disease (p. 19.53). The disease usually referred to as **histiocytosis X** (p. 18.15) is of uncertain nature but is probably non-neoplastic.

Tumours of T lymphocytes

As mentioned earlier, a small number of tumours within the lymphocytic/lymphoblastic or immunoblastic categories are of T-cell derivation. As immunological marker techniques have become more widely applied, however, it has become apparent that T-cell tumours are much more common than has generally been realised and cannot readily be accommodated within existing classification systems. As noted below, some of these recently described T-cell tumours arise in lymph nodes but many are extra-nodal and tend in particular to involve the skin.

The term **T-zone lymphoma** has been applied to perhaps the most common nodal tumour arising in adults from peripheral (i.e. post-thymic) T lymphocytes. It is only moderately aggressive, and classifiable as low grade. Microscopically, the neoplastic infiltrate is pleomorphic with small lymphoid cells predominating, and there is pronounced proliferation of venules resembling those seen in normal T-zones: moreover, (like other T lymphomas) the infiltrate occupies nodal T zones leaving the B-cell areas isolated but initially intact, i.e. the reverse of follicular lymphoma (p. 18.24).

Lympho-epithelioid-cell lymphoma (Lennert's lymphoma) is another distinctive lymph-node neoplasm usually arising in old people. It is often associated with systemic symptoms e.g. fever and weight loss, and has a poor prognosis, mean survival being usually less than 2 years. Microscopically, affected nodes show loss of normal architecture due to an infiltrate of small lymphoid cells and immunoblasts accompanied by conspicuous foci of epithelioid histiocytes. Eosinophils may also be numerous. While some patients with this nodal picture eventually develop Hodgkin's disease, in other instances the condition evolves into an unequivocal T-cell neoplasm, sometimes of immunoblastic type.

The **multilobated T cell tumour** illustrates several of the features which typify this group of neoplasms. This remarkable tumour mainly affects older people and most often arises as a localised, sometimes large mass in the skin or other extra nodal sites (e.g. bone, gonads). Histologically the tumour cells are large and possess bizarre lobulated nuclei without prominent nucleoli. Despite this alarming appearance the tumour responds well to local therapy and many patients have survived for over 5 years.

As mentioned earlier, T cell tumours are unusually common in Japan, and perhaps the most notable of these is the **adult T-cell leukaemia/lymphoma syndrome.** This aggressive tumour mainly affects middle-aged adults and is characterised by generalised lymphadenopathy, hepatosplenomegaly, and often skin lesions and a terminal leukaemic blood picture. Hypercalcaemia has also been a feature in some cases. The tumour cells show pronounced irregularity of nuclear outline, and appear to belong to the helper cell sub-group of T cells. Within Japan the tumour is largely restricted to the South-Western islands of Kyushu and Shikoku, and there is firm evidence that its development is associated with an oncogenic retrovirus, human T-cell leukaemia virus, type I (HTLV—I) (p. 13.7) prevalent in this area. Clusters of this unusual tumour have also been found in the Carribean area and elsewhere.

Lymph node tumour metastases

It must be emphasised that lymphatic spread and formation of metastatic tumours in the lymph nodes is an extremely important feature of all forms of carcinoma (p. 12.23) with the exception of basal cell carcinoma of the skin. Usually the draining nodes are enlarged first, but eventually more distant nodal metastases commonly develop. Most types of sarcoma tend to spread especially by the bloodstream, but lymph node involvement is by no means rare, particularly in rhabdomyosarcoma and synovial sarcomas.

The Thymus

The development of the thymus and the advances in our understanding of its major role in the immune response are described in Chapter 6, while the immune deficiencies resulting from defective thymic development are considered on pp. 7.34–5. The changes in the thymus in myasthenia gravis, and their possible significance, are dealt with on p. 21.76. It remains to provide a brief account of thymic tumours.

Tumours of the thymus

Primary thymomas are of several types, all of which are rare.

Epithelial and lymphocytic tumours. Tumours containing both epithelial cells and lymphocytes are least uncommon. They usually consist of nodules, and may be predominantly epithelial, predominantly lymphocytic or may show widely differing ratios of the two cell types in different parts of the tumour and sometimes within single nodules. The epithelial cells may be plump and ovoid, spindle-shaped or rounded, or they may show acinar formation and resemble tumours of the endocrine glands, and two or more types of epithelium may be present in the same tumour. These tumours may be encapsulated and intersected by dense fibrous stroma, or may extend locally to involve the adjacent tissues, including the major blood vessels, pleura, lung and pericardium. Most tumours are symptomless, and are detected incidentally by x-ray, or cause pressure symptoms, but not uncommonly a thymoma is accompanied by **myasthenia gravis,** or less commonly by **systemic lupus erythematosus, hypogammaglobulinaemia** or **pure red-cell aplasia.** The significance of these associations is not known, but it is noteworthy that the last two may respond to removal of the tumour, while the response of myasthenia gravis is more variable (p. 21.76).

Very rarely, tumours of mixed epithelial-lymphocytic type, or purely epithelial tumours, are anaplastic and more highly malignant, and squamous-cell carcinoma has been observed.

Teratoma also occurs in the thymus, and may be wholly well-differentiated or have poorly-differentiated areas.

Seminoma of the thymus resembles closely the commoner testicular tumour, and is highly radio-sensitive.

Lymphoid neoplasms may originate in the thymus. The condition sometimes termed *granulomatous thy-*

moma is the nodular sclerosing form of Hodgkin's disease involving the thymus and often the mediastinal lymph nodes. *Sternberg's tumour* (p. 18.25) appears to originate, at least in some instances, in the thymus, which may be involved in various other forms of lymphoma.

References and Further Reading

Chilcote, R.R., Bachner, R.L. and Hammond, D. (1976). Septicaemia and meningitis in children splenectomised for Hodgkin's disease. *New England Journal of Medicine* **295,** 798–800.

Lennert, K. (1978). *Malignant lymphomas other than Hodgkin's disease*. pp. 833. Springer-Verlag.

Lennert, K. (1981) *Histopathology of non-Hodgkin's lymphomas*. (Based on the Kiel classification) Springer-Verlag, Berlin.

Lukes, R.J. (1971). Criteria for involvement of lymph nodes, bone marrow, spleen and liver in Hodgkin's disease. *Cancer Research*, **31,** 1753–69.

Lukes, R.J. and Collins, R.D. (1977). Lukes-Collins classification and its significance. *Cancer Treatment Reports*, **61,** 971–9.

Robb-Smith, A.H.T. and Taylor, C.R. (1951). *Lymph node biopsy. A diagnostic atlas*. pp. 308. Miller Heyden, London.

Sommers, S.C. and Rosen, P.P. (Eds.) (1973). *Malig-·nant lymphomas. A Pathology Annual Monograph*. pp. 333. Appleton-Century Crofts, Norwalk, Connecticut.

Stein, H., Gerdes, J., Schwab, U., Lemke, H., Mason, D.Y., Ziegler, A., Schienle, W. and Diehl, V. (1982). Identification of Hodgkin and Sternberg-Reed cells as a unique cell type derived from a newly-detected small-cell population. *International Journal of Cancer*, **30,** 445–59.

Stuart, A.E., Stansfeld, A.G. and Lauder, I. (Eds). (1981). *Lymphomas other than Hodgkin's disease*. pp. 69. Oxford University Press, Oxford, etc.

Wright, D.H. and Isaacson, P.G. (1983). *Biopsy pathology of the lymphoreticular system*. pp. 337. Chapman and Hall, London. (An excellent practical account of lymph node pathology with a good bibliography).

Yunis, J.J., Oken, M.M., Kaplan, M.E., Ensrud, K.M., Howe, R.R. and Theologides, A. (1982). Distinctive chromosomal abnormalities in histologic subtypes of non-Hodgkin's lymphoma. *New England Journal of Medicine*, **307,** 1231–6.

19

Alimentary Tract

I: The Oral Cavity, Salivary Glands and Oropharynx

The oral cavity

In general, the tissues of the mouth are subject to the same types of lesion found in other sites but these often show distinctive features peculiar to the mouth. In addition there are a number of specific lesions related to the teeth and their supporting structures.

The most frequent diseases in the mouth are dental caries and non-specific chronic inflammation of the soft tissues immediately related to the teeth. The principal aetiological agents in both of these diseases are the oral bacteria. The bacterial flora of the mouth is complex. Bacteria in the mouth are found in saliva, adherent to the epithelium and also in adherent deposits on tooth surfaces. These deposits are *dental plaque* consisting of bacteria in an organic matrix mainly of bacterial but also of salivary origin. Calcium salts may be deposited in dental plaque to form hard, adherent *dental calculus.*

The teeth

Teeth consist of three specialised calcified tissues (Fig. 19.1): the **dentine** which consists of a thick layer of calcified collagenous tissue surrounding the soft tissues of the pulp, the **enamel**, which forms the hard outer layer of the crown, and is non-cellular, consisting largely of calcium apatite crystals with a delicate organic matrix, and thirdly the **cementum**, which over-

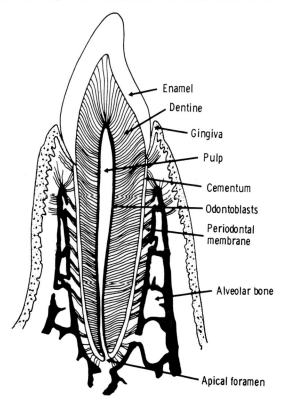

Fig. 19.1 Cross section of an anterior tooth and related tissues.

lies the dentine of the root(s). At the apex of each root is an apical foramen through which vessels and nerves enter the pulp.

19.1

Developmental abnormalities. Tooth development and eruption of the first dentition and then the second dentition begin at about 3 months of intrauterine life and continue until the early 20s. During this period many developmental abnormalities can occur in the number of teeth, in their form and colour, in the structure of individual tooth elements and the times of eruption and shedding of teeth. These abnormalities result from various factors, both genetic and environmental. An example of iatrogenic disease is the unsightly permanent staining of the calcified dental tissues caused by administration of some tetracyclines during tooth development.

Dental caries is the progressive destruction, by bacteria and their products, of the calcified tissues of the teeth exposed to the oral environment. Caries itself, and consequent inflammation of the tooth pulp, are the commonest causes of tooth loss up to middle age.

Dental caries usually starts in two principal areas of the tooth, the fissures on the occlusal or biting surfaces of posterior teeth and the areas between teeth (*interproximal caries*). Both of these are areas of relative stagnation (p. 8.3) in which plaque is likely to accumulate because of lack of friction from normal chewing and from contact with a mucosal surface. The bacteria within the plaque produce various organic acids. The amount of acid produced and the resulting pH depend on a number of factors, among which the thickness of the plaque and the concentration of dietary sugars appear to be particularly important. The initial attack upon enamel (Fig. 19.2) is by the acid, which produces decalcification. At first this is a painless process, but, as the lesion extends through the enamel, dentine is involved and the pain of toothache starts. Bacteria do not enter the enamel until decalcification has so weakened the structure that breakdown has occurred to form a cavity. At this stage the acid conditions within the cavity particularly favour the growth of *Lactobacilli*, which appear to be the main organisms involved in dentine caries. The organisms initially penetrate the dentinal tubules, but then cause softening and distortion of the dentine by a combination of decalcification and proteolytic breakdown of the collagen matrix (Fig. 19.3). The carious dentine becomes yellow by absorption of pigment from bacterial metabolic products and from the mouth; the

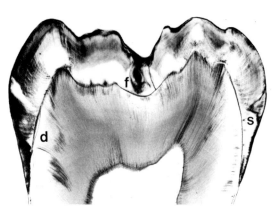

Fig. 19.2 Ground section of a molar tooth crown showing early smooth surface enamel caries (s), fissure caries (f) and early dentine caries deep to enamel caries (d). × 6.

process then extends through the dentine towards the dental pulp.

Dental caries may also start at the neck of

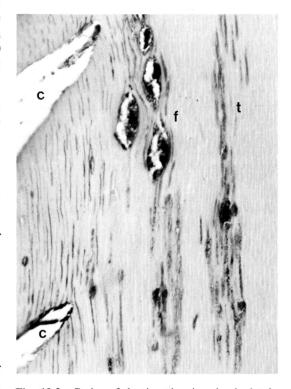

Fig. 19.3 Caries of dentine showing dentinal tubules with bacteria (t) which in places have accumulated in liquefaction foci (f) and in other areas spread along the incremental growth lines giving dentine clefts (c). × 110.

the tooth either by involving the cementum and then the dentine, or, if cementum is deficient, by directly attacking the dentine. This form of caries is more common in older patients in whom recession of the gingiva is common.

In the very early stages of enamel caries, the damage due to acid attack of enamel is reversible, but thereafter the process of caries of enamel and dentine is progressive except in unusual circumstances where the area becomes self-cleaning and the lesions may be arrested.

Lesions of the dental pulp. The dental pulp is a vascular connective tissue confined within the rigid pulp chamber and root canals in the dentine. The most frequent and clinically significant lesions of the pulp are inflammatory lesions (*pulpitis*) due to the extension of the carious process into dentine and eventually to the pulp. Physical injury, e.g. heat and chemical irritation from filling materials, may also give rise to inflammation in the pulp.

Pulpitis may be acute or chronic. The pathological processes of acute pulpitis are the same as in other acute inflammatory lesions. Because these changes are occurring within the rigid confines of the pulp chamber there is increase in pressure due to inflammatory exudate. Consequently acute pulpitis is very painful and may proceed quickly to necrosis of the pulp.

If the insult to the pulp is less severe, chronic pulpitis may result: it is characterised by infiltration of lymphocytes and plasma cells and there is loss of specialised cells such as odontoblasts. The pulp may eventually undergo necrosis, which is often symptomless. Clinically the non-vital tooth lacks lustre and may be discoloured by the leaching of products of the necrotic pulp into the dentine. In children, a large carious cavity penetrating quickly to the pulp may result in a large opening into the pulp chamber, leading to open pulpitis from which exudate can drain. A mass of granulation tissue forms in the pulp and may extend, as a *pulp polyp*, into the carious cavity.

Periodontal disease

Acute inflammation of the gingiva can arise from various physical, chemical and infective causes. *Acute ulceromembranous gingivitis (Vincent's infection)* is a distinctive condition in which there is necrosis of the interdental papillae with variable spread to other parts of the gingiva. It is characterised by a localised overgrowth of two commensal organisms, *Fusobacterium fusiforme* and *Borrelia vincenti* but the exact relationship of these to the disease is not clear. In particularly susceptible individuals such as grossly under-nourished children, infection may spread to the soft tissues of the cheek and lips and cause gross tissue destruction: this gangrenous lesion is known as **cancrum oris** or **noma**.

Chronic inflammation is very common in the periodontal tissues and is the most frequent cause of tooth loss in older individuals. A number of local and systemic factors are involved, but of these the most important is the *bacterial plaque around the neck of the tooth*.

For clinical convenience the lesions are divided into **chronic gingivitis** where the disease is confined to the gingiva and **chronic periodontitis** where the process involves the deeper tissues, causing retraction towards the root apex of the part of the gingiva attached to the tooth. As in most examples of chronic inflammation, there is both tissue destruction and proliferation of new tissue in attempted repair, but there is a net tissue loss. Many mechanisms of tissue destruction have been described involving polymorphonuclear leucocytes, macrophages and both humoral and cell mediated immune mechanisms. It is probable that all of these are operative in different situations. The later stages of the disease involve the alveolar bone supporting the teeth. Osteoclastic resorption occurs and progresses to the formation of areas of deepening of the gingival sulcus, termed *periodontal pockets*: these contain a mixture of necrotic tissue and anaerobic bacterial plaque. Infrequently there is an acute exacerbation of infection in such pockets and a *periodontal abscess* can arise.

Periapical lesions. A variety of lesions can occur in the tissues related to the root apices of teeth. The most frequent of these arise from spread of infection from pulpitis, through the apical foramina of the tooth, to reach the periodontal membrane. This can result in an acute **periapical abscess**, a very painful condition which may be accompanied by cervical lymphadenopathy and generalised fever and malaise. Pus tracks through the adjacent bone and, after the periosteum is breached, a soft tissue abscess—a **gumboil**—develops and later discharges.

More frequently periapical infection follows a low grade pulpitis and a **periapical granuloma** develops. This consists of a mass of granulation tissue heavily infiltrated with chronic inflammatory cells. There is resorption of surrounding bone, seen radiographically as a periapical radiolucency (Fig. 19.4). Acute exacerbation of a periapical granuloma may result in an acute periapical abscess and conversely a periapical granuloma can develop after an acute periapical abscess has pointed and drained.

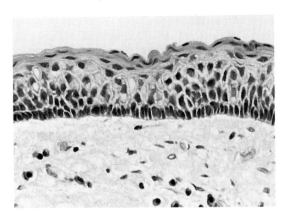

Fig. 19.5 Lining of an odontogenic keratocyst showing a thin regular parakeratinised epithelium with a distinctive columnar basal cell layer. × 140.

Epithelial-lined cysts of the jaws

A number of different types occur; they can be classified into *odontogenic cysts*, in which the epithelium is derived from the dental epithelial tissues, and *fissural cysts* which arise in areas of fusion of embryonic processes.

Odontogenic cysts may be further subdivided into *inflammatory* and *developmental cysts* and categorised by their position in relation to the teeth. The commonest is the *dental cyst* (synonyms, *radicular* or *periapical cyst*) which is an inflammatory cyst developing from a periapical granuloma. Epithelial remnants related to the root are stimulated to grow and cyst formation occurs. If the affected tooth is extracted, the cyst may be left in the bone and remain as a *residual cyst*. The most frequent of the developmental odontogenic cysts is the *dentigerous cyst* which arises in the reduced enamel epithelium around the crown of a tooth which has failed to erupt. Closely related is the *eruption cyst* which presents as a bluish fluctuant swelling overlying the crown of an erupting tooth.

The odontogenic cysts described above are lined by non-keratinised stratified squamous epithelium which may include a few mucus-secreting cells. These cysts are usually symptomless unless infected and can grow to several centimetres with considerable bone destruction. They must be differentiated from the *odontogenic keratocyst* (synonym—*primordial cyst*) which has a distinctive keratinised stratified squamous epithelial lining (Fig. 19.5). Its relationship to the teeth is variable but frequently it is not directly related to any one tooth. It occurs anywhere in the jaws, the most common site being in the mandibular molar area, often extending up into the vertical ramus of the mandible. The importance of this cyst lies in the frequency with which it recurs after attempted surgical removal, because of the friable nature of the lining and the presence of related small daughter cysts.

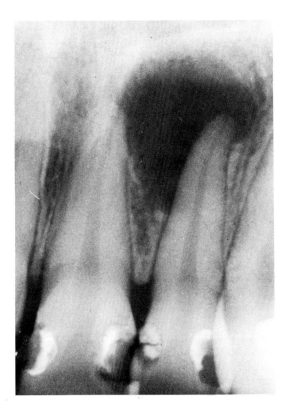

Fig. 19.4 Radiograph of upper anterior teeth with large restorations. The upper lateral incisor is non-vital and a radiolucency is present in the bone around the apex of the tooth.

Fissural cysts. The *nasopalatine cyst* arises in the nasopalatine canal in the midline of the anterior part of the hard palate. It may be entirely within the bone or present as a palatal swelling. A similar type, the *nasolabial cyst*, occurs in the upper lip below the ala of the nose, but this is within the soft tissues. The fissural cysts are usually lined by epithelium with numerous mucus secreting cells, but areas of non-keratinised stratified squamous epithelium may also be present.

Oral mucosa

The oral epithelium is conventionally divided into three structural varieties. (*a*) The loose, mobile mucosa of the cheeks, lips, floor of mouth, ventral surface of tongue and soft palate is known as *lining mucosa* and is non-keratinised: (*b*) The mucosa of the hard palate and gingivae, and the alveolar mucosa which covers the edentulous ridges after tooth loss, is *masticatory mucosa* and is keratinised: (*c*) The specialised lining of the dorsum of the tongue is keratinised *gustatory epithelium*. Although the oral epithelia are grouped into these three types, there is wide variation in histological appearances even within individual types. The supporting connective tissues also show wide variation between the loose corium of lining mucosa and the dense mucoperiosteum of the hard palate.

The oral mucosa is subjected to numerous physical insults and is exposed to vast numbers of micro-organisms, and to food and other material introduced into the mouth. Oral epithelium has a high rate of cell turnover. In almost all lesions of oral mucosa, physical trauma and infection will play a role, and this may be superimposed upon a previously normal or an abnormal mucosa. It is not surprising that these circumstances produce complex changes in disease which are not yet fully documented or understood.

Developmental abnormalities of oral epithelium. Apart from Fordyce's disease—the presence of pale yellowish sebaceous glands in the lining mucosa, especially of the cheeks—developmental abnormalities of oral mucosa are rare.

Infections. Oral mucosa is frequently subject to infection, both as a primary event or superimposed upon some preceding disease.

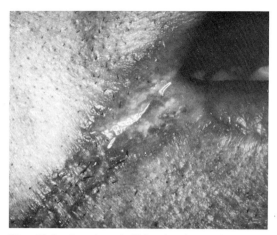

Fig. 19.6 Angular cheilitis showing typical moist skin fissuring.

Fungal infection is usually due to *Candida sp.* which are part of the oral flora of over half the population. *Candida albicans* is the most frequent of these and the lesions have been categorised into several types. *Thrush* is an acute condition found most often in young children or debilitated adults and is characterised by detachable white fungal plaques on the epithelium. *Chronic atrophic candidiasis* is found under upper dentures. The mucosa is a fiery red due to an inflammatory reaction to fungi which are mainly in the interstices of the fitting surface of the denture. Alternatively candidal hyphae may be found in adherent hyperkeratotic lesions as *chronic hyperplastic candidiasis (candidal leucoplakia)*. Persistent oral candidal infections are a frequent problem in patients with AIDS.

Angular cheilitis (Fig. 19.6) is a painful cracking at the angles of the mouth often of multifactorial aetiology. With the loss of natural teeth and muscle tone, folds occur which may be moistened by saliva. Infection with *Candida albicans* and *Staphylococcus aureus* is frequent. Underlying nutritional deficiencies, notably of the B group of vitamins and of iron, can predispose to the condition.

Virus infections. The most frequent viral infection of oral epithelium is caused by *herpes simplex* virus. This occurs in the primary form as *acute herpetic gingivo-stomatitis* characterised by extensive painful ulceration and occasionally generalised upset. *Secondary or recurrent herpetic lesions* are more frequent, especially at mucocutaneous junctions round the lips and nose, where the initially vesicular

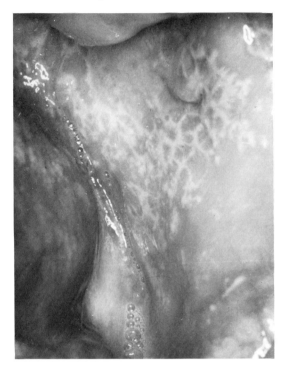

Fig. 19.7 Lichen planus of the cheek mucosa showing a reticular pattern of keratinised striae.

phase is followed by ulceration and crusting. Measles virus also produces vesicular lesions of the mucosa which then ulcerate: these are known as Koplik's spots.

Dermatoses. A number of diseases can involve the skin and mucosae. The skin manifestations of these diseases are discussed in Chapter 27. The oral mucosal features are similar, but frequently not so clearcut, making diagnosis more difficult. Lichen planus (Fig. 19.7) is the most frequent of the dermatoses which affect the mouth. Other examples include pemphigus, benign mucous membrane pemphigoid, erythema multiforme and lupus erythematosus.

Recurrent oral ulceration (Aphthous ulceration). Recurrent ulcers, either singly or in crops, are a common and troublesome problem. In many cases these are of unknown aetiology, but in some patients they are associated with vitamin B group deficiencies, iron deficiency, or various food allergies.

Leucoplakia. Leucoplakia is a clinical descriptive term commonly used to describe a white patch or patches on the oral mucosa which cannot be attributed to a specific disease, such as lichen planus or lupus erythematosus. It is not a pathological entity.

The term covers a variety of histological changes. It is, however, commonly due to keratinisation of a normally unkeratinised site or hyperkeratosis of a site where keratin is normally present. In many cases the aetiology is quite unknown, although chronic irritation from smoking, particularly pipe smoking, is a contributory cause in some. Histologically the viable cell layers of the epithelium may show acanthosis or atrophy and a variable inflammatory infiltrate is present. In most cases there is no epithelial dysplasia, but a small proportion do show dysplasia and can proceed to squamous-cell carcinoma. It is now generally agreed that this is unusual: for example, in a large series of patients followed up carefully, malignancy developed in 4% during a 20-year period. In certain sites, however, leucoplakia has been shown to be more prone to become malignant, particularly in elderly people. These are the floor of the mouth and the ventral surface and lateral margins of the tongue. Leucoplakia arising on an atrophic epithelium or showing as areas of white upon an erythematous background (*speckled leucoplakias*) is also more likely to proceed to carcinoma. Speckled leucoplakias often appear to be associated with superficial infestation by *Candida albicans*.

Pigmentation. Melanin pigmentation, especially of the gingiva, is frequent in coloured races but is infrequent in whites. Melanin pigmentation of the lips and buccal mucosae occurs in Addison's disease. Perioral melanin pigmentation is a feature of the rare Peutz-Jeghers syndrome (p. 19.61).

Ingestion of various heavy metals can give rise to dark blue or black pigmented lines around the gum margins, where the pigment is deposited in soft tissues as sulphides following reaction with bacterial products from the dental plaque.

Soft tissue swellings

Fibrous overgrowths of the oral mucosa are a common response to chronic irritation. These may occur on labial or buccal mucosa when they are best designated simply as *fibrous overgrowths*, although the older term *fibroepithelial*

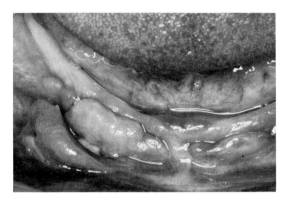

Fig. 19.8 Denture-induced hyperplasia of the lower labial sulcus with folds of fibrous overgrowth provoked by the margin of an old ill-fitting denture.

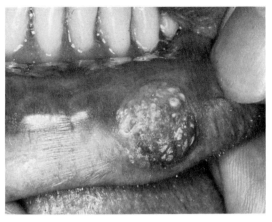

Fig. 19.9 Small exophytic squamous-cell carcinoma of the lower lip.

polyps may still be used. A frequent site is in relation to the margins of old and ill-fitting dentures where the term denture-induced hyperplasia is used (Fig. 19.8).

An **epulis** is a localised swelling on the gingiva. The common type is a reaction to chronic irritation, e.g. from dental calculus or the rough margin of a carious cavity or filling; it consists of a mass of highly cellular fibrous tissue frequently with metaplastic bone formation. Less commonly, such lesions consist of highly vascular granulation tissue and are then described as **pyogenic granulomas**: this may occur during pregnancy—*pregnancy epulis.*

Giant cell epulis is a distinctive lesion consisting of numerous multinucleated giant cells in a vascular stroma. The giant cell epulis is a superficial lesion with minimal bone involvement, but intra-osseous lesions, such as *central giant cell granuloma* or *osteitis fibrosa cystica* may mimic a giant cell epulis if they extend to involve the gingival soft tissues.

Haemangiomas and less frequently **lymphangiomas** can arise in the oral mucosa and submucosa.

Tumours of the oral mucosa

Tumours arise from any of the tissues of the oral mucosa, but the most frequent neoplasms are epithelial. **Squamous cell papilloma** may occur at any site on the oral mucosa. The most frequent malignant tumour is **squamous-cell carcinoma**, which accounts for more than 90%

of oral malignancies. Despite the fact that early recognition should be possible, many oral cancers have a bad prognosis because the tumours are not recognised and treated when small. Although squamous-cell carcinoma can occur at any oral site, more than half the lesions involve either the lower lip (Fig. 19.9) or the lateral border of the tongue (Fig. 19.10). Carcinoma of the lower lip is much more frequent in males and exposure to sunlight appears to be an important causal factor. The lesion is most often seen as an ulcer which fails to heal. Histologically it is usually a well-differentiated squamous carcinoma which shows slow local spread and involves lymph nodes relatively late.

Intra-oral carcinomas as a generalisation have a poorer prognosis the further posteriorly in the mouth they arise. Although some appear

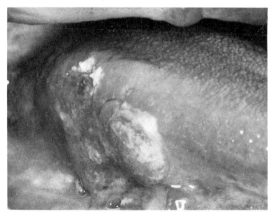

Fig. 19.10 Squamous cell carcinoma of the lateral margin of the tongue and lingual sulcus.

to develop from recognised premalignant lesions, over three-quarters of carcinomas develop in clinically normal mucosa. The earliest lesions are red rather than white and are symptomless. As successful treatment is dependent upon early diagnosis, it is important that lesions of the oral mucosa which do not relate to obvious causes, or which fail to respond to the removal of obvious causes, be examined microscopically.

Other tumours occur rarely in the mouth. They include malignant lymphomas of the tonsils and palate, tumours of the minor salivary glands and the usually-benign granular cell myoblastoma.

Odontogenic tumours. The lesions designated odontogenic tumours are a group of several rare lesions, of widely differing pathology, derived from the dental soft and hard tissues. Some of these lesions are neoplasms but several are hamartomas. The most important of the odontogenic neoplasms is the *ameloblastoma* which is an epithelial neoplasm of distinctive appearance (Fig. 19.11). Ameloblastomas are most frequent in the molar region of the mandible and are locally aggressive, often producing extensive bone destruction. When the tumour mass contains enamel and dentine the term *odontoma* is used. A complex odontoma consists of a disorganised mass of dental tissues, whereas a compound odontoma consists of numerous small teeth.

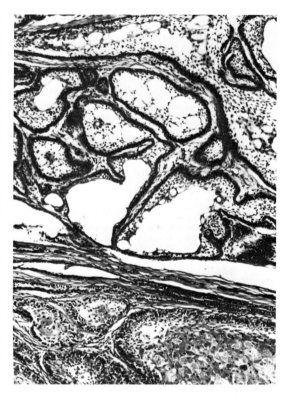

Fig. 19.11 Ameloblastoma, showing the proliferated epithelium in spaces enclosed in a well-defined stroma. In places, the epithelium forms a loose network. The appearances resemble the enamel organ. The lower part of the field shows a histological variant of an ameloblastoma in which granular cells are present.

The salivary glands

These include the three pairs of major glands—parotid, submandibular and sublingual—and numerous intra-oral minor salivary glands.

The commonest acute inflammatory lesion of the salivary glands is **mumps**. This viral infection has an incubation period of 3 weeks and infected individuals secrete the virus in their saliva for about a week before the main symptom of painful salivary gland swelling is evident and for just over a week thereafter. Both parotid glands are usually involved and sometimes also the submandibular. The salivary enlargement usually subsides without permanent damage to the glands. Mumps may be accompanied by orchitis or pancreatitis, both of which are more prone to result in some degree of atrophy. Mumps virus is also a relatively frequent cause of aseptic meningitis (pp. 21.30–31).

Suppurative parotitis is due to infection by pyogenic cocci and occurs as a postoperative complication in dehydrated patients. It may also occur in elderly debilitated patients, sometimes as a sequel to septicaemia.

Chronic sialadenitis can occur in either the parotid or submandibular glands. In the latter it is often associated with salivary calculi. Duct obstruction leads to atrophy with marked acinar loss and interstitial fibrosis (Fig. 19.12).

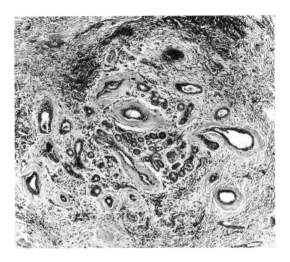

Fig. 19.12 Atrophy and fibrosis of submandibular gland with chronic inflammatory infiltration, resulting from duct obstruction. × 55.

The most frequent lesion of minor salivary glands is a mucocele. This is seen, especially in the lower lip and presents as a bluish, slowly enlarging swelling due to leakage of mucus from a damaged duct. Histologically there is pooling of mucus in soft tissues, surrounded by granulation tissue. A larger variant of this lesion occurs in the floor of the mouth involving sublingual glands and is known as a *ranula*.

Auto-immune sialadenitis. Chronic inflammation of the salivary and/or lacrimal glands, often accompanied by the presence in the serum of auto-antibodies to the duct epithelium of those glands, occurs in middle and old age, particularly in women. Usually the inflammation is focal, centred around the ducts, and symptomless; rarely it is associated with enlargement of one or more of the glands and is sufficiently extensive to cause deficiency of salivary and/or lacrimal secretion (the sicca syndrome), with consequent severe dental caries and/or chronic conjunctivitis. Histologically there is destruction of the intraglandular ducts, often with hyperplasia of the duct epithelium to form masses containing pale-staining hyaline material and dense infiltration with lymphocytes and plasma cells (Fig. 19.13). The glandular tissue shows various degrees of atrophy, perhaps due to duct obstruction. Although it has the features of an organ-specific auto-immune disease, the condition is not usually associated with other members of this group (p 7.24), but rather with the connective tissue diseases, particularly rheumatoid arthritis, a combination known as *Sjøgren's syndrome*.

Uveo-parotid fever. This is one of the important lesions of sarcoidosis (p. 9.26) in which iridocyclitis and parotid swelling occur, sometimes involving the facial nerve and causing paralysis. The glands may be considerably enlarged due to the presence of chronic inflammatory infiltrates in which sarcoid follicles are found.

Salivary gland tumours

These tumours are not very common, but notably variable in histology and often difficult to treat. Approximately 80% occur in the parotid and 10% each in the submandibular and minor salivary glands. Very few occur in the sublingual glands. About 20% of salivary gland

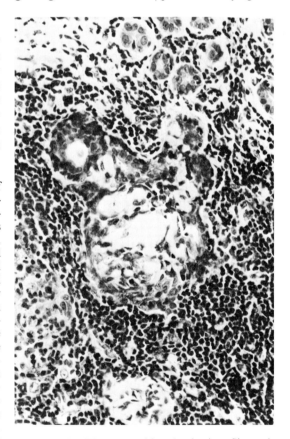

Fig. 19.13 The parotid gland in Sjøgren's syndrome, showing heavy infiltration with lymphocytes, loss of glandular tissue and proliferation of duct epithelium to form a cellular mass containing foci of pale-staining hyaline material. × 320.

tumours are malignant, the proportion being higher in tumours of the minor glands. Theories to explain the histological diversity are numerous, and none satisfactory. Similar tumours occur in the lacrimal, nasal and sweat glands.

Pleomorphic salivary adenoma (PSA). Over two-thirds are of this type. They form firm slow-growing nodules, apparently well defined (Fig. 19.14). Most characteristically they consist of an epithelial element made up of small ducts and cysts surrounded by more or less solid masses of cells which probably correspond to myoepithelium of the normal gland, and which stream off into the stroma (Fig. 19.15). This stroma is usually infiltrated with connective-tissue mucin ('myxoid') and in about one case in seven shows metaplasia to cartilage: it was this combination of epithelial tissue with cartilage that gave rise to the old name of *'mixed parotid tumour'*. These tumours are benign and do not metastasise, but they often recur (sometimes after decades). This is largely due to the fact that small outgrowths of the tumour often protrude through the capsule and are left behind if close excision is done, while wide excision is made difficult by the facial nerve and

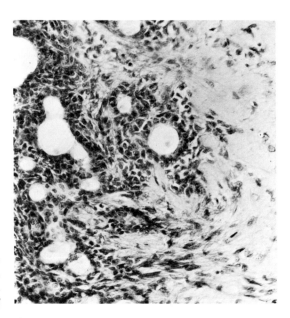

Fig. 19.15 Pleomorphic salivary adenoma, showing gland-like epithelial structures, from which cells appear to be streaming off into the connective tissue stroma. × 200.

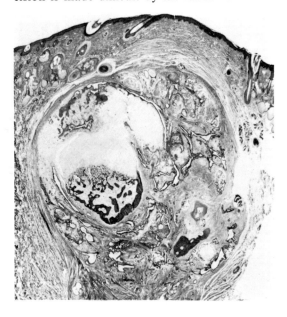

Fig. 19.14 A small pleomorphic salivary adenoma of the lower lip. The tumour is roughly rounded and sharply defined. The pale part of the mushroom-shaped area within it is cartilage, which shows formation of bone trabeculae, seen as dark areas. × 7.

other important structures. Occasionally a frank carcinoma arises in a pre-existing PSA.

Adenolymphoma (Fig. 19.16), the second commonest tumour, is basically a papillary cystadenoma, with a characteristic two-layered epithelium of tall pink-staining (mitochondrion-rich) cells, and with abundant lymphoid tissue filling the stroma. In distinction from all other tumours of these glands, they occur chiefly in older men, are almost entirely limited to the parotids, may be multiple and bilateral, and are *always benign*. Adenolymphoma is sometimes classified with the **monomorphic tumours** of the salivary glands. As the name suggests, these lack the variety of structure of the pleomorphic **adenomas**, although several different patterns exist.

Acinic-cell tumours are usually well circumscribed but tend to invade locally.

Muco-epidermoid tumours may be either benign or malignant. The degree of differentiation is some guide, but even well-differentiated examples may metastasise.

Adenoid cystic carcinoma is the commonest malignant tumour, and, though slow-growing and slower to metastasise, is often widely infiltrative and difficult to eradicate. It consists of masses of small dark-staining cells which show a characteristic sieve-like or 'cribriform' pattern (Fig. 19.17) and has a particularly striking tendency to infiltrate along nerves.

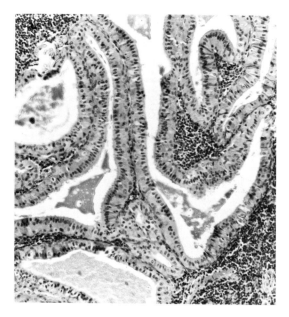

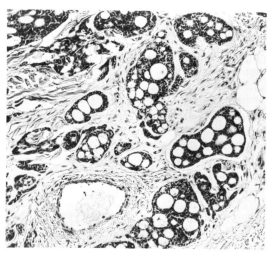

Fig. 19.17 Adenoid cystic carcinoma showing the characteristic architecture. × 90.

Fig. 19.16 Adenolymphoma of the parotid gland, showing the papillary architecture, with lymphoid stroma. × 130.

Besides the varieties already mentioned, occasional ordinary **adenocarcinomas** and even **squamous-cell carcinomas** occur, and **malignant lymphomas** (sometimes apparently arising in Sjøgren's lesions of long standing) are also not very rare.

Oropharynx

Tonsillitis. Acute tonsillitis is a common cause of sore throat. Haemolytic streptococci are the commonest infecting agents and give rise to acute inflammatory swelling with purulent exudate in the tonsillar crypts—*follicular tonsillitis*. The infection occasionally extends more deeply and involves the whole tonsil and adjacent tissues with frank suppuration; this is known as *quinsy*. From such a lesion streptococcal cellulitis may spread widely into the neck—*Ludwig's angina*—or even into the mediastinum or may give rise to a retropharyngeal abscess.

Acute streptococcal tonsillitis occurring alone or in scarlet fever is the usual antecedent infection in rheumatic fever and post-streptococcal glomerulonephritis. Chronic enlargement of the tonsils and adjacent lymphoid tissue commonly results from colonisation by one or other of the many adenoviruses.

Vincent's angina is a painful necrotic ulcerating lesion on the fauces characterised by a patch of yellowish-white false membrane surrounded by an area of acute inflammation, and may be difficult to distinguish from diphtheria (see below). In common with acute ulceromembranous gingivitis (p. 19.3) it is thought to be due to the symbiotic action of fusiform bacilli and the spirochaete *Borrelia vincenti*.

Blood dyscrasias. Swelling, haemorrhage and ulceration of the gingivae occur in the acute leukaemias, particularly in the monocytic form, and necrotic ulceration occurs on the fauces, pharynx and larynx in various conditions characterised by extreme reduction in the number of circulating polymorphonuclear leucocytes, i.e. in *agranulocytosis* (p. 17.13).

Dipththeria is an acute inflammation which affects most frequently the fauces, soft palate and tonsils, but may also attack the nose, or the larynx and trachea; it occurs chiefly in young children, but may also affect adults. The causal organism, *Corynebacterium diphtheriae*, exists in three main forms, *mitis*, *intermedius* and *gravis*, and infections with the last type tend to be more severely toxic and also to show greater local inflammatory reaction. The organisms remain strictly localised at the site of infection and the systemic effects are due to the formation and absorption of a powerful exotoxin which may cause myocardial damage and toxic fatty change in the organs; the mechanism of cellular injury is outlined on p. 3.10. The local lesions are characterised by the formation on the affected surfaces of a false membrane composed of fibrin and leucocytes. In the fauces, palate and tonsils the stratified squamous epithelium becomes permeated by exudate which forms a fibrinous coagulum in which the epithelium is incorporated; it then undergoes extensive necrosis under the influence of the diphtheria toxin. The whole false membrane is dull greyish-yellow and it can be detached only with difficulty owing to the attachment of the dead epithelium to the underlying tissues. When it is removed a bleeding connective tissue surface is laid bare. In *gravis* infections, membrane formation may be less obvious but inflammatory congestion and swelling are more marked and the cervical lymph nodes may be much swollen.

Diphtheria of the nasopharynx and of the larynx is described on p. 16.5.

Immunisation programmes are largely responsible for the present low incidence of diphtheria in many parts of the world.

Tumours of the oropharynx

Benign tumours. The least uncommon is *squamous papilloma*, which occasionally recurs after removal but rarely progresses to malignancy. *Lymphangiomas* occur, usually in the tonsillar regon.

Malignant tumours. Squamous-cell carcinoma and lymphomas occur in approximately equal numbers and together account for about one-third of extracranial malignant tumours of the head and neck (excluding skin tumours). Squamous-cell carcinoma develops most often in the tonsillar region in elderly men and is usually of well-differentiated type, although some are anaplastic. It usually ulcerates and becomes infected and death often results from aspiration bronchopneumonia. *Lymphomas* are of various types and arise in the lymphoid tissue of Waldeyer's ring.

Tumours of the nasopharynx are described on pp. 16.4–5.

II: Oesophagus

The oesophagus is a muscular tube, lined by squamous epithelium and adapted to bear without injury the rapid passing of food over its surface. It has marked powers of resistance and is a rare site of primary bacterial invasion, but damage to the mucosa of the lower end from regurgitated gastric juice is fairly common. Oesophageal obstruction can arise from various lesions, the most important being carcinoma of the oesophagus and invasion by bronchial carcinoma.

Circulatory disturbances

Oesophageal varices. The submucosal veins in the lower oesophagus and cardia of the stomach communicate with both the portal and systemic venous systems. In cases of portal hypertension, most frequently due to *hepatic cirrhosis*, these veins become distinctly varicose (Fig. 19.18): they may rupture, causing severe and often fatal haemorrhage.

Other causes of oesophageal haemorrhage. *Peptic reflux oesophagitis* (p. 19.13), particularly with ulceration, is a cause of bleeding of the lower oesophagus, and haemorrhage can also occur from *laceration of the mucosa at the cardia* during vomiting (p. 19.14). Rarely severe haemorrhage occurs as a result of impaction of a sharp *foreign body*, e.g. a fish bone, in the oesophagus: suppuration and ulceration develop and may involve the aorta or other large vessel: an *ulcerated oesophageal carcinoma* may similarly cause haemorrhage. Rarely an *aortic aneurysm* ruptures into the oesophagus.

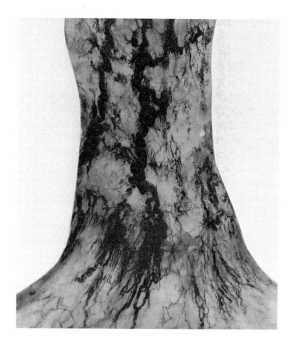

Fig. 19.18 Oesophagus and cardiac end of stomach, showing large dilated varicose veins from a case of cirrhosis of the liver.

Inflammatory conditions

As already mentioned, primary infections of the oesophagus are rare. Occasionally the lesion of diphtheria extends into, or arises primarily in, the oesophagus. In the rare but distinctive form of disseminated herpes simplex infection encountered in early infancy, the virus sometimes gains entry through the oesophagus. The characteristic lesion associated with South American trypanosomiasis (Chagas' disease) is described below.

'**Opportunistic infections**' (p. 8.1) may, however, occur in the oesophagus in states of debility or reduced immunity, and are often caused by organisms normally of low virulence. **Thrush**, caused by the yeast-like fungus *Candida albicans*, is the most common infection of this type and is characterised by the formation of irregularly raised opaque whitish patches consisting of swollen and sodden epithelium infiltrated by the septate mycelial threads and spores of the fungus (Fig. 19.19). The infection may have spread from the mouth or throat and can extend more distally in the gastrointestinal tract or even invade the bloodstream to produce generalised lesions. In adults, herpes sim-

plex oesophagitis may complicate diabetes mellitus or states of immunosuppression.

Oesophagitis can arise from non-infective causes. The most common example of this is *peptic oesophagitis* caused by regurgitation of gastric juice from the stomach (see below). The accidental or intentional swallowing of corrosive or irritating fluids can cause severe, even fatal, injury to the oesophagus. Concentrated strong acids or alkalis, for example, produce extensive necrosis and sloughing of the oesophageal wall. More dilute solutions lead to superficial destruction followed by inflammatory changes. If the patient survives, scarring may result in fibrous stricture.

Peptic or reflux oesophagitis. This important clinical disturbance is caused by a defect in the mechanism which normally prevents reflux of gastric juice into the lower oesophagus. This mechanism is not completely understood but appears to depend on the strength and competence of the intrinsic sphincter at the lower end of the oesophagus. Sphincter tone is controlled partly by gastrin. The attachment of the cardio-oesophageal junction to the diaphragmatic hiatus and the maintenance of the cardio-oesophageal angle (probably by a muscular sling extending over the body of the stomach) may also have a supportive role. The anti-reflux mechanism tends to become defective if there is an increase in intra-abdominal pressure, due for example to obesity or

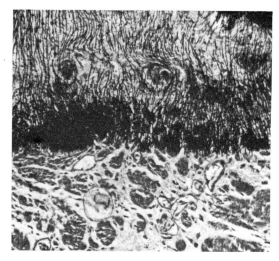

Fig. 19.19 Thrush of oesophagus, showing mycelial threads penetrating the wall. × 115.

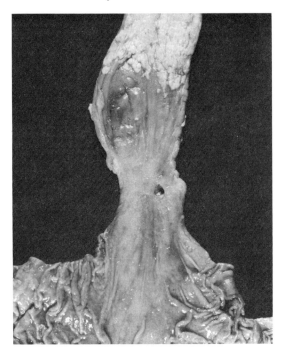

Fig. 19.20 Sliding hiatus hernia with chronic peptic ulceration in Barrett's syndrome.

pregnancy, and particularly if this is associated with acid hypersecretion in the stomach and low levels of serum gastrin. These factors tend to be associated also with the development of the **sliding type of hiatus hernia**, i.e. the herniation of the upper part of the stomach with its peritoneal covering through the diaphragmatic hiatus (Fig. 19.20), but the clinical importance of this condition is doubtful.

Reflux of gastric juice damages the squamous epithelium of the lower oesophagus. Initially there is elongation of the connective tissue papillae and infiltration of polymorphs: later, superficial ulceration develops which, if it persists, leads to marked fibrosis in the deeper layers of the oesophageal wall. Only in cases of severe continuous reflux does peptic ulceration of the squamous epithelium of the lower oesophagus penetrate as deeply as it does in the stomach (p. 19.23). The main clinical consequences of these pathological phenomena are oesophageal pain, usually readily recognisable as 'heartburn', but sometimes resembling angina pectoris (p. 15.8), haemorrhage sometimes leading to iron-deficiency anaemia, and stricture of the lower oesophagus.

Peptic oesophagitis is usually made worse by lying flat, and symptoms of it are very common in hospital patients.

Diagnosis of peptic oesophagitis at autopsy is not easy, for considerable digestion of the lower oesophagus can occur after death, the wall being discoloured, soft and shreddy, and often perforated. Accordingly, the diagnosis of peptic oesophagitis at autopsy requires histological confirmation of an inflammatory reaction.

Barrett's syndrome. The stricture formation associated with recurrent reflux oesophagitis tends to extend up the oesophagus as time passes, and the squamous epithelium distal to the stricture may undergo metaplastic change, being replaced by epithelium of intestinal or gastric type. It is now recognised that this is a pre-malignant condition, since it may be succeeded by dysplasia which may progress to adenocarcinoma.

Rupture of the oesophagus

This unusual condition occurs in previously healthy men, usually when a heavy meal has been followed by violent vomiting. The lesion takes the form of a longitudinal slit (Fig. 19.21), most often in the left posterior position, just above the diaphragm. The acid gastric contents are discharged into the pleural cavity directly or after first distending the posterior mediastinum. The appearance of the lesion indicates that it is brought about by sudden overdistension of the lower oesophagus in the act of vomiting, but digestion by the strongly acid gastric juice may also be a factor. Peptic ulceration of stomach or duodenum is often present.

Severe vomiting, usually associated with heavy alcohol intake, may also lead to brisk haematemesis as a result of laceration of the mucosa in the vicinity of the cardia. The damage, however, usually affects the gastric rather than the oesophageal mucosa. (Mallory-Weiss syndrome.)

Oesophageal obstruction

Obstruction of the oesophagus usually has an *organic* basis. In some instances, however, a pri-

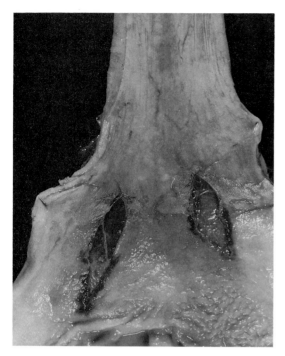

Fig. 19.21 Spontaneous rupture of the oesophagus. Two longitudinal tears are present, involving the lower end of the oesophagus and adjacent cardia of the stomach. × 0.7

mary organic lesion cannot be recognised and the obstruction is apparently due to *muscular dysfunction ('functional obstruction')*.

Organic obstruction

This may arise in a number of different ways. (1) The lumen of the oesophagus may actually be occluded, usually by tumour, either benign or malignant, although occasionally by a foreign body. (2) Disease within the wall of the oesophagus may lead to stenosis of the lumen; again malignant tumours are most often implicated. Fibrous stricture may, however, arise as a complication of hiatus hernia, the swallowing of corrosive or scalding fluids, trauma, or as a congenital defect. (3) The oesophagus may be compressed from outside, e.g. by a mediastinal tumour or cyst, aortic aneurysm, enlargement of the left atrium following mitral stenosis, congenital malformation of the great vessels, or pharyngeal diverticulum. (4) Diseases affecting the neuromuscular co-ordination of the oesophagus may interfere with normal deglutition.

Progressive systemic sclerosis and Chagas' disease are suitably included in this group, and also disorders of the central nervous system which interfere with deglutition.

Progressive systemic sclerosis. This is a connective tissue disease (p. 23.62) which may produce widespread systemic lesions, the skin of the hands and face (acrosclerosis) and the kidneys being especially affected. Dysphagia is not uncommon, and is due to replacement of the oesophageal musculature by fibrous tissue which, if diffuse, leads to pronounced interference with peristaltic activity. Shortening of the oesophagus causing reflux oesophagitis may be an additional complication.

Chagas' disease (South America trypanosomiasis). This disease, caused by the protozoon *Trypanosoma cruzi*, is described on p. 28.12. In the oesophagus, there may be widespread destruction of the ganglia of the myenteric plexus, leading to disturbance of peristalsis and the development of a clinical picture very similar to that of achalasia (see below).

'Functional' obstruction

The most important 'functional' disturbance is *achalasia of the oesophagus*, although other functional disorders have been described, e.g. diffuse spasm, sometimes associated with organic lesions of the gastro-intestinal tract, especially peptic ulcer, gall-bladder disease and hiatus hernia. Dysphagia may also occur from dysfunction of the upper end of the oesophagus in anaemic women (Plummer–Vinson syndrome, p. 17.42): the constriction can be visualised radiologically and by oesophagoscopy, and is sometimes described by the vague term *oesophageal web*: since it is not seen at autopsy, and is usually cured by treating the anaemia, it appears to be due to muscle spasm.

Achalasia of the oesophagus. In this condition there is pronounced narrowing of the terminal part of the oesophagus with dilatation proximally. It usually develops in early adult life and leads to dysphagia and regurgitation of food; later there may be more serious obstruction. Oesophageal narrowing is usually at the diaphragmatic level and marked dilatation of the oesophagus results (Fig. 19.22), with compensatory muscular hypertrophy of the wall. The narrowing was formerly attributed to muscular spasm, hence the term *'cardiospasm'*; there is

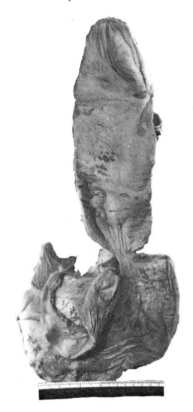

Fig. 19.22   Achalasia of oesophagus. Note the great dilatation with numerous superficial ulcers. ×0·25.

probably, however, a primary disturbance of motility with defective transmission of peristaltic waves to the cardia and subsequent failure of relaxation of the cardiac sphincter. The cause of this disturbance remains uncertain. Degenerative changes have been described in the myenteric ganglia, and it is probable that achalasia is an acquired abnormality of autonomic innervation; the close similarity to the oesophageal disturbance in Chagas' disease supports this hypothesis. Incision of the oesophageal wall through to the mucosa at the level of obstruction (Heller's operation) appears to be the most satisfactory form of surgical treatment in severe cases.

Diverticula

Two varieties of local dilatation are observed in the oesophagus, namely the *pulsion diverticulum* and the *traction diverticulum*.

The pulsion diverticulum is caused by forcible distension during the act of swallowing. It is usually not noticeable till early adult life but may be due to a congenital weakness or deficiency in the muscle of the inferior constrictor of the pharynx; it is therefore more correctly termed a *pharyngeal* pouch or diverticulum. Once a diverticulum has formed, as may result from repeated stretching of the deficiency in the wall during swallowing of food, it tends to become distended with food and gradually extends downwards behind the wall of the oesophagus, tilting the tube forwards so that the mouth of the sac comes to lie in line with the upper pharynx. The sac ultimately becomes permanently distended by food and may compress and obstruct the adjacent oesophagus, with consequent severe dysphagia and weight loss.* Such a diverticulum is lined by mucous membrane supported by connective tissue, but its wall usually contains no muscle; it becomes ulcerated. Less commonly, a diverticulum occurs anteriorly and bulges between the trachea and the oesophagus.

The traction diverticulum of the oesophagus is produced by the contraction of connective tissue pulling the wall outwards, usually by the adhesion to the wall of the tube of a mass of calcified tuberculous lymph nodes or occasionally a mass of silicotic nodes. A pouch with a sharp apex is the result, and this is stretched and increased both by further scarring and by the movements of the oesophagus. Ulceration of the diverticulum may occur and may lead to perforation, resulting in gangrenous mediastinitis which may extend to the pleura and other parts.

Rarely a diverticulum occurs opposite the bifurcation of the trachea as a congenital abnormality, arising in the same way as a communication between the oesophagus and trachea (see p. 19.18). Such diverticula are sometimes lined by columnar epithelium.

Tumours

Benign tumours. These are all rare. Lipoma, fibroma and leiomyoma may all occur, leiomy-

---

* 'Bloody' Judge Jeffries had a pharyngeal pouch, the discomfort of which may have contributed to the severity of his sentences.

oma probably being the least rare and occasionally reaching a large size. Benign tumours tend to project into the lumen as polyps.

Malignant tumours

Carcinoma of the oesophagus. Carcinoma is by far the commonest malignant tumour in the oesophagus. It occurs usually after the age of 45, and is much commoner in men than in women. The commonest site is at the level of the bifurcation of the trachea, the lower and upper ends being next in order of frequency. There is, however, a distinct sex difference in the sites of incidence. About three-quarters of cases of cancer in the hypopharynx and upper end of the oesophagus occur in women, whereas over 80% of cancers elsewhere in the oesophagus occur in men.

Oesophageal carcinoma shows remarkable geographical variation in incidence. Although not uncommon in this country its incidence is much greater in certain parts of Central Asia and China. In these high incidence areas poor nutritional status, deficiency of trace elements in soil, fungal contamination of grain and the ingestion of plant nitrosamines have all been incriminated. Hot and spicy food may also contribute in some areas (e.g. Curaçao). Little is known about the causation of oesophageal cancer in Western Europe and North America apart from a possible association with heavy alcohol intake and pipe and cigar smoking. The long-suspected relationship of iron-deficiency anaemia and dysphagia with post-cricoid carcinoma in women has never been firmly established. Other local factors, such as the Barrett syndrome (p. 19.14), achalasia and longstanding strictures (especially those following ingestion of carbolic acid), are also important.

Naked-eye appearances. There are two chief types. *Scirrhous carcinoma* grows round the tube and induces a fibrous reaction, causing progressively severe stenosis. The *soft* or *encephaloid* type involves a greater length of the oesophagus, forms irregular projections into the lumen and thus tends to cause occlusion (Fig. 19.23). At the same time, the destruction of the muscular tissue by infiltration interferes with contraction. The tumour may spread upwards and downwards in the submucous tissue, and forms secondary nodules which raise the

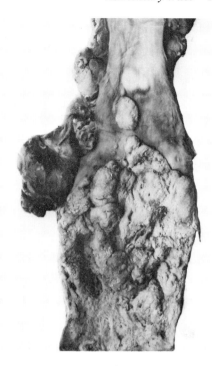

Fig. 19.23 Extensive ulcerating carcinoma in middle part of oesophagus.

mucosa, giving a false appearance of multifocal origin.

In addition to causing obstruction, the tumour may spread to the trachea or a bronchus, and ulcerate through the wall. Infected fluids are then likely to pass down the bronchi and cause *aspiration pneumonia*. Rarely ulceration into the aorta may result in fatal haemorrhage. Metastases also occur in the local lymph nodes, and occasionally also in the internal organs, especially the liver; but death is usually caused by oesophageal obstruction.

Microscopic appearances. In nearly all cases the tumour is a poorly keratinised squamous carcinoma; rarely it resembles oat-cell bronchial carcinoma. Adenocarcinoma is less common but may arise as a complication of Barrett's syndrome (p. 19.14). Many 'oesophageal' adenocarcinomas are, however, of gastric origin. Tumours arising from the oesophageal glands are uncommon; they present the features of mucoepidermoid or adenoid cystic carcinomas found in the salivary glands (p. 19.10 *et seq.*).

Sarcoma is rare. It resembles the softer varieties of carcinoma, but its growth may be more massive. Rhabdomyosarcoma of the oesophagus is extremely rare.

Congenital abnormalities

In addition to stenosis or dilatation, already mentioned, there may be various degrees of atresia of the oesophagus. The commonest of these is a condition in which the upper part forms a blind sac which is separated from the lower part, while the latter is patent and communicates with the trachea closely above its bifurcation. Sometimes the oesophagus is patent throughout, but there is a small communication with the trachea, through which food may pass into the trachea and cause a suppurative or necrotising pneumonia. A congenital diverticulum is a lesser degree of this malformation.

III: Stomach

The two most important pathological conditions in the stomach are peptic ulcer and carcinoma. Bacterial infection as a cause of serious disease in the stomach is comparatively rare. Gastric juice rapidly destroys most vegetative bacteria entering with food, and when digestion has been completed, and the stomach contents pass on to the intestine, the stomach soon returns to a state of virtual sterility. Nevertheless ingested tubercle bacilli, *Salmonellae*, *Brucellae* and dysentery bacilli can all successfully evade the chemical barrier of the gastric secretion and no doubt more easily if there is defective acid secretion or stasis. Acute inflammation of the gastric mucosa may be due to swallowing irritating fluids or food contaminated with bacterial, e.g. staphylococcal, toxins. It is also likely that the stomach can be affected by some of the enteroviruses and perhaps other viruses also.

Chronic gastritis of the acid-secreting mucosa has the features of an organ-specific auto-immune disease. The chronic inflammation which frequently occurs in the antral mucosa appears to be due to agents which damage the surface epithelium, such as bile and alcohol.

Acute gastritis

This term is quite often applied to the acute gastric symptoms which arise during the course of infective fevers or following dietary indiscretion or stress. The diagnosis of acute gastritis, however, is basically histological, and rests upon the demonstration in gastric biopsies of acute inflammatory changes in the mucosa, and apart from occasional reports of such changes in acute alcoholism or following ingestion of staphylococcal enterotoxin, these changes have seldom been observed in clinical practice. It is, none the less, known that non-steroidal anti-inflammatory agents (especially aspirin) are capable of causing a variety of acute gastric lesions which may culminate in gastric erosions (see below) or even frank ulceration. Such lesions are now well recognised as a cause of gastric haemorrhage with, on occasion, melaena or even frank haematemesis. Sometimes drug-induced mucosal damage is accompanied by extensive haemorrhage into the mucosa, a severe condition known as **acute haemorrhagic gastritis**. This may also complicate shock-like states following trauma or surgical procedures, and has been attributed to the back diffusion of hydrogen ions through a damaged mucosal surface.

Corrosive gastritis. The ingestion of strong acid or alkali leads to variable destruction of gastric tissue usually associated with haemorrhage and sometimes with perforation. There may be marked gastric scarring should the patient survive. Acid tends to produce coagulative tissue necrosis, whereas alkali more often causes tissue liquefaction. Mild acids, e.g. oxalic or acetic, and arsenic, produce more superficial mucosal ulceration and gastritis. Some chemicals, e.g. phenol or mercuric chloride, actually fix the gastric tissues. For details, special works on toxicology should be consulted.

Acute bacterial gastritis. As mentioned earlier, bacterial infection is an unusual cause of acute gastritis, but *acute infective gastritis*, together with acute enteritis, is seen in 'food poisoning' due to *Salmonellae* and in *Yersinia* infections (p. 19.50). Rarely, extensive suppuration in the submucosa and muscle layer may develop when pyogenic bacteria, especially streptococci, gain entrance from an ulcerated carcinoma or from injury by a foreign body (phlegmonous gastritis).

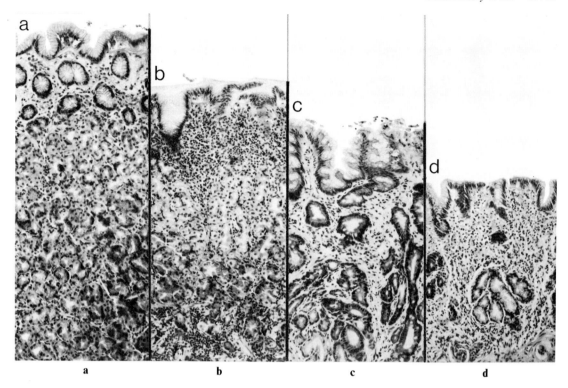

Fig. 19.24   Chronic gastritis of acid-secreting mucosa. All × 100. (**a**) Normal mucosa. (**b**) Superficial gastritis and atrophic gastritis affecting the deep part of the mucosa. (**c**) Complete loss of parietal and chief cells with intestinal metaplasia. (**d**) Complete atrophic gastritis. The remaining glands are of simple mucus-secreting type. In (**b**), (**c**) and (**d**), the full thickness of the mucosa is shown.

Chronic gastritis

Chronic non-specific gastritis. Modern endoscopic biopsy techniques have revealed that chronic inflammatory changes are common in the gastric mucosa and become increasingly so with advancing age. With the few exceptions described on pp. 19.20-21, these changes lack diagnostically specific pathological features. *Macroscopically*, chronic gastritis is unimpressive if it can be identified at all: it is essentially a histological concept, hence the importance of endoscopic biopsy in its recognition. None the less, the condition has important clinical implications.

Histologically, chronic non-specific gastritis varies in severity. Its mildest expression is known as chronic superficial gastritis, the main feature of which is the infiltration by plasma cells and lymphocytes of the superficial foveolar zone of the lamina propria surrounding the gastric pits, which may become slightly elongated and tortuous (Fig. 19.24b). In more severe cases, the inflammatory changes extend more deeply to involve the gastric glands which become progressively damaged with resultant thinning of the mucosa (Fig. 19.24c), hence the term **chronic atrophic gastritis**. Eventually, the inflammatory process may subside, but leaves a gross depletion of the glandular component of the mucosa——**gastric atrophy** (Fig. 19.24). The epithelial damage of chronic gastritis is often associated with metaplastic change, and in particular *intestinal metaplasia*, in which the gastric epithelium is replaced by cells of intestinal type such as enterocytes, goblet cells and Paneth cells. In the body of the stomach the specialised parietal and zymogenic cells may be replaced initially by more simple mucous glands (*pseudopyloric metaplasia*).

Chronic non-specific gastritis exists in two main forms. In **Type I** the lesions usually affect mainly the body of the stomach diffusely, with widespread destruction of the zymogenic and

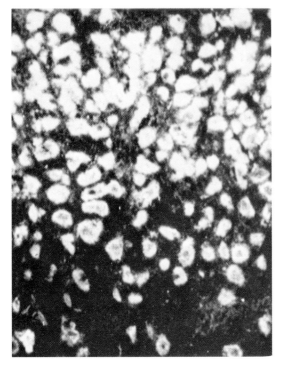

Fig. 19.25 Indirect immunofluorescence test for parietal-cell antibody. The parietal cells fluoresce brightly, indicating the presence of the antibody in the serum being tested.

parietal cells. This results in progressive reduction in the secretion of pepsin and acid, with the ultimate development of complete achylia of which the absence of acid secretion (*achlorhydria*) is the most readily detectable clinically. A more serious consequence however, is impaired secretion of intrinsic factor (IF) which in some cases at least, leads to *malabsorption of vitamin B_{12}, and the development of the most important form of megaloblastic anaemia, pernicious anaemia* (p. 17.39). In spite of its name, Type I chronic gastritis is a good example of an organ-specific auto-immune disease (p. 7.24). It is in part at least genetically determined and is commonly associated with auto-immune disease of other organs such as the thyroid and adrenal. Anti-gastric antibodies can be detected in the serum in many cases (Fig. 19.25); in patients with pernicious anaemia the incidence of serum antibodies to parietal cells is over 90% and antibodies to IF can also be found in the serum of over 50% of cases. Furthermore, IF antibodies, some of which are directed against the vitamin B_{12} binding site, may be found in the

gastric juice and play an important part in inhibiting the absorption of B_{12} and precipitating the development of megaloblastic anaemia. Minor degrees of Type I chronic gastritis are very common, as reflected by the occurrence of parietal cell antibodies in about 10% of apparently normal individuals over the age of 50 years in this country. The role of anti-gastric antibodies in causing damage to the gastric mucosa is debatable (p. 7.26). Type I chronic gastritis seldom produces symptoms referable to the stomach, but may be complicated by gastric neoplasia (p. 19.27). In pernicious anaemia, the incidence of carcinoma is three to four times that of the comparable normal population; malignant lymphoma may also develop and multiple carcinoid tumours (p. 19.30) have also been reported.

Type II chronic gastritis is seen more often in endoscopic biopsies than Type I. The lesions tend to be patchy and occur mainly in the antrum or at the junction of antrum and body. Some reduction in acid secretion is usual but is seldom severe, and absorption of vitamin B_{12} is adequate unless the patient has had a previous partial gastrectomy. While the causation of this form of gastritis is far from clear, it is suspected that damage to the surface epithelium, mediated, for example, by reflux of bile or the prolonged ingestion of irritant substances such as aspirin-type analgesics or alcohol, is involved in most cases, the back-diffusion of hydrogen ions being the ultimate common mechanism triggered by these disparate agencies. Type II chronic gastritis may have an important role in the pathogenesis of peptic ulcer (p. 19.26) and may contribute to the development of gastric carcinoma (p. 19.27). Type II chronic gastritis may cause dyspeptic symptoms, which appear to be associated with the superimposition of acute inflammatory changes with infiltration of poplymorphs, etc. in the superficial part of the mucosa (*active gastritis*) upon the chronic changes described above.

Other types of chronic gastritis

Granulomatous gastritis. The presence of a sarcoid reaction in the gastric mucosa or deeper tissues sometimes occurs without apparent reason, but it may be a manifestation of sarcoidosis (p. 9.26) or of tuberculous origin. Sometimes it complicates peptic ulceration or gastric carcinoma, and there is always the possibility that it represents an unusual expression of Crohn's disease (p. 19.33). Tuberculous ulcers sometimes develop in the stomach in patients with advanced pulmonary tuberculosis.

Hypertrophic gastritis. This rather ill-defined term is applied to lesions in which there is macroscopic enlargement of gastric rugae. This may be due to the increase in parietal cell mass that results from gastrin-producing tumours (p. 20.65) or is found in some patients with duodenal ulcers. The most important cause, however, is *Ménétrièr's disease* in which there is marked thickening of the gastric mucosa due chiefly to elongation and tortuosity of the foveolae. The aetiology is not clear. The main clinical effect is loss of protein into the gastric lumen and hypoalbuminaemia.

Gastric erosions

An erosion may be defined as an ulcer of the gastric wall which is limited to the superficial part of the mucosa and heals without scar formation. Acute erosions are usually multiple (Fig. 19.26), and develop as part of the clinical spectrum of acute gastritis, especially the haemorrhagic variant (p. 19.18). They are particularly associated with the ingestion of aspirin-type anti-inflammatory agents, and are a cause of gastric haemorrhage. Histologically, erosions are characterised by small foci or sometimes more diffuse areas of necrosis and loss of the superficial mucosa, deposition of fibrin, neutrophil infiltration and haemorrhage

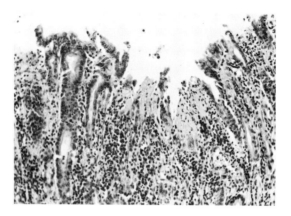

Fig. 19.27 Acute erosive gastritis. There is superficial loss of the surface epithelium with fibrinoid necrosis and polymorph infiltration. × 205.

(Fig. 19.27). Recently, a more chronic type of erosion has been described in which foci of epithelial necrosis become surrounded by swollen, inflamed gastric mucosa showing marked elongation of the gastric pits (foveolar hyperplasia): they may be of allergic origin and can persist for several months.

Peptic ulceration

This term is applied to a form of ulceration which develops for reasons as yet unknown in epithelial-lined surfaces exposed to the acid secretion of the gastric glands. The sites most often affected are the stomach itself, the duodenal bulb and the distal part of the oesophagus (p. 19.14). Less often, peptic ulceration is seen in the more distal parts of the duodenum, in the jejunum adjacent to the pylorus and in the ileum close to foci of gastric metaplasia in a Meckel's diverticulum (p. 19.67).

Two main types of peptic ulcer are recognised: **acute ulcers**, which destroy the lamina muscularis mucosae but do not extend more deeply than the submucosa, and **chronic ulcers** which completely penetrate the muscularis propria. The term *subacute* is sometimes used to describe ulcers which have only partially penetrated the muscularis propria, and presumably represent a developing phase of the chronic ulcer. The terms 'acute' and 'chronic' ulcers also have a temporal connotation, although acute ulcers may progress to chronic ulcers, and

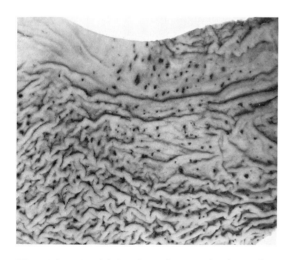

Fig. 19.26 Multiple minute haemorrhagic erosions of the gastric mucosa. × 0·75.

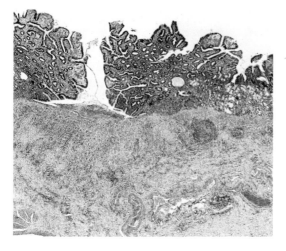

Fig. 19.28 A small acute peptic ulcer which has penetrated superficially into the submucosa. × 12.

some peptic ulcers are capable of penetrating the muscularis propria very rapidly: this seems to have been the case with the so-called *acute perforating ulcers* which were observed in young women at the turn of the century, but are now seen only rarely. While it is obviously true that a chronic ulcer must have passed through an acute stage, there are distinct differences between the clinical and epidemiological features of acute and chronic peptic ulcers.

Acute peptic ulcers may arise at any age from childhood onwards and usually present by causing upper gastro-intestinal haemorrhage. They generally develop under conditions of stress, for example following severe burns (*Curling's ulcer*), sepsis or traumatic shock, and may also complicate intracranial trauma or surgical operations (*Cushing's ulcer*). They may also be related to the ingestion of drugs, particularly aspirin-type anti-inflammatory agents. In all these circumstances, acute ulcers may be associated with erosions (see above) or haemorrhagic gastritis (p. 19.18). The acute perforating ulcer mentioned above seems to have been associated with the abdominal constriction generated by the tight corsets fashionable in Victorian times. It should be mentioned, however, that drug-induced ulcers may also bring about rapid perforation. Macroscopically, acute ulcers occur mainly in (any part of) the stomach, but also in the proximal duodenum. They are usually multiple and only occasionally exceed 1 cm in diameter. Healing occurs without significant scarring. The histological appearances of the ulcerated surface resembles that of the chronic type (see below). By definition, the ulcerative process does not extend beyond the submucosa (Fig. 19.28) except in the, now rare, acute perforating type: even so, the erosion of a submucosal artery may lead to severe haemorrhage (Fig. 19.29).

Chronic peptic ulcer

This occurs in adult life, and is very common in developed countries. About 8% of adults in the UK develop a chronic peptic ulcer at one time or another. Overall, males are much more often affected than females, and develop ulcers in the duodenal bulb or less often in the prepyloric region of the stomach. In females, ulceration usually occurs more proximally in the stomach. It is thus evident that duodenal ulcer is more common than gastric ulcer and is overwhelmingly a disease of males (in Scotland <10 to 1). For gastric ulcer, there is only a slight male preponderance.

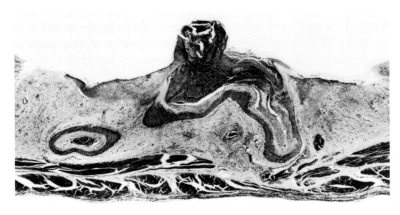

Fig. 19.29 Superficial acute ulcer of stomach which has eroded an artery and caused fatal haemorrhage. × 10.

The incidence of chronic peptic ulcer has varied greatly over the last century. Before 1900 chronic duodenal ulcer was almost unknown; thereafter its incidence increased dramatically to reach a peak in 1920–30, since when it has fallen slightly. The changes in incidence of chronic gastric ulcer have been similar. People born towards the end of the nineteenth century appear to have been exceptionally prone to develop peptic ulcer, and have retained this susceptibility over the years. Subsequent generations seem to have been less seriously affected.

Macroscopic features. Chronic peptic ulcers usually occur as single lesions: occasionally two ulcers are found, and rarely more than that. Sometimes duodenal and gastric ulcers are associated, the former usually developing first. Most chronic ulcers measure less than 3 cm in diameter but gastric ulcers occasionally grow much larger, usually in old people, and may exceed 10 cm across. Ulcers in the duodenum are usually restricted to the first 3 cm, developing with equal frequency on the anterior and posterior walls, and very occasionally on both——'*kissing ulcers*'. Most gastric ulcers arise in the lesser curvature at the junction between antrum and body (c.f. chronic gastritis p. 19.19). This level is extremely variable: it may be close to the cardia, particularly in females, and this accounts for the occurrence of some gastric ulcers high on the lesser curve. When peptic ulcers are found outside these zones, the possibility of some unusual predisposing factor

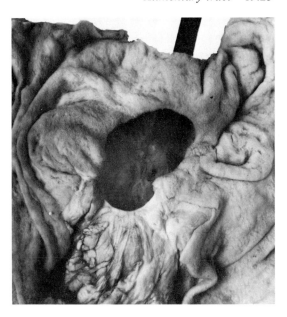

Fig. 19.31 Large chronic ulcer of duodenum just beyond the pylorus. The ulcer had perforated at the margin, as indicated by the pointer. × 0·8.

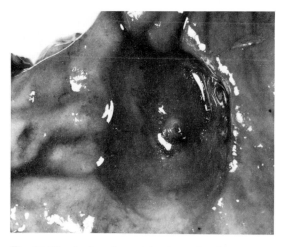

Fig. 19.30 A chronic gastric ulcer, showing an eroded artery from which fatal haemorrhage occurred. × 2.

e.g. gastrinoma (p. 20.65) should be considered. Chronic peptic ulcers are usually round or oval, with sharply defined, deeply shelving margins, giving the lesions a characteristic punched-out appearance (Figs. 19.30, 19.31). The mucosa usually appears normal up to the ulcer margin: it is not raised (c.f. an ulcerated cancer) and in gastric ulcers the mucosal folds typically extend almost to the very edge of the ulcer crater, unlike ulcerated cancers which tend to show blurring of the surrounding mucosal architecture. While the base of a chronic ulcer is usually formed by the thickened serosal coat of the duodenum or stomach, the ulceration may extend into adjacent organs such as the liver and pancreas. When an ulcer involves the colon, a gastro-colic fistula may develop. There have even been instances in which the heart wall has been eroded by an ulcer arising in a portion of the stomach which has herniated into the thoracic cavity.

Microscopic features. The wall of a peptic ulcer presents a distinctive appearance. On the ulcer surface there is a layer of neutrophil polymorphs, most of which are dead and partially digested by peptic activity and appear as amorphous haematoxyphilic bodies. Merging with this layer is a zone of fibrinoid necrosis which is intensely eosinophilic. Underlying this is an

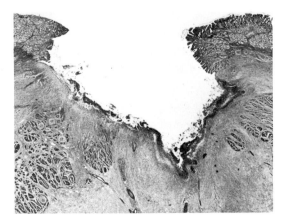

Fig. 19.32 Chronic gastric ulcer at later stage, showing breach of muscular coat. × 7.

organising zone of granulation tissue of variable thickness, showing active proliferation of fibroblasts and endothelial cells. Deeper still, the granulation tissue has matured into fibrous scar tissue, which radiates widely from the ulcer base and laterally replaces the muscularis propria for a variable distance (Fig. 19.32). Arteries incorporated into the ulcer base commonly show endarteritis obliterans (Fig. 14.3, p. 14.2) unless the ulcerative process has been unusually rapid. An infiltrate of lymphocytes, plasma cells, macrophages and eosinophils is observed in the ulcer base. These cells may be surprisingly sparse, but occasionally lymphocytic infiltration is heavy and extends laterally from the ulcer margin, when the lesion may be mistaken for an ulcerated lymphoma. More rarely, the adjacent mucosa shows a granulomatous reaction.

The mucosa at the margin of chronic ulcers shows a combination of regenerative activity and inflammatory changes. In the stomach these changes take the form of chronic atrophic gastritis invariably accompanied by intestinal metaplasia and superficial neutrophil infiltration (*active gastritis*, p. 19.20). Similar but less well defined inflammatory changes are observed in the duodenal mucosa surrounding peptic ulcers; in particular, neutrophil infiltration is found in relationship to the surface epithelium of duodenal villi (*active duodenitis*). Foci of gastric metaplasia in the villous epithelium are also prominent and are thought to indicate high acid levels in the duodenal lumen. Active duodenitis also occurs in the absence of peptic ulceration,

but it is uncertain whether it gives rise to clinical dyspepsia.

The healing of a chronic peptic ulcer is initiated by re-epithelialisation of the ulcerating surface and may be remarkably complete, but some scarring of the underlying submucosa and muscularis propria invariably persists.

Results and complications of peptic ulceration

(1) Healing and scarring. Acute peptic ulcers usually undergo healing without a visible scar. Healing is the rule also in the subacute type and is common in chronic ulcers, even when large, as is shown by the common autopsy finding of contracted scars in the ulcer-prone sites. If the ulcer has been superficial, the scar may be merely a small depression with a smooth whitish surface, but if it has penetrated more deeply there is often a radiating indrawing of the surrounding mucous membrane, so that a stellate appearance results. Scarring of an ulcer at or near the pylorus commonly results in **pyloric stenosis**, with its consequent effects (p. 19.55).

Stenosis of the duodenum or pyloric antrum by the scarring of chronic ulcers has similar effects, and ulcers higher up on the lesser curvature of the stomach may, by scarring and contraction, produce the deformity of 'hour glass' stomach.

(2) Perforation. When an ulcer perforates rapidly (Fig. 19.33), gastric contents escape

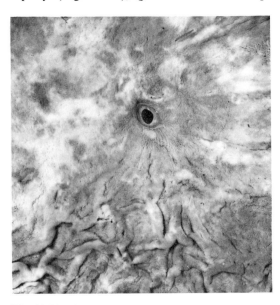

Fig. 19.33 Acute perforating ulcer. × 1.

either into the general peritoneal cavity or into the lesser sac. The pain, abdominal rigidity and symptoms of collapse which follow are usually dramatic and are caused by the acid gastric contents; these are virtually sterile at first, but without prompt surgical treatment, organisms soon flourish and **acute peritonitis** results. Air from the stomach comes to lie between the liver and diaphragm where it is visible radiologically. After successful surgical treatment of the perforation, there is a risk that infected material lodged between the liver and diaphragm may become sealed off by fibrinous exudate and cause a **subphrenic abscess** which may later infect the pleura. Occasionally a localised peritoneal abscess develops around the site of a perforation without general peritonitis. Perforation of deep ulcers which progress slowly is often prevented by local obliteration of the peritoneal sac by fibrinous exudate and then fibrosis between the two layers. When this happens the advancing ulceration can extend into adjacent organs, e.g. the liver and pancreas, without causing peritonitis. In the duodenum, ulcers situated anteriorly perforate most frequently. As the name implies 'acute perforating ulcers' progress rapidly to perforation (Fig. 19.33) but they are now uncommon.

(3) **Haemorrhage** is common and varies greatly in degree. Minor but continued loss of blood is caused by the erosion of small blood vessels in the base of an ulcer, and may only be detected by testing for occult blood in the faeces. It may present as iron-deficiency anaemia (p. 17.41). More severe bleeding, giving rise to 'coffee-ground' vomit or 'tarry' stools (melaena) is usually due to involvement of a larger submucosal artery in the base of an acute ulcer (Fig. 19.29). The most dramatic form of haemorrhage, however, is caused by a rapidly penetrating chronic ulcer eroding a major artery lying outside the gastric or duodenal wall (Fig. 19.30). Ulcers of the lesser curvature may involve the left gastric artery, and posteriorly-sited duodenal ulcers, the gastro-duodenal artery. Haemorrhage may be severe, causing haematemesis and sometimes death. Arteries involved in the base of more slowly progressing peptic ulcers are liable to bleed less or not at all owing to reduction or occlusion of their lumina by endarteritis obliterans (Fig. 14.3, p. 14.2). Rarely, involvement of an artery causes an aneurysm which may rupture.

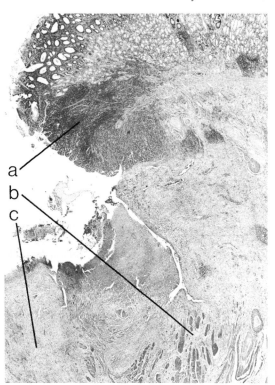

Fig. 19.34 Ulcer-cancer of stomach. A chronic peptic ulcer showing the characteristic complete breach of the muscle coat. A focus of early carcinoma was detected microscopically at (**a**) in the overhanging margin of the ulcer crater: (**b**) muscle coat: (**c**) fibrous base of ulcer.

(4) **Development of carcinoma.** Although carcinoma sometimes develops in a chronic gastric ulcer, its frequency has probably been overestimated in the past. One reason for this lies in the difficulty in distinguishing between a chronic peptic ulcer which has undergone malignant change and a carcinoma which has ulcerated. Complete interruption of the muscle coat is good evidence of pre-existing chronic peptic ulceration (Fig. 19.34).

Cancer develops in the continuously regenerating epithelium at the ulcer margin (Fig. 19.34) and tends to encircle the ulcer crater, spreading outwards into the submucosa and muscular coat, but not usually invading far into the fibrous ulcer floor. By contrast, a carcinoma developing without peptic ulceration often invades the muscular coat but practically never destroys it entirely and even in advanced cases remains of muscle are to be found between cancer cells. Another important point is that irregular growth and displacement of epithelium at the margin of a peptic ulcer may give a false impression of malignant change.

Taking these factors into consideration, it is unlikely that cancer develops in more than 1% of chronic gastric ulcers. There is, however, an increased risk of carcinoma developing in a stomach with a chronic peptic ulcer because of the associated chronic gastritis (p. 19.24). *Carcinoma does not arise in chronic duodenal ulcers.*

Aetiology of peptic ulcers

In addition to the important morphological differences between acute and chronic peptic ulcers, they differ also in their aetiology. Acute ulcers tend to develop under conditions of stress (p. 19.22), probably because stress can cause acid hypersecretion.

Chronic peptic ulceration is of more complex aetiology and still largely unexplained. The possible importance of **genetic factors** in the pathogenesis is suggested by its occurrence in some families and by a relatively high incidence of duodenal ulceration in individuals who do not secrete blood-group substances into the gastric juice and belong to blood group O. **Environmental factors** must be responsible for the changing incidence of peptic ulcer during this century and for 'epidemics' of the disease which may be localised or affect certain age groups in the community. Geographical variations in incidence also emphasise the importance of environment. Peptic ulcer is essentially a disease of developed, industrialised communities. Factors such as dietary habits, drugs (especially aspirin) and occupational or social stresses may be important. Cigarette smoking is also a contributory factor, especially in gastric ulcer, and may account for the association between peptic ulcer and chronic bronchitis.

It seems necessary to explain firstly the development of a mucosal lesion, and secondly why it does not heal like a wound made in a normal stomach. Local ischaemia due to thrombosis, embolus or vascular spasm has been postulated as a cause of the initial injury, but lacks supporting evidence.

The only entirely consistent finding associated with peptic ulceration is the presence of gastric acid, which is undoubtedly a causal factor. *Peptic ulcer does not develop in patients with histamine-fast achlorhydria and is caused by interference with the capacity of the gastro-intestinal mucosa to resist digestion by gastric acid,* due either to impaired mucosal resistance or to hypersecretion of gastric juice, or possibly both. The nature of the mucosal defence mechanism is complex and depends among other things upon the secretion of mucus and the presence of inhibitors of gastric secretion. Interference with these protective factors appears to be of particular importance in the pathogenesis of **gastric ulcer**, in which gastric secretion may be normal but is often reduced by chronic gastritis. There is also evidence that dietary factors may be of particular importance in the pathogenesis of gastric ulcer.

By contrast, gastric hypersecretion appears to be the major causal factor of **duodenal ulcer**; some of those affected have an increased parietal-cell mass, while in others, the acid secretory capacity is normal but the acid response to meals is exaggerated, possibly as a result of a defect in the feedback mechanism which controls gastric secretion (Sircus, 1979).

Although the role of humoral stimulants of gastric secretion in the pathogenesis of peptic ulcer in general is uncertain, excess of such substances is capable of causing a fulminating ulcer diathesis. This occurs in the Zollinger–Ellison syndrome (p. 20.65) in which a single or multiple pancreatic islet-cell tumours secrete large amounts of gastrin. In these cases, peptic ulceration takes place not only in the common sites but also in unusual areas, e.g. the greater curvature of the stomach and distal duodenum. There is evidence that a raised level of blood calcium promotes an increase in gastric secretion, and this may account for the high incidence of peptic ulceration in patients with hyperparathyroidism. The Zollinger–Ellison syndrome can occur as a part of one of the multiple endocrine neoplasia syndromes (p. 26.41).

Dilatation of the stomach

This may result from obstruction, usually at or near the pylorus and most often caused by the scarring associated with gastric or duodenal ulceration (p. 19.24), by gastric carcinoma, or, in infants, by congenital pyloric hypertrophy (p.

19.31). Such obstruction causes repeated vomiting and may lead to serious metabolic effects, e.g. hypokalaemic alkalosis (p. 19.55). Various degrees of muscular hypertrophy occur in the stomach wall proximal to the obstruction, but chronic dilatation eventually develops, and is often associated with chronic gastritis, mucosal atrophy and greatly reduced acid secretion. In such cases, various saprophytic bacteria and fungi may grow in the retained gastric contents, with production of gas, etc. from fermentation.

Occasionally, acute dilatation takes place in the absence of obstruction. This is usually a complication of surgery, similar to paralytic ileus (p. 19.56), but has been observed as a consequence of diabetic coma.

Tumours

Benign tumours. The stomach is an uncommon site of benign tumours, adenoma and leiomyoma being the least rare.

Gastric adenoma is a polypoid tumour, usually single; like the polypoid adenomas of the colon (p. 19.62) these tumours show various grades of tubular or villous differentiation and may progress to adenocarcinoma, particularly those which exceed 1 cm in diameter. Hyperplastic and regenerative polyps are much commoner, and most often contain both foveolar and glandular cell components: *hyperplastic polyp* seems a better name for them than the suggested one of 'hyperplasiogenous polyp'.

Leiomyoma may also protrude into the lumen; usually it is small and symptomless, but the larger examples commonly undergo deep central ulceration and may bleed profusely into the lumen. A substantial minority are of clear-cell or epithelioid appearance (leiomyoblastoma) and show features suggestive of malignancy, but metastasis is uncommon.

Gastric carcinoma

Despite a steady fall in incidence over the past 50 or so years, this is still one of the most common internal malignancies in many parts of the world (Table 12.3, p. 12.16), and in global terms is probably still the commonest fatal tumour. The prognosis is poor; the 5-year survival rate is 5–10% in most countries and has shown little improvement.

Epidemiology. Gastric carcinoma shows considerable geographical variation in incidence, even within individual countries. It is generally rare in tropical Africa, but extremely common in Japan, Chile, some parts of Central Asia, and in Finland and Iceland. Most other countries occupy an intermediate position. The incidence increases sharply with age, is everywhere greater in males than in females, and is extremely high in some families.

Causal factors are largely unknown. Not surprisingly, many dietary components have been suspected, but none has been incriminated. One possibility is that nitrates and nitrites in the diet may be converted to carcinogenic nitrosamines by the various bacteria which colonise the stomach in chronic gastritis with achlorhydria (see below). There may also be a genetic predisposition, for there is a slightly increased risk in people of blood group A: this does not, however, account for the geographical and familial variations mentioned above.

Premalignant lesions. There is no doubt that some polypoid adenomas become malignant, although hyperplastic polyps (see above) seldom do so. The incidence of gastric carcinoma is increased by about ten times in individuals with atrophic gastritis, including that accompanied by pernicious anaemia. There is some evidence that the pre-malignant feature of atrophic gastritis is intestinal metaplasia (p. 19.19), particularly the partial form in which goblet cells are associated with atypical mucin-secreting cells rather than with enterocytes (as in the complete form). The relationship of peptic ulceration to carcinoma is discussed on p. 19.25. Following partial gastrectomy for gastric ulceration, there is an increased risk of gastric cancer in the residual tissue, because chronic gastritis is always present. Finally, there is evidence that Ménétrier's disease (p. 19.21) predisposes to carcinoma.

Macroscopic features

Carcinomas may develop in any part of the stomach, but most occur in the distal third. Tumours arising in the cardiac region and involving the lower oesophagus are, however, by no means uncommon. The tumour may form a large irregular sessile mass which projects into

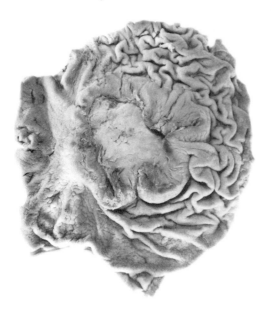

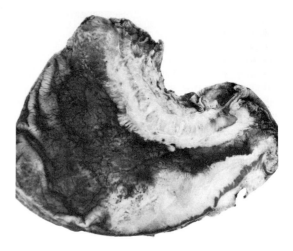

Fig. 19.37 Mucoid carcinoma at pylorus, showing great infiltration and thickening of the wall (anterior part of stomach viewed from behind). × 0·5.

Fig. 19.35 Ulcerating scirrhous carcinoma of stomach, with thickened, raised margin and ulcerated base.

the lumen and commonly undergoes necrosis and infection. In a second, *ulcerative form*, the tumour invades deeply into the stomach wall and ulcerates, appearing as an ulcer with an irregular necrotic base and raised margins (Fig. 19.35). Third, the wall of the stomach may be extensively infiltrated by cancer cells, often of signet-ring type (p. 19.30) and accompanied by

an intense desmoplastic reaction which causes diffuse thickening of the wall—*diffuse carcinoma, linitis plastica* or *leather-bottle stomach* (Fig. 19.36). Less commonly, carcinoma may spread extensively in the mucosa without invading the underlying tissues, forming the *superficial spreading type*. If abundant mucin is secreted by the tumour cells, gastric carcinoma may present the gelatinous appearance of *mucous (colloid) carcinoma* (Fig. 19.37).

The appearance of *early gastric cancer* is becoming more widely recognised by use of

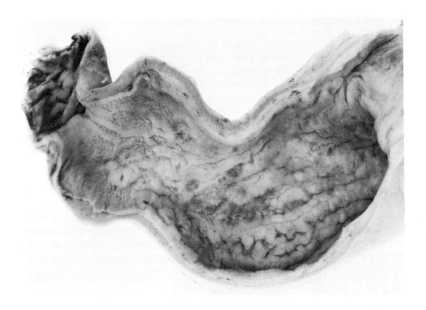

Fig. 19.36 Diffuse carcinoma of stomach. Note the general thickening of the wall without a localised tumour mass and with little ulceration. × 0·7.

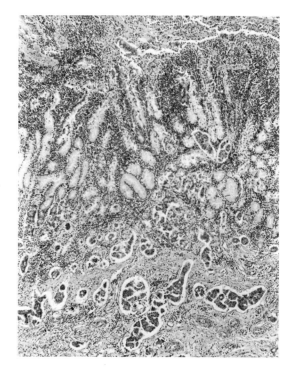

Fig. 19.38 Stomach wall, showing infiltration of lymphatics by carcinoma cells, which, in places, are growing upwards through the muscularis mucosae into the mucosa. Note the severe chronic gastritis. × 30.

endoscopic techniques, especially in Japan. Cytological techniques in expert hands may also be of value in the early detection of gastric carcinoma.

Spread of gastric carcinoma. *Local spread* is usually prominent. The muscularis is infiltrated most extensively in the *ulcerative* and *diffuse* types and involvement of the oesophageal and duodenal muscle coat is common. The duodenal mucosa is rarely invaded, but the oesophageal mucosa is often involved by tumours of the fundus or cardia. In the ulcerated type, the gastric wall is penetrated early, with direct extension to adjacent structures such as the greater and lesser omentum, liver, pancreas, spleen, diaphragm and abdominal wall. Invasion of the peritoneum may lead to *transcoelomic spread:* numerous minute nodules may be scattered throughout the peritoneal cavity and the greater omentum may be converted to a hard, palpable contracted mass in the epigastrium. The ovaries may be involved via the peritoneum and sometimes present the character-

istic microscopic features of the *'Krukenberg tumour'* (p. 24.25).

Lymphatic spread is early and frequent and often determines whether surgical removal is possible. The tumour spreads to the wide network of submucosal lymphatics (Fig. 19.38) and through the muscularis to the serosal lymphatics and thence to the para-gastric lymph nodes, which are usually the first to be involved. Retrograde spread into the mucosa may occur from the submucosal lymphatics to form numerous mucosal nodules, giving a false impression of multifocal origin. Lymphatic spread is often extensive, especially in diffuse carcinoma, involving lymphatics in the omentum, mesentery and wall of the intestine; it may take the form of extensive permeation (p. 19.72) with or without formation of tumour nodules. Lymph node metastases are usual in the upper abdomen, and more distant nodes may also be involved.

Blood spread occurs by the portal venous sys-

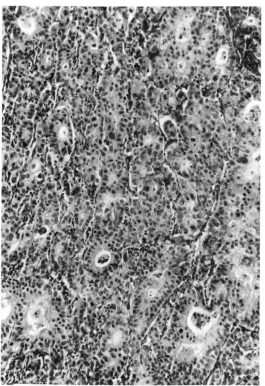

Fig. 19.39 Adenocarcinoma of the stomach showing formation of acini but also solid, poorly differentiated areas. × 130.

tem, usually resulting in early metastasis to the liver, and eventually to the lungs. Various other organs, including the brain and bones, may be involved. Blood spread is less common in mucous cancer, and is unusual in the diffuse type, although in the latter the liver is sometimes involved by lymphatic permeation.

Microscopic appearances. In most cases the tumour is a mucin-secreting **adenocarcinoma**, often rather poorly differentiated (Fig. 19.39). In areas of high incidence it is thought to arise usually from the metaplastic 'intestinal' epithelium of the gastric mucosa in chronic gastritis (p. 19.19). Some, however, are composed of solid masses of anaplastic cells. Mixed patterns are observed in both ulcerative and fungating tumours. In the diffuse type the cells often occur singly or in small groups throughout the fibrosed gastric wall: they may be small and difficult to recognise, but 'signet-ring' cells can usually be seen (Fig. 19.40) and confirm the diagnosis of cancer. In the mucous type, the cells are bathed in extracellular mucin (Fig. 12.31, p. 12.20).

Associated conditions. Achlorhydria or hypochlorhydria is usual in gastric carcinoma, and in many cases is due to the chronic gastritis which precedes or accompanies the tumour.

Achlorhydria, necrosis and ulceration of the tumour and stasis due to pyloric obstruction all provide conditions in which various bacteria, yeasts and fungi grow, and doubtless contribute to the *anorexia* and *cachexia* of gastric cancer. There is usually some degree of *anaemia*, which may be of *'secondary' type, due to infection of the tumour, or to iron-deficiency* from bleeding: *macrocytic anaemia* is a rare association and due to atrophic gastritis, i.e. pernicious anaemia. When gastric carcinoma becomes widespread it may be associated with a low-grade *microangiopathic haemolytic anaemia*, possibly caused by permeation of tumour mucin into vessel walls and widespread microvascular thrombosis. This type of anaemia is often accompanied by a leucoerythroblastic blood picture due to bone-marrow metastases.

Cancer of the stomach is one of the tumours sometimes accompanied, or even preceded, by *acanthosis nigricans*, which consists of multiple warty hyperkeratotic patches of the skin, especially about the folds or flexures.

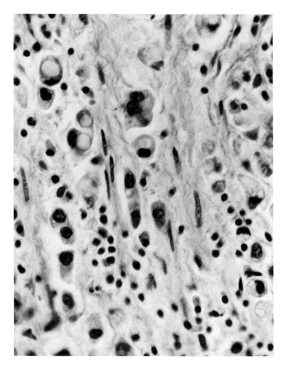

Fig. 19.40 Diffuse type of carcinoma in muscular coat of stomach. The cells are irregularly scattered, some contain mucous globules and others showing atrophic change. × 600.

Other malignant tumours of the stomach

Various types of sarcoma may arise in the stomach, but these constitute less than 5% of malignant gastric neoplasms.

Leiomyosarcoma (p. 12.34) is perhaps the commonest of these. It tends to be more localised than carcinoma and usually forms a large fungating mass projecting into the lumen.

Malignant lymphoma is usually of follicle-centre-cell or immunoblastic type; it may form a localised mass or infiltrate more diffusely, causing enormous thickening of the whole gastric wall. When localised to the stomach, the prognosis after surgery is better than for carcinoma.

Carcinoid tumours may also arise occasionally in the stomach, but differ from the commoner carcinoids of the intestine both in morphology and in their secretory effects (p. 19.59). They appear to be commoner in patients with pernicious anaemia.

Congenital abnormalities

The most important is **stenosis of the pylorus**. It is not uncommon; symptoms develop usually about 2 to 3 weeks after birth, and persistent vomiting may lead to death. The stenosis is associated with muscular hypertrophy of the wall at the pylorus, and this may extend back into the pyloric canal, gradually fading off, or may form a more localised, discrete band (Fig. 19.41). The circular muscle fibres are especially increased, and narrowing of the lumen is sometimes severe. The hypertrophy may be produced by spasmodic contraction at the pylorus, but the cause is not really known. A degree of concordance in siblings, and especially in twins, suggests a genetic predisposition, but the occurrence in families does not fit with a monogenic inheritance and the condition is six times commoner in male than in female infants. Relief of the obstruction by incision of the hypertrophied muscle is usually necessary and effective. Occasionally some degree of congenital pyloric stenosis may persist into adult life, and if it causes symptoms is liable to be mistaken for carcinoma.

Diverticula occur in the pyloric and fundal regions of the stomach, but they are rare. Occasionally the stomach is congenitally narrowed about the middle, producing the so-called 'hour-glass' contraction, but

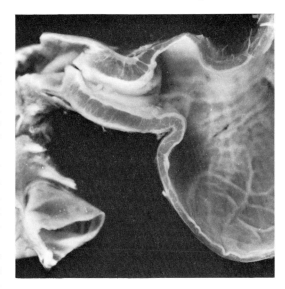

Fig. 19.41 Congenital stenosis of pylorus. The anterior wall at the pylorus has been cut away to show the greatly hypertrophied muscle at the pyloric antrum. × 1·2.

this occurs more frequently as the result of scarring around a chronic gastric ulcer (p. 19.24). Persistent vomiting and failure of a neonate to thrive may also be due to congenital deficiency in the enzymes necessary for the metabolism of the sugars—galactose, lactose or sucrose—and these rare conditions may be mistaken for congenital pyloric stenosis.

IV: The Intestines

The pathology of the intestine is influenced considerably by the normal presence of bacteria in its lumen: lesions of the intestinal wall, whether due to ischaemia, neoplasia or of unknown cause, e.g. Crohn's disease or ulcerative colitis, are prone to undergo secondary bacterial infection, with the usual forms of inflammatory response. In addition, various pathogenic bacteria and parasites find a suitable environment in the intestine, and **infection** is much more important than in the stomach. Extensive mucosal lesions, particularly in the small intestine, can result in **malabsorption syndromes**, and a large number of conditions can cause **intestinal obstruction**. Finally, **carcinoma** is very common in the colon and rectum, but rare in the small intestine.

Although the small and large intestines each have their own specific diseases, these are relatively few, and most pathological processes affect them both similarly. For that reason the intestine is considered as a whole in most of the account which follows.

Ischaemic disease

Ischaemic lesions of the intestine vary greatly in extent, severity and causation. The most dramatic is classic **haemorrhagic infarction** which leads to gangrene and is usually caused by occlusion of the superior mesenteric artery (SMA) by thrombosis or embolism; less often it is due to thrombosis of the superior mesenteric vein. Infarction usually involves the area supplied by the occluded vessel, but may be less extensive if there is efficient anastomotic support from adjacent vessels. Severe narrowing of the SMA by atheroma does not as a rule lead to infarction but if associated with similar stenosis of the coeliac axis may cause the syndrome of **abdominal angina** which is characterised by postprandial pain (so severe that it may cause fear of food), weight loss and sometimes malabsorption.

Ischaemic disease may, however, be more focal in distribution and not clearly related in extent to the supply of a major vessel. Such **focal lesions** may occur in the small or large bowel. They are sometimes due to disease of small blood vessels, and in particular to the arteritis of rheumatoid arthritis, polyarteritis nodosa or systemic lupus erythematosus (pp. 14.26–28). Another cause of focal ischaemia is inadequate perfusion of intestinal arteries. The splenic flexure of the large bowel is the area most likely to be affected in this way. This site is supplied by the inferior mesenteric artery, the origin of which is often narrowed or occluded by atheroma, and may be destroyed by surgical operations such as aortic bifurcation graft performed for aortic aneurysm. Surprisingly, occlusion of such a major vessel may not have serious consequences if there are effective anastomotic vessels linking the SMA and the superior haemorrhoidal artery. Even so, this watershed zone is vulnerable to hypoperfusion during episodes of generalised circulatory embarrassment as in acute (or exacerbations of chronic) cardiac failure. The effects of this depend on the duration of hypoperfusion and vary from slight mucosal damage which produces little more than an episode of rectal bleeding and heals completely, to full-thickness necrosis of the colonic wall with subsequent gangrene. Occasionally, necrosis of the mucosa and submucosa is followed by healing with scarring and formation of a stricture. In such cases, the mucosal damage is exploited by commensal bacteria in the intestine and inflammatory changes develop (Fig. 19.42), hence the term **ischaemic colitis** and the difficulty sometimes encountered in distinguishing it from primary inflammatory bowel disease.

Ischaemic change may develop in the large bowel proximal to obstructive lesions, especially carcinoma, presumably because the increased intraluminal pressure interferes with mucosal perfusion. 'Stercoral' ulceration (p. 19.56) may sometimes be produced in this way.

The term **ischaemic enterocolitis** is applied to multiple randomly distributed foci of ischaemic damage involving both the small and large intestine. This may occur in congestive cardiac failure, uraemia, endotoxic or post-traumatic, shock. The exact mechanisms operating in such

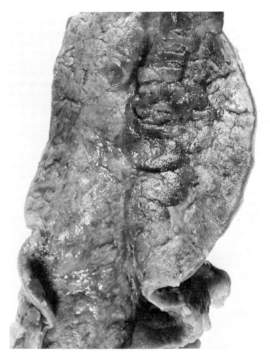

Fig. 19.42 Ischaemic colitis in an elderly woman. The lesion was multifocal in the transverse and descending colon. The area illustrated shows pseudomembranous inflammation, but there were older lesions with submucosal fibrosis and narrowing. Although ischaemic, the exact causation of such lesions is not clear (*see text*).

states are mostly unknown, but spasm of intestinal vessels complicating hypotension or disseminated intravascular coagulation (p. 17.67) may be involved in some cases. A variant of this condition is encountered in newborn infants and is termed **neonatal necrotising entero-**

colitis. The cause is unknown: premature infants are especially affected, and it has been suggested that hypoxia during the neonatal period is an important factor. Clostridial infection has also been implicated in some cases.

Inflammatory conditions of uncertain aetiology

Inflammatory lesions are very common in both the large and small intestines. Some are clearly of infective nature (p. 19.43), but some are of unknown cause, and as infections come increasingly under control this latter group assumes greater importance: it is commonly termed **inflammatory bowel disease** (IBD) and the two most important examples are Crohn's disease and ulcerative colitis. In addition, inflammation occurs commonly in the appendix and in relation to diverticula. The intestine may also be inadvertently damaged by drugs or irradiation treatment of disease elsewhere.

and distal extension into the caecum and ascending colon is common. The colon may also be involved primarily, especially in the older age groups, and many cases of segmental or right-sided forms of colitis, previously classified as cases of ulcerative colitis (p. 19.36), are, in fact, examples of Crohn's disease. The lesion is characterised by intense oedematous thickening of the bowel wall, the submucosa being especially involved, and there is marked narrowing of the lumen (Fig. 19.43). Ulceration of the oedematous mucosa is invariable and often assumes a linear form to produce the typical 'cobblestone' appearance (Fig. 19.44). Fissures

Crohn's disease

This is a chronic granulomatous inflammatory disease of unknown cause. The lesions may involve any part of the alimentary tract, from mouth to anus, but the distal ileum is most often affected——hence the earlier name, *regional enteritis*.

Clinical features. Young adults of both sexes are most frequently affected, and there is some evidence of familial incidence, although this is not striking. The symptoms are ill-defined at first, mild diarrhoea and vague abdominal pain being the usual complaints. Later, subacute or chronic intestinal obstruction develops and may require excision of the narrowed segment of bowel. The disease runs a prolonged course, with long remissions, and recurrence after operation occurs in about 50% of cases. Malabsorption and protein-losing enteropathy can result from repeated and extensive involvement of the small intestine.

Naked-eye appearances. The changes are most often observed in the distal ileum. 'Skip lesions' separated from the main lesion by apparently healthy bowel are sometimes found,

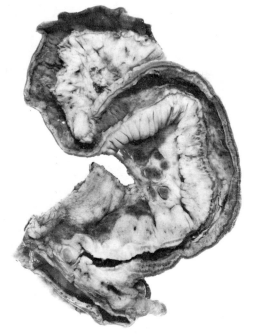

Fig. 19.43 Crohn's disease, showing diffuse thickening of the wall of the lower part of the ileum, with narrowing of its lumen.

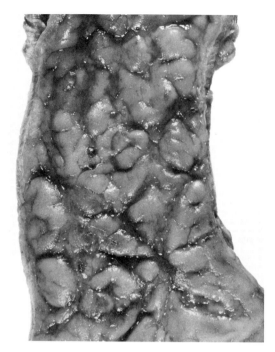

Fig. 19.44   The ileum in Crohn's disease, showing the 'cobblestone' appearance of the fissured, oedematous mucosa.

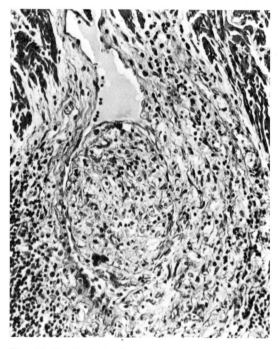

Fig. 19.45   Crohn's disease, showing a granulomatous lesion occluding a lymphatic in the muscle coat of the ileum. × 200.

penetrating the entire thickness of the bowel wall, and sometimes developing into fistulas opening into adjacent loops of intestine or the urinary bladder, are characteristic. The mesentery is usually thickened and oedematous and the regional lymph nodes conspicuously enlarged.

Microscopic appearances. It is characteristic of Crohn's disease that the *inflammatory changes extend throughout the entire thickness of the bowel wall* (*c.f. ulcerative colitis, below*). The most constant change is focal lymphocytic infiltration, usually most prominent in the submucosa. Of greater diagnostic value, however, is the presence, in about 60% of cases, of *epithelioid-cell granulomas* which resemble closely those of sarcoidosis: they may occur in all the layers of the bowel wall and even in the mesentery and mesenteric lymph nodes. Sometimes they arise in relation to lymphoid aggregates, but more often they are found in and around lymphatic channels (Fig. 19.45). Lymphatic obstruction and dilatation are, however, almost always found in early cases, and lymphatic obstruction is thought to be of primary importance in the pathogenesis of the disease. Certainly this accounts for the *marked oedema* which is always most conspicuous in the submucosa (Fig. 19.46) and is mainly responsible for the thickening of the bowel wall and mesentery in the early stages of the disease. *Fibrosis*, however, becomes increasingly prominent in more chronic cases. The mucosal changes, such as *ulceration* and subsequent *metaplasia* to pyloric type glands, are mainly due to *secondary infection* of the lesions. The increasing use of endoscopic biopsy techniques has shown that granulomas are by no means rare in the mucosa, especially in the colon, and commonly develop in close relationship to the crypts of Lieberkuhn (Fig. 19.47). A further change of diagnostic value is the presence of *fissures* which arise from ulcer bases and may penetrate the whole thickness of the bowel wall. Microscopically, they are lined by granulation tissue with foci of suppuration due to secondary bacterial infection. Although the destructive inflammatory lesions of Crohn's disease are usually of patchy distribution, it has been demonstrated recently that mucosal inflammation may be diffuse, at least in the colon.

Aetiology. There is no convincing evidence that Crohn's disease is related to sarcoidosis

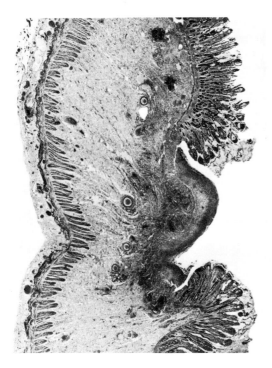

Fig. 19.46 Crohn's disease showing oedematous thickening, especially of the submucosa, with focal inflammatory infiltration and ulceration. × 12.

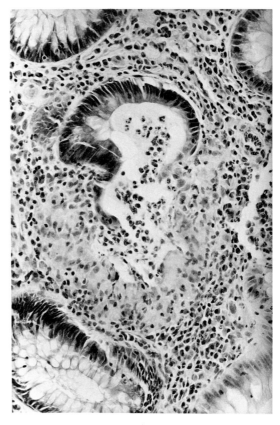

Fig. 19.47 Crohn's disease, showing disruption of a crypt of the colonic mucosa and an associated epithelioid-cell granuloma. × 200.

(p. 9.26), which rarely affects the intestinal tract. It is of interest, however, that as in sarcoidosis, abnormalities of cell-mediated immunity have been reported and in some instances the disease has been found to respond to the therapeutic use of immunosuppressive drugs such as aza-thioprine. There is a possibility that Crohn's disease is caused by hypersensitivity to a particular type of micro-organism, possibly a virus, and that susceptibility to the disease has an immunological basis.

Complications. As mentioned above, surgical resection of narrowed bowel may be necessary, but the risks of fistula formation in relation to the surgical wound and of recurrence of the disease are considerable. Spontaneous peri-anal fistulas are not uncommon and may develop early, especially in the colonic form of the disease: the detection of epithelioid-cell granulomas in the wall of such fistulas is of diagnostic help. Iron-deficiency anaemia is common, and occasionally a macrocytic anaemia results from interference with vitamin B_{12} absorption, which takes place exclusively in the ileum. Other features of malabsorption syndrome (p. 19.51)

may develop, especially in diffuse jejuno-ileal forms of the disease. As in ulcerative colitis, systemic complications may occur. These include arthritis, uveitis and skin lesions. It is now recognised that there is an increased risk of carcinoma in both the small and large intestine in patients with Crohn's disease.

Ulcerative colitis

This condition, of unknown cause, is particularly serious and by no means uncommon. It behaves as a distinct clinical and pathological entity, although it may be difficult to distinguish, particularly in the early stages, from other inflammatory diseases of the colon, notably Crohn's disease.

Clinical features. The disease mainly affects young adults of both sexes and is characterised by episodes of diarrhoea with the passage of blood per rectum. Malaise, anorexia and weight loss vary greatly in degree. Most cases follow a chronic relapsing course with exacerbations and remissions. Some are mild and possibly self-limiting, but a few run a more severe, continuous course and fulminating rapidly fatal forms are by no means rare.

Naked-eye appearances. Ulcerative colitis typically involves the sigmoid colon and rectum either alone or in continuity with the remainder of the colon. The entire colon is affected in about half of the cases, and in such instances the terminal ileum may also be inflamed. In some cases the proximal colon, with or without the terminal ileum, is principally affected. It is now recognised, however, that many such 'segmental' or 'right-sided' forms of colitis are examples of Crohn's disease (p. 19.33) and others may have an ischaemic origin.

In its early phases, sigmoidoscopy shows the

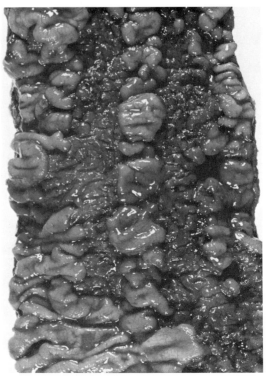

Fig. 19.49 The colon in chronic ulcerative colitis. The mucosa is extensively ulcerated and the surviving portions are swollen and hyperplastic with many undermined bridges of mucosa. × 0·8.

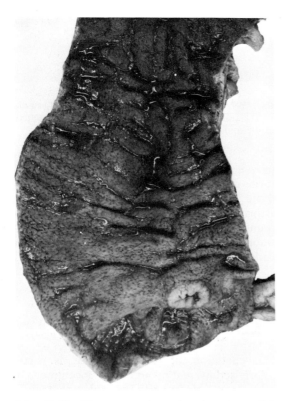

Fig. 19.48 The caecum in early ulcerative colitis with intense congestion, haemorrhage and multiple pin-point ulcers of mucosa. The appendicular orifice is shown, and in this case is not affected. × 0·7.

colonic mucosa to be deeply congested, velvety in appearance, and to bleed easily (Fig. 19.48). Punctate erosions herald the onset of ulceration, which usually begins in the rectum or sigmoid and is found initially at the tips of the mucosal folds overlying the longitudinal muscle bands. Later the ulcers coalesce, giving rise to large irregular areas of mucosal denudation associated with extensive muco-purulent discharge and haemorrhage. Between the ulcers, especially in chronic cases, the surviving mucosa becomes swollen and hyperplastic (Fig. 19.49) and in some instances numerous polypoid excrescences are seen, a condition known as *pseudo-polyposis*. Attempts at healing take place during remissions, but fibrous thickening and stenosis of the lumen are relatively uncommon. During relapses, the colon is spastic and the early loss of the normal sacculation produces a characteristic radiological appearance.

In severe cases or during exacerbations the colon may become greatly dilated—*'toxic dila-*

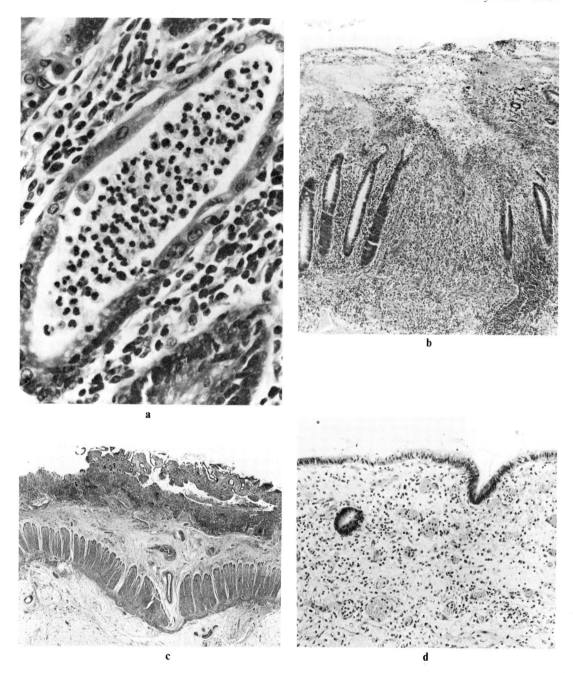

Fig. 19.50 Ulcerative colitis. (**a**) Crypt abscess. × 425. (**b**) Early mucosal ulceration with purulent exudate. × 70. (**c**) Chronic stage: complete loss of mucosa on the left, with undermining of surviving mucosa on the right. × 13. (**d**) Healing stage showing granulation tissue covered by a simple mucosa. × 115.

tation' (see below) and the stretched wall may perforate.

Microscopic appearances. Unlike Crohn's disease, it is the mucosa which is primarily in-

volved in ulcerative colitis. During active phases it is congested and densely infiltrated with leucocytes, especially plasma cells. The formation of *crypt abscesses* (Fig. 19.50a), characterised by accumulation of neutrophils, eosinophils, red cells and mucus within crypt lumina, is a conspicuous feature, although by no means specific for ulcerative colitis (see Fig. 19.47). The epithelial lining of the crypts degenerates and ultimately breaks down, releasing infected material into the lamina propria mucosae. This lesion leads to the appearance of frank ulceration (Fig. 19.50*b*), which is produced by the coalescence of ruptured crypt abscesses in the deeper parts of the mucosa. The base of the ulcers is formed by vascular granulation tissue (Fig. 19.50*c*) containing large numbers of macrophages, plasma cells and lymphocytes, the latter becoming increasingly conspicuous in chronic cases. Ulceration seldom extends more deeply than the submucosa, but the muscularis propria may be involved in severe cases and this may contribute to the development of toxic dilatation (see below). An important feature of such severe cases is the herniation of inflamed mucosa through the lamina muscularis mucosae: this phenomenon may lead to extensive submucosal suppuration (lacunar abscesses) and when the overlying mucosa disintegrates large areas of deeply penetrative ulceration develop. The pseudo-polyps observed in chronic cases consist of islands of surviving hyperplastic mucosa and tags of granulation tissue; they are not true polypoid adenomas (p. 19.63), although carcinoma is a common complication in longstanding cases. Surface reepithelialisation of ulcerated areas may take place but the healed mucosa contains few glands (Fig. 19.50*d*). An increase in Paneth cells in the crypts of Lieberkühn is noted especially in the proximal colon. This is probably metaplastic in nature, and may be associated in severe cases with gastric metaplasia.

Complications. The most urgent of **local complications** is *perforation of the colon*, which is usually associated with pronounced dilatation of the colon ('*toxic dilatation*'). This complication may be due to superimposed infection, or precipitated by the use of antispasmodic drugs. *Peri-anal fistulae* may be troublesome in some cases. Although simple fibrous strictures are uncommon, it is now recognised that the development of *carcinoma* of the colon is a considerable risk. It occurs most commonly in cases in which the entire colon is involved, the onset is early in life and the disease has been active for 10 years or more (see p. 19.65); the risk is such as to

provide an indication for total colectomy in some instances.

By repeated biopsy, it is possible to detect the development of premalignant epithelial dysplasia (Fig. 12.10, p. 12.8), which usually starts in a flat (as opposed to polypoid) mucosa: the changes include nuclear pleomorphism, hyperchromatism, loss of polarity and increased mitotic activity in the epithelial cells (Morson, 1978).

The various **systemic complications** include fever and leucocytosis, and debilitating diarrhoea with haemorrhage and exudation leads to protein depletion and anaemia. Arthritis, iridocyclitis and skin lesions, such as erythema nodosum and pyoderma gangrenosum, are seen in a proportion of cases. There appears to be an association between joint disease, especially ankylosing spondylitis, and chronic inflammatory disease of the intestine. Liver disease, of which chronic pericholangitis is the most characteristic and frank cirrhosis the most severe, is not infrequent in ulcerative colitis.

Aetiology. The cause of ulcerative colitis remains an unsolved problem. The disease is commonest in affluent societies and shows a familial incidence. No specific micro-organism has been isolated, although it is notable that certain types of colonic infection, especially amoebiasis (p. 28.14) may closely resemble ulcerative colitis pathologically. *A search for Entamoeba histolytica and other known pathogens should always be undertaken in suspected cases.* The possibility that ulcerative colitis has an immunological basis is tenuous. Antibodies which react with colonic epithelium (and also with *Esch. coli* 0119 B14) are present in the serum in some cases, and there is evidence also of cell-mediated immunity to colonic epithelium, but these findings have not been shown to be specific for ulcerative colitis, and may be secondary phenomena.

Other non-specific intestinal lesions

Eosinophilic gastro-enteritis. In this disease segments of the stomach or small intestine are extensively infiltrated by eosinophils and often markedly oedematous. When the submucosa is mainly affected, obstructive symptoms predominate; if the mucosa is involved there may be malabsorption or protein-losing enteropathy. It is probably an allergic reaction to dietary constituents or metazoan parasites and is often accompanied by eosinophil leucocytosis.

Inflammatory fibroid polyp is a term applied to certain localised lesions of stomach or small bowel, in which exuberant granulation tissue accompanied by eosinophilic infiltration produces a mass which protrudes into the lumen of the gut and may cause intussusception. The cause is not known.

Non-specific ulcers of the intestine. Solitary ulcers of a non-specific nature are occasionally encountered both in the small bowel and colon. In most instances the causation is unknown. Recently, however, it has been suggested that administration of enteric-coated tablets of potassium chloride in association with the diuretic chlorothiazide is responsible in some instances.

Solitary ulcer of the rectum. This term is used to describe a recurrent ulcerative condition, which usually affects young adults and presents a distinctive appearance in rectal biopsies. The mucosa shows variable inflammatory change with irregular superficial ulceration, and fibro-muscular thickening of the lamina propria. There may also be displacement of crypt epithelium into the submucosa with subsequent cyst formation. These changes are thought to be related to muscular spasm possibly related to chronic straining at stool, and have also been observed in association with rectal prolapse.

Colitis cystica profunda. This rare condition is to be regarded more as a pathological phenomenon than as a distinct disease entity. It is caused by the displacement of epithelium into the colonic submucosa with subsequent cyst formation. It is commonly a consequence of mucosal inflammation and may be observed in the vicinity of solitary ulcers (see above). Cyst formation in the mucosa (*colitis cystica superficialis*) has been described in pellagra and in malabsorption states.

Cronkite-Canada syndrome. In this rare and usually fatal condition, diffuse gastro-intestinal polyposis is associated with skin pigmentation, alopecia and atrophy of the nails. There may be severe diarrhoea, vomiting and enteric protein loss. A notable feature is the presence of microscopic mucus retention cysts in the intestinal mucosa. Infective and toxic causal agents have been postulated, but it is probably of nutritional origin.

Functional disorders of the colon. In clinical practice it is by no means uncommon to encounter patients who have constipation, mucous stool and lower abdominal pain, in whom organic lesions cannot be demonstrated.

'Mucous colitis', in which membranous structures composed of inspissated mucus are passed by the bowel, is probably a variant of this syndrome.

Although a variety of names has been attached to such states, the term 'irritable colon syndrome' is most commonly employed, and finds justification in the fact that the colon may be found to exhibit unusual irritability or hypermotility. The causation is obscure—indeed this syndrome may possibly include more than one disease entity—although previous organic disease, for example dysentery, psychological disturbance and dietary indiscretion might be involved.

Acute appendicitis

This lesion is of the highest importance because of its frequency and serious complications. Individuals of either sex and of virtually any age may be affected but the disease is commonest in children and young adults.

Naked-eye appearances. The condition occurs in three forms: *simple acute, suppurative* and *gangrenous* appendicitis. The first two of these types are different degrees of severity of the same condition; the third has special features of its own. Perforation may occur in both suppurative and gangrenous types.

In all cases the whole thickness of the wall is involved. In the earlier stages of simple or suppurative appendicitis the appendix is swollen, tense and markedly congested, and there may be a little fibrin on the surface (Fig. 19.51). When the appendix is cut across, the mucosa bulges owing to the swelling, and turbid exudate may escape from the lumen.

In other cases the changes are of greater severity. The primary inflammatory lesion may progress to a small abscess in the wall, and this may perforate. There may occur also more general suppuration and necrosis with multiple abscesses and perforations. The presence of a concretion (*faecolith*) in the lumen may predispose to perforation because, in acute appendicitis, the swollen wall becomes stretched over the concretion with consequent ischaemia and gangrene.

Gangrenous appendicitis (Fig. 19.51) is due to acute appendicitis complicated by thrombosis of the veins in the meso-appendix, with consequent haemorrhage and arrest of the circulation. In some cases, however, gangrene develops early and rapidly and affects the whole appendix apart from any vascular lesion: in such cases, gangrene is due to obstruction at the outlet of the appendix and distension with faecal material, or to the presence of a faecolith

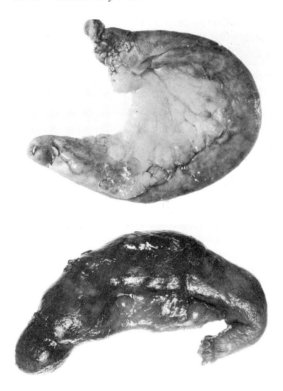

Fig. 19.51 Acute appendicitis. *Above*, showing swelling and congestion and dulling of the serosal surface by fibrin. *Below*, gangrenous appendicitis, showing swelling, haemorrhage and fibrin deposition.

(see above). Experimentally a closed portion of small intestine filled with faecal material becomes gangrenous within a short time, and many cases of so-called fulminating, i.e. gangrenous, appendicitis are of this nature. The great danger of gangrenous appendicitis is the early development of general peritonitis due to mixed bacterial infection, including anaerobes.

Microscopic appearances. In most cases of acute appendicitis, there is an acute inflammatory reaction involving the entire thickness of the appendicular wall, with a fibrinopurulent exudate on the peritoneal surface. This inflammatory reaction probably originates from a focus of mucosal ulceration, possibly in the deeper parts of the epithelial crypts with subsequent extension into the lamina propria (Fig. 19.52). Several foci of inflammation are sometimes observed, but the changes are usually most marked in the distal part (i.e. the blind end) of the appendix. Sometimes the inflam-

mation is localised and can easily be missed on cursory examination. In some patients with an appendicitis-like syndrome the only changes seen are pus cells in the appendicular lumen, associated with either foci of polymorph infiltration in the superficial parts of the mucosa, or occasional crypt abscesses. The clinical significance of such limited forms of appendicitis is debatable since similar changes are sometimes seen in appendices removed prophylactically during the course of some other operation, e.g. hysterectomy.

Clinical features. Acute appendicitis presents typically as colicky abdominal pain in the umbilical region, due to spasmodic contractions of the inflamed appendix. This is followed by a continuous 'burning' pain, tenderness and rigidity of the abdominal muscles, in the vicinity of the appendix. These latter features are due to irritation of the parietal peritoneum by the inflamed appendiceal serosa, and they may be inconspicuous or absent when the appendix is retrocaecal. Vomiting, pyrexia, increased pulse rate and neutrophil leucocytosis are inconstant features.

The diagnosis of acute appendicitis is often difficult and gangrenous appendicitis may be accompanied by remarkably slight clinical upset. The

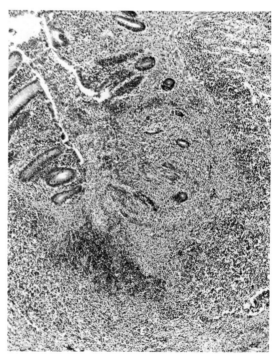

Fig. 19.52 Acute appendicitis, showing a local ulcerative lesion in mucosa with commencing abscess formation beneath. × 60.

results of delay in removing an acutely inflamed appendix (see below) are so serious that exploratory laparotomy is often necessary in cases where the diagnosis is far from certain.

Complications. Acute appendicitis gives rise to important complications. In some cases there is merely a slight amount of fibrinous exudate on the surface, which does not spread and may afterwards become organised, resulting in local adhesions. In others, a localised collection of pus may form around the appendix—**appendix abscess**. Sometimes an escaped concretion is present in the pus. The pus may track upwards alongside the caecum and ascending colon and between the surface of the liver and the diaphragm. Alternatively, an abscess may develop in, or extend into, the pelvic cavity. Such abscesses may be persistent, with increasing surrounding fibrosis, or they may discharge, e.g. from the pelvis into the rectum. In other cases, **generalised peritonitis** may develop, and this can happen very rapidly in gangrenous appendicitis. Other complications of appendicitis are due to infection of the veins. There may be a local septic phlebitis, and from this emboli may be carried to the liver, where they set up secondary abscesses. Rarely, a spreading thrombosis with secondary suppuration may extend up the portal vein—*portal pylephlebitis* (p. 20.37).

Aetiology. Although the lesions of acute appendicitis are due to *bacterial infection*, the factors which trigger it off are still largely unknown. There is even uncertainty about which organisms primarily invade the wall, although there is no doubt that the important effects are caused by coliform bacilli, streptococci and anaerobic bacteria, all of which are normally present in the lumen. It seems certain, however, that *obstruction* of the appendicular lumen is involved in many cases and, as already mentioned, gangrenous appendicitis is often produced in this way. Less easy to explain is the cause of the obstruction; foreign bodies and intestinal parasites, e.g. *Oxyuris vermicularis*, have been blamed from time to time, but in many cases are absent. A more promising suggestion is that obstruction is caused, particularly in childhood, by swelling of the appendicular lymphoid tissue, due possibly to viral infection, or, as has recently been demonstrated, by infection with *Yersinia enterocolitica*, an organism also known to produce acute mesenteric lymphadenitis (which incidentally can mimic acute appendicitis clinically). The part played by faecal concretions, or faecoliths, which are hard masses of faeces mixed with mucus and occasionally calcium salts, is difficult to assess, since these are commonly found even in normal appendices. As explained above, a *concretion* is likely to cause ischaemia and gangrene in an acutely inflamed appendix. It is notable that appendicitis, like diverticular disease (see below), is essentially a disease of developed countries, and it might well be that, as Burkitt has claimed, refined diets lacking in roughage are of importance in its pathogenesis.

Recurrent and chronic appendicitis and mucocele of the appendix. Recurrent acute appendicitis is not unusual in cases where the initial attack has been relatively mild and has been treated conservatively. If there is no history of an acute attack, recurrent abdominal pain without localising symptoms is unlikely to be due to appendicitis.

Fibrous thickening of the wall of the appendix, especially in young people, may be a consequence of acute inflammation. Occasionally, fibrosis may be the result of persistent chronic infection—the so-called *chronic appendicitis*—and there may be no history of an acute attack. It is conceivable that mild attacks of abdominal pain in the region of the appendix are due to this ('appendicular dyspepsia'). It should be emphasised, however, that in older individuals asymptomatic appendicular fibrosis is extremely common and can almost be regarded as a normal ageing process.

A common result of a localised lesion of the appendix is obliteration of the lumen at that point, whilst elsewhere the mucosa may be comparatively well preserved. This may be readily explained by the commonly focal nature of acute appendicitis. When localised obliteration is present, dilatation of the distal portion of the lumen may follow (Fig. 19.53). This may be slight, or there may be a cyst-like enlargement filled with mucus—**mucocele**.

Occasionally a mucocele ruptures and the mucus leaks into the peritoneum, where it becomes organised, resulting in peritoneal adhesions. The condition known as *pseudomyxoma peritonei* may be produced in this way; it is more likely, however, that serious forms of this condition, in which mucus-secreting cells seed throughout the peritoneum, are due to mucus-secreting neoplasms of the appendix.

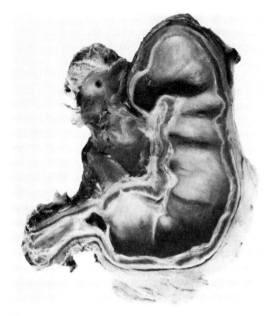

Fig. 19.53 Chronic appendicitis with obliteration at the proximal end and mucocele of the distal portion.

Another quite common lesion is a *diverticulum*, which may project on the surface of the appendix, and is due to distension of part of the wall in which the muscle coat has been weakened, possibly by previous inflammation.

Diverticular disease

A diverticulum consists of protrusion of the mucous and submucous coats through the muscle of the wall: the projecting pouch has no muscle coat, and is properly called a 'false diverticulum', in contrast to a true diverticulum, e.g. Meckel's (p. 19.67), which has a complete layer of muscle like the bowel.

(a) Small intestine. Diverticula are uncommon in the small bowel. The duodenum is most often involved, followed by the jejunum and ileum in that order. The diverticula may be single or multiple and are invariably found along the mesenteric border of the bowel in close relationship to the entry-sites of the blood vessels. They may enlarge to over 3 cm in diameter.

Pathological effects. Small-bowel diverticula are seldom encountered before adult life; they probably cause abdominal symptoms more often than is generally realised. Frank inflammatory change, haemorrhage and obstruction are, however, rare complications. More often malabsorption similar to that in the 'blind-loop syndrome' (p. 19.54) is the principal feature: it is caused mainly by abnormal and excessive bacterial proliferation in the diverticula. Bacterial uptake of vitamin B_{12} before it can reach its main absorptive site in the distal ileum leads to vitamin B_{12} deficiency and megaloblastic anaemia, and it is probable that bacteria are also responsible for the steatorrhoea which is sometimes observed. Oral broad-spectrum antibiotics lead to improvement in both vitamin B_{12} and fat absorption.

(b) Colon. Multiple diverticula of the colon are very common in later adult life: in this country about one person in ten is affected, although in only 20% of cases does the condition produce symptoms. The sigmoid colon is most often involved, although diverticula may occur at a higher level, including the caecum. Characteristically they lie in two rows between the mesenteric and the anti-mesenteric taeniae and are related to the entry of blood vessels into the colonic wall. They commonly extend into the appendices epiploicae. Small depressions at first, they enlarge and become spherical or flask-shaped (Fig. 19.54), usually less than 1 cm in diameter. Diverticula frequently contain inspissated faeces and it is notable that muscle hypertrophy and thickening of the peri-colic fat are commonly observed in the adjacent bowel.

Pathological effects. Inflammatory change in the diverticula (*diverticulitis*) is the common cause of clinical symptoms, which are usually encountered in the older age groups. Acute inflammation leads to a syndrome resembling appendicitis with localisation of pain to the left side of the abdomen. This condition may progress to peri-colic abscess formation and even to free perforation into the peritoneal cavity and acute peritonitis. The development of fistulae between the colon and adjacent organs, especially the bladder, is not uncommon. More chronic diverticulitis leads to fibrous thickening of the colonic wall with some degree of intestinal obstruction, and the lesion may be mistaken macroscopically for carcinoma. There is no evidence that diverticular disease is a precancerous condition. Rarely severe rectal haemorrhage occurs, probably due to erosion of blood vessels in the diverticular wall.

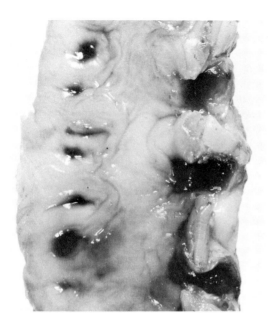

Fig. 19.54 Part of the sigmoid colon cut open to show the mucosal surface in diverticulosis. There are two longitudinal rows of diverticula: those on the right have been opened and can be seen to herniate through the muscle coat of the bowel.

Aetiology. It is generally accepted that diverticula are caused by high pressure within the bowel lumen leading to protrusion of the mucosa through points of weakness in the bowel wall. The latter are usually related to the entry of blood vessels from the mesocolon. Recent studies suggest that, at least in the colon, diverticula are associated with the generation of localised areas of unusually high intraluminal pressure by abnormal segmental contraction of the bowel musculature, and that the muscle hypertrophy related to diverticula is a morphological expression of this effect. It is notable that diverticular disease is mainly restricted to developed societies and the consumption of refined foods lacking in vegetable fibre may be the most important aetiological factor.

Intestinal infections

Many inflammatory conditions of the intestines, both acute and chronic, are produced by bacilli of the typhoid-coli group the most serious lesions being produced by *Salmonella typhi* and organisms of the *paratyphoid group*. The food-poisoning bacilli (*Salmonella typhimurium* etc.) cause acute diffuse mucosal inflammation of the small or large intestine. The *dysentery bacilli* affect chiefly the large intestine and cause both acute and chronic lesions. In all these cases, and also in *cholera*, infection is acquired by ingesting the specific micro-organisms in food or water contaminated by the excreta of cases of the disease or of carriers of the infection. Contamination by handling of food, or by the activities of flies, gives rise to sporadic cases or small outbreaks, but major epidemics are virtually always due to seepage of sewage into water supplies. An additional source of infection in food poisoning by *Salmonellae* is the soiling of food by the faeces of infected mice or rats. Bacteria of the genus *Campylobacter* have recently been implicated in outbreaks of infective diarrhoea, as have *rotaviruses* in infantile gastro-enteritis (p. 19.49). Chronic infections of the intestines are caused by *Myco. tuberculosis*, *Actinomyces israelii* and *Entamoeba histolytica*. Many *viruses* that produce no apparent lesion of the gut are nevertheless excreted in the faeces and are invasive when ingested, e.g. poliovirus and Coxsackieviruses.

The enteric fevers

This term is used to describe the illnesses caused by acute infections with *S. typhi* (typhoid fever) or *S. paratyphi* (paratyphoid fever).

Typhoid fever

This disease is caused by the Gram − ve bacillus *Salmonella typhi*. Corresponding with the clinical illness there are inflammatory changes and necrosis in the lymphoid tissue of the bowel, followed by healing.

Course. After an incubation period of about two weeks, the ingested organisms, which have already invaded the lymphoid tissues of the small intestine, enter the bloodstream, probably via the lymphatics. Bacteraemia is accompanied by progressive fever of insidious onset, sometimes with a 'staircase' rise: after a further week the characteristic rose spots appear in the skin. In the first week of the fever blood cultures are usually positive, thus confirming the diagnosis. About the end of ten days, immunity begins to develop and the organisms disappear from the bloodstream. Thereafter they persist in the liver and biliary passages and re-enter the small intestine in large numbers from the bile so that they are then readily detected in the faeces. During the bacteraemic phase, the lymphoid tissues of the gut and draining lymph nodes become acutely inflamed and progress through the stages described below. It is significant that the gallbladder bile is invariably infected during the bacteraemic phase, and the wall of the viscus may become inflamed, producing a typhoid cholecystitis. These phases in the distribution of the organisms are of decisive importance in the bacteriological diagnosis of the disease. The

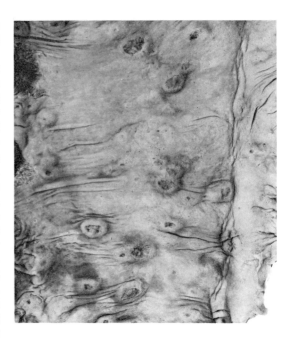

Fig. 19.56   Colon in typhoid fever showing swelling and ulceration of the lymphoid follicles.

course may be modified considerably by previous immunisation, and diagnosis may then be difficult both clinically and bacteriologically.

Naked-eye appearances. Re-infection of the lymphoid tissue of the gut by organisms in the bile leads to the development of lesions which are usually most marked in the Peyer's patches of the distal ileum, although solitary lymphoid follicles more proximally and distally are also affected. The lymphoid patches initially show an inflammatory swelling which is followed, usually about the tenth day of the illness, by necrosis and subsequent ulceration (Figs. 19.55, 19.56). Healing usually begins about the end of the third week and is complete by the fifth week in uncomplicated cases. The ulcers have a yellowish-brown or black colour, correspond in shape and extent to the lymphoid patches, and tend to have soft, shreddy, undermined margins. Healing of these ulcerated lesions leaves a smooth silky scar which never shows any tendency towards stricture formation. *Severe haemorrhage* sometimes occurs from these necrotic ulcerated lesions, although a more serious complication resulting from extensive necrosis is *perforation of the small bowel* with usually fatal generalised peritonitis. Clinically this latter event is seldom accompanied by the dramatic

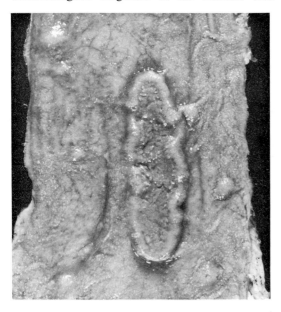

Fig. 19.55   The lower ileum in typhoid fever, showing necrosis and ulceration of the Peyer's patches and solitary lymphoid follicles.

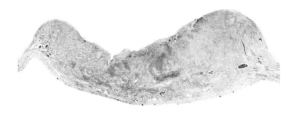

Fig. 19.57 Peyer's patch in the early stage of typhoid fever, showing the marked inflammatory swelling and commencing necrosis. × 5.

symptoms associated with gastroduodenal perforation, possibly because the alkaline intestinal contents have less irritant effect on the peritoneal cavity.

Microscopic appearances. The early changes are those of acute inflammation, but neutrophil polymorphs are absent. The enlargement of the Peyer's patches (Fig. 19.57) is thus due to congestion, oedema and the infiltration of inflammatory cells, predominantly lymphocytes, plasma cells and macrophages. Haemorrhage and fibrinous exudation often contribute to the inflammatory swelling. These inflammatory changes may extend deeply to involve the muscularis propria (Fig. 8.4, p. 8.15) and even the serosal coat. As the inflammatory lesion progresses, patchy necrosis develops with extensive nuclear karyorrhexis and the surrounding macrophages, sometimes called typhoid histiocytes, typically ingest the nuclear debris as well as extravasated red cells. The development of necrosis may well represent a delayed hypersensitivity reaction to bacterial antigens. Polymorphs are only seen in relation to ulceration and secondary infection. The **mesenteric lymph nodes** are commonly enlarged and show changes closely similar to those in the Peyer's patches (Figs. 18.4, p. 18.9 and 3.31, p. 3.31). The development of focal necrosis can lead to softening and rupture of the lymph node with subsequent peritonitis.

Associated lesions. The most characteristic change in the blood is a low leucocyte count—usually below $4 \times 10^9/l$ (4000/μl)—due to a decrease of neutrophil polymorphs: this is associated with diminished granulopoiesis in the bone marrow. Similarly the *spleen* (p. 18.4), although commonly enlarged, contains few neutrophils, contrary to what might be ex-

pected in a severe bacterial infection. Typhoid fever is associated with a great variety of lesions which are widely distributed and may arise during the course of the disease or later: they are due to endotoxaemia (p. 8.7) and bacteraemia.

Endotoxaemia may be responsible for the fever and produces degenerative changes in several organs, e.g. myocardial damage, which may precipitate heart failure, and focal necrosis of the abdominal muscles (Zenker's degeneration), which is characteristic. The liver and kidneys also show toxic injury. Typhoid endotoxaemia probably also impairs resistance to invasion by other bacteria and the well recognised development of *laryngitis, bronchitis* (sometimes an early symptom) and *pneumonia* may well be due to this. **Bacteraemia** brings about acute enlargement of the spleen and probably accounts for the characteristic rose-coloured spots in the skin. In some patients, infection persists in the gallbladder, with or without cholecystitis, and less commonly in the urinary tract. This is the pathological basis of the **carrier state**, since *patients thus affected excrete bacilli in the faeces or in the urine for varying periods and are commonly the source of outbreaks of typhoid fever*. Other lesions produced by circulating bacilli include endocarditis, meningitis and arthritis. Periostitis and osteomyelitis may develop after the acute illness, even years later. Perichondritis involving the costal and laryngeal cartilages are also well recognised complications.

Paratyphoid infections

Infections caused by the paratyphoid organism are not uncommon, paratyphoid B being the most frequent of the enteric fevers in West Europe. In some cases the disease has the general features of typhoid, though usually less severe. There is a similar involvement of the lymphoid tissue, especially the Peyer's patches and solitary follicles of the small intestine, with swelling of mesenteric nodes and spleen; but the necrotic and ulcerative processes are less marked and usually limited to the lower part of the ileum. In other cases a generalised mucosal inflammatory reaction is found, and there is little implication of the lymphoid tissue; sometimes enteritis is associated with marked gastritis. The 'carrier' condition may result also from paratyphoid infections, as has been described above in typhoid fever.

Other Salmonella infections

Many species of *Salmonellae* have been implicated in local outbreaks of bacillary food infection throughout the world. The most important of these are *S. enteritidis* and *S. typhimurium*. Such organisms produce an *acute gastro-enteritis* with fever, vomiting and diarrhoea developing 12–14 hours after eating the contaminated food. In most cases recovery is complete, but death from water and electrolyte depletion may occur in severe cases. It is also becoming increasingly recognised that *acute colitis* may be due to salmonellae (Day *et al.*, 1978).

Cholera

This disease is caused by *Vibrio cholerae* or its subtypes and is a classical example of a waterborne infection capable of causing explosive epidemics. Profuse watery diarrhoea is the outstanding clinical feature and the stools are often described as having a colourless 'rice-water' appearance. Diarrhoea leads to the loss of about 30 litres of fluid during an illness lasting 3–6 days, and the depletion of water and electrolytes, especially sodium and potassium, is extremely severe and often fatal.

It was formerly believed, from autopsy studies, that cholera caused an intense necrotising inflammation of the mucosa of the small intestine. Intestinal biopsies have shown, however, that the changes are minimal, and that inflammation, if present, is extremely mild. *Vibrio cholerae* is present in large numbers in the lumen, but does not invade the mucosa, and causes diarrhoea by producing an exotoxin which increases the net flow of fluid and electrolytes from the plasma into the lumen of the gut, particularly in the jejunum. The mechanism differs from that of inflammatory exudation, and the fluid has a low protein content. It is probable that cholera toxin exerts its effect by stimulating adenyl cyclase activity, thus increasing adenosine monophosphate which affects the equilibrium of fluid and electrolytes

between the mucosal cell and gut lumen. Oral administration of glucose and electrolyte solutions has been shown to be of great therapeutic value. Although the organisms are largely confined to the intestinal tract, they can become established in the gallbladder and lead to a carrier state which, although usually of short duration, may last as long as four years. It has also become apparent that the number of cases of cholera is far exceeded by the number of individuals who become infected and excrete the vibrio without developing the disease.

The **El Tor vibrio**, first isolated in Sinai, is closely related to *V. cholerae* and has been responsible for recent outbreaks of a cholera-like illness in various parts of the world.

Tuberculosis

Intestinal tuberculosis was formerly common, but in many countries the incidence is now low, partly because infection of milk by bovine tubercle bacilli has been eliminated, and partly as a consequence of the falling incidence of pulmonary tuberculosis. Three main forms of intestinal tuberculosis are recognised.

(a) Primary infection. The small bowel was formerly a common site for the primary tuberculous complex in children who had ingested cow's milk containing bovine tubercle bacilli. As elsewhere, the site of entrance of the organisms is inconspicuous, although this probably means that the lesion has been minute and has not spread, rather than that the bacilli have invaded without producing any lesion. The prominent change is produced in the mesenteric lymph nodes, which become greatly enlarged and caseous (tabes mesenterica). In favourable circumstances, the condition remains localised, and the calcified mesenteric nodes still quite often observed in the elderly represent the result of intestinal infection in early life. Occasionally, however, the disease spreads from the nodes to the peritoneal cavity leading to tuberculous peritonitis (p. 19.70).

(b) Secondary infection. Intestinal lesions used to be a common complication of open pulmonary tuberculosis, especially in children. This secondary form of intestinal tuberculosis, caused by swallowing sputum containing tubercle bacilli, causes ulcers of the intestine, but

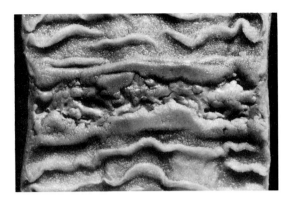

Fig. 19.58 Tuberculosis of the ileum causing transverse ulceration.

with only slight involvement of the mesenteric lymph nodes.

The small intestine is the common site of the lesions, which usually occur in the Peyer's patches or solitary lymphoid follicles. Initially, caseating tubercles develop in the mucosa and the submucosa, and subsequent mucosal breakdown leads to the formation of small ulcers, which become progressively enlarged by direct spread of the organisms to adjacent parts of the mucosa. Ultimately large ulcers are produced and these tend to extend by spread of infection along the lymphatics, transversely to the longitudinal axis of the bowel; sometimes indeed they encircle the gut (Fig. 19.58). The larger ulcers have an irregular outline, undermined edges and raised nodular margins (Fig. 19.59). The floor is uneven or granular and may be coated by caseous material, but tubercles are rarely visible. The serous coat overlying the ulcer is often thickened and opaque and the presence of visible tubercles along the lines of serosal lymphatics may be of diagnostic value.

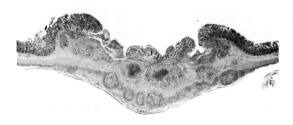

Fig. 19.59 Small tuberculous ulcer of small intestine with thickened and irregular margins and floor. Note the tubercles beneath the serosal surface: these are often visible at laparotomy. × 6.

Histologically, the tuberculous lesions are similar to those observed elsewhere: the ulceration extends through the mucosa into the submucous layer and there may be varying degrees of fibrous replacement of the muscular coat. Tubercles are usually found throughout the entire thickness of the bowel and in the related mesenteric lymph nodes, although the nodes are seldom as grossly affected as in the primary form.

Tuberculous ulceration rarely causes gross haemorrhage, and perforation into the peritoneal cavity is uncommon. The formation of fistulae between adjacent loops of bowel, initiated by the development of adhesions, may, however, lead to short-circuiting of bowel contents and malabsorption: the effects thus contrast with those of typhoid ulceration. The peritoneum may show frank tuberculous lesions (p. 19.70) or simply multiple fibrous adhesions which may cause mechanical obstruction of the bowel.

(c) 'Hyperplastic caecal tuberculosis'. This is usually secondary to pulmonary tuberculosis and is now rare in Europe and North America. It consists of gross fibrous thickening of the wall of a length of the caecum or ascending colon with ulceration of the surface and caseating tubercle follicles. Because it causes obstruction and is sometimes palpable, the lesion may be clinically suggestive of carcinoma. Pathologically, it may be confused with Crohn's disease affecting the caecum, and demonstration of tubercle bacilli by microscopy, culture or animal inoculation is important in order to make the differential diagnosis between the two conditions.

The **appendix** is occasionally affected in cases of intestinal tuberculosis. The changes are similar to those in the intestine and in some cases a faecal fistula develops following appendicectomy. More often, however, this sequence is attributable to Crohn's disease.

The dysenteries

The term dysentery was originally used to denote conditions of severe inflammation and ulceration of the colon, with diarrhoea, tenesmus and the passage of blood and mucus in the stools. Two main types of dysentery are distinguished, namely, *bacillary* and *amoebic*.

Bacillary dysentery

Bacillary dysentery is produced by bacilli of the *Shigella* species, of which there are several varieties, distinguishable by their serological and fermentative reactions. The mildest type is usually caused by *Shigella sonnei*, and in children is often called ileocolitis; more severe infections are caused by *Sh. flexneri*, and the most severe tropical form by *Sh. dysenteriae* (*Sh. shigae*), which produces a powerful exotoxin. The lesion is essentially inflammation of variable intensity in the colon, though the lower end of the ileum is sometimes also affected.

In mild cases the main features are intense mucosal inflammation with oedema, haemorrhage and excess mucus secretion. There may be some fibrinous exudation on the mucosal surface, but this is much more marked in severe cases in which there is extensive pseudomembrane formation with mucosal necrosis, and subsequent ulceration. The ulcers extend in an irregular manner and tend to have shredded margins. It is usual for healing to take place after the acute phase and the re-epithelialised ulcers assume a smooth and even appearance in contrast to the surrounding mucosa. The disease may, however, be prolonged and relapses are quite frequent. Such subacute or chronic cases are characterised by repeated ulceration and healing and can lead to polypoid mucosal irregularity with fibrous scarring and subsequent stenosis of the bowel. Bacillary dysentery may also be complicated by pyogenic bacterial infection of the portal venous system and focal suppuration in the liver.

Microscopically, the colonic mucosa shows intense inflammatory reaction in the lamina propria and polymorphs can be seen surrounding the mucosal crypts and invading the epithelial surfaces. The appearances resemble early ulcerative colitis (p. 19.37). The presence of numerous polymorphs admixed with red cells and mucus in the faeces is of presumptive diagnostic value.

Amoebic dysentery

This is caused by *Entamoeba histolytica* and is described on p. 28.14. It is only rarely acquired in temperate climates except in people who have acquired it in tropical and subtropical countries. Like ulcerative colitis, Crohn's dis-

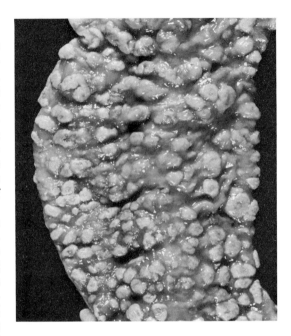

Fig. 19.60 Pseudomembranous colitis, showing the typical discrete raised patches of pseudomembrane and normal intervening mucosa. × 0·7.

ease and ischaemic colitis, it causes chronic ulceration of the colon and rectum and accurate diagnosis is extremely important as the treatment is quite different.

Antibiotic-associated pseudomembranous colitis

It is becoming increasingly recognised that various antibiotics, especially those of the clindamycin–lincomycin group and ampicillin, may be complicated by diarrhoea, and in many cases pathological changes can be found in the colon and occasionally also the distal ileum. In severe cases, which may be complicated by circulatory collapse and may be fatal, this takes the form of *pseudomembranous colitis*, characterised macroscopically by the appearance of raised yellowish-white plaques on the colonic mucosa (Fig. 19.60), which otherwise appears normal or at most slightly congested.

Histologically this disease process is initiated by focal damage to the intestinal epithelium with underlying acute inflammation. Subsequently a prominent adherent exudate or 'pseudomembrane', consisting of strands of fibrin and mucus with enmeshed neutrophils, arises from these foci of damage (Fig. 19.61). In severe cases the underlying mucosa shows progressive necrosis and crypt dilatation.

Recent studies have shown that pseudomembranous colitis of this kind is due to the action of exotoxin produced by *Clostridium difficile* under the promoting influence of antibiotics (p. 8.4). It now seems unlikely that similar pathological changes are caused by staphylococcal superinfection, although staphylococci can produce more widespread severe inflammatory changes in the intestinal mucosa.

Pseudomembrane formation may also be seen in association with other intestinal disturbances such as ischaemic disease (p. 19.32) and bacillary dysentery (p. 19.48).

Actinomycosis

As a path of entry for the branching, colony-forming Gram + ve bacterium *Actinomyces israelii*, the intestine comes next to the mouth in order of frequency. The lesions consist of suppuration and ulceration (p. 9.32) of the wall of the gut, with a tendency to spread to involve the peritoneum or adjacent loops of gut, abdominal wall, etc. with formation of sinuses and fistulas. The wall of the appendix seems to be the most common portal of entry; acute appendicitis may result and appendicectomy is liable to be followed by local recurrence and formation of fistulas. In some cases, the infection spreads beyond the appendix, usually to the wall of the caecum, before causing localising symptoms. In the peritoneum, loculated abscesses between the coils of intestine may discharge into the bowel. Diagnosis can usually be made by finding colonies of *Actinomyces* on microscopic examination. Secondary actinomycotic abscesses may occur in the liver.

Intestinal schistosomiasis

This disease, which is common in various tropical and subtropical parts of Africa and other countries, is produced by the dioecious trematode, *Schistosoma mansoni*. It is described on p. 28.26.

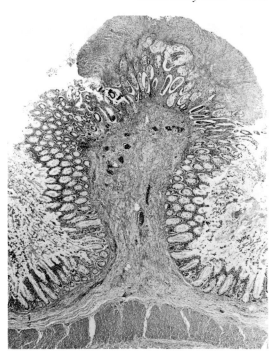

Fig. 19.61 Pseudomembranous colitis, showing one of the lesions. The mucosal glands are dilated and undergoing necrosis beneath the pseudomembrane. The thrombosis of submucosal blood vessels is a late event. × 12.

Gastro-enteritis of infancy

This infection, which can become epidemic in nurseries, carries a high mortality, usually attributable to fluid and electrolyte depletion resulting from diarrhoea and vomiting, in infants under 2 years of age. Despite this, the pathological changes are seldom impressive, although intestinal mucosal biopsies have shown epithelial damage associated with some increased leucocytic infiltration in the lamina propria and moderate degrees of villous atrophy. Indeed, villous atrophy may persist for some weeks after the acute episode and produce transient malabsorption. In fatal cases the liver often shows marked fatty change. The pathogenesis is sometimes uncertain but some serological types of *Escherichia coli* (for example 0111, 055 and 0119) are commonly blamed. Recently, virus particles have been demonstrated by electron microscopy, both in duodenal biopsies and in the faeces, in a substantial proportion of cases in which pathogenic bacteria have not

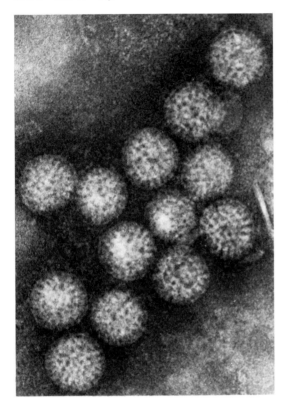

Fig. 19.62 Human rotavirus in a direct electron micrograph of centrifuged faecal extract. The complete virus particles, with the outer surface layer, are illustrated. × 200 000. (Professor C. R. Madeley, Department of Virology, University of Newcastle upon Tyne.)

been isolated. Of the various types which have been described, the best recognised are the *rotaviruses*, so called because of their cart-wheel morphology (Fig. 19.62).

Other specific intestinal infections

Yersinial disease. Bacteria of the genus *Yersinia*, especially *Y. enterocolitica* and *Y. pseudotuberculosis*, are capable of producing a variety of acute inflammatory lesions in the alimentary tract. These organisms have a predilection for the gut-associated lymphoid tissue, and are responsible for some cases of acute ileitis, acute appendicitis (p. 19.41) and acute mesenteric adenitis, any of which may be associated with acute pharyngitis. Histologically the characteristic feature of these infections is the development of foci of suppuration within lymphoid aggregates and in the case of *Y. pseudotuberculosis* those lesions may be surrounded by a mantle of macrophages, resembling closely the lesion of lymphogranuloma venereum (p. 25.3).

Clostridial disease. It is well recognised that some self-limiting cases of *food poisoning* are due to the ingestion of food contaminated by *Cl. welchii*. In malnourished individuals, however, the ingestion of heavily contaminated food may produce a severe and often fatal form of *necrotising enteritis*. This has been observed, especially in children, in E. Africa and New Guinea, where it is known as 'pig-bel' since it follows the consumption of infected porcine offal at wedding feasts. The most dramatic form of clostridial disease is *botulism*, which is caused by the ingestion of improperly cooked food in which *Cl. botulinum* has been permitted to grow and produce a powerful exotoxin capable of producing muscular weakness and paralysis. Death commonly results from respiratory paralysis and aspiration pneumonia.

Staphylococcal disease. Some of the most dramatic forms of *food poisoning* are due to the ingestion of food contaminated with staphylococcal enterotoxin, which is capable of producing acute gastroenteritis. Fortunately it is self-limiting. Staphylococcal *infection* may be implicated in some cases of antibiotic associated diarrhoea.

Campylobacter infections. It has recently been shown that infections with the vibrio-like organisms of the Campylobacter genus are often responsible for infective diarrhoea. The inflammatory lesions are sometimes found in the small intestine but an acute colitis is a commoner finding.

Sexually-transmitted disease. It is becoming increasingly recognised that a wide variety of infections of the distal large intestine can be caused by sexual contact (pp. 25.1–5). This occurs in both sexes, but especially among the active male homosexual population. Of particular importance in this respect are syphilitic and gonorrhoeal forms of proctitis, and most cases of chlamydial infection, such as lymphogranuloma venereum (LGV, p. 25.3) and chlamydial proctitis in males probably arise in this way. The latter is a distinctive granulomatous proctitis not unlike early Crohn's disease (p. 19.34). In females with LGV the distal large bowel may become involved as a result of lymphatic spread of the infection from the genital tract, the most notable outcome of this being the lesion known as inflammatory stricture of the rectum.

The malabsorption syndrome

The products of digestion of food are absorbed almost exclusively from the small intestine, and accordingly most extensive pathological processes in the small intestine interfere with this important function to some degree. The absorption of some nutrients may be restricted to certain relatively well-defined parts of the small bowel; iron, for example, is absorbed mainly from the duodenum and vitamin B12 from the distal ileum. Depending thus upon the extent, site and nature of the disease process, the absorption of some constituents of the diet may be affected more than others. In severe cases, all nutrients including protein, fat, carbohydrates, vitamins, minerals and even water may fail to be adequately absorbed. Failure to absorb fat is the most prominent feature in most cases and on it depend some of the other deficiencies.

Clinical features. The clinical manifestations of malabsorption vary accordingly. The most common symptom is chronic diarrhoea; the stools are pale, bulky and foul-smelling and contain an excess of fat (**steatorrhoea**) and of nitrogenous material. In severe cases, loss of weight, muscle wasting, dehydration and hypotension are prominent features. Hypoglycaemia with abnormally low glucose tolerance curve indicates failure of carbohydrate uptake. Hypoproteinaemia, associated with oedema, may be the result not only of impaired amino-acid absorption, but also of protein leakage into the bowel lumen (**protein-losing enteropathy**)—a feature of many gastro-intestinal diseases. Vitamin deficiencies are common, and symptoms of beri-beri, pellagra, scurvy and rickets in children, may be presenting features of the syndrome. Anaemia frequently dominates the clinical picture; usually it is microcytic and attributed to iron deficiency but macrocytic anaemia following failure to absorb vitamin B12 or folic acid is by no means unusual. It is rare for all of those features to be noted together, and any one deficiency may predominate; biochemical tests, however, usually reveal more extensive malabsorption than is clinically evident.

Peroral intestinal biopsy. This technique, now widely used, is of great help in the diagnosis and investigation of malabsorptive disturbances. Biopsy makes it possible to assess not only the morphological state of the mucosa but also the enzyme content of the absorptive epithelium and the bacterial content of the intestinal lumen.

Under the dissecting microscope, the normal jejunal mucosa has tall, slender finger-shaped villi interspersed with occasional broader leaf-shaped villi, which are more conspicuous in the duodenum. The villi measure about $400\,\mu m$ in height and usually account for about 70% of the total mucosal thickness. In tropical residents, however, the villi are more often leaf-shaped and may even fuse to form short ridges. Histologically, moreover, they appear shorter and broader than their temperate counterparts. The cause of this geographical variation in jejunal morphology is not known.

The absorptive epithelial cells lining the villi are formed in the crypts of Lieberkühn and gradually ascend the villi before being extruded into the lumen after a life-span of about 3 days. These cells are the principal source of the digestive enzymes of the succus entericus, and the final stage in the digestion of many nutrients takes place in the vicinity of the innumerable microvilli which form the epithelial surface. Malabsorptive disturbance may be caused by deficiency of intestinal enzymes, especially the disaccharidases.

Villous atrophy (Fig. 19.63) is the commonest pathological change in mucosal pattern. In the *partial* form (PVA) the villi show extensive fusion with the formation of long ridges or convolutions; histologically they appear shorter and broader than normal, although the crypts are enlarged and hyperplastic. The villous epithelium often shows degenerative change, and there is little doubt that the fundamental disturbance is a shortening of the life-span of these cells with compensatory hyperplasia of the generative crypt cells. There is often increased cellular infiltration in the lamina propria, plasma cells being most conspicuous. In the more severe *subtotal* form (SVA) villous fusion is more advanced and the mucosa appears completely flat both under the dissecting microscope and histologically. Epithelial degenerative changes are also more prominent.

Villous atrophy is not a specific change. It is, however, characteristic of the two major primary malabsorption disorders, namely **tropical sprue** and **coeliac disease**, the latter being by far the commonest cause of severe villous atrophy in temperate climates. Less often it is found following gastro-enteritis in

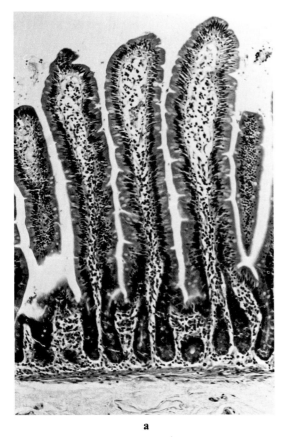

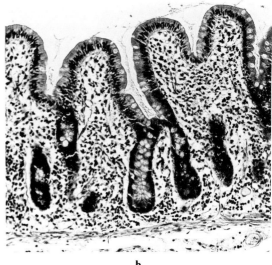

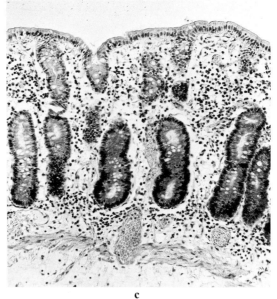

Fig. 19.63   Villous atrophy of jejunum: (a) normal jejunal mucosa; (b) partial villous atrophy; (c) subtotal villous atrophy. × 150. (Material obtained by peroral biopsy.)

childhood. Some degree of villous atrophy is also commonly associated with some forms of **agammaglobulinaemia**, although this has been attributed to complicating giardiasis. In the tropics, kwashiorkor (p. 20.8) is a recognised cause of villous atrophy. Minor villous changes have also been described in many other diseases, although the association is inconstant and of dubious significance.

Malabsorption occurs also in **Whipple's disease** (see below) and in **intestinal amyloidosis** (p. 11.4). The appearances of these conditions are unmistakable in biopsies and congenital agammaglobulinaemia can

be recognised by absence of plasma cells in the lamina propria. In the rare **intestinal lymphangiectasia**, there is diffuse dilatation of mucosal lymphatics which is associated with malabsorption of fat, lymphopenia and protein-losing enteropathy (p. 19.51). **Congenital absence of β-lipoprotein** produces a complex syndrome in which there is a curious spiny abnormality of red cells (acanthocytosis), cerebellar dysfunction, retinal abnormality and fat malabsorption: distension of villous epithelial cells by neutral fat, in an otherwise normal intestinal biopsy, is the diagnostic feature. It is unusual for Crohn's disease or tumour to be detected by biopsy techniques, although the rare, so-called Mediterranean type of intestinal lymphoma produces a typical appearance (p. 19.62). Intestinal parasites capable of causing malabsorption, e.g. *Giardia lamblia* (p. 28.16), can be detected by intestinal biopsy and also in the stools.

Primary malabsorptive disorders

This group includes *coeliac disease* (idiopathic steatorrhoea or gluten enteropathy), *tropical sprue* and the rare *Whipple's disease*.

Coeliac disease is one of the most important causes of intestinal malabsorption in temperate climates and includes both the childhood form of the disease and the adult condition formerly called *idiopathic steatorrhoea*. In both forms, malabsorption is characteristically associated with severe diffuse abnormalities of the intestinal mucosa, and *withdrawal of the wheat protein gluten from the diet brings about both clinical and morphological remission*. The mucosa shows **villous atrophy** (see above) which is most marked and usually subtotal in the proximal jejunum, and becomes progressively less severe, i.e. partial, more distally. There is an associated heavy infiltration of the lamina propria with plasma cells and a marked increase in the number of lymphocytes between the surface epithelial cells. In some cases, especially those with a poor response to therapy, there is collagen deposition beneath the epithelial surface, but American workers regard this as a disease entity ('*collagenous sprue*') distinct from coeliac disease. Withdrawal of dietary gluten leads to a reversal of the mucosal changes, initially in the distal small bowel and later in the upper jejunum which, particularly in adults, may never revert entirely to normal. It seems clear that gluten is in some way responsible for the mucosal damage, but the mechanism involved is not known. Coeliac disease has a strong familial tendency and patients have a strikingly high incidence of histocompatibility antigens HLA-B8 and DW3. While an inherited enzyme defect cannot be discounted as a causative factor, it seems more likely that coeliac disease is caused by a genetically-determined abnormal immune response to gluten. Certainly the nature of the mucosal inflammatory reaction is consistent with this and antibodies and cell-mediated immunity to α-gliadin, a constituent of gluten, and antibody to reticulin fibres, are commonly demonstrable. There is also evidence of impaired immune responsiveness to various exogenous antigens and *splenic atrophy* is commonly observed in adult patients (p. 18.3).

It is now recognised that many, if not most patients with the skin disease *dermatitis herpetiformis* (p. 27.13) also have coeliac disease, although for reasons as yet unclear, the intestinal lesions tend to be mild and patchy. Of more serious consequence is the increased incidence of neoplasia in coeliac disease. In the small intestine, *carcinoma* is 80 times more frequent than in the general population. Even so, by far the most common intestinal neoplasm arising in coeliac disease is *malignant histiocytosis of the intestine* or MHI (p. 19.62). It is seldom possible to detect this tumour in a random jejunal biopsy, but its development may be suspected if the jejunal mucosa shows foci of crypt damage or surface erosion caused by invasion of the epithelium by atypical histiocytes. Such lesions are not seen in uncomplicated coeliac disease. The unexplained development of ulceration in coeliac disease or in a mucosa showing subtotal villous atrophy (*ulcerative jejunitis*) should also be regarded with suspicion, for in many such instances MHI ultimately develops. The incidence of some extra-intestinal tumours, most notably *osophageal carcinoma*, is also increased in coeliac disease.

Tropical sprue is a disease encountered in certain areas in the tropics and sub-tropics, Africa being an exception. There is malabsorption resulting in severe emaciation and chronic diarrhoea, and macrocytic anaemia from deficiency of B_{12}, folate or both. Villous atrophy, usually partial and less often subtotal, is the characteristic change found at jejunal biopsy. This lesion, and the malabsorptive disturbance, are relieved by removal of the patient from the tropical environment and by oral broad-spectrum antibiotics, but a gluten-free diet has little or no beneficial effect. Folic acid may also cause some improvement. The cause of the disease remains uncertain, but abnormal bacterial colonisation of the upper small bowel is probably involved.

Whipple's disease. This rare and interesting disease affects mostly adult males in middle age. Malabsorption is usually the presenting feature, although other signs and symptoms such as generalised lymphadenopathy, arthropathy, skin pigmentation and chronic

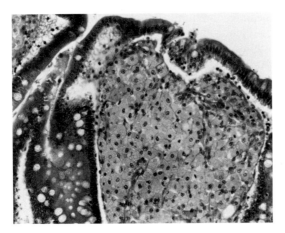

Fig. 19.64 Whipple's disease of small intestine, showing infiltration of the mucosa with granular macrophages. × 230.

cough may be encountered. Jejunal biopsy is diagnostic: the mucosal lamina propria is stuffed with large granular macrophages containing glycoprotein which stains strongly with the periodic acid-Schiff technique for mucopolysaccharides (Fig. 19.64). The regional lymph nodes, and occasionally other tissues, e.g. brain and heart valves, contain similar cells. Neutral fat accumulates in lymphatic channels. Electron microscopy has demonstrated that the abnormal glycoprotein within macrophages consists of unidentified bacteria and bacterial debris. Moreover, the disease responds to oral antibiotics. It would, however, be premature to assert that Whipple's disease is a form of specific infection, especially in view of the age and sex incidence.

Secondary malabsorption

Many disease processes can interfere with absorption. Most of these are discussed elsewhere, and only a brief account will be given here. Classification is most rationally based upon the mechanism thought to be mainly involved in causing malabsorption, although it should be appreciated that more than one mechanism may be operating in any individual disease.

(a) Chronic intestinal disease may cause malabsorption if extensive areas of the mucosa are affected. Examples include Crohn's disease, tuberculosis, tumours (especially malignant lymphoma), amyloidosis, radiation injury and connective tissue disorders such as systemic sclerosis.

(b) Abnormal bacterial proliferation in the small bowel interferes not only with the absorption of vitamin B_{12} but also to some extent with fat absorption. It results from stasis in the intestinal lumen, especially that produced by short-circuit operations which leave stagnant loops of bowel **(the blind-loop syndrome)**. Stasis occurs also in jejunal diverticulosis (p. 19.42), in chronic intestinal obstruction, and in the blind loop resulting from some techniques of partial gastrectomy; malabsorption may complicate these conditions.

(c) Other mechanisms which may cause malabsorption include *biochemical defects* such as disaccharidase deficiency, agammaglobulinaemia and abetalipoproteinaemia; *endocrine disturbances*, including the carcinoid syndrome (p. 19.60) and the Zollinger–Ellison syndrome (p. 20.65); *lymphatic obstruction*, congenital or acquired, e.g. as a result of tuberculosis or tumour; *circulatory disturbances*, especially mesenteric vascular insufficiency; and *drug therapy*, e.g. phenindione, neomycin.

(d) Inadequate digestion must always be considered as a cause of malabsorption and may be due to disease of the liver and biliary tract or to exocrine pancreatic insufficiency. Malabsorption following gastro-jejunostomy, alone or with partial gastrectomy, is largely a consequence of disordered digestion. There is inadequate mixing of food with pancreatic enzymes and bile as a result of interference with the normal anatomical relationships.

Pyloric obstruction and intestinal obstruction (ileus)

Passage of intestinal contents is dependent on the patency, viability and normal contractions of the gut. Accordingly, 'obstruction' may result from *mechanical compression or occlusion* of the intestine, from *ischaemia*, and from *neurological disturbances* interfering with contractility. The effects of obstruction depend on whether it is sudden or gradual, complete or partial, and on its level in the gut.

The following are the chief **mechanical causes** of intestinal obstruction:

(*a*) *Constriction from outside*—for example, by a hernial sac, by special conditions such as volvulus or intussusception, or by fibrous peritoneal adhesions. This is the commonest cause of acute mechanical obstruction.

(*b*) *Stenosis caused by thickening and contraction of the wall* is produced by diverticular disease, ischaemic stricture, Crohn's disease, tuberculosis and, of course, primary or secondary malignant tumours, most commonly carcinoma of the colon. The obstruction from these causes is usually incomplete and chronic, but complete obstruction may supervene by impaction of inspissated faecal masses in the narrowed portion of bowel.

(*c*) *Actual obstruction of the lumen.* This may result from impaction of a large gallstone or other foreign body or by the growth of a tumour into the lumen, usually malignant but sometimes a benign polyp.

(*d*) *Pressure from outside*, for example by a large tumour in the pelvis; obstruction is not often complete from such a cause.

The nervous type of obstruction is called *paralytic or adynamic ileus* and may occur after handling of the intestines at operation, or it may result from peritonitis. The principal **vascular lesion producing obstruction** is occlusion of the mesenteric vessels by embolism or thrombosis. In the type of mechanical obstruction seen in group (*a*) above, vascular obstruction is commonly superadded and the subsequent course is then modified. When the blood supply is intact the obstruction is said to be **simple**; when it is seriously impaired the term **strangulation** is applied.

A length of strangulated gut rapidly becomes haemorrhagic and necrotic. Bacteria proliferate in its bloodstained contents and invade the necrotic wall, producing **gangrene.** Toxaemia is very severe and may be fatal before the distended gangrenous loop ruptures.

The results of intestinal obstruction

The site of the obstruction is important in determining both the effects and the prognosis. High intestinal obstruction is in general more acute in onset, more rapid in its progress and more likely to be complete than low intestinal obstruction which is usually of slow onset, is often incomplete and is less rapidly fatal.

Acute obstruction. When a portion of the small intestine is suddenly obstructed, e.g. by passing under a fibrous peritoneal band, the part above contracts actively for a time and then passes into a condition of paralytic distension. There are probably both increased secretion from the wall and diminished absorption, and thus the bowel becomes distended with fluid in which there is abundant growth of bacteria. The fluid is passed back to the stomach by antiperistalsis and is vomited. Its exact composition depends on the site of the obstruction, but since nearly 8 litres of fluid are secreted into the gut daily, of which all but 100 ml are normally reabsorbed, the volume of fluid available for loss by vomiting or by pooling in the gut is obviously considerable.

If the obstruction is at the **pylorus** or **duodenum** the fluid lost is predominantly acid in reaction with a high Cl^- content. This results in a depletion of plasma chloride, and the urinary excretion of chlorides is then diminished or absent. Since sodium, the ion which normally balances the Cl^- ion, is not lost, carbonic acid is retained to take the place of the lost chloride and the plasma bicarbonate content therefore rises. This state of *alkalosis* is shown clinically by drowsiness and slow shallow respiration and can be demonstrated on analysis by a rise in the CO_2 combining power. A further complication is the development of *tetany* due to a fall in the ionised serum calcium, as a result of the alkalosis. Extracellular potassium deficiency may be superadded—*hypokalaemic alkalosis*. If the fluid loss is great enough, oliguria and *extrarenal uraemia* may follow, the blood urea being markedly raised terminally.

Obstruction in the **jejunum** results in the loss by vomiting of a fluid which contains saliva, gastric juice, bile, pancreatic juice and succus entericus. This leads to depletion of Na^+, K^+, and Cl^-. The CO_2 combining power remains normal, without marked disturbance of the acid-base balance. Although in high obstruction there is a tendency towards acidosis, it is the loss of fluid and electrolytes that leads rapidly to a fall in blood volume, dehydration, haemoconcentration and finally death. Fluid and electrolyte replacement is therefore essential to prolong life until surgical intervention can be undertaken.

Chronic obstruction. In **low intestinal obstruction** the absorptive area of the gut proximally is extensive, and depletion of water and electrolytes is often delayed. Ultimately, however, dehydration due to vomiting does take place and the vomitus becomes brown and foul-smelling—the so-called faecal or stercoral vomit. The dominant and dangerous factor in this form of obstruction is distension of the gut with fluid and with gas mainly derived from swallowed air. Prolonged increase of intraluminal pressure impairs the viability of the bowel wall, with subsequent diffusion of toxic bacterial products into the peritoneal cavity where they are absorbed and produce toxaemia and death. Relief of distension by intubation is thus critically important and sustains life until surgical intervention can be undertaken. The fluid lost by intubation is predominantly alkaline and this leads to acidosis and a low CO_2 combining power. Parenteral infusion of normal saline should thus be supplemented by lactate or carbonate. A further complicating factor is potassium depletion which leads to weakness and muscular paresis and may superimpose a state of adynamic ileus on the existing obstructive lesion (see below). In this context it must be appreciated that potassium is an intracellular ion and the plasma level does not reflect accurately the state of the cells. Caution must therefore be exercised in interpreting the biochemical analysis of the plasma as a basis for potassium replacement. In partial chronic obstruction, prolonged intermittent gut distension leads to hypertrophy of the bowel muscle proximal to the obstructive lesion. Also the pressure of faecal accumulation impairs mucosal viability and predisposes to bacterial invasion which leads to the formation of a mucosal exudate and ultimately to mucosal breakdown and ulceration. This so-called *stercoral ulceration* can take place some distance proximal to the obstruction and sometimes leads to perforation and faecal peritonitis. The effects of chronic stricture, especially in the colon, are aggravated if the regurgitation of faecal material proximally is prevented, for example by an all too competent ileo-caecal valve (closed loop obstruction). In this situation stercoral ulceration is likely to occur in the caecum even when the stricture is in the distal colon, and the caecum may rupture.

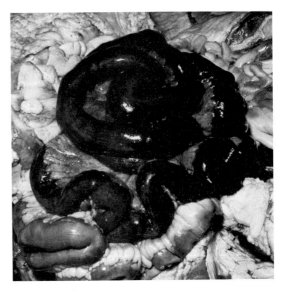

Fig. 19.65 Haemorrhagic infarction of the small intestine due to thrombosis of the superior mesenteric artery. The infarcted bowel is black and would soon have become gangrenous.

Vascular causes of obstruction

Apart from strangulation these are chiefly embolism of thrombosis of the superior mesenteric artery, but thrombosis of the mesenteric veins will produce the same result. This is sometimes seen when a thrombus occluding the portal vein extends backwards to obstruct the mouths of the splenic and superior mesenteric veins.

Haemorrhagic infarction with gangrene of a segment of bowel quickly supervenes (Fig. 19.65), and death follows from toxic absorption and peritonitis.

Neural causes of obstruction

Paralytic ileus. In this condition the motor activity of the bowel is impaired without the presence of a physical obstruction. Sometimes it is due to over-activity of the sympathetic nervous system, and may then be relieved by antagonistic drugs, but in other cases toxic damage to the bowel muscle causes the paralysis. Lowering of the potassium level of the plasma greatly aggravates the condition. It is seen most often in association with peritonitis or it may follow operations on the abdomen, frequently of a minor nature. It may result also from intestinal infections or severe toxaemia.

The whole intestine may be affected and may become greatly distended. The condition is serious and if untreated will result in death in much the same way as in acute mechanical obstruction. Following intubation and drainage of the distended bowel, its contractility may return, particularly if electrolyte and fluid balance can be restored.

Hirschsprung's disease. This is a rare congenital condition characterised by an enormous accumulation of faeces in the greatly enlarged colon which comes to occupy much of the swollen abdomen. There may be periods of weeks or months without defaecation, and repeated attacks of obstruction. The distension may extend as far as the caecum, but at first affects mainly the lower colon. The grossly hypertrophied and dilated colon tapers rather abruptly into a narrow rectal segment joining sigmoid to anus. In the narrowed segment, there is congenital absence of the para-sympathetic ganglion cells of both Auerbach's and Meissner's plexuses, extending for a distance of 5–20 cm below the dilated sigmoid, i.e. corresponding to the narrow segment of rectum. In consequence there is overaction of the sympathetic, which normally inhibits the propulsive contraction of the intestinal wall and stimulates contraction of the internal anal sphincter. The disease is thus one of neuromuscular inco-ordination. While lumbar sympathectomy has proved helpful in some cases, the results have not always been permanent and excision of the defective narrow segment and anastomosis of the sigmoid to the anus has proved more effective.

Hernia

This term is applied to any protrusion of a portion of viscus outside its natural cavity. Protrusion of the bowel usually occurs in a pouch of the peritoneum, which projects on the surface of the body, forming an **external hernia**. The term **internal hernia** is applied when the swelling does not present to an external surface. Two major factors are involved in the formation of a hernia—local weakness and increased pressure. *Local weakness* is usually congenital, notably at the umbilicus or the inguinal canal; occasionally it results from the stretching of the scar of an operation wound—**incisional hernia**. *Increased intra-abdominal pressure* is usually caused by muscular exertion, coughing and straining at stool.

External hernias. The commonest are the *inguinal, femoral* and *umbilical hernias*. Those arising at other sites in the abdominal wall are termed *ventral hernias. Inguinal hernias* are of two types, *indirect*, where the hernia follows the inguinal canal lateral to the inferior epigastric artery, and *direct*, which passes medial to the artery and projects though the external abdominal ring. The femoral hernia passes under Poupart's ligament medial to the femoral vessels. Examples of **internal hernia** are seen when the protrusion occurs through an aperture in the diaphragm, through the foramen of Winslow, or into a pouch in the jejuno-duodenal fossa, the pouch then passing behind the peritoneum. The common external hernias usually contain a loop of small intestine, though in the larger ones omentum or other structures may also be present. So long as it is possible to return the contents into the abdominal cavity, the hernia is termed **reducible**. When this is impossible owing either to the bulk of the contents or to adhesions which have formed within the hernial sac, the hernia is termed **impacted**.

The most serious result of hernia is strangulation, i.e. obstruction of the blood flow through the herniated gut. This may occur by the addition of a fresh loop of bowel to the sac or by accumulation of faeces and gas. Strangulation may develop when the hernia is first formed, a portion of bowel being forced into a tight aperture; this is not uncommon in a femoral hernia. The changes following strangulation have already been described (p. 19.55).

Intussusception

In this condition a length of intestine is invaginated into the portion below. This usually has serious consequences and presents clinically as an acute surgical emergency. An exception to this is the multiple form observed quite often at autopsy, particularly in children dying from various causes, and presumably due to irregular bowel contraction around the time of death (agonal intussusception). The clinically important forms are also most often observed in infancy and early childhood. This is probably because the intestinal lymphoid tissue, especially in the distal ileum, is prone to undergo swelling in childhood, and because it protrudes into the intestinal lumen, is propelled distally by peristaltic activity, drawing the adjacent

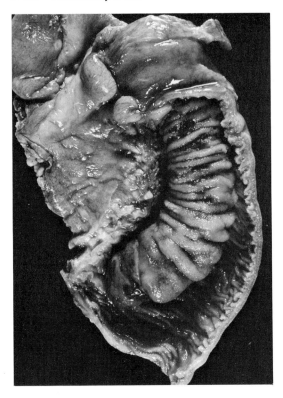

Fig. 19.66 Intussusception of the small intestine. The ensheathing section of gut has been cut open to show the invaginated loop, which is passing downward. The invaginated loop shows early haemorrhagic necrosis at the apex (near lower margin of excision) and near the entrance (at the top of the photograph).

bowel with it. Viruses of the ECHO or adenovirus groups may be responsible for the lymphoid swelling and have been isolated from the intestinal contents and mesenteric lymph nodes in children with intussusception. An inverted Meckel's diverticulum projecting into the intestinal lumen also predisposes to intussusception, and in adults polypoid intestinal tumours are the usual cause.

Naked-eye appearances. In intussusception of the ordinary type three layers of bowel are seen on section, two layers formed by the doubling of the invaginated length of bowel, and one layer consisting of the wall of the bowel into which the invagination has occurred. Thus it consists of an entering tube, a returning tube and an ensheathing tube (Fig. 19.66). The commonest site is at the ileocaecal valve, and usually the valve forms the apex of the intus-

susception and is passed along the large intestine. The apex may ultimately reach the rectum, and the whole lesion forms a fairly firm sausage-shaped mass, which is palpable during life. This type of intussusception is called **ileocaecal**. More rarely the small intestine is passed through the ileocaecal valve into the colon— **ileocolic** type—and there may also be combinations of those two types with more complicated invaginations. For example, the ileocaecal valve may be passed along for only a short distance, so that the tip of the appendix may be still visible, and then coils of the small intestine may be passed down through the valve and firmly impacted. Intussusception also occurs in the small intestine or the transverse colon, but it is comparatively rare. Intussusception of the appendix has been recorded, but it is very rare; it occurs chiefly in children.

Results. The important effects of intussusception are interference with the blood supply and mechanical obstruction of the bowel. The vessels of the invaginated part are stretched and also compressed; venous obstruction, oedema and extensive haemorrhage result. Accordingly the passage per anum of a mixture of blood and mucus is a common sign of intussusception, but pure blood may be passed. Unless the intussusception can be reduced (i.e. reversed), the haemorrhagic, ischaemic bowel becomes infarcted and gangrenous, and in most cases death results from obstruction or general peritonitis unless early excision is performed. In some cases, however, the serosa of the invaginated bowel becomes glued by fibrinous exudate at its point of entry, to the serosa of the ensheathing bowel: general peritonitis is thus prevented and the gangrenous invaginated bowel may then slough off and be passed in fragments along the lower bowel. The fibrinous serosal adhesions organise. In this way, natural amputation and union may restore the continuity of the gut and effect cure.

Volvulus

In this condition a loop of bowel is twisted or rotated through 180° or more, so that the lumen is effectively obstructed at the point of twisting and the venous drainage is prejudiced. It occurs particularly in the sigmoid colon (Fig. 19.67), especially when this is heavily loaded with faeces and the mesocolon is unusually

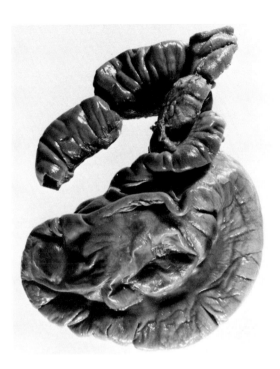

Fig. 19.67 Volvulus of sigmoid colon.

long. The twisted loop becomes increasingly distended with gas and fluid and blood flow is further impaired. The wall of the gut becomes congested, haemorrhagic and ultimately gangrenous. In some cases a portion of bowel is found to be enormously distended, filling a large part of the abdominal cavity. Volvulus of the small intestine may occur also, but it is less common; the favouring conditions are the same, and sometimes the approximation of the ends of the loop is due to local adhesions around calcified mesenteric lymph nodes. In children, however, volvulus of the small bowel is much commoner than in adults. More rarely two loops of intestine become intertwined and then the symptoms are very severe.

Intestinal obstruction by foreign bodies

The most common cause of this type of obstruction is a large composite gallstone, which has entered the duodenum through a fistulous track developing between gallbladder and bowel; commonly there is little or no history of symptoms to indicate cholelithiasis. The calculus passes along the intestine but may become impacted, usually about a metre proximal to the ileocaecal valve. Even the largest stone is smaller than the diameter of the fully relaxed bowel, so muscle spasm must contribute to the impaction. Unmasticated food may act similarly, for example obstruction of the ileum by a mass of dried fruit. Gastro-enterostomy predisposes to the passage of large masses of undigested food into the intestine, and thus to obstruction.

Tumours of the Intestines

Small intestine

For reasons which are obscure, the small bowel has a surprisingly low incidence of clinically important tumours. Epithelial neoplasms of the small bowel, for example, account for less than 2 per cent of all intestinal (including colonic) tumours. Nevertheless the tumours that do arise form an interesting group.

Carcinoid tumour (argentaffinoma)

This arises from specialised cells which are located within the epithelial surface of the gastro-intestinal tract, and belong to the widely distributed family of cells with a paracrine (local endocrine) function sometimes termed **apud cells**, an acronym derived from the property common to all cells of the system, namely, **a**mine-**p**recursor **u**ptake and **d**ecarboxylation (p. 12.43). While tumours arising from these endocrine cells have been given the generic name **apudoma**, those occurring in the gut are more commonly called **carcinoid tumours**, because in the appendix (their commonest site of origin) they are clinically benign despite an appearance of infiltration resembling carcinoma. Both in the appendix and in the ileum, which is also a common primary site, carcinoid tumours arise from the most distinctive intestinal representative of the apud system, namely the *argentaffin cell*, so named because of its capacity to form cytoplasmic deposits of metallic silver from silver salts. This histologically demonstrable property is related to its secretion of 5-hydroxy-tryptamine (5HT). Carcinoids only rarely occur in the stomach and large intestine, and in these sites they may arise from a different member of the apud system, since the cells often fail to show the argentaffin reaction unless a reducing agent is added (argyrophilia). Carcinoid tumours are usually found by chance in or near the tip of appendices removed surgically, often for acute appendicitis. Although sometimes only a few millimetres in diameter, they can occlude the distal lumen of the appendix and have a distinctive yellowish-brown colour.

In the small intestine, especially in the lower ileum, carcinoids are commonly multiple. They form small button-like swellings in the mucosa, one or more of which shows deep penetration of the muscular wall which may be locally hypertrophied (Fig. 19.68). Unlike those in the appendix, ileal carcinoids are malignant and often spread widely by the lymphatics. They cause intestinal obstruction and frequently metastasise to the mesenteric lymph nodes and liver. Both the primary tumour and its metastases grow very slowly.

Microscopically, carcinoid tumours consist of small clear cells, closely packed in alveolar formations (Fig. 19.69), throughout the whole thickness of the appendicular or ileal wall. The yellowish colour is due to lipids, some of which are doubly refracting. As stated above, the tumour cells contain granules which reduce silver salts—hence the term 'argentaffinoma'. In the appendix, carcinoid tumours are commonly related to old inflammatory lesions and the cells are often associated with proliferated nerve fibres. *In a recently recognised form of carcinoid of the appendix the tumour cells secrete mucin ('goblet-cell carcinoid'). This form is malignant and behaves like ileal carcinoids.*

The carcinoid syndrome. Large hepatic secondary growths of carcinoid tumours are sometimes, but not invariably, accompanied by attacks of flushing of the face, diarrhoea and bronchospasm. There may also be pulmonary stenosis. These effects are due to the secretion of large amounts of 5HT and other compounds by metastatic tumour cells in the liver. 5HT is inactivated by amine oxidase in the liver cells, and so long as the tumour is confined to the

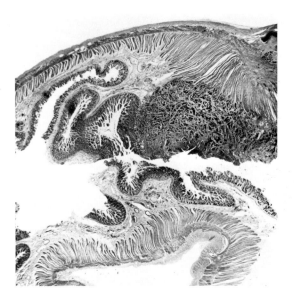

Fig. 19.68   Carcinoid tumour of ileum, seen as the darkly-stained tissue invading the circular muscle coat, which is greatly hypertrophied, and causing stenosis. There were hepatic metastases and the carcinoid syndrome developed. × 2·5.

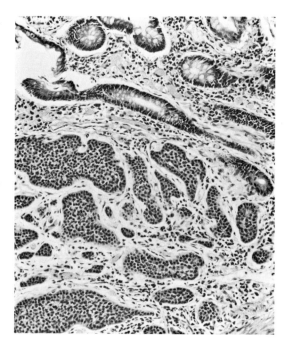

Fig. 19.69   Carcinoid tumour of ileum, showing clumps of small polygonal epithelial cells infiltrating the mucosa. × 125.

drainage area of the portal circulation systemic effects are not produced. Hepatic metastases, however, set free 5HT into the systemic circulation. In man, 5HT is vasoconstrictor and a smooth-muscle stimulant; it may also stimulate fibroblastic proliferation and so cause the subendocardial fibrosis in the right atrium and ventricle and the pulmonary stenosis which is a late feature of the syndrome. The left side of the heart is less often involved, since 5HT is inactivated also in the lungs. Excessive diversion of tryptophane to the metabolism of massive secondary deposits may induce symptoms of pellagra. 5HT is converted by the enzyme amine-oxidase to 5-hydroxyindoleacetic acid (5HIAA), which is excreted in the urine where its quantitative estimation affords a valuable clinical test for the presence of large argentaffin tumours. The flushing attacks are often precipitated by alcohol or sympathetic stimulation: they are not due to 5HT, but probably to kallikrein, which is also secreted by the tumour cells, and activates the kinin system (p. 4.18).

Carcinoids ('adenomas') of the bronchi (p. 16.70) secrete 5-hydroxytryptophane, possibly because they lack the enzyme decarboxylase required to convert this substance to 5HT. Carcinoids of the stomach may also secrete histamine in addition to 5HT and kallikrein. Colonic carcinoid tumours rarely give rise to the syndrome.

Other tumours of the small intestine

Connective tissue tumours. Members of this group, such as leiomyoma, lymphangioma and lipoma, are quite common but seldom cause symptoms unless they protrude into the intestinal lumen and produce intussusception. Occasionally a leiomyoma ulcerates and leads to intestinal blood loss and iron-deficiency anaemia. *Leiomyosarcoma*, the only malignant tumour of this group that is at all common, presents clinically like its benign variant but tends to recur after operation and sometimes metastasises to the liver. The behaviour of smooth muscle tumours of the gut often belies their histological appearances, and it is very difficult to classify them as benign or malignant.

The Peutz-Jeghers syndrome. This interesting hereditary disorder is transmitted as a Mendelian dominant of high penetrance. Multiple epithelial-lined highly differentiated polyps are found in the small intestine, especially the jejunum, and are associated with melanotic pigmented spots on the lips and oral mucosa, and sometimes on the fingers and toes. The polyps cause recurring attacks of intussusception and sometimes iron deficiency anaemia due to blood loss, but rarely undergo malignant transformation. Grossly, they may be sessile or pedunculated and resemble the neoplastic polyps of the large intestine, but the epithelium consists of a mixture of the several normal cell types found in the small intestine, and they have a branching muscular stroma derived from the muscularis mucosae. Because of these features they are regarded as hamartomas (p. 12.47) rather than true neoplasms. Single polyps of this type, without other features of the syndrome, also occur in the stomach and large intestine (Morson, 1978).

Carcinoma. This is surprisingly uncommon in the small bowel, being rather less frequently encountered than lymphoid tumours. Length for length, the proximal parts of the small bowel are more often affected than the distal. In appearance and behaviour, carcinomas of the small intestine are very similar to those of the colon (p. 19.65). Intestinal obstruction and the effects of haemorrhage are the most common modes of presentation, but diagnosis is not often made early enough to allow curative excision. The causal factors are usually unknown, but carcinoma may arise as a complication of coeliac disease (p. 19.53) or surgical blind loops. There is also an increased incidence of small bowel carcinoma in Crohn's disease (p. 19.35), and the tumour may be difficult to diagnose in a length of intestine already thickened and stenosed. Histologically the tumour may show a curious 'endometrioid' infiltrative pattern with widely separated neoplastic glands deep in the gut wall. There may also be extensive dysplastic change in the overlying mucosa.

Lymphomas of the small intestine

Most intestinal lymphomas have morphological features similar to those arising in lymph nodes (p. 18.16). Many are of follicle-centre-cell type, the most characteristic variant being the condition described as **lymphomatous polyposis**. In this condition, the gastro-intestinal tract is beset by multiple polypoid tumours which are usually centrocytic in type; extra-intestinal spread and

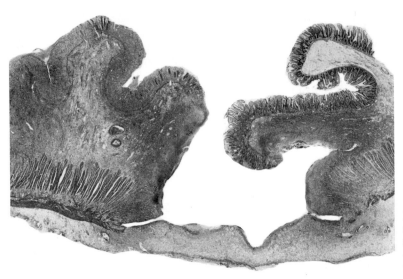

Fig. 19.70 Malignant histiocytosis, showing deep but sharply localised ulceration of the wall of the small intestine. × 6·5.

leukaemia may eventually develop. More localised centroblastic or immunoblastic tumours also occur especially in the ileum, and in children and young adults a particularly aggressive intestinal **lymphoblastic lymphoma** resembling Burkitt's tumour (p. 18.26) is well recognised.

Another important tumour in this category is the condition known as **malignant histiocytosis of the intestine (MHI)**, which rarely occurs except as a complication of coeliac disease (p. 19.53). This tumour arises in the mucosa of the upper small intestine and is commonly multifocal. It may cause intestinal obstruction or, more characteristically, ulceration (Fig. 19.70) and sometimes perforation. Histologically, the tumour may be difficult to recognise; it may resemble an inflammatory ulcer because the tumour cells are often accompanied by numerous plasma cells or eosinophil leucocytes. The neoplastic process may remain localised to the small bowel for a long time, but usually spreads at an early stage to the sinusoids of the lymph nodes, liver, spleen and bone marrow. It is this pattern of spread, which resembles that seen in other forms of malignant histiocytosis, which gives the tumour its name.

In the littoral of the eastern Mediterranean, and occasionally elsewhere in tropical or subtropical zones, a peculiar form of lymphoproliferative disease (sometimes referred to incorrectly as *Mediterranean lymphoma*) occurs in the small intestine. Initially the mucosa of the small bowel is diffusely infiltrated by plasma cells and severe malabsorption is noted clinically. In many instances, the heavy chain of IgA can be found serologically (**alpha chain disease**——p. 17.62). There is still doubt as to whether this initial phase, which is commonly fatal, is truly neoplastic, but it can certainly evolve into an unequivocally neoplastic process in which the plasma cells are focally replaced by follicle-centre cells. Chronic intestinal infection or parasitisation has been incriminated in the causation of this disease.

Large intestine

Although connective tissue tumours and lymphomas are rare in the large intestine, both benign and malignant epithelial tumours are all too common and constitute a major problem in terms of management and prevention.

Benign neoplastic polyps (adenomas)

These tumours are the commonest types of polyp of the colon and rectum. They present a spectrum of macroscopic and microscopic appearances, and are classified as *tubular, tubulovillous* and *villous adenomas*. In spite of these names, the cells of all these tumours show various degrees of dysplasia (atypia) and *they all have a tendency to undergo malignant change to adenocarcinoma*. A general account of these tumours is provided on pp. 12.14–15.

Tubular adenoma is usually a small (less than

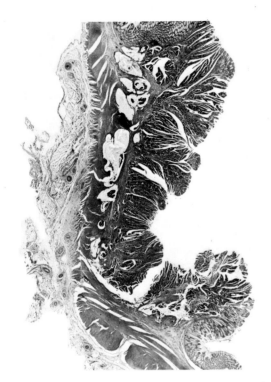

Fig. 19.71 Villous adenoma of rectum. There is malignant infiltration of the wall by mucoid carcinoma. × 3.

1 cm diameter) pedunculated nodule with a smoothly lobulated surface (Fig. 19.74). Microscopically (Figs. 12.20, 12.21, p. 12.14) it is seen to consist of closely-packed neoplastic epithelial tubules resembling the tubular glands of colonic mucosa but less regular in size and shape and lined by closely-packed epithelial cells.

Villous adenoma is really a papilloma but is now included, rather illogically, with the adenomas (World Health Organization Classification) because of the occurrence of all gradations between villous and tubular tumours. The villous adenoma is usually over 1 cm in diameter when detected and is typically a sessile papillary tumour composed of numerous fronds which project into the gut lumen (Fig. 19.71). Each frond consists of a fine vascular stromal core covered by a layer of epithelium.

Tubulo-villous adenoma presents features of both the above adenomas, having a mixed tubular and villous structure in various proportions. In most instances the tubules lie deep to blunt, short villi.

Adenomas may be single or multiple and one

or more is found incidentally in about 10% of autopsies. They are also found in about 25% of colons excised for carcinoma. Adenomas less than 1 cm in diameter are widely distributed throughout the large intestine and epidemiologically have a world-wide incidence. Larger adenomas, however, have an anatomical distribution and epidemiology similar to that of carcinoma (see below). Villous adenomas have a predilection for the rectum and sometimes secrete sufficient albuminous or potassium-rich fluid to cause hypoalbuminaemia or hypokalaemia. Otherwise, colorectal adenomas are usually symptomless, but sometimes give rise to melaena and very rarely to intussusception. Their predisposition to undergo carcinomatous change is reflected in the various degrees of cellular aberration of their epithelium, including pleomorphism, nuclear hyperchromasia, loss of polarity, crowding of cells and an increase in mitoses. Tumour size also correlates with malignant transformation, and villous adenomas, regardless of size, have a greater tendency to become malignant.

Confirmation that excision of a colorectal adenoma is complete requires careful histological examination of the excision margin, which should include the adjacent normal colonic mucosa around the base of the tumour.

Adenomatosis (polyposis) coli. This hereditary disorder is usually transmitted as a Mendelian dominant but in some families either with very low penetrance or as a recessive character. It is characterised by the development of at least a hundred, and often many more, adenomatous polyps in the large intestine (Fig. 19.72). The condition does not usually appear until late childhood or early adult life. Since each of the polyps appears to share the predisposition to become malignant, carcinoma of the colon is almost inevitable, usually about 15 years after the development of adenomatosis. The adenomas themselves may be symptomless for many years and frequently the presenting features are caused by the development of one or more carcinomas.

Other polypoid lesions

Non-neoplastic polyps occur in the large bowel, and are not to be confused with the true tumours already described. The **metaplastic polyp** is a small, raised, pale, sessile lesion and

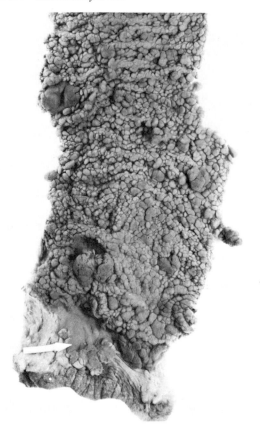

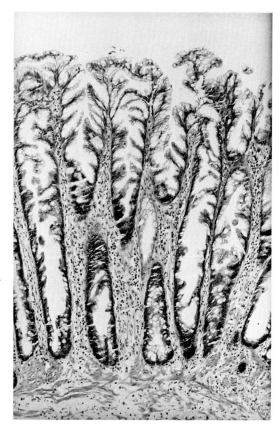

Fig. 19.73 Part of a metaplastic polyp of the colon, showing the typical papilliform appearance of the lining epithelium of the crypts. × 50.

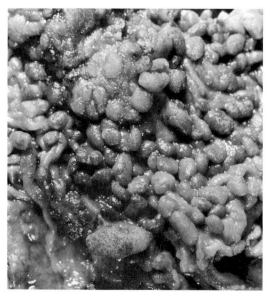

Fig. 19.72 Polyposis coli. *Above*, innumerable small polyps and several larger ones are present. Two small cancers have developed just above the anal margin. × 0·5. *Below*, showing the appearance of the individual polyps. × 2·5.

is not uncommon in middle or later adult life. Histologically there is localised papilliform hyperplasia of the epithelium lining the surface and upper parts of the crypts (Fig. 19.73). This lesion lacks the dysplasia of the adenomatous polyps and does not appear to be premalignant. **Hamartomatous polyps** of the Peutz-Jeghers type (p. 19.61) are found occasionally in the colon. In childhood, globular polypoid lesions, sometimes quite large, are encountered in the rectum: histologically they consist of intensely inflamed mucosa in which the crypts are markedly dilated and cystic, and are frequently ulcerated. These so-called **juvenile polyps** do not show epithelial dedifferentiation and may be hamartomatous in nature. Apart from adenomatosis coli, true colonic adenomas are seldom observed in children. Finally, mention must be made of the condition known as **benign lymphoid polyposis of the rectum**, in which multiple polypi, consisting of masses of lymphoid tissue, showing numerous germinal centres and covered by normal rectal epithelium, develop in the rectum, especially in young women. The condition is of unknown causation but, as the name implies, does not have malignant potential.

Carcinoma of the large intestine

This is one of the commoner malignant tumours. It occurs mainly among older people. The rectum is the commonest site, especially in males; next follows the sigmoid colon, the caecum and ileo-caecal valve and the flexures. The overall incidence is about the same for males and females.

Aetiology is largely unknown, although carcinoma of the large bowel is principally a disease of urban communities, low-fibre diet being a possible aetiological factor. It has also been suggested that Western diets encourage the growth of certain (mainly anaerobic) bacteria capable of converting the faecal bile acids into carcinogens.

It is generally believed that, in most instances, colorectal carcinoma develops from an adenomatous polyp, as described above. In adenomatosis coli, where hundreds of such polyps are present, the development of carcinoma is almost invariable, usually 10–15 years after the appearance of the polyps. Colorectal cancer is also an important complication of ulcerative colitis (see p. 19.38), the risk being greatest in patients with extensive, active ulcerative colitis of early onset and long duration: after 10 years the risk rises to about 10% and after 20 years it increases to about 40%. Another predisposing cause is Crohn's disease, although here the risk is only slightly increased. In ulcerative colitis, Crohn's disease and adenomatosis coli, the tendency for the development of carcinoma 10–15 years after onset means that it may occur in relatively young people.

Naked-eye appearances. When carcinoma begins in an adenomatous polyp, infiltration of the stalk and base occurs so that the tumour appears like a button fixed to the bowel wall; subsequently the centre breaks down leaving a necrotic ulcer with raised everted ('rolled') edges (Fig. 19.74). The base is then fixed to the muscular coat, which is ultimately breached by progressive ulceration. Spread in the submu-

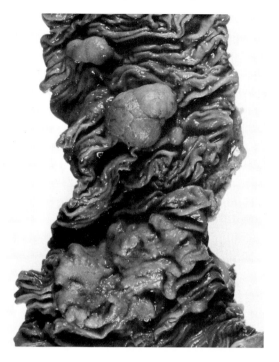

Fig. 19.74 Part of the caecum and ascending colon showing two tubular adenomas (*above*), the larger of which has the typical smoothly lobulated surface. The ulcerated carcinoma (*below*) has originated in a third adenoma.

cous and subserous lymphatics also occurs so that the tumour gradually encircles the bowel wall. The majority of cancers of the colon are scirrhous, and cause contraction and stricture; some, however, are soft and fungating, and others are mucous and appear gelatinous. The more slowly growing types especially tend to encircle the bowel, forming a ring-shaped growth and thus producing narrowing or complete obstruction. The bowel above the obstruction undergoes great, sometimes enormous dilatation, while its wall becomes hypertrophied (Fig. 19.75). The raised intraluminal pressure may interfere with mucosal blood flow and an ischaemic enterocolitis, sometimes with pseudomembrane formation, may develop proximal to the tumour. In other cases, frank ulceration occurs, especially in the caecum (so-called *stercoral ulceration*): perforation and peritonitis may result. Some cancers grow mainly as a projection into the lumen, forming a soft, irregular, sessile mass which usually undergoes necrosis, infection and ulceration (Fig. 19.76) and

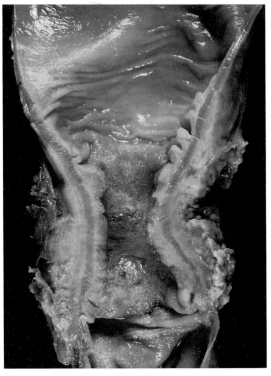

Fig. 19.75 Carcinoma of the descending colon. The tumour has ulcerated and caused obstruction, with consequent dilatation of the colon proximally and hypertrophy of the muscle coat. × 1.

eventually obstructs the bowel. The mucoid type may, as in the stomach, lead to widespread infiltration and thickening of the wall, and often spreads to the peritoneum.

Microscopic appearances. Practically all intestinal cancers are adenocarcinomas, some being highly differentiated, while others are anaplastic (Fig. 12.7, p. 12.7), including those in patients with ulcerative colitis.

Spread and prognosis. These tumours tend to spread circumferentially in the wall of the large intestine and also directly through the wall to the serosa. Occasionally extensive spread occurs in the peritoneal cavity. Lymphatic spread, with metastases in the paracolic lymph nodes, often occurs quite early, while blood spread to the liver or elsewhere is usually relatively late. Using *Duke's staging*, patients in whom the tumour is confined to the intestinal wall (stage A) have a cure rate approaching 100%, unless the tumour has penetrated the whole thickness of the wall (stage B), when the cure rate falls to

70%. Lymph-node metastases (stage C) reduce the cure rate to approximately 30%.

Colonic carcinomas are among the tumours which secrete a glycoprotein (**carcino–embryonic antigen** or **CEA**) which is produced also by normal fetal endodermal tissues (p. 12.44). Detection of CEA in the serum has not provided a reliable diagnostic test, for it is present in trace amounts in the serum of normal subjects and in increased amounts in various types of cancer, in inflammatory bowel disease and in some other non-neoplastic conditions. Nevertheless, assay of CEA may be helpful in the management of patients with carcinoma, for the level falls after removal of the tumour and a subsequent increase suggests recurrence or metastases.

Other malignant tumours

Malignant lymphomas occur, particularly in the caecum and rectum, but are less common than in the small intestine. They may form a large mass and cause obstruction (Fig. 19.77) or ulcerate and sometimes perforate. Leiomyosarcoma is rare.

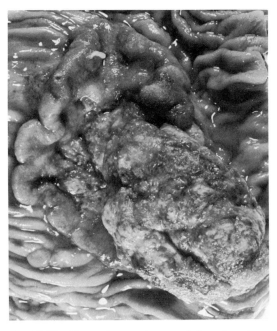

Fig. 19.76 Fungating carcinoma of the colon showing ulceration. Note the raised margin of the ulcer.

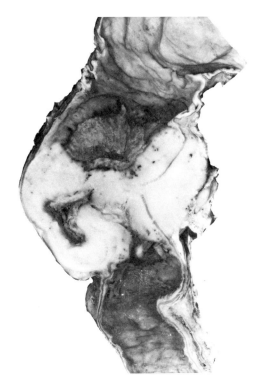

Fig. 19.77 Malignant lymphoma of the ileo-caecal region.

Tumours of the anal canal

Malignant tumours are uncommon. Most are *squamous carcinomas*, often with a 'basaloid' pattern, i.e. resembling rodent ulcer of the skin: some show a mixture of squamous and mucin-secreting elements (*muco-epidermoid carcinoma*). These tumours all tend to metastasise to both pelvic and inguinal nodes, and the prognosis is then poor. *Malignant melanoma* also occurs in the anal canal, where it is almost always fatal.

Secondary tumours of the intestines

Apart from invasion by peritoneal and lymphatic spread, intestinal metastases are extremely uncommon, though metastatic melanoma is seen occasionally, and lymphoid neoplasms of the thyroid (p. 26.26) have a notable tendency to metastasise to the gut. The peritoneum is a common site for secondary carcinoma (p. 19.71) and the bowel may become invaded from the serous surface with consequent narrowing of the lumen.

Congenital Abnormalities

The commonest of these is the **Meckel's diverticulum**, which represents the proximal end of the omphalomesenteric duct. The diverticulum usually measures about 2–3 cm in length, and is narrower than the small intestine (Fig. 19.78). Occasionally it is adherent at the umbilicus and in some cases a fistula is present; or again, there may be obstruction at the proximal end, sometimes merely by a fold, and accumulation of mucus occurs so that an *enterocyst* results. A Meckel's diverticulum rarely leads to any serious results, but when it is adherent it may cause volvulus of the small intestine or, even more serious, strangulation. Acute inflammation of a Meckel's diverticulum presents features similar to those of acute appendicitis, and requires similar surgical treatment. Sometimes heterotopic acid-secreting gastric mucosa is present and may lead to peptic ulceration of the diverticulum with perforation or haemor-

rhage. In the adult the diverticulum occurs usually about a metre above the ileo-caecal valve, and at about half that distance in young children. Carcinoma has very rarely been observed to develop in the apex of a Meckel's diverticulum.

Stenosis or actual **atresia** may occasionally occur in the intestines. In the small intestine, the commonest site is at the orifice of the common bile duct or at the ileo-caecal valve. Part of the intestine may be absent, usually along with other malformations. The commonest site of atresia, however, is at the lower end of the rectum. Sometimes a dimple in the skin, representing the anus, is separated from the lower end of the rectum by a thin layer of tissue—the condition being known as **imperforate anus**. In other cases of atresia of the lower end of the rectum, however, the lower end of the bowel communicates with the bladder or urethra in the male and with the vagina in the female.

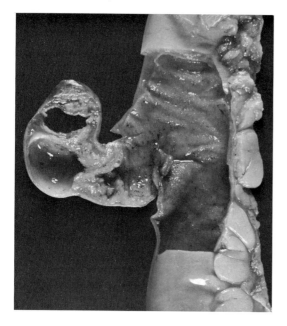

Fig. 19.78 Meckel's diverticulum. In this instance there was pancreatic tissue in the wall and a cystic space. (Dr. John S. Currie.)

V: The Peritoneum

Acute peritonitis

Because it contains the gastro-intestinal tract, with its heavy bacterial flora, the peritoneal cavity is liable to bacterial infection, and because of its potential volume and large surface area, acute bacterial infection of the whole peritoneal cavity is a severe, often fatal condition. It is therefore not surprising that the cavity is guarded by potent defence mechanisms. Like other serosal membranes, there are a large number of readily available macrophages in or on the mesothelial lining. These cells are particularly numerous in the omentum, in which they are aggregated in visible 'milk spots'. Even the mild irritation of perfusion by 'physiological' solutions, as in peritoneal dialysis, releases huge numbers of macrophages into the cavity. This phenomenon does not, of course, exclude the usual emigration of polymorphs and subsequently monocytes from the venules in the inflamed peritoneal surfaces. A second impor-

tant defence mechanism is localisation of an infected focus by the omentum and adjacent viscera. These tissues become glued together by fibrin deposition on their surfaces and so tend to wall off the site of infection from the rest of the cavity.

Causes. Acute bacterial peritonitis is nearly always due to infection from one of the abdominal viscera, in most instances the gastro-intestinal tract. Any breach in the integrity or viability of the wall of the tract is likely to cause local or general peritonitis. The list of causes is thus long. The commonest in Western countries is *acute appendicitis*, but *perforation of a peptic ulcer* and *acute diverticulitis of the colon* are also frequent causes. Others include *perforation of typhoid ulcers*, usually in the ileum; rupture of the large intestine proximal to an *obstruction* or in *severe ulcerative colitis*; penetrating abdominal wounds; perforation of an *ulcerated tumour* of the intestine, particularly a *lymphoma*; devitalisation of the gut due to *mesenteric vascular* *thrombosis*; or *strangulation* of part of the gut by herniation, volvulus, etc.

Acute peritonitis can also arise from an acutely infected gallbladder, either by rupture of the wall or spread of the bacteria through it. Acute haemorrhagic pancreatitis, acute salpingitis and acute cystitis may also result in peritonitis. Haematogenous peritonitis is relatively uncommon.

Appearances. The features of acute peritonitis depend on the types of bacteria responsible and the nature of the causal lesion. When the infection is due to escape of bacteria from the gut, the infection is likely to be a mixed one, although one or other species of bacteria may predominate. *Escherichia coli* infection is extremely common, either alone or associated with the other species. Various streptococci, including anaerobes, and *Clostridium welchii*, *Bacteroides*, and various Gram −ve bacilli are all encountered. Pneumococcal peritonitis used to be encountered as an apparently primary phenomenon in young girls, but is not often seen now in developed countries.

When virulent bacteria enter the peritoneum, or when heavy infection occurs, as in perforation of an ulcer or gangrenous appendicitis, general peritonitis is likely to result. With less virulent bacteria or more gradual infection, the spread may be limited, either by rapid elimination of the bacteria or by formation of fibrinous adhesions around the infected site.

In **generalised peritonitis**, the surfaces are inflamed and the exudate varies in amount and appearance. In haemolytic streptococcal peritonitis, formerly a common puerperal infection, there may be only a little serous or haemorrhagic exudate. With coliform bacilli and the other bacteria mentioned above, exudate is usually more abundant and turbid or frankly purulent, and there is usually a deposit of fibrin on the serosal surfaces. When peritonitis has resulted from perforation of a peptic ulcer, there may be accumulation of air beneath the diaphragm, detectable by radiography: the leakage of acid gastric juice results in a haemorrhagic exudate, and this is seen also when there has been leakage of bile. In acute haemorrhagic pancreatitis the affected surfaces show fat necrosis and the exudate is haemorrhagic: the changes may be generalised or limited to the lesser sac.

The appearances of **localised peritonitis** depend on the causal organisms and the site affected. If infection is mild, it may resolve without suppuration, although there may be residual adhesions; this is seen when gonococcal salpingitis progresses to pelvic peritonitis. Frequently, however, local acute peritonitis results in suppuration as, for example, when an acutely inflamed appendix becomes surrounded by omentum, loops of gut, etc., and a peri-appendicular abscess results: this may occur also in relation to an acutely inflamed diverticulum, or when perforation of a peptic ulcer occurs in the lesser sac.

General peritonitis may be overcome, and yet leave residual foci of infection, e.g. a collection of pus in the pelvis or between the liver and diaphragm (*subphrenic abscess*) walled off by adhesions between adjacent structures.

Effects. Acute generalised peritonitis is an extremely serious, often fatal condition, firstly because the cavity is so large and has such a great surface area from which toxins are absorbed, and secondly because the intestines bathed in bacterial toxins are very likely to develop *paralytic ileus* (p. 19.56). These factors result in *severe toxaemia* and also *gross dehydration* and disturbance of electrolyte and acid-base balances from loss of fluid into the peritoneal exudate and paralysed gut, and by vomiting. The result is a combination of *septic and hypovolaemic shock* which is very likely to be fatal unless effectively treated. In many instances, bacteraemia or septicaemia develops.

Recovery may be complicated by residual abscesses, as mentioned above, or by organisation of deposited fibrin to form fibrous adhesions between loops of gut (Fig. 19.79) and the parietal peritoneum, etc.: such adhesions carry a risk of subsequent intestinal obstruction by kinking of the gut or internal hernia.

Chronic peritonitis

As stated above, abscess formation may result from localised or generalised peritonitis, and may persist for weeks or months unless drained. As elsewhere, the persistent abscess becomes enclosed in dense fibrous tissue, which may interfere with the function of the loops of intestine usually forming the wall.

Tuberculous peritonitis is now uncommon in developed countries. It may be general or localised. The origin of the generalised type may be a caseous mesenteric lymph node, or the bacilli may reach the peritoneum from a tuberculous Fallopian tube, either directly through its covering or by way of its abdominal opening. In other cases where no gross lesion can be found, the infection is probably by the bloodstream, a small focus forming from which dissemination afterwards occurs. The appearances vary widely in different cases. There may be an eruption of minute grey tubercles all over the peritoneum, with or without a sero-fibrinous effusion. The omentum is often extensively involved and forms a large mass across the upper part of the abdomen. In other cases, there may be caseation, either in scattered foci or diffusely. Lastly, cases are encountered in which the tubercles are comparatively scanty and where the chief result is formation of adhesions, sometimes with serous effusion between them. When chronic tuberculous peritonitis is associated with ulcers of the intestine, ulceration between adjacent loops of the bowel may lead to the formation of multiple fistulae, and may result in the malabsorption syndrome.

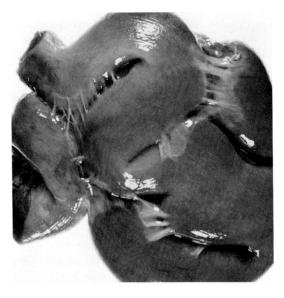

Fig. 19.79 Fibrous adhesions between loops of small intestine, resulting from organisation of fibrin deposited during acute peritonitis.

Non-bacterial peritonitis

As already mentioned, acute peritonitis results from the irritant effect of gastric juice or bile when these escape into the peritoneal cavity, and also from leaking pancreatic enzymes in acute pancreatitis. All these conditions are, however, likely to be complicated by acute bacterial peritonitis.

There are a number of miscellaneous conditions in which chronic peritonitis or fibrous thickening of the peritoneum occurs in the absence of bacterial infection.

The former use of *talc*, and more recently *starch*, to lubricate surgical gloves led, in some instances, to the development of a granulomatous peritoneal reaction with consequent fibrous adhesions. Peritoneal involvement by *carcinoma*, e.g. from the stomach, colon or ovary, often results in an inflammatory exudate and adhesions (see below). The term *chronic hyperplastic peritonitis* is sometimes used to describe hyaline fibrous thickening of the visceral peritoneum, often over the liver and spleen, but sometimes also the omentum and mesentery. It is usually accompanied by ascites. The term 'sugar-iced liver' (Zuckergussleber) has been applied: in appearance, it resembles the hyaline pleural plaques attributable to inhalation of asbestos, and indeed this may be the cause in some cases. Hyaline thickening involving all the serous sacs is sometimes called *Concato's disease*, while involvement of the pericardium and hepatic peritoneum is termed *Pick's disease*. Very striking thickening of the posterior peritoneum may also occur in the carcinoid syndrome, possibly due to a desmoplastic effect of 5HT (p. 19.61).

Retroperitoneal fibrosis

In this condition, there is extensive formation of fibrous tissue retroperitoneally. It tends to cause trouble by constricting the ureters. While the aetiology is not known, the condition has been associated with Riedel's thyroiditis, and also with taking the drug methysergide.

Ascites

Serous effusion into the peritoneum occurs in cases of general oedema of both the cardiac and renal types, and is sometimes abundant; some fluid may accumulate also in severe anaemias

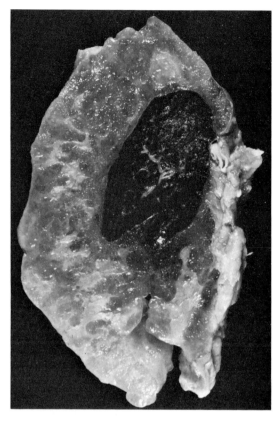

Fig. 19.80 Section of the spleen embedded in a large mass of mucoid carcinoma.

and wasting diseases. The most severe ascites, however, results from portal obstruction, and the accumulation of fluid often leads to enormous distension of the abdomen: the commonest cause is cirrhosis of the liver, and in cases which develop primary liver cancer, thrombosis of the portal vein often occurs, the ascitic fluid then accumulating very rapidly and becoming bloodstained. Endophlebitis of the hepatic veins (Budd-Chiari syndrome) is also accompanied by gross ascites. In the above conditions the fluid is a transudate and there is no formation of fibrin in the peritoneum, but in cases of portal cirrhosis it is not uncommon for a mild infection to become superadded, and occasionally tuberculous peritonitis. Accumulation of inflammatory exudate is, of course, a prominent feature of acute peritonitis, and occurs in some cases of tuberculous peritonitis. Peritoneal carcinomatosis also commonly induces an inflammatory, sometimes haemorrhagic, exudate.

Tumours

Primary tumours of the peritoneum are rare, and in most cases they take origin not from the serous layer but from some adjacent structure. For example, *lipoma* may arise from the appendices epiploicae; *fibroma* takes origin from the connective tissue and sometimes from the sheaths of the nerves in *neurofibromatosis*; and *lymphangioma* occasionally arises from the lymphatics of the mesentery. *Mesothelioma* of the peritoneum presents features like those of mesothelioma of the pleura but is less frequent, and the same caution in the interpretation of the appearances is required. In both situations there is an association with inhalation of asbestos (p. 16.72).

Secondary tumours of the peritoneum are comparatively common, especially in cases of gastric and ovarian carcinoma. They may be extremely numerous and very minute and may be mistaken macroscopically for tubercles. As mentioned above, they may induce a haemorrhagic inflammatory exudate; or there may be larger nodules and diffuse infiltration. The

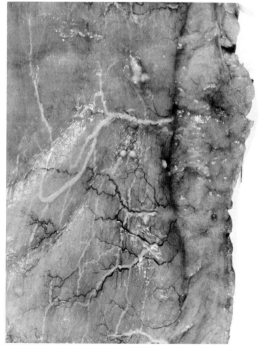

Fig. 19.81 Permeation of lymphatics in the serosa of of the small intestine by gastric carcinoma cells. × 2·5.

omentum is very frequently involved and becomes contracted into a hard irregular mass. In some cases of cancer the chief lesion is a very diffuse infiltration with thickening of the serous layers, but with little nodular formation; by such a process the mesentery may become greatly thickened and shrunken. This often results from *linitis plastica* of the stomach, and is accompanied by marked ascites. In mucoid carcinoma the peritoneum is sometimes overgrown by enormous soft translucent tumour masses (Fig. 19.80). Metastases of melanoma are not infrequent and the peritoneum may be studded with enormous numbers of small black nodules; these tend to be specially numerous in the omentum and mesentery.

As in the other serous cavities, the lining cells may desquamate and multiply in ascitic fluid, sometimes developing bizarre morphological features which make them very difficult to distinguish from cancer cells.

Extensive lymphatic permeation by carcinoma is often readily seen in the peritoneum (Fig. 19.81).

References and Further Reading

Day, D. W., Mandal, B. K. and Morson, B. C. (1978). The rectal biopsy appearances in Salmonella colitis. *Histopathology* **2,** 117–31.

Lee, F. D. and Toner, P. G. (1980). *Biopsy Pathology of the Small Intestine*, pp. 188. Chapman and Hall, London.

Morson, B. C. (1978). *The Pathogenesis of Colorectal Cancer*, pp. 164. Saunders, Philadelphia, London and Toronto.

Morson, B. C. and Dawson, I. P. M. (1979). *Gastrointestinal Pathology*, 2nd edn., pp. 805. Blackwell Scientific, Oxford, London, Edinburgh and Melbourne.

Riddell, R. H. *et al.* (1983). Dysplasia in inflammatory bowel disease. Standard classification with provisional clinical applications. *Human Pathology*, **14,** 931–68.

Sircus, W. (1979). The enigma of peptic ulcer. *Scottish Medical Journal* **24,** 31–7.

Sobin, L. H., Thomas, L. B., Percy, Constance and Henson, D. E. (Eds.) (1978). *A Coded Compendium of the International Histological Classification of Tumours*, pp. 116. World Health Organization, Geneva.

Whitehead, R. (1979). *Mucosal Biopsy of the Gastrointestinal Tract*, 2nd Edn., pp. 202. Saunders, London.

Wright, R. (Ed.) (1980). *Recent Advances in Gastrointestinal Pathology*, pp. 374. Saunders, Philadelphia, London and Toronto.

20

Liver, Biliary Tract and Pancreas

The Liver

The anatomical unit: The structural unit of the liver has long been considered to be the lobule, arranged around a central hepatic venule and with portal tracts at its periphery (Fig. 20.1a). In fact, the lobule forms a unit only in so far as blood from it drains into one central venule. It receives portal venous and hepatic arterial blood from several portal tracts, and its bile drains into several small bile ducts. On the basis of elegant microcirculatory studies, Rappaport and his colleagues (1954) have defined the basic structural unit as the **simple acinus** (Fig. 20.1b); this is the parenchyma receiving blood from a single terminal portal venule and hepatic arteriole (termed together the *axial vessels* of the acinus) and passing its bile into a single small duct in the same portal tract. The simple acinus lies between two hepatic ('centrilobular') venules into which its blood drains.

The simple acinus is subdivided into three zones (Fig. 20.1b). The hepatocytes in zone 1 (**periportal zone**) are those nearest to the axial vessels: they receive blood rich in nutrients and oxygen and are metabolically more active than cells in the other zones. Zones 2 (**mid-zone**) and 3 (**perivenular zone**) are more peripheral to the axial blood supply; the cells of zone 3 are metabolically least active, are most susceptible to hypoxic damage and are at the microcirculatory periphery of the acinus. The three or more simple acini relating to the preterminal branches of a portal venule and hepatic arteriole together form a **complex acinus** (Fig. 20.2a), the central part or core of which is made up of zones 1 of the simple acini, the intermediate part of zones 2, while zones 3 are peripheral and continuous with zones 3 of adjacent complex acini (Fig.

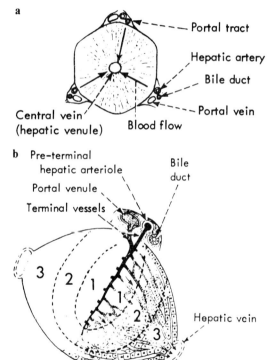

Fig. 20.1 (a) Diagrammatic illustration of the hepatic lobule arranged around a single central (hepatic) vein into which its blood flows. (b) Diagrammatic illustration of the simple acinus arranged around the terminal branches of the hepatic artery, showing its blood draining into two hepatic vein branches.

20.2b). Finally, aggregates of three or four complex acini, deriving their blood supply from a single portal vein branch and hepatic arterial branch, are termed **acinar agglomerates.**

Although the three zones of the simple acinus

20.1

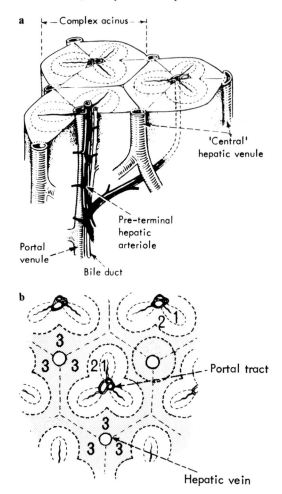

a — Complex acinus —

'Central'
hepatic venule

Pre-terminal
hepatic
arteriole

Portal
venule

Bile duct

b

Portal tract

Hepatic vein

Fig. 20.2 (a) Diagrammatic illustration of the complex acinus comprising three simple acini but deriving its blood from a single pre-terminal branch of the hepatic artery. (b) Diagrammatic illustration showing the relationship between adjacent complex acini, and how there is continuity between zones 3, i.e. the microcirculatory periphery of the acini.

correspond loosely to the peripheral, mid-zonal and centrilobular zones of the traditional lobule, study of Fig. 20.1 will make it clear that the correspondence is inexact. Lesions of hepatocytes which are influenced by their relationship to axial vessels and differences in their metabolic activities are more readily understood and described on the basis of the acinar concept. In practice this applies to most lesions of hepatocytes, and although in previous chapters we have adhered to the traditional concept of the lobule, which is still widely used, we shall

refer in this chapter to the acinus as the anatomical and functional hepatic unit.

Pathophysiology

The liver has a very large number of important physiological functions. It is involved in the intermediary metabolism of proteins, carbohydrates and fats, in the synthesis of a number of plasma proteins such as albumin and fibrinogen, the production of various enzymes and the formation and secretion of bile. It is also responsible for the detoxication of endogenously produced waste products or exogenously derived toxins and drugs, and in the storage of proteins, glycogen, various vitamins and metals. Accordingly, the liver is liable to injury from a variety of causes, and injury to it may have profound metabolic effects.

The major causes of liver disease

Injury from metabolic disturbances. In experimental animals specific dietary deficiencies can produce fatty liver and liver cell necrosis. Similarly in man, protein malnutrition, e.g. in kwashiorkor, can produce marked fatty change and there is evidence that malnutrition may considerably exacerbate other forms of injury. Specific enzyme deficiencies may cause various hepatic storage diseases (p. 20.8) or failure of biliary secretion (p. 20.54).

Injury from toxins and poisons. The liver cell is especially liable to injury because of its function of taking up and dealing with many metabolites, toxic substances, drugs and poisons. The vast number of chemicals used industrially and pharmacologically provide an ever-increasing hazard to the liver, particularly as it has been shown that certain chemicals are harmless to most individuals, but can cause extensive liver damage in individuals with a special susceptibility, as yet unpredictable. A wide spectrum of hepatotoxic effects may be produced by the numerous drugs now in clinical use (p. 20.44). The liver also receives blood draining the gastro-intestinal tract, and is exposed to poisons and toxins absorbed from the gut.

Lesions of the biliary tract affect the liver in two ways. Biliary obstruction, if sufficiently prolonged, results in biliary cirrhosis, and the bile ducts are also the most common route of bacterial infection of the liver.

Certain virus infections damage the liver severely, causing acute hepatitis with extensive necrosis of liver cells. They include Type A (infectious hepatitis), Type B (serum hepatitis) and Type 'non-A:non-B'. Progression to chronic hepatitis is a complication of Type B and Type non-A:non-B.

Hypoxia. Owing to their active and complex metabolism, liver cells are readily injured by hypoxia, as in shock, venous congestion or anaemia. However the dual blood supply to the liver affords some protection against hypoxic injury; the portal venous supply provides 70% of oxygen requirements.

Tumours. Primary tumours of the liver are relatively uncommon in this country though of great frequency in parts of Africa and the Far East; they are commonly associated with cirrhosis. The liver is a very common site of metastatic carcinoma, particularly from primary tumours of the gastro-intestinal tract.

Pathological effects of disturbed hepatic function

Disturbances of function resulting from lesions of the liver and biliary tract are varied and complex in their effects. They may be considered under three major headings: hepatocellular failure, portal hypertension and biliary obstruction. These are described more fully later in this chapter, but brief summaries of their main features are helpful at this point.

Hepatocellular failure arises when total liver cell function falls below the minimum required to maintain a physiological state. It results from loss of a large number of liver cells from various causes, and/or from impaired function of liver cells, usually attributable to chronic interference with hepatic blood flow; both factors may be involved, especially in hepatic cirrhosis. The more important effects include: **(a) changes in nitrogen metabolism** with a rise in the blood level of toxic nitrogenous compounds produced by bacteria in the gut and normally metabolised by the liver cells; these compounds affect especially the central nervous system, causing hepatic encephalopathy which consists of neuropsychiatric and locomotor disturbances,

delirium, convulsions and sometimes 'hepatic coma'; **(b) failure to remove bilirubin** from the blood, to conjugate it and excrete it in the bile; **(c) failure to produce plasma proteins** in normal amounts, particularly albumin, but also fibrinogen, prothrombin and various other clotting factors; **(d) hormonal disturbances** attributable to interference with hepatic metabolism of various steroid and other hormones; **(e) circulatory disturbances** of obscure nature, with cyanosis and a hypervolaemic hyperkinetic circulation; **(f) functional renal failure** (*the hepato-renal syndrome*). The precise mechanisms of this are not fully understood but the evidence suggests that humoral factors released as a result of severe liver cell injury impair proximal tubular function, resulting in renal failure but without any evident morphological change.

Portal hypertension. This is caused by obstruction to the blood flow through the liver. As a result, veins which provide an anastomosis between the portal and systemic systems enlarge and some of the portal blood is shunted directly into the systemic circulation instead of passing through the liver. Some of these dilated anastomotic channels, notably in the submucosa of the oesophagus, may rupture and bleed; furthermore the bypassing of the liver increases the blood level of toxic compounds absorbed from the gut, thus aggravating the effect of hepatocellular failure on the central nervous system and other organs.

Biliary obstruction. This results from obstruction of the common hepatic or common bile duct or from stagnation of bile in the biliary canaliculi without major duct obstruction. The effects include: (*a*) re-absorption of conjugated bilirubin into the blood, producing **obstructive jaundice**; (*b*) re-absorption of other constituents of bile, such as bile acids and cholesterol; (*c*) malabsorption of fats and fat-soluble vitamins because of the lack of bile salts in the intestine, producing **steatorrhoea** and effects arising from the **deficiency of vitamins A, D, E and K**; (*d*) prolonged cholestasis resulting in **liver cell necrosis** and eventually in **cirrhosis**. Secondary bacterial infection of the biliary tract—*ascending cholangitis*—is an important complication of major duct obstruction.

Circulatory Disturbances

The total hepatic blood flow is approximately 1·5 litres per minute, three-quarters of the blood being supplied by the portal vein and one-quarter by the hepatic artery. Thus, although hepatic arterial blood has a higher oxygen saturation (95%) than portal vein blood (85%), the latter normally provides approximately 70% of the hepatic oxygen requirement. Mixing of the two blood supplies takes place in the liver sinusoids, blood flow through which is controlled by sphincters at their portal and venular ends: flow of arterial blood into the sinusoids may be intermittent, with consequent variations in the proportion of arterial and portal venous blood.

Hepatic arterial obstruction

The hepatic artery is rarely severely obstructed by disease. Fatal infarction has followed accidental ligation of the main trunk or its branch to the right lobe, but in other instances adequate collateral circulation has prevented this. Obstruction of smaller intrahepatic branches is usually without effect because of adequate collateral circulation. However, local infarction may occur in polyarteritis nodosa and has also been described in acute bacterial endocarditis.

Portal venous obstruction

The normal portal venous pressure is 7 mm of mercury, and the *most important effect of portal venous obstruction, whatever the site or cause, is portal hypertension* (p. 20.34). Impairment of the portal venous blood flow can arise from obstruction of the hepatic veins, hepatic sinusoids, intrahepatic portal vein branches, or of the portal vein itself. *The commonest and most important cause of obstruction is hepatic cirrhosis.* Other intrahepatic causes include congenital hepatic fibrosis (p. 20.43), schistosomiasis (p. 28.25) and metastatic or primary carcinoma of the liver. The portal venous pressure may also rise transiently in acute hepatitis——viral and alcoholic——due to sinusoidal compression by the swollen liver cells.

Obstruction of the portal vein itself is uncommon. It can result from thrombosis, which may occur apparently spontaneously or may complicate (a) umbilical sepsis in the neonatal period, (b) intra-abdominal sepsis, (c) direct invasion by tumour, (d) myeloproliferative disorders, (e) splenectomy, especially in a patient with a normal pre-operative platelet count, and (f) portal hypertension. Obstruction of the portal vein without thrombosis may result from pressure by tumours in or around the porta hepatis.

The effects of *complete portal vein obstruction* depend on the site. If it is in the portal vein alone, nothing dramatic happens, but when it extends to occlude the ostium of the splenic vein, then the blood cannot drain via the splenic and gastro-oesophageal anastomoses and venous infarction of the bowel follows. In patients surviving portal venous thrombosis, new vascular channels develop in the portal fissure, so that a cavernous type of tissue is formed. *Occlusion of a branch of the portal vein* may sometimes be followed by 'red infarction' (Fig. 20.3), especially when venous congestion is also present. Such lesions, however, are not complete infarcts but are due to sinusoidal engorgement and atrophy of liver cells (p. 10.26).

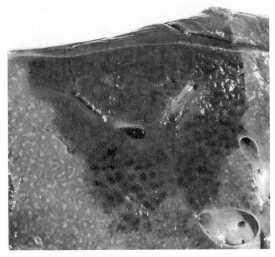

Fig. 20.3 Subcapsular 'red infarct' of the liver.

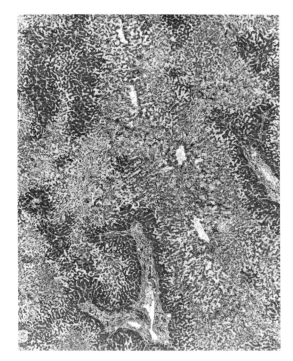

Fig. 20.4 Liver in Budd–Chiari syndrome due, in this instance, to carcinomatous obstruction of the inferior vena cava; there is extensive perivenular hepatocyte necrosis and haemorrhage, and prominent sinusoidal dilatation. × 28.

Hepatic venous obstruction

Obstruction of the major hepatic veins, clinically producing the Budd–Chiari syndrome, is rare. In many instances it is due to endophlebitis with superadded thrombosis, the aetiology being unknown. Compression by tumour masses or direct spread of tumour in the hepatic vein or the terminal inferior vena cava predisposes to thrombotic venous occlusion, and spontaneous thrombosis of these vessels may occur in myeloproliferative disorders or in thrombophlebitis migrans. Intense engorgement of the liver results, with sinusoidal dilatation, perivenular congestion and haemorrhage, and atrophy and necrosis of liver cells (Fig. 20.4). Ascites is usually severe, and death results from hepatocellular failure.

Veno-occlusive disease of the liver occurs in Jamaica and certain other tropical countries, probably as a result of drinking various plant or herbal medicines—'bush teas'. The active agents are alkaloids of the pyrrolizidine group present in plants of the genera *Senecio* (ragwort), *Crotalaria* and *Heliotropium*. Liver damage also occurs in animals that eat these plants, and has been produced experimentally. Changes are seen first around the hepatic venules with obliteration of sinusoids and hepatocellular injury. Later the hepatic vein radicles show sub-intimal oedema and progressive fibrosis, which may proceed to complete occlusion (Fig. 20.5). Death may result from liver failure in acute cases, but a chronic stage may develop with perivenular fibrosis and nodular hyperplasia progressing to cirrhosis. A similar condition may result from irradiation of the liver, and has also been associated with certain drugs, e.g. oral contraceptive steroids and urethane.

Circulatory disturbances due to systemic disease

Acute circulatory failure and shock. In cardiac, hypovolaemic and bacteraemic shock the cir-

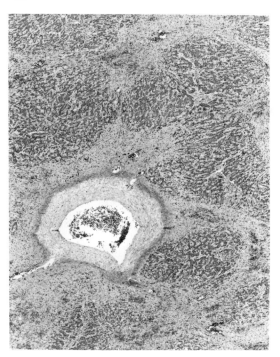

Fig. 20.5 Liver in veno-occlusive disease. There is extensive perivenular hepatocyte loss with replacement fibrosis and marked intimal fibrosis of the hepatic vein branch. × 28.

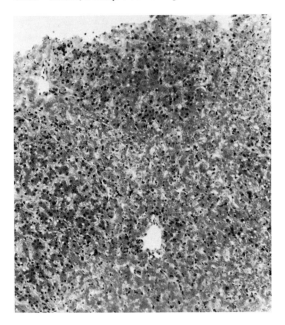

Fig. 20.6   Liver in acute circulatory failure: note the perivenular necrosis of hepatocytes extending in a radiate pattern and producing bridging necrosis between adjacent branches of hepatic veins. × 80.

culation through the liver is impaired. This results from a fall in both hepatic arterial and portal venous blood flow as part of the general circulatory failure. Initially the microcirculatory periphery (zone 3) of the acinus is injured, but involvement of zones 2 and 1 may occur in prolonged shock. Ischaemic hepatocyte necrosis (Fig. 20.6) of varying distribution patterns results, surrounding which there is usually an acute inflammatory reaction with infiltration of polymorphs. Biochemically these changes are reflected by elevations of serum aminotransferases, which are sometimes as high as in acute viral hepatitis, and by variable increases in serum bilirubin levels.

Venous congestion. In the systemic venous congestion of *acute cardiac failure* the liver is enlarged, often tender, and microscopy shows sinusoidal dilatation and congestion in the perivenular areas. *In chronic cardiac failure* the changes are more marked (p. 10.3), with liver

cell loss resulting from the continued effects of hypoxia and compression by the dilated sinusoids. Clinically there may be mild jaundice, moderate or sometimes marked elevation of the serum aminotransferase levels and also a reduced rate of hepatic inactivation of various drugs. In very prolonged venous congestion, perivenular hepatocyte loss may be fairly extensive. In some instances compensatory liver cell hyperplasia may occur with nodule formation and only minimal fibrosis—*nodular regenerative hyperplasia*. Sometimes replacement fibrosis takes place and fibrous septa link adjacent hepatic venous branches, resulting in architectural disorganisation (Fig. 20.7): although still called 'cardiac cirrhosis' this seldom, if ever, progresses to a true cirrhosis. The prognosis in hepatic venous congestion is that of the cardiac disease causing it.

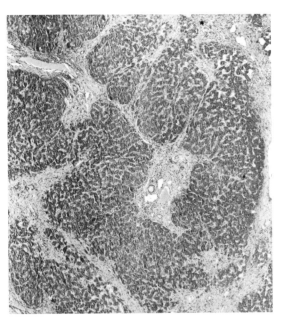

Fig. 20.7   Liver in chronic venous congestion: perivenular fibrosis has occurred with septate linkage between hepatic vein branches. Note the large portal tract (*central*) surrounded by surviving hepatic parenchyma. This corresponds to so-called cardiac cirrhosis. × 40.

Degenerations and Metabolic Disorders

Atrophy

The chief cause of general atrophy of the liver is starvation, in which it becomes shrunken and brown. This is seen also in senility. The cells, especially in the perivenular zones, are shrunken, and often contain granules of lipofuscin (p. 11.19).

Pressure atrophy occurs around tumours and cysts in the liver, in sinusoidal congestion (see Fig. 10.1, p. 10.4) and amyloidosis (see Fig. 11.4, p. 11.3), and focal atrophy is widespread in cirrhosis. The so-called cough furrows are due to localised atrophy caused by the pressure of diaphragmatic contraction during coughing and are of no importance.

Hyperplasia and hypertrophy

These occur commonly as a compensatory process, the liver cells both multiplying and enlarging, and often becoming multinucleate. These processes are prominent where there has been extensive liver cell necrosis, e.g. in viral or drug-induced hepatitis (Fig. 20.8), and in cirrhosis. The changes are often focal and the surrounding liver tissue may be compressed and atrophic. Hyperplasia and hypertrophy occur in the residual liver following experimental partial hepatectomy. Even when as much as two-thirds of the liver are removed, the weight of the organ may be restored within a few weeks. In fact, restoration occurs so rapidly that attempts to study diminished hepatic function by this method have usually failed.

Fatty change

Lipid metabolism is outlined in Chapter 3 (pp. 3.7 *et seq*). Because of their central role in fat metabolism, the liver cells are particularly prone to undergo fatty change, i.e. to accumulate in their cytoplasm droplets consisting mainly of neutral fat, and in adults a minor degree of fatty change is probably within physiological limits. In *pathological obesity* (p. 3.8) severe fatty change occurs in the liver, the

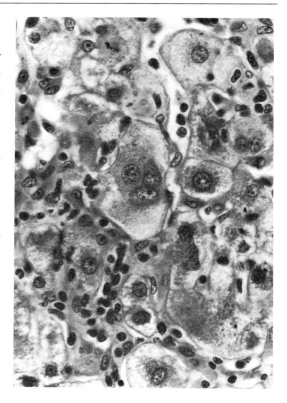

Fig. 20.8 Multinucleated liver cells, in the stage of recovery after acute hepatitis. × 450.

accumulation of fat beginning and being greatest in periportal hepatocytes (Fig. 3.9, p. 3.7). The liver cells, in addition to taking up a high proportion of dietary fat absorbed from the intestine and fatty acids released from the depots, are also active in the synthesis of fat from glucose and amino acids. The relative importance of these processes depends on the amounts of carbohydrate, fat and protein in the diet.

In addition to the causes of general fatty change—hypoxia, starvation and wasting disease, and numerous chemical and bacterial toxins—fatty change in the liver may also result from chronic malnutrition, alcohol abuse (p. 20.22) and in the rare conditions of acute fatty liver of pregnancy (p. 20.44) and Reye's syndrome (p. 20.43).

Fatty change in chronic malnutrition is a controversial topic of some importance because of the prevalence of malnutrition in many parts

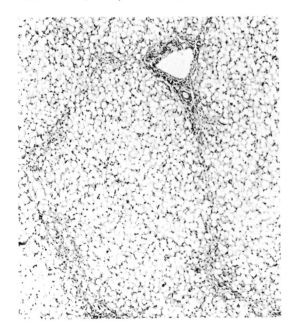

Fig. 20.9 Fatty liver in kwashiorkor. In addition to vacuolation of each liver cell by a large globule of fat, there is an apparent increase in fibrous tissue, seen as fine strands running through the parenchyma. × 40. (Preparation kindly lent by Professor R. S. Patrick.)

of the world. Severe malnutrition gives rise to a syndrome termed *kwashiorkor*, which affects infants and young children in many parts of southern and central Africa, in tropical America, and extensively in the Far East. The syndrome is a complex one, attributable to a diet severely deficient in high-grade protein, less deficient in total calories, and with additional features due to vitamin deficiencies. Growth is impaired, the liver is severely fatty (Fig. 20.9), the pancreas is atrophic, the plasma albumin is low and there is nutritional oedema. It seems likely that the fatty liver is the result of impaired lipoprotein synthesis due to the protein deficiency, perhaps aggravated by inadequate carbohydrate intake. There is no evidence that the fatty liver in malnutrition progresses to cirrhosis.

Haemosiderosis

Haemosiderin pigment gives a blue staining reaction with prussian blue stain (Perls' reaction).

The normal adult liver contains approximately 0·3 g of iron, but more than half of this is in the form of ferritin, and the amount of haemosiderin is not sufficient to give a prussian blue reaction (p. 11.15). In infancy the liver normally gives an iron reaction and this becomes more marked in wasting conditions of children.

Excess iron deposition occurs (a) in primary haemochromatosis (p. 11.16); (b) in conditions of excessive blood destruction, e.g. haemolytic anaemias of all types; (c) following multiple blood transfusions in some chronic blood disorders; (d) in alcoholic liver disease and (e) from ingestion of excessive amounts of iron, either in medicines or in the diet. This is common in the South African Bantu whose staple diet of porridge is prepared in iron pots. Excessive iron deposits in the liver may involve only the parenchymal cells in the early stages of primary haemochromatosis, whereas in the other conditions of iron overload both parenchymal cell and Kupffer cell siderosis occur. The haemosiderin appears as brownish-yellow granules in the liver cells. Deposits initially tend to be more marked in the periportal hepatocytes. Subsequently there may be diffuse hepatocellular deposition.

Amyloid disease

The liver is involved in approximately 50% of cases of primary and secondary amyloidosis, but is less frequently involved in myeloma-associated amyloid. The SAA protein (p. 11.6) is synthesised by liver cells. The amyloid deposits affect the hepatic artery branches and/or the perisinusoidal space, compressing neighbouring hepatocytes (see Fig. 11.4, p. 11.3). Amyloid disease only rarely causes hepatocellular dysfunction.

Glycogen storage diseases

Glycogen storage diseases (pp. 3.11, 3.16) result from enzyme defects, and the ultimate diagnosis depends on the demonstration of the specific defect. The liver cells are involved in Types I, II, III, IV, VI and VIII, and the intracellular site of glycogen storage varies in the different types: light and electron microscopy thus reveal diagnostically useful changes. Hepatocellular adenomas may develop in Type I and cirrhosis in Type IV.

Excess of glycogen accumulates also in other metabolic disturbances, e.g. in diabetes mellitus. The electron-microscopic appearances of glycogen are shown on p. 3.16.

Lipid storage diseases

In these conditions abnormal amounts of *lipids* (other than triglyceride fats) accumulate, mainly in cells of the mononuclear-phagocyte system, the Kupffer cells being consistently involved in Gaucher's disease (cerebroside accumulation) and Niemann–Pick disease (sphingomyelin). Hypercholesterolaemic lipid storage diseases rarely affect the liver.

Other metabolic disorders

Many other inherited metabolic disorders affect the liver, and involvement is severe in some, e.g. galactosaemia, alpha-1-antitrypsin deficiency, Wilson's disease and erythropoietic protoporphyria. Although these conditions are rare, preventive measures or treatment may be helpful and so clinical awareness and early recognition are important.

Liver Cell Necrosis

Necrosis of liver cells, of greater or lesser extent, occurs in many diseases of the liver, and also in many other conditions, such as severe infections, wasting diseases and cardiac failure, in which liver cell injury is neither the most important nor the most characteristic feature. Infarction (p. 10.26) needs no further description here.

Necrosis may affect: **(a) single scattered liver cells** which die one by one (*necrobiosis or apoptosis* (p. 3.29)). Single liver cells may also undergo 'acidophilic' or 'eosinophilic' necrosis; these are recognised as eosinophilic granular cells with a pyknotic nucleus which is eventually extruded leaving the *acidophilic* or 'Councilman' body; **(b) small groups of hepatocytes,** irregularly distributed (*focal necrosis*) in relation to which macrophages and lymphocytes may accumulate. Such foci may result from many types of liver injury, but are common in severe toxaemia, particularly when due to infections within the portal drainage area. Focal necrosis also occurs in acute viral and drug-induced hepatitis; **(c) large groups of hepatocytes** (*confluent necrosis*) as in severe viral hepatitis, drug-induced and acute ischaemic liver injury. In severe viral hepatitis, confluent necrosis may extend between contiguous hepatic venules or between hepatic venules and portal tracts ('central-central' and 'central-portal' bridging necrosis); **(d) extensive areas of the liver** (*massive hepatic necrosis*), which represents a more severe degree of confluent necrosis and may be a sequel to viral hepatitis or drug injury. Clinically, it results in fulminant acute hepatocellular failure with a mortality approaching 80%.

The factors which determine the topographical distribution of hepatic necrosis are not known but presumably include the zonal differences in enzyme distribution, cell metabolism and quality of blood supply. Ischaemic injury affects the perivenular zones of the acini (Fig. 20.6) as do many drugs and toxins, e.g. alcohol and paracetamol. Other agents produce periportal injury, e.g., phosphorus, while yellow fever characteristically affects zone 2 of the acinus, producing a 'mid-zonal' pattern of necrosis.

Massive liver cell necrosis is described later as a complication of viral hepatitis, and 'piecemeal necrosis' is defined as a characteristic feature in many forms of chronic hepatitis.

Hepatitis

Hepatitis literally means any inflammatory lesion of the liver. In practice the term is not used for focal lesions, such as an abscess, but only when there is diffuse involvement of the liver. This may be either acute or chronic, and in some instances acute and chronic hepatitis may be present simultaneously.

Hepatitis may be further classified on an aetiological basis, and some types are best dealt with under separate headings, e.g. alcoholic hepatitis, drug-induced hepatitis, and chronic hepatitis in Wilson's disease, haemochromatosis and biliary disease. Cirrhosis represents a late, irreversible and progressive stage of chronic hepatitis, and it also will be discussed separately (p. 20.26).

In this section we deal with (i) *acute viral hepatitis* due to the well-recognised hepatitis A virus (HAV), hepatitis B virus (HBV), the more recently recognised hepatitis non-Anon-B viruses and other acute virus and virus-like infections; and with (ii) *chronic hepatitis*, often of unknown cause, and sub-classified into chronic persistent and chronic active types.

Acute viral hepatitis

This is an acute infection characterised by diffuse hepatitis with widespread liver cell necrosis. There are two well-characterised types, A and B, and a less-well characterised non-Anon-B type which may, however, include a number of different virus infections.

Hepatitis A (infectious hepatitis) is a naturally acquired infection, has an incubation period of 15–40 days, and occurs endemically and as epidemics. The infective agent is a picornavirus and associated 27 nm particles occur in the blood and faeces during early infection and have been demonstrated in the liver-cell cytoplasm in experimental animals. In contrast to HBV, only one serotype of hepatitis A has been identified in world-wide studies. The highest natural incidence occurs in children under 15, boys and girls being equally affected, with a higher frequency in the lower socio-economic classes. It is estimated that 50–75% of the community may be infected during epidemics, but

in most of them the infection is anicteric and often subclinical. Faeces and blood become infected 3–4 weeks after exposure to the virus, and remain infective for about 3 weeks. Specific immunity is established after recovery from hepatitis A and protective IgG class antibody is demonstrable in the serum. The demonstration of IgM class antibody serologically establishes the diagnosis during the acute phase. Active immunisation is still not possible, but passive immunisation with pooled human IgG has been shown to prevent clinical disease.

Hepatitis B (Serum hepatitis) has an incubation period of 50–180 days; it is most frequently transmitted by blood and blood products, but may also be transmitted by intimate physical contact e.g. from mother to child and sexually. It is a particular hazard among male homosexuals, intravenous drug addicts and patients treated by renal dialysis. The disease occurs in any age group; it is more severe than hepatitis A, with a higher mortality, and infection may result also in the development of a carrier state or in progression to chronic liver disease.

In 1964, Blumberg and his colleagues described a lipoprotein complex in the blood of an Australian aborigine, using as antibody the serum of a much-transfused haemophiliac. This complex they called **Australia (Au) antigen**; subsequently it was shown by them (1967) and others to be particularly associated with cases of serum hepatitis. It is now known to be hepatitis B virus surface antigen (see below), and is demonstrable by various serological techniques of which solid phase radioimmunoassay and enzyme-linked immunoassay (ELISA) are the most sensitive.

Electron microscopy (Fig. 20.10) shows two morphologically distinct viral components which are also known to represent two serologically distinct antigens. The 42 nm Dane particle is regarded as the complete infective virion of HBV. The central core of the Dane particle, hepatitis B core antigen (**HBcAg**), contains DNA polymerase, circular double-stranded DNA, and protein antigens; the core antigen is equivalent to the nucleocapsid antigen of other viruses. Viral replication occurs in the liver cell nuclei, and core particles may appear free within the liver cell cytoplasm, but are demon-

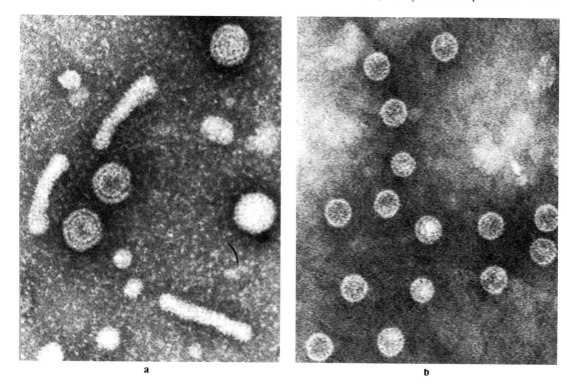

Fig. 20.10 Electron micrographs showing the morphological forms of the HB Ag. (**a**) This shows the small spheres and tubular structures (20 nm diameter) together with the larger double-shelled Dane particles (42 nm diameter). The small spheres, tubules and outer coat of the Dane particle comprise HBsAg. The inner part of the Dane particle is HBcAg. × 300 000. (**b**) A preparation of purified core particles—HBcAg. × 300 000. (Dr June Almeida.)

strable in the serum only within complete Dane particles. The outer envelope of the Dane particle is antigenically distinct from HBcAg, and is referred to as hepatitis B surface antigen (**HBsAg**). It is produced in excess in the liver cell cytoplasm and appears in the serum, both as the coating material of Dane particles and also as 20 nm spherical particles and tubular structures (Fig. 20.10). A third antigen, 'e' antigen (**HBeAg**) is closely related to Dane particle formation and its presence therefore correlates with infectivity. The nature of this antigen is uncertain, but serological testing for HBeAg and antibody is of considerable prognostic value.

HBsAg is not serologically homogeneous, and various antigenic markers have been described. All **subtypes** contain three such antigens, 'a', 'd' or 'y', 'w' or 'r'. These subtypes— adw, adr, ayw, and ayr—do not appear to differ in their clinical effects, but are of considerable value in epidemiological studies.

The distribution of the HB antigens within the liver cells has been demonstrated by immunofluorescence techniques, direct electron microscopy and immuno-electron microscopy. HBcAg is found mostly in the nuclei (Fig. 20.11) and to a lesser extent in the cytoplasm; it always acquires a surface antigen coating before entry into the serum. Excess of HBcAg in the nucleus may occasionally be recognisable by light microscopy as 'sanded nuclei', containing a granular eosinophilic inclusion (Fig. 20.11). HBsAg is found exclusively in the liver cell cytoplasm; it is present in the smooth endoplasmic reticulum, and the cytoplasmic deposits produce characteristic 'ground-glass' hepatocytes (Fig. 20.12) which are readily recognisable on routine haematoxylin and eosin or trichrome stains, but are rendered more conspicuous by orcein or by aldehyde thionine. It should be emphasised that the liver-cell distribution of these antigens has been demonstrated mainly in chronic carriers of hepatitis **B** or

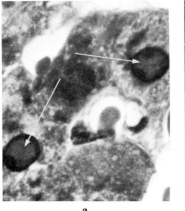
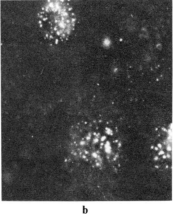
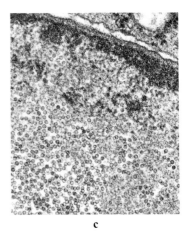

a   b   c

Fig. 20.11 Hepatitis B core antigen. (**a**) Nuclear excess of antigen producing 'sanded nuclei' (*arrows*). × 150. (**b**) Specific immunofluorescence for core antigen: note the granular nature of the intranuclear deposits. (**c**) Intranuclear core particles demonstrated by electron microscopy: the nuclear membrane runs transversely across the upper part of the illustration. × 43 000. (Professor L. Bianchi, University of Basel, Switzerland.)

patients with chronic hepatitis as a sequel to the acute infection. 'Sanded' nuclei and 'ground-glass' hepatocytes are not seen in the acute clinical attack.

The patterns of antigen and antibody response in the acute classical attack, with elimination of the virus and full clinical recovery, are shown in Fig. 20.13a. The development of antibody to HBsAg (HBsAb) appears to be delayed, but it is regarded as the protective antibody. While recovery with elimination of the virus is the outcome in most patients, about 5% develop chronic hepatitis and progress to cirrhosis and about 5% become chronic carriers; the pattern of antigen and antibody responses in these patients is shown in Fig. 20.13a. Fail-

ure to produce HBsAb and persistence of HBeAg is associated with chronic active hepatitis. The chronic carrier produces HBeAb, but there is persistence of HBsAg and a failure to produce HBsAb; such a carrier state may develop after a period of chronic active liver disease (Fig. 20.13b) with so-called sero-conversion to HBeAb positive and cessation of viral replication. The host factors which determine these sequelae are not fully understood, but they are more likely to occur in males.

The incidence of carriers in the community shows marked geographic variation, being of the order of 0.1% in this country, whereas in parts of Africa and South-East Asia it is as high as 20%. Vertical transmission from mother to

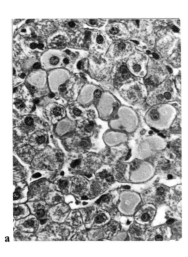
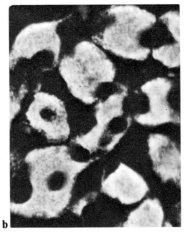

a   b

Fig. 20.12 Hepatitis B surface antigen. (**a**) Cytoplasmic excess of antigen producing 'ground-glass hepatocytes' with an intracytoplasmic homogeneous inclusion. Masson's trichrome. × 250. (**b**) Specific immunofluorescence for surface antigen showing uniform cytoplasmic staining; the nuclei are negative. (Fig. 20.12b, Professor L. Bianchi, University of Basel, Switzerland.)

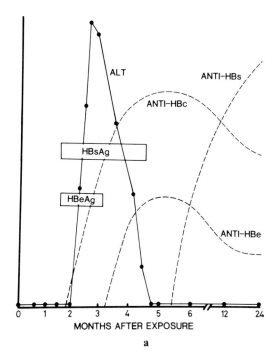

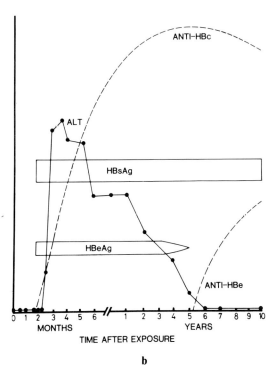

Fig. 20.13 Humoral responses in hepatitis B infections (see text). (**a**) With clinical recovery and viral elimination (**b**) Chronic infection with continued viral replications. (ALT - alanine aminotransferase). Units on the vertical axis are arbitrary.

child in the early weeks of life is an important mode of infection in countries with high carrier rates.

The Delta agent. Initially discovered by Rizetto and his colleagues in 1977, this has now been shown to be a defective RNA virus which requires HBV for its replication. The infective particle contains the RNA coated with HBsAg material. Antigen and antibody can be detected in serum by radio- or enzyme-linked immunoassay; antigen can be detected in the liver by immunohistochemistry, and is present mainly in liver-cell nuclei with smaller amounts in the cytoplasm. This agent, which occurs on a worldwide basis, modifies both acute and chronic HB infections; it can be acquired simultaneously with HB (co-infection) or it may secondarily infect patients with chronic HBs antigenaemia. In both events the clinical illness, now called hepatitis D, is more severe and the liver injury more extensive.

The main significance of the discovery of HBV and its complicated antigen/antibody systems has been as follows: (a) it allows screening of potential blood donors and may thus reduce the incidence of direct transmission of hepatitis **B**; (b) it has resulted in specific diagnostic and retrospective tests for infection and this has greatly increased our knowledge of the epidemiology of the disease and of its clinical behaviour; (c) it has provided information on the possible relationships of HBV to chronic liver disease and hepatocellular carcinoma; (d) of most importance, however, has been the development of vaccines to provide active immunisation against the virus. Various preparations of HBsAg material have now been shown to be effective vaccines, the production of HBsAb affording protection against the virus. The widespread future use of these vaccines may result in eradication of the disease.

Hepatitis non-Anon-B (NANB) was first described following blood transfusion after serological exclusion of other known hepatitis viruses and with the demonstration of a transmissible agent which induces hepatitis in chimpanzees. Prospective studies have indicated that it is now responsible for more than 70% of post-transfusion hepatitis. At least two types of NANB hepatitis have been postulated. However the infective agent(s) have not been identified nor have antigenic markers been detected. Carrier states occur, and there is evidence of an

Table 20.1   Comparative aspects of A, B and non-A non-B viral hepatitis

	Hepatitis A (HAV)	Hepatitis B (HBV)	Hepatitis non-A non-B (NANB)
Mode of spread	Oro-faecal (parenteral)	Parenteral (oro-faecal and sexual)	Parenteral ? others
Incubation period (days)	15–40	50–180	10–90
Age affected	Younger age groups	Any age	Any age
Clinical episode	Mild: mortality rate 1% or less	Severe: mortality rate variable up to 15%	May be severe; tendency for clinical fluctuation
Virus and type	RNA picornavirus 27 nm; HA Ag	DNA hepadnavirus*	Not yet identified
Carrier states and chronic hepatitis	No	Yes**	Yes†
Transmissible experimentally to	Marmoset, Chimpanzee	Chimpanzee	Chimpanzee

*See test for discussion of antigen/antibody systems   † Chronic sequelae prominent
**Association also with hepatocellular carcinoma (p. 13.17).

increased risk of progression to chronic hepatitis following the acute disease.

Clinical and biochemical features

The clinical and biochemical features of the three types are very similar. Their features are compared in Table 20.1.

The early clinical features are severe nausea, anorexia, intolerance of fat, often retching, vomiting and fever. A 'serum-sickness-like' syndrome may be seen, with arthralgia and occasionally skin rashes. There is often epigastric pain and the liver is enlarged, tender and the site of a dull ache. Jaundice develops 3 to 9 days after this prodromal illness and reaches a peak in 10 days, during which period the stools are pale and the urine dark. The spleen is palpably enlarged in a third of patients. These features subside in 2–6 weeks but full clinical recovery may take several more weeks. An initial leucopenia is seen in the pre-icteric stage, succeeded by a lymphocytosis with, in a small proportion of cases, atypical lymphocytes resembling those found in infectious mononucleosis. The serum bilirubin level is between 80 and 250 μmol/litre (4–12 mg/dl) and this is mainly in the conjugated form. Serum alkaline phosphatase levels do not usually exceed 30 King-Armstrong units/dl. Serum aspartate aminotransferase (SGOT) and alanine aminotransferase (SGPT) levels may reach levels greatly in excess of 1000 iu/litre early in the disease and then fall rapidly with

the onset of jaundice. The one-stage prothrombin time is usually prolonged, and this measurement provides the best single indication of the severity of the hepatitis.

Most patients recover completely from an attack. Mortality rates are lower in hepatitis A than in B, but vary in different communities and outbreaks from 1 to 20%; there is now some evidence that NANB may be the most frequent type of fulminant viral hepatitis and with the lowest survival rates. In very severe cases, death results acutely from fulminant liver failure due to massive hepatic necrosis. The hepatitis may progress, sometimes with fluctuations in severity, and cause death from liver failure in 3–8 weeks: this occurs more frequently in females. In some cases jaundice is deeper and persists for weeks or even months— *cholestatic hepatitis*—but eventually with complete recovery. The development of chronic carrier states and of chronic active hepatitis and cirrhosis are discussed later. The so-called *posthepatitis syndrome* with vague features—undue fatigue, dyspepsia and hepatic pain—occurs in a small number of patients.

Pathological changes

Classical acute hepatitis. The mechanisms of the liver cell injury are not understood but may vary for the different types of virus. There is diffuse hepatic involvement but the changes are usually more severe in the perivenular (acinar zone 3) areas. These comprise acute

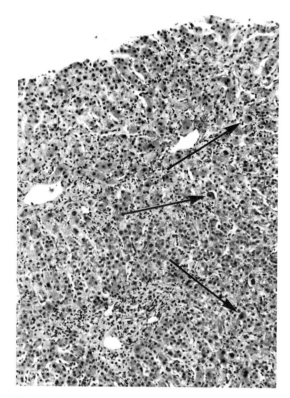

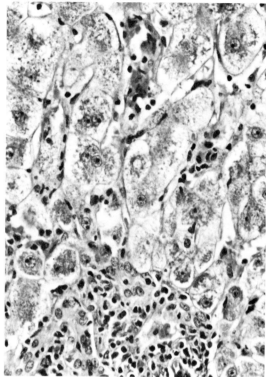

Fig. 20.14 Liver in viral hepatitis. There is a moderately intense mononuclear cell infiltrate of the portal tract (*lower centre*), and a more intense diffuse parenchymal cell infiltrate with liver cell degeneration and a number of acidophilic bodies (*arrowed*). × 120.

Fig. 20.15 Liver in viral hepatitis showing swelling of liver cells and foci of liver cell necrosis. Note also the portal tract inflammation (*lower centre*). (Professor R. S. Patrick.) × 465.

degenerative changes in scattered hepatocytes accompanied by a predominantly mononuclear cell infiltrate of the portal tracts and parenchyma, Kupffer cell reactive hyperplasia and varying degrees of hepatocyte regenerative activity (Fig. 20.14).

There is great variation in the degree of injury of individual liver cells: many cells appear normal, but there may be single or focal hepatocellular necrosis. The cells may be enlarged, with granular cytoplasm tending to be condensed round the nucleus—ballooning degeneration (Fig. 20.15); others show acidophilic degeneration, with shrinkage of the cells, increased cytoplasmic eosinophilia, pyknosis and eventual extrusion of the nucleus, leaving the acidophilic or Councilman body (Fig. 20.16). With necrosis and eventual lysis of single cells or groups of cells, there is disruption of liver cell plates, but the reticulin framework remains intact. An inflammatory infiltrate,

mainly of lymphocytes, very occasional plasma cells and a few polymorphs, is intimately related to the liver cell necrosis and is also a regular finding in the portal tracts. Kupffer cells show reactive hyperplasia; many contain phagocytosed cellular debris, bile pigment and lipofuscin granules, and they contribute to the striking increase in cellularity so characteristic of the histological appearance. Biliary stasis is usually not severe but intracytoplasmic bile pigment granules and occasional bile thrombi are seen. Electron microscopy shows irregular swelling of the endoplasmic reticulum of hepatocytes to form vesicles, detachment of the membrane-associated ribosomes and enlarged phagosomes containing altered mitochondria and organelle debris. None of these electron-microscopic changes is specific.

The acute liver cell injury is brief, and before the attack has subsided clinically, hypertrophy and hyperplasia are seen among surviving

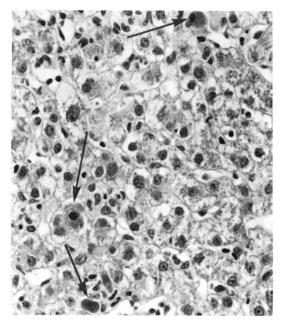

Fig. 20.16   Liver in viral hepatitis: perivenular area showing a number of ballooned hepatocytes, a diffuse mononuclear infiltrate, and a number of acidophilic (Councilman) bodies (*arrowed*) one of which lies free in a sinusoid. × 360.

hepatocytes with the formation of binucleate and multinucleate cells (Fig. 20.8).

Necrosis gradually diminishes and phagocytic activity by Kupffer cells becomes more marked as regression occurs.

Acute viral hepatitis with bridging necrosis. In these cases the features of classical acute hepatitis are seen but there is more extensive loss of liver cells. Confluent necrosis occurs particularly in acinar zone 3; lysis of injured hepatocytes produces an empty reticulin pattern which later collapses, forming a loose meshwork or septum heavily infiltrated with lymphocytes and macrophages (Fig. 20.17). Such extensive lesions may result in fulminant hepatic failure. Survival depends on the regenerative power of the spared parenchyma, and with survival there is usually a restoration of normal architecture.

Acute hepatitis with massive (panacinar) necrosis. This may occur in all three types of viral hepatitis. There is confluent necrosis of all or nearly all the parenchymal cells in large areas of the liver, often more extensive in the left lobe. When almost the whole of the paren-

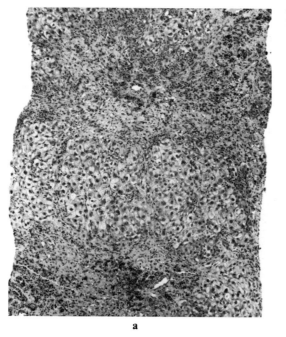

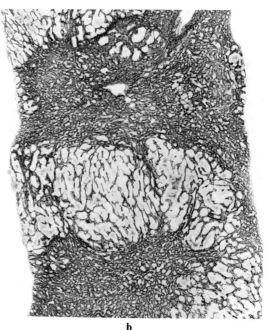

a   b

Fig. 20.17   Liver in viral hepatitis: acute Type B infection with bridging necrosis. Note the extensive confluent necrosis of liver cells, producing collapse of the reticulin framework. Full uneventful recovery occurred in this patient. (**a**) H & E. × 60. (**b**) Gordon and Sweets' reticulin. × 60.

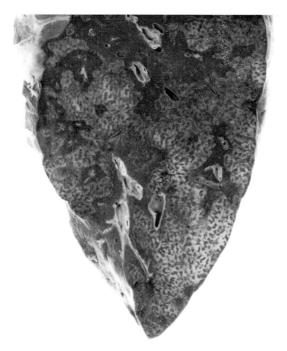

Fig. 20.18 Massive necrosis of liver three weeks after the onset of jaundice. Note the irregular dark areas from which the dead liver cells have been absorbed, and the portions showing persisting liver structure which were deeply jaundiced. These latter areas had undergone necrosis shortly before death.

chyma is destroyed, death results from fulminant hepatic failure.

Massive liver cell necrosis may occur as an unusual complication in acute viral hepatitis. When death occurs within a few days, i.e. before autolysis of the dead liver cells, the liver is approximately normal in size and is strikingly yellow owing to bile-staining. Subsequently the dead cells disappear, the affected parts of the liver become shrunken, soft and red due to sinusoidal congestion and local haemorrhage (Fig. 20.18). If the patient survives for weeks or months, proliferation of the surviving parenchyma produces pale nodules varying in size to over a centimetre, and scarring occurs in the area of liver cell loss. These changes result in a shrunken nodular liver—*post-necrotic scarring* or *multiple nodular hyperplasia*. The variation in size of nodules and the breadth of intervening fibrous tissue bands are much greater than in cirrhosis (Fig. 20.19). The prognosis is still poor, and death may result from a recurrence

of massive necrosis, from chronic hepatocellular failure, or from portal hypertension.

Certain chemicals used therapeutically and in industry may also produce massive liver cell necrosis in a small proportion of individuals at risk. The patterns of massive necrosis due to viral hepatitis, drugs or chemicals are microscopically similar. Initially there is extensive liver cell death, with only a few surviving periportal hepatocytes, and with little inflammatory cell reaction (Fig. 20.20). Subsequently there is extensive autolysis of dead cells with consequent collapse of the reticulin framework (Fig. 20.21). There is a moderately intense mononuclear cell infiltrate, and after a few days fibrosis and hepatocyte regeneration may be noted.

It is not clear why massive hepatic necrosis occurs in some cases of viral hepatitis, usually a fairly benign condition, or following thera-

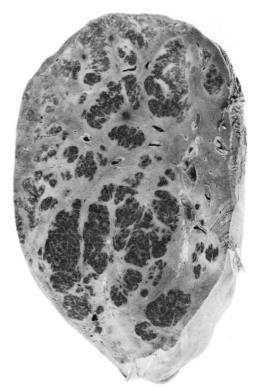

Fig. 20.19 Massive necrosis of liver with fatal recurrence. The pale areas consist of fibrous tissue, the liver cells having undergone necrosis in the initial attack and subsequent autolysis. The dark areas consist of tissue in which the liver cells survived the initial attack, but were destroyed in a rapidly fatal recurrence.

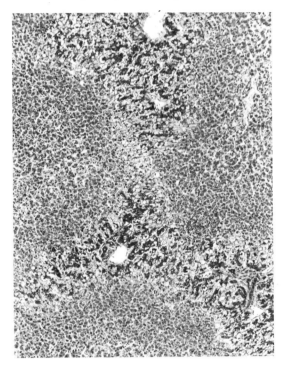

Fig. 20.20   Massive liver cell necrosis in paracetamol overdosage: the hepatocytes in the periportal zones have survived and appear darkly stained. × 60.

peutic doses of various drugs in certain susceptible individuals. While there are reports that acute viral hepatitis may run a more severe course in malnourished people, there is little evidence that this is a factor in massive hepatic necrosis in this country.

Hepatitis due to other viruses

Acute hepatitis may occur as an unusual complication of *rubella* or of *herpes simplex* in infancy and childhood, but rarely in adults. In *infectious mononucleosis* due to the Epstein–Barr virus, abnormal lymphoid cells may accumulate in the portal tracts and sinusoids, and a mild form of clinical hepatitis may occur with focal liver cell necrosis and slight cholestasis. *Cytomegalovirus* hepatitis is a feature of the generalised form of infection with this virus, which occurs in neonates infected *in utero*. In older children and adults, this virus can cause hepatitis closely resembling acute viral hepatitis A or B and sometimes occurring as part of an illness resembling infectious mono-

nucleosis, particularly in immunosuppressed patients.

Yellow fever, caused by a Group B arbovirus, occurs sporadically and in epidemics in certain parts of Africa and tropical America. The disease occurs in monkeys and is transmitted to man by the bite of *Aedes aegyptii* and certain other mosquitoes. It varies in severity from a mild unsuspected febrile illness to a fatal combination of fulminant massive hepatic necrosis, acute renal failure and marrow depression with leucopenia and thrombocytopenia. The hepatic lesion consists of mid-zonal necrosis and fatty infiltration in mild cases. Acidophilic liver cell necrosis is prominent, producing the classical Councilman body. The kidneys show proximal tubular necrosis.

Chronic hepatitis

Chronic hepatitis may be conveniently defined as inflammation of the liver continuing without

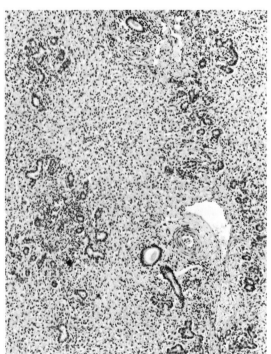

Fig. 20.21   Massive liver cell necrosis: there are virtually no surviving hepatocytes and the parenchyma comprises dilated capillary-like structures. Some bile duct proliferation is seen around portal tracts. × 75.

improvement for at least six months. It is a primary disease of liver and can be viral, drug-induced or of unknown aetiology.

Chronic inflammation is also a feature of Wilson's disease, longstanding biliary obstruction, alcohol-induced liver injury and other metabolic disorders; while these conditions may also be associated with morphological features similar to those about to be described, and also run a chronic course, they are not usually included in the definition of chronic hepatitis.

Chronic hepatitis has been subdivided into a relatively benign form, **chronic persistent hepatitis**, in which the inflammation is confined to the portal areas, and a more aggressive form, **chronic active hepatitis,** in which there is portal and parenchymal involvement with progressive fibrosis ending in cirrhosis. These definitions are based on morphological criteria, and have replaced former terms such as subacute hepatitis, lupoid hepatitis, juvenile cirrhosis, etc. The clinical and pathological features of chronic hepatitis will first be outlined, and aetiological mechanisms will then be discussed.

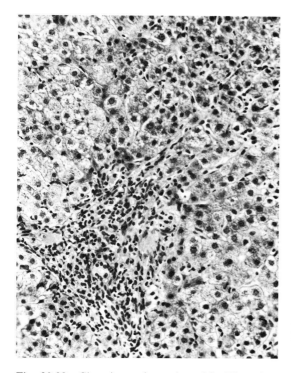

Fig. 20.22 Chronic persistent hepatitis. There is a mononuclear cell infiltrate confined to the portal tract in the lower left quadrant with little or no involvement of the hepatic parenchyma. × 205.

Chronic persistent hepatitis

This is a mild disease, with a benign course, and characterised clinically by symptoms of fatigue, malaise, vague upper abdominal pain and sometimes intolerance of dietary fat. The liver may be tender and slightly enlarged. Biochemical tests show a moderate elevation of aminotransferase levels, but levels of IgG are within the normal range.

Liver biopsy shows a moderately intense mononuclear cell infiltrate of the portal tracts, with a normal architecture, intact limiting plates, little or no significant increase in portal fibrous tissue and only minimal parenchymal cell necrosis (Fig. 20.22).

This entity is thought to be a sequel to a subclinical or clinical attack of acute viral hepatitis. Although progression to cirrhosis has not been reported, transition to chronic active hepatitis has been described in a few cases, and cases of chronic active hepatitis have changed to a pattern of chronic persistent hepatitis following treatment.

Chronic active hepatitis

Clinical features. Without treatment, this condition usually progresses to cirrhosis, although some cases may subside spontaneously. In our experience there is a female to male preponderance of 3 to 1, but it is well recognised that HB-associated chronic active hepatitis (see below) is more common in males. The condition occurs mainly between 20 and 50 years of age, but is seen also in older people. The onset may be acute in about a third of patients and indistinguishable from an acute viral hepatitis, or it may be insidious with non-specific symptoms of anorexia, tiredness, vague upper abdominal pain and often amenorrhoea. There may be evidence of hepatocellular failure, but the disease tends to fluctuate in severity. There is hepatomegaly, and often splenomegaly which precedes the development of any portal hypertension.

Additional features include arthralgia, skin rashes, pleural effusions, thrombocytopenia, leucopenia and proteinuria attributable to glomerular lesions; they occur in various degrees and combinations. Some patients also may have chronic inflammatory bowel disease, chronic thyroiditis, Sjøgren's syndrome, and other diseases of possible auto-immune aetiology.

Biochemical tests show elevations of aminotransferase levels, usually over 100 iu/litre. The occurrence and degree of jaundice varies; when present it is usually associated with a moderate

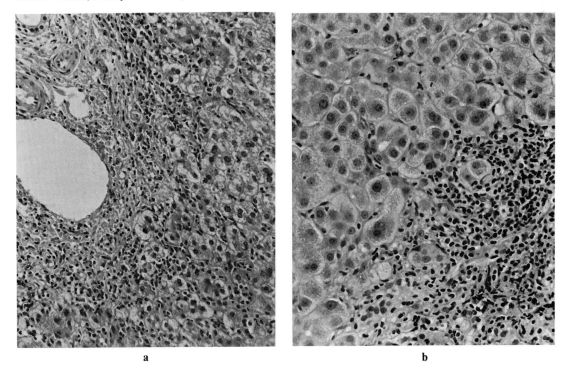

a   b

Fig. 20.23   Chronic active hepatitis with piecemeal necrosis. (**a**) Note the irregular margin (limiting plate) between the portal tract fibrous tissue and periportal liver cells, some of which are swollen and vacuolated and are being entrapped and surrounded by chronic inflammatory cells. × 300. (**b**) In this area of piecemeal necrosis entrapped liver cells, some of which show degenerative changes, are seen within a predominantly lymphocytic infiltrate which is extending out from the fibrous septum running across the right lower quadrant. Note the pseudoglandular pattern adopted by some regenerating liver cells. × 340.

rise of the serum alkaline phosphatase level. Hyperglobulinaemia, predominantly of IgG, is a frequent finding. In the later stages, more advanced changes of hepatocellular dysfunction and cirrhosis are manifest, e.g. hypoalbuminaemia and prolongation of the prothrombin time.

Morphologically, chronic active hepatitis is a continuing progressive inflammation with liver-cell degeneration and necrosis accompanied by fibrosis of variable extent and distribution, progressing to cirrhosis in a proportion of cases. The liver may be of normal size or enlarged. For a long time the surface is smooth but eventually it becomes nodular. The most significant histological lesion is **piecemeal necrosis** (Fig. 20.23), which is defined as 'the destruction of liver cells at an interface between parenchyma and connective tissue, together with a predominantly lymphocytic or plasma cell infiltrate' (Bianchi *et al.*, 1977). The inflammatory cells infiltrate between liver cells which show *feathery degeneration* (swelling and

irregular cytoplasmic vacuolation) and eventual necrosis. Fibrosis occurs early, and when regenerative activity occurs groups of hepatocytes surrounded by fibrous tissue produce pseudoglandular rosettes (Fig. 20.23b).

Histologically, two broad categories of chronic active hepatitis are recognised. (a) Chronic active hepatitis with predominantly portal and periportal inflammation and piecemeal necrosis affecting the periportal hepatocytes. Extension of this necrosis and accompanying fibrosis results in fibrous septa linking portal tracts, and there is also extension into the parenchyma producing progressive distortion of the normal architecture (Fig. 20.24). (b) Chronic active hepatitis with bridging hepatic necrosis; in this form hepatic necrosis and fibrosis extend between adjacent hepatic veins and between hepatic veins and portal tracts; there is also piecemeal necrosis of hepatocytes at the margins of the septa (Fig. 20.25). Both forms usually progress to a macronodular

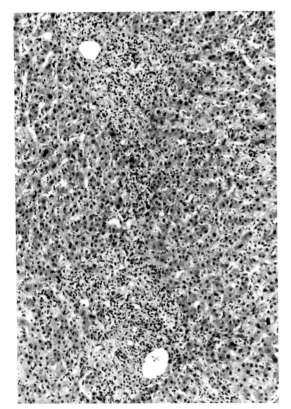

Fig. 20.24 Chronic active hepatitis: the inflammation here is predominantly portal and periportal with early portal–portal bridging: there is also diffuse inflammation within the parenchyma. × 120.

cirrhosis, but this tends to develop more rapidly in (b) than in (a).

In both groups the features of acute hepatitis may be superimposed, particularly during clinical relapse, and this produces a more generalised parenchymal involvement. When chronic active hepatitis is a sequel to hepatitis B infection then 'ground-glass' hepatocytes (p. 20.12) may be identified. Remission may occur spontaneously, with greatly reduced intensity of the inflammatory and destructive processes, and may also be produced by treatment with corticosteroids and azathioprine. The prognosis, however, is variable. About 50% of patients survive longer than 5 years, but recent reports suggest that this figure is increased by better therapeutic management.

Recently a *chronic 'lobular' hepatitis* has been described in which the histological features are indistinguishable from those of acute viral hepatitis, but

these appearances persist for years. The diagnosis is based on serial biopsy in patients with biochemical evidence of hepatitis. It is not known whether progressive fibrosis occurs. Some are HB-associated, but in others a non-A non-B aetiology is suspected.

The aetiology of chronic active hepatitis is controversial. HB antigen studies have shown that about 6% of patients with acute hepatitis B fail to eliminate the virus and progress to chronic active hepatitis with persistence of HBsAg in the serum and of both surface and core antigens in the liver. A chronic course occurs also in some cases of non-A non-B, but not in hepatitis A. *There is thus a virus-associated type of chronic active hepatitis.* In a proportion of patients (60% of ours) *auto-antibodies* are found in the serum. These include antinuclear factors, and smooth muscle antibodies: rheumatoid factor and microsomal antibody are less frequent. None of these antibodies is specific for chronic active hepatitis, and there is no evidence that they are of aetiological

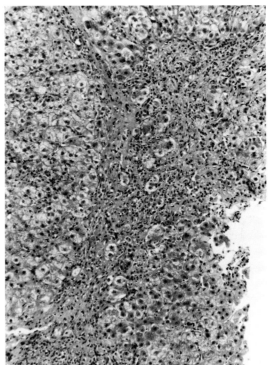

Fig. 20.25 Chronic active hepatitis with bridging septa causing architectural distortion; there is well-marked piecemeal necrosis at the fibrous/parenchymal interface. × 120.

significance. Currently the auto-antibody-associated disease is termed '*lupoid hepatitis*'. There is usually no evidence of hepatitis B infection in such cases, and lupoid hepatitis is included by many in the group of auto-immune diseases although future studies may show non Anon B virus(es) to be causal in some patients.

The elevation of serum immunoglobulin levels, the lymphocyte and plasma cell infiltrate in the liver, and the clinical response to immuno-suppressive therapy all suggest that immune mechanisms are important in the pathogenesis of this disease. The differences in incidence relating to sex, the development of the disease in only a small percentage of hepatitis B patients,

its rare occurrence in association with certain drugs (methyldopa and isoniazid) and the increased incidence of the HLA antigens A1 and B8 in patients with 'lupoid' hepatitis, also indicate that individual host factors are important. The cause of the persistence of viral infection in some cases is not known. The possible mechanisms of auto-immunisation are discussed on pp. 7.27–29. It seems that in both groups (viral and lupoid) the liver cells are the target of an aberrant and aggressive immune reaction, but the interplay between host factors and possible viral, drug or other aetiological agents remains obscure.

Alcoholic Liver Disease

The changes in the liver brought about by high alcohol consumption include *fatty liver, alcoholic hepatitis, hepatic fibrosis* and *cirrhosis*. Fatty change alone is considered to be a reversible disorder although when it is very severe, cholestasis and hepatocellular failure may develop; alcoholic hepatitis is considered to be the precursor of cirrhosis. *Excess alcohol consumption alone has now been shown to produce these hepatic lesions in man without any other obvious nutritional abnormality, and their degree and severity are related to the amount and duration of alcohol abuse.* This is supported by the experimental production of fatty liver and cirrhosis in baboons on a nutritionally adequate diet. However, dietary imbalance and nutritional deficiencies, particularly of protein, may accompany alcohol abuse, and may aggravate the hepatotoxic effects of alcohol.

Alcoholic fatty liver

Under controlled conditions, alcohol administration has been shown to produce hepatic fatty change regularly in man. After a single dose of alcohol, the fatty acids which accumulate in the liver are derived from fat depots, whereas with chronic alcohol intake they are predominantly of dietary origin, mobilisation of fat from adipose tissues being inhibited in this state, prob-

ably by acetate circulating as an end product of alcohol metabolism.

The relationships between alcohol metabolism and accumulation of fat in the hepatocyte are outlined in Fig. 20.26. Alcohol is broken down mainly by oxidation by alcohol dehydrogenase (ADH) in the cell sap. This results in the generation of hydrogen ions, and is reflected by an increase in the reduced nicotinamide adenine dinucleotide:nicotinamide adenine dinucleotide ratio (NADH:NAD), with a resultant change in reduction–oxidation (redox) potential. Some alcohol is also metabolised by microsomal enzymes in the smooth endoplasmic reticulum (SER), this pathway being known as the microsomal ethanol oxidising system (MEOS): it is dependent on the reduced form of NAD phosphate (NADPH), or an NADPH generating system. Normally it is thought that the ADH:MEOS ratio for alcohol metabolism is approximately 3:1, but in chronic alcohol abuse with an increase in SER a greater amount may be metabolised via the MEOS.

This increase in the SER is a well-recognised feature of alcoholic liver damage, and it seems likely that induction of a number of microsomal enzyme systems may accompany this increase in SER and contribute to some of the other effects of alcohol on hepatocyte fat metabolism. In addition, the mitochondria are damaged by alcohol: they become swollen, sometimes markedly so, producing giant forms

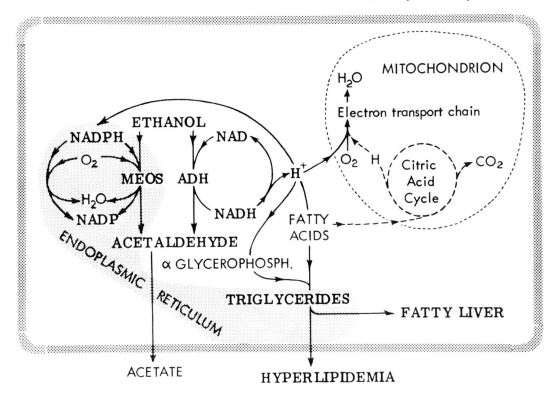

Fig. 20.26 Alcohol metabolism and fatty change in the liver cell, schematic representation. ADH = alcohol dehydrogenase; MEOS = microsomal ethanol oxidising system. Pathways that are decreased by alcohol are represented by interrupted lines. (Modified after and printed with permission from Professor C. S. Lieber.)

with disorganisation of the cristae, associated with increased fragility and permeability of the mitochondrial membrane.

The cumulative effects of these changes on hepatocyte fat metabolism are as follows: (a) increased lipogenesis *per se*; (b) accumulation of fatty acids, mainly because the NADH:NAD redox changes inhibit their oxidation via the citric acid cycle; this is aggravated by the direct damage to mitochondria. In addition there is an increase in the concentration of α-glycerophosphate and this results in trapping of fatty acids in the hepatocytes. These fatty acids are then esterified in the endoplasmic reticulum to triglycerides, some of which accumulate in the hepatocytes. In addition, however, increased lipoprotein synthesis occurs in the SER and some of these triglycerides are thus transported into the circulation, producing hyperlipidaemia; (c) cholesterol esters also accumulate, and there is evidence that this is partly due to increased cholesterol production in the SER and partly to a reduced cholesterol catabolic rate.

The mechanisms thus combine to produce hepatic fatty change, which can be detected after only two days of excess alcohol. Similarly, stopping alcohol results in a rapid mobilisation of the stored fat.

Alcoholic hepatitis and cirrhosis

In contrast to our understanding of alcohol-induced fatty liver, the metabolic events that lead to the development of alcoholic hepatitis and cirrhosis are still not understood. Both the volume of alcohol and the duration of alcohol abuse relate to the development of these lesions. Estimates suggest that a daily consumption of more than 100 g of alcohol (5 large whiskies, 5 pints of beer or 1 bottle of wine) represents a hepatotoxic level of alcohol abuse. However, there are undefined host factors which determine susceptibility. Clinical evidence suggests that alcoholic hepatitis develops after

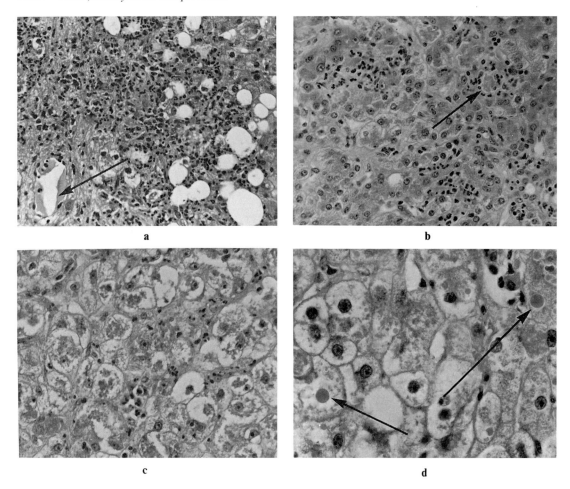

Fig. 20.27   Alcoholic hepatitis. (**a**) The perivenular distribution of the lesion is evident (hepatic vein arrowed). There is extensive liver cell necrosis with an inflammatory cell infiltrate. ×150. (**b**) Foci of liver cell necrosis with a neutrophil polymorph infiltrate, these cells in some areas (arrow) arranging themselves around Mallory-body containing liver cells. ×270. (**c**) There is marked ballooning degeneration of hepatocytes and a number of Mallory-bodies are present; a few neutrophil polymorphs are also seen. ×270. (**d**) Giant mitochondria (arrowed) within liver cells. ×350.

3 to 5 years of sustained alcohol abuse but this occurs in only about 35% of chronic alcoholics; in turn only one-third of these (i.e. 12% of alcoholics) progress to cirrhosis. Females, however, may be at greater risk, developing alcoholic hepatitis with smaller daily amounts and over a shorter period of abuse.

In alcoholic hepatitis there is ballooning degeneration and necrosis of hepatocytes, associated with a neutrophil polymorph reaction (Fig. 20.27b). Fatty change is usually also present. Characteristically the hepatitis develops around the hepatic vein branches (Fig. 20.27a). Amorphous irregular eosinophilic ag-

gregates of **Mallory's hyalin** (Mallory bodies— Fig. 20.27c) are seen within the cytoplasm of some hepatocytes; it has a fibrillar pattern on electron microscopy and represents an accumulation of intermediate filaments in the damaged cells. Giant mitochondria may also be noted (Fig. 20.27d). Fibrosis is an early feature, showing a striking pericellular distribution and, with continued liver cell loss, producing fibrous septa with replacement of the parenchyma and obliteration of sinusoids. In some instances the changes progress rapidly with diffuse parenchymal involvement, an intense polymorph infiltration, peripheral leucocytosis, and portal hyper-

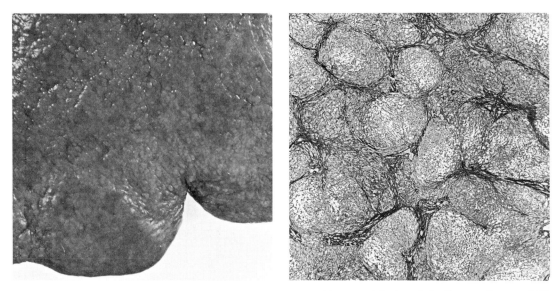

Fig. 20.28 Micronodular cirrhosis. *Left*, showing the fine uniform nodularity of the liver surface. × 0·75. *Right*, microscopy shows regular nodular regeneration: the hepatocytes in many of the nodules show marked fatty change. (Gordon and Sweets' reticulin.) × 20.

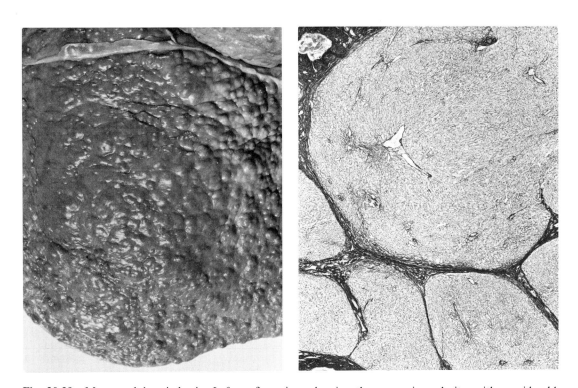

Fig. 20.29 Macronodular cirrhosis. *Left*, surface view, showing the coarse irregularity, with considerable variation of nodular size. × 0·75. *Right*, microscopy shows the variation in nodular size. (Gordon and Sweets' reticulin.) × 20.

tension with progressive ascites and hepato-cellular failure develop.

With continuing alcoholic hepatitis there is progressive fibrosis and scarring; fibrous septa extend and form links between contiguous perivenular areas and between perivenular areas and portal tracts. The liver architecture is increasingly distorted, fibrous contraction occurs and eventually a regular micronodular cirrhosis is established (Fig. 20.28). If there is still further parenchymal cell loss and fibrosis, with accompanying nodular regeneration, the end-stage liver may show a mixed or macronodular cirrhosis.

Hepatic fibrosis

Alcohol may also produce perivenular and pericellular fibrosis without an accompanying hepatitis. This lesion may also progress and proceed to cirrhosis.

Cirrhosis

Definition. Cirrhosis is a condition involving the entire liver in which the parenchyma is changed into a large number of nodules separated from one another by irregular branching and anastomosing sheets of fibrous tissue. It results from long-continued loss of liver cells, with a persistent inflammatory reaction accompanied by fibrosis and compensatory hyperplasia. The progressive loss and regeneration of liver cells occurs focally and leads to disruption of the normal architecture, so that the portal tracts and hepatic veins are spaced irregularly in the nodules of surviving parenchyma, as well as being embedded in the fibrous septa. The condition is irreversible and the fibrosis and architectural distortion interfere with the flow of blood through the liver, with the result that, in most cases, loss of liver cells continues, even in the absence of the original cytotoxic agent (e.g. alcohol) and death usually results from hepatocellular failure, portal hypertension, or a combination of both.

It is important to emphasise that the changes of cirrhosis affect the whole liver. Localised scarring caused, for example, by syphilitic gummas, is not included within the term cirrhosis; nor are mild degrees of more generalised hepatic fibrosis unaccompanied by loss of lobular architecture.

Pathological features

The liver may be of normal size or enlarged if there is fatty change of the liver cells or excessive development of hyperplastic regenerating nodules. Usually, however, it shrinks as the disease progresses, due to loss of liver cells exceeding regeneration, and terminally may weigh less than 1 kg. The surface is diffusely nodular and on section the parenchyma is seen to be divided up everywhere into rounded nodules, separated by bands of fibrous tissue (Figs. 20.28, 20.29). The colour varies considerably, depending on whether or not there is severe fatty change, on the presence or absence of cholestasis, and on the degree of congestion. Recently-divided liver cells are deficient in lipochrome, and the nodules are thus often paler than normal liver parenchyma.

Microscopy of the nodules shows loss of normal architecture, the portal tracts and hepatic veins having lost their regular spacing. This is associated with foci of liver cell atrophy and loss, and foci of hypertrophy and hyperplasia, so that in some parts of a nodule the cells are small, and in others they are enlarged and include binucleate forms (Fig. 20.30).

The fibrous tissue runs in septa between parenchymal nodules: it may contain fine or dense collagen fibres, and varies in its vascularity depending on the duration of the cirrhotic process. It tends to involve the portal tracts, but also envelops hepatic veins. Some nodules are partially divided by incomplete septa extending into them. Collagen develops in relation to damaged liver cells, which presumably stimulate its production by fibroblasts or the perisinusoidal cells of Ito. Fibroblasts are not, however, conspicuous in early experimentally-induced cirrhosis. Commonly, single and small groups of liver cells are entrapped within the fibrous septa. Increased numbers of small bile duct elements are also present in the fibrous tissue—so-called 'ductular proliferation' (Fig. 20.31). Cholestasis is not usually marked (except in biliary cirrhosis, p. 20.29), but is seen focally in some cases and may develop terminally in hepatocellular failure.

Lymphocytes, and less commonly plasma cells, infiltrate the connective tissue and less frequently the parenchymal nodules. The infiltrates vary considerably in degree from case to case, and may be focal. Feathery degeneration of liver cells (p. 20.20) may be observed especially at the margins of the nodules, and this, particularly if associated with heavy lymphocytic infiltration, is an indication that the cirrhotic process is progressing actively. In autopsy material there is often extensive recent liver cell necrosis, attributable to terminal failure of the circulation.

Classification of cirrhosis

The differentiation of cirrhosis into various types has some clinical significance, and elucidation of the causes of cirrhosis, and thus eventually its prevention, are dependent on distinguishing between various types. Cirrhosis may be classified on an aetiological basis or on the morphological appearances of the liver.

The morphological divisions are into a **micronodular** or regular cirrhosis in which the nodules are of approximately the same size, i.e. up to 3 mm in diameter, a **macronodular** or irregular cirrhosis in which the nodules are of variable size and may range up to 1 cm in diameter, and a **mixed** type in which both small and large nodules are present (Figs. 20.28, 20.29). The value of this classification is doubtful, and in our experience the correlation between aetiological factors and the morphology of the cirrhosis is poor. In the end-stage liver the pattern is most frequently a mixed one, and this is dependent on a balance between the degree of continued liver injury and the regenerative capacity of the liver, and is probably also a function of time. Examination of biopsy material, however, reveals features which correlate with aetiological factors, and it now

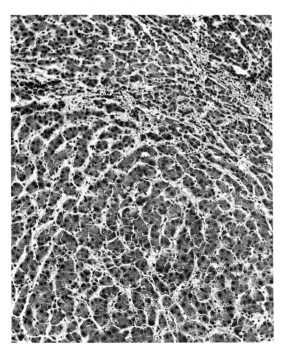

Fig. 20.30 Cirrhosis of liver, showing hypertrophy of the liver cells in part of a nodule, and stretching and atrophy of the adjacent cells in upper part of field. × 90.

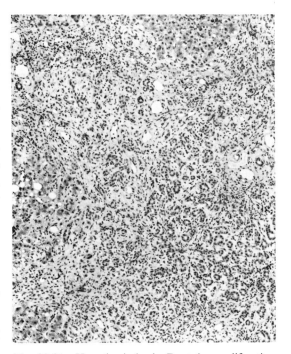

Fig. 20.31 Hepatic cirrhosis. Ductular proliferation in fibrous septa. × 80.

Table 20.2   Classification of cirrhosis

Acquired

  Alcoholic

  Post-hepatitic or post-viral

  Of unknown aetiology

    Cryptogenic
    Indian childhood cirrhosis

  Biliary cirrhosis

    Primary (of unknown aetiology)
    Secondary (due to bile duct obstruction)

Congenital

  Inborn errors of metabolism

    Haemochromatosis
    Thalassaemia
    Wilson's disease
    Alpha 1-antitrypsin deficiency
    Galactosaemia
    Type IV glycogen storage disease
    Tyrosinosis
    Fructose intolerance

seems appropriate to give an aetiological classification (Table 20.2) and describe the pathological features most commonly found in each type.

In our experience in this country, alcoholic cirrhosis comprises 30–35% of all cases of cirrhosis, post-viral 15–20%, 40–45% are cryptogenic and the remainder form a miscellaneous group. The features of some of these will now be briefly outlined.

Alcoholic cirrhosis

The pathological features have already been described. Alcoholic cirrhosis is commoner in men than in women, and develops mainly between 40 and 70 years of age, although recently younger cases have occurred, reflecting alterations in social drinking habits.

The degree of fatty change in the liver tends to diminish as the disease progresses. Reduction in size of the liver is usually slight, the weight being 1·2 kg or more. The early pattern of the cirrhosis is micronodular with loss of acinar architecture (Fig. 20.28), but with further liver-cell loss and nodular hyperplasia the liver may show a mixed or a predominantly macronodular appearance.

The margins between nodules and fibrous septa are in most places fairly regular, the septa are narrow and composed of mature connective tissue, bile duct proliferation is slight, and lymphocytic infiltration is usually not heavy. The presence of Mallory's hyalin (Fig. 20.27c) is a useful diagnostic marker; it is, however, seen also in Wilson's disease, Indian childhood cirrhosis and in primary biliary cirrhosis.

Hepatic encephalopathy is less common than in post-viral cirrhosis. Additional but inconstant features include muscle wasting, anaemia, vitamin B and C deficiency, polyneuritis, alcoholic gastritis and peptic ulceration, chronic pancreatitis, Dupuytren's contracture and the mental changes of chronic alcoholism.

It is important to recognise this type of cirrhosis because it progresses more slowly than most other types, and improvement may result from abstinence from alcohol.

Post-viral (post-hepatitic) cirrhosis

The liver is usually smaller than in alcoholic cirrhosis, and fatty infiltration is slight or absent. It may be reduced to about 1 kg and the pattern of cirrhosis is usually macronodular (Fig. 20.29). The normal architecture is not completely lost, and can be detected in parts of some of the nodules. The liver cells vary considerably in size, multiple and large nuclei being common. In places the margin between nodules and fibrous septa is irregular. Where there is piecemeal necrosis and the septa are heavily infiltrated with lymphocytes this is regarded as indicating continuing activity.

Post-hepatitic cirrhosis is commoner in women than in men, and occurs usually at a younger age than alcoholic cirrhosis, although the range is wide. In those cases which result from chronic active hepatitis, many of the additional features of this condition may persist. For example, the spleen is often palpable at an early stage, there may be skin rashes, arthropathy, leucopenia, etc., the serum IgG level may be high and there may be various auto-antibodies. The disease has a poor prognosis, progressive portal hypertension and hepatocellular failure usually being more rapid than in alcoholic cirrhosis. There is also a higher incidence of liver cell carcinoma, especially where there is associated persistent HB antigenaemia.

Cryptogenic cirrhosis

Morphologically this group is a heterogeneous one. Most cases show a macronodular pattern, but micronodular and mixed patterns are also observed.

Biliary cirrhosis

Long-continued cholestasis, whether of extra- or intra-hepatic origin, can lead to cirrhosis from the harmful effect of retained bile upon the hepatocytes, often aggravated, in patients with major duct obstruction, by ascending bacterial cholangitis. Two varieties are recognised.

(*a*) *Primary biliary cirrhosis* in which a non-suppurative destructive process of unknown aetiology affects intrahepatic bile ducts.

(*b*) *Secondary biliary cirrhosis* resulting from prolonged mechanical obstruction of the larger biliary passages.

Primary biliary cirrhosis. This is an uncommon condition, occurring predominantly in middle-aged women, the female preponderance being 8 or 9 to 1. Clinically, the onset is insidious, frequently with pruritus and sometimes with a period of vague ill-health before jaundice appears. There is usually a marked degree of hepatomegaly. The level of jaundice may fluctuate, and is initially usually mild. The serum alkaline phosphatase level is disproportionately high when compared with the increase in conjugated bilirubin. Serum aminotransferase levels are mildly raised and cholesterol levels may be markedly elevated. After a duration varying from months to many years, death results from liver failure or complications of portal hypertension. In long-standing cases malabsorption develops, and there may be osteomalacia and osteoporosis. There may also be features of secondary hypersplenism with varying degrees of leucopenia, thrombocytopenia and anaemia.

Although the clinical and biochemical features are those of obstructive jaundice, the large intrahepatic and extrahepatic bile ducts are patent. The most conspicuous change is an infiltration of lymphocytes and plasma cells in and around the epithelium of the smaller (50 μm or less) intrahepatic bile ducts. The epithelium shows degenerative changes in some areas and becomes heaped up in others (Fig. 20.32), and there is gradual destruction and loss of these smaller bile ducts. Macrophage granulo-

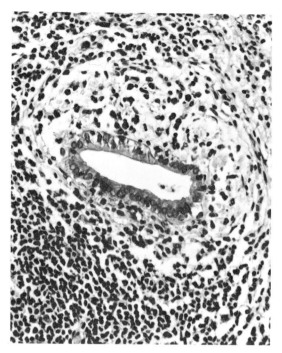

Fig. 20.32 Primary biliary cirrhosis, showing an intrahepatic bile duct with surrounding inflammatory reaction. The duct epithelium is unduly basophilic with vacuolation of the cells lining the upper margin. × 350.

mas are found in about one-third of the cases and may be intimately related to bile ducts (Fig. 20.33). Later the chronic inflammatory cell infiltrate extends to involve the periportal parenchyma, and this is accompanied by portal fibrosis and cholestasis, usually most marked in the periportal areas. Accumulation of protein-bound copper in the periportal liver cells is a late feature and is due to impaired excretion of copper in the bile. Eventually irregular loss and nodular regeneration of liver cells complete the picture of cirrhosis, usually of a micronodular pattern. Mallory's hyalin, affecting periportal hepatocytes, is seen in 25% of cases.

Aetiology. In this disease the initial lesion is an inflammatory destructive process involving septal and interlobular bile ducts. Later, parenchymal cell necrosis is superadded, probably due to cholestasis, and progresses to cirrhosis. In nearly all cases the serum contains, in high titre, an antibody which reacts with a non-organ specific mitochondrial antigen. Demonstration of this antibody by indirect immuno-

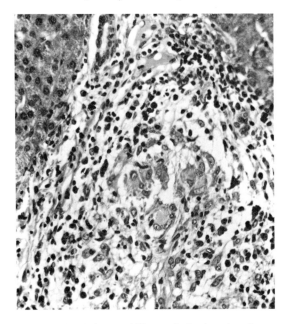

Fig. 20.33 Primary biliary cirrhosis, showing a granuloma with formation of giant cells, lying in a portal area which is heavily infiltrated with lymphoid cells. × 350.

fluorescence provides a valuable confirmatory diagnostic test. The lymphocytic and plasma-cell infiltration of the portal tracts and bile duct epithelium, the occurrence of the mitochondrial antibody and the commonly elevated serum IgM levels, raise the probability that immune reactions are involved in this disease. Catabolism of some of the complement components is increased and there is evidence of circulating immune complexes in most cases. Sensitisation to an antigen present in bile has been demonstrated in some patients, but its significance is not yet known.

Secondary (obstructive) biliary cirrhosis. Unrelieved obstruction to the outflow of bile from the liver from any cause results, in time, in secondary biliary cirrhosis. The rate of development of cirrhosis is extremely variable, and depends partly on the degree of obstruction. In some cases, and particularly when obstruction is due to gallstones, an ascending bacterial cholangitis is superadded and, if severe, leads to necrosis and abscess formation (Fig. 20.34). In obstruction due to neoplasms, e.g. cancer of the head of the pancreas, the period of survival is limited and death usually results before cirrhosis has developed.

The early changes following biliary obstruction consist of cholestasis, bile accumulation developing in the hepatocytes, bile canaliculi and Kupffer cells, particularly in the perivenular zones (Fig. 20.35), and in the small bile ducts. Subsequently the larger bile ducts become dilated and filled with concentrated bile. After weeks or months a progressive inflammatory reaction develops in the portal tracts, which become oedematous and infiltrated with lymphocytes, plasma cells and significant numbers of polymorphs (Fig. 20.36). Bile duct proliferation develops, and there is fibroblast proliferation and development of fibrous septa extending irregularly into the parenchyma and linking up with adjacent portal tracts. Periductal fibrosis is often also a feature.

Single or small groups of liver cells become pigmented, swollen and show feathery degeneration. Aggregates of such necrotic cells may form distinct **'bile infarcts'**. Rupture of canals of Hering adjacent to the portal tracts may occur with escape of bile to form **bile lakes**. Biliary granulomas may also be a feature. Loss of liver cells and fibrosis result eventually in disturbance of architecture and, together with the development of regenerating nodules, progress to a micronodular cirrhosis. Possibly because the cholestasis interferes with their function, the hepatocytes show marked hyper-

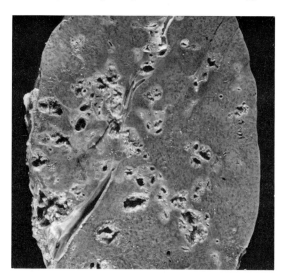

Fig. 20.34 Liver slice from a case of large duct obstruction and ascending cholangitis: numerous abscesses, some of which show central breakdown, are present in the parenchyma.

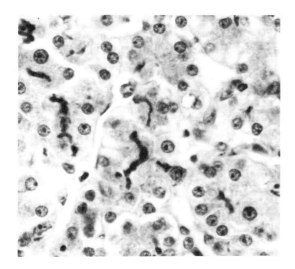

Fig. 20.35 Perivenular cholestasis in early extra-hepatic obstruction. × 390.

plasia, and consequently the liver is enlarged: it is also firm from the increase in fibrous tissue, deeply jaundiced and the surface is usually finely nodular. Portal hypertension may eventually supervene, but death results more often from liver failure or intercurrent infection.

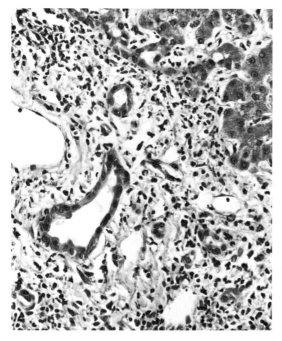

Fig. 20.36 Extra-hepatic obstruction with oedema of the portal area, a prominent neutrophil infiltrate, some of which is closely related to the bile ducts, and early duct proliferation. × 250.

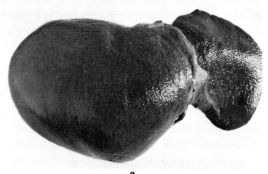

a

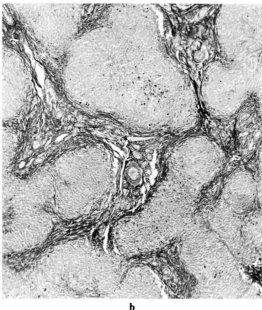

b

Fig. 20.37 Secondary biliary cirrhosis. The liver of a child with congenital atresia of the biliary tract. (**a**) uniform fine nodularity of the surface. × 0·7. (**b**) micronodular cirrhosis with cholestasis. × 25. (Dr A. M. MacDonald.)

In man, the best example of pure obstructive biliary cirrhosis without infection is seen in congenital biliary atresia (Fig. 20.37) which may involve either the extrahepatic or intrahepatic biliary tree. In the extrahepatic variety there is marked jaundice and death occurs within a few months of birth. Patchy atresia of smaller intrahepatic bile ducts sometimes has a more prolonged course with survival into early adult life: secondary biliary cirrhosis develops, as described above.

In recent years a condition known as **primary**

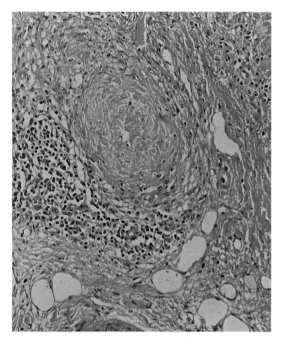

Fig. 20.38 Primary sclerosing cholangitis. In this portal tract the bile duct has been replaced by a dense whorl of fibrous tissue. × 210.

sclerosing cholangitis has been increasingly recognised. This disease shows a male preponderance of 3:1 and in 70% of cases is associated with chronic inflammatory bowel disease, especially ulcerative colitis. It is characterised by a chronic non-suppurative destruction of bile ducts in which there is progressive periductal fibrosis with eventual obliteration of bile ducts (Fig. 20.38). Over a variable period there is progression to cirrhosis, the pattern resembling that seen in primary biliary cirrhosis, and with Mallory bodies and copper retention also developing. The aetiology is not known and the association with ulcerative colitis is obscure.

Congenital cirrhosis

Many of the metabolic abnormalities listed in Table 20.2 can cause cirrhosis in childhood. In addition, there are other causes of cirrhosis in childhood, e.g. *Indian childhood cirrhosis* which is common in 1–3 year-olds in that country. It is of unknown aetiology, but gross accumulation of copper in the liver cells has been demonstrated. Biliary cirrhosis may result from congenital intra- or extra-hepatic biliary atresia,

and from cystic fibrosis (p. 20.60).

Wilson's disease (Hepatolenticular degeneration) is an inherited disorder of copper metabolism determined by a pair of autosomal recessive genes, and with a prevalence of 1 per 200 000 of the population. Increasing amounts of copper accumulate in and damage the liver, the lenticular nuclei, the kidneys and the eyes. The aetiological biochemical abnormality in Wilson's disease is found in the liver: there is an increase in the hepatic lysosomal copper concentration presumed to be due to defective excretion of copper via the bile. This defect is associated in most patients with reduced hepatic synthesis of the serum copper glycoprotein, caeruloplasmin. The accumulation of copper in the liver begins in infancy, and in time excess amounts diffuse from liver to blood and accumulate in and damage other target organs.

In the liver, fatty change, hepatocellular necrosis and fibrosis, sometimes morphologically resembling chronic active hepatitis, and with Mallory's hyalin in a proportion of cases, progress at variable rates to produce a macronodular cirrhosis. The changes in the nervous system are described on page 21.43. There is excess urinary copper excretion, and defective tubular absorption leads to amino-aciduria. In the eyes, deposits of copper in Descemet's membrane of the cornea produce the diagnostic Kayser-Fleischer rings. Treatment with D-penicillamine by increasing urinary copper excretion is of considerable clinical value.

Haemochromatosis. A general account of this disease, and of other conditions causing gross iron overload, is given on pp. 11.16–19. The liver is the major organ affected, but iron deposition and fibrosis of the pancreas and other viscera is also present. There is a characteristic pattern of hepatic fibrosis, and in the later stages a micronodular cirrhosis is established. Excess iron deposits are present in hepatocytes, Kupffer cells, portal-tract macrophages and in bile duct epithelium. Increased amounts of lipofuscin are also present in hepatocytes.

The development of cirrhosis and the intensity of iron deposition are not closely correlated. However, the iron deposition is considered to be fibrogenic, and removal of iron by repeated venesection results in some reduction of the fibrosis. There is an increased incidence of primary carcinoma of the liver in both treated and untreated patients.

Pathogenesis of cirrhosis

Cirrhosis results from long-continued loss of liver cells, accompanied by compensatory liver cell hyperplasia and nodule formation, and by chronic inflammation and progressive replacement fibrosis, i.e. chronic hepatitis. It is, in fact, the outcome of prolonged hepatocellular necrosis. *Eventually the irregular liver cell hyperplasia and fibrosis interfere with blood flow to such an extent that, whatever the initial cause of the injury, hepatocyte loss continues as a result of ischaemia and the changes become progressive, leading to death from hepatocellular failure and/or portal hypertension* (Fig. 20.39). In

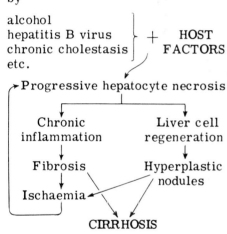

Fig. 20.39 The pathogenesis of cirrhosis.

experimental animals liver cell injury, e.g. by CCl$_4$, is followed by replacement of any liver cells destroyed and a return to normality. This also occurs after repeated liver injury unless the CCl$_4$ is administered at intervals of less than 10 days, when complete regeneration does not occur and the lesion progresses to cirrhosis (Fig. 20.40).

The possible aetiological factors in human cirrhosis have already been enumerated, but in over 40% of cases in this country none of these factors can be incriminated and the aetiology remains unknown. Whereas in secondary biliary cirrhosis the progression to cirrhosis is predictable, in alcohol abuse only 10% of patients develop cirrhosis. Similarly, in acute Type B viral hepatitis only a small percentage progress

to chronic active hepatitis and cirrhosis (p. 20.21). In others the chronic hepatitis is subclinical and after some years of apparent well-being the patients present with manifestations of cirrhosis.

In cryptogenic cirrhosis there is, by definition, no history of any previous acute liver disease and the stage of morphological progressive chronic hepatitis has been clinically silent. While some such cases are probably the result of an episode of viral hepatitis, more sensitive tests for evidence of previous virus infection must be developed before this relationship can be elucidated.

It is now generally accepted that, in spite of apparently contrary experimental evidence in rats, malnutrition *per se* is not a cause of cirrhosis in man, although it may be a contributory factor and may aggravate the effects of alcohol abuse and of viral hepatitis.

The sequence of events in the development of cirrhosis is summarised diagrammatically in Fig. 20.39. Predisposing factors, such as known metabolic defects, may explain occasional cases, but usually the nature of such factors is not clear. The progression from an acute to a chronic hepatitis may be due to persistence of

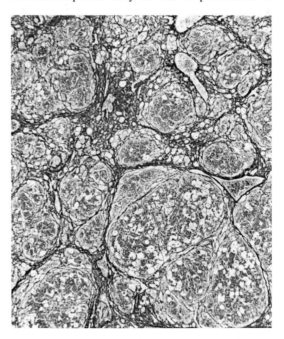

Fig. 20.40 Cirrhosis produced in a rat by repeated inhalation of carbon tetrachloride. Gordon and Sweets' reticulin. × 40.

the aetiological agent, as has been shown in some cases of type B viral hepatitis, or may be the result of auto-immunisation or some other cytotoxic immunological reaction, as has been postulated in some cases of chronic active hepatitis and in primary biliary cirrhosis. Similarly the factors responsible for initiating hepatic fibrosis also remain obscure, but the importance of the fibrosis in the progression of the cirrhosis and in the development of the secondary effects of cirrhosis is not in doubt. Fibrosis is a feature of chronic inflammation of any sort and so is to be expected in chronic hepatitis.

Effects of cirrhosis

Cirrhosis has two important effects, **portal hypertension** and **hepatocellular failure** which are described below. It is the major cause of these two conditions, particularly when they occur together. **Liver-cell carcinoma** arises in 10–15% of all cirrhotic patients in this country, the incidence varying with sex and with different aetiological types of cirrhosis.

Portal Hypertension and Hepatocellular Failure

Portal hypertension

The normal portal venous pressure is 7 mm of mercury. Portal hypertension occurs when there is interference with the blood flow within the liver or obstruction of the portal vein (p. 20.4). The obstruction may be **post-sinusoidal** as in cirrhosis, veno-occlusive disease, hepatic vein obstruction, alcoholic hepatitis and congestive cardiac failure, or **pre-sinusoidal** as in schistosomiasis, congenital hepatic fibrosis and portal vein obstruction. Massive splenomegaly with increased splenic blood flow can also cause portal hypertension in the absence of obstruction. Effects of portal hypertension result from some of the portal blood by-passing the liver and entering the systemic veins at sites of portal-systemic anastomosis. In cirrhosis, in addition,some of the blood which does enter the liver does not perfuse the liver cells adequately and is shunted into the hepatic veins.

Portal-systemic anastomoses at the following sites become enlarged, with varicosity of the veins.

(i) in the lower oesophagus and upper gastric fundus, between the left gastric vein (portal) and the azygos minor vein (systemic).

(ii) in the lower rectum and anus, between the superior haemorrhoidal (portal) and the middle and inferior haemorrhoidal veins (systemic).

(iii) in the falciform ligament between the left branch of the portal vein and the superficial veins of the anterior abdominal wall, via the para-umbilical veins.

(iv) at points of contact between abdominal viscera and the posterior abdominal wall.

The most important anastomoses are those at the gastro-oesophageal junction, where **spontaneous rupture of the large submucosal varices** (see Fig. 19.18, p. 19.13) results in bleeding which may be fatal and also contributes to the development of hepatocellular failure (see below).

Portal hypertension results in **splenomegaly,** due primarily to passive congestion, but often with lymphoid hyperplasia. *Hypersplenism* (p. 17.32) may result in anaemia, thrombocytopenia and granulocytopenia. Focal haemorrhages may occur in the spleen and produce siderotic fibrotic nodules (Gamna-Gandy bodies). Portal hypertension is a major factor in the production of **ascites** (p. 19.70). Portacaval, lienorenal or other surgical shunt procedures may be carried out to reduce the hypertension and thus the risk of bleeding from oesophageal varices. These procedures, however, are of limited value in patients with portal hypertension and cirrhosis, for they increase the danger of hepatic encephalopathy (see below).

Hepatocellular failure (liver failure)

Although the liver has a large functional reserve and a high regenerative capacity when injured, liver insufficiency, manifested by failure of the liver cells to perform adequately their various functions, occurs both in patients with severe acute liver injury and in advanced cases of chronic liver disease. **Acute liver failure** occurs in severe viral hepatitis, as an adverse reaction to certain drugs, as a result of drug overdose or poisoning by certain hepatotoxic chemicals, in massive liver cell necrosis of unknown cause, and occasionally in severe fatty infiltration of the liver. Hepatic failure results directly from the parenchymal cell injury and is a manifestation of the degree of hepatocellular damage. **Chronic liver failure** is most often due to cirrhosis. It may occur even in patients with a relatively large amount of surviving liver tissue, and is attributable in part to the interference with hepatic blood flow which results from the disturbed architecture and fibrosis of the liver. Acute on chronic hepatic failure may be precipitated by factors such as gastro-intestinal bleeding, the use of diuretic or narcotic drugs, bacterial infection, paracentesis, portacaval shunt and other surgical operations.

Because of the multiple functions of the liver, acute or chronic hepatic insufficiency gives rise to a complex syndrome, which includes neurological disturbances, jaundice, defects of blood coagulation and renal failure. Additional features include ascites and oedema, endocrine and circulatory disturbances, but these occur mainly in chronic failure. The mechanisms involved in these manifestations of liver failure are discussed below.

Neurological disturbances comprise mental confusion with apathy, disorientation or excitement, a coarse flapping tremor and muscular rigidity, and finally coma. These are accompanied by characteristic changes in the electro-encephalogram and by a number of biochemical abnormalities. All these features are reversible, and morphological changes have been observed only in the astrocytes, the nuclei of which are enlarged, sometimes to 25 μm in diameter; the chromatin is condensed around the nuclear membrane, and the nucleolus is unduly conspicuous. In occasional cases, however, progressive brain damage may occur. In acute liver failure, cerebral oedema is often a significant contributory cause of death.

The neurological disorder is probably due to a metabolic disturbance, for it is potentially fully reversible: it is of multifactorial aetiology and in individual cases the following factors are probably involved in various combinations.

(i) Failure of the liver to remove potentially toxic agents: in particular, nitrogenous bacterial metabolites absorbed from the gut may avoid detoxication in the liver, due to liver cell loss and/or portasystemic by-pass of the liver. An increased nitrogen load from a high protein intake or haemorrhage from oesophageal varices often precipitates hepatic encephalopathy. In most cases there is an increased level of ammonia in the blood, but the levels correlate only approximately with the depth of coma; moreover the clinical features of ammonia toxicity as seen in urea-cycle enzyme deficiencies are different from those of hepatic encephalopathy. Other metabolic products of intestinal origin have also been implicated; false neurotransmitters, such as octopamine, may replace true transmitters in the brain; gamma-aminobutyric acid (GABA), an inhibitory neurotransmitter, has produced many of the features of hepatic encephalopathies in experimental animals and its significance is currently under investigation in man. Increase in serum aromatic amino acids, and/or a decrease in branched-chain amino acids, increase in serum short-chain fatty acids and mercaptans, may be important.

(ii) Increased cerebral sensitivity to a variety of agents, possibly due to interference with oxidative metabolism via the citric acid cycle and consequent ATP depletion.

(iii) Changes in vascular permeability, particularly affecting the blood–brain barrier.

(iv) The hypotension, anoxia and electrolyte disturbances which accompany hepatic failure.

(v) Loss of (unidentified) factors normally produced by liver cells and regarded as essential for normal neuronal function.

The nature of the functional neuronal changes in hepatic encephalopathy is even less certain.

Jaundice is usual in acute hepatocellular failure, its severity reflecting the degree of hepatocellular damage. In very severe cases, however, death may result before jaundice has become conspicuous. In chronic failure the degree and type of jaundice depends upon the nature of the liver disease. In secondary biliary cirrhosis, obstructive jaundice precedes and accompanies the development of hepatic dysfunction. In other cirrhoses, jaundice is a late but bad prognostic sign, and is usually only of mild or moderate degree. The precise mechanisms of the hyperbilirubinaemia are uncertain, but are considered to be most likely due to failure of hepatocytes to excrete bilirubin.

Coagulation defects result primarily from defective synthesis of a number of coagulation factors by the liver (p. 17.67). There may also be thrombocytopenia (accompanied sometimes by anaemia and leucopenia) due to hypersplenism, and, particularly in acute failure, disseminated intravascular coagulation with consumption of clotting factors (p. 17.68).

Renal failure may develop in both acute and chronic hepatic failure. Acute renal failure may result from hypotension due to bleeding from oesophageal varices. Impairment of renal function without morphological damage may also occur terminally in hepatic failure: this is characterised by reduced glomerular filtration rate and progressive oliguria, but without a fall in urine osmolarity. The mechanisms remain uncertain but the renal failure is reversible with improvement in hepatic function.

Ascites and oedema. Ascites does not result from hepatocellular failure unless there is also portal hypertension, as in cirrhosis. In chronic liver failure there is diminished production of plasma albumin, with a consequent fall in plasma osmotic pressure. The portal hypertension increases the intravascular hydrostatic pressure in the microvasculature of the gut, and in addition there is leakage of hepatic lymph because of obstruction to its outflow from the liver. Secondary hyperaldosteronism (p. 10.37) occurs in some cases, and may, by inducing sodium retention, aggravate the oedema and ascites. The causation of secondary hyperaldosteronism, and why it occurs in some cases and not others, is not clear. Peripheral oedema is due mainly to the fall in plasma osmotic pressure.

Endocrine disturbances. In chronic liver failure there is, in both sexes, a tendency to depression of libido, sterility and loss of body hair. In men, the testes are frequently atrophic, and occasionally one or both breasts are enlarged (*gynaecomastia*). These effects result from failure of hepatic inactivation of oestrogens, which have a stimulating effect upon the breast and may also suppress the production of pituitary gonadotrophin, thus explaining the testicular atrophy. The exact mechanisms of the menstrual irregularities, secondary amenorrhoea and breast atrophy which occur in women are not clear. Two well-known vascular changes in liver failure are exaggerated mottling, due to patchy congestion, of the skin of the palms—the so-called '*liver palms*'—and the development in the superior vena caval drainage area of small leashes of dilated vessels in the superficial dermis, radiating out from a central arteriole—the '*spider naevus*'. Both these features may occur in normal pregnancy and probably have a hormonal basis.

Circulatory disturbances. A hyperkinetic circulation characterised by peripheral vasodilatation and an increase in circulation rate, cardiac output and blood volume may occur in hepatic failure. This may possibly result from circulating vaso-active substances or may be due to impaired sympathetic responsiveness. Cyanosis with arterial hypoxia is not uncommon and finger clubbing develops in a small percentage of patients.

Other features. In hepatocellular failure, particularly when acute, the breath has a peculiar sweetish smell termed '*foetor hepaticus*', possibly due to failure of the liver to detoxify substances absorbed from the gut. *Fever* is also common in acute failure, but profound *hypothermia* has been described in chronic failure. *Bacteraemia*, particularly with coliform organisms, is also a complication. General ill-health with anorexia, wasting and vomiting is common.

Non-Viral Infections of the Liver

The common virus infections of the liver have been dealt with on p. 20.10 *et seq.* Accordingly this account deals with infections by bacteria and protozoa, and infestation by metazoan parasites.

Pyogenic infections. Because of improvements in diagnostic facilities and the earlier use of antibiotics, pyogenic infection of the liver is less common than it used to be, and when it does occur it is usually due to extension of bacteria within the biliary duct system—**ascending cholangitis.** *Escherichia coli,* either alone or with other bacteria, is the commonest causal organism. Bile duct obstruction is the most important predisposing cause, and because bacterial infection commonly accompanies stones, obstruction by a stone is especially liable to be complicated by suppurating cholangitis. The process extends into the liver tissue, giving rise to multiple abscesses in which the pus is characteristically bile-stained.

Multiple abscess formation in the liver also results from suppurative phlebitis affecting the veins around a septic focus in the abdomen or pelvis, e.g. acute appendicitis, diverticulitis of the colon, or infected haemorrhoids: the infection may reach the liver by **septic emboli** or by **portal pylephlebitis.** Umbilical sepsis in the neonate sometimes spreads to the intrahepatic portal vein radicles via the umbilical vein.

Abscesses may also develop in the liver in septicaemia or pyaemia, but these are less frequent and less important than in various other organs.

Actinomycosis. Actinomycosis occurs in and around the appendix, from where it may extend to the liver by the portal venous system or by direct spread. Multiple abscesses form in the liver separated by granulation and fibrous tissue, and produce a honeycomb appearance. The abscesses contain thick greenish-yellow pus, and the characteristic yellowish or greyish sulphur granules, which comprise aggregates of the branching filaments of the causal organism—*Actinomyces israeli* (p. 9.32).

Leptospirosis. The spirochaete *Leptospira icterohaemorrhagiae* causes endemic chronic renal infection in rats, and can survive in water or damp conditions for some time after excretion in rat urine. It can penetrate the intact human skin or may gain entry via the respira-

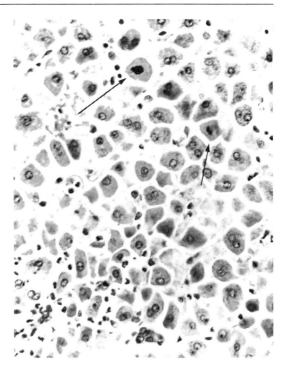

Fig. 20.41 Liver in Weil's disease: post-mortem liver showing separation and rounding of hepatocytes, proliferative activity (*arrows*) and focal liver cell necrosis with a related inflammatory cell infiltrate (*lower left*). × 400.

tory or oral routes, and after an incubation period of 10–15 days causes an intense febrile illness (**Weil's disease**) with conjunctivitis, renal tubular damage, a haemorrhagic tendency, jaundice, focal myocardial and skeletal muscle necrosis and often a mild lymphocytic meningitis. The disease occurs chiefly in sewer workers, agricultural workers and fish handlers. Various other leptospira, including *L. canicola* from dogs, can cause a similar but usually milder disease in man.

Liver biopsy may show liver cell degeneration, prominent mitotic activity of the hepatocytes and sometimes focal necrosis, cholestasis and haemorrhages. In some cases, however, the changes are slight. After death, the liver cells are often rounded and separated from another (Fig. 20.41). This may be a post-mortem change but it is certainly seen when autopsy has been performed within a few hours of death (as in Fig. 20.41), and is helpful in suggesting the diagnosis.

The mortality rate is about 15%. Death may occur in the first week, when haemorrhagic consolidation of the lungs may be the most conspicuous lesion. Later, death is usually due to renal failure, which in these patients is almost always accompanied by evident hepatic involvement.

Syphilis. The liver is frequently affected in both congenital and acquired syphilis. In **congenital syphilis,** the commonest lesion is a diffuse interstitial pericellular fibrosis, proliferating fibroblasts extending between the sinusoidal endothelium and the liver cells producing compression or ischaemic atrophy of the hepatocytes. A dense interstitial mononuclear cell infiltrate is also present. Miliary gummas (p. 9.31) are not uncommon. In fatal cases, spirochaetes are usually abundant throughout the liver. In **acquired syphilis,** a diffuse hepatitis, sometimes with miliary granulomas, may occur in the secondary stage. Hepatic gummas were a common feature of tertiary syphilis before effective treatment became available. They were typically rounded, might be multiple and became very large (>10 cm). Healing usually occurred even without treatment, and scarring was extensive, producing gross distortion of the liver— *hepar lobatum.*

Relapsing fever. This is a spirochaetal disease, caused by various species of *Borrelia.* It may be louse- or tick-borne. Large epidemics have occurred in the past and sporadic outbreaks are encountered in various parts of the world. Jaundice occurs in severe infections, accompanied by biochemical evidence of liver cell injury. In fatal cases there is perivenular necrosis and a moderate generalised inflammation of the liver.

Tuberculosis. Tuberculous lesions are less common in the liver than in most other organs. In generalised tuberculosis miliary tubercles occur, and are distributed irregularly in the parenchyma: sometimes they are large enough to be visible to the naked eye and may have a caseous bile-stained centre. Rarely, a few large caseous lesions result from blood spread, and may be identifiable only by the finding of tubercle bacilli. Tuberculous cholangitis is extremely rare, and probably results from ulceration of a tuberculous nodule of the liver into a bile duct.

Other causes of tubercle-like granulomas in the liver. Lesions resembling tubercle follicles occur in the liver in several non-tuberculous conditions. They consist of aggregates of epithelioid cells, often with one or more multinucleated giant cells which may contain various cytoplasmic inclusions, and show little or no central necrosis. Such lesions occur in most cases of sarcoidosis and brucellosis, and are seen frequently in tuberculoid leprosy and histoplasmosis; they occur sometimes in secondary syphilis and in chronic berylliosis due to inhalation of beryllium compounds. Tubercle-like follicles are seen also in rather less than 40% of liver biopsies from patients with early primary biliary cirrhosis and around impacted ova in schistosomiasis. Occasionally granulomas are found incidentally in the liver in individuals not obviously suffering from tuberculosis or any of the above conditions; their significance is unknown.

Parasitic infestations

Hepatic amoebiasis. This is a complication of amoebic dysentery (p. 28.14), brought about by amoebae (*Entamoeba histolytica*) entering colonic venules and passing by the portal vein to the liver, which they then colonise. Liver lesions may be the presenting clinical feature, or may occur only many years after the colonic lesions have apparently subsided. They consist of one or more cavities termed **tropical abscesses,** and are described on p. 28.15.

Malaria. In the incubation period, malarial parasites develop within hepatocytes (p. 28.3) but they do not bring about permanent hepatic damage. In the stage of blood infection, colonised erythrocytes are phagocytosed by Kupffer cells, which show marked hypertrophy and hyperplasia and contain abundant dark brown granules or 'malarial pigment'. Relapses of *Plasmodium vivax* and *ovale* malaria have been shown to result from the persistence of these parasites in the liver cells, sometimes for many years.

Kala-azar (Visceral leishmaniasis) is described on p. 28.9. The liver is usually enlarged, and there is hyperplasia of the Kupffer cells which are distended by large numbers of Leishmann–Donovan bodies (see Fig. 28.12, p. 28.9). There may be some fibrosis, but cirrhosis does not result.

Schistosomiasis. Infestation of the liver by *Schistosoma mansoni* is described on p. 28.25. In endemic areas it is an important cause of portal venous hypertension.

Hydatid disease. The formation of hydatid

cysts in the liver and other organs is caused by the tapeworm *Echinococcus granulosus*. These lesions are described on p. 28.33.

Clonorchiasis and fascioliasis result from invasion of the biliary tree by the larvae of the Chinese liver fluke (*Opisthorcis sinensis*) and the sheep fluke (*Fasciola hepatica*) respectively. The effects of these parasites on the liver are described on pp. 28.29–30.

Ascariasis, i.e. infestation of the intestine by the roundworm *Ascaris lumbricoides* is widely distributed throughout the world, but is particularly prevalent in Africa and the Far East. It commonly affects children, and in over a third of cases is associated with direct invasion of the common bile duct, producing obstruction and cholangitis (p. 28.40).

Tumours of the Liver

Benign tumours

Benign tumours of the liver are rare, comprising approximately 5% of all hepatic neoplasms. They include: (*a*) **liver cell adenomas,** which bear a close microscopic resemblance to normal liver tissue, the cells forming regular trabeculae two or three cells thick. Bile canaliculi are present and appear normal but bile ducts are absent. These tumours are usually very vascular and are not always encapsulated. An increased incidence of these tumours has been found in women using oral contraceptive pills and a causal association is now accepted; (*b*) **bile duct adenomas** are very rare and are usually an incidental finding. These are less than 1 cm in diameter, and are composed of small bile duct elements in a fibrous stroma. Intrahepatic bile duct *cystadenomas* are also rare, but sometimes large, tumours; (*c*) **haemangiomas,** usually cavernous, dark purple owing to the contained blood, and sharply demarcated from the surrounding hepatic tissue, are not uncommon. Most are less than 2 cm in diameter, but some are larger. They are usually superficial and may be mistaken for infarcts by the casual observer.

Malignant tumours

Liver cell carcinomas account for approximately 85% of primary malignant tumours of the liver, bile duct carcinomas for approximately 5–10%, and the remainder are relatively rare tumours including haemangiosarcomas, hepatoblastomas, and mesenchymal tumours.

Liver cell (hepatocellular) carcinoma

This tumour shows marked geographic variation in incidence. In this country it is present in less than 1% of all autopsies, whereas in parts of Africa and Far East Asia it is 5–6 times more common. In both low- and high-incidence areas 80–90% of cases occur in males, and the tumour supervenes on cirrhosis (predominantly of macronodular type) in 70–80% of cases. In cases without pre-existing cirrhosis, the male:female ratio is 2:1. *In low-incidence areas* the tumour arises usually after the age of 50, and while the incidence of cirrhosis is often high the proportion of cases in which malignancy supervenes is low, estimates varying from 5 to 15%: the tumour develops as a late complication of long-established cirrhosis. By contrast, *in high-incidence areas* the tumour arises in a much younger age group. The incidence of cirrhosis in these areas is uncertain; it appears to be high, but not high enough to explain the high frequency of liver cell carcinoma; in such areas there is a much greater risk of tumours supervening in cirrhosis, some estimates being as high as 50%, and clinical features of the tumour and of cirrhosis often present virtually simultaneously. The tumour cells secrete α-fetoprotein and levels in excess of 10 ng/ml are found in the serum in 85% of cases.

Aetiological factors

The precise relationship between cirrhosis and liver cell carcinoma is uncertain. Whereas we have previously subscribed to the view that the cirrhosis was a premalignant lesion, neoplasia

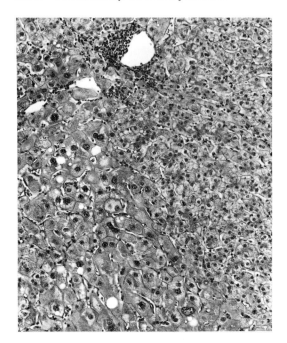

Fig. 20.42 Liver cell dysplasia: there is a focal increase in liver cell size, with nuclear pleomorphism and some binucleate and multinucleate cells. This section was from the right lobe of liver in a patient with a liver cell carcinoma in the left lobe. × 80.

supervening on the longstanding and continued hyperplasia of the cirrhotic liver, we feel that, on the basis of the epidemiological facts just presented, two other possibilities must be considered. These are (i) that both the cirrhosis and the tumour are caused by one agent, and (ii) that the cirrhotic liver is peculiarly predisposed to the carcinogenic effects of a variety of microbiological and/or chemical agents.

There is growing evidence of an association between HBV infection and liver cell carcinoma: i) there is a close correlation between the distribution of HBs antigenaemia and liver cell carcinoma; ii) serological markers of hepatitis B infection (e.g. HBsAg or HBcAb) have been detected in 80-90% of patients with tumour even in some areas with a low overall incidence of liver cell carcinoma; iii) liver cell carcinoma occurs more frequently in HB-associated cirrhosis. Liver cell dysplasia (Fig. 20.42) regarded as a premalignant change is a common feature of cirrhosis in high incidence areas and shows a significant association with HBs antigenaemia; iv) prospective studies of chronic HBsAg carriers have shown the relative risk of tumour

to be 200 times greater than in non-carriers. In high carrier-rate areas, transmission of HB infection from mother to child has been demonstrated and such early infection could be a factor in the observed early development of liver cell cancer; v) integrated DNA sequences of HBV have been shown in tumour cells and in liver cancer cell-lines secreting HBsAg. Thus the evidence for an association between virus and tumour is indeed strong. However, a direct oncogenic role for HBV is not established and

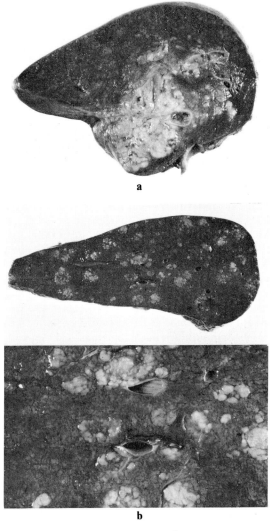

Fig. 20.43 Liver cell carcinoma. (**a**) arising as a single large mass and with evident permeation of surrounding portal vein branches. (**b**) arising as multicentric foci throughout the liver (shown also at higher magnification).

the HBV infection could be acting as a promoter.

Experimentally, liver cell carcinoma has been produced in rats by feeding with mouldy peanuts, and this has been attributed to *aflatoxins* which are products of the mould *Aspergillus flavus*. These and other *mycotoxins* and *plant toxins* may contaminate stored foods and cereals, and this may explain in part the geographical variation in incidence in man. *Chemical carcinogens*, notably *o*-aminoazotoluene and *p*-dimethylaminoazobenzene (butter yellow) produce liver tumours in experimental animals without an intervening cirrhosis (p. 13.19), the incidence being increased by a diet low in protein or deficient in cystine and methionine. Accordingly *protein deficiency* may be synergistic in promoting the development of liver cell cancer in man, and may help to explain geographic variations in incidence. Recent attention has been focussed on the possible role of *nitrosamines*, compounds which can be synthesised from nitrites and secondary amines in the gastro-intestinal tract, and which produce experimental liver tumours. Nitrites (and nitrates) are common food additives, and the possibility that some nitrosamines are carcinogenic for man has been raised.

Macroscopically the tumour may form a single large mass (Fig. 20.43a), often sharply defined, with central necrosis, haemorrhage and irregular bile-staining. In other cases the tumour is apparently multicentric (Fig. 20.43b), and there is also a type in which extensive nodular infiltration involves a considerable part of the liver. Extensive permeation of intrahepatic portal vein branches is a common feature; extrahepatic metastases occur in less than half the cases, mostly in the lungs and lymph nodes.

Microscopically the tumour cells closely resemble hepatocytes, their arrangement being more or less trabecular, and with intervening sinusoids (Fig. 20.44). Canaliculi, sometimes containing bile, may be seen.

Bile duct carcinoma (cholangiocarcinoma)

Primary tumours composed of cells resembling biliary epithelium (Fig. 20.45) are much less common than liver cell tumours. They are not usually associated with cirrhosis, and there is no difference in sex incidence. In the Far East,

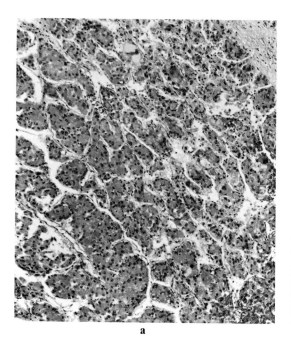
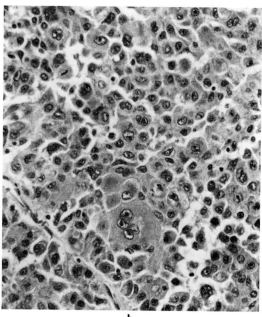

a   b

Fig. 20.44 Liver-cell carcinoma. (**a**) trabecular arrangement with endothelial-lined blood vessels separating the aggregates of tumour cells. × 75. (**b**) individual tumour cells resembling hepatocytes with some binucleate and giant cell forms. × 250.

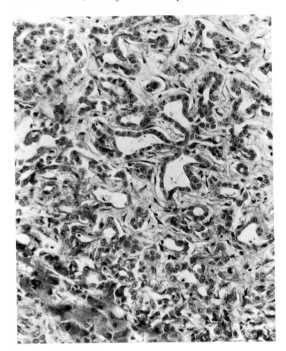

Fig. 20.45 Bile duct carcinoma—an adenocarcinomatous pattern resembling bile ducts, with a related fibrous reaction. × 200.

where these are relatively frequent, about 65% of cases are associated with infestation by the liver flukes *Clonorchis sinensis* or *Opisthorchis viverrini*.

Hepatoblastoma and haemangiosarcoma

These are both very rare. Hepatoblastomas are congenital tumours of childhood and are composed of mixtures of epithelial and mesenchymal elements. Haemangiosarcomas are angioformative tumours: they have previously been associated with exposure to thorotrast and chronic exposure to arsenic and more recently the tumour has been shown to be associated with exposure to vinyl chloride monomer.

Secondary tumours

The liver is a very common site of secondary carcinomas of all kinds, notably from the gastro-intestinal tract, lung and breast. Secondary carcinoma may develop as one or two main masses, but often the whole organ is permeated by tumour nodules (Fig. 20.46). The liver becomes enlarged and its surface is beset with

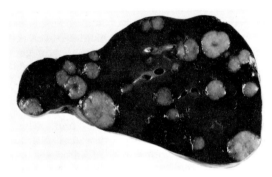

Fig. 20.46 Multiple secondary deposits in liver from a primary carcinoma of oesophagus.

nodular elevations, some of which may show umbilication owing to central necrosis. The organ may come to weigh 5 kg or more. Intrahepatic cholestasis and jaundice may develop from pressure on bile duct radicles.

Sarcomas also frequently metastasise to the liver, and may produce marked hepatomegaly. Leukaemic infiltration and metastatic spread by malignant lymphoid neoplasms are common.

Other Disorders of the Liver

Liver diseases in childhood: congenital malformations

Many of the forms of liver disease which can occur in childhood are dealt with elsewhere. They include the congenital forms of cirrhosis, Indian childhood cirrhosis, biliary cirrhosis due to bile duct atresia or as a complication of fibrocystic disease of the pancreas, congenital syphilis, and the various metabolic storage diseases in which there may be hepatic involvement. There remain a few miscellaneous conditions which merit a brief description.

Neonatal hepatitis. This is a presumed virus infection of the liver and is sometimes familial. Cytomegalovirus, hepatitis B, herpes simplex and rubella viruses are all possible causes, while some metabolic disorders, e.g. galactosaemia and alpha-1-antitrypsin deficiency, and also biliary atresia, may produce a histological picture of hepatitis. Diffuse giant cell transformation of liver cells, often with 30–40 nuclei, is a striking feature of neonatal hepatitis (Fig. 20.47).

Reye's syndrome affects children up to 10 years old. A mild upper respiratory infection is followed by convulsions, vomiting, fever, coma and sometimes death. There may be hypoglycaemia and raised serum ammonia levels. The aetiology is uncertain, and while viral infection is suspected, the profound metabolic disturbances are unexplained. The liver is usually enlarged and shows very severe microvesicular fatty change (Fig. 20.48), which is seen also in other viscera.

Cystic disease of the liver. Congenital cysts in the liver are rare and are usually associated with cystic disease of the kidneys; the latter condition, however, occurs much more commonly alone. The cysts vary greatly in size and number; the liver may be studded with them, there may be only a few, or they may comprise microscopic hamartomatous lesions—*von Meyenburg complexes*. They usually contain a clear fluid, have a cuboidal epithelial lining, and probably originate from the bile ducts.

Congenital hepatic fibrosis. This is regarded by some workers as a form of cystic disease of the liver. It may be familial and is sometimes accompanied by cystic disease of the kidneys. Bands of dense fibrous tissue extend irregularly throughout the liver, but the normal architec-

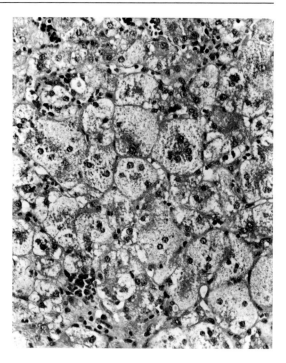

Fig. 20.47   Neonatal hepatitis: many of the liver cells are enlarged and multinucleate forms are evident: there is also intrasinusoidal extra-medullary haemopoiesis. × 190.

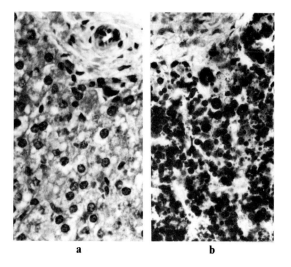

a   b

Fig. 20.48   Liver in Reye's syndrome: there is a severe degree of microvesicular fatty change. **(a)** H & E. × 250. **(b)** Oil Red O × 250.

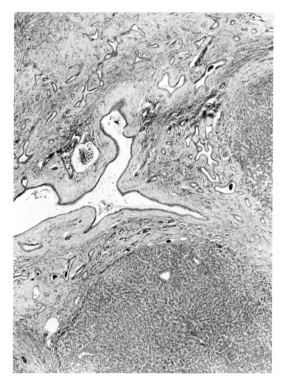

Fig. 20.49 Congenital hepatic fibrosis: wide fibrous septum within which are numerous mature bile duct elements, some of which contain inspissated bile. × 30.

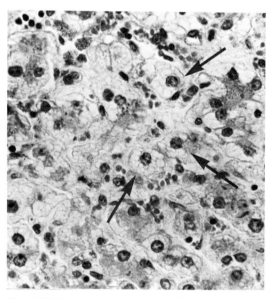

Fig. 20.50 Acute fatty liver of pregnancy: the hepatocytes are enlarged and contain multilocular droplets of fat arranged circumferentially round the nucleus (arrows). × 400.

ture is preserved between these. Within the fibrous bands there are numerous mature bile duct elements lined by cuboidal epithelium (Fig. 20.49). Affected individuals present in childhood or early adult life with portal hypertension, and when this is relieved surgically the prognosis is usually good because hepatocellular function is normal (c.f. cirrhosis). However, there appears to be an increased susceptibility to cholangitis.

Focal nodular hyperplasia. This is a benign hamartomatous lesion in which there is a focal aggregation of hyperplastic liver cell nodules separated by fibrous septa, and which may be mistaken for tumour. The lesion is usually functionally and histologically benign, although a few instances of portal hypertension have been reported where the lesion has arisen in the region of the porta hepatis.

Liver disease in pregnancy

Pregnancy may modify the clinical course of certain hepatic diseases. *Massive hepatic necrosis*, possibly viral, occurs more frequently in pregnancy, particularly in the last trimester.

A benign form of **intrahepatic cholestasis** may recur with each pregnancy and is probably due to increased levels of steroid hormones.

Acute fatty liver of pregnancy occurs usually in the last trimester, and is commonly fatal. There is widespread fatty accumulation in hepatocytes, but of an unusual appearance (Fig. 20.50). A similar morphologic appearance may occur with tetracycline toxicity, and the lesion appears to result from depressed hepatocyte protein synthesis with resultant accumulation of fat.

Liver in eclampsia. The liver is not usually injured in eclampsia, but in fatal cases there are often foci of periportal necrosis and haemorrhage with fibrin thrombi within related portal capillaries and sinusoids and plasmatic vasculosis (p. 11.7) of hepatic artery branches (Fig. 20.51). These lesions are probably ischaemic and due to hepatic involvement in the disseminated intravascular coagulation now regarded as of pathogenic significance in the hypertension of pregnancy.

Drug and toxic liver injury

The liver plays a central role in the metabolism of many drugs and chemicals, and drug-

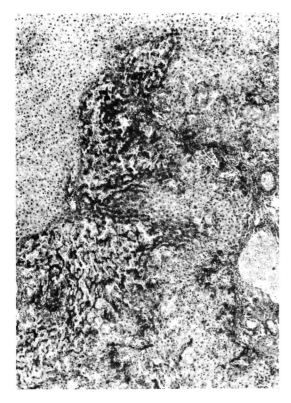

Fig. 20.51 Liver in eclampsia, showing necrotic liver cells separated by fibrin (darkly stained) and haemorrhage. × 75.

induced hepatic injury is now one of the commonest forms of iatrogenic disease. Indeed, *in any patient presenting with liver disease or with unexplained jaundice, the possibility of a drug-induced lesion should always be considered.* Many of the pathological features already described in this chapter can be reproduced by drugs—hepatocellular injury and necrosis (sometimes massive), both acute and chronic hepatitis, hepatic fibrosis and cirrhosis, vascular injury, hepatic neoplasia, and cholestasis by various mechanisms. It is not proposed to list the drugs which have hepatotoxic side-effects but merely to outline the hepatic disease patterns which may occur and to give examples of those drugs or agents which may produce them.

As with drug reactions in general, those affecting the liver may be divided into two main classes: (a) those which are *predictable*, i.e. they occur in most individuals taking the drugs in sufficient amount, the severity being related to the dose of the drug; they usually have similar effects in experimental animals and may either cause direct structural injury to liver cell components (membranes, etc.), or interfere with liver cell metabolism and result in secondary structural damage; (b) those which are *unpredictable* or *idiosyncratic*, i.e. they occur in only a proportion of individuals taking the drug, and are usually not dose-related; similar lesions are not produced regularly in experimental animals, and injury may be the result of host hypersensitivity or due to some individual metabolic aberration which renders a particular drug toxic.

Hepatocellular injury and necrosis. Fatty change may occur with tetracycline and in phosphorus poisoning; many drugs can produce focal necrosis, and massive necrosis can be caused by various industrial agents, including chlorinated hydrocarbons such as carbon tetrachloride and, seen increasingly in this country, by paracetamol overdosage. The poisonous mushroom *Amanita phalloides* also causes massive hepatic necrosis.

Hepatitis. Acute drug-induced hepatitis closely resembles classical viral hepatitis, and may be virtually indistinguishable in liver biopsy. Isoniazid, halothane and methyldopa are examples and in severe cases fulminant hepatic failure results from massive liver cell necrosis. With methyldopa and isoniazid progression to a condition resembling chronic active hepatitis has been described.

Cirrhosis has resulted from the prolonged use of methotrexate, e.g. for the treatment of leukaemia or psoriasis.

Vascular injury. Veno-occlusive disease due to pyrrollizidine alkaloids has been described earlier: urethane and radiotherapy may each cause a similar lesion, while hepatic vein thrombosis has been associated with the use of contraceptive steroids. Anabolic and contraceptive steroids may also produce periportal sinusoidal dilatation, and a rare condition *peliosis hepatis* (seen also in patients with advanced tuberculosis) in which blood-containing cysts up to 1 cm in diameter form, usually in the perivenular zones.

Hepatic neoplasia. An increased incidence of adenoma of the liver has resulted from the use of contraceptive steroids: regression after withdrawal of the drug suggests, however, that it is not a true tumour. Long-term use of anabolic (and possibly contraceptive steroids) is currently suspected of increasing the risk of liver-cell carcinoma. Thorotrast, once used extensively in angiography, carries a serious risk of liver-cell and bile-duct carcinomas and also haemangiosarcoma of the liver, which has recently been associated also with exposure to vinyl chloride monomer.

Jaundice occurs in most drug-induced liver-cell injuries, and may be a prominent feature, for example in **intrahepatic cholestasis** which results regularly from *high dosage* of C17-alkylated anabolic and contraceptive steroids and as an idiosyncratic reaction to chlorpromazine

and other drugs of the phenothiazine group. **Unconjugated hyperbilirubinaemia** may result from drug-induced haemolysis or from interference with conjugation of bilirubin in the liver, e.g. by novobiocin.

It is clear that many drugs are potential hepatotoxins and, in addition, many chemicals used in industrial processes may have hepatotoxic and possibly carcinogenic effects. The need for continued surveillance for such effects cannot be over-emphasised, and a careful occupational and drug history should be taken in patients with liver disease.

The Gallbladder and Bile Ducts

Function of the gallbladder

The relatively watery bile from the liver is stored in the gallbladder and concentrated by the absorption of water and electrolytes. Accordingly, with the addition of mucin from the mucosa, gallbladder bile becomes thick and mucoid. The normal structure of the mucosa is well suited to this absorptive function (Fig. 20.52). This concentrating ability of the gallbladder facilitates its radiological examination, in that certain iodine-containing compounds taken orally or administered intravenously are excreted and concentrated in the bile and, being radio-opaque, allow the gallbladder and the extrahepatic biliary system to be visualised.

The gallbladder bile is discharged into the duodenum in response to the entry into the duodenum of food, particularly fatty foods. When the food enters the duodenum the gallbladder discharges a proportion of its contents, and thereafter only small quantities are passed at intervals: there is always a relatively large amount of bile retained in the gallbladder. Between these periods of discharge there is probably a steady flow of hepatic bile into the gallbladder where it is concentrated.

The release of bile into the duodenum is due to contraction of the gallbladder accompanied by relaxation of the sphincter of Oddi. This is mediated humorally by cholecystokinin which is secreted by the duodenum in response to the presence there of fatty food.

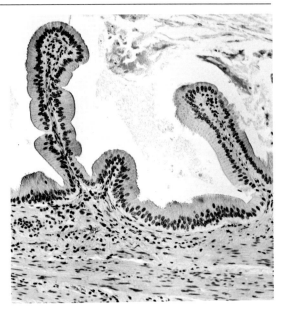

Fig. 20.52 Normal human gallbladder, showing delicate villous folds of mucosa covered by tall columnar epithelium. × 180.

Gallstones (Cholelithiasis)

Gallstones are formed from constituents of the bile—cholesterol, bile pigments and calcium salts—in various proportions, along with other organic material. They form usually in the gallbladder, but may also develop in the extrahepatic biliary tree and occasionally within intrahepatic ducts.

There is marked geographic variation in incidence, cholesterol stones being uncommon in developing countries. There is a very high incidence in North American Indians. Gallstones are commonest in late adult life, in women, especially multiparous, and in association with diabetes and obesity; the use of oral contraceptives may accelerate the development of gallstones. In patients who have undergone ileal resection there is an increased tendency for stone formation due to a decrease in the bile-acid pool.

Pathogenesis

The exact mechansims of stone formation remain debatable, and it seems likely that changes in the composition of the bile, local factors in the gallbladder and biliary tract infection are predisposing causes.

Composition of the bile. Cholesterol is the main constituent of most gallstones. It is synthesised in the liver and excreted in the bile, where it is kept in solution by the formation of micelles comprising cholesterol, phospholipids and bile salts. The phospholipids, also insoluble in water, are mainly (96%) lecithins and small amounts of lysolecithin and phosphatidyl ethanolamine. The primary bile acids are synthesised in the liver from cholesterol, the most important ones being cholic acid and chenodeoxycholic acid: they are secreted in the bile as conjugates of the amino acids glycine and taurine, the glycine/taurine conjugate ratio being 3 to 1. In the colon the primary bile acids are dehydroxylated to form the secondary bile acids, deoxycholic and lithocholic acid. These major bile acids, together with other minor ones, constitute the bile-acid pool, approximately 2–4 g in man, and more than 85% of this is reabsorbed daily from the distal small intestine and colon and re-cycled. The primary bile acids act as detergents in the bile and thus help to keep the cholesterol and phospholipids in true solution as mixed micelles. The ratio of cholesterol to bile acids and phospholipids determines cholesterol solubility.

Gallstones tend to form when there is a relative excess of cholesterol to bile acids and phospholipids—so-called '*lithogenic bile*'. This may result either from an increase in bile cholesterol or a decrease in the bile-acid pool: these changes are commonly found in patients with gallstones, but are unexplained.

Local factors in the gallbladder. These must have some part to play in the actual precipitation of stones. Not all patients with cholesterol stones secrete lithogenic bile. The parts played in stone formation by the gallbladder mucosa, the mucus and glycoprotein which it secretes, and the effects of local stasis are not known. There may also be a feedback effect on bile composition from the gallbladder and lithogenic bile shows a return to more normal composition following cholecystectomy.

Infections. It is doubtful whether infection is involved in the formation of cholesterol or pigment stones. The bile is sterile in most patients with such stones. Infection may, however, enhance the effects of local factors already mentioned and thus contribute to increase in size of stones and the formation of additional and mixed ones.

Types of stone

Stones containing predominantly cholesterol are by far the commonest, whereas bile pigment stones and calcium carbonate stones are comparatively rare.

Cholesterol stones can be classified as *mixed* or *laminated*, *pure*, and *combination or compound cholesterol* stones (Fig. 20.53).

Mixed or *laminated gallstones*. These, the commonest type, are always multiple and often very numerous (Fig. 20.53c). They are sometimes associated with and secondary to a solitary cholesterol stone. They vary greatly in size—from 1 cm or more in diameter to the size of sand grains, are irregular in shape and often faceted. On section they have a distinctly laminated structure, dark brown and paler layers alternating. These layers consist chiefly of cholesterol and bile pigment respectively, both containing also an admixture of calcium salts and organic material. The layers are thicker at the angles. The faceting is due to growth of the stones in contact with one another. Their colour varies greatly from white, grey, brownish-yellow, pinkish, brown or almost black according to the nature of the covering layer and the stage of oxidation of the bile pigment. Mixed gallstones occur in very variable numbers; occasionally there may be hundreds of small stones. They may lie free in the bile, which may be mixed with inflammatory

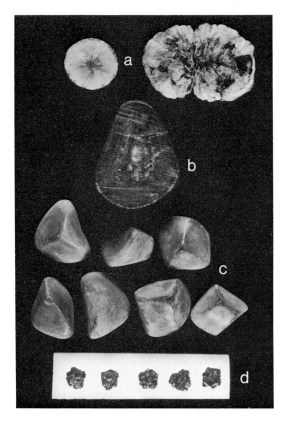

Fig. 20.53 Types of gallstones. (**a**) Two cholesterol stones; (**b**) Combination stone: a cholesterol core coated by laminated surface deposits of mixed composition; (**c**) multiple faceted mixed stones; (**d**) bile-pigment stones.

cium salts, the pigment causing the darker markings (Fig. 20.53b). This is due to a secondary deposit, which occurs when the gallbladder wall becomes inflamed by superadded bacterial infection. Stones of this class may be called *combination* or *compound cholesterol stones*. They constitute the largest gallstones. Occasionally a contracted gallbladder contains two or three barrel-shaped combination cholesterol stones placed end to end.

Bile pigment stones. Such stones are usually multiple, black, irregular in form or occasionally somewhat stellate (Fig. 20.53d). They are composed chiefly of bile pigment, and may be friable or hard. They are often present in chronic haemolytic anaemias and are due to excess of bile pigment in the bile, but are encountered also occasionally in the absence of increased red cell destruction. The gallbladder usually appears normal.

exudate or pus, or they may be tightly packed together within a contracted gallbladder with a thickened wall (Fig. 20.54).

The pure cholesterol stone is usually solitary, oval, and may reach over 3 cm in length. It is pale yellow or almost white, soapy to the touch and of low specific gravity, often floating in water. Some are almost transparent with a frankly crystalline surface (Fig. 20.53a). When broken across, the stone shows a crystalline structure composed of sheaves of cholesterol crystals which radiate outwards from the centre. The core is sometimes dark owing to the incorporation of bile pigment between the crystals, but there is no break in the continuity of their formation, and no trace of lamination. Some specimens of solitary cholesterol stones, however, have a laminated cortex (i.e. concentric deposits) composed of bile pigment and cal-

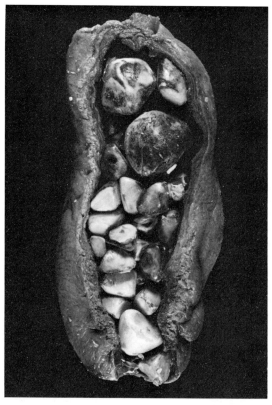

Fig. 20.54 Gallbladder filled with numerous gallstones of mixed type. The wall is thickened and fibrosed due to chronic cholecystitis.

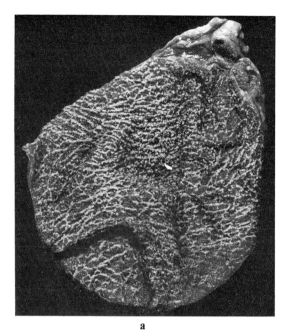
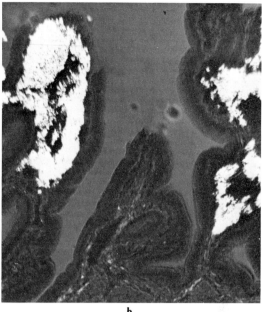

a   b

Fig. 20.55 Cholesterosis of gallbladder. (**a**) the characteristic macroscopic pattern of 'strawberry gallbladder'. (**b**) deposits of cholesterol esters in papillae, viewed by polarised light. × 90. (Professor W. A. Mackey.)

Calcium carbonate stones. These also are rare. They are multiple, small, pale yellowish and fairly hard.

Cholesterosis of the gallbladder

This unimportant condition results from the patchy deposition of doubly refractile cholesterol esters within mucosal macrophages. This produces distinct yellowish flecking of the mucosa giving the appearance of so-called 'strawberry gallbladder' (Fig. 20.55). The lipid deposits may increase in size to form polypoidal nodules. It is associated with cholesterol stones, solitary or mulberry, in one-third of cases.

Cholecystitis

Inflammation of the gallbladder is one of the commonest causes of abdominal pain, and frequently necessitates cholecystectomy.

Acute cholecystitis

Acute cholecystitis is nearly always associated with the presence of stones. It has been shown repeatedly that in the early stages of acute cholecystitis, bacteria cannot usually be cultured from the gallbladder. It is therefore thought that the initial inflammation is chemically induced. Obstruction to the outflow of bile due to a stone results in the bile becoming over-concentrated and this produces an irritant effect with consequent inflammation. Secondary bacterial infection may then occur, aggravating the inflammatory reaction. The organisms are thought to reach the gallbladder via the lymphatics, and are most commonly *Esch. coli.* or *Strep. faecalis.* Acute cholecystitis rarely occurs in the absence of stones, and is then usually associated with a source of infection elsewhere.

Pathologically, acute cholecystitis may be merely a mild catarrhal inflammation, or more severe—fibrinous, pseudo-membranous, haemorrhagic or suppurative. These more severe types occur especially when there is continued obstruction of the cystic duct either by stone or by superadded inflammatory oedema and exudate. The lumen may then become filled with pus—*empyema of the gallbladder*. Abscesses may also form in the wall, or there may even be necrosis or gangrene of the wall with rupture into the peritoneal cavity. In acute cholecystitis, fibrin deposition on the serosal surface may be

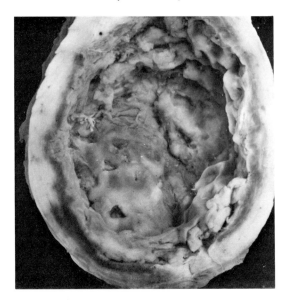

Fig. 20.56 Chronic cholecystitis, showing great thickening of wall. The gallbladder was packed with small rounded stones.

organised, resulting in fibrosis and adhesions. The condition is often recurrent and may become chronic.

Chronic cholecystitis

This may result from repeated attacks of acute cholecystitis. In many patients, however, the disease is one of insidious onset, accompanied by dyspeptic symptoms or biliary colic. Gallstones are almost always present. The gallbladder wall is shrunken and shows marked fibrous thickening (Fig. 20.56). The lining is irregular, and there may be distinct pouches, especially when numerous stones are present. The contents may be clear, turbid or frankly purulent. The lining epithelium sometimes extends normally as downgrowths between the muscle bundles to form gland-like structures known as *Rokitansky–Aschoff sinuses*. This becomes much more marked in some cases of chronic cholecystitis, and there may be multiple complex epithelial overgrowths within the wall, which have occasionally been mistaken for adenocarcinoma (Fig. 20.57). Previously referred to as 'cholecystitis glandularis proliferans', the condition is now known as *adenomyomatosis of the gallbladder* and is benign. It may rarely occur in the absence of stones, and produce inflammation and symptoms resembling biliary colic.

Complications of cholelithiasis and cholecystitis

Gallstones and infections of the gallbladder are so intimately related that the complications associated with them are best considered together. Some of these have been referred to already.

Gallstones, single or multiple, may lead to no noticeable symptoms—so-called silent stones. When a stone becomes impacted in Hartmann's pouch or in the cystic duct, great distension of the gallbladder results: the bile pigments are absorbed and the contents become clear and mucoid—mucocele of the gallbladder (Fig. 20.58). In the presence of infection, however, the contents become turbid or purulent— empyema of the gallbladder. Inflammation of the wall may progress to necrosis, with escape of the contents into the peritoneal cavity producing localised or generalised peritonitis.

Stones may also obstruct the common bile

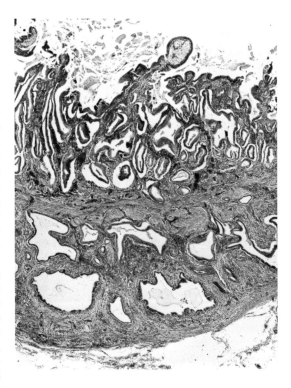

Fig. 20.57 Chronic cholecystitis showing extensive penetration of fundus of gallbladder by epithelial-lined spaces lying between muscle and serosa (Rokitansky–Aschoff sinuses). × 20.

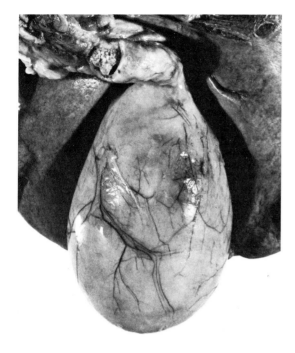

Fig. 20.58 Mucocele of the gallbladder. A stone is impacted in the cystic duct producing distension of the gallbladder, the contents of which have become clear and mucoid. Note how this accentuates the vascular markings on the serosa.

duct, producing biliary colic, extrahepatic obstruction and jaundice (p. 20.55). If the stone remains loose in the duct, the jaundice may be intermittent. Secondary bacterial infection is common, resulting in ascending cholangitis. In only a small proportion of cases does obstruction of the bile duct by stones lead to secondary biliary cirrhosis.

In chronic cholecystitis the wall becomes thickened and may be contracted over a mass of closely packed stones: there are often adhesions around the gallbladder and a stone or stones may ulcerate in one of several directions. A large stone of the compound cholesterol type may, for example, ulcerate through into the duodenum or less frequently into the colon. It may pass along the bowel, or may become arrested at some part of the small intestine, chiefly by contraction of the muscular coat, and may produce acute intestinal obstruction, which is then termed *gallstone ileus*. Ulceration into the portal vein with the setting up of portal pyaemia has been recorded.

Lastly, the irritation produced by gallstones may lead to carcinoma of the gallbladder, or, more rarely, of the large ducts.

Tumours of the biliary tract

Benign tumours, such as fibroma, lipoma and papilloma, are all very rare. Rarely, a large papilloma may obstruct the outflow with much distension of the gallbladder.

Carcinoma of the gallbladder is uncommon, and gallstones are an important factor in its causation, being present in fully 80% of cases of cancer. The commonest site is the fundus and next is the neck of the gallbladder. It is usually of the slowly-growing, infiltrating type, but sometimes it is a soft growth with a tendency to necrosis. Occasionally the gallbladder may be practically destroyed and its cavity represented by a small irregular space in which gallstones may be present. It may invade the liver (Fig. 20.59) and may also give rise to numerous metastases. In most cases it is an adenocarcinoma, sometimes a cancer of spheroidal-cell or mucoid type. Squamous-cell carcinoma, arising secondarily to metaplasia of the lining epithelium, also occurs.

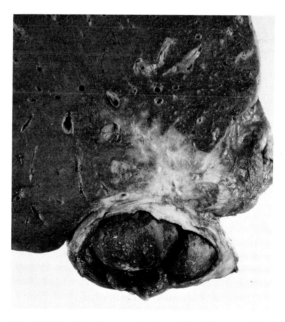

Fig. 20.59 Carcinoma of the gallbladder spreading directly into the overlying liver.

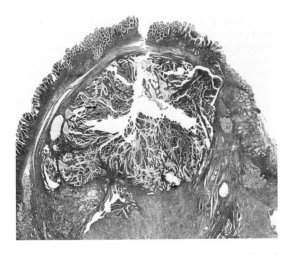

Fig. 20.60 Primary carcinoma of the ampulla of Vater causing obstructive jaundice. × 6.

Carcinoma occurs also in the *large bile ducts* and is usually a small and slowly growing tumour. The two commonest sites are the lower end of the common bile duct (Fig. 20.60) and the junction of the cystic and hepatic ducts, the latter being more frequent; this site is also commonly involved by secondary lymphatic spread from carcinoma of the gallbladder.

Of the very many individuals who develop gallstones, less than 2% develop carcinoma of the gallbladder; the incidence of bile-duct carcinoma is also low, although it is often not possible to determine whether a tumour around the ampulla has originated from bile duct or pancreas.

Congenital anomalies

A large number of abnormalities of the gallbladder have been described and may affect its size, shape, position, relation to the liver, etc. Gallstones may occur more frequently at a younger age in association with these anomalities.

Varying degrees of extrahepatic *biliary atresia* may occur and may result in secondary biliary cirrhosis. The rare *choledochal cyst* comprises a sac-like dilatation of a part or all of the biliary tract, and is associated with jaundice and cholangitis.

Jaundice

Staining of the tissues with bilirubin or bilirubin complexes is known as **jaundice** or **icterus.** When the serum level of these pigments exceeds about 34 μmol/litre (2 mg/dl), generalised jaundice develops. According to the severity and duration of the condition the skin and conjunctiva present various degrees of yellow staining up to deep orange colour and in very chronic cases it becomes olive-green owing to formation of biliverdin. The internal organs also are pigmented except the brain and spinal cord, which are not usually affected. In *icterus gravis neonatorum*, however, there may be bile staining of areas in the central nervous system, usually localised to the grey matter of the basal nuclei—the so-called *kernicterus*—but sometimes affecting the cortex (p. 21.44). The presence of the pigment in the blood in a case of marked jaundice is readily shown by the colour of the serum. Bile pigment may also be excreted in the urine and in the sweat; the tears, however, are not coloured, nor are the saliva, gastric juice or bile-duct epithelial secretion.

When the cause of the jaundice has been removed the skin may remain stained for some time after the serum bilirubin level has returned to normal, owing to the strong affinity of the elastic tissue for bilirubin. A rise of serum bilirubin from the normal level of 3–14 μmol/litre (0.2–0.8 mg/dl) up to 34 μmol/litre (2 mg/dl) is not usually accompanied by visible jaundice, but is sometimes called 'latent jaundice'. The term 'localised jaundice' is seldom used but it is seen around a bruise, the escaped haemoglobin being broken down to bilirubin.

Before considering further the features and types of jaundice, it is necessary to give an outline of the normal bile pigment metabolism.

Bile pigment metabolism

More than 80% of the bile pigment is derived from the breakdown of effete mature red cells. Approximately 6 g of haemoglobin are broken down daily, mainly in macrophages, in man chiefly in the spleen, bone-marrow and liver, and the steps have already been described (p. 11.11). The remaining 20% is derived in part from non-haemoglobin haem-containing pigments, e.g. myoglobin, catalase and cytochromes, and in part from ineffective erythropoiesis during red cell maturation (p. 17.35). Excessive production of this latter erythropoietic component may occur in thalassaemia, congenital porphyria and in dyserythropoietic or shunt hyperbilirubinaemia. Approximately 300 mg of bilirubin are produced daily.

Following release from macrophages, bilirubin (sometimes called **unconjugated bilirubin** to distinguish it from bilirubin glucuronides—see below) circulates in the plasma and is preferentially taken up by the hepatocytes. Within these it is conjugated with glucuronic acid, a reaction catalysed by the enzyme uridine diphosphate glucuronyl transferase. Both mono- and diglucuronide conjugates are formed, and possibly also sulphate and carbohydrate conjugates whose importance is uncertain. These conjugates are water soluble, and are referred to as **conjugated bilirubin**; they are rapidly excreted directly into the bile canaliculi and hence pass into the bile. Conjugated bilirubin is converted in the intestine into **stercobilinogen,** the normal brown faecal pigment. A small fraction of the stercobilinogen is re-absorbed from the gut, and most of this passes back to the liver where it is re-excreted into the bile—the entero-hepatic circulation of bile pigment. A minute amount (1–3 mg daily) of the re-absorbed stercobilinogen is excreted in the urine as **urobilinogen.**

To understand the clinical, biochemical and morbid anatomical features of the different types of jaundice, it is necessary to appreciate that *unconjugated bilirubin is water-insoluble and remains in solution in the plasma only as a rather firm complex with albumin. Consequently, it does not readily pass through capillary walls, and its increase in the plasma is not accompanied by bilirubinuria.* Nevertheless, unconjugated bilirubin is capable of staining the tissues, although the form in which it escapes from the plasma

remains unknown. *Another feature of unconjugated bilirubin is its solubility in lipids, which may explain the bilirubin-staining of the brain in neonates with high plasma levels of unconjugated bilirubin. The brain damage which may result is due to the toxic effects of bilirubin on nerve cells. By contrast, conjugated bilirubin is water-soluble, and increased levels in the plasma are always accompanied by its appearance in the urine: it is relatively insoluble in lipids and causes neither staining of, nor damage to, the central nervous system.*

The biochemical estimation of serum bilirubin employs the **van den Bergh reaction.** When Ehrlich's diazo reagent, a mixture of sulphanilic acid and sodium nitrite, is added to a solution of bilirubin, the pigment becomes diazotised to give a blue-violet compound which can be assayed colorimetrically. Conjugated bilirubin gives an *immediate* or *direct* reaction, and the *total* bilirubin is then measured after treatment with alcohol which splits the unconjugated or indirect-reacting bilirubin from its bilirubin-albumin complex.

Classification of jaundice

Jaundice may result from:

(1) Increased bilirubin production.
(2) Interference with hepatic uptake of bilirubin.
(3) Interference with hepatic conjugation of bilirubin.
(4) Interference with hepatic excretion of bilirubin.
(5) Combinations of 2–4 resulting from reduction in functional hepatic cell mass.

While it is of diagnostic and therapeutic importance to determine which of the above five factors is responsible for the development of jaundice, in practice it is found that more than one factor is often concerned. For example, the anaemia resulting from increased red cell destruction may cause liver cell injury, as also does prolonged obstruction of the biliary tract, whether or not accompanied by infection. Thus *jaundice is frequently attributable to more than one factor, and diagnosis of the underlying condition is sometimes very difficult.*

(1) Increased bilirubin production

(a) Haemolytic (acholuric) jaundice. This is not uncommon and is due to increased red cell destruction, either acute or chronic (see p. 17.19), with consequent production in the macrophage system of increased amounts of bilirubin, up to 1·5 g daily. Normally, the liver is capable of extracting, conjugating and excreting such large amounts of bilirubin, and jaundice is thus latent or mild. The agent causing the haemolysis may, however, also damage the liver, or the anaemia resulting from haemolysis may depress liver function, and in these circumstances jaundice is more pronounced. In infants, the rate of red cell destruction is relatively high, and the liver is deficient in the enzymes necessary for conjugation of bilirubin, particularly when birth is premature. Accordingly, *icterus neonatorum* is a common condition, and is likely to be especially severe in infants with haemolytic anaemia due to maternal iso-antibodies (p. 17.30). Exchange blood transfusions may be necessary to keep the plasma bilirubin below 250 μmol/l (15 mg/dl), the level at which there is a real danger of brain damage from kernicterus (p. 21.44).

In haemolytic jaundice, most of the bilirubin in the plasma is unconjugated, and thus bile pigment is absent from the urine (*acholuric jaundice*). The amount of urobilinogen in the urine is, however, usually much increased. The faeces are dark from the excessive amounts of bile pigment excreted.

(b) Dyserythropoietic (shunt) hyperbilirubinaemia. This is associated with ineffective or abnormal red cell maturation resulting in the premature destruction of erythrocyte precursors in the marrow: there is an unconjugated bilirubinaemia but with a normal peripheral blood red cell survival time. The disease is rare, familial and the mode of inheritance is not defined.

(2) Interference with hepatic uptake of bilirubin

Gilbert's disease. Although rare, this is the commonest form of familial non-haemolytic acholuric jaundice. It is apparently due to a 'dominant' defect of a single autosomal gene which impairs either transport of bilirubin to the liver, or uptake of bilirubin by the liver. Mild intermittent acholuric jaundice results. The condition is, however, rather poorly defined.

(3) Interference with hepatic conjugation of bilirubin

(a) Physiological or neonatal jaundice. This is a common condition, particularly in premature babies. It is due to relative deficiency of glucuronyl transferase in the neonatal liver. The jaundice usually improves 2–3 weeks post-partum as the enzyme attains normal levels.

(b) Inherited defective bilirubin conjugation. In the very rare *Crigler-Najjar syndrome*, deficiency of glucuronyl transferase results in very high levels of unconjugated bilirubin. In Type I, in which the enzyme is absent, kernicterus within the first two years of life is the usual cause of death, whereas in Type II, with a variably reduced enzyme activity, normal survival may occur.

(4) Interference with hepatic excretion of bilirubin

(a) Intrahepatic inherited. In the rare *Dubin-Johnson syndrome*, there is a partial failure of the liver cells to secrete conjugated bilirubin into the bile canaliculi, and as a consequence conjugated bilirubin is regurgitated into the blood and intermittent jaundice results. The other constituents of the bile are secreted normally, and the serum alkaline phosphatase level is not raised. A curious feature is accumulation of granules of brown pigment in hepatocyte lysosomes, as yet of uncertain nature but possibly melanin-like. Little or no disability results from this syndrome, which is believed to be due to a single gene defect with 'dominant' transmission. A second, and genetically related, condition is the *Rotor syndrome* in which there is failure to secrete conjugated bilirubin but no accumulation of brown pigment in the liver cells.

In a further rare condition—*benign idiopathic recurrent intrahepatic cholestasis*—multiple recurrent attacks of cholestasis occur in the absence of large duct obstruction, the jaundice persisting for some months, but without producing any evidence of progressive or permanent liver damage. An intrahepatic cholestatic syndrome may also occur in pregnancy; in an affected female it usually occurs in all pregnancies; it tends to be familial and is entirely benign.

Byler disease is a rare autosomal recessive form of intrahepatic cholestasis which progresses to cirrhosis and death in infancy.

(b) Intrahepatic acquired. This occurs in primary biliary cirrhosis, and also as a complication of therapy with certain drugs (p. 20.46).

Drug-induced cholestasis occurs as an idiosyncrasy in a small proportion of patients taking phenothiazine derivatives, notably chlorpromazine, and appears unrelated to dosage. It is reversible, at least in most cases, on discontinuing the drug. Cholestasis results also from administration of methyltestosterone and certain other C17-alkyl-substituted testosterones, and does not depend upon idiosyncrasy, being produced regularly by a sufficient dosage of such compounds.

(c) Extrahepatic biliary obstruction is the commonest cause of jaundice in middle and old age: it is termed **obstructive jaundice.** Major duct obstruction is caused chiefly by gallstones lodging in the common bile duct, and by carcinoma of the head of the pancreas or of the lower end of the common bile duct. Less commonly, it arises from scarring of bile ducts due to previous inflammation and ulceration by gallstones, and from accidental injury or ligations of the common bile duct during operations in this area. Other causes include congenital malformations of the major duct system, and involvement of the ducts in tumours or tuberculosis affecting the lymph nodes and surrounding tissues in the portal fissure.

When due to gallstones, the obstruction may be sudden and complete, or intermittent if the stone or stones move along the common bile duct; it is often accompanied by biliary colic. In carcinomatous involvement or scarring of the ducts, obstruction, and hence jaundice, are usually of more gradual onset, progressive and often painless. As in all forms of obstructive jaundice the serum alkaline phosphatase is greatly raised.

Apart from jaundice and its effects, major duct obstruction, particularly if caused by gallstones, is likely to be complicated by superadded suppurative cholangitis, and in unrelieved obstruction the patient does not usually survive long enough to develop secondary biliary cirrhosis (p. 20.30).

(5) Reduction in functional hepatic cell mass (hepatocellular or toxic jaundice)

This type of jaundice is also common. It results from damage to liver cells, e.g. by viruses, bacterial or hepatocellular toxins. It is a feature of the various forms of viral hepatitis and leptospirosis (Weil's disease), where the organisms are actually present in the liver, and it occurs occasionally in typhus, pneumonia, septicaemia, relapsing fever, smallpox etc. It is seen also in some forms of snake bite, in poisoning with various chemicals and toxins—trinitrotoluene, phosphorus, amanitine and amanita toxin from various fungi, etc. Except in biliary cirrhosis, jaundice is usually a late complication of hepatic cirrhosis, and is then likely to be attributable to liver cell necrosis and hepatocellular failure.

Two factors are concerned in the production of hepatocellular jaundice: (*a*) damage to the liver cells may interfere with the passage of bile along the bile canaliculi: in other words, a degree of intrahepatic cholestasis arises. Focal necrosis or swelling of the liver cells, and disorganisation of the liver cell plates and fibrosis (as in cirrhosis), may thus cause focal cholestasis; (*b*) removal of unconjugated bilirubin from the blood, its conjugation and discharge into the bile canaliculi, may all be impaired as a result of liver cell injury. The relative importance of these two factors varies in different cases, and may also change, as liver cell injury progresses, in the individual case.

The Pancreas

Introduction

The pancreas is often thought of as two separate organs—an exocrine one concerned with digestion, and an endocrine one concerned with the metabolism of carbohydrate, fat and protein. Their association within one gland is simply regarded as fortuitous. However, knowledge of the embryology, anatomy, physiology and pathology of the pancreas all militate against this simplistic approach.

Embryology. Dorsal and ventral pancreatic buds develop independently from the foregut. They fuse to give a single organ in which there is usually union of the duct systems of the two buds. The ventral bud eventually forms about one-tenth of the pancreas identifiable as a 'lobe' in the postero-inferior part of the pancreatic

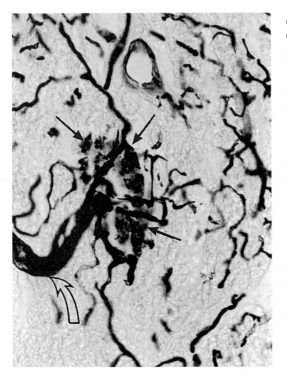

Fig. 20.61 Section of pancreas after injection of the blood vessels with India ink. The B cells of the islets have been stained black by the immunoperoxidase technique. The periphery of an islet is marked by straight arrows. An arteriole (curved arrow) breaks up into sinusoids which supply the islet and drain into capillaries which supply the surrounding exocrine tissue. × 120.

head. In early fetal life the pancreas comprises a series of branching ductules from which are derived both acinar tissue and islet cells. Thus the whole pancreas, exocrine and endocrine, is derived from foregut endoderm. This conclusion is supported by much experimental research.

Structure. Connective tissue septa divide the pancreas into lobules. Within the lobule the secretory unit is the acinus, the cells of which have cytoplasmic zymogen granules—membrane-bound sacs containing digestive enzymes. The secretory products drain via intralobular and interlobular ducts to the main pancreatic duct. The anatomy of the pancreatic blood supply is interesting. Most lobules receive a single arterial branch, and within lobules containing islets much of the circulation passes by arterioles to the islets, the exocrine tissue being supplied by a portal system of capillaries which

drain the blood from the sinusoids of the islets (Fig. 20.61). The pancreatic acini around islets are thus exposed to very high levels of islet hormones—possibly several hundred times higher than the levels in the systemic circulation. Most of the endocrine cells are grouped together into islets, although individual endocrine cells can be found in duct epithelium and among acini. In the adult pancreas, islets in that part derived from the dorsal bud (superior anterior part of head, body and tail of the pancreas), consist of 82% insulin-secreting (B) cells, 13% glucagon-secreting (A) cells, 4% somatostatin-secreting (D) cells and 1% pancreatic polypeptide-secreting (PP) cells. By contrast, in the part derived from the ventral bud, islets are composed of 18% B cells, 1% A cells, 2% D cells and 79% PP cells. Not surprisingly, this part of the pancreas is termed the *PP-rich lobe* and the remainder is called the *glucagon-rich lobe* (Fig. 20.62). Because of the greater density of islets in the former, PP cells constitute 36% of all the endocrine cells in the pancreas.

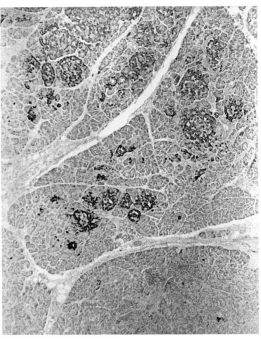

Fig. 20.62 This shows the junction between the PP-rich lobe (top) and the glucagon-rich lobe (bottom). Note the high density of islets in the PP-rich lobe. (Immunoperoxidase technique using antibody directed against pancreatic polypeptide.) × 50.

Functional aspects. The exocrine pancreas is now known to secrete about 20 digestive enzymes, prominent among which are trypsin, elastase, amylase, lipase and phospholipase. Most are secreted in inactive forms and are activated in the duodenum. Bicarbonate is secreted by the duct epithelium.

In addition to its systemic effects, which are discussed later, insulin is a major trophic hormone for the exocrine pancreas, increasing the rate of DNA and protein synthesis in acinar tissue. *Weight for weight the exocrine pancreas synthesises considerably more protein (mainly enzymes) than any other tissue in the body.* (Eight times more than liver, for example.) Since one of the main actions of insulin in all cells of the body is to stimulate protein synthesis, it is interesting to speculate that the islets, with their distinctive blood supply which ensures very high levels of insulin in the exocrine capillaries, have evolved to aid the massive protein synthesis requirements of the exocrine pancreas. Pancreatic polypeptide is also a trophic hormone for the exocrine pancreas, while glucagon and somatostatin have an inhibitory effect.

Pancreatitis

Pancreatitis is classified into acute and chronic forms which appear to be two distinct entities. Acute pancreatitis rarely proceeds to the chronic form even when it recurs several times, although the course of chronic pancreatitis is frequently punctuated by acute exacerbations.

Acute pancreatitis

This is defined simply as acute inflammation in the pancreas. It is usually associated with necrosis of intrapancreatic fat and acini. If there is macroscopic haemorrhage in the pancreas the term *acute haemorrhagic pancreatitis* is used, but this is probably simply the severe end of a spectrum of changes.

Clinical features. The onset is often sudden with abdominal pain, vomiting and collapse and may easily be confused clinically with perforation of a peptic ulcer. The diagnosis is confirmed by demonstrating a serum amylase level greater than 1200 iu/l. Two-thirds of patients

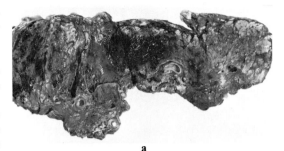

a

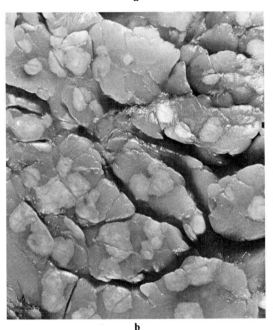

b

Fig. 20.63 (a) Acute haemorrhagic pancreatitis. × 0·6. (b) Part of the greater omentum from the same case, showing pale patches of fat necrosis. × 1·7.

admitted to hospital have a mild illness which settles readily with nasogastric suction and intravenous fluids. Severe pancreatitis, characterised by shock, hypocalcaemia, hypoxaemia and hyperglycaemia, is less common and carries a 50% mortality rate.

Macroscopic changes. The abdominal findings in severe cases are acute peritonitis with bloodstained ascitic fluid and white flecks of fat necrosis on the omentum (Fig. 20.63b) and surface of the pancreas. The cut surface of the pancreas usually shows further flecks of necrotic tissue, possibly in combination with haemorrhage which may be confluent, resulting in a firm black necrotic mass (Fig. 20.63a).

Microscopic changes. There appear to be two

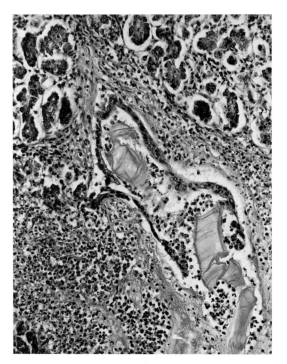

Fig. 20.64 Acute pancreatitis, showing periductal necrosis. An interlobular duct is dilated by protein-rich concretions. The surrounding acini are necrotic and there is an acute inflammatory infiltrate in and around the ducts. × 180.

quite distinct initial lesions. In some cases, necrosis and an acute inflammatory infiltrate appear first within and around excretory ducts (**periductal necrosis**—Fig. 20.64). In others, inflammation develops at the periphery of pancreatic lobules (**perilobular necrosis**—Fig. 20.65). These two patterns can be correlated with aetiology (see below). The excretory ducts are surrounded by a venous plexus, and in cases with initial periductal necrosis, there may be escape of pancreatic enzymes causing autodigestion of vessels and secondary thrombosis. If such thrombosis is widespread, extensive infarction may occur with coagulative necrosis of entire lobules and intervening ducts and blood vessels (**panlobular necrosis**): this corresponds with macroscopic **acute haemorrhagic pancreatitis**, and is commonly complicated by super-added bacterial infection of the necrotic pancreas and peritoneum. The bacteria are usually *Esch. coli* and other gut commensals.

Aetiology. (a) *Periductal necrosis*. In Western countries, over 80% of clinically observed cases

are associated either with the presence of biliary calculi or with alcohol abuse. The initial pathological event in either case is ductal inflammation and periductal necrosis. In '**gallstone pancreatitis**', the initiating event appears to be the passage of a gallstone into the common bile duct, resulting in temporary obstruction of the pancreatic duct at the ampulla of Vater. If such patients are treated surgically within 48 hours of the onset of gallstone pancreatitis, impacted gallstones are found at the ampulla in over 70% of cases. It has also been shown by operative cholangiography that there is reflux of contrast material from the bile duct into the pancreatic duct, signifying a common exit channel in 67% of patients with gallstone pancreatitis, but in only 18% of patients with gallstones but without pancreatitis. Thus *reflux of bile into an obstructed pancreatic duct is the likely initial event*. Normal bile alone does not damage the pancreatic duct, but infected bile or bile pre-incubated with trypsin causes ductal inflammation and necrosis when infused into the pancreatic duct at physiological pressure. Both

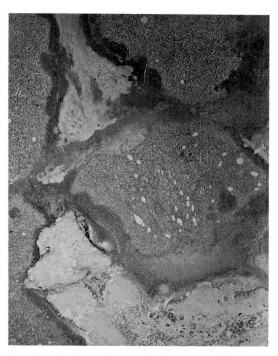

Fig. 20.65 Acute haemorrhagic pancreatitis, showing necrosis of the peripheral parts of the lobules. (The necrotic tissue is mostly darker staining than the surviving tissue.) × 18.

infection and trypsin convert primary bile salts into secondary bile salts, which are toxic to pancreatic duct epithelium. Bile is infected in at least 40% of cases of gallstone pancreatitis, and in the presence of an obstructing stone, bile which has refluxed into the pancreas can be altered by pancreatic trypsin.

Alcoholic pancreatitis also appears to be initiated by ductal inflammation but the mechanisms involved are uncertain.

(b) *Perilobular necrosis*. In those cases of pancreatitis where only perilobular necrosis is found, the pancreatitis appears to result from ischaemia. It will be remembered that pancreatic lobules receive a single arterial branch and thus during prolonged hypotension the periphery of the lobule is prone to ischaemic damage. This form of pancreatitis may complicate shock from any cause and is the form seen in pancreatitis secondary to hypothermia. Hypothermia is associated with diminished prostacyclin synthesis resulting in an increased thrombotic tendency, and this, in combination with hypotension, may precipitate perilobular thrombosis and necrosis in the pancreas.

Rarer causes of acute pancreatitis include direct pancreatic trauma, Polya type gastrectomy, exploration of the common bile duct and viral (notably mumps) infection. The incidence is also increased in hyperparathyroidism and in diabetes mellitus. Lack of pathological material in these conditions has precluded study of the pathogenetic mechanisms.

Complications of acute pancreatitis

(a) **Systemic.** Severe acute pancreatitis is complicated by chemical peritonitis which, even in the absence of superadded bacterial peritonitis, can cause death from endotoxic shock due to escape of intestinal endotoxin into the circulation. Release of pancreatic enzymes into the blood may also contribute to the shock syndrome.

(b) **Local.** Sepsis in a necrotic pancreas may result in widespread suppuration or a **pancreatic abscess**. Another local effect is the formation of a **pseudocyst**—a localised collection of pancreatic juice and necrotic debris resulting from disruption of the pancreatic ductal drainage. It is lined by granulation tissue and commonly forms in the lesser sac.

Chronic pancreatitis

Chronic pancreatitis, known also as *relapsing chronic pancreatitis* if the clinical evolution is punctuated by acute exacerbations, is characterised by the persistence of pancreatic damage, even if the primary cause of the pancreatitis is eradicated (see below). There is obviously a grey area clinically and pathologically between recurrent acute pancreatitis and relapsing chronic pancreatitis but in the former the patient is well between attacks and chronic pancreatitis does not usually ensue.

Clinically, most patients present with severe, erratic abdominal pain, perhaps accompanied by weight loss and jaundice. Steatorrhoea and diabetes are later manifestations, but may be presenting features in patients with painless disease. Plain abdominal radiographs may show diffuse pancreatic calcification, and endoscopic retrograde pancreatography will usually show strictures and distortions of the pancreatic ducts and also the presence of pancreatic calculi in the ducts.

Macroscopically the pancreas is usually enlarged and firm, and the cut surface shows a smooth grey appearance with loss of normal lobulation. This change is the result of diffuse fibrosis. The main ducts are often focally dilated, sometimes forming cysts which contain calcific stones.

Microscopically, early lesions consist of ductal strictures and luminal concretions, with fibrosis of the areas of pancreas drained by the stenosed ducts (Figs 20.66, 20.67). The remaining pancreas is normal. Later the change in the pancreas becomes more diffuse with generalised fibrosis. Islets are involved only in the late stages.

Aetiology. Most cases of chronic pancreatitis are related to alcohol abuse. Epidemiologically, the disease is found in individuals who persistently drink large amounts of alcohol daily, accompanied by a high-protein diet. Alcohol increases the protein concentration in pancreatic juice with subsequent precipitation of concretions in the ducts: these tend to cause ulceration of the ductal epithelium which heals by scar tissue and stricture formation. The area of pancreas drained by a stenosed duct undergoes atrophy and fibrosis.

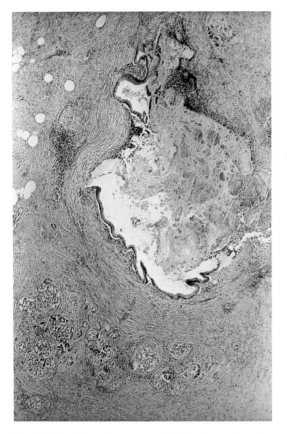

Fig. 20.66 Chronic pancreatitis showing ulceration and dilatation of a duct and periductal fibrosis. Note the loss of acini but preservation of islets. × 24.

Cystic fibrosis

This disease is due to a generalised abnormality of exocrine gland secretion involving pancreas, bowel, bronchi, biliary tree and sweat glands. In the newborn it may give rise to intestinal obstruction by inspissated meconium (*meconium ileus*). In older children, malabsorption due to exocrine pancreatic failure and chronic suppurative lung disease are the main features and the principal causes of death. There is an increased sodium chloride content of the sweat of affected individuals and this provides a useful diagnostic test. Attempts are being made to diagnose cystic fibrosis prenatally by measuring the concentrations of various microvillous membrane enzymes in amniotic fluid, but such tests are not yet reliable.

Cystic fibrosis occurs in one per 2000 live births among Caucasians, in whom it is the commonest disease determined by a single gene defect. The inheritance is autosomal recessive, approximately one in 25 of the population being heterozygous for the abnormal gene. The biochemical nature of the defect is not known.

The changes in the affected glandular organs are due to obstruction of the ducts by inspissated secretion, with secondary parenchymal injury. The pancreas is always affected. Microscopically, inter- and intra-lobular ducts are dilated and filled with concretions and there is secondary acinar atrophy and fibrosis (Fig. 20.68). These features are reminiscent of chronic pancreatitis, but the changes in cystic fibrosis occur diffusely throughout the pancreas from the outset, while in chronic pancreatitis the changes are initially patchy and only later become confluent. Obstruction of small bronchi is complicated by secondary bacterial infections and results in bronchiectasis (p. 16.14) and recurrent bronchopneumonia. Other pathological findings include a predominantly subcapsular portal fibrosis in the liver with biliary concretions, and occlusion of the vas deferens.

Tumours of the exocrine pancreas

Apart from carcinoma, pancreatic tumours are rare. Fibroma, lipoma, lymphangioma, adenoma and cystadenoma have been described. **Cystadenomas** of the pancreas are often large and multiloculated. When they are lined by a non-mucin-secreting epithelium which contains glycogen they are invariably benign. Some of the mucin-secreting multicystic tumours may be malignant, and are termed cystadenocarcinomas.

Carcinoma has doubled in incidence in the UK during the last 50 years. The increase in the USA has been even higher and it now ranks second only to colorectal carcinoma among alimentary tract cancers in that country. It is commoner in males than females and increases progressively in incidence after the age of 50 years. Epidemiologically it has been linked to smoking, a high-fat, high-protein diet, and possibly diabetes. There is no association with chronic pancreatitis or alcohol abuse. Sixty-five per cent of tumours are situated in the head of the pancreas where they usually obstruct the

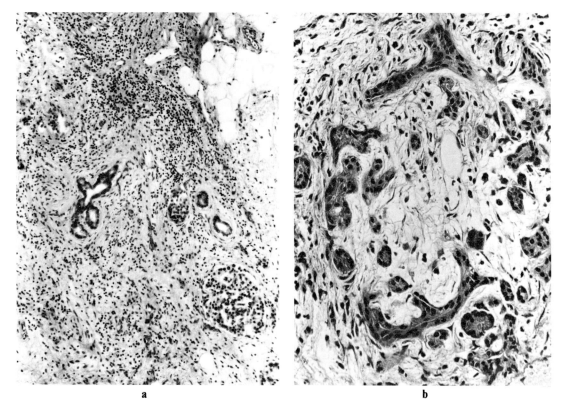

Fig. 20.67 (a) Chronic pancreatitis with diffuse fibrous replacement of exocrine pancreas: a surviving islet is present (*lower right*) and there is a chronic inflammatory cell infiltrate of the interstitium. × 100. (b) Chronic pancreatitis: surviving acinar elements in fibrous tissue showing compression and distortion. × 250.

common bile duct, causing obstructive jaundice, sometimes before spread has occurred. By contrast, carcinoma arising in the body or tail of the pancreas is usually clinically silent until there are multiple metastases. Pancreatic cancer may also present with bizarre clinical effects due to unexplained venous thrombosis, peripheral neuropathy (p. 21.44) or myopathy (p. 21.76). Histologically, the tumour is usually a scirrhous adenocarcinoma (Fig. 20.69). It frequently obstructs the main pancreatic duct, and exocrine pancreatic tissue distal to the obstruction becomes atrophic with some associated chronic inflammation: biopsy of such tissue adjacent to the tumour may suggest an erroneous diagnosis of chronic pancreatitis. The tumour itself, with its small acini in a fibrous stroma, can also cause difficulties in distinction from chronic pancreatitis (*c.f.* Figs. 20.67 and 20.69). The presence of perineural tumour invasion, which is common in pancreatic carcinoma, is, however, diagnostic of malignancy.

Congenital abnormalities

Annular pancreas is a rare condition in which pancreatic tissue completely surrounds the second part of duodenum. About 50% of such cases present in infancy with duodenal obstruction, and in these cases ectopic pancreatic tissue is also found within the muscular wall of the duodenum.

Foci of ectopic pancreatic tissue, which may be single or multiple, are occasionally found in the submucosa of the jejunum, duodenum, stomach, or Meckel's diverticulum.

Diabetes mellitus

Diabetes is not a single disease but the pathological and metabolic state caused by inadequate insulin action: a feature common to all types is glucose intolerance. It is defined clinically

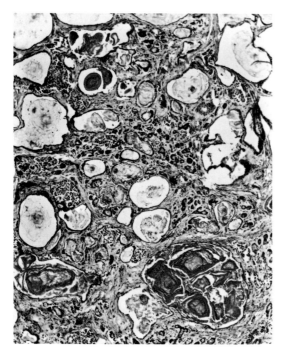

Fig. 20.68 Fibrocystic disease of the pancreas. The ducts are filled with eosinophilic laminated secretion; the acini are either markedly atrophied or much dilated. × 50. (Professor G. L. Montgomery.)

as either a fasting plasma glucose level greater than 7.8 mmol/l (140 mg/dl) or a 2-hour post-prandial plasma glucose greater than 11 mmol/l (200 mg/dl).

Insulin is a major anabolic hormone. It promotes the uptake of glucose by cells and the formation of intracellular glycogen from glucose. It stimulates cells to utilise amino acids for protein synthesis rather than for gluconeogenesis and it promotes the uptake of free fatty acids (FFA) by adipose tissue. Insulin lack therefore results in a general catabolic state with loss of weight, hyperglycaemia, diminished protein synthesis, increased gluconeogenesis, and hyperlipidaemia due to lipolysis in adipose tissue. Although the renal threshold is usually raised, there is heavy glycosuria which results in an osmotic diuresis, causing dehydration and thirst. In the liver, excess FFA are converted via acetyl-CoA into ketone bodies which, in the absence of available glucose, are metabolised for cellular energy. The ketone bodies (aceto-acetic acid, β-hydroxybutyric acid and acetone) dissociate to produce hydrogen ions, with a resulting metabolic acidosis (keto-

acidosis). This complex of metabolic disturbances produces hyperosmolarity, hypovolaemia, acidosis and electrolyte imbalance, which have serious effects on the functions of neurones and result in one form of **diabetic coma—keto-acidotic coma**. The other major form, **hyperosmolar non-ketotic coma**, results from massive dehydration and profound hyperglycaemia in the absence of keto-acidosis. Relative or absolute overdosage with insulin causes **hypoglycaemic effects**, including coma which, unless treated, may be fatal.

Classification of diabetes. There are two major forms of diabetes (types I and II), and a number of specific diseases in which diabetes occurs as a secondary event (p. 20.64).

Type I diabetes (Insulin-dependent diabetes)

This is characterised by reduced pancreatic insulin secretion. The patient is usually under 25 years at presentation, is wasted and may develop keto-acidosis. Insulin is required for maintenance treatment.

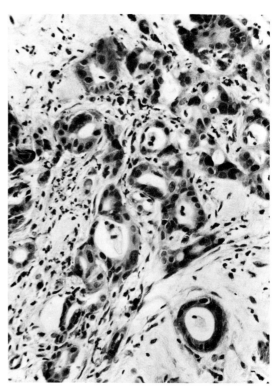

Fig. 20.69 Adenocarcinoma of pancreas, showing a regular acinar pattern and with a related scirrhous reaction. × 250.

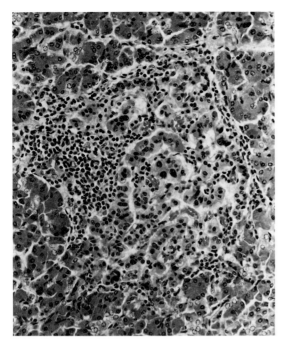

Fig. 20.70 Insulitis in an early case of type I diabetes. There is a lymphocytic infiltrate affecting this insulin-secreting islet. The polyploid endocrine cells are B cells. × 210.

Aetiology. There is evidence that type I diabetes is caused by destruction of B cells accompanied by inflammation of the islets (insulitis), and that genetic factors, auto-immunity and possibly viral infection are involved.

(*a*) *Genetic factors.* Ninety-eight per cent of patients possess either HLA-DR3 (relative risk × 5), HLA-DR4 (relative risk × 7) or both antigens (relative risk × 14). Fifty per cent of patients are DR3, DR4 heterozygotes. It is clear from this evidence that there is a marked genetic link in the aetiology of type I diabetes. However, the concordance rate between identical twins is only 40%, indicating the involvement also of non-genetic factors.

(*b*) *Immunological features.* At presentation, at least 85% of type I diabetic patients have circulating *cytoplasmic* islet-cell antibodies. These antibodies, which are directed against A and D cells as well as B cells, are present up to five years before the clinical onset, suggesting a prolonged latent period for the disease. Islet cell *surface* antibodies are also present at diagnosis and these, together with complement, have been shown *in vitro* to lyse B cells preferentially. Patients with type I diabetes are five times more

likely to have thyroid and gastric parietal cell auto-antibodies than the normal population and forty times more likely to have auto-antibodies directed against adrenal cortex. These findings support the inclusion of type I diabetes in the group of organ specific auto-immune diseases.

Type I diabetes sometimes follows an upper respiratory tract viral infection, but the significance of the association is uncertain.

(*c*) *Islet changes.* In patients dying shortly after the onset, the majority of islets have been shown by immunofluorescence and immunoperoxidase studies to be deficient in B cells but have a normal complement of A, D and PP cells. **Insulitis**, with heavy lymphocytic infiltration in and around the islets (Fig. 20.70) may be present and is more commonly seen in islets containing residual B cells. This finding supports the possibility of a specific, immunologically mediated destruction of B cells as the cause of type I diabetes.

In conclusion, type I diabetes occurs in individuals with a hereditary susceptibility to the development of organ-specific auto-immune diseases, of which insulitis and loss of B cells may be a manifestation. Environmental factors are also involved, but they have not been identified: viral infection (coxsackie B, mumps and rubella viruses are under suspicion) may act as a trigger, and ingested toxins may also possibly be involved.

Type II diabetes (Non-insulin-dependent diabetes)

In this type, insulin secretion is not obviously reduced. The patient is usually over 40 years of age at presentation and 80% are obese. Keto-acidosis is not a feature but hyperosmolar non-ketotic coma may be a complication. Administration of insulin is not required for maintenance therapy. Type II diabetes is ten times commoner than type I.

Aetiology. The concordance rate for this type of diabetes in identical twins is close to 100%, and hereditary factors obviously play a major aetiological role. However, there is no known HLA linkage nor any recognisable Mendelian form of inheritance. Islet-cell antibodies are not found and insulitis is not present. The available evidence suggests that the islets are normal at the onset or show features suggestive of insulin hypersecretion. Insulin initiates many of it actions by combination with specific surface receptors which are present on the surface of most cells in the body. The concentration of insulin receptors on cell surfaces has been shown to be reduced by about 50% in type II diabetes, although those present are of normal affinity. Reduction of weight by dieting increases the concentration of cell receptors in obese diabetics and their glucose tolerance improves. However, it is not yet known whether the reduction in receptor concentration is of pathogenic importance or merely an epiphenomenon.

Complications of diabetes

Coma due to lack of diabetic control is now a relatively rare cause of death, and the mortality and morbidity of diabetes are now due mainly to its complications.

Cardiovascular complications. It is customary to speak of diabetic macro-angiopathy, most commonly affecting large muscular arteries, and diabetic micro-angiopathy, affecting arterioles and capillaries. The former is simply **atheroma**, which tends to develop early and become severe in diabetics of either sex. In consequence, myocardial infarction, cardiovascular disease, and peripheral vascular disease are unduly common and account for 80% of adult (mostly type II) diabetic deaths. In diabetic patients with peripheral vascular disease, the small muscular arteries of the lower leg and foot are commonly affected. Thus a toe may be gangrenous in the presence of normal femoral and popliteal pulses due to the fact that relatively small vessels are narrowed by atheroma. In **diabetic micro-angiopathy** two types of lesion have been described: (**a**), a thickening of the basement membrane or an accumulation of basement membrane-like material in capillaries, and (**b**), endothelial cell proliferation together with basement membrane thickening. The cause of the micro-angiopathy is uncertain but it affects diabetics of all types, appears to be related to the duration of the disease, and is probably precipitated partly by poor diabetic control. It is responsible for diabetic retinopathy (p. 21.82) and diabetic nephropathy (p. 22.39). The latter is the commonest cause of death in patients with type I diabetes and diabetic retinopathy is the commonest cause of blindness under the age of 65 years in developed countries.

Infections. There is an increased susceptibility to bacterial and fungal infections. Boils, carbuncles and urinary tract infections, sometimes complicated by pyelonephritis and renal papillary necrosis, are of frequent occurrence and may precipitate diabetic coma. Diabetics have an increased risk of tuberculosis, especially of the lungs, and, unless treated, the disease tends to progress rapidly.

Other pathological effects. Trophic disturbances, such as ulceration of the fingers or toes and neuropathic arthropathy (p. 23.51), may develop as complications of diabetic peripheral neuropathy. It is noteworthy that atheroma, diabetic micro-angiopathy, peripheral neuropathy and susceptibility to infections all tend to promote gangrene of the extremities in diabetes. Diabetic mothers show an increased liability to pre-eclamptic toxaemia, and pregnancy aggravates the diabetic state. The babies of diabetic mothers are usually above normal weight but paradoxically they experience disorders similar to those occurring in premature babies.

Other causes of diabetes

Secondary diabetes may complicate chronic pancreatitis, haemochromatosis, acromegaly, hypercortisolism (Cushing's syndrome or administration of glucocorticoids or ACTH), glucagon-secreting tumours and phaeochromocytoma. Lesions of the brain can also cause hyperglycaemia and glycosuria, possibly by disturbing the hypothalamus. Acute hyperglycaemia can also occur in severe acute pancreatitis. The usual complications of diabetes are encountered in patients with longstanding secondary diabetes, e.g. in haemochromatosis.

Endocrine-exocrine interactions in pancreatic pathololgy

The pancreas in longstanding type I diabetes is atrophic and reduced in weight. The pancreatic polypeptide-rich lobe (p. 20.56) is normal in size but there is acinar atrophy and a two-thirdsreduction in the weight of the rest of the pancreas in such patients. This morphological abnormality is matched by a 70% reduction in exocrine secretory capacity. This change in type

I diabetics is explicable in terms of the islet-exocrine portal vascular arrangement (p. 20.56) which results in exposure of the normal exocrine pancreas to very high levels of islet hormones. In type I diabetes, where there is a drastic reduction in insulin-secreting B cells, the acinar tissue in the glucagon-rich lobe will be bathed in high levels of glucagon and somatostatin, both of which inhibit exocrine function. By contrast, in the PP-rich lobe the main hormone in exocrine capillaries will be pancreatic polypeptide, which, like insulin, is a trophic hormone for the exocrine pancreas.

While pancreatic endocrine failure (type I diabetes) leads to exocrine dysfunction, so also exocrine failure can be complicated by diabetes. Cystic fibrosis and chronic pancreatitis are the most common causes of exocrine failure and in both there is an increased incidence of diabetes, which requires insulin therapy. It used to be thought that the diabetes in these diseases was simply the result of destruction of islets, but residual B cell-containing islets are usually plentiful. Under normal circumstances several hormones, prominent among which is gastric inhibitory polypeptide (GIP), are released from cells in the duodenal and jejunal mucosa in response to absorption of glucose and triglycerides from the lumen. GIP stimulates pancreatic B cells to secrete insulin. In exocrine pancreatic failure there is maldigestion and thus malabsorption which results in chronically low levels of GIP and diminished insulin secretion. This may play a causal role in the diabetes, since the addition of oral pancreatic extract to the diet restores GIP secretion and reverses the diabetic state. Lack of stimulation of islet B cells by GIP in postoperative parenteral nutrition may explain the beneficial effect of adding insulin to the intravenous infusion, and also the increased incidence of diabetes in coeliac disease.

Hyperfunction of the endocrine pancreas

This is usually the result of a hormone-secreting adenoma or carcinoma of islet-cell type. Rarely, hyperplasia of the islets appears to be the cause. An islet-cell tumour is usually a solitary discrete

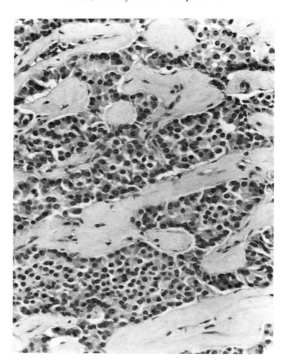

Fig. 20.71 A pancreatic islet-cell tumour showing the cords and clusters of tumour cells. The stroma contains amyloid material. × 230.

nodule embedded in the pancreas. Microscopically the tumour cells closely resemble normal islet cells, and form cords or clusters separated by fibrous stroma (Fig. 20.71). Distinction between benign and malignant tumours on a morphological basis is often difficult. For practical purposes, the tumours are most appropriately described in relation to the principal hormone which they produce.

Insulinoma. This is the commonest islet cell tumour and is associated clinically with recurrent attacks of hypoglycaemia, which may result in confusion, mania, dizziness or coma. These effects are reversed by taking glucose or excision of the tumour. Insulinomas are rarely malignant.

Gastrinoma. Although gastrin is normally produced only by G cells in the stomach and duodenum, 90% of gastrinomas arise in the pancreas. In the resulting **Zollinger–Ellison Syndrome**, persistent hypersecretion of acid gastric juice causes multiple peptic ulcers which are refractory to medical treatment and which may occur even in the jejunum. Most gastrinomas are malignant. In the multiple endocrine neoplasia type 1 (MEN 1) syndrome, adenomas of the parathyroids, pituitary, adrenal cortex and pancreas may be present in association with peptic ulceration. The pancreatic tumour in this rare hereditary syndrome is usually a gastrinoma.

Other islet-cell tumours are much less common, and may produce one or more of the following hormones. (1) **Glucagon** resulting in diabetes accompanied by peculiar skin manifestations; (2) **Vasoactive intestinal peptide (VIP)**, causing watery diarrhoea, hypokalaemia and achlorhydria—'**WDHA**' or **Verner-Morri-** **son syndrome**; (3) **Inappropriate (ectopic) hormones** resulting in the carcinoid syndrome, Cushing's syndrome, etc.

Idiopathic hypoglycaemia of infancy. In this rare condition there is an apparent increase of insulin secretion in the absence of an insulinoma or convincing hyperplasia of islet B cells. One report has suggested that this syndrome is due to a relative deficiency of somatostatin-secreting D cells, which normally inhibit insulin secretion. The standard treatment is pancreatic resection.

References and Further Reading

Liver and biliary tract

Bassendine, M. F. (1984). Hepatitis B virus and liver cell carcinoma. In *Recent Advances in Histopathology*, No. 12. Anthony, P. P. and MacSween, R. N. M. (Eds), pp. 137–46. Churchill Livingstone, Edinburgh.

Bianchi, L., De Groote, J., Desmet, V. J., Gedigk, P., Korb, G., Popper, H., Poulsen, H., Scheuer, P. J., Schmid, M., Thaler, H. and Wepler, W. (1977). Acute and chronic hepatitis revisited. *Lancet* **ii**, 914–19.

Blumberg, B. S. (1964). Polymorphism of serum proteins and the development of iso-precipitins in transfused patients. *Bulletin of the New York Academy of Medicine* **40**, 377–86.

Blumberg, B. S., Gerstley, B. J. S., Hungerford, D. A., London, W. I. and Sutnick, A. I. (1967). A serum antigen (Australia antigen) in Down's syndrome, leukaemia and hepatitis. *Annals of Internal Medicine* **66**, 924–31.

MacSween, R. N. M. (1984). Primary sclerosing cholangitis. In *Recent Advances in Histopathology*, No. 12. Anthony, P. P. and MacSween, R. N. M. (Eds), pp. 158–67. Churchill Livingstone, Edinburgh.

MacSween, R. N. M., Anthony, P. P. and Scheuer, P. J. (Eds). (1979) *Pathology of the Liver*, pp. 458. Churchill Livingstone, Edinburgh.

Rappaport, A. M., Borowy, Z. J., Lougheed, W. M. and Lotto, W. N. (1954). Subdivision of hexagonal liver lobules into a structural and functional unit; role in hepatic physiology and pathology. *Anatomical Record* **119**, 11–34.

Rizetto, M. (1983). The Delta agent. *Hepatology* **3**, 729–737.

Scheuer, P. J. (1984). Viral hepatitis. In *Recent Advances in Histopathology*, No. 12. Anthony, P. P. and MacSween, R. N. M. (Eds), pp. 129–37. Churchill Livingstone, Edinburgh.

Pancreas

Bliss, M. (1983). *The discovery of insulin*, pp. 304. Paul Harris Publishing, Edinburgh.

Foulis, A. K. (1984). Acute Pancreatitis. In *Recent Advances in Histopathology*, No. 12. Anthony, P. P. and MacSween, R. N. M. (Eds), pp. 188–96. Churchill Livingstone, Edinburgh.

Foulis, A. K. and Stewart, J. A. (1984). The pancreas in recent-onset Type I (insulin dependent) diabetes mellitus: insulin content of islets, insulitis and associated changes in the exocrine acinar tissue. *Diabetologia*, **26**, 456–61.

Henderson, J. R., Daniel, P. M., and Fraser, P. A. (1981) The pancreas as a single organ: the influence of the endocrine upon the exocrine part of the gland. *Gut* **22**, 158–67.

Howat, H. T. and Sarles, H. (Eds) (1979). *The exocrine pancreas*, pp. 540. Saunders, Eastbourne.

Klöppel, G. and Heitz, P. U. (1984) *Pancreatic Pathology*, pp. 239. Churchill Livingstone, Edinburgh.

Volk, B. W. and Wellmann, K. F. (1977). *The diabetic pancreas*, pp. 599. Plenum Press, New York.

21

The Nervous System and Voluntary Muscles

I: The Brain

The nervous system is composed of two types of tissue both of which are involved in varying degree in disease processes. The first consists of the highly specialised **nerve cells (neurons)** with their processes and also the **neuroglial cells**, all of which are of neuroectodermal origin. The second comprises the meninges, the blood vessels and their supporting connective tissue, all derived from mesoderm, and phagocytic cells (microglia): it is similar in many respects to corresponding tissue found in other systems of the body. Some diseases of the nervous system are similar to those observed in other organs—for example, inflammation, diseases of the blood vessels and tumours. Others are primary diseases of the neuron involving its cell body, its axon or its myelin sheath and in this group the aetiology is often obscure. Even in those diseases where the primary damage is to the neuron, the most conspicuous pathological abnormalities are often reactive changes in the neuroglia, the microglia (p. 21.5) or the blood vessels. Indeed quite severe derangement of neuronal function may occur in the absence of obvious structural abnormalities in neurons.

As in other organs, particular functions of the nervous system have been ascribed to the various specialised cells. These specific functions are,· to a large extent, mediated by proteins, many of which may be unique to the nervous system. Immunohistochemical techniques are proving most valuable to detect and characterise these proteins, e.g. glial fibrillary acidic protein which is a major component of the astroglial fibre and the basic and proteolipid proteins of myelin.

Applied anatomy

The arrangement of the meninges and the distribution of the cerebrospinal fluid (CSF) influence the spread of pathological processes. The dura mater acts as the periosteum to the cranial bones but it can be stripped from the skull, e.g. by haemorrhage into the potential **extradural space** secondary to tearing of a meningeal blood vessel by a fracture of the skull. The dura and the outer surface of the arachnoid are normally in contact but the **subdural space** can more readily be distended by blood or pus than the extradural space. The arachnoid forms a continuous sheet in contact with the dura, while the pia follows the convolutions of the brain. The space between the pia and arachnoid, known as the **subarachnoid space**, is traversed by delicate trabeculae of connective tissue into a series of intercommunicating spaces filled with CSF. Apart from the cisterna magna and the cisterns at the base of the brain, the subarachnoid space is broadest in the sulci. **The major cerebral arteries and veins** run in the subarachnoid space, and from the arteries small **nutrient vessels** pass into the cortex. The nutrient arteries to the basal ganglia and other deep structures enter the base of the brain at the **perforated areas**.

21.1

As an artery penetrates the brain it carries a sheath of pia with it, the resulting potential perivascular space (often known as the **Virchow-Robin space**) between the vessel wall and the invaginated pia being continuous with the subarachnoid space. As the vessels become smaller the two layers fuse to form a reticular perivascular sheath which can be followed as far as precapillary vessels but not to the capillaries themselves. **The foot processes of astrocytes** form a cuff in apposition to and completely surrounding the Virchow-Robin space and the capillaries of the brain.

Micro-organisms and their toxins readily spread throughout the subarachnoid space, which may become filled with inflammatory exudate. The inflammatory process may then spread into the brain around the nutrient blood vessels which become surrounded by collections of leucocytes. The ventricular system communicates with the subarachnoid space by means of the exit foramina in the roof (Magendie) and lateral recesses (Luschka) of the fourth ventricle. Cerebrospinal fluid passes freely through these foramina and, in certain disease processes, so also do blood, pus, micro-organisms or, more rarely, tumour cells. The circulation of the CSF is dealt with in greater detail in relation to hydrocephalus (p. 21.9).

Examination of the CSF often provides valuable information about diseases of the nervous system. Specimens are ordinarily obtained by lumbar puncture, but ventricular or cisternal puncture may sometimes be indicated. The pressure of the CSF should always be measured, as either an increase or a decrease may be of diagnostic value. Microbiological, serological, cytological and biochemical investigations on the CSF are routine procedures.

Normal CSF is clear and colourless, does not coagulate and has a specific gravity of 1.006. It contains 0·15–0·45 g/litre protein, 2·8–4·4 mmol/litre (50–80 mg/100 ml) glucose, approximately 128 mmol/litre sodium and 128 mmol/litre chloride. A few mononuclear cells may be found in normal fluid but rarely more than 4 per μl. (See Table 21.1, pp. 21.46–47.)

The Reactions of the Nervous System to Disease

Neurons

The neuron (Fig. 21.1) is one of the most complex and specialised cells in the body, and since it is incapable of dividing after the first few weeks of extra-uterine life, any brain damage involving loss of neurons is structurally irreversible. While the chemical diversity of neurons can be explored by immunohistochemical techniques, an adequate picture of the structure and function of neurons is provided only by the use of multiple histological and biochemical techniques. Such methods show a neuron to consist of three main parts, the **perikaryon** or cell body from which extend the **dendrites** and the **axon**. The perikarya are the main constituents of grey matter, in which they tend to be arranged in layers, as in the cerebral cortex, or in aggregates, as in the basal ganglia. A particularly conspicuous feature in the perikarya, especially those of large neurons, is the presence of **Nissl granules**, which are rich in RNA and are composed of stacks of rough endoplasmic reticulum and intervening groups of free ribosomes. Silver stains demonstrate neurofibrils in the cytoplasm, while *microtubules* and *neurofilaments* (10 nm in diameter) can be identified with the electron microscope. *Mitochondria* are numerous in dendrites and in the pre-synaptic region. *Lysozomes* are also found. A particularly characteristic feature in large neurons is a progressive increase in their content of *lipofuscin* with age. Some neurons, however, particularly those in the ventral horns of the spinal cord (Fig. 21.1a) and in the inferior olivary nuclei, contain large amounts of lipofuscin even in early adult life; others e.g. those in the substantia nigra and the pigmented nucleus of the pons, contain *neuromelanin*. Various substances (neurotransmitters, proteins and cell organelles) are transported in the fast and slow phases of *axoplasmic flow* from the cell body along the

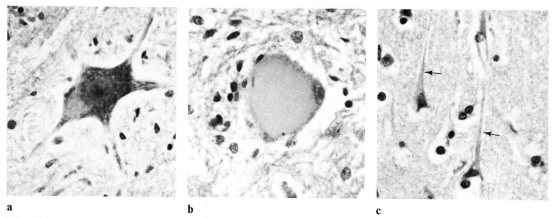

a   b   c

Fig. 21.1a Normal motor neuron in ventral horn of spinal cord. The dark granules within the cytoplasm are the Nissl granules. The pale area is the region occupied by lipofuscin. **b.** Similar neuron showing the features of central chromatolysis. Note the pale homogeneous cytoplasm and the eccentric nucleus. **c.** Neurons showing the features of ischaemic cell change. They are shrunken and contain dark hyperchromatic nuclei. All × 400.

axons and dendrites to synapses. There is also a retrograde axoplasmic flow of material from the periphery towards the perikaryon.

Reactions of the neuron to disease take several forms. **Central chromatolysis** occurs in the perikaryon between 5 to 8 days after the axon has been severed. It can also occur as a response to certain virus infections and in some deficiencies of the vitamin B group. Initially the cell body swells and becomes spherical, the nucleus becomes eccentric and the Nissl granules break down into dust-like particles before disappearing altogether, although a few may persist at the margin of the cell (Fig. 21.1b). The cytoplasm becomes pale and homogeneous. Recent studies have shown that this response to injury is accompanied by an increase in protein synthesis and it is therefore considered to be a *regenerative* phenomenon. When it is due to damage to a peripheral (cranial or spinal) nerve, central chromatolysis is sometimes reversible. By contrast, effective regeneration does not occur in the central nervous system (CNS) and **retrograde degeneration** of the axon results. Following axonal transection, both the proximal and distal ends of the severed axon swell to form axonal bulbs: these may be found within 3–6 hours of injury, may persist for up to 60 days, and are thought to be due to continuance of axoplasmic flow in both directions.

Neurons require a constant supply of oxygen and glucose and if this is inadequate they undergo a series of changes termed **the ischaemic cell process**. Mitochondria become swollen, the perikaryon shrinks and often becomes triangular in shape, Nissl granules disappear, the cytoplasm becomes intensely eosinophilic and the nucleus pyknotic (Fig. 21.1c). A characteristic feature of recent neuronal necrosis is the presence of small dark granules, known as encrustations, on the surface of the perikaryon and its dendrites. Some neurons, particularly the Purkinje cells of the cerebellum, appear to react in a different manner: the Nissl substance disappears, the cytoplasm becomes pale and swollen, and the nucleus becomes pyknotic. Dead neurons are removed by phagocytes. Moderate neuronal loss is very difficult to recognise histologically unless there are also some reactive changes in the neuroglia.

Another common change in neurons is **simple atrophy**. This occurs in many of the slowly progressive degenerative diseases such as motor neuron disease (p. 21.52). The nerve cells appear smaller than normal and lipofuscin accumulates in the cytoplasm.

There are many other less common changes in neurons, e.g. the presence of *inclusion bodies* in certain virus infections and in Parkinsonism, **neurofibrillary degeneration** in some types of dementia, and distension of the cytoplasm with lipid-laden lysozomes in certain inborn errors of metabolism, but these will be dealt with later.

When the perikaryon of a myelinated neuron is destroyed by trauma, infarction, etc., its axon and myelin sheath break down by the process of **Wallerian degeneration**. This is also seen when a peripheral nerve is transected. The axon *distal* to the point of transection shrinks and becomes irregular and then breaks up into fragments which are later absorbed. At the same time the myelin sheath is broken down into simpler lipids and, ultimately, neutral fat. Globules of lipid may be seen 3 or 4 days after damage to the axon and thereafter the fatty globules are taken up and gradually degraded by macrophages. The Schwann cells proliferate to form cords of cells within endoneural tubes. Retrograde degeneration of the *proximal* part of the axon usually extends for one or two segments above the level of transection, and the perikaryon undergoes central chromatolysis (see above). An essentially similar type of degeneration occurs in axons within the CNS when they are transected. When large tracts are affected, lipid-laden macrophages may be present for many months.

Wallerian degeneration of the long tracts in the spinal cord is dealt with in more detail on p. 21.48. It should be noted here that two principal types of staining technique are used to demonstrate loss of myelin. The first of these—the *Marchi technique*—is used as a positive technique to demonstrate recent breakdown of myelin within the preceding 2–3 months: the unsaturated fatty acids formed during this process are stained black, while normal myelin remains unstained. Later, however, when most of the breakdown products have been removed, demyelinated areas are best demonstrated by their pallor with conventional stains for myelin, e.g. the *Weigert-Pal method* and its modifications: negative techniques of this type are used also to demonstrate loss of myelin in conditions other than Wallerian degeneration, e.g. multiple sclerosis (p. 21.38).

Repair of neural tissue is described on p. 5.20. It should, however, be emphasised that, *while the axons of peripheral nerves can regenerate, particularly if the endoneural tubes remain, there is no structurally significant regeneration of axons in the CNS*. In both these circumstances, however, there is often some recovery of function which may in part be ascribed to *plasticity*, surviving neurons forming new contacts with neurons which have lost their afferent connections.

Another form of secondary degeneration is **trans-neuronal** or **trans-synaptic atrophy**. This occurs in neurons whose principal afferent connections have been destroyed: examples are atrophy of the neurons in the external geniculate body after lesions in the retina or optic nerves, or in the nucleus gracilis and nucleus cuneatus when the posterior columns of the spinal cord have degenerated. Trans-synaptic degeneration is sometimes 'retrograde', i.e. it can occur in cells whose axons make synaptic connections with cells which have been destroyed.

Cerebral atrophy

Diffuse atrophy of the brain (weight less than 1200 g) is due to a progressive loss of tissue, particularly of the cerebral cortex. When the process is advanced, the convolutions become more rounded and firmer than normal and the sulci widen, so that there is an excess of CSF in the subarachnoid space. The meninges, especially over the vertex, may become thickened and opalescent, while the surface of the hemispheres often appears gelatinous because of the increase of CSF in the subarachnoid space.

The full extent of the atrophy is often not obvious until the meninges have been stripped from the surface of the brain. As the neuronal loss is accompanied by the disappearance of their axons and myelin sheaths, the white matter also shrinks and this is accompanied by enlargement of the ventricles. The histological changes underlying atrophy vary with the many different causes, e.g. senile and pre-senile dementia, ischaemia, subacute encephalitis and, to a more limited degree, as part of the changes in old age, but the two constant abnormalities are **loss of neurons and reactive gliosis**.

Neuroglia

The neuroglia include astrocytes, oligodendrocytes and ependymal cells, all of which are of neuro-ectodermal origin.

Astrocytes are stellate cells with numerous fine branching processes. These processes are characterised electron-microscopically by the presence of intracellular 10 nm glial fibres, a major component of which is glial fibrillary acidic protein. During development, proliferating neuroblasts migrate along a template provided by astrocytes, while in post-natal life astrocytes, in addition to being the principal supporting tissue of the CNS, are concerned with the regulation, amongst other things, of extracellular fluid and electrolytes. *Protoplasmic astrocytes* and *fibrillary astrocytes* may be distinguished. Normally, the former are found mainly in the grey matter and the latter in white matter and beneath the pia. Both forms are attached to the walls of blood vessels by one or more swellings—the so-called *foot processes.* Similar expansions unite the fibres to the pia.

In general, reactions of astrocytes correspond to those of fibroblasts in other tissues. They are less susceptible to injury than neurons, but when injury is severe, as in an infarct or an acute inflammatory lesion, they undergo necrosis and disintegration. In less severe injury, the initial response of astrocytes is to enlarge, proliferate and produce additional glial fibres. This reaction, termed **gliosis**, occurs in almost all conditions where there is damage to the central nervous system. In the later stages the cell bodies shrink and all that can be seen is a dense network of glial fibrils—*fibrillary gliosis.* Basophilic circular bodies, known as *corpora amylaceae*, accumulate and the brain tissue is firmer than normal and may have a grey translucent appearance.

Oligodendrocytes, so named because of their few short processes, are small cells with a darkly staining nucleus resembling that of a lymphocyte. They are very numerous and are seen as perineuronal satellites in the grey matter and as rows of closely-apposed nuclei between bundles of myelinated nerve fibres—*the interfascicular oligodendroglia.*

Oligodendrocytes play an important role in both the formation and maintenance of myelin, and loss of interfascicular oligodendrocytes in some of the leucodystrophies (p. 21.42) appears to precede obvious degeneration of myelin. Very little is known about the causes or significance of reactive changes in the oligodendrocytes apart from the *acute swelling* which occurs in many toxic processes and the proliferation of perineuronal satellites (*satellitosis*) around degenerating neurons.

Ependymal cells form a single layer of cells lining the ventricular system and the central canal of the spinal cord. They are columnar and have a ciliated free (luminal) surface, immediately deep to which there is a line of small oval bodies known as *blepharoplasts.* In some regions of the hypothalamus, specialised ependymal cells have long processes extending to adjacent blood vessels. The function of the cilia on the ventricular surface of the ependyma is not fully understood but their movement is synchronised, suggesting that they play a role in the circulation of the cerebrospinal fluid (CSF). Recent studies have shown that the ependyma is not a barrier to the movement of fluid in either direction between the ventricles and extracellular 'space' of the brain.

Ependymal cells show few reactive changes. For example, when the ventricles enlarge as in hydrocephalus, the ependyma is stretched and then broken, but the ependymal cells do not proliferate to fill the defects. A common but non-specific reaction to chronic irritation is the appearance of numerous small excrescences on the ventricular surface—*granular ependymitis*; they consist of focal proliferations of subependymal astrocytes (Fig. 21.2).

Microglia

Microglial cells belong to the mononuclear-phagocyte system (p. 4.33). They are small and have an elongated hyperchromatic nucleus, scanty cytoplasm and delicate cytoplasmic processes. They are derived from monocytes which emigrate from the small blood vessels and invade the neural tissue from the pia shortly before birth. They often lie close to blood vessels and, though normally inconspicuous, are capable of enlarging and becoming active macrophages. It is, however, not known what proportions of the macrophages seen in various lesions of the CNS are derived from microglia,

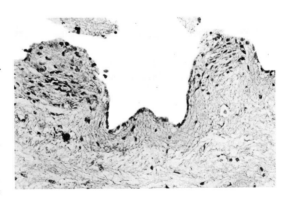

Fig. 21.2 Granular ependymitis in the floor of the fourth ventricle. × 112.

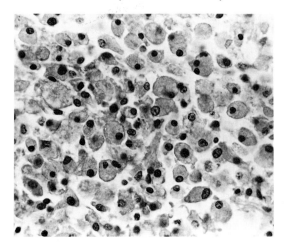

Fig. 21.3 Lipid-laden phagocytes in a cerebral infarct. × 510.

from perivascular stem cells, and from circulating monocytes.

As in other tissues, macrophages are seen in the CNS where there is tissue destruction, and they become laden with myelin breakdown products to appear as *lipophages* or *foamy macrophages*. Such cells may be present for some months after necrosis of brain tissue, e.g. in infarcts (Fig. 21.3). When neurons are killed selectively, for example by hypoxia or by viruses, they become surrounded by macrophages, and sometimes neutrophil polymorphs,

and undergo phagocytosis. This is known as *neuronophagia* (Fig. 21.41, p. 21.35), a feature which must be distinguished from non-specific satellitosis by oligodendroglia.

In some conditions, e.g. subacute encephalitis, microglia increase in length and become slightly thicker than normal, and are known as 'rod cells'.

Blood vessels

While gliosis readily occurs when there is any damage to the brain, *production of fibrous tissue is seen only when the injury is severe enough to damage blood vessels*. For instance, when suppuration occurs within the brain, fibroblastic proliferation along with the formation of new blood vessels leads to the production of a distinct capsule around the abscess cavity. Gliosis occurs within and around the fibrous capsule and this combined glial and fibroblastic response is often called a *gliomesodermal reaction*. Necrosis unaccompanied by bacterial infection, e.g. infarction, induces a reaction in which gliosis predominates, although some fibrous tissue is formed. *Proliferation of capillaries is the rule around infarcts, abscesses, etc.*, and in relation to rapidly growing cerebral tumours.

The Pathology of Intracranial Expanding Lesions

Various pathological processes, such as tumour, haematoma, or a massive recent cerebral infarct, cause an increase in the bulk of the brain. *As the brain is enclosed within the rigid cranium, there is very little free space to accommodate these various expanding lesions with the result that they ultimately produce an **increase in intracranial pressure***. Extracerebral intracranial expanding lesions, such as an extradural or subdural haematoma or a meningioma, have the same effect. There is, however, a period of **spatial compensation** during which the intracranial pressure remains within normal limits. This compensation is brought about principally by a reduction in the volume of CSF both within the ventricles and within the subarachnoid

space, by a reduction in the volume of blood within the intracranial veins, and less commonly by pressure atrophy of brain tissue. When all the available space has been utilised *there is a critical point at which a further slight increase in the volume of the intracranial contents causes an abrupt increase of intracranial pressure and deterioration, often rapid, in the patient's condition*. Near this critical point, arteriolar vasodilatation due to even a short period of increased arterial P_{CO_2} may be sufficient to produce this effect. Clearly the compensatory mechanisms will fail more rapidly when the lesion is expanding rapidly, e.g. an intracerebral haematoma, than one of similar size that has developed slowly, e.g. a meningioma, allow-

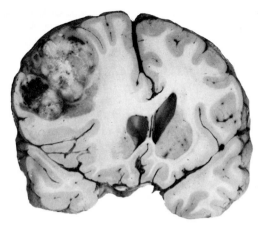

Fig. 21.4 Increased intracranial pressure due to frontal lobe tumour. Note displacement of the lateral ventricles, midline shift and supracallosal hernia.

ing time for the occurrence of local pressure atrophy and loss of brain tissue. Expanding lesions also cause distortion of the brain and it must be emphasised that *distortion and displacement of the brain and any associated increase in intracranial pressure are often of greater significance with regard to the immediate survival of the patient than the nature of the lesion or the amount of cerebral tissue destroyed by it.*

In a **supratentorial intracerebral expanding lesion**, the sequence of changes in the brain follows a fairly standard pattern. As the lesion expands, so also does the hemisphere. The CSF in the subarachnoid space is displaced and the convolutions become flattened against the dura, the sulci are progressively narrowed and at autopsy the surface of the brain looks dryer than normal. CSF is also displaced from the ventricular system with the result that the lateral ventricle on the same side as the lesion becomes smaller while the contralateral ventricle may become larger. Further expansion of the affected hemisphere leads to distortion of the brain and a lateral shift of the midline structures, notably the interventricular septum, the anterior cerebral arteries and the third ventricle (Fig. 21.4). Such displacement is readily seen radiologically by ventriculography, carotid arteriography or CT scanning. Depending to some extent on the site of the expanding lesion, internal herniae then develop. Thus the cingulate gyrus frequently herniates under the free margin of the falx cerebri above the corpus callosum—the so-called **supracallosal** or **subfalcine**

hernia (Fig. 21.4). However, the most important hernia associated with a supratentorial expanding lesion is a **tentorial hernia**, in which the medial part of the ipsilateral temporal lobe is squeezed through the tentorial opening (Fig. 21.5). The herniated brain tissue compresses and displaces the midbrain, which is pushed against the contralateral rigid edge of the tentorium. The pressure is often sufficient to produce a distinct groove (*Kernohan's notch*) on the surface of the midbrain at this point. As a result of the inevitable *plugging of the tentorial opening*, the supratentorial intracranial pressure becomes higher than the infratentorial pressure, and this is associated with a rapid deterioration of the patient's clinical state. *Compression of the aqueduct* may also block the free flow of CSF from the lateral ventricles and this further increases the supratentorial pressure.

Other features associated with a tentorial hernia are caudal displacement of the brain-

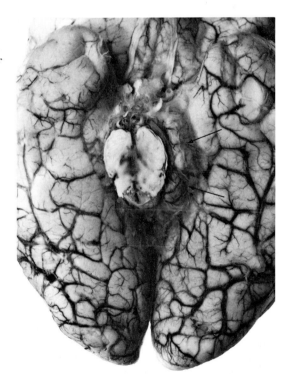

Fig. 21.5 Increased intracranial pressure due to a supratentorial tumour. Note displacement of brainstem and medial and downward displacement of the medial part of the temporal lobe—a tentorial hernia. The deep groove (*arrows*) indicates the position of the edge of the tentorium.

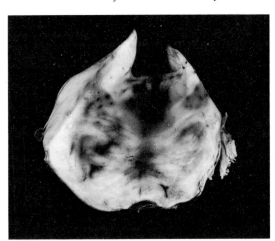

Fig. 21.6 Secondary haemorrhage into the pons caused by increased intracranial pressure.

stem, compression of the third and sixth cranial nerves with resultant disturbances of eye movement and pupillary reflexes and, less commonly, infarction of the ipsilateral medial occipital cortex due to selective compression of the posterior cerebral artery over the tentorium. A common terminal event in raised intracranial pressure is **haemorrhage into the midbrain and pons** (Fig. 21.6), usually involving the tegmentum adjacent to the midline, and thought to be due to a combination of caudal displacement of the brainstem, obstruction to venous drainage and stretching of arteries.

Similar abnormalities are brought about by extracerebral intracranial expanding lesions. In more diffuse increases in the volume of the brain, as in generalised cerebral oedema, both lateral ventricles and the third ventricle are reduced in size, and there may be bilateral tentorial herniae. A frequent clinical sign of raised intracranial pressure is **papilloedema** due to compression of the retinal vein where it traverses the subarachnoid space in the optic nerve sheath.

A supratentorial expanding lesion may also cause a **tonsillar hernia (cerebellar cone)**, i.e. impaction of the cerebellar tonsils in the foramen magnum (Fig. 21.7) but this type of hernia is more constant in **subtentorial expanding lesions**. The tonsils compress the medulla and interfere with the function of the vital centres within it, particularly the respiratory centre. By obstructing the flow of CSF through the fourth ventricle and the exit foramina, such herniation may

further increase the intracranial pressure so that a vicious circle is set up.

In a patient with an intracranial expanding lesion, lumbar puncture can precipitate cerebellar coning or tentorial herniation, with serious consequences. Even if only a small amount of CSF is withdrawn, more may leak into the spinal extradural space via the puncture wound in the meninges. *Lumbar puncture is therefore contraindicated in a patient with suspected increased intracranial pressure until the presence of an intracranial expanding lesion has been excluded.* An exception to the rule is a suspected case of bacterial meningitis, when lumbar puncture is an essential step in establishing the diagnosis (p. 21.24).

Prolonged increase in intracranial pressure may result in erosion of the posterior clinoid processes and, in children, thinning of the inner table of the skull over the convolutions, producing the so-called convolutional markings or beaten-brass appearance.

The clinical features of raised intracranial pressure include headache, vomiting, a raised systolic blood pressure with a slow pulse and high pulse pressure, and diminished consciousness passing into coma. Ophthalmoscopy reveals papilloedema.

Brain swelling

This term is now applied to an increase in volume of the brain due to oedema and/or vaso-

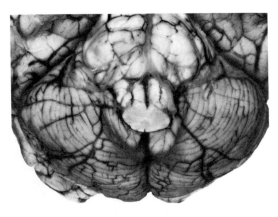

Fig. 21.7 Increased intracranial pressure. Tonsillar hernia resulting from a diffuse astrocytoma of the pons.

dilatation. Such an increase often makes an important contribution to increased intracranial pressure. **Vasodilatation** alone may occur in states of hypoxia or hypercapnia or result from the loss of vasomotor tone, which may complicate acute brain damage and may be a major factor contributing to brain swelling in acute head injuries (p. 21.15).

Cerebral oedema is classified, in current jargon, as *vasogenic* and *cytotoxic*. *Vasogenic oedema* corresponds to oedema elsewhere resulting from increased filtration pressure and/or permeability of the capillaries and venules (pp. 4.5–13). It is often prominent in the tissue around cerebral contusions, recent infarcts, a brain abscess and some tumours. The oedema fluid is mainly interstitial, the cut surface appearing pale, swollen, glistening and wetter than normally. Microscopy shows separation of tissue elements by the oedema fluid, and astrocytes may be swollen.

In *cytotoxic oedema*, which is less common, the fluid is intracellular. It occurs in some metabolic derangements and following acute hypoxia, and can be produced experimentally by various noxious agents such as triethyltin. In cytotoxic oedema there is basically a disturbance of cellular osmoregulation; the blood-brain barrier to proteins remains relatively intact and the oedema is intracellular.

Hydrocephalus

Hydrocephalus denotes an increase in the amount of CSF within the skull, and by far the commonest cause of **primary hydrocephalus** is obstruction to the flow of CSF. **Secondary hydrocephalus** is a compensatory increase of CSF following loss of neural tissue, e.g. from cerebral atrophy, and is less important because there is no increase in the total volume of the intracranial contents and so no rise in intracranial pressure. The increase of CSF may be in the ventricles, in the subarachnoid space or in both.

Source and circulation of CSF

The main source of CSF is the choroid plexuses of the ventricles but some may be formed on the surface of the brain and spinal cord, for it is known that ionic exchange between blood and CSF can occur widely and is not restricted to the choroid plexuses. The total volume of the CSF is about 120–150 ml and it is renewed several times per day. The fluid formed in the lateral ventricles passes by the foramina of Monro to the third ventricle and then by the aqueduct of Sylvius to the fourth ventricle. It then passes through the foramina of Magendie and Luschka in the roof and lateral recesses respectively of the fourth ventricle to reach the subarachnoid space of the cisterna magna and basal cisterns. Thereafter it spreads through the subarachnoid space over the surface of the brain and spinal cord and is absorbed into the blood through the arachnoid granulations (arachnoid villi) which project into the dural venous sinuses (Fig. 21.8).

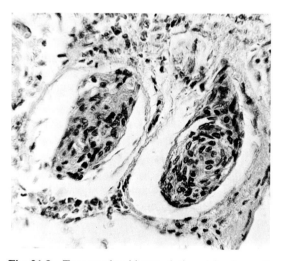

Fig. 21.8 Two arachnoid granulations lying in small dural veins.

Primary hydrocephalus

This is most often caused by obstruction to the free flow of CSF. Obstruction is most likely to occur where the channel is narrow, e.g. in the aqueduct or at the exit foramina of the fourth ventricle, but it may also occur in the subarachnoid space itself.

Obstruction to the flow of CSF results in expansion of that part of the CSF pathway which lies proximal to the obstruction. Thus, if the obstruction is in the third ventricle, both lateral ventricles enlarge symmetrically; if at the exit foramina in the fourth ventricle, the entire ventricular system enlarges. Obstruction at any of the above sites results in **non-communicating hydrocephalus,** i.e. the CSF cannot pass from the ventricular system to the subarachnoid space. By contrast, when the obstruction is in the subarachnoid space at the base of the brain, the entire ventricular system again enlarges but hydrocephalus is of **communicating** type. The site of obstruction in primary hydrocephalus can be detected by withdrawing CSF, injecting air into the lumbar subarachnoid space or into the ventricle, and following its distribution by x-rays on moving the patient into various positions. Alternatively, CSF may be withdrawn from the ventricles and radio-opaque fluid injected.

It is convenient to divide obstructive hydrocephalus into **congenital** and **acquired** types, but the distinction is not always clear-cut. Other causes of primary hydrocephalus are increased production or impaired absorption of CSF. Increased production is rare but may contribute to the hydrocephalus associated with a secreting papillary tumour of the choroid plexus (Fig. 21.67, p. 21.58). Decreased absorption of CSF is theoretically possible, but its occurrence in man is controversial.

Congenital hydrocephalus

This condition may so enlarge the fetal head as to interfere with birth. More often it is only slight at birth and increases afterwards. The head may become enormously enlarged and tends to become quadrangular, the vertex becomes flattened and the frontal bone projects over the orbits. The sutures are greatly widened and the fontanelles enlarged. There is a corresponding enlargement of the brain, the convo-

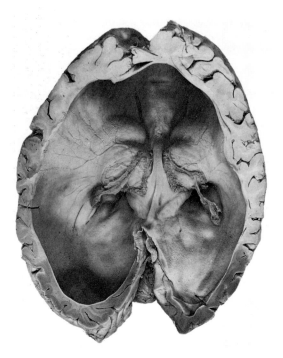

Fig. 21.9 Section of brain in congenital hydrocephalus, showing enormous dilatation of the lateral ventricles.

lutions being broadened and flattened and the sulci shallow. Distension of the lateral ventricles may be considerable, with corresponding thinning of the brain tissue around them (Fig. 21.9). If the third ventricle is involved its floor becomes greatly ballooned and extremely thin. It is remarkable how the brain can adapt itself to its altered shape and although considerable interference with mental function is usual, in a very few cases the child may be surprisingly intelligent.

One of the commoner causes of congenital hydrocephalus is the **Arnold–Chiari malformation** (Fig. 21.10): this consists of a tongue-like prolongation of the inferior cerebellar vermis through the foramen magnum and lying dorsal to the greatly elongated medulla. The lower part of the fourth ventricle lies in the upper part of the vertebral canal and the foramen magnum is blocked by the displaced tissue from the posterior fossa. Cerebrospinal fluid can flow out of the main exit foramina in the fourth ventricle and the hydrocephalus is therefore of communicating type (see above), but as the CSF is unable to re-enter the cranial cavity it cannot reach the main sites of reabsorption.

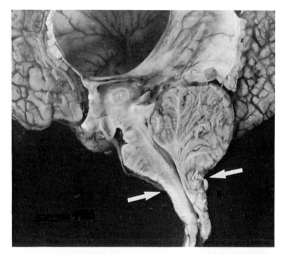

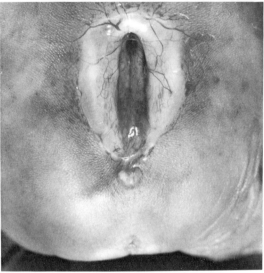

Fig. 21.10 The Arnold-Chiari malformation (*above*). Note the hydrocephalus, 'z-shaped' deformity of the brainstem and protrusion of the inferior part of the cerebellum as a tongue-like mass through the foramen magnum (*arrows*). Meningomyelocele (*below*) is almost always present. (Dr A. A. M. Gibson.)

The entire ventricular system thus becomes grossly enlarged. A **meningomyelocele** (p. 21.47) is an almost invariable accompaniment of the Arnold–Chiari malformation, and other features include a small posterior fossa, a poorly developed tentorium cerebelli and fusion and 'beaking' of the colliculi.

Other relatively common congenital abnormalities causing hydrocephalus are faulty development of the aqueduct and atresia of the foramina of Luschka and Magendie. In the former, hydrocephalus is confined to the lateral and third ventricles; in the latter there is in addition dilatation of the aqueduct and fourth ventricle. The ballooning of the roof of the fourth ventricle in these latter cases is usually severe enough to distort the inferior surface of the cerebellum.

Congenital hydrocephalus occurs also in the absence of any apparent developmental malformation. One cause of this is intra-uterine meningitis or ventriculitis, e.g. due to toxoplasmosis in which the inflammatory process produces obliterative changes in the subarachnoid space or in the ventricular system, particularly in the aqueduct. It seems likely, too, that some cases of hydrocephalus which are apparently congenital are caused by neonatal meningitis or subarachnoid haemorrhage resulting from cerebral birth injury, organisation of either of which may lead to obliteration of the subarachnoid space and obstruction to the flow of CSF.

Acquired hydrocephalus

Any expanding lesion within the skull, e.g. a tumour, abscess or haematoma, can obstruct the flow of CSF, but the effects of the lesion depend less on its nature than on its location. Even a small lesion in a vital site, e.g. adjacent to a foramen of Monro or close to the aqueduct, will cause hydrocephalus, whereas larger lesions elsewhere in the cerebral hemispheres may not interfere with the circulation of CSF. In general, *expanding lesions in the posterior fossa are particularly prone to cause hydrocephalus because they readily compress the aqueduct and the fourth ventricle.* Common examples are a tumour of the acoustic nerve, a meningioma or a tumour in the fourth ventricle. Acquired obstruction of the exit foramina or of the subarachnoid space is almost always due to acute pyogenic or subacute (e.g. tuberculous) meningitis. The subarachnoid space is at least partly occluded by exudate. If the inflammation does not resolve, organisation leads to obliteration of the subarachnoid space, particularly in the basal cisterns (Fig. 21.11) and around the midbrain, which is closely embraced by the rigid tentorium cerebelli. Organisation and obstruction are most likely to occur if treatment is delayed or inadequate.

A relatively uncommon cause of hydro-

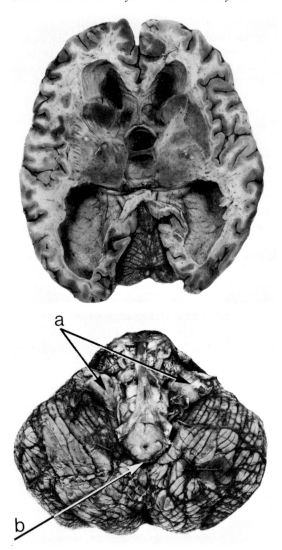

cephalus occurring after early childhood is progressive gliosis around the aqueduct. The aetiology of this is obscure but it is probably a hamartomatous proliferation (p. 12.47) of astrocytes.

Secondary hydrocephalus

Symmetrical enlargement of the ventricles may be secondary to a generalised reduction in the amount of brain tissue. If there is only local loss of cerebral tissue, the adjacent ventricle enlarges; a common example of this is enlargement of one lateral ventricle following adjacent infarction (Fig. 21.18, p. 21.18).

A syndrome characterised by dementia, a disturbance of gait and hydrocephalus, apparently without increased intracranial pressure, is usually referred to as '**normal pressure hydrocephalus**' but a better term would be intermittent hydrocephalus, for monitoring of the ventricular fluid pressure has shown that there may be significant rises during sleep. Some patients with this syndrome improve if a ventriculoperitoneal shunt operation is undertaken.

Fig. 21.11 Hydrocephalus due to occlusion of the foramina of Luschka **(a)** and Magendie **(b)** by fibrous adhesions.

Head Injury

In the United Kingdom, trauma is responsible for more deaths in all age groups under 45 than any other single cause, and *brain damage resulting from a head injury is the most important factor contributing to death or serious incapacity due to trauma.* In civilian practice most head injuries are of the *non-missile* type where the head suddenly accelerates or decelerates. This is associated with transient distortion of the

skull, which may fracture, and linear or rotational movements of the brain within the skull which produce **primary brain damage**, such as focal contusions and diffuse damage to nerve fibres. The clinical manifestations range from mild concussion to coma persisting until death. Other damage directly attributable to injury may be **delayed**, i.e. the process is initiated at the moment of injury but the clinical manifestations may not become apparent for some hours or even days: the commonest of these are intracranial haemorrhage and brain swelling which are sometimes referred to as **primary complications** of the head injury. **Secondary complications** include brain damage attributable to raised intracranial pressure and distortion of the brain, ischaemic or hypoxic brain damage, or infection.

Fracture of the skull

There is a tendency to exaggerate the importance of a fracture of the skull, for many patients with simple fractures may have suffered no significant brain damage, while *about 20% of fatal head injuries do not have a fracture*. A fracture, however, does indicate that the blow has probably been of considerable force and that there is a greater likelihood of brain damage and particularly of haemorrhage. There are some specific features associated with fractures which are important. Thus a fracture may be depressed, causing local pressure on the brain, and if there is also a laceration of the scalp the fracture is a potential source of subsequent intracranial sepsis. Any fracture of the base of the skull provides a potential source of infection from the nasal passages, the paranasal sinuses or the middle ear. The presence of such a fracture may be shown by a CSF rhinorrhoea or otorrhoea. Other complications of a fracture are laceration of a meningeal artery leading to the formation of an extradural haematoma (see below), or injury to the carotid artery within the cavernous sinus giving rise to a caroticocavernous fistula.

(1) Primary brain damage

Contusions and lacerations are the commonest form of focal brain damage directly attributable to injury. They may occur at the site of impact, particularly if there is a depressed fracture, but in any non-missile head injury they tend to involve the frontal poles, the orbital gyri, the temporal poles and the inferior and lateral surfaces of the anterior halves of the temporal lobes (Fig. 21.12). These regions are vulnerable

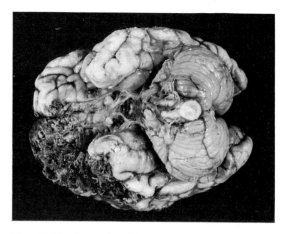

Fig. 21.12 Acute head injury, showing contusions of the frontal and temporal poles.

because movement of the brain within the skull brings them into forcible contact with bony protuberances in the base of the skull. Contusions are usually asymmetrical and they may be more extensive on the side opposite the one that has suffered the impact ('*contre coup*' injury): thus severe frontal contusion may occur in association with an occipital impact. The reverse is very rare because the inner surface of the occipital bone is smooth. Contusions may be superficial, when they tend to occur in the crests of the gyri, but they may extend through the full thickness of the cortex into the adjacent white matter and be associated with some intracerebral haemorrhage and oedema. Old healed contusions are represented by golden-brown shrunken areas of gliosis which have such a characteristic distribution and appearance that it is often possible at autopsy to diagnose previous head injury with certainty.

Diffuse axonal injury. Nerve fibres are torn at the moment of injury as a result of shear strains produced by movement, particularly rotational, of the brain within the skull. This type of brain damage may occur in the absence of obvious contusions, and if the patient dies soon after the injury the only macroscopic abnormality may be small haemorrhagic lesions in the corpus callosum and in the dorso-lateral quadrant of the rostral brainstem. The striking microscopical abnormality is the presence of *axonal retraction balls*, extruded axoplasm at the point of axonal injury, in all parts of the brain (Fig. 21.13). Some patients with this type of brain damage who experience no further

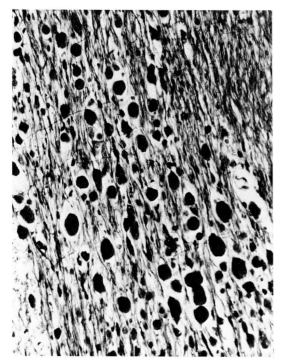

Fig. 21.13   Diffuse axonal injury. Axonal retraction balls in the pons of a patient who survived 10 days after a head injury. (Palmgren.) × 320.

complications of their injury may survive in a 'vegetative' state for up to a year or so. At autopsy, dissection shows ventricular enlargement due to a reduction in the white matter, and small shrunken cystic lesions in the corpus callosum and in the dorso-lateral quadrant of the rostral brainstem, i.e. where haemorrhagic lesions are seen in patients who die shortly after their injury. Microscopy shows Wallerian-type degeneration in the cerebral and cerebellar hemispheres, the brainstem and the spinal cord. Although the clinical features of axonal injury are often referred to as *primary brainstem injury*, the damage is diffuse.

(2) Primary complications

Intracranial haemorrhage

Extradural haematoma results from haemorrhage from a meningeal vessel, usually the middle meningeal artery. As the haematoma develops, it gradually strips the dura from the skull to form a large ovoid mass (Fig. 21.14)

that progressively compresses the adjacent brain. Although the tear in the meningeal artery is usually caused by a fracture of the skull, it sometimes occurs without fracture, particularly in children. The initial injury is often apparently mild, and many patients, whether or not they lose consciousness immediately after the injury, experience a lucid interval of some hours before developing headache and becoming drowsy. As the haematoma enlarges the patient lapses into coma and may die from the effects of raised intracranial pressure unless the haematoma is evacuated. Extradural haematomas occasionally occur in the frontal or the parietal regions, or within the posterior fossa.

Subdural haematoma results from laceration of small 'bridging' veins which traverse the subdural space or of larger veins running into the main venous sinuses. In contrast to extradural haematoma, which usually remains localised, the blood tends to spread diffusely over one or both hemispheres.

Acute subdural haematoma is a common autopsy finding if death has occurred soon after a head injury. The haematoma forms a thin

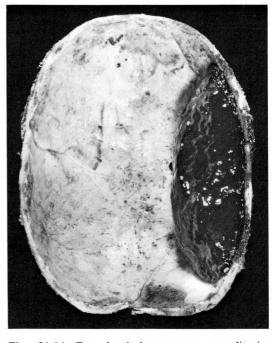

Fig. 21.14   Extradural haematoma complicating fracture of the skull. The specimen shows the under-surface of the vault of the cranium from which the dura has been removed.

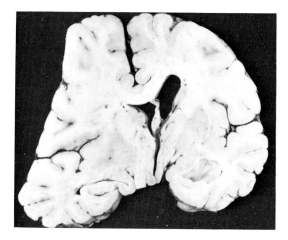

Fig. 21.15 Severe distortion of the brain caused by a chronic subdural haematoma.

layer and may not have contributed significantly to death, for such patients often have extensive contusions and lacerations of the brain. In some cases, however, an acute subdural haematoma may be much larger and unless surgically evacuated can produce coma and death from raised intracranial pressure. Some patients with acute subdural haematoma experience a lucid interval similar to that classically associated with extradural haematoma.

Chronic subdural haematoma present weeks or months after an apparently trivial head injury. Indeed many patients deny any history of head injury. The precise aetiology is not clear but the clot is gradually organised and so becomes encapsulated in a fibrous membrane. It enlarges slowly, probably as a result of repeated small haemorrhages. Because chronic subdural haematoma is particularly common in old people who already have some cerebral atrophy and because the haematoma expands very slowly, it may become very large—often 2–3 cm thick—before symptoms appear. In untreated cases, however, death is usually due to brain damage secondary to increased intracranial pressure (Fig. 21.15). Chronic subdural haematoma is not uncommonly bilateral.

Intracerebral haemorrhage following injury is usually associated with contusions of the brain and so traumatic haematomas are most often seen in the frontal and in the temporal lobes. They are often multiple and vary greatly in size. They may also occur deep within the hemispheres where they are presumably due to shear strains affecting small vessels at the moment of injury.

(3) Secondary complications

Not all of the brain damage found in fatal head injury is directly attributable to the injury. If an intracranial haematoma develops, much of the brain damage is due to **raised intracranial pressure** and distortion of the brain (p. 21.7).

Brain swelling (p. 21.8) is a further factor that may contribute to a high intracranial pressure in a head-injured patient. Thus there is almost always some swelling around contusions and lacerations but there may be diffuse swelling of both hemispheres, particularly in children. In patients with an acute subdural haematoma, there is often diffuse swelling throughout the affected cerebral hemisphere(s).

Hypoxic brain damage is frequently observed in patients dying from non-missile head injury. Some of the causes of this are well recognised, e.g. cardiorespiratory arrest or status epilepticus, the latter being particularly frequent in children. Other hypoxic brain damage may be a direct consequence of raised intracranial pressure, but there remains a fairly large group of cases who develop focal infarction in the cerebral cortex or in the basal nuclei, the pathogenesis of which is not clearly understood.

Infection results from the entrance of bacteria through a compound fracture of the vault or base of the skull. It usually presents as **meningitis** and its onset is not restricted to the early post-traumatic period, because a small traumatic fistula from the subarachnoid space to one of the major air sinuses in the base of the skull may persist. **Intracranial abscess** is a rarer complication and is usually secondary to a penetrating injury.

Clinical features of head injury

Since the pathogenesis of brain damage due to a head injury is complex, the clinical spectrum is wide. Primary brain damage is the beginning of an evolving process which may range from progressive improvement without complications, as in most patients with so-called concussion, to death. The period of disturbed consciousness and the interval between the injury and the return of continuous memory—**post-traumatic amnesia**—are probably closely related to the degree of diffuse brain damage: if this is mild, the patient may only be transiently dazed; if it is severe the patient will remain in a vegetative state until death. By contrast, focal contusions, may have relatively mild clinical effects and even severe cerebral contusions may cause little or no permanent cerebral dysfunction. But even if the initial injury appears only trivial, primary or secondary complications may develop, e.g. intracranial haematoma, raised intracranial pressure, hypoxic brain damage or infection. Thus in a personally studied series of 151 patients with fatal non-missile head injuries, who had been referred to a neurosurgical unit because their neurological state had been causing concern, 58 were found to have talked at some time after their injury, i.e. they had apparently recovered in some measure after their injury, only to deteriorate and die later. *The management of head-injured patients has therefore to be based on the knowledge that complications occur only too frequently, and that at least some of these are avoidable.*

Head injury is an important cause of **symptomatic epilepsy**. About 10% of patients admitted to hospital with a non-missile head injury develop fits. These tend to occur in the first week after injury (*early epilepsy*) or are delayed for 2–3 months or more after the injury (*late epilepsy*). Early epilepsy occurs more commonly after severe or complicated head injuries, although children under 5 may develop it after apparently trivial injuries. Factors predisposing to late epilepsy include a depressed fracture and an acute intracranial haematoma. Fits are less liable to recur in patients with early epilepsy than in those who develop late epilepsy. With missile (i.e. penetrating) head injuries, the incidence of epilepsy is about 45%.

Trauma to the spinal cord

Injuries of the spinal cord, like those of the brain, are of all degrees of severity. In cases of fracture-dislocation, bullet wounds, etc., the cord may be directly lacerated, or even torn across. Apart from such extreme cases, the cord may be damaged by acute flexion or extension of the neck, when haemorrhage may occur outside or inside the dura or within the spinal cord itself. There may also be infarction of the cord. Haemorrhage occurs especially immediately dorsal to the grey commissure, and tends to extend upwards and downwards through several segments. In cases of haemorrhage into the cord, or *haematomyelia*, the blood is broken down and ultimately an elongated pigmented encapsulated cavity may result, which may simulate syringomyelia (p. 21.53). Transverse lesions of the cord are described on pp. 21.48–51.

Circulatory Disturbances

Cerebrovascular disease (*stroke*) is a major health problem, accounting for about 10% of all deaths, and of those who survive some 50% remain severely disabled. The incidence rises with age, about 80% occurring in patients over 65. About 85% of *strokes* are due to ischaemic brain damage (cerebral infarction) while 15% are due to spontaneous intracranial haemorrhage (intracerebral and subarachnoid). A number of major predisposing factors have been identified, notably those which predispose to atheroma, thrombosis and systemic embolism. Hypertension is of particular importance, especially in predisposing to intracerebral and probably subarachnoid haemorrhage.

Ischaemic brain damage

The brain receives its blood supply from the internal carotid and vertebral arteries via the major intracranial cerebral arteries. A **cerebral infarct** occurs when the blood flow to any part of the brain falls below the critical level necessary to maintain the viability of brain tissue and, as elsewhere, consists of a patch of tissue within which all the cellular elements have undergone ischaemic necrosis. An infarct may be of any size from a small discrete lesion in the grey or white matter to necrosis of a large part of the brain. Infarction may occur in any part of the brain but the commonest site is in the middle cerebral arterial territory. Reduction in blood flow may result in the death of only the most susceptible cells, i.e. the neurons, but usually it is more severe producing necrosis also of the neuroglial cells and, slightly less commonly, of microglia and blood vessels also. These changes, in which some tissue cells and blood vessels survive the ischaemia, are not true infarcts (see above) but it is reasonable to describe such changes as *partial infarction*. Infarction may result not only from occlusion of a cerebral artery, but also from an episode of severe hypotension or transient cardiac arrest in the absence of arterial disease: usually, however, there is stenosis and/or occlusion of one or more major arteries. The critical reduction in the blood flow to a particular region of the brain need last for between only 10 and 15 minutes to produce an infarct. If the reduction is transient, flow through the infarct may return to normal. When the cerebral circulation is already compromised by pre-existing arterial stenosis, infarction is particularly liable to occur in any hypotensive state, e.g. following myocardial infarction.

It is estimated that 30–60% of infarcts are *embolic* in origin. Cerebral emboli may arise from vegetations of infective endocarditis, from mural thrombus in patients with arrhythmias or a myocardial infarct, or from atheromatous plaques in the large arteries in the neck. Infarction may also result from *air, nitrogen* and *fat embolism*, which are described in pp. 10.20–22.

Another important local cause of an inadequate cerebral blood flow is *atheroma*: this may result only in stenosis, but the artery may become occluded by *thrombus* forming on an atheromatous plaque. Other less common vascular diseases leading to a reduced arterial lumen with or without thrombosis are *arteritis* (e.g. polyarteritis nodosa or the arteritis of tuberculous meningitis or syphilitic endarteritis). A small proportion of cerebral infarcts result from the arterial occlusion which occurs in various blood diseases, notably polycythaemia rubra vera, essential thrombocythaemia, sickle-cell disease and other haemoglobino-pathies.

The size of the infarct depends to a considerable extent on the degree of occlusive arterial disease and the available collateral circulation. Collateral channels exist between the major cerebral arteries on the surface of the brain and in the circle of Willis, but the arteries within the brain are end arteries (p. 10.23). Depending on the site of the vascular occlusion, an infarct may affect the whole or part of a major arterial territory, e.g. of the middle cerebral artery. If, however, the blood flow through two adjacent arterial territories is reduced, infarction may occur in the *boundary zone* between them.

Arterial occlusion

Cerebral infarction may result from occlusion of arteries within the cranium or in the neck. The commonest intracranial site of occlusion is the middle cerebral artery. Atheromatous narrowing or occlusion may occur in any part of the common carotid or vertebral arteries, but the commonest site is at the origin of an internal carotid artery, and infarction results only if the collateral circulation is or becomes inadequate: the usual site of such infarction is in the distribution of the middle cerebral artery on the same side. In some cases, thrombosis extends along the internal carotid artery into the middle and anterior cerebral arteries to produce infarction of a large part of the cerebral hemisphere. When the vertebral arteries are the more severely atheromatous or are occluded, ischaemic changes occur characteristically in the brainstem, the cerebellum, and the parts of the cerebral hemispheres supplied by the posterior cerebral arteries, i.e. the occipital lobes. Cerebral infarction is often the result of a combination of systemic circulatory insufficiency and stenosis of the extracranial and/or cerebral arteries by atheroma.

Structural changes in a cerebral infarct. These depend upon the size of the lesion and on the survival time. A cerebral infarct may be *pale* or *haemorrhagic* (p. 10.24). An intensely haemorrhagic infarct may superficially resemble a haematoma, but the distinctive feature is the preservation of the intrinsic architecture of the infarcted tissue (Fig. 21.16). A pale infarct less than 24 hours old may be difficult to identify

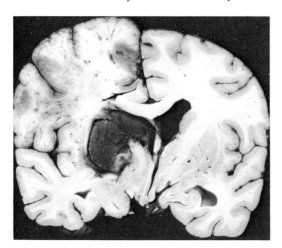

Fig. 21.16 Recent infarct in left cerebral hemisphere. The basal ganglia show the features of haemorrhagic infarction; the posterior part of the frontal lobe above the Sylvian fissure shows those of pale infarction. Note that the affected hemisphere is swollen and that there is displacement of the midline structures to the right.

macroscopically but thereafter the dead tissue becomes slightly soft and swollen and there is loss of the normal sharp definition between the affected grey and white matter. At this stage, histological examination will show ischaemic necrosis of neurons, pallor of myelin staining and sometimes infiltration of polymorphs around the necrotic vessel walls. If the infarct is large, oedema of the surrounding brain tissue may produce the typical features of an acutely expanding intracranial lesion, with raised intracranial pressure (p. 21.7). Within a few days, the infarct becomes distinctly soft and the dead tissue disintegrates (Fig. 21.17); hence a cerebral infarct is often referred to as a '**softening**'. Microscopic examination at this stage will show macrophages filled with globules of lipid produced by the breakdown of myelin (Fig. 21.3, p. 21.6) and, around the dead tissue, enlarged astrocytes and early capillary proliferation. During the following weeks the dead tissue is removed, lipid phagocytes become scanty, and a fibrillary gliosis occurs, often with a little fine fibrosis. The lesion ultimately becomes shrunken and cystic (Fig. 21.18), and the cysts are often traversed by small vessels and glial fibrils. If the infarct has been haemorrhagic, some of the phagocytes will contain haemosiderin and the cyst walls appear brown. Shrinkage of an infarct in a cerebral hemisphere is usually

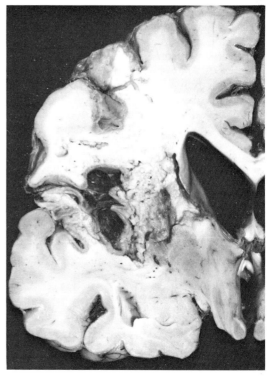

Fig. 21.17 Infarct of a week's duration in the left cerebral hemisphere. The dead tissue is disintegrating and there is already some shrinkage of the affected cortex.

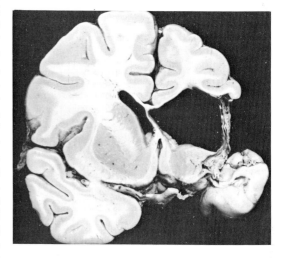

Fig. 21.18 Infarct of several years' duration in the right cerebral hemisphere. The dead tissue has been completely removed. The lateral ventricle is separated from the surface of the brain by a narrow web of tissue composed of leptomeninges, ependyma and a few glial fibrils.

accompanied by enlargement of the adjacent lateral ventricle (Fig. 21.18). The meninges overlying an old cortical infarct are thickened and opaque and underneath there is usually an adherent layer of brownish/yellow cortical tissue composed of enlarged astrocytes and occasional lipid phagocytes. Beneath this the cortex is usually cystic and traversed by strands of thick astrocytic fibres. A consequence of infarction is Wallerian degeneration of the nerve fibres that have been interrupted. Thus, if the infarct involves the internal capsule, there is progressive degeneration and shrinkage of the corresponding pyramidal tract in the brainstem and spinal cord.

Venous obstruction

This may result from either occlusion of the cerebral veins or thrombosis in one of the large dural sinuses. Thrombosis may be *primary* (non-infectious or marantic), or *secondary* to pyogenic infection (septic thrombosis). *Primary thrombosis* is most frequent in poorly nourished and dehydrated children during the course of acute infections, e.g. gastro-enteritis, but it may occur in adults where predisposing factors include congestive cardiac failure and conditions which cause shock or hypercoagulability of the blood. There is also an increased incidence in pregnancy and the puerperium. The commonest site of thrombosis is the superior sagittal sinus and, when obstruction is complete, intense engorgement of the superficial veins occurs. There may also be irregular zones of intensely haemorrhagic infarction in the parasagittal parts of the cerebral hemispheres. In thrombosis of the straight sinus, similar haemorrhagic areas occur in the walls of the third ventricle. *Septic thrombosis* is the result of direct spread of organisms in open head injuries or from an adjacent septic lesion, such as chronic suppurative otitis media. As in septic venous thrombosis elsewhere (p. 9.8), the thrombus is digested by polymorphs and pyaemia may result.

Cardiac arrest

Neurons are highly dependent on a continuous supply of oxygen and glucose, without which consciousness is lost within a few seconds. The supply of oxygen depends upon pulmonary function and on the cerebral blood flow which, in turn, depends on the *cerebral perfusion pressure*, i.e. the difference between the systemic arterial pressure and the cerebral venous pressure. *The vitally important cerebral blood flow is controlled by an autoregulatory mechanism which maintains a relatively constant blood flow in spite of changes in perfusion pressure.* Autoregulation is affected mainly by changes in the cerebrovascular resistance, i.e. tone of the cerebral arterioles, which dilate when arterial pressure falls and constrict when arterial pressure increases. In consequence, blood flow is maintained within normal limits even when the systemic arterial pressure falls as low as 50 mmHg, provided the subject is in the prone position. At arterial pressures lower than this, the cerebral blood flow falls rapidly. Autoregulation may be impaired in chronic hypertension, in hypoxic or hypercapnic states, and in a wide range of acute conditions producing brain damage, e.g. head injuries and strokes.

Because of the susceptibility of neurons to hypoxia, the vital factor determining the immediate and ultimate outcome in such medical emergencies as cardiorespiratory arrest, a severe episode of hypotension, carbon monoxide intoxication or status epilepticus, is whether or not satisfactory resuscitation can be achieved before the occurrence of irreversible brain damage. Severe hypoglycaemia has an essentially similar effect because neurons require also a continuous supply of glucose. The neuronal damage in the above emergencies varies in its distribution: when some circulation is maintained, as in a severe but transient episode of hypotension, it tends to be focal and most marked in the boundary zones between major arterial territories. Diffuse neuronal damage occurs in more generalised disturbances of the supply of oxygen and/or glucose to the brain, as in cardiac arrest, status epilepticus, carbon monoxide poisoning and severe hypoglycaemia.

Many patients suffer severe diffuse brain damage after a cardiac arrest and die within a few days after the episode; the brain may appear entirely normal macroscopically. Provided the patient has survived for more than about 12 hours, however, microscopic examination will disclose widespread and severe neuronal necrosis. There are minor variations in the distribution of neuronal damage but the nerve cells most susceptible to oxygen deprivation are those in the Ammon's horns (hippocampus), in the third, fifth and sixth layers of the cerebral cortex (particularly within the sulci of the posterior halves of the cerebral hemispheres), in certain of the basal nuclei, and the Purkinje cells of the cerebellum. After a few days the dead neurons disappear and reactive changes in astrocytes, microglia and capillaries become intense. If the patient survives for more than a few weeks, the affected regions become shrunken and cystic as in a conventional infarct.

Spontaneous intracranial haemorrhage

The two common types of spontaneous intracranial haemorrhage are primary intracerebral haemorrhage and subarachnoid haemorrhage.

Intracerebral haemorrhage

Primary intracerebral haemorrhage occurs mostly in patients with hypertension and is due to *rupture of one of the numerous microaneurysms* found in the brain tissue of most people with hypertension (p. 14.33).

The commonest site of hypertensive intracerebral haemorrhage is in the region of the basal ganglia and the internal capsule (Fig. 21.19). Other common sites are the pons (Fig. 21.20) and the cerebellum. Subcortical haemorrhage also occurs but is rare. The haematoma usually increases in size rapidly, causes severe local destruction of tissue, and produces a sud-

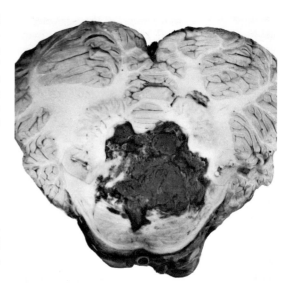

Fig. 21.20 Hypertensive haemorrhage into the pons.

den rise in intracranial pressure and rapid distortion and herniation of the brain (p. 21.7). The blood may rupture into the ventricles or through the surface of the brain directly into the subarachnoid space. The clinical onset is usually sudden and patients with large intracerebral haematomas rarely survive for more than 36 hours, death being precipitated by secondary haemorrhage into the brainstem as a result of raised intracranial pressure.

The appearance of the haematoma at autopsy varies with its duration. A recent haematoma is composed of ordinary dark red clot. If the haematoma is not large enough to be rapidly fatal, its periphery has a brownish colour after about a week, and there are early reactive changes in capillaries and astrocytes in the adjacent brain. This brownish colour then spreads throughout the entire haematoma, while gliosis leads to the formation of a poorly defined capsule. If the patient survives, the clot is ultimately completely removed by macrophages and replaced by yellow fluid to form a so-called apoplectic cyst (Fig. 21.21).

Spontaneous subarachnoid haemorrhage

This is nearly always caused by rupture of a so-called berry aneurysm on one of the major cerebral arteries. These aneurysms (described on p. 14.32) occur most often at the bifurcation of a middle cerebral artery within the Sylvian

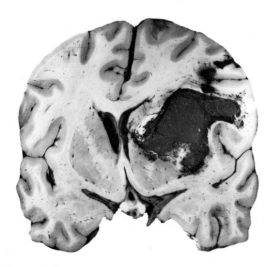

Fig. 21.19 Large haematoma in basal ganglia, resulting from chronic hypertension.

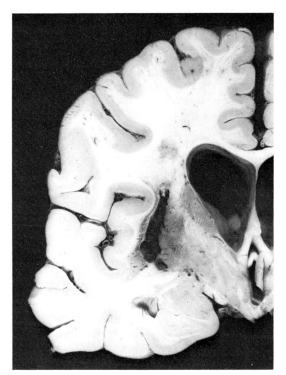

Fig. 21.21 Apoplectic cyst on left side of brain. The cyst is centred on the external capsule and the outer part of the lentiform nucleus.

fissure, at the junction of the anterior communicating artery with an anterior cerebral artery, and at the junction of a posterior communicating artery with an internal carotid artery. They may also occur on the basilar artery and its branches. About 10 to 15% of patients who present with symptoms due to an aneurysm are found to have multiple (usually two or three) aneurysms.

When a berry aneurysm ruptures, the escaping blood may be limited to the immediate vicinity of the aneurysm, but frequently it spreads extensively through the subarachnoid space. Blood may also track into the brain to produce an intracerebral haematoma (Fig. 21.22), and if the aneurysm is embedded in brain tissue, intracerebral haemorrhage may occur without any subarachnoid haemorrhage.

Anterior communicating aneurysms tend to burst into the frontal lobe, while posterior communicating aneurysms and middle cerebral aneurysms commonly rupture into the temporal lobe. Thus, patients with ruptured intracranial aneurysms may have the clinical and patho-

logical features of an acute expanding lesion in addition to subarachnoid haemorrhage. Such intracerebral haematomas often rupture into the ventricles.

Another complication of a ruptured aneurysm is **infarction**, most commonly in the region of the brain supplied by the affected artery. This is probably partly attributable to arterial spasm, which causes a reduction in local cerebral blood flow, and the swelling which occurs around a recent infarct (p. 21.18) may cause further displacement and distortion of the brain.

In many fatal cases of ruptured berry aneurysm there is a history of a previous small subarachnoid haemorrhage, and in such cases examination of the brain may reveal the presence of altered blood pigment in the meninges adjacent to the aneurysm. Subarachnoid haemorrhage due to rupture of a berry aneurysm is a serious condition and 25% of patients die within a few hours. If untreated, many of the patients will die from complications of the first haemorrhage or as a result of a second or subsequent bleed.

Rarer causes of intracranial aneurysm are infected emboli (*mycotic aneurysms*—p. 10.20) and atheroma.

It should be emphasised that subarachnoid haemorrhage and ruptured intracranial aneurysm are not inevitably associated; the former may be the result of an acute head injury or haemorrhage from a vascular malfor-

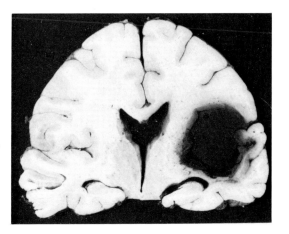

Fig. 21.22 Ruptured aneurysm. Haemorrhage from an aneurysm on the middle cerebral artery has produced a haematoma in the Sylvian fissure and in the adjacent brain.

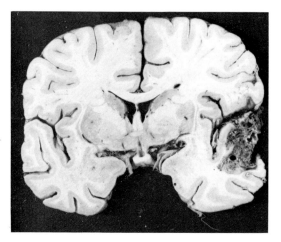

Fig. 21.23   Vascular malformation. There is a plexi-form mass of vessels in the superficial part of the temporal lobe.

mation (see below) or it may be secondary to a primary intracerebral haemorrhage tracking into the ventricles or directly to the surface of the brain. A ruptured berry aneurysm may cause an intracerebral haematoma or a cerebral infarct without any significant subarachnoid haemorrhage.

Other causes of spontaneous intracranial haemorrhage

Probably the commonest of these is rupture of a **vascular malformation**, which may range in size from a small capillary angioma to a massive lesion composed of large, often thick-walled vascular channels (Fig. 21.23). They usually occur on the surface of the brain or spinal cord but sometimes lie deep in the brain. Rupture may produce a large intracerebral haematoma which is rapidly fatal, but a more frequent result is mild subarachnoid haemorrhage. Many of these lesions are compatible with long survival, sometimes punctuated with episodes of subarachnoid haemorrhage.

Other causes of spontaneous intracranial haemorrhage include **haemorrhage into tumours** and **haemorrhagic diseases** (p. 17.62). For example, cerebral haemorrhage is a common fatal complication in acute leukaemia.

Spontaneous intracerebral haemorrhage sometimes occurs **without obvious cause** in normotensive subjects: the pathogenesis is not clear but it may be due to rupture of one of the occasional micro-aneurysms found in normotensive subjects (p. 14.33), or to rupture of a small vascular malformation too small to be detected at autopsy.

Bacterial Infections of the Nervous System

The brain and spinal cord are relatively well protected from bacteria, and infections of the nervous system are not particularly common. But once micro-organisms have gained access to the nervous system, the infection may spread rapidly by way of the CSF pathway. The severity of the clinical illness depends on the virulence of the infecting agent and the susceptibility of the host, but many micro-organisms which are relatively non-pathogenic elsewhere in the body may cause serious and often fatal infection of the nervous system.

Inflammation of the meninges—**meningitis**—and inflammation of the brain—**encephalitis**—will be considered separately because, although both are usually present in any severe inflammatory process, one is almost always much more severe than the other.

Meningitis

Meningitis may involve the dura—**pachymeningitis**—or the pia and the arachnoid—**leptomeningitis**. The latter is by far the commoner, and the term **meningitis** is often used instead of leptomeningitis.

Pachymeningitis

Acute inflammation of the dura is practically always due to extension of inflammation from the bones of the skull. The underlying infection may be chronic suppurative otitis media or mastoiditis, or the infection may be a sequel to a compound fracture of the skull. When pyogenic organisms spread from the bone, suppuration occurs between bone and dura and an **extradural abscess** may form. The dura becomes swollen and softened, and the infection may penetrate through it and spread widely over the hemisphere to form a **subdural abscess**. The organisms may also spread to the subarachnoid space, setting up either localised or general **leptomeningitis**. Further effects of spread, such as the production of cerebral abscess, are described below. The dura is occasionally the site of gummatous lesions in syphilis (p. 21.28).

Widespread use of antibiotics has greatly reduced the incidence of these various types of pachymeningitis.

Meningitis (leptomeningitis)

Acute pyogenic meningitis

This is caused by infection of the subarachnoid space. The pia-arachnoid membrane becomes inflamed and exudate is added to the CSF, which is a good culture medium for many bacteria.

Unless treated early, acute bacterial meningitis is often fatal from the severity of the infection, or results in severe disability. *It is thus a medical emergency requiring urgent antibiotic therapy.*

Causal organisms are many and varied. The commonest are *Neisseria meningitidis*, *Strep. pneumoniae* and the haemophilus group, while *Escherichia coli* is common in infants. Less common are *Strep. pyogenes*, *Staph. aureus*, the colon-typhi group and *Bacillus anthracis*.

It must be emphasised that tuberculous, leptospiral, syphilitic and fungal meningitis may simulate closely acute pyogenic meningitis and the distinction can often be made only by bacteriological examination of the CSF. Acute viral meningitis (p. 21.30) is also clinically similar but usually milder than bacterial meningitis.

Routes of infection. (*a*) *By the bloodstream.* Most cases of meningitis are of haematogenous origin. In meningococcal meningitis (*cerebrospinal fever*), for example, infection is spread by droplet infection from nasopharyngeal carriers. Spread is favoured by poor hygienic conditions, especially overcrowding, and thus the disease tends to occur in epidemic form among recruits in overcrowded barracks, refugees in camps, etc. In susceptible persons the meningococci

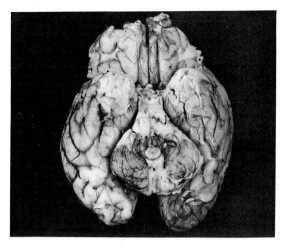

Fig. 21.24   Purulent meningitis. Large amounts of pus are seen at the base of the brain.

pass from the nasopharynx to the meninges by the bloodstream and during epidemics cases of fatal meningococcal septicaemia can occur without meningitis, death sometimes occurring within a few hours of infection. A characteristic feature of meningococcal septicaemia is haemorrhagic rash.

(*b*) *From an adjacent lesion.* Meningitis may

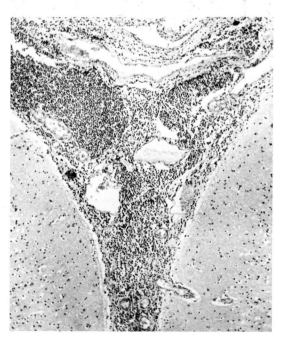

Fig. 21.25   Acute pneumococcal meningitis: section of cerebral cortex showing distension of the subarachnoid space with purulent exudate. × 55.

result from spread of infections in the middle ear or in any of the air sinuses in the base of the skull. It is also a fairly common complication of a compound fracture of the skull, particularly fractures of the base involving the nasopharynx or air sinuses.

(*c*) *Iatrogenic infection* can occur from the introduction of micro-organisms at operation or by lumbar puncture with non-sterile instruments. This is rare, but as the infecting agents are introduced directly into the subarachnoid space, a generalised meningitis rapidly ensues.

Structural changes. Exudate accumulates in the subarachnoid space and is most easily seen where the space is wide, i.e. within sulci and at the base of the brain, where it accumulates around the optic chiasma and in the adjacent cisterns (Figs 21.24, 21.25). It varies markedly in appearance, even in the same type of infection. There may merely be excess of turbid fluid in the sulci, or the exudate may be abundant, yellowish and fibrinous or purulent. Some degree of hydrocephalus is common because deposition of fibrin interferes with the flow of CSF.

The inflammation frequently extends into the ventricles: they contain turbid CSF and a coating of fibrin is seen on their walls and on the choroid plexuses. Exudate is also abundant in the spinal subarachnoid space, particularly on the dorsal surface of the cord.

Diagnosis. *The CSF must be examined as soon as possible whenever meningitis is suspected, even if there is some clinical evidence of increased intracranial pressure* (p. 21.6), for this is the only means by which the diagnosis can be established and the causal agent identified. The CSF is usually turbid and may be distinctly purulent. Microscopic examination shows it to contain numerous neutrophil leucocytes. The protein content is raised and the sugar reduced or absent (Table 21.1, pp. 21.46–47). The causal organisms are often apparent, although in some cases they can be detected only by culture.

Treatment. Vigorous early treatment with an appropriate antibiotic usually results in resolution of the infection with little or no residual damage. Late or inadequate treatment may allow progression of the disease to a subacute or chronic phase. Formerly this was not uncommon in young children, particularly with meningococcal meningitis, and the disease was then referred to as *posterior basal meningitis*. The meninges become thickened and oedematous and organisation of fibrin deposits leads to obliteration of the foramina in the roof of the fourth ventricle and/or some degree of obstruction in the subarachnoid space, and consequent hydrocephalus (p. 21.10). Various cranial nerves may be involved with resulting paralyses. Similar chronic changes can occur in the spinal meninges with widespread involvement of nerve roots. Bacteria are usually scanty in such chronic cases. Closely similar structural changes may be brought about by the tubercle bacillus (see p. 21.26).

Bacterial encephalitis

In bacterial meningitis, the brain tissue adjacent to the pia-arachnoid (including the perivascular space) shows various degrees of acute inflammatory change, and there may even be foci of suppuration in the superficial brain tissue. Apart from this, bacterial encephalitis usually takes the form of a *brain abscess*.

Brain abscess

The causative organisms include the common pyogenic cocci and many others—anaerobic streptococci, diphtheroids and coliforms, etc.

Routes of infection

As in meningitis, they reach the brain by direct spread from a local infection or by the blood.

Direct spread of bacteria is usually a consequence of pyogenic infection in the bones or sinuses of the skull or of a compound fracture. The most important cause is chronic suppurative otitis media or mastoiditis. The bone is eroded by a chronic osteitis and infection reaches the dura to produce an *extradural* or a *subdural abscess* (p. 21.23). The infection extends to the leptomeninges but generalised meningitis is often prevented by local adhesions. The bac-

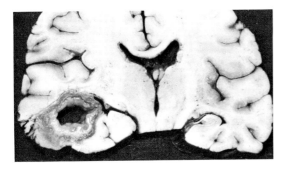

Fig. 21.26 Cerebral abscess. There is an encapsulated abscess in the left temporal lobe, secondary to chronic suppurative otitis media.

teria may, however, invade and cause septic thrombosis of small veins which pass from the brain to the venous sinuses. By this route, infection can spread deeply into the brain and produce a brain abscess.

If the middle ear infection spreads upwards through the tegmen tympani, the abscess occurs in the temporal lobe (Fig. 21.26). If infection spreads from the mastoid antrum, or from the middle ear, to the posterior aspect of the petrous bone, the abscess occurs in the cerebellum; in such cases the sigmoid sinus may be involved and thrombosed. In some cases with chronic middle ear disease, abscesses may be found both in the temporal lobe and in the cerebellum.

As in other tissues, an abscess in the brain becomes limited by a pyogenic membrane which, unless the infection extends very rapidly to involve the meninges or ventricles, soon becomes a well-defined capsule composed of young connective tissue, new capillaries, enlarged astrocytes and lipid phagocytes. In the adjacent cerebral tissue there are varying degrees of oedema, reactive gliosis and infiltration by lymphocytes and plasma cells, particularly in the perivascular spaces. The symptoms of an abscess are often vague and by the time the diagnosis is made it may contain thick greenish-yellow pus commonly with a foul odour because of the mixed bacterial flora. An abscess may remain latent for some months, but it commonly enlarges and becomes multilocular, and finally may rupture into a ventricle or the subarachnoid space.

Otitis media and mastoiditis. Disease of the middle ear, mastoid antrum and air cells, re-sulting from spread of infection along the Eustachian tube from the pharynx, is commoner in children than in adults. It often starts as a complication of streptococcal tonsillitis, but in infants pneumococci are often responsible. Mixed infections are also common. Acute suppurative inflammation of the lining of the tympanic cavity develops and, if this progresses, the mucous membrane is destroyed and replaced by a layer of granulation tissue; the tympanic membrane is often perforated, allowing access to a very mixed bacterial flora. The bone becomes eroded by osteitis and infection may reach the dura, giving rise to local pachymeningitis, acute leptomeningitis, cerebral abscess, sinus thrombosis, etc. A similar sequence may follow acute suppuration in the frontal sinus, the resulting abscess being in the frontal lobe, but this is uncommon.

Septic sinus thrombosis results from spread of pyogenic infection to the wall of a sinus, most frequently to the sigmoid sinus from the mastoid or middle ear. The process is similar to septic venous thrombosis (p. 9.8) with infection and sometimes suppuration of the thrombus. Extension of thrombosis into the jugular vein often prevents the dissemination of septic emboli from the sinus, so that pyaemia is unusual.

The risk of brain abscess and other complications of otitis media has been greatly reduced since the widespread use of antibiotics.

Haematogenous abscesses occur most frequently in the parietal lobes but may appear in any part of the brain and are often multiple. When solitary they may become large and develop a thick gliomesodermal capsule before being diagnosed. The source of the septic embolus may be anywhere in the body but the primary site is often in the lung. In the past, there was a particularly close association between **suppurative bronchiectasis** and brain abscess, but fortunately infection in bronchiectasis can now usually be adequately controlled by antibiotics. Individuals with congenital cyanotic heart disease are, however, still prone to develop a brain abscess. Multiple small acute abscesses occur in **pyaemia**, while in a patient dying with **infective endocarditis** numerous small perivascular haemorrhagic inflammatory foci are commonly found in the brain.

Yeasts and fungi are rarer causes of haematogenous brain abscess (p. 21.30).

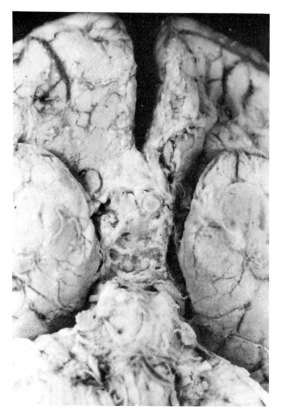

Fig. 21.27 Tuberculous meningitis, showing exudate which obscures structures at base of brain. A few tubercles can be seen on the frontal lobes.

Tuberculosis

Involvement of the nervous system is a not uncommon feature of tuberculosis. It is always secondary to tuberculosis elsewhere in the body and usually presents as a *subacute meningitis*. Less commonly it takes the form of a *tuberculoma*.

Tuberculous meningitis. The bacilli reach the brain by the bloodstream: this may be simply one manifestation of miliary tuberculosis, usually in association with a primary complex, but sometimes it is a complication of chronic pulmonary or renal tuberculosis in adults. Another mode of infection is by way of a small haematogenous caseous lesion in the cortex of the brain. Less commonly the infection may spread to the meninges by direct spread from tuberculosis of a vertebral body.

On reaching the meninges the bacilli proliferate and spread throughout the subarachnoid space where their presence induces a diffuse meningitis characterised by both exudation and the formation of tubercles. At first the CSF is clear or faintly turbid, but later the exudate in the subarachnoid space becomes thick and gelatinous or caseous (Fig. 21.27). As is usual in meningitis, the exudate is most abundant in the basal cisterns and in the sulci: the exudate itself, and deposited fibrin, obscure the surface features of the base of the brain, the brainstem and the cord. Tubercles are seen most readily when the exudate is still thin: they appear as grey nodules, 1–2 mm in diameter, adjacent to the blood vessels in the subarachnoid space (Fig. 21.28).

Microscopically, the subarachnoid space may at first contain many polymorphonuclear leucocytes but these are soon replaced by macrophages, lymphocytes and desquamated pia-arachnoid lining cells. Fibrin is deposited in the subarachnoid space and may later undergo organisation. The tubercles are seen to be poorly formed rounded cellular aggregates with central caseation: the cells are mainly macrophages which show incomplete transformation to epithelioid cells, while giant cells are relatively small or absent.

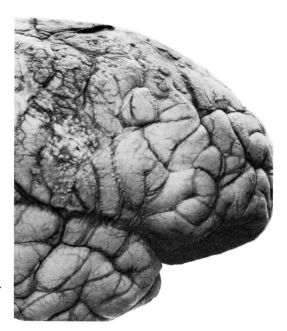

Fig. 21.28 Tuberculous meningitis: localised eruption of tubercles on the surface of the hemisphere in the region of the Sylvian fissure.

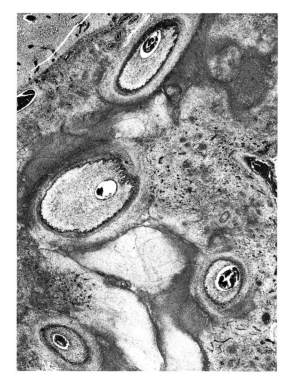

Fig. 21.29 Cerebral arteries in chronic tuberculous meningitis, showing obliterative endarteritis. × 15.

At an early stage, the arteries and veins in the subarachnoid space are involved in an intense acute necrotising vasculitis with polymorph infiltration and deposition of fibrin in their walls. Later, and particularly in prolonged cases where treatment has been started relatively late, there is an intense reactive endarteritis obliterans (Fig. 21.29). In consequence, there is quite often focal infarction of the adjacent superficial brain tissue and of cranial and spinal nerves, resulting in various focal neurological signs.

Some degree of hydrocephalus is an almost invariable accompaniment of tuberculous meningitis because the tough exudate readily obstructs the free flow of CSF.

The CSF in tuberculous meningitis is under increased pressure. It may be clear but more often has an opalescent appearance. A fine fibrin web may appear on standing. The number of cells is raised, often to over 200 per μl: usually they are mostly lymphocytes with a few macrophages, but polymorphs may be present and may occasionally exceed the lymphocytes, especially in the earliest stages of the disease. The protein is increased and the glucose and chlorides are diminished. Tubercle bacilli can usually be found on microscopic examination of the centrifuged deposit or of the fibrin web which forms in the fluid on standing.

Appropriate antibiotics should be administered to all suspected cases, even when tubercle bacilli cannot be found in the CSF. Delay in starting treatment may allow the pathological changes to progress to a point from which return to normal is impossible.

Tuberculomas are frequently encountered in regions where tuberculosis is still common, and in some localities they account for a considerable proportion of all intracranial expanding lesions. They occur particularly in children and young adults and may be multiple. The commonest sites are the cerebellum (Fig. 21.30) and brainstem. They are composed of firm, dull yellow, caseous material with a grey fibrous, or more highly vascular, red capsule.

Syphilis

Syphilitic lesions of the central nervous system used to be common and serious. They fall into two groups. Firstly, lesions occurring in the late secondary and tertiary stages, which involve connective tissues and the blood vessels; these comprise meningitis, gummas and endarteritis, either singly or combined. Secondly, *neurosyphilis*, which includes tabes dorsalis and general paralysis of the insane; these occur much later than the tertiary stage, and involve the neural tissue directly.

Syphilitic meningitis is a chronic condition which may involve the dura, the leptomeninges,

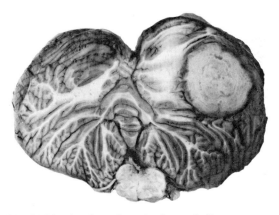

Fig. 21.30 A tuberculoma in the cerebellum.

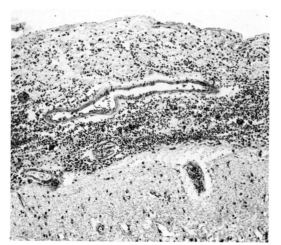

Fig. 21.31 Syphilitic leptomeningitis, showing thickening and lymphocytic infiltration of the pia-arachnoid. × 50.

or both. *Syphilitic leptomeningitis* most commonly affects the pia-arachnoid over the base of the brain. The affected meninges are diffusely thickened and gelatinous, and there may be patches of gummatous necrosis. Various cranial nerves, especially the optic and oculomotor nerves, become involved. The process may obstruct the foramina of the fourth ventricle and cause hydrocephalus.

Microscopy shows a fibroblastic reaction and a heavy infiltrate of lymphocytes and plasma cells (Fig. 21.31) and commonly endarteritis obliterans (Fig. 21.32) with consequent focal infarction in the adjacent cortex. Cellular infiltration occurs round the small penetrating vessels and there is gliosis in the outer layers of the cortex.

Similar lesions occur in the spinal meninges, in which endarteritis and infarction of the cord are prominent. The rare *hypertrophic cervical pachymeningitis* is produced mainly by syphilis: the dura and arachnoid are thickened and adherent, gliosis occurs in the spinal cord, and the nerve roots may be compressed and undergo atrophy.

Meningeal gummas may be multiple in syphilitic meningitis. Gummas of the dura are usually flattened and may cover a large part of a hemisphere (Fig. 21.33): they may erode the skull and/or compress the adjacent brain tissue.

Neurosyphilis

This includes two conditions, *general paralysis of the insane* and *tabes dorsalis*, which occur in a small proportion of patients some years after the tertiary lesions and usually 5–20 years after contracting syphilis. They affect men much more often than women and may occur together. They may also occur in congenital syphilis, usually from 10 years of age onwards. The changes in the neural tissue in these conditions are not due to vascular disease.

General paralysis of the insane (GPI) is a subacute encephalitis with widespread lesions in the nervous system; the resulting symptoms are motor, sensory and psychiatric. *Treponema pallidum* has been demonstrated in the brain, and the Wassermann reaction is usually positive in both blood and CSF.

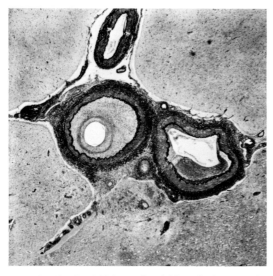

Fig. 21.32 Syphilitic endarteritis of the anterior cerebral arteries. There is also a well-marked syphilitic meningitis. Multiple small infarcts were present in both hemispheres. × 28.

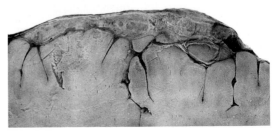

Fig. 21.33 Section of hemisphere showing a large gummatous mass arising in the dura. × 0.5.

Structural changes are most marked in the frontal lobes, where the gyri are atrophic and the sulci widened, with a corresponding increase in CSF. The pia and the arachnoid are thickened and opaque and are unduly adherent to the brain. There may be chronic subdural haematomas. The ventricles are enlarged as a result of cerebral atrophy (secondary hydrocephalus) and there is a granular ependymitis (Fig. 21.2, p. 21.5).

Microscopically, the cortical grey matter is much more cellular than normal, although the number of neurons in it is greatly reduced. The cells include lymphocytes and plasma cells, which are most numerous in the space around the small nutrient vessels, and rod cells (p. 21.6), many of which contain granules of haemosiderin, and which are sometimes conspicuous also in the deep tissues. There is a general increase in glial fibres, while enlarged fibrillary astrocytes are conspicuous, particularly in the superficial cortex and around small blood vessels. Gliosis may extend to the white matter. With effective treatment, the inflammation subsides, leaving residual gliosis, both general and cortical, and loss of nerve cells.

Cerebrospinal fluid. The cells are usually increased to over 50 per μl—mostly lymphocytes but with some macrophages and plasma cells. Protein, particularly IgG, is usually much increased. On immuno-electrophoresis, much of the IgG in the CSF separates into a number of discrete bands, indicating its production in the CNS by plasma cells derived from a small number of B-cell clones. The Lange test gives a paretic pattern (Table 21.1, pp. 21.46–47) and the CSF almost invariably gives a positive Wassermann reaction.

Tabes dorsalis (locomotor ataxia). The lesion in this late syphilitic disorder is a slowly progressive degeneration of the posterior roots of the spinal nerves and secondary degeneration in the posterior columns of the spinal cord. The posterior roots entering the lumbar enlargement of the cord are mainly or solely affected in most cases, but in some the cervical enlargement is affected (*cervical tabes*).

In sections stained by the Weigert-Pal method (Fig. 21.34) the posterior roots, posterior horns and posterior columns all appear pale from loss of myelinated fibres. At higher levels in the cord the posterior roots appear relatively or completely normal, and the posterior column degeneration is confined to the medial (gracile) tract as in ascending degenera-

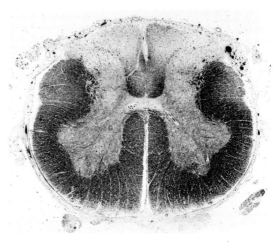

Fig. 21.34 Tabes dorsalis: section through lumbar enlargement of cord, showing degeneration in the posterior roots and posterior columns. × 8. (Weigert-Pal method.)

tions in general (p. 21.49). Degenerative changes may involve the sensory cranial nerves, and involvement of the optic nerves with visual loss is common.

Clinically, there is early loss of proprioceptive sense in muscles and joints in the lower limbs, with loss of co-ordination and ataxia. The posterior root lesion also interrupts the spinal reflex arc, with absence of the knee-jerk, etc. and loss of muscle tone with a characteristic stamping gait. There is also loss of pain sense, and consequent trophic changes are common, e.g. deep ulceration of the soles of the feet, and neuropathic arthropathy (*Charcot's disease*—p. 23.51). Some common clinical features are not satisfactorily explained, for example, the *Argyll-Robertson phenomenon* in which the pupils contract normally during accommodation but not in response to light, abdominal crises which simulate acute surgical emergencies and attacks of 'stabbing pain' in the lower limbs.

In *cervical tabes* the pathological changes are similar and result mainly in disturbances of function in the upper limbs.

The CSF in tabes shows an increase of cells, usually to over 50 per μl; they are mainly lymphocytes but with some macrophages. The protein is normal or slightly raised and, as in GPI, IgG is usually raised and of oligoclonal origin. The Lange test usually gives a luetic reaction (Table 21.1, pp. 21.46–47) and the Wassermann reaction is usually positive.

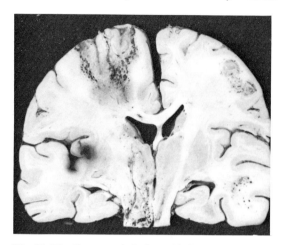

Fig. 21.35   Opportunistic fungal infection. There are several acute haemorrhagic lesions. The causal fungus was *Candida albicans*.

Fungal infections

Fungal infections of the nervous system are invariably secondary to infection elsewhere in the body but lesions at the portal of entry may be small and readily overlooked. The brain, therefore, may appear to be the only organ involved. In other cases, infection of the nervous system may simply be one of the manifestations of a generalised infection. Some fungi, e.g. *Cryptococcus neoformans* and *Coccidioides immitis*, may produce disease in man in the absence of predisposing factors other than increased exposure to the particular fungus. Apart from cryptococcosis (torulosis), these infections are extremely rare in Britain. Both meningitis and brain abscesses caused by fungi are, however, encountered with increasing frequency as opportunistic infections in patients with depressed immunity (p. 7.32 *et seq.*).

Cryptococcosis. The commonest clinical presentation of infection with *Cryptococcus neoformans* (p. 9.37) is as a subacute meningitis. The exudate in the subarachnoid space is rather gelatinous and usually contains masses of encapsulated cryptococci. Flask-shaped cysts filled with cryptococci in the superficial layers of the cortex are frequently found. Inflammatory changes in the brain and subarachnoid space are often remarkably mild but occasionally there is a granulomatous reaction very similar to that seen in tuberculous meningitis.

Opportunistic fungal infections. These are caused mainly by *Candida albicans*, *Aspergillus fumigatus* and *Nocardia asteroides*. They generally produce multiple brain abscesses of various sizes (Fig. 21.35). In the acute stages the abscesses may resemble haemorrhagic infarcts but later they usually become encapsulated. Candida may also cause a florid meningitis. Histological examination usually discloses abundant fungus, particularly at the edges of the abscesses. Accurate identification, however, depends on culture. *Mucormycosis* is a rarer opportunistic infection. It has a particular predilection for uncontrolled diabetic patients. Infection usually commences in the paranasal sinuses and spreads directly into the anterior fossa of the skull to produce selective involvement of the frontal lobes.

Parasitic diseases

Protozoa which cause lesions of the nervous system include *Plasmodium falciparum* (cerebral malaria), *Toxoplasma gondii* (toxoplasmosis), the amoebae *Entamoeba histolytica* ('tropical abscess') and *Naegleri fowleri* (meningo-encephalitis), and various trypanosomes ('sleeping sickness'). **Metazoa** which may involve the nervous system include the tapeworms *Taenia solium* (cysticercosis) and *Echinococcus granulosus* (hydatid disease).

Diseases caused by most of these parasites occur mainly in the tropics and sub-tropics, although some are encountered increasingly elsewhere as a result of increased travel and migration, and toxoplasmosis is world-wide. They are described in Chapter 28.

Viral Infections of the Nervous System

Most patients with a viral infection of the CNS present as cases of either *'aseptic' leptomeningitis* or *encephalitis*, although some degree of both (meningo-encephalitis) is often present. In some types of encephalitis due, for example, to the polioviruses (i.e. viruses which destroy neurons), the most severe lesions occur in the spinal cord, where there is selective involvement of motor neurons, presenting clinically as paralysis. Viral meningitis (e.g. in mumps) is the commonest clinical illness but relatively little is known about its pathology since it is rarely fatal. By contrast, encephalitis usually causes severe and frequently fatal brain damage.

Acute viral diseases of the nervous system have long been recognised but only relatively recently has the nature of **persistent viral infections,** e.g. subacute sclerosing panencephalitis (p. 21.36), and **slow viral infections**, e.g. kuru (p. 21.37), been appreciated.

Pathogenesis

Most viruses reach the nervous system by way of the bloodstream, i.e. there is a viraemia, often after primary replication of the virus in lymphoid tissue. They may enter the body by various routes, e.g. infection of the skin, or mucous membranes (herpes simplex virus), by the alimentary tract (enteroviruses), through injured skin (B virus of monkeys), or by the bite of an arthropod (arboviruses). A few viruses reach the nervous system by travelling along peripheral nerves (e.g. rabies virus).

Symptoms of virus infections of the nervous system frequently occur late, when viraemia is subsiding and circulating antibody has appeared. This suggests that at least a proportion of the brain damage is brought about by immunological reactions to viral antigens in the nervous system.

Only a small proportion of individuals infected by potentially *neurotropic viruses* (i.e. viruses with a predilection for the nervous system) develop clinical evidence of neurological disease.

Viruses of the herpes group

The nervous system may be affected by at least four viruses in the herpes group—herpes simplex, varicella-zoster, B virus of monkeys and cytomegalovirus. All are DNA viruses of similar morphology.

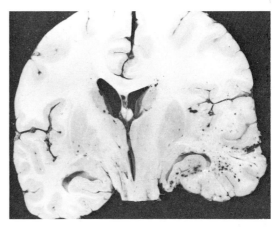

Fig. 21.36 Acute necrotising encephalitis due to herpes simplex virus. Within the swollen right temporal lobe there are many small haemorrhagic foci.

Herpes simplex virus infection

This causes three types of disease in the CNS. The most severe is *acute necrotising encephalitis*, the commonest type of acute encephalitis in Western Europe. The others consist of *foci of necrosis* throughout the brain associated with similar lesions in other organs and tissues in disseminated herpes simplex virus infection in infants, and *aseptic meningitis* (see above).

Acute necrotising encephalitis is fulminating and often rapidly fatal. The lesions consist of widespread, large irregular-shaped patches of necrosis, readily visible at autopsy. They are bilateral but asymmetrical and involve the temporal lobes most severely. At autopsy, there is usually flattening of the convolutions and raised intracranial pressure, while the more severely affected temporal lobe is soft, swollen and often focally haemorrhagic (Fig. 21.36). There is often also an ipsilateral tentorial hernia (see p. 21.7). Necrosis usually occurs also in the insulae and in the cingulate gyri. *Microscopic examination* shows diffuse infiltration of the meninges and perivascular spaces by lymphocytes and plasma cells and, where necrosis has occurred, there are numerous plasma cells and macrophages in the affected brain tissue. In the cortex adjacent to the zones of necrosis, intranuclear inclusion bodies may be found within neurons and astrocytes in some cases (Fig. 21.37a) and the virus particles can be seen by electron microscopy (Fig. 21.37b). Neuronophagia is seen widely throughout the brain and spinal cord. The diagnosis of herpes simplex

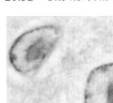

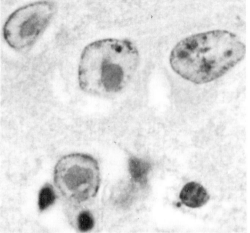

Fig. 21.37a Acute necrotising encephalitis. Note the presence of intranuclear inclusion bodies. × 1200.

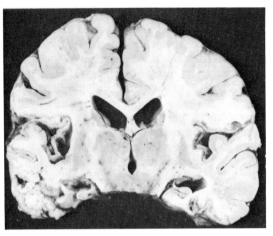

Fig. 21.38 Acute necrotising encephalitis. This patient survived for several weeks. The affected regions are now shrunken and focally cystic. The left temporal lobe is more severely affected than the right one.

Herpes zoster

This is a disease of adults, caused by the varicella-zoster (v-z) virus that also causes varicella (chickenpox). During the illness there is often a rise in the antibody titre against the virus to levels above those commonly seen in varicella. Adults with herpes zoster sometimes infect susceptible children, who develop varicella. The reverse, however, is very rare, and it appears that herpes zoster is the result of recrudescence of a latent infection with v-z virus in a partially immune subject. Herpes zoster results from acute inflammation of a posterior root ganglion, most commonly one of the lower cervical or dorsal ganglia. In one type of herpes zoster the Gasserian ganglion is affected. Pain and hyperalgesia occur along the course of the nerve related to the affected ganglion, followed by erythema and the formation of vesicles containing a serous or haemorrhagic exudate. The acutely inflamed ganglion is swollen by haemorrhagic exudate and heavily infiltrated with lymphocytes, while the nerve cells show various degrees of acute injury (Fig. 21.39): many of them undergo necrosis while in other areas they appear almost normal. The inflammatory process may extend into the dorso-lateral quadrant of the spinal cord at the level of the affected ganglion. Central chromatolysis is commonly seen in the neurons of the anterior horn and there may be paresis.

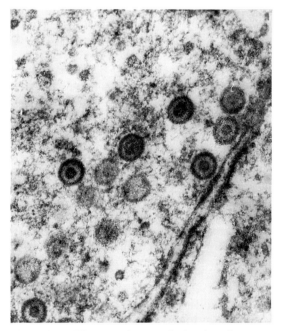

Fig. 21.37b Electron micrograph showing virus particles within the nucleus of a neuron in a case of herpes encephalitis. × 82 000.

encephalitis during life rests on the isolation of virus from a brain biopsy or demonstration of an increasing ratio of CSF/serum antibody titres: virus cannot usually be isolated from the CSF. If the patient survives the acute phase, the necrotic tissue becomes shrunken and cystic (Fig. 21.38).

with paralysis of cranial nerves and the respiratory muscles, usually progressing to coma and death within two weeks. Histological examination shows a *multifocal necrotising encephalitis* affecting grey and white matter, sometimes with a particular predilection for the spinal cord.

Cytomegalovirus

Involvement of the nervous system by cytomegalovirus is mainly due to infection acquired *in utero*. In the neonate it presents as an acute, often severe, *disseminated necrotising encephalomyelitis* with selective involvement of periventricular tissue. Cytomegalic inclusions may be found in various types of cell. Survivors are almost always mentally retarded; the principal abnormalities in the brain are hydrocephalus and periventricular calcification. Infection early in pregnancy may lead to developmental malformations such as microgyria (p. 21.47). Severe disease does not invariably result from fetal infection; mild or asymptomatic infection is also seen, but even the mild infection may lead to some degree of mental impairment.

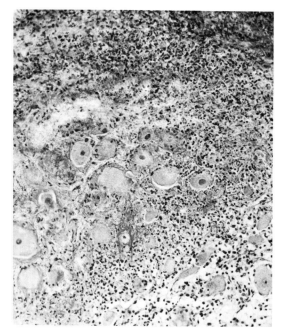

Fig. 21.39 Section of posterior root ganglion in herpes zoster, showing inflammatory infiltration and destruction of nerve cells. × 160.

The nerve cell injury is followed by Wallerian degeneration (shown by Marchi's method) along the nerve fibres to their peripheral distribution, and also proximally through the posterior nerve roots and for a distance upwards in the posterior columns of the cord. Later, secondary fibrosis occurs in the inflamed root ganglia.

What produces reactivation of the latent virus is not clear, but physical trauma to the affected part seems to be a fairly frequent precipitating factor. Immunological disturbances may also be involved, for herpes zoster is common in patients with a malignant lymphoma, in whom the lesions may become disseminated with a *generalised varicelliform rash*, particularly in patients treated with cytotoxic drugs or corticosteroids. In such cases there may also be a *multifocal necrotising encephalomyelitis*.

B-virus encephalomyelitis

B virus is a natural parasite of monkeys in which it causes stomatitis and viraemia. Transmission to man is by a monkey bite or by contamination of a skin wound by saliva or tissues from an infected monkey. The human disease is an acute encephalomyelitis

Enteroviruses

The most important enteroviruses are the polioviruses, coxsackie and ECHO viruses. All are small RNA viruses. They are a frequent cause of *aseptic meningitis* but they may also cause *paralytic disease*, e.g. acute anterior poliomyelitis, which is classically associated with the polioviruses, but is caused occasionally by other enteroviruses, particularly Coxsackie A7. Indeed, in countries where a vigorous poliovirus immunisation programme has been undertaken, coxsackie virus may now be a commoner cause of paralytic disease than the polioviruses. Overt paralysis probably occurs in no more than about 1% of individuals infected with the most pathogenic poliovirus—type I.

Acute anterior poliomyelitis

This is an acute encephalomyelitis affecting especially severely the anterior horns of the spinal cord, and leading to destruction of the motor neurons, with corresponding paralysis and subsequent atrophy of the related muscles.

Epidemiology and virology. Before the introduction of poliovaccine, this was the commonest acute viral encephalomyelitis. It may occur sporadically but also in both major and minor epidemics. Three types of poliovirus have been distinguished and immunity to one type does not protect against the others. Most cases of paralytic poliomyelitis are caused by type I virus.

In man the natural route of infection is by the mouth and the virus replicates in the epithelium of the alimentary tract. It is often present in the naso-pharyngeal secretions of a person suffering from the disease but is most readily isolated from the faeces, where it may persist for long after the acute illness. There is an early viraemia and the infection reaches the central nervous system by crossing the blood–brain barrier.

In the past, endemic poliomyelitis affected young children almost exclusively. In the large epidemics of paralytic disease which swept through countries with a high standard of living (and hygiene) in the years before and just after World War II, there were however proportionately more cases in adults. *The infectivity rate of poliovirus is high but most of those infected develop either no symptoms or only a mild febrile illness.* Only a few develop severe neurological lesions. The development of paralytic disease is partly determined by factors such as muscular fatigue during the initial stage of the illness, or by local tissue damage, e.g. by intramuscular injections, such as those used in the immunisation of children by combined prophylactics, especially those containing alum. Infected adults are more likely than children to develop paralysis. The occurrence of epidemics of paralytic disease in countries with high standards of hygiene was attributable to the relatively low incidence of infection in childhood, adults encountering the virus for the first time being at greater risk of developing severe, paralytic disease. By contrast, in countries with poor standards of hygiene, most people encounter the infection in childhood, and so the risk of paralytic disease is less.

Structural changes. The virus selectively attacks the neurons in the ventral horns of the spinal cord, particularly in the lumbar and cervical enlargements, which are affected asymmetrically. Macroscopic examination in an acute case reveals little beyond congestion of the meninges over the affected part of the cord and of the ventral horns which may be necrotic and haemorrhagic.

Microscopic examination reveals extensive inflammatory infiltration of the leptomeninges, with lymphocytes, plasma cells, and some neutrophil polymorphs but no fibrin. The infiltrate extends along the perforating vessels, especially branches of the anterior spinal arteries (Fig. 21.40).

In the anterior horns there is intense congestion and oedema along with the cellular infiltration; some of the smallest vessels may be thrombosed and there may be capillary

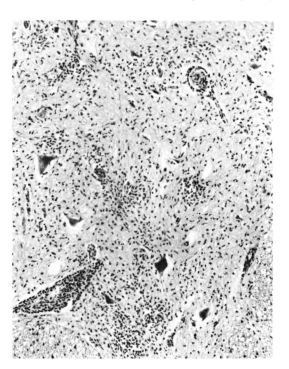

Fig. 21.40 Ventral horn of lumbar cord in poliomyelitis fatal on the 5th day. Note the perivascular cuffing, the general inflammatory infiltration and neuronophagia of dead nerve cells.

haemorrhages. Some of the nerve cells undergo acute necrosis, and are removed by phagocytes (Fig. 21.41). If the nerve cell dies, disintegration of its axon and myelin sheath follows. Other nerve cells show varying degrees of central chromatolysis, although some appear normal or nearly so. The adjacent white matter usually shows only perivascular cuffing by mononuclear cells.

Sometimes the virus affects the motor nuclei in the medulla, causing *acute bulbar paralysis*. There may also be involvement of neurons in

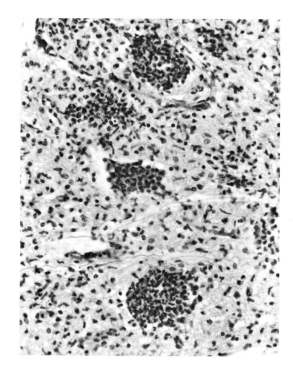

Fig. 21.41 Ventral horn of lumbar cord in acute poliomyelitis (5th day). Each of the dense cellular aggregates is a dead neuron which is obscured by polymorphs and macrophages (neuronophagia).

the motor and pre-motor areas of the cerebral cortex.

Effects. Neuronal injury stops within a few days, but the infiltrate of lymphocytes and plasma cells may persist for some months. In the acute illness, there is paralysis of the muscles supplied by damaged neurons. Since many of the less severely injured neurons recover, the paralysis may improve considerably. The destructive lesions in the cord are followed by removal of the degenerated tissue by macrophages, with subsequent gliosis. Gradually the affected parts shrink, and if the lesion has been severe, the ventral horns become very small, and the anterior nerve roots thin. The permanently affected muscle fibres undergo typical neurogenic atrophy (Fig. 21.88, p. 21.72). Owing to the unopposed action of the unaffected muscles, deformities of the limbs, including various forms of club-foot etc., develop. The bones in the affected limbs may show atrophy, being reduced both in thickness and in density (Fig. 3.18, p. 3.21).

Rabies

Rabies is still a major problem in Central and Eastern Europe, in India and in some parts of North and South America. Its incidence in animals is increasing in Europe. The virus enters the body in the saliva of biting animals and reaches the CNS by travelling along peripheral nerves. The major reservoirs of the virus are the fox, the skunk, the jackal and the bat, although most human cases result from the bite of a rabid dog or cat. The incubation period of the disease in man is usually between one and two months: rabies may be of the restless type, corresponding to the 'furious' rabies of dogs, or, much less commonly, of the paralytic type. Spasm of the muscles of swallowing on attempting to drink water is a prominent and early symptom, and accounts for the old name, *hydrophobia*.

At autopsy, the brain and cord may appear grossly normal or congested. Microscopy shows a diffuse acute encephalomyelitis in which various degrees of neuronal injury, up to necrosis and neuronophagia, are accompanied by congestion, perivascular cuffing with lymphocytes and plasma cells, and aggregation of macrophages. A characteristic feature are the **Negri bodies**—large, sharply defined, round or oval acidophilic inclusion bodies, one or more of which may be seen in the cytoplasm of individual neurons. They are usually most conspicuous in the pyramidal cells of the hippocampus and in Purkinje cells in the cerebellum. Negri bodies consist of nucleocapsid viral material which may be demonstrated by immunofluorescence; the virus spreads centrifugally from the central nervous system along peripheral nerves and invades many tissues; it may be detected immunohistologically in a skin biopsy or in corneal cells.

In classical rabies the dorsal root ganglia, lower brainstem and hypothalamus are principally affected. In the paralytic form, abnormalities are more severe in the lower parts of the spinal cord and in the medulla.

When someone is bitten by a dog suspected of having rabies, the animal should not be killed, for its survival for a week excludes the diagnosis. Rabies can be diagnosed in animals by the histological identification of Negri bodies in the brain.

Other viral infections

Arboviruses

Arboviruses are RNA viruses that are transmitted from host to host by blood-sucking insects (**ar**thropod-**bo**rne viruses). They multiply in both vertebrate and invertebrate hosts. An arthropod vector is infected by sucking blood from a vertebrate and, after an incubation period, the virus reaches the salivary gland of the arthropod whose bite infects a new host: after an interval during which viral replication occurs, there is a period of viraemia during which other arthropods may bite and become infected. Man is not the natural host for any arbovirus but during periods of epizootic spread among the natural hosts (usually wild birds and small mammals), he may become infected.

Several arboviruses can cause severe encephalitis in man, e.g. *St Louis encephalitis, Eastern and Western equine encephalomyelitis* and *Japanese B encephalitis*, all of which are mosquito-borne. The structural changes are in general those of a disseminated encephalitis, sometimes with focal necrosis in vessel walls. Tick-borne arboviruses are responsible for *Russian spring-summer encephalitis* and *louping ill*.

Encephalitis lethargica

This was the first pandemic encephalitis in modern times, and its sudden appearance, rapid pandemic spread and subsequent disappearance are not the least of its mysterious features since its cause was never established. It is however generally accepted that the disease was a virus encephalitis. A small epidemic with a mortality rate of about 50% occurred in Vienna in the winter of 1916–17. The disease then spread through Western Europe, and reached North America towards the end of 1918. The epidemic reached its peak in Britain in 1924. It had virtually disappeared from there by 1926.

The symptoms were those of an acute generalised encephalitis, often with disturbed sleep rhythm and extreme lethargy by day. The mortality averaged about 25%. A high proportion of patients who survived developed permanent Parkinsonism (see p. 21.45).

If the patient died in the acute stages of the disease, there was characteristically intense congestion of the meninges, the cerebral cortex, the basal ganglia and the brainstem. Microscopical examination showed infiltration of the meninges and perivascular cuffing by lymphocytes and plasma cells (Fig. 21.42) and sometimes haemorrhages into perivascular sheaths and adjacent tissue. Thrombosis of small vessels was sometimes present. Although many nerve

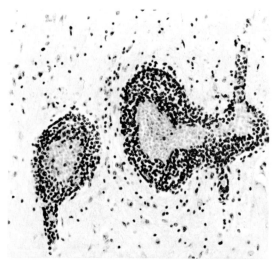

Fig. 21.42   Section of posterior part of medulla in encephalitis lethargica, showing the extensive perivascular infiltration by lymphocytes and plasma cells. × 170.

cells showed evidence of chromatolysis, neuronophagia was slight.

Subacute sclerosing panencephalitis (SSPE)

This is a **persistent virus infection** of the nervous system caused by the measles virus, which can be detected in brain biopsies. It is a rare form of prolonged encephalitis, occurring mainly between the ages of 4 and 20 years, and usually fatal in 6 weeks to 6 months. In the early stages there are personality changes and intellectual deterioration, followed by a stage of periodic involuntary movements and finally profound dementia and decerebrate rigidity.

SSPE occurs some years after an apparently uncomplicated attack of measles. Its pathogenesis is not understood, but it appears to be due to reactivation of measles virus which has remained latent in the brain since the time of primary infection. There are high levels of both IgM and IgG classes of antibodies to measles virus in the blood and CSF. The CSF antibody levels are not only higher than the serum levels, but on immuno-electrophoresis of the CSF they separate into distinct bands, indicating that antibody-producing plasma cells in the CNS are derived from a small number of B lymphocyte clones.

In measles and some other virus infections, cell-mediated immunity to various antigens is reduced. It is not known what role this plays in SSPE.

At autopsy, the brain may appear almost normal, but the white matter is often abnormally firm. Microscopic examination shows the features of a subacute meningo-encephalitis with widespread cuffing of vessels throughout the brain with lymphocytes and plasma cells. Neuronophagia is common, and varying numbers of residual neurons contain intra-nuclear and/or cytoplasmic inclusion bodies. There is also considerable gliosis in the white matter.

Subacute spongiform encephalopathy

The discovery and investigation of **kuru** has been one of the most dramatic occurrences in the entire field of diseases of the nervous system in the past two decades. It is a subacute disease of the brain charac-terised by microcystic degeneration in the grey mat-ter, referred to as *status spongiosus*, associated with loss of neurons and a great excess of hypertrophied astrocytes. These changes are particularly severe in the cerebellar system. Kuru is restricted to the Fore tribe and their tribal neighbours in the Eastern High-lands of New Guinea. Its peculiar importance is that it was the first progressive degenerative disease of the nervous system of man to be transmitted to another animal, first the chimpanzee but later to other pri-mates, by injecting extracts of brain tissue from patients with the disease. It is therefore now classi-fied as a **slow virus infection** although the agent, which is filterable and capable of replicating, has not been identified. Cannibalism was the primary mode of transmission, and the incidence of the disease has subsided since this practice ceased.

A second progressive degenerative disease of the nervous system, **Creutzfeldt-Jakob disease**, has been shown to be transmissible to other primates (and accidentally to man). It is a progressive dementia of world-wide distribution, again characterised by sta-tus spongiosus and astrocytosis. Kuru and Creutz-feldt-Jakob disease along with two transmissible di-seases of the nervous system in animals (*scrapie* of

sheep and *mink encephalopathy* which are both caused by the same agent), are now classified as *subacute spongiform encephalopathies*. All of these conditions appear to be due to slow viruses, have an exception-ally long incubation period, and have an unremitting and always fatal progressive course. The transmiss-ible agents have so far not been shown to be antigenic in that antibody has not yet been demonstrated.

Progressive multifocal leukoencephalopathy (PML)

This condition is an opportunistic infection caused by a papovavirus (JC virus) morpho-logically similar to polyoma virus. As its name implies, PML is characterised by multiple foci of degeneration in the brain, particularly in the white matter.

The most characteristic macroscopic feature is the presence of multiple small grey foci distributed widely but usually asymmetrically in the white mat-ter. These foci can coalesce to form large grey areas which may become cystic. Microscopy shows multiple foci of demyelination accompanied by lipo-phages, abnormal oligodendrocytes with large hyper-chromatic nuclei containing ill-defined inclusion bodies, and usually large and bizarre astrocytes. Most patients who develop the disease already have a disseminated malignant lymphoid neoplasm or leukaemia and it has been suggested that the virus may remain latent following a symptomless primary infection. Antibody to the virus is common in the community and PML occurs when immunological deficiency develops, due to the lymphoma or to immunosuppressive therapy.

Demyelinating Diseases

The cardinal feature of these disorders is destruction of myelin with relative preservation of axons. They are quite distinct from genetic disorders of myelin formation—*dysmyelination* (p. 21.42), and from diseases causing breakdown of myelin secondary to neuronal destruction—*Wallerian degeneration* (p. 21.4). The group includes acute conditions associated with considerable inflammatory exudation—**acute disseminated perivenous encephalomyelitis** and **acute haemorrhagic leukoencephalitis**—and chronic disorders in which there is conspicuous fibrillary gliosis in the demyelinated areas, the

most important being **multiple** or **disseminated sclerosis**. Forms intermediate in both clinical and pathological features are not uncommon.

Acute disseminated perivenous encephalomyelitis

This disease, also known as post-infectious encephalitis, develops as an unusual sequel to (a) various acute virus diseases such as measles, rubella or varicella; (b) respiratory infections presumed to be viral, and (c) primary vaccina-tion against smallpox (post-vaccinial encephal-itis) and anti-rabies inoculation (p. 21.35). The onset is often sudden, occurring between 5 and 14 days after the clinical onset of the initial infection: the prognosis is generally good.

The lesions in the nervous system are mainly around small venules throughout the brain and spinal cord, but often affect most severely the ventral half of the pons, the deeper layers of the cerebral cortex, the thalamus and the white matter of the cerebral hemispheres. The brain usually appears normal macroscopically but the characteristic histological features are perivenular demyelination (Fig. 21.43) associated with

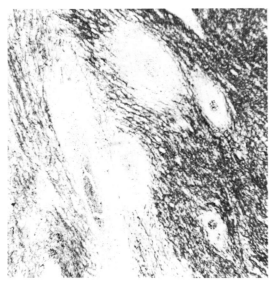

Fig. 21.43 Acute demyelinating encephalomyelitis following measles. A section showing perivascular demyelination in the white matter of the brain. (Loyez stain: myelin stained black.) × 60.

inflammatory oedema and perivenular infiltration mainly by neutrophil polymorphs in the acute stage and later by lymphocytes and macrophages. Demyelination occurs very rapidly, being sometimes almost complete within 4 days. Axons are relatively unaffected and there may be a slight increase of lymphocytes and macrophages in the meninges. The lesions are therefore quite different, both in character and distribution, from those of acute viral encephalitis due to the presence of a known virus in the central nervous system.

Aetiology

It is widely accepted that acute disseminated perivenous encephalomyelitis represents a delayed hypersensitivity reaction in the CNS in which the precipitating virus infection leads to the development of an auto-immune response against neural tissue antigen(s). The possibility of an immune reaction against virus, or virus-infected cells, cannot, however, be completely excluded as the cause.

Acute haemorrhagic leukoencephalitis

This relatively uncommon disease may also occur as a sequel to any one of several possible viral infections and it may also complicate septic shock, treatment with various drugs, and various other diseases assumed to be hypersensitivity reactions, e.g. asthma and acute glomerulonephritis. The course is rapid and usually fatal within a few days. At autopsy the brain is swollen and there are numerous petechial haemorrhages, particularly in the white matter, the macroscopic appearances being very similar to those observed in cerebral fat embolism or cerebral malaria.

Microscopic examination shows focal necrosis of the walls of venules and arterioles, perivascular 'ball and ring' haemorrhages, and perivascular demyelination, often with infiltration first by neutrophil polymorphs and later by lymphocytes and macrophages, cerebral oedema and an inflammatory exudate in the meninges. Some consider the condition to be a hyperacute variant of acute disseminated perivenous encephalomyelitis, and to be caused by the deposition of immune complexes and activation of complement.

Multiple (Disseminated) sclerosis (MS)

This fairly common disease is characterised by patchy demyelination and gliosis of the brain and cord. It usually starts before 50 years of age and most often in adolescents and young adults. Typically, the course is episodic, acute attacks of demyelination occurring at irregular intervals, and resulting in increasing disability. In some cases, however, the intervening periods of remission extend over years, and the rate of progress and severity vary considerably. In many cases, the disease becomes relentlessly progressive in the later stages, but occasionally is steadily progressive from the start. A common early symptom is an acute unilateral **optic neuritis** which progresses to some degree of optic atrophy: other symptoms and signs include sensory disturbances, pareses and bladder dysfunction.

Structural changes

The clinical features of MS are caused by patchy demyelination of irregular distribution in the brain and spinal cord, the area of demyelination being referred to as a **plaque**. Acute lesions are yellowish and soft; they are rounded or irregularly shaped and measure 10 mm or so across.

Microscopically, the changes are those of acute demyelination with infiltration by lipid-containing macrophages and perivascular cuffing by lymphocytes and plasma cells. As the plaque ages, the cellular infiltration subsides and vascular thickening and gliosis occur, but without much contraction or distortion. The partial clinical recovery from the disabling effects of the acute lesions is probably due to subsidence of inflammatory oedema in and around the acute lesions since the demyelinated axons may persist and function for a long time. Many of the axons eventually undergo Wallerian degeneration. The nerve cells in a plaque usually show little or no abnormality. Old plaques are firm, grey and slightly translucent. They are readily visible in the unstained brain

or cord (Fig. 21.44) and are seen as conspicuous pale areas in sections stained by the Weigert-Pal method, which demonstrates complete loss of myelin and a fairly sharp line of demarcation from the adjacent normal tissue (Fig. 21.45). Smaller plaques, up to a few millimetres across, are usually round or oval; larger ones are irregular, and may result from the confluence of smaller plaques. In a typical case with a prolonged episodic course, most of the lesions seen at autopsy are old: they vary greatly in number, size and distribution, but are usually most easily seen in the white matter of the cerebrum, particularly at the angles of the lateral ventricles and at the junction of the cortex and white

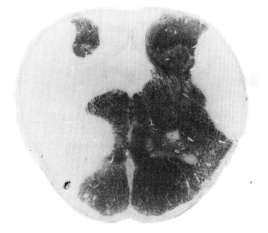

Fig. 21.45 Multiple sclerosis. Section through the lower part of the medulla. The demyelinated plaques appear pale. (Weigert–Pal method.)

matter. Plaques do, however, occur in the cortex and central grey matter. They are common in the brainstem, particularly around the aqueduct and fourth ventricle, and in the spinal cord. If there is a history of retrobulbar neuritis, a plaque can usually be found in the optic nerve.

The CSF in MS may contain more than 5 lymphocytes per μl, particularly during an acute episode, and lipid-containing macrophages and plasma cells may also be present. The protein levels may be normal or slightly increased; IgG is often moderately increased and, as stated below, may be oligoclonal: the demonstration of a 'paretic' reaction in the Lange colloidal gold test is a less sensitive indication of changes in the protein content.

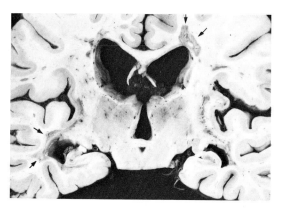

Fig. 21.44 Multiple sclerosis. There are several well-defined round or oval grey plaques of demyelination in each cerebral hemisphere and a group of coalescent plaques (*arrows*).

Aetiology

Genetic and environmental factors both appear to be of importance in MS. Genetic factors are suggested by a 70% incidence of the HLA antigen DW2 in patients (cf 16% in the general population), and slightly increased incidences of HLA-A3 and B7. Epidemiological studies point to an environmental factor being of importance in childhood, for there are considerable differences in the incidence of MS in various parts of the world, and people who migrate from one area to another after the age of about 14 retain the incidence of their childhood locality. There is an increasing incidence of MS among siblings (particularly twins) and parents of patients with the disease, but it is not known whether this is attributable to genetic or environmental factors or to a combination of both.

There is evidence of an immune reaction in MS, notably an increase of lymphocytes in the CSF, and of lymphocytes and plasma cells in the acute lesions. As in subacute sclerosing panencephalitis, neurosyphilis and the Guillain-Barré syndrome, immuno-eletrophoresis of the CSF demonstrates bands of homogeneous IgG, indicating IgG production by plasma cells derived from a small number of B lymphocyte clones. These immunological factors could be interpreted as indicating either a response to a neurotropic virus or an auto-immune response to a neural tissue component, as in experimental auto-allergic encephalomyelitits (see below). In support of a viral infection, the titres of antibody to measles virus are relatively high in both the serum and CSF, and antibodies to some other viruses are also raised. Isolation of various viruses from MS tissue has indeed been reported, and virus-like particles have been detected by electron microscopy in MS tissue, but the findings are conflicting and no persistent pattern has emerged. Nor does the disease resemble known persistent or slow virus infections of the CNS in man or animals (p. 21.37). Current investigations using genetic probes may prove to be more rewarding. In support of an auto-immune aetiology, antibodies which, together with complement, cause demyelination of cultures of neural tissue, have been detected in the serum of MS patients. However, they occur also in various non-demyelinating diseases and, despite many studies, the evidence is inconclusive. Also, acute demyelination complicating rabies prophylaxis in man (see below) and in experimental allergic encephalomyelitis (both of which appear to have an auto-immune pathogenesis) occurs as a single acute episode and is perivenular, in contrast to the recurrent episodes of MS, in which plaques are much larger and show no obvious relationship to small vessels.

Experimental auto-allergic encephalomyelitis (EAE) is produced in various species of animal by the injection of homogenised neural tissue, of the same or a different species, emulsified in Freund's adjuvant (p. 6.30). The disease develops after a latent period of 10 days or more, is believed to be due to the development of an immune response to neural tissue antigen in the inoculum, and a subsequent immunological reaction with the animal's own neural tissue. The antigen is a basic protein present in myelin and an encephalitogenic fragment has been isolated and synthesised but differs for different species. The presence of antibody in the serum does not correlate well with the occurrence of the disease, and there is strong evidence that the lesions result from a delayed auto-hypersensitivity reaction in which sensitised lymphocytes and possibly macrophages react directly with the encephalitogenic components of myelin.

In some species the changes are similar to those of acute disseminated perivenous encephalomyelitis in man, which develops 10 days or so after the predisposing virus infection, and may be caused by a similar immunological reaction (p. 21.38). Although EAE can be induced by one injection of antigen in Freund's adjuvant, its production in monkeys without the use of Freund's adjuvant requires many injections. An acute demyelinating encephalitis of similar nature sometimes results in man from multiple injections of anti-rabies vaccine prepared from infected rabbit spinal cord tissue. Use of vaccine prepared from infected duck embryo appears to avoid this complication.

As mentioned earlier, acute perivenous encephalomyelitis and EAE are monophasic illnesses, whereas multiple sclerosis is essentially a chronic relapsing condition. There are, however, certain similarities between acute perivenous encephalomyelitis and MS and recently a chronic relapsing model of EAE has been described in which the pathology is very similar to that of MS.

In conclusion, the lesions of MS present features suggestive of an immunological reaction, but there is no convincing evidence pointing to either a virus or a component of brain tissue as the antigen. Claims that the lesions result from a biochemical disturbance or a toxin have also been made, but they too lack strong supporting evidence.

Variants of multiple sclerosis include *neuromyelitis optica* (*Devic type*) and *sudanophilic diffuse sclerosis*.

Neuromyelitis optica is a disease of adults characterised by rapid loss of vision and the development of paraplegia. As in MS, extensive demyelinating lesions develop in the brain and cord, but particularly in the optic nerves. The disease is commonly preceded by fever; it runs a more acute course than MS and the lesions are more severely destructive, but the two diseases cannot be sharply distinguished.

Sudanophilic diffuse sclerosis This condition is a severe and usually acute progressive form of demyelinating disease, usually of childhood and not to be confused with a leukodystrophy (p. 21.42). There is widespread degeneration of the cerebral white matter, notably in the occipital lobes (hence the common occurrence of early visual impairment), but any part of the cerebral hemispheres, cerebellum or brainstem may be affected. Typically, the subcortical arcuate fibres are spared and stand out as a conspicuous white band in the affected areas. In Weigert-Pal preparations, demyelination is seen to be less sharply demarcated than in MS and shades off marginally into normal white matter. In the affected areas, macrophages filled with sudanophilic lipid are abundant while the degree of fibrillary gliosis varies with the duration of the disease. Axons are usually lost in the lesions but, apart from occasional neurons showing central chromatolysis, the grey matter is normal.

Other disorders of the central nervous system

Lysosomal disorders

The general features and examples of these disorders have been described on pp. 3.14–15, 18.7 They result from genetically determined deficiencies of particular lysosomal enzymes which play an essential role in the degradation of various normal metabolites or cell break-down products. In consequence, the undegraded material accumulates in, and causes gross enlargement of, the lysosomes of certain cells; the distribution depends on the particular enzyme deficiency. Some of these disorders affect neurons, which become enlarged with a ballooned appearance. The stored material can be detected histochemically, and electron microscopy demonstrates grossly enlarged lysosomes containing non-metabolisable residue, in some instances presenting highly distinctive morphological features diagnostic of a specific disorder. In the early stages, the storage leads to neuronal dysfunction. Ultimately the affected cells die and disappear and in these conditions which affect the nervous system there is atrophy of the brain and gliosis in grey and white matter. Clinically there is retardation or progressive deterioration of mental and motor functions, apathy, lassitude, spastic or flaccid paralysis, fits, often visual disturbances, and ultimately coma and death.

Diagnosis by assay of the relevant lysosomal enzymes in blood, urine, leucocytes or cultured skin fibroblasts is now often possible and has reduced the need for diagnostic biopsy of the brain, nerves, etc. Based on the observed enzyme defects, there are more than 20 known lysosomal storage disorders that can be divided for convenience into two main groups: those that affect neurons (*neuronal storage diseases*), and those that affect the white matter (*leukodystrophies*). In some diseases there is also involvement of other tissues.

Neuronal storage disorders

Principal amongst these are the *gangliosidoses* and the *mucopolysaccharidoses*. One of the commonest gangliosidosis affecting especially the neurons is *Tay Sach's* disease, the classical infantile type of amaurotic familial idiocy. A particularly characteristic sign of this disease (but not restricted to it) is the cherry red spot at the macula due to retinal involvement. Since the abnormal metabolite is ganglioside G_{M2}, this condition is best termed **G_{M2} gangliosidosis**. The missing enzyme is hexosaminidase A and the greatly enlarged lysosomes filled with ganglioside have highly distinctive electron-microscopic appearances: they are known as *membranous cytoplasmic bodies*.

In the *mucopolysaccharidoses* there is a disturbance of glycosaminoglycan metabolism in which there is often considerable overlap in the patterns of involvement of the viscera and brain. Recognised subdivisions of this condition include the *Hunter*, *Hurler* and *Morquio's syndromes* (p. 11.9).

Other neuronal storage disorders include *Gaucher's disease* (deficiency of glucocerebroside β-glucosidase—p. 18.7). *Niemann-Pick disease* (deficiency of sphyngomyelinase—p. 18.7) and a group of conditions affecting infants, older children and occasionally adults in which there is an accumulation of excessive amounts of ceroid material.

Leukodystrophies

This complex group of rare diseases has in common diffuse demyelination and gliosis of the white matter of the cerebral hemispheres, and sometimes also in the cerebellum, the brainstem and the spinal cord. Most forms are genetically determined and occur in childhood: they have also been regarded as *dysmyelinating* diseases in the belief that the myelin is biochemically abnormal before it degenerates. Other cases, however, are apparently non-familial, start in adult life and show inflammatory changes in addition to demyelination.

Some cases of *sudanophilic leukodystrophy* in males are associated with adrenal insufficiency which may precede or accompany the onset of the neurological illness, or may remain subclinical. In the disease known as *adrenoleukodystrophy* the single most reliable test to establish the diagnosis is adrenal biopsy. A characteristic feature is the presence of ballooned vacuolated cortical cells containing linear lamellar bodies with distinctive fine structural features. Similar cytoplasmic occlusions occur in the brain. It has been suggested that the overwhelming majority of males with sudanophilic leukodystrophy are really cases of adrenoleukodystrophy. The cases occurring in males without adrenal changes and in females may represent a variant of multiple sclerosis. The term *Schilder's disease* has been used in the past for leukodystrophy of sudanophilic type. If the term has to be retained, it should now be restricted to cases of adrenoleukodystrophy.

There is an accumulation of metachromatic material within the central nervous system and peripheral nerves in *metachromatic leukodystrophy*. This is a rare familial disease occurring mainly in children between 2 and 5 years of age but not confined to this age group. It is progressive and tends to run a course of one or two years. The basic defect is a genetically-determined deficiency of arylsulphatase. In contrast to myelin destruction in other diseases, myelin is not broken down into neutral fat or cholesterol esters but into metachromatic material containing sulphatides which are PAS+ve and stain brown by cresyl violet or thionine in an acid solution. At autopsy the brain feels unusually firm, and the white matter may be somewhat greyer and more translucent than normal. The subcortical arcuate fibres are usually not spared. Microscopic examination demonstrates widespread loss of myelin in the white matter, the fibre systems which mature last being the most severely affected. Demyelinated areas contain large quantities of intracellular and extracellular metachromatic lipid material which can only be demonstrated satisfactorily in frozen sections. Sudanophilic lipid is present in only small amounts in perivascular phagocytes. The metachromatic material is not restricted to white matter, being demonstrable in neurons and peripheral nerves. It may also be present in other tissues, e.g. liver, pancreas, adrenal and kidney.

A rarer type of leukodystrophy is *Krabbe's disease* (p. 3.14) in which there is deficiency of the enzyme galactocerebroside β-galactosidase, resulting in changes confined to the nervous system. The striking histological feature is the presence of large fused multinucleated macrophages known as *globoid cells*.

Other inborn errors of metabolism

Even though they are not common, these conditions make a considerable contribution to the morbidity and mortality of children. *Neonatal hypothyroidism, phenylketonuria* and *galactosaemia* are the most important of these because they can be detected by screening tests in infants, and brain damage can be prevented or reduced either by replacement therapy or by exclusion of the precursor substances from the diet.

There is increasing evidence that **phenylketonuria** is not a single disease entity but encompasses a heterogeneous collection of disorders that are now referred to as *hyperphenylalaninaemias*. Not unexpectedly, there is genetic heterogeneity, the condition being characterised by one of several defects of phenylalanine hydroxylase activity (which converts phenylalanine to tyrosine), with consequent accumulation of phenylalanine in the blood and tissues and excretion of phenyl-pyruvic acid in the urine. Epileptiform fits, severe mental deficiency and some failure of myelination are the principal findings.

In **galactosaemia** there is hepatosplenomegaly, cataract and mental retardation associated with inability to metabolise galactose because of the absence of the enzyme galactose-1-phosphate uridyl transferase. Galactose-1-phosphate accumulates in the tissues, rises to toxic levels and is excreted in the urine.

Disorders of fructose metabolism have also been recognised, as has brain damage in the **glycogen storage disorders** (p. 3.16), particularly when there is a deficiency of glucose-6-phosphatase.

Despite the severe mental derangement, no specific pathological abnormality has been recognised in the brain in these serious conditions. As in most enzyme

The nervous system and voluntary muscles

disorders, the defective enzyme may be absent or produced in an abnormal form.

Hepatolenticular degeneration (*Wilson's disease*). In this condition (p. 20.32), cirrhosis of the liver is accompanied by brain changes, mainly in the putamen and caudate nucleus, which become soft, shrunken, and ultimately cystic. Neuronal loss is accompanied by a fibrillary gliosis and the occurrence of large astrocytes with strikingly vesicular, swollen nuclei. These are termed *Alzheimer astrocytes*: they are found in cases of chronic liver failure of any cause and may be widely distributed throughout the grey matter. The lesions in the nervous system in hepatolenticular degeneration are due to metabolic disturbances resulting partly from the deposition of copper. A greenish-brown discoloration of the cornea near the limbus (known as the *Kayser-Fleischer ring*) is also due to the deposition of copper. The resulting symptoms are mainly muscular tremors and spasticity.

Acquired metabolic disturbances

One of the more common is acquired hepato-cerebral degeneration in which the signs and symptoms of hepatic encephalopathy develop in patients with liver failure. The acute forms are associated with massive liver cell necrosis and the principal abnormality in the brain is the occurrence of Alzheimer astrocytes (see above). A chronic form may occur in individuals with cirrhosis of the liver and a large porto-systemic venous shunt. Alzheimer astrocytes again occur in the brain but there may also be microcystic degeneration in the basal ganglia and in the deeper layers of the cerebral cortex.

Vitamin B$_1$ (thiamine) deficiency. In addition to causing an axonopathy (p. 21.68), vitamin B$_1$ deficiency sometimes presents as the **Wernicke-Korsakoff syndrome** (Wernicke's encephalopathy). The deficiency may be chronic, as in chronic alcoholism or prolonged malnutrition, or it may be acute, e.g. as a complication of persistent vomiting. Wernicke's encephalopathy caused by an acute vitamin B deficiency is probably much commoner than is generally recognised, but **chronic alcoholism** remains the commonest underlying cause in a well-nourished community. The disorder was common among prisoners-of-war in the Far East during the Second World War and was attributed to an acute dietary deficiency.

Clinically, the onset is acute or subacute: the clinical features include disturbances of consciousness, ophthalmoplegia, nystagmus, and ataxia with, if untreated, terminal coma. The blood pyruvate level is raised and if the deficiency state is chronic there is usually also a peripheral neuropathy. In acutely fatal cases there are numerous petechial haemorrhages in the mamillary bodies, in the floor and walls of the third ventricle, around the aqueduct, in the midbrain and in the floor of the fourth ventricle. The anterior nuclei of the thalamus may also be involved. In subacute cases, macroscopic abnormalities may be restricted to slight granularity and blurring of structural features in the affected areas. Microscopy shows dilatation and proliferation of capillaries and small haemorrhages: the parenchyma stains palely and there are various degrees of reactive change in astrocytes and microglia. Neurons are relatively spared.

Improvement following the administration of the vitamin B group may be dramatic, but a good clinical recovery is unlikely if the mamillary bodies are already structurally damaged before treatment is started. They become shrunken and often have a brownish discoloration on section. Such patients usually have a persistent psychosis of Korsakoff type.

Other alcohol-related disorders of the nervous system include the **fetal alcohol syndrome**, which is thought to be due to a direct cytotoxic effect of alcohol on the developing brain. **In adults**, alcoholism is associated with *cerebral atrophy*, *degeneration of the cerebellum*, and *demyelination of the pons* (*central pontine myelinolysis*) *and of the corpus callosum* (*Marchiafava-Bignami disease*). Most of the patients are likely to be deficient in multiple vitamins, due partly to the restricted diet and partly to deficient absorption from the alimentary canal because of associated gastro-intestinal disturbances.

Deficiency of vitamin B$_{12}$ causes *subacute combined degeneration of the cord* (p. 21.53).

Various chemicals are toxic to the nervous system. These include, for example, both the organic and inorganic forms of *lead, mercury, tin,* and various industrial agents such as *solvents* and *pesticides*.

Kernicterus. When severe **jaundice** occurs in

infancy it carries the risk of brain injury: necrosis of neurons and bile staining are seen particularly in the hippocampus and basal nuclei (*kernicterus* or *nuclear jaundice*) and sometimes in the cerebral cortex, and are followed by gliosis. If not fatal, the brain injury is likely to cause choreo-athetosis, spasticity and often mental deficiency. The condition is particularly likely to occur when the plasma level of unconjugated bilirubin exceeds 250 μmol/litre (15 mg/100 ml), and by far the commonest cause of this in full-term Caucasian infants is haemolytic anaemia due to fetal-maternal Rh incompatibility (p. 17.30). In some other ethnic groups, haemolysis due to G-6-PD deficiency is an important cause (p. 17.25). Other causal factors include functional immaturity of the liver in premature infants, liver injury of various kinds and genetically determined defects in bilirubin conjugation (p. 20.54). Hypoxia during labour or at birth, or due to severe anaemia, may be contributory factors and the administration of excess vitamin K analogues (for haemorrhagic disease in the newborn) tends to aggravate haemolysis and so may increase the jaundice.

In the fetus, bilirubin is excreted by the placenta, so jaundice becomes severe only after birth. This can be minimised by an exchange blood transfusion (p. 17.30).

Disorders of the nervous system in cancer

The nervous system may be implicated by malignant tumours arising elsewhere by direct or metastatic invasion of the brain, spinal cord and peripheral nerves, or by compression of the cord by extradural tumour. **Indirect (paraneoplastic** or **non-metastatic) effects** also occur in the nervous system, the commonest being a *peripheral neuropathy* (p. 21.67) which may be predominantly motor or sensory, or of mixed type. Other conditions in this group are a **myasthenic syndrome** (p. 21.76), a **diffuse encephalomyelitis** characterised by perivascular cuffing by lymphocytes and affecting particularly the medial parts of the temporal lobes—**limbic encephalitis**, and **subacute cerebellar atrophy** characterised by a severe loss of Purkinje cells and degeneration of the long motor and sensory tracts in the spinal cord. These changes are found most often in, but not confined to, patients with bronchial carcinoma. Neurological symptoms not infrequently precede local ones caused by the tumour itself. In longstanding malignant lymphomas and in widespread involvement of the lymphoreticular tissues by other conditions, e.g. carcinomatosis or sarcoidosis, the brain may show many irregularly distributed areas of demyelination and an unusually severe degree of astrocytic hyperplasia. The term *progressive multifocal leukoencephalopathy* is applied to this condition (p. 21.37).

The dementias

Dementia is a generalised disturbance of higher mental functions in an otherwise alert patient. It may be brought about by more or less extensive destruction or disorganisation of the cortex, white matter and subcortical (nuclear) structures, either singly or in combination, by one or more pathological processes. The causes of dementia are therefore numerous but a classification has been evolved into (**a**) *the primary organic dementias* in which the principal damage occurs in the cerebral cortex (in some cases there is associated extrapyramidal and spinal tract degeneration), and (**b**) *secondary dementias* resulting from some other primary abnormality in the brain, e.g. a deeply seated tumour or diffuse processes such as general paralysis of the insane, toxic and metabolic disturbances, various infections, and hydrocephalus. By far the commonest type of secondary dementia, however, is that produced by *ischaemic brain damage*, and called *multi-infarct* or *arteriopathic dementia*.

Primary organic dementias

These conditions are usually relentlessly and slowly progressive, and have fairly specific pathological features. Common to all is *cortical atrophy*, the gyri becoming rounder and firmer than normal and the sulci wider, and *secondary hydrocephalus*.

Alzheimer's disease and senile dementia. Most older people with dementia are thought to fall into this category. These two types of dementia show the same pathological features but Alzheimer's disease is the term used when the onset

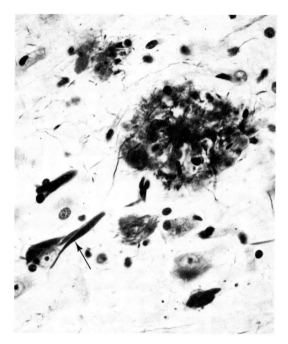

Fig. 21.46 Alzheimer's disease. Note the presence of a typical senile plaque composed of filamentous and granular material. A neurofibrillary tangle is seen in a neuron (*arrow*). King's amyloid stain. × 250.

is presenile (before the age of 60). The pathological findings represent a gross exaggeration of those of the normal ageing processes of the brain, and death usually occurs a few years after the onset. Cortical atrophy is widespread but more conspicuous in the frontal and temporal poles. Microscopy reveals a generalised loss of neurons, reactive gliosis and vast numbers of senile (Alzheimer) plaques in the cortical grey matter (Fig. 21.46), composed of masses of small argyrophilic granules and filaments often with a core of amyloid material. In addition, there are tangles of coarse neurofibrils (*Alzheimer's neurofibrillary change*) in many of the large nerve cells of the cerebral cortex. It has been established recently that the levels of many biochemical cell markers are reduced in the brain in Alzheimer's disease. There is, however, a relatively severe loss of choline-acetyl transferase, suggesting a selective loss or dysfunction of cholinergic neurons.

Pick's disease. This is much less common than Alzheimer's disease. It is classified as a presenile dementia due to cortical atrophy from loss of neurons, particularly in the frontal and temporal lobes, giving the brain a distinctive macroscopic appearance. The consequent degeneration of axis cylinders probably accounts for the loss of myelin, the reactive gliosis and considerable shrinkage of the underlying white matter. Some of the surviving neurons are greatly swollen by a globular mass of intracellular argyrophilic material.

Huntington's chorea. This disease of middle adult life is characterised by coarse choreiform movements, progressive mental deterioration and, in some cases, striatal rigidity. It is believed to be inherited by an autosomal dominant gene. In addition to widespread cortical atrophy, there is particularly severe atrophy and loss of nerve cells in the caudate nucleus and putamen.

The dementia occurring in association with hepatolenticular degeneration (p. 21.43), *Creutzfeld-Jacob disease* (p. 21.37) and *normal pressure hydrocephalus* (p. 21.12) are also often grouped under the heading of primary organic dementias.

Secondary dementias

These are many, but by far the commonest type is **multi-infarct dementia** which often has a rapid and step-wise course. Most patients are over 60 and hypertensive. Widespread atheroma of the major cerebral arteries results in repeated cerebral infarction. The distribution of the infarcts does not appear to correlate with the development of dementia, and it seems likely that the dementia occurs after a certain volume of the brain—perhaps about 100 ml—has been destroyed. The ventricles are usually enlarged symmetrically if there are multiple small infarcts in each hemisphere, and asymmetrically if the infarcts involve mainly one hemisphere.

The psychoses

In many quite common psychiatric disturbances, including schizophrenia and the involutional psychoses, there are no identifiable structural abnormalities in the brain. They are therefore still classified as functional disorders.

Parkinsonism (paralysis agitans)

This is a common disease of the elderly which affects men more often than women. It develops

Table 21.1 The Cerebrospinal Fluid

	Normal	Acute pyogenic meningitis	Tuberculous meningitis	*Acute virus infection with meningo-encephalitis
Pressure (horizontal posture)	60–150 mmH$_2$O	Probably to 200 mm or more	Increased to as much as 300 mm or more	Increased sometimes to 250 mm
Appearance	Clear and colourless	Turbid or frankly purulent	Clear or slightly opalescent. A fine fibrin coagulum may form on standing	Clear or slightly opalescent
Cell content per μl	0–4 leucocytes (all lymphocytes)	Markedly raised 500–5000 polymorphs at first, mononuclears* later	Increased up to 500 mononuclears; some polymorphs at first	Increased 50–500 mononuclears; some polymorphs at first
Protein g/litre	0·15–0·45	0·5–2·0 average; up to 10	0·5–3 usually; if spinal block present, may rise to over 10	0·5–2·0; 0·5–1·0 in paralytic polio
Glucose mg/100 ml (mmol/litre)	50–80 (2·8–4·4)	Absent or greatly reduced	Decreased to 20—30 (1—1·5)	Normal
Bacteriology	Sterile	Causative organisms present; type confirmed by culture	Tubercle bacilli in fibrin coagulum or in deposit. Positive cultures usually obtained	Sterile
Lange's colloidal gold test	Normal, i.e. 0000000000	May be normal or meningitic, e.g. 0012344320	Normal or meningitic	Normal or meningitic. Weak paretic or luetic in poliomyelitis
Wassermann	Negative	Negative	Negative	Negative

*'Mononuclears' is used here to indicate lymphocytes and monocytes

gradually and, if untreated, is permanent and tends to get worse. The predominant clinical features are involuntary tremor and muscular rigidity: the fixed facial expression, dribbling of saliva and tottering gait are characteristic and are brought about by a selective and progressive destruction of the pigmented dopaminergic neurons in the substantia nigra and the locus ceruleus of the brainstem. The destruction of neurons is of unknown cause and is accompanied by granules of pigment lying free in the parenchyma and within macrophages, and also some fibrillary gliosis. Frequently some of the residual pigmented neurons contain large intracytoplasmic inclusions known as *Lewy bodies*. In advanced cases, depigmentation of the substantia nigra is readily apparent macroscopically. A similar clinical syndrome may sometimes occur in association with small infarcts in the rostral brainstem or follow poisoning by manganese or carbon monoxide; the pathological changes are as noted above. Parkinsonism was also a sequel to the *encephalitis lethargica* (p. 21.36) of unknown aetiology which occurred in pandemic form during 1919–1926.

Developmental abnormalities

Congenital defects of the brain are many and the anatomical changes are often complex; only the main ones are summarised here. **Anencephaly** is a condition in which there is a deficiency of the cranial vault with absence of the brain, although there is often a small sac with the remains of cerebral tissue on the exposed and rudimentary base of the skull. The condition, which is incompatible with life, is sometimes associated with non-closure of the spinal canal or *rachischisis* (see below).

Occasionally there is a deficiency in the cranial bones and a sac-like protrusion is present. This occurs in the line of a suture, is often median and usually occipital, but sometimes lateral, e.g. at the side of an orbit or the nose. The sac is lined in some instances by the meninges and contains only CSF—**meningocele**. In other cases the sac is lined by neural tissue and sometimes, when the defect is posterior, may contain a considerable part of the cerebrum—**encephalocele**. The term **micrencephaly**

in health and in certain diseases

General paralysis of the insane	Tabes dorsalis	Multiple sclerosis	Subarachnoid haemorrhage	Complete spinal block (Froin's syndrome)
Normal	Normal	Normal	Raised often to 300 mm or more	Low: CSF may have to be actively withdrawn
Normal	Normal	Normal	Frankly bloodstained: on centrifugation, supernatant is yellow	Yellow, opalescent and tends to clot
Up to 100 (mononuclears)	Up to 50–100 (mononuclears)	Slight increase to 20–100 (mononuclears)	Many red cells and some leucocytes	Slight increase of mononuclears
0·5–1·0 Oligoclonal IgG	0·3–0·6 Oligoclonal IgG	0·3–0·6 Oligoclonal IgG	Normal in the early stages. Slight rise later	More than 30
Normal	Normal	Normal	Normal	Normal
Sterile	Sterile	Sterile	Sterile	Sterile
Paretic, e.g. 5544321000	Luetic, e.g. 123321000	Paretic, rarely luetic or may be normal	Normal	Meningitic
Positive	Positive in 80% of cases	Negative	Negative	Negative

means a congenitally small brain. There is deficiency in the convolutions, and the sulci are imperfectly formed; it is associated with severe mental retardation. The whole brain may be abnormal, but usually the cerebellum and brainstem are less affected than the cerebrum. In other cases, there is a local defect in growth, often associated with a small size of the convolutions or *microgyria*. Some virus infections, e.g. cytomegalovirus (p. 21.33) can cause microgyria, but the cause of most cases of micrencephaly is not known. The term **porencephaly** is applied when part of the brain is replaced by a collection of fluid, covered by meninges and sometimes in communication with the ventricles. In the *primary type*, which results from failure of growth of the brain, the edges of the defect are usually smooth. The condition is occasionally bilateral and sometimes accompanied by other defects. In the *secondary form*, the lesion is supposed to be the result of encephalitis, e.g. toxoplasmosis, or of interference with the blood supply during intrauterine life, and a somewhat similar condition may result from injury at the time of birth.

Spinal cord defects. These are of particular interest because of their frequency and their seriousness. Fortunately, their intrauterine detection, made possible by an elevated α-fetoprotein in the amniotic fluid in 90% of cases, has allowed therapeutic abortion and greatly reduced the incidence of these malformations.

Failure of closure of the embryonic neural canal results in a series of abnormalities known as **spina bifida**: they are usually associated with maldevelopment of the laminae of the vertebrae (*rachischisis*). If the vertebral defect is covered by dura and skin, the term *spina bifida occulta* is applied: sometimes there is excessive growth of hair over the lesion. More often, however, there is a distinct rounded projection over the site of the defect, which is known as *spina bifida cystica*.

The usual position of spina bifida is in the lumbo-sacral region and in all cases the spinal cord extends to a lower level than is normal. In the commonest form, the spinal cord is adherent to the posterior wall of the sac and the term **meningomyelocele** is applied. The dura is absent in the sac, over which there is often an area where the skin is deficient (Fig. 21.10, p. 21.11).

At this point there is a smooth membrane in which the spinal cord is incorporated, the cord being open posteriorly, with the openings of the central canal visible as one or two small depressions. The spinal nerves are spread out on the inner lining of the sac. The more severe forms of this variant are almost invariably associated with hydrocephalus and the **Arnold-Chiari malformation** (p. 21.10). In another rarer form, the space containing the fluid is a distension of the central canal and is lined by ependyma. In this form, termed **myelocystocele** or **syringomyelocele**, the spinal cord has closed posteriorly, the abnormality having arisen later in development than the previous form. In a third and least common variety, the sac is lined by a hernial protrusion of the arachnoid, and the spinal cord lies normally in relation to the vertebrae: this is called **meningocele**.

Paraplegia and urinary tract infections determine the generally poor progress of these patients, who seldom achieve adulthood despite early surgical repair of the spina bifida and treatment of the hydrocephalus that usually accompanies the more severe malformations.

In **spina bifida occulta**, where there is no swelling to indicate the defect, the overlying skin usually shows abnormalities in appearance and there is sometimes excessive growth of hair on it.

Diastematomyelia is the term applied when the cord is split into two by a fibrous or bony spur projecting into the vertebral canal.

Tuberous sclerosis. In this disorder there are multiple foci of hyperplasia of neuroglia and nerve cells in the cortex of the brain and in the subependymal tissue, in association with rhabdomyoma of the heart muscle (p. 15.45), adenoma sebaceum and other congenital abnormalities. In a few cases one or more of the glial foci give rise to a distinctive subependymal giant-celled type of astrocytoma.

II: The Spinal Cord

The tissue of the spinal cord is similar to that of the brain but the relative frequencies of various lesions are very different. Specific diseases of the spinal cord are described later but so-called *transverse lesions* and the consequent ascending and descending Wallerian degeneration within the cord will be dealt with first.

Transverse lesions

These occur when partial or complete interruption of the cord is produced by local disease or trauma. **Slowly progressive effects** may be produced by *pressure on the cord by extrinsic tumours* in the extradural space, e.g. metastatic carcinoma (Fig. 21.47) or lymphoid neoplasm, or in the subdural space, e.g. meningioma (Fig. 21.76, p. 21.61) or schwannoma. *Intrinsic tumours*, e.g. astrocytoma and ependymoma, are rarer causes. *Tuberculosis* is still a common cause in various parts of the world. It leads to angular curvature of the spine, cold abscesses and granulomatous masses (p. 23.8) any of which can cause pressure on the cord; this may

be so severe that infarction of the cord may occur at this level. **Acute transverse lesions** may be due to *trauma*, usually a fracture-dislocation of the vertebrae, *infarction* when the circulation through the anterior spinal artery is impeded, *haemorrhage*, usually from a vascular malformation, *acute myelitis* (see below) or acute *demyelination* as in neuromyelitis optica (p. 21.41).

An inevitable consequence of a total or partial transverse lesion of the cord, besides the local damage, is the development of **ascending and descending Wallerian degeneration** in the interrupted tracts of the spinal cord. Degeneration occurs in those fibres that are separated from their cell bodies by the lesion and is best demonstrated by the Marchi technique (p. 21.4). The degenerating fibres appear black from about a week after onset (Fig. 21.48). The method is applicable until the degenerated myelin has disappeared—that is, for 3 months or so. In older lesions, the Weigert-Pal method, which stains the normal myelin black, should be used since, when the degenerate myelin has become absorbed, the affected tract appears as a pale area (Fig. 21.50).

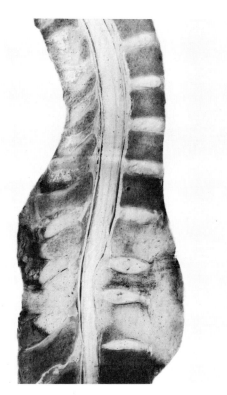

Fig. 21.47 Sagittal section of the vertebral column in lower cervical–upper dorsal region, showing metastatic tumour pressing on the cord.

Ascending degeneration

If we take as an example a comparatively recent lesion in the lower thoracic spine, the ascending degenerations found in a section taken a few segments above the lesion (Fig. 21.48) involve the posterior columns (with the exception of a small area dorsal to the grey commissure where there are chiefly commissural fibres) and the spino-thalamic and spino-cerebellar tracts. In the cervical region, however, the degeneration in the posterior columns is practically confined to the gracile tracts (Fig. 21.49) because the cuneate tract is composed of ascending fibres that have joined the cord above the level of the lesion. Degeneration of the affected axons ascends up to the cuneate and gracile nuclei in the medulla. Ascending degeneration in the posterior spino-cerebellar tract extends up to the inferior cerebellar peduncle and into the cerebellum, and in the anterior spino-cerebellar tract to the middle lobe of the cerebellum. In old lesions, loss of myelin (Figs. 21.50 and 21.51) and reactive gliosis are more conspicuous in the posterior columns because the inflow of normal myelinated fibres proximal to the lesion masks the loss of myelinated fibres in the spino-cerebellar and spino-thalamic tracts.

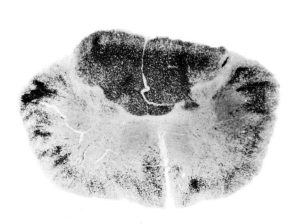

Fig. 21.48 Immediately above the lesion. The whole of the posterior columns and antero-lateral ascending tracts are degenerating.

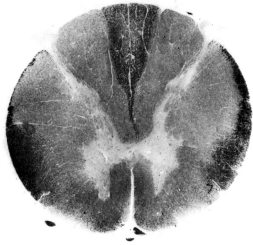

Fig. 21.49 Cervical region. There are fewer degenerating fibres because of the inflow of fibres above the level of the lesion.

Figures 21.48 and 21.49 Ascending degeneration above a recent transverse lesion in the lower dorsal region, stained by Marchi's method: the degenerating fibres appear black.

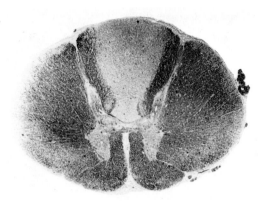

Fig. 21.50   A short distance above the lesion.

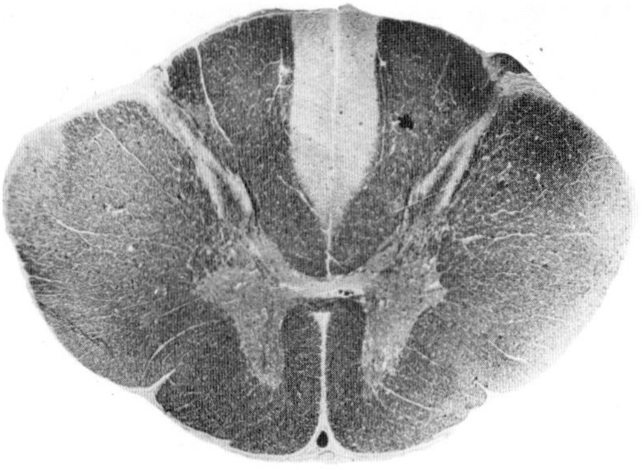

Fig. 21.51   Cervical region. Degeneration appears to be confined to the gracile tract.

Figures 21.50 and 21.51   Ascending degeneration above an old transverse lesion in the dorsal region, stained by the Weigert–Pal method. The degenerated fibres appear pale.

Descending degeneration

This occurs distal to a transverse lesion in the cord, and as a result of lesions in certain parts of the brain. In a section taken distal to a *transverse lesion* of the cord the most marked degeneration is in the crossed (lateral) and uncrossed (anterior) pyramidal tracts unless the lesion is low in the cord where the uncrossed tract is no longer present.

The commonest example due to a *lesion of the brain* is destruction of the motor fibres in the internal capsule by infarction. There is degeneration of the crossed pyramidal tract on the opposite side (Fig. 21.52) and of the uncrossed pyramidal tract on the same side. As the uncrossed pyramidal tract does not usually extend below the upper thoracic segments, its degeneration will not be seen in sections of the lower thoracic cord (Fig. 21.53).

In compression of the spinal cord by a gross lesion which also blocks the subarachnoid space, the CSF below the block becomes altered. There is a great increase in protein concentration and the fluid coagulates rapidly after withdrawal; it is often yellow (xanthochromia). There may also be a slight increase in lymphocytes. These changes are grouped under

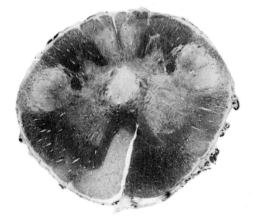

Fig. 21.52   Medulla. The pyramid on one side is degenerated.

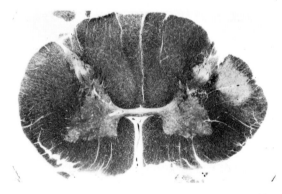

Fig. 21.53   Thoracic region. The crossed pyramidal tract on one side is degenerated.

Figures 21.52 and 21.53   Descending degeneration. Transverse sections through medulla and spinal cord showing descending degeneration from an old lesion of one internal capsule. Stained by Weigert–Pal method: degenerated fibres appear pale.

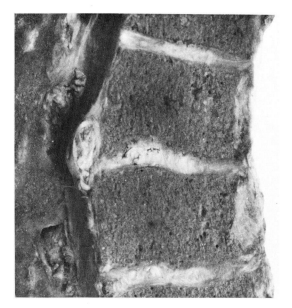

Fig. 21.54 Sagittal section of vertebral column, showing ruptured disc protruding beneath the posterior longitudinal ligament.

the term 'Froin's syndrome' (see Table 21.1, pp. 21.46–47).

Prolapsed intervertebral disc

This is a common cause of compression of the nerve roots and more rarely causes compression of the cord. The intervertebral disc consists of a central nodule of semifluid matrix, the nucleus pulposus, surrounded by a ring of fibrous tissue and fibrocartilage, the annulus fibrosus. The posterior segment of the annulus is thinner and less firmly attached to bone and, following unusual stress, part of the matrix of the nucleus pulposus may herniate through it (Fig. 21.54). The lesion, often termed 'slipped disc', may occur after slight injury and symptoms depend on the direction taken by the extruded matrix. It usually tracks postero-laterally around the expansion of the posterior longitudinal ligament, appearing at one side and compressing the spinal nerve root in the intervertebral foramen. Disc protrusions almost always occur in the lumbar spine and L5–S1, L4–L5 and L3–L4 discs are affected in that order of frequency: they also occur occasionally in the cervical spine, principally in C5–C6 and C6–7 discs. If the protrusion is small, localised pain is produced by irritation of the posterior longitudinal ligament; if larger, there may also be root pain due to pressure on nerves leaving the spinal canal, producing the clinical signs and symptoms of **sciatica**. A single midline posterior disc protrusion may compress the spinal cord or obstruct the anterior spinal artery, and is a rare but important cause of permanent damage to the spinal cord if surgical treatment is delayed. When there are several protrusions, as in **cervical spondylosis**, the resulting compression may impair the circulation and variable effects of ischaemia of the spinal cord may result. There may be cavitation of the cord and loss of nerve cells in the severely affected areas, the condition being known as *spondylotic myelopathy*. Even in cervical spondylosis, however, nerve root compression is commoner than myelopathy.

Acute myelitis

This uncommon condition, by definition an acute inflammation of the cord, is more a clinical syndrome than a precise pathological entity. It is usually of acute or subacute onset and is characterised by flaccid paralysis and sensory loss, either of which may be total or partial, below the level of the lesion. A considerable length of the cord may be affected — *diffuse myelitis*, or the lesion may be confined to one or two segments — *transverse myelitis*. These terms, however, tend to be used for any pathological process, other than external pressure or tumour, which causes damage to the grey and white matter of the cord.

Causes. Acute demyelination (p. 21.39), and infarction of the cord due to impaired circulation through the anterior spinal artery, are probably the commonest causes. In some cases of infarction of the lumbo-sacral cord in adults, there are numerous hyalinised vessels within the cord: this condition is known as *subacute necrotic myelitis*. Other causes of transverse myelitis are acute disseminated encephalomyelitis (p. 21.37), spontaneous haematomyelia (probably from a vascular malformation) and, more rarely, bacterial infections.

Structural changes. The appearances of the cord vary with the underlying pathological process. In general, however, the affected part of the cord is swollen and soft, the normal architectural markings are blurred and there may be foci of haemorrhage.

If the patient survives the acute stage, there may be some restoration of function. More often the affected part of the cord becomes shrunken, cystic and gliosed, there is ascending and descending degeneration, and the patient is permanently paraplegic.

Lesions of the motor neuron

The main acute disease of lower motor neurons, *acute anterior poliomyelitis*, has already been described (p. 21.33). Chronic progressive degenerative disease of the motor neurons is usually referred to as *motor neuron disease*.

Motor neuron disease

In this disease there is a relentless and progressive degeneration of motor neurons of unknown aetiology. The brunt of the damage may fall on the lower motor neurons in the spinal cord (*progressive muscular atrophy*) or on the cranial nerve nuclei in the brainstem (*progressive bulbar palsy*). Some degeneration of upper motor neurons (in the cerebral cortex) is usual and may be prominent (*amyotrophic lateral sclerosis*). These three variants of *motor neuron disease* occur in middle and late adult life, and are much more frequent in men than in women.

Progressive muscular atrophy. In this variant there is a progressive degeneration of the neurons in the anterior horns of the spinal cord. It usually starts in the cervical enlargement in the neurons controlling the small muscles of the hand. The affected muscles show fibrillary twitchings, followed by gradual atrophy with corresponding weakness. The thenar and hypothenar eminences become markedly wasted, the interossei also become involved, and the hand assumes a characteristic claw-like form. Involvement then extends to the muscles of the arm and shoulder girdle. Terminally the symptoms of bulbar paralysis may appear. In the anterior horns there is gradual atrophy and loss of neurons. Gliosis may occur but is usually not marked. The anterior spinal nerve roots become wasted, particularly in the cervical region and in the cauda equina, and appear grey and thin to the naked eye, while in the related muscles there is neurogenic atrophy (Fig. 21.90, p. 21.73).

Progressive bulbar palsy. This variant of motor neuron disease may appear first, or may follow spinal involvement. There is progressive paralysis and wasting of the muscles of the tongue, lips, jaws, larynx and pharynx; death often occurs by involvement of the respiratory centre, or by foreign matter entering the lungs through the paralysed larynx. The lesions are in the medulla and are of the same nature as those in the cord. They are usually most marked in the hypoglossal and spinal accesory nuclei, but occur also in the nuclei of the vagus and facial nerves and in the nucleus of the motor part of the trigeminal nerve. Along with the changes in the brainstem there is varying involvement of the nerve cells in the anterior horns and of the pyramidal fibres.

Amyotrophic lateral sclerosis. In cases where there is considerable degeneration of upper motor neurons, there is loss of nerve fibres in the cortico-spinal tracts and consequently various degrees of spasticity. When this is marked, the clinical syndrome is usually called amyotrophic lateral sclerosis. In addition to the atrophic changes in the anterior horns, there is widespread sclerosis and loss of myelin in the lateral and anterior white columns, especially the pyramidal tracts (Fig. 21.55). The changes in the pyramidal fibres usually start first and are most marked at their lower extremities, the process then extending upwards. Atrophic changes, corresponding to those in the anterior horns, occur in the motor cells of the cerebral cortex and here also many disappear.

No sharply dividing line can be drawn between these variants of motor neuron disease. Their names merely emphasise that in any one case, the early stages of the disease may have a particular distribution. In the terminal stages there is often widespread involvement of motor neurons in the brainstem and in the spinal cord, and involvement of the lateral and ventral white columns in the spinal cord.

Friedreich's ataxia

In this disease there is atrophy in both motor and sensory tracts. It often affects more than one member of a family, and so is sometimes called **familial ataxia**; rarely it occurs in successive generations. Isolated cases also occur. It usually begins in childhood and the chief symptoms are ataxia with muscular weakness. Lateral curvature of the spine and talipes equinus often develop, and nystagmus and disturbance of speech are also common. In such cases, the spinal cord is found to be relatively thin and there is degeneration in the posterior and lateral columns

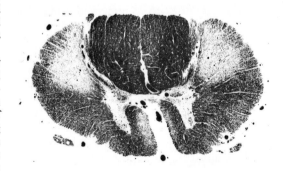

Fig. 21.55 Amyotrophic lateral sclerosis. Section of the spinal cord, showing degeneration in the lateral and anterior columns and preservation of the posterior columns. There is selectively severe involvement of the crossed pyramidal tracts. (Weigert–Pal method.)

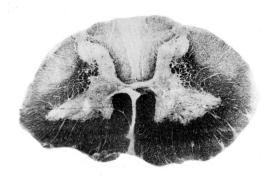

Fig. 21.56 Section of spinal cord in Friedreich's ataxia, showing degeneration in posterior and lateral columns. (Weigert–Pal method.)

(Fig. 21.56). The posterior roots also show degeneration, especially the fibres within the cord, and involvement of the roots and posterior columns may be present in the cervical region as well as lower down; the cells in the posterior root ganglia, however, are little altered. In the lateral columns the pyramidal fibres are degenerate, most markedly at lower levels. The posterior spino-cerebellar tracts are similarly affected, and the cells of the thoracic nucleus show degenerative changes. There may be some degeneration also in the anterior spino-cerebellar and spino-thalamic tracts. The nature of the disease is obscure. Friedreich's ataxia and *Marie's hereditary cerebellar ataxia* are probably related: the two conditions sometimes overlap and intermediate forms occur, but each affected family presents its own variant. Friedreich's ataxia is frequently associated with a chronic progressive myocarditis, in which focal coagulative necrosis of the muscle fibres is followed by replacement fibrosis.

Other lesions of the spinal cord

Subacute combined degeneration

Since highly effective purified preparations of vitamin B_{12} have been available for treatment of pernicious anaemia (p. 17.37), this complication is now uncommon. Similar lesions have been found even more rarely in some other chronic diseases, e.g. malabsorption syndromes, leukaemia, diabetes and carcinoma. *Subacute combined degeneration may develop in the 'pre-anaemic stage' of pernicious anaemia.* The administration of vitamin B_{12} in adequate doses is completely effective in preventing the development of neural lesions.

The anatomical changes consist of degeneration in the dorsal and lateral columns of the spinal cord (Fig. 21.57). The process appears to start, and to be most severe and extensive, in the lower thoracic region and then extends upwards and downwards. In the involved segments the degenerate myelin is removed by phagocytes which migrate to the perivascular sheaths. In untreated cases there is practically no glial proliferation and the degenerated areas present an open spongy appearance. With long survival on B_{12} treatment, however, some gliosis eventually occurs in pre-existing lesions. The degeneration in the motor tracts may ascend through the internal capsule and degenerative changes may be seen in the Betz cells of the cortex. The symptoms depend on the degree and extent of tract involvement, and consist mainly of ataxia and spasticity. *In view of its progressive, disabling nature, and the arresting effects of B_{12} therapy, early diagnosis is of the utmost importance.*

Syringomyelia

This is a rare condition in which a cyst-like space or spaces develop within the cord, containing fluid and enclosed by neuroglia. There is considerable controversy over its nature and pathogenesis. In the past, it was distinguished from hydromyelia (dilatation of the central canal of the spinal cord) on the basis that syringomyelic cavities first appear dorsal to the central canal. There is, however, increasing evidence that, in most cases, syringomyelia is caused by CSF being propelled through a valve-like opening between the caudal extremity of the fourth ventricle and the central canal, i.e. that the cavity is a greatly distended central canal. Individuals with this type of syringomyelia also tend to have a mild developmental abnormality at the cranio-cervical junction, the cerebellar tonsils protruding further through the foramen magnum than usual. Whatever its pathogenesis, however, the structural abnormalities in the cord

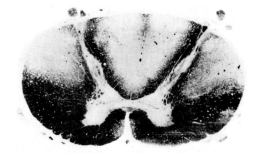

Fig. 21.57 Subacute combined degeneration, showing conspicuous degeneration in both lateral and posterior columns. (Weigert–Pal method.)

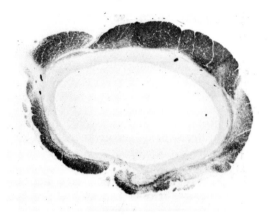

Fig. 21.58   Syringomyelia: junction between cervical and thoracic portion. (Weigert–Pal method.)

are fairly stereotyped. The cavity usually extends through several segments of the cervical cord (Fig. 21.58) and, as it enlarges, the cord becomes swollen and feels somewhat soft. Microscopically, the tissue around the cavity is seen to consist of enlarged astrocytes and coarse astrocytic fibrils. Occasionally syringomyelia occurs in association with tumours affecting the spinal cord.

Effects. These are due principally to destruction of the cord by the enlarging cavity. The first fibres to be affected are the decussating sensory fibres conveying the sensations of heat and pain: the resulting defect, known as *dissociated anaesthesia*, is a selective insensibility to heat and pain in the region corresponding to the involved segments of the spinal cord. A neuropathic arthritis occurs, closely similar to that in tabes (p. 21.29), but, as syringomyelia is usually in the cervical region, the joints of the upper limbs are chiefly involved. Trophic lesions also occur in the skin; they include vesicles, ulceration and painless whitlows. As the cavity enlarges it ultimately affects the lateral white columns leading to spastic paraplegia, the ventral grey horns leading to neurogenic atrophy of muscles, and the posterior white columns leading to even greater disturbances of sensation.

Barotrauma, etc.

Lesions of the spinal cord are one of the more serious features of **acute decompression sickness**. This and related non-thrombotic embolic phenomena, notably **air embolism** and **fat embolism** are described on pp. 10.20–22.

Developmental abnormalities of the spinal cord are described on pp. 21.46–48.

Tumours of the Nervous System

Many tumours of the nervous system arise intrinsically in neural tissue, i.e. they are neuro-ectodermal tumours (mainly gliomas). Others arise from the meninges (meningioma) or from cranial and spinal nerve roots (schwannoma). The brain is also a common site of metastatic carcinoma, and finally there are many relatively rare tumours of the nervous system.

Primary tumours of the CNS occur in 4–5 per 100 000 of the general population. Up to the age of 15 years, they are the second commonest form of cancer, being exceeded only by leukaemia. In adults they account for about 2% of primary malignant tumours (excluding basal-cell carcinoma of the skin).

Of 1500 consecutive cases of intracranial tumour investigated in the Institute of Neurological Sciences in Glasgow, 67% were of neuro-ectodermal origin, 17% were meningiomas and 4% were schwannomas of the cranial nerves. The remaining 12% were a miscellaneous group including vascular tumours and malformations. During the same period, 400 patients investigated for suspected intracranial tumours were found to have metastatic tumours. In a general hospital autopsy service, the proportion of patients with secondary carcinoma is much greater.

Intracranial tumours may produce **local effects** which will depend on their site, e.g. focal (Jacksonian) epilepsy, paralysis, defects of the visual fields, and also behave as **expanding intracranial lesions** with the effects described on pp. 21.6–8. An important feature is oedema of the surrounding brain tissue, which usually responds dramatically to steroid therapy.

Biopsy through a burr-hole in the skull and examination of smear preparations is invaluable in the immediate identification of brain tumours.

Tumours of neuro-ectodermal origin

These include all the tumours which arise from the primitive medullary epithelium. In the CNS these cells consist of the neuroglia (astrocytes, oligodendrocytes and ependymal cells) and the nerve cells. Most neuro-ectodermal tumours are of neuroglial origin and are known collectively as the **gliomas**: they account for about 45% of all intracranial tumours.

Gliomas

Some gliomas are mature tumours composed of cells that resemble closely astrocytes, oligodendrocytes or ependymal cells, the respective tumours being called **astrocytoma, oligodendroglioma** and **ependymoma**. Secondly, there are tumours in which only a proportion of the cells are of this type, the others being pleomorphic and less well differentiated: these are referred to as the **anaplastic variants** of these tumours.

As in other tissues, the general rule usually applies that the more primitive or undifferentiated the cells are, the more rapid is their growth, but in contrast to tumours in other tissues, gliomas cannot be divided into benign and malignant types, for *all gliomas, whether composed of highly or poorly differentiated cells, infiltrate the adjacent brain tissue and are never truly sharply demarcated or encapsulated.* Paradoxically the rapidly growing anaplastic forms often appear to be the better demarcated, because they also compress and push aside surrounding tissues. Another feature of gliomas is that, *like all primary intracranial tumours, they virtually never metastasise beyond the CNS unless craniotomy has been performed and then only rarely.* They may however be disseminated by the CSF to other parts of the CNS. The individual gliomas thus differ mainly in their degree of cellular differentiation and rate of growth.

Astrocytoma. This is by far the commonest type of glioma. A well-differentiated astrocytoma is a slowly growing whitish tumour, usually poorly defined at its margin where it merges with the surrounding tissue. Some contain abundant glial fibres and are tough, almost rubbery: others have scanty glial fibres and are soft. Cystic change is common (Fig. 21.59)

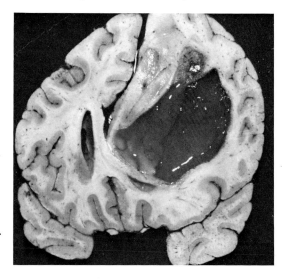

Fig. 21.59 Cystic astrocytoma in the right frontal lobe. Tumour tissue is identifiable adjacent to the upper pole of the cyst.

particularly in the cerebellar astrocytoma of childhood.

In a *fibrillary astrocytoma*, microscopic examination shows unevenly distributed and often loosely arranged elongated cells separated by glial fibrils (Fig. 21.60). Even in the absence of gross cystic change there are often numerous

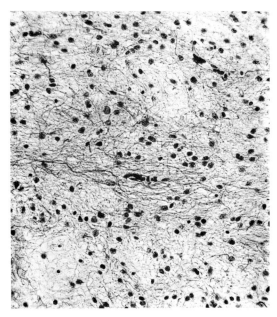

Fig. 21.60 Astrocytoma of relatively low cellularity showing well formed glial fibrils (PTAH). × 260.

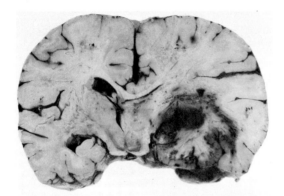

Fig. 21.61 Glioblastoma multiforme of temporal lobe. Note the well-defined margin and haemorrhagic areas within the tumour. There is a pronounced midline shift, virtual obliteration of the lateral ventricle and a supracallosal hernia (see p. 21.7).

microcysts. Sometimes the brain tissue is diffusely permeated by tumour astrocytes, often with remarkable preservation of nerve cells and fibres. The edge of this type of tumour often defies recognition with the naked eye. It is known as *diffuse astrocytoma* or *gliomatosis cerebri* and is particularly common in the brainstem and spinal cord. Other rarer forms of astrocytoma are composed of protoplasmic astrocytes or swollen, so-called gemistocytic astrocytes.

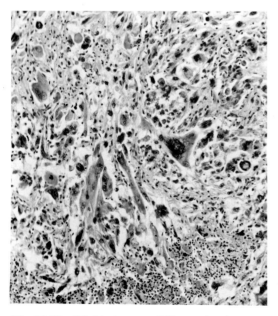

Fig. 21.62 Glioblastoma multiforme showing many aberrant giant cells. × 110.

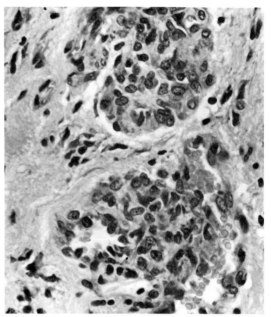

Fig. 21.63 Glomeruloid endothelial proliferation in glioblastoma. × 390.

All astrocytomas display a marked tendency to become *anaplastic* : this may be restricted to one part of the tumour or it may be multifocal. To the naked eye the anaplastic areas are haemorrhagic and necrotic and often appear to have a relatively well-defined edge. The microscopic features of these areas are similar to those of glioblastoma multiforme.

The term **glioblastoma multiforme** may be used for astrocytomas that are highly anaplastic throughout. Such tumours occur in adults, most frequently in the cerebral hemispheres, forming a rapidly growing, apparently relatively well-defined mass with extensive necrosis and haemorrhage. It produces considerable distortion of the brain and often a rapid increase in intracranial pressure (Figs. 21.4, p. 21.7 and 21.61).

Microscopically a glioblastoma multiforme is richly cellular in the areas that are not necrotic and there are great variations in cell type ranging from closely packed masses of small anaplastic cells to pleomorphic giant cells (Fig. 21.62). Mitoses are often frequent and glial fibrils extremely scanty. Small vessels in and around the tumour may show curious bud-like or 'glomeruloid' endothelial proliferations (Fig. 21.63). Necrosis is usually extensive and fre-

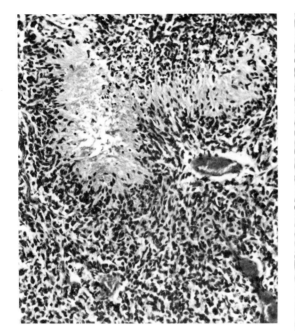

Fig. 21.64 Glioblastoma multiforme, showing a common pattern of central necrosis with peripheral palisading of spindle-shaped cells. × 130.

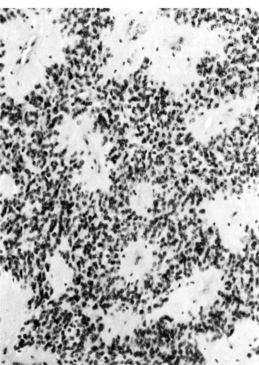

Fig. 21.65 Ependymoma. Note the characteristic perivascular fibrillary haloes. × 125.

quently elongated tumour cells form a palisade around necrotic foci (Fig. 21.64).

Ependymoma. This not uncommon tumour is most frequently encountered in children, usually in the fourth ventricle but it occurs also in the other ventricles. The tumour cells often have a distinctly epithelial appearance and they are characteristically orientated around small blood vessels but are separated from them by an eosinophilic fibrillary band (Fig. 21.65). Less frequently columnar cells form small canaliculi (Fig. 21.66), and near the free edge of these cells there may be small rod-shaped blepharoplasts. Ependymomas may also become anaplastic as shown by the occurrence of cellular pleomorphism and poor differentiation, haemorrhage and necrosis. Closely related to the ependymoma is the *papillary tumour of the choroid plexus*. This is also most often seen in children, forming a rounded bulky tumour usually in one lateral ventricle. The papillae have a vascular connective tissue core covered by columnar epithelium very similar in appearance to normal choroid plexus epithelium (Fig. 21.67). It frequently causes hydrocephalus.

A curious tumour, the *myxopapillary ependymoma*, arises from the filum terminale in adults. It is slowly

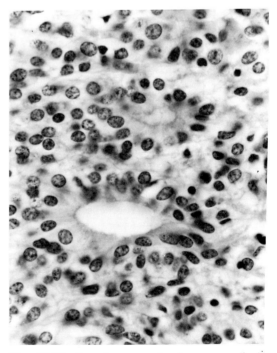

Fig. 21.66 Ependymoma showing a canaliculus lined by columnar cells. × 480.

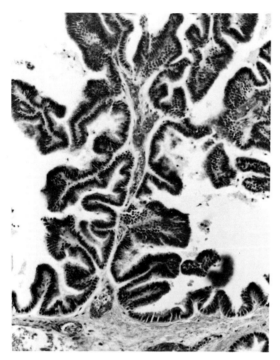

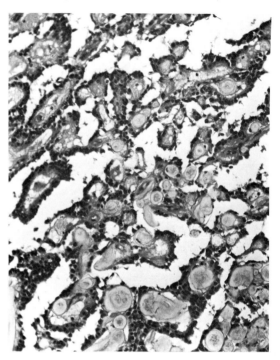

Fig. 21.67   Papillary tumour of the choroid plexus, showing delicate papillary processes covered by cuboidal epithelium. × 200.

Fig. 21.68   Myxopapillary ependymoma, a papillary structure with very gelatinous stroma, covered by a mainly cuboidal epithelium. × 125.

growing, markedly gelatinous, and gradually ensheathes the nerve roots of the cauda equina and the caudal part of the spinal cord. The stroma consists of a central vascular core surrounded by mucoid connective tissue and covered in places by cuboidal epithelium (Fig. 21.68); elsewhere the covering cells may form a network between the papillae. This tumour may cause pressure atrophy of the adjacent bones and may even invade them; it is then liable to be mistaken for a chordoma (p. 23.39).

Oligodendroglioma. In our experience this glioma is rarer than ependymoma. It occurs in the cerebral hemispheres, is slowly growing, rather gelatinous and commonly exhibits numerous small foci of calcification which may be seen radiologically. The cells are uniform, small and rounded, like normal oligodendroglial cells, with somewhat clear cytoplasm and distinct cell-membranes (Fig. 21.69). Cell processes are small and difficult to demonstrate. As with other gliomas, anaplastic change may occur in these tumours.

The above tumours are the commonest types of glioma: other clearly defined variants have not been mentioned because they are rare. Not all gliomas can be placed in a specific category. Indeed a comprehensive microscopic examina-

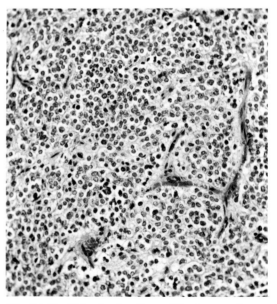

Fig. 21.69   Oligodendroglioma. The tumour is very cellular, the cells being round or oval with distinct cell boundaries. × 125.

tion of any glioma may result in the identification of various types of tumour within it and the name applied comes to depend on the most prominent element. In some gliomas both astrocytomatous and oligodendrogliomatous elements are conspicuous. Furthermore each main division exists as a spectrum; at one end there is a mature well-differentiated tumour composed of cells resembling normal glial cells, while at the other there is a highly anaplastic and poorly differentiated tumour. *As all gliomas infiltrate into the adjacent brain, particularly the better differentiated types, total surgical excision is rarely feasible*: radiotherapy is also at best palliative and the ultimate prognosis for a patient with a glioma is usually poor.

Tumours of the neuron series

These include tumours composed of primitive cells, namely *medulloblastoma, neuroblastoma* and *retinoblastoma* (p. 21.86), and tumours containing large ganglion cells, namely *ganglioneuroma* and *ganglioglioma*. The latter types, however, occur very rarely within the central nervous system.

Medulloblastoma. This is the commonest nerve cell tumour of the CNS: it occurs most often in childhood, is a poorly differentiated and rapidly growing cellular tumour and originates in the cerebellum. It forms a soft greyish-white mass protruding into the fourth ventricle and commonly spreads over the surface of the cerebellum as a thin sheet that obscures the normal surface architecture. Seeding of tumour cells by the CSF is usual, and may result in diffuse meningeal tumour or be restricted to small secondary nodules on the nerve roots of the cauda equina. Retrograde spread to the third and lateral ventricles is also common.

Microscopically, its cells are either spherical with little cytoplasm and no fibrils, or somewhat triangular, like short carrots, and arranged around blood vessels and also as rosettes without a central cavity (Fig. 21.70).

Neuroblastoma and ganglioneuroma. These, in general, are tumours derived from ganglion cells or their precursors in sites outwith the central nervous system. The majority arise in the adrenal medulla or in sympathetic ganglia but they may also arise in the more distal ganglia of the parasympathetic system. *Neuroblastoma*

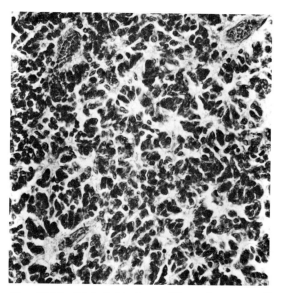

Fig. 21.70 Medulloblastoma. The cells are small and closely packed, but form poorly defined rosettes. × 285.

(sometimes known as sympathicoblastoma) is a primitive, highly malignant tumour whereas *ganglioneuroma* is a mature benign tumour: tumours of an intermediate or mixed character are also encountered.

Neuroblastoma is mainly a tumour of childhood, usually of children under 4 years of age. The commonest sites are the adrenal medulla and the retroperitoneal tissues. A neuroblastoma of the adrenal gland forms a bulky soft cellular and haemorrhagic tumour with extensive necrosis, which destroys the adrenal, spreads rapidly to the upper abdominal lymph nodes, to the liver and notably to the skeleton, secondary tumours in the skull being especially frequent.

Microscopically, the cells are small, round or oval, with little cytoplasm. In many parts they are irregularly arranged, while in places they may form small ball-like masses of cells which sometimes show further differentiation into rings or rosettes, consisting of radially-arranged cells with central cytoplasmic fibrillary projections (Fig. 21.71) which are stained by silver impregnation methods, although not so strongly as nerve fibrils. These structures are closely similar to the clumps of neuroblasts which grow out to form the sympathetic system: they are readily seen in the fetal adrenal when it is becoming invaded by neuroblasts

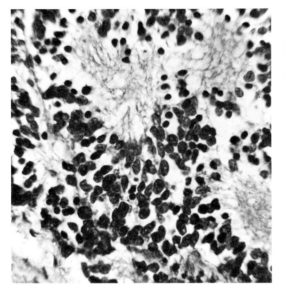

Fig. 21.71 Neuroblastoma. Many of the cells are carrot-shaped and are arranged in well-defined rosettes, the centres of which contain the fine fibrils prolonged from the tapering cells. × 425.

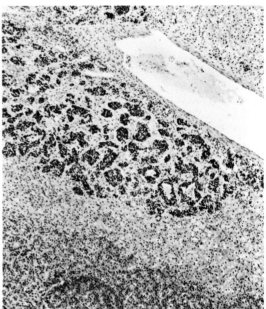

Fig. 21.72 Adrenal medulla of an infant of 9 months, showing masses of undiffentiated neuroblasts. × 60.

which form the medulla of the gland. Rests of undifferentiated neuroblasts are occasionally found in the adrenal medulla in infancy (Fig. 21.72). Some neuroblastomas show partial differentiation, the cells resembling immature neurons.

Ganglioneuroma. This tumour affects older age groups than neuroblastoma and occurs more often in the posterior mediastinum than in the abdomen. It is usually firm, encapsulated like a benign tumour and of rounded or irregular outline. It contains well-formed ganglionic nerve cells, irregularly arranged in a finely fibrillar stroma, and also smaller cells of various forms (Fig. 21.73). There are usually also a large number of nerve fibres, both myelinated and non-myelinated. The tumour is usually benign, but occasionally it is associated with a cellular malignant neuroblastoma.

Neuroblastomas and tumours containing well-differentiated neurons are rare in the CNS: the latter contain also neoplastic neuroglial elements and so are more accurately termed *gangliogliomas* than ganglioneuromas.

The common origin of some of these various tumours is emphasised by the fact that neuroblastic and ganglionic tumours unconnected with the adrenals, e.g. in the thorax, may secrete pressor substances, notably dopamine and noradrenaline, causing severe hypertension.

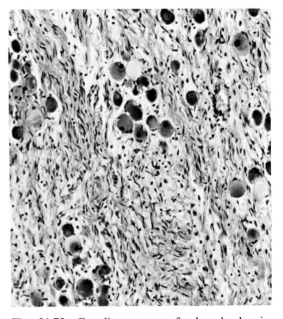

Fig. 21.73 Ganglioneuroma of adrenal, showing abundant mature ganglion cells and non-myelinated nerve fibres.

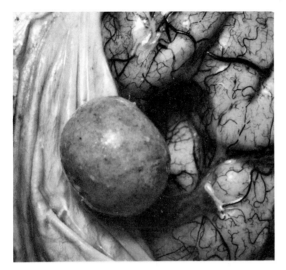

Fig. 21.74 Meningioma attached to dura mater, showing the typical depression of the cerebral cortex from which the tumour is readily withdrawn. × 1·4.

Tumours of the meninges

The common tumour in this group is the *meningioma*. It is a tumour of the arachnoid and most probably originates from the arachnoid granulations (Fig. 21.8, p. 21.9).

Meningiomas account for between 15–20% of intracranial tumours: they are solid lobulated growths, well demarcated from the brain tissue into which they project, forming a depression: they are usually firmly attached by a broad base to the dura. They tend to arise adjacent to the major venous sinuses, commonly parasagittally (Fig. 21.74), or from the base of the skull, often in the region of the olfactory groove when the

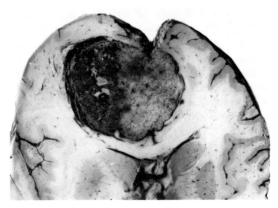

Fig. 21.75 Large meningioma between the frontal lobes.

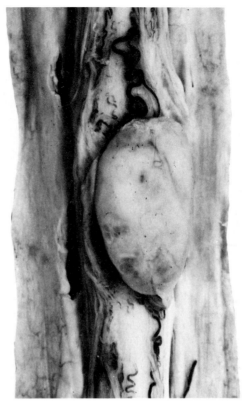

Fig. 21.76 Spinal meningioma compressing the cord. × 1·5.

meningioma projects into the fissure between the frontal lobes (Fig. 21.75). Another common site is the sphenoidal ridge. Rarely a meningioma may arise from the tela choroidea and appear as an intraventricular tumour. Meningiomas may be soft or hard and gritty (see below). Most are benign and can be removed successfully. Some, however, infiltrate the overlying bone, which may be greatly thickened. Very occasionally meningiomas metastasise (mostly to the lungs): this may occur following spread into the soft tissues of the scalp after craniotomy, but occasionally from invasion of a venous sinus.

Spinal meningiomas have similar general features, but, owing to their situation, are smaller (Fig. 21.76). They are intradural tumours which arise most frequently on the postero-lateral aspect of the cord, and the disturbances at first are chiefly sensory—pain, paraesthesia, etc. Later, various effects up to complete paraplegia may result from pressure on the cord.

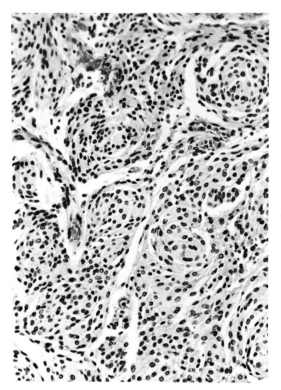

Fig. 21.77 Section of meningioma of common cellular type showing the arrangement of cells and fibres in whorls. × 220.

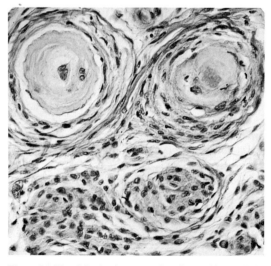

Fig. 21.78 Meningioma, showing fibrocellular masses with concentric arrangement and formation of psammoma bodies. × 350.

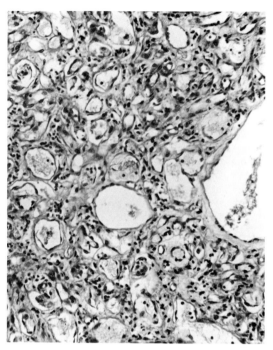

Fig. 21.79 Haemangioblastoma of the cerebellum in a case of Lindau's disease. × 130.

Microscopically meningiomas show considerable variation. The most common variety is composed of fibrocellular tissue with a somewhat whorled appearance owing to the concentric arrangement of the cells (Fig. 21.77). The centres of some of the whorls contain small blood vessels, but others undergo hyaline change and become calcified, resulting in a hard gritty tumour containing numerous spherical calcified particles—*psammoma bodies* (Fig. 21. 78). In the more cellular varieties the whorls are composed of rather plump spindle-shaped cells resembling endothelium, but all degrees of transition to the fibrous types are encountered.

Sarcoma very occasionally arises from the meninges and extends widely over its surface. Occasionally a primary *malignant melanoma* occurs as a diffusely spreading tumour in the meninges.

Tumours of vascular origin

Tumours of vascular origin are uncommon, forming about 2% of cerebral tumours. They are divided into *angiomatous malformations*, and the *haemangioblastomas*. The former are not true tumours but are similar to vascular hamartomas elsewhere. They may be chiefly capillary, venous, or arterio-venous, and their principal importance is as a cause of intracranial haemorrhage (p. 21.22).

Haemangioblastomas are true tumours arising from vascular elements. They occur most frequently in the cerebellum and are composed of vascular channels or spaces (Fig. 21.79), among which there is a large accumulation of lipid-laden cells with an abundant network of reticulin fibres among them. There is a marked tendency to cyst formation, one or more large spaces being surrounded by compressed, gliosed brain tissue; the tumour is seen as a nodule in the cyst wall. In **Lindau's disease** a haemangioblastoma of the brain is accompanied by non-vascular cysts in the pancreas (p. 14.40) or kidneys, and adenomas in the kidneys or adrenals.

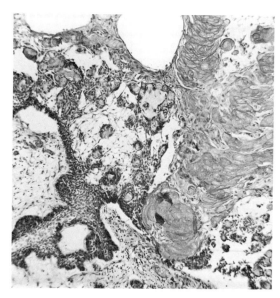

Fig. 21.80 Craniopharyngioma, showing partly squamous, partly 'adamantinomatous' structure. Note the stellate reticulum within the epithelial bands. × 130.

Developmental tumours and cysts

Dermoid and epidermoid cysts, which present clinically as tumours, occasionally affect the nervous system and occur especially at the base of the brain, in the vertebral canal, and in the bones of the skull. An *epidermoid cyst* is well encapsulated, and has a whitish and rather shining appearance (pearly tumour) and rather dry, crumbling contents. The wall is thin and is composed of cells of squamous epithelial type from which keratinised squames are shed into the interior where they accumulate, together with crystals of cholesterol, and thus distend the cyst. In *dermoid cysts*, hairs and sebaceous glands are present. Midline dermoid and epidermoid cysts in the posterior fossa and in the vertebral canal are sometimes connected to the skin surface by a sinus. The opening on the skin may be very small but the sinus provides a route by which the cyst may become infected. *Inclusion epidermoid cysts* in the region of the cauda equina can result from repeated lumbar puncture during childhood.

A somewhat similar partly cystic tumour, is found in children and adults in the region of the pituitary stalk, compressing the gland in the sella turcica and pressing upwards into the third ventricle. These rare suprasellar tumours probably arise from nests of epidermoid cells derived from the pars tuberalis and they are known as **suprasellar cysts** or **craniopharyngiomas**. Their lining epithelium is in part squamous, but there is also a partial differentiation towards stellate reticulum resembling enamel organ (Fig. 21.80), and the name **adamantinoma** is sometimes applied. The wall is usually partially calcified. The chief clinical features are disturbances of vision and of hypophyseal function (p. 26.8). True *Rathke pouch cysts* are intrasellar.

Teratomas are rare intracranial tumours, their chief site being the pineal, where, in boys, their occurrence may be associated with precocious sexual development. They may be well differentiated but more often are of the germinoma type, the histological features being indistinguishable from those of seminoma (p. 25.14).

Metastatic tumours

Metastatic tumours are very common in the brain and may produce symptoms suggestive of a primary brain tumour before the real origin, e.g. a bronchial carcinoma, is suspected. Metastatic deposits are typically multiple and usually sharply circumscribed. The tumour cells tend to spread along the perivascular spaces, ensheathing the blood vessels. Sometimes metastatic carcinoma spreads diffusely throughout the subarachnoid space (*meningeal carcinomatosis*) and the clinical features may be those of a subacute meningitis, but it is usually possible to identify tumour cells in the CSF. The brain may also be infiltrated directly or compressed by tumours arising in the naso-pharynx, or by a chordoma growing from the basiphenoid. Secondary tumours within the dura of the spinal cord are rare, but extradural spinal metastases are common.

Tumours of nerve roots and peripheral nerves

These may be solitary or multiple, the latter being especially associated with neurofibroma-tosis, a disorder inherited as an autosomal dominant. Tumours of nerves are believed to originate from Schwann cells, but some contain a large amount of collagen; hence the sub-division into **schwannoma** and **neurofibroma.** They do, however, exist as a spectrum, ranging from a discrete paraneural schwannoma at one end to a poorly delineated plexiform neurofibroma at the other.

Schwannoma (Neurilemmoma). This is typi-cally a rounded or lobulated, often partly cystic, well circumscribed and encapsulated tumour arising from a nerve. These tumours may be intracranial, intraspinal or peripheral. Within the cranium the commonest site of ori-gin is the vestibular portion of the acoustic nerve, but they also occur in association with the trigeminal nerve. An acoustic schwannoma (**'acoustic neuroma'**) takes origin just within the internal auditory meatus, which it invariably expands; and the enlargement may be visible radiologically. The tumour fills the cerebello-pontine angle (Fig. 21.81) and eventually produces severe distortion and displacement of the adjacent brain and some degree of hydro-cephalus from compression of the fourth ventricle. When bilateral, they are usually associated with von Recklinghausen's neuro-fibromatosis (see below). In the spinal canal, schwannomas occur as intradural tumours on the dorsal nerve roots, mostly in the thor-acic region. Their main effect is to compress the spinal cord, but they may extend through the intervertebral foramen to produce a much larger intrathoracic portion. On peripheral nerves they may occur as isolated single nodules or they may be multiple. The nerve fibres tend to be spread over the surface, espe-

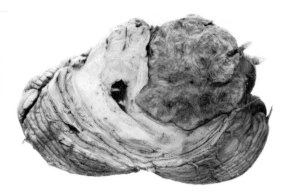

Fig. 21.81 Large schwannoma of the auditory nerve in the cerebello-pontine angle, which has caused great displacement of the adjacent structures.

cially at one side, and are not incorporated in the tumour.

Microscopic examination shows the tumour to consist of fibro-cellular bundles in a whorled pattern; within the fasciculi, the cells are closely arranged in parallel fashion with their rod-shaped nuclei forming a characteristic 'palisade' (Fig. 21.82). In other areas the tumour may be of looser texture or even cystic and contain

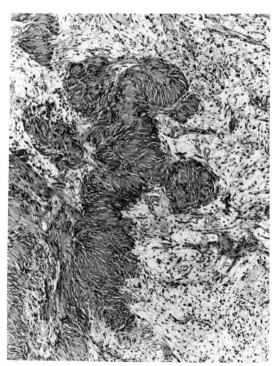

Fig. 21.82 Schwannoma of acoustic nerve, showing whorling and palisading of cells. × 65.

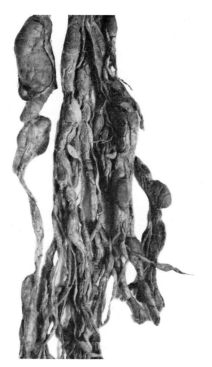

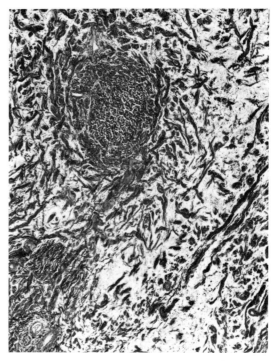

Fig. 21.83 Plexiform neuroma of the sciatic nerve and its branches. Note the numerous nodules of various sizes and forms.

Fig. 21.84 Plexiform neurofibroma showing nerve fibres and loosely arranged interlacing connective tissue bundles. × 120.

large numbers of fat-laden foamy cells between the fasciculi. The softer and more cellular tumours are prone to repeated local recurrence, and occasionally become frankly sarcomatous.

Neurofibroma may present as a fusiform swelling on a single nerve, but more often a group of nerves are extensively affected by numerous oval and irregular swellings—**plexiform neurofibroma** (Fig. 21.83). If subcutaneous nerves are affected, as not uncommonly occurs in the scalp and neck, the overlying skin becomes firm and nodular and may appear convoluted.

Histological examination shows the nerve to be expanded by large elongated and spindle-shaped cells often separated by mucoid matrix (Fig. 21.84). Residual nerve fibres can be identified in neurofibromas. There is a tendency for local recurrence after excision, and sarcomatous change is not unusual.

In **neurofibromatosis ('von Recklinghausen's disease')**, nodules of various sizes, sometimes numbering hundreds, occur along small nerve branches, especially of the skin, but also in some cases along the visceral branches of the sympathetic. Tumours sometimes arise also from the spinal nerves and their roots within the spinal canal, leading to compression of the spinal cord. The connective tissue of the nodules varies, but is often dense and hyaline; nerve fibres can be traced running through it. Neurofibromatosis is usually associated with multiple pigmented patches in the skin, and lastly, there is occasionally a localised general thickening of the tissues, with nodulation and folding of the skin—a sort of local elephantiasis, to which the name *elephantiasis neuromatosa* has been applied.

III: The Peripheral Nerves

Normal nerve structure

Two main types of nerve fibres are found in peripheral nerve, myelinated and non-myelinated. Up to ten non-myelinated axons (0.2–3 μm diameter) invaginate a Schwann cell. Myelinated axons (1–15 μm diameter) lie singly within a chain of Schwann cells, each of which forms a myelin sheath around the axon. The boundaries between each Schwann cell on the myelinated fibre are clearly demarcated as *nodes of Ranvier*. The axons of myelinated fibres arise from neurons in the posterior root ganglia and in the anterior grey horn of the spinal cord. Non-myelinated axons arise from neurons in the posterior root ganglia and in the autonomic ganglia.

In addition to electric transmission, the axon is intimately involved in the transport of organelles, nutrients and metabolic products both to and from the perikaryon and the periphery (p. 21.2).

Groups of intermingled unmyelinated and myelinated fibres, each enclosed in an *endoneural sheath*, constitute a fascicle. Each fascicle is surrounded by the *perineurium*, which is a major diffusion barrier similar to the blood–brain barrier. Groups of fascicles are bound together by the *epineurium* to form the peripheral nerve.

Degenerative changes in peripheral nerves

There are two main types of nerve fibre degeneration, (a) axonal degeneration and (b) segmental demyelination. In most of the clinical neuropathies both types occur, but usually one type predominates.

(a) Axonal degeneration. In this type of degeneration, described on p. 21.3, axon death leads to secondary breakdown of the myelin sheath. Axonal death may be caused by disorders of the peripheral axon or the perikaryon. In focal injury to the peripheral nerve there is total degeneration of the axon and myelin distal to the site of injury (*Wallerian degeneration*). If the lesion is distal, the nerve cell body undergoes transient swelling and breakdown of the endoplasmic reticulum (*chromatolysis*) but recovers to support *regeneration* of the damaged axon (p. 5.20). However, if the lesion is proximal or involves the nerve cell body, irreversible nerve cell death may occur. Provided the connective tissue of the endoneural tubes is preserved, the prognosis for recovery is good. However, if the lesion transects the nerve, many axonal sprouts may not reach the distal stump, and form a *traumatic neuroma*. When axonal degeneration occurs due to diseases other than trauma, the term *axonal neuropathy* or *axonopathy* are used. In many such disorders the transport function of the axon is disrupted, leading to abnormalities starting at the most distant part of the axon, the pathological process then extending back (*retrograde degeneration*) to the cell body ('*dying back*' neuropathies).

(b) Segmental demyelination. This occurs when the Schwann cell and myelin sheath are damaged, leaving the axon relatively intact. The process is usually patchy. Schwann cells are capable of division and remyelination occurs provided the cause of the Schwann cell death is removed. The demyelinated internode is usually replaced by two or more Schwann cells leading to a decrease in internodal length in this segment.

Investigation of peripheral nerve disease

The investigative techniques employed in peripheral nerve disorders include electrophysiology and nerve biopsy. Due to the complex structure and the length of the peripheral nerves, each technique has major limitations.

Electrophysiology. The speed of conduction along motor and sensory nerves and the magnitude of the evoked nerve action potential are measured. In general, demyelinating neuropathies are associated with a *reduced conduction velocity* and axonal neuropathies with a *fall in the amplitude of the evoked nerve action potential*.

However, these techniques assess only the myelinated fibres of large diameter and provide no information on fine, including non-myelinated, fibres. Normal electrophysiology does not therefore exclude disorder of a peripheral nerve.

Nerve biopsy. *Removal of a length of nerve will denervate part of the body, and it is therefore impor-*

tant that the information expected from biopsy is *sufficiently important to justify the procedure*. Very little information can usually be obtained from conventionally-stained paraffin-embedded sections and special techniques are necessary to justify the biopsy.

Single fibres are studied in teased preparations to measure the internodal length, which is decreased in remyelinated fibres (see above). Semi-thin plastic-embedded and electron-microscopic sections are used for quantitative studies and to observe the general morphological changes. Quantitative studies provide information on the numbers and diameters of myelinated and non-myelinated fibres present and thus help to detect selective involvement or loss of a particular type.

Classification of neuropathies

Disorders of the peripheral nerves are classified into *symmetrical generalised polyneuropathy*, *focal and multifocal neuropathies* and *genetically-determined neuropathies*.

Symmetrical generalised polyneuropathy

This is subdivided, on the basis of the primary pathological change, into *neuronopathy, myelinopathy* and *axonopathy*: this subdivision is supported by differences in the symptomatology of the three groups.

Neuronopathy

This describes conditions in which the primary pathological change occurs in the perikaryon. Either the motor neurons or the primary sensory neurons may be involved. Anterior horn cell involvement is seen in *poliomyelitis*: dorsal root ganglion involvement is seen in *herpes zoster*.

Subacute sensory neuropathy develops in association with carcinoma and is the most common non-infective neuronopathy. Clinically, the onset is rapid or subacute. Symmetrical sensory loss can occur anywhere in the limbs and trunk and facial sensory loss is common. The deep tendon reflexes are lost and CSF protein is variably increased. Nerve conduction velocities are normal in motor nerves and conduction is slowed or absent in sensory nerves.

The cause of the neuronal damage is unknown. Recovery is variable, depending on the extent of neuronal loss.

Myelinopathy

This describes conditions where the primary pathological process is segmental demyelination with preservation of axons. Demyelination starts at a node of Ranvier and may be patchy or confined to one segment of the nerve fibre. The spinal roots are usually involved and this accounts for the raised CSF protein, which is a feature of demyelinating neuropathies. During recovery, the Schwann cells divide and form short internodes of thin myelin. If subsequent repeated demyelination occurs, the dividing Schwann cells fail to attach to an axon and migrate to form rings (onion bulbs) around the axon. This process is characteristic of chronic myelinopathies.

Clinically, the disease may develop in a few hours or over days or weeks. Motor weakness is much more evident than sensory signs, although early sensory symptoms are common. The weakness usually begins distally and spreads centrally and cranial nerves may become involved. The deep tendon reflexes are absent and nerve conduction velocities show marked slowing. The CSF protein is raised without a marked rise in cell count. Recovery depends on successful remyelination and is usually good.

Acute infectious polyneuropathy (*Guillain-Barré syndrome*) is the commonest myelinopathy and is characterised by a progressive ascending paraplegia. About two-thirds of patients give a history of prior infection, usually of the upper respiratory tract. The disease can occur at any age. About 50% of patients reach maximum disability in the first week and most of the remainder by the third week. Approximately one-third of patients develop respiratory failure due to weakness of the diaphragm and intercostal muscles, and may require prolonged artificial ventilation. In some patients, cranial nerve involvement develops. Sensory symptoms and signs are seen in about 20% of cases. Autonomic neuropathy, with sphincter disturbance and cardiac arrythmias, may also develop. Between 80 and 90% of patients recover completely. A small percentage have relapses and a few are left with permanent weakness.

Axonopathy

This is the most common effect of toxins and metabolic diseases on the peripheral nerves. The primary pathology is distal in the axon and progresses back to the cell body ('dying-back'). When the axon breaks down there is secondary demyelination (Fig. 21.85). Clinically the onset is insidious, producing a glove and stocking sensory loss and distal muscle weakness. Sensory symptoms usually precede motor loss. The ankle reflexes are lost early. Nerve conduction velocities are slightly or moderately slowed and the CSF protein is normal.

Recovery depends on axonal regeneration and is therefore slow (p. 5.20) and often incomplete.

Axonopathy may complicate diabetes, uraemia, porphyria and cancer. It occurs also in deficiency of thiamine (nutritional and alcoholic) or of pyridoxine; also as a toxic effect of drugs (e.g. nitrofurantoin, diphenylhydantoin, isoniazide, perhexiline maleate, vincristine and cisplatin) and of chemicals used in industry (e.g. organophosphorus, lead, thallium and hexacarbons).

Focal and multifocal neuropathies

These disorders are produced by trauma (e.g. entrapment), ischaemia and infiltration of individual nerves (e.g. in leprosy and in amyloid disease). The primary pathological reaction is *Wallerian degeneration*, with loss of both axon and myelin sheath below the level of the lesion. In most patients, motor and sensory symptoms develop simultaneously.

Genetically-determined neuropathies

Hereditary motor sensory neuropathies (HMSN) are subdivided, on the basis of the

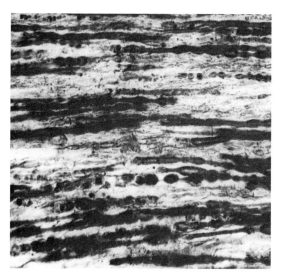

Fig. 21.85 Longitudinal section of peripheral nerve in alcoholic neuropathy showing degeneration of myelin sheaths. (Marchi method.) × about 400.

major pathological process, into three major groups.

HMSN I (*peroneal muscular atrophy* or *Charcot–Marie–Tooth disease*) is usually an autosomal dominant condition, the patients showing distal weakness and wasting in the legs with absent tendon reflexes. The disease is slowly progressive, but may produce only minor disability.

The pathological feature of this condition is demyelination. In attempted remyelination, the Schwann cells do not become attached to an axon but form concentric rings around the axon—'onion bulb formation' (see above): it may be detected clinically as palpably thickened nerves.

HMSN II The clinical features are similar to those of HMSN I. Inheritance is autosomal and may be either dominant or recessive. The abnormality is thought to be in the perikaryon and results in an axonopathy.

HMSN III (*Dejerine–Sottas disease*). This is a disorder of childhood in which severe demyelination is often associated with skeletal deformity. It is inherited as an autosomal recessive condition. The pathological features are similar to HMSN I.

IV: Voluntary Muscles

Striated skeletal muscle comprises 40–50% of the weight of the body. Although it is specifically designed to convert chemical energy into mechanical work, muscle also has major functions as a store of energy-rich compounds and protein and plays an important role in the general metabolism of the body.

Normal structure

An individual muscle consists of bundles of fibres within a connective tissue framework. This can be divided into three components, the *endomysium* which separates the individual muscle fibres, the *perimysium* which envelops bundles of fibres and the *epimysium* which ensheaths the whole muscle. Individual muscle fibres are elongated multinuclear syncytia with diameters 10–100 μm and up to 10 cm long. The muscle nuclei lie at the periphery of the fibre, under the plasma membrane (*sarcolemma*), which is enclosed in a basal lamina. Cross-striations, seen in longitudinal sections, result from the parallel arrangement of thick (myosin) and thin (actin) filaments. During contraction these filaments slide between each other.

The individual motor unit comprises the anterior horn cell and its peripheral nerve fibre, the neuromuscular junction, and the myofibres supplied by it. Disease states can occur from lesions at any level of the motor unit. The number of myofibres receiving their nerve supply from a single anterior horn cell determines the size of the motor unit: in general, the more delicate the function to be performed, the smaller the size of the unit. Myofibres are of type 1 and type 2 and all the muscle fibres in a motor unit are of the same type which is determined by the parent anterior horn cell. *Type 1* (*slow* or *red*) *fibres* are highly resistant to fatigue: they are rich in mitochondria and contain a relatively high ratio of lipid to glycogen. These fibres are adapted for posture-maintaining contractions. In contrast, *type 2* (*fast* or *white*) *fibres* are rich in myofibrillar ATPase activity compared to mitochondria, and contain a high ratio of glycogen to lipid. They are specialised for fine rapid movement. Both fibre types are found in all skeletal muscle, but their proportion varies according to the main function of the muscle.

The fibres of a motor unit do not form a discrete group, but are intermingled with fibres of adjacent units (Fig. 21.87).

Reactive changes

The basic pathological reactions of the muscle cell are similar to those of other cells, but the specialised development of the contractile apparatus, and the fact that the fibre is a syncytium formed by fusion of myoblasts, both influence the reactions of the cell to injury or disease.

Atrophy occurs when a muscle loses its nerve supply: this may result from death of the anterior horn cell (as in poliomyelitis), from peripheral nerve damage or from lesions of the specialised neuromuscular junction (as in myasthenia gravis). Some degree of atrophy is also seen in response to lack of use of the muscle, notably where a fractured limb is immobilised: type 2 fibres are mainly affected.

Hypertrophy occurs physiologically as a response to increased workload. Hypertrophy of individual scattered fibres is seen as a compensatory response to loss of fibres, notably in the denervating conditions: the hypertrophied fibres may appear to have split longitudinally and may have central nuclei (*myotubes*—see 'hypertrophy' below). Generalised hypertrophy of muscle fibres occurs in the rare myotonia congenita.

Necrosis of muscle, ischaemic necrosis. Muscle has an extensive collateral circulation and thus infarction is a rare event except as part of ischaemic 'gangrene' of the leg. Ischaemic necrosis of healthy muscle may, however, occur (a) when a major arterial supply is interrupted e.g. in Volkmann's ischaemic contracture following trauma to the elbow, (b) in thrombosis of multiple intramuscular vessels as in polyarteritis nodosa, and (c) following unaccustomed strenuous exercise, especially in the anterior tibial group of muscles. Muscle swelling following strenuous and unaccustomed exercise may lead to reduction of the blood supply and subsequent necrosis which further increases the swelling. Following ischaemic necrosis, muscle regeneration is patchy and fibrosis develops.

'Toxic' necrosis (*Zenker's or waxy degenera-*

tion) occurs in severe toxaemia and is seen most often affecting groups of fibres in the muscles of the anterior abdominal wall in typhoid fever, but it occurs also in acute viral infections, where the causal factors are not known. The affected fibres have a pale hyaline, waxy appearance and there is remarkably little reaction.

Segmental necrosis affects usually short lengths of individual fibres. It has many causes but is due fundamentally to loss of integrity of the plasmalemma (plasma membrane) with consequent ingress of calcium ions in excess. This interferes with mitochondrial function and so loss of the energy required for normal metabolism. Autolytic changes and disorganisation result, and macrophages enter the affected length of fibre and remove the debris. Foci of necrosis and regeneration may be seen in the same fibres.

Focal subfibre necrosis is a process in which patches of sarcoplasm within a fibre undergo necrosis and autophagocytosis, leaving residual bodies containing lipofuscin. Restoration is incomplete and regeneration by myoblasts does not occur.

Necrosis in infections is described below under 'infective myositis'.

Regeneration. Following damage to voluntary muscle fibres, their capacity to regenerate depends mainly on whether loss of fibres is accompanied by destruction or loss of basement membrane and endomysium. When these are lost, little effective regeneration of a fibre occurs, but if they remain intact there may be considerable regeneration. Proliferation of satellite stem cells provides mononuclear myoblasts which fuse to form a new fibre: initially this has a row of central rounded nuclei and is known as a myotube. The nuclei then migrate to the periphery and the fibre assumes its adult form. Myotubes may form alongside one another within the endomysial tube, resulting in apparent 'split' muscle fibres.

Infective myositis

Viral myositis most commonly affects children under the age of 10 years and is usually seen during influenza epidemics. Pain and weakness of the calf muscles develop 48 hours following the onset of generalised symptoms. Muscle biopsy shows acute segmental necrosis with a prominent inflammatory infiltrate. Other groups of muscles are rarely involved. The illness is benign and total recovery is to be expected. Severe post-viral rhabdomyolysis and myoglobinuria may be seen in younger children.

Pyogenic myositis is rare in developed countries but is relatively common in the tropics and subtropics. The commonest infecting organism is *Staphylococcus aureus* and some cases are due to spread from an overlying skin infection, but in many there is no obvious source of infection. The *quadriceps and glutei* are most often affected, but any muscle may be involved. Intense local pain with swelling is the classical clinical presentation. The changes are those of acute inflammation with intense interstitial oedema, progressing to necrosis and suppuration. Without treatment, haematogenous spread is common. Treatment consists of drainage and antibiotics. Recovery of muscle function is good.

Gas gangrene. In severe trauma of muscle, particularly when the wound is contaminated by soil or other foreign material, there is a risk of gas gangrene, most often caused by *Clostridium welchii*. The features are described on p. 9.11.

Trichinosis. Infection with *Trichinella spiralis* is described on p. 28.46.

Neuromuscular disorders

This term includes a large group of diseases in which impaired function of motor units (p. 21.69) presents clinically as weakness. Some are neurogenic, i.e. result from lesions of the lower motor neurons and their nerve fibres: others arise from defects of the neuromuscular junction or of the muscle fibres themselves. By convention, the term *atrophy* is applied to neuromuscular disease when the cause is neurogenic. The term *myopathy* is used for disorders of the muscle fibres, and *dystrophy* is applied to genetically determined myopathies in which there are degenerative changes in the muscle fibres without evidence of a storage disorder.

As a general rule, when clinical examination shows bilateral symmetry of muscle involvement the patient is likely to have myopathy, while asymmetric and selective involvement of muscles is likely to be of neurogenic origin.

Methods of investigation. Clinical investigation is based on careful clinical examination to determine the pattern of muscle weakness. Electrophysiological studies are used to test the function of the peripheral nerve and to sample muscle fibre reactions. These tests are subject to sample error and are used as a guide to further investigation.

The serum creatine kinase is used as an index of muscle fibre damage, being markedly elevated when there is necrosis.

Biopsy is usually performed on large proximal limb muscles (e.g. quadriceps or biceps). A muscle which is *severely* involved by the disease should usually be avoided because the basic pathological process may not be apparent in end-stage muscle. Biopsies are obtained by the 'open' or 'needle' techniques. The major advantage of the latter is that it is repeatable and allows the disease process to be followed sequentially. The application of histochemical techniques to the study of fresh frozen muscle biopsy samples has greatly enhanced understanding of the neuromuscular diseases. Some disorders previously thought to be single entities have been shown to be pathologically heterogeneous. Diseases due to defects in energy pathways (*the metabolic myopathies*) have been identified and specific defects in myofibre development (e.g. *myotubular myopathy*) and in fibre type distribution (*fibre type disproportion*) have been shown to be the cause of many cases of the 'floppy infant' syndrome.

Classification. A classification of neuromuscular disorders was provided in 1968 by the World Federation of Neurology. Many of the diseases included are inherited disorders of motor neurons, and diseases in which the cause of motor neuron injury was known, e.g. poliomyelitis, were excluded. A simplified classification is given in Table 21.2. The terms 'limb-girdle' and 'facioscapulohumeral' are best used to indicate the distribution of muscle weakness

at the time of examination and not as indicating specific types of myopathy.

Table 21.2 Classification of neuromuscular disorders

Motor neuron disease (described on p. 21.52)
X-linked muscular dystrophy (Duchenne and
  Becker dystrophies)
Spinal muscular atrophy
Inflammatory myopathy
Metabolic myopathy
Myotonic disorders
Periodic paralyses
Congenital myopathy
Toxic and drug-induced myopathy
Myasthenia gravis and other disorders of the
  neuromuscular junctions

The commoner neuromuscular disorders are motor neuron disease (amyotrophic lateral sclerosis, etc.) which is described on p. 21.52, Duchenne muscular dystrophy, spinal muscular atrophy, the polymyositis/dermatomyositis complex and myasthenia gravis.

X-linked muscular dystrophy

Duchenne muscular dystrophy is the commonest genetic myopathy, with an incidence of 20–30/100 000 live-born males. Inheritance is X-linked, the disease being manifest in males and carried by females. Some cases arise by mutation in the absence of a family history. Affected males present before the age of 5 years with delayed development of motor function, notably waddling gait and inability to run. Due to weakness of the pelvic-girdle muscles these children are unable to rise easily from the floor and use their arms to push the trunk into the upright position (Gower's manoeuvre). The majority of boys are confined to a wheelchair by 13 years of age and death due to respiratory failure occurs usually in the late teens.

Pathological changes in muscle depend on the age of the child at the time of biopsy. Up to 1 year the predominant finding is the presence of frequent hyaline (pre-necrotic) and necrotic fibres with adequate regeneration (Fig. 21.86 *upper*), but as regenerative capacity declines, there is progressive replacement of the muscle fibres by adipose and fibrous tissue (Fig. 21.86 *lower*).

Current research suggests that the genetically-determined abnormality is a defect

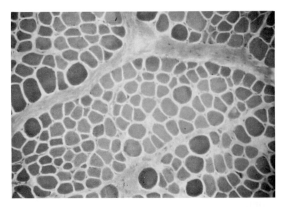

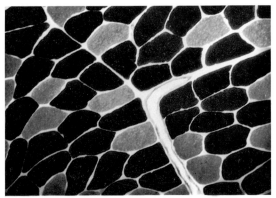

Fig. 21.87   Section of normal muscle showing intermingling of types 1 and 2 fibres. (Frozen section stained for myofibrillar ATPase: type 2 fibres appear darker than type 1.) × 250.

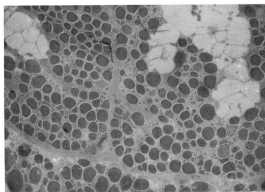

Fig. 21.86   Duchenne muscular dystrophy. *Upper*, at early stage, showing necrotic and pre-necrotic fibres. *Lower*, later stage with atrophic fibres and replacement by fatty and fibrous tissue. × 120.

of the muscle sarcolemma which permits the ingress of excess calcium ions, leading to muscle necrosis.

The serum creatine kinase is markedly elevated (10 000–20 000 iu/l) in the early years and tends to fall in the teens.

Becker muscular dystrophy. In its clinicopathological features (including X-linked inheritance) this resembles Duchenne muscular dystrophy but the course is much more benign. The age of onset is from 3–20 years, death occurring between 30 and 60 years.

Spinal muscular atrophy (SMA or neurogenic muscular weakness)

Weakness and wasting in SMA is due to loss of anterior horn cells with secondary involvement of the muscle fibres in their motor units. Because the fibres from different motor units are normally intermingled (Fig. 21.87) denerv-

ation of a single motor unit results in the presence of small and ribbon-like atrophic fibres scattered between normal muscle fibres (Fig. 21.88). This process is referred to as *disseminated neurogenic atrophy*.

In a normal muscle fibre, responsiveness to acetylcholine is limited to the end-plate zone. In response to denervation, all of the sarcolemma becomes responsive to acetyl choline. This appears to stimulate the formation of collateral sprouts from intact nerve terminal branches, which annexe the recently denervated fibres. The fibres then redevelop to normal size and take on the histochemical features of the fibre type determined by the new nerve. This leads to grouping of fibre types with loss of the normal checkerboard appearance (Fig. 21.89).

When an enlarged motor unit is affected,

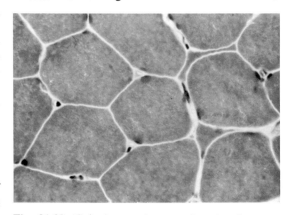

Fig. 21.88   Spinal muscular atrophy, showing two inconspicuous atrophic muscle fibres lying among normal fibres. × 400.

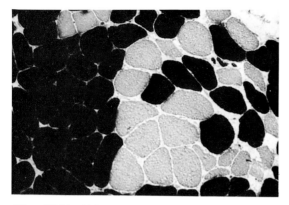

Fig. 21.89 Spinal muscular atrophy, showing grouping of type 2 fibres resulting from re-innervation and regeneration of denervated fibres. (Frozen section stained for myofibrillar ATPase: type 2 fibres darkly stained.) × 250.

groups of atrophic fibres are seen (Fig. 21.90). Eventually re-innervation is no longer possible and the atrophic fibres appear small and rounded, with densely stained nuclei. Secondary 'myopathic' changes are seen in the biopsy at this stage, with fibre 'splitting', hypertrophy, internal migration of nuclei and excess fatty and fibrous tissue.

Inheritance of SMA may be autosomal dominant or recessive, but sporadic cases also occur. The disease varies in severity in different families.

The cause of the loss of anterior horn cells is unknown. The clinical syndromes of SMA depend on the rate of denervation: when this is rapid, re-innervation is incomplete and the disease runs a short course (*progressive infantile SMA*). When denervation slows down and re-innervation is more effective, the disease progresses more slowly (*chronic childhood SMA*). When denervation is slow and re-innervation is effective, *adolescent or adult-onset SMA develops.*

Adolescent and adult-onset SMA presents with asymmetrical selective weakness in a limb-girdle or facioscapulohumeral distribution, often with hypertrophy of distal lower limb muscles. The course of the disease is slow with long periods of stability. Abnormalities of cardiac conduction are seen in some cases.

Progressive infantile SMA (*Acute Werdnig-Hoffman disease*) may develop at any time in the first five months of life. The infant is profoundly hypotonic with severe generalised weakness and respiratory difficulty. The course is progressive, leading to death within two years.

Chronic childhood SMA (*Kugelberg-Welander syndrome*) may present in early childhood with a rapidly progressive course which then arrests, the child surviving for many years despite the inability to walk, sit or stand unaided. In other cases, the disease starts in later childhood and progresses in a stepwise manner with periods of deterioration, in which denervation takes place faster than re-innervation, and long periods of stability in which re-innervation keeps pace with denervation. Weakness of the paraspinal muscles during growth leads to scoliosis, and death occurs between 20 and 30 years from respiratory failure.

Inflammatory myopathy

Polymyositis/dermatomyositis complex (PM/DM). Symmetrical progressive limb-girdle weakness is the cardinal presenting clinical feature of PM/DM in the child or adult. In childhood, DM is seen more commonly than PM, but the similarities in the clinicopathological features, the course of the disease and the response to therapy, suggest that the disease is of the same nature in children and adults.

Patients with PM/DM present with proximal weakness which progresses slowly over months. Muscle pain, frequently described as aching and increased by exercise, is common. Raynaud's disease and swallowing difficulties are seen in some patients. A heliotrope rash develops around the eyes, across the bridge of the nose, over the dorsal aspect of the joints of the hands and often on the extensor surface of the thighs.

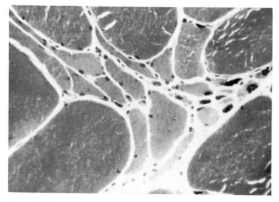

Fig. 21.90 Spinal muscular atrophy. Re-innervation has resulted in grouping of fibres of a motor unit. Subsequent denervation has resulted in atrophy of the grouped fibres. × 600.

Patients may present with focal disease which subsequently assumes a limb-girdle or occasionally a facioscapulohumeral distribution.

In approximately 75% of cases, PM/DM is primary ('uncomplicated'). In 17% of cases it is associated with a connective tissue disease (usually systemic lupus erythematosus or rheumatoid arthritis), and in about 8% with a carcinoma. The aetiology is unknown, but recent evidence indicates that abnormalities of cell-mediated immune responses are an important factor.

Pathologically, there is widespread patchy necrosis and inflammation, often affecting the peripheral fibres of muscle fascicles (Fig. 21.91). Fibres in various stages of regeneration are seen. The inflammatory infiltrate, which is often perimysial, is composed of lymphocytes, macrophages and eosinophils.

Treatment for DM/PM is with steroids and immunosuppression, treatment being continued for up to 5 years. The prognosis for uncomplicated PM/DM is good. The prognosis for PM/DM associated with connective tissue disease or carcinoma is that of the underlying disease.

Granulomatous myositis

Granulomatous inflammation of muscle usually occurs as a feature of systemic diseases, particularly sarcoidosis, polyarteritis nodosa and Wegener's granuloma. Muscle biopsy is often useful in providing a tissue diagnosis in these disorders.

Metabolic myopathies

This group of disorders is due to defects in intermediary metabolism in the muscle cell. They are subdivided into disorders of glycolysis or glycogen synthesis, of oxidative and/or lipid metabolism and of mitochondrial function.

Despite their varied aetiology, the clinical presentation is similar, either as a progressive myopathy or exercise-induced muscle pain and cramp which may or may not be associated with episodic weakness.

Glycogen storage diseases. Brief comments on these diseases are given on pp. 3.15–17 and 20.8. Type 2 (acid maltase deficiency), type 3 (debrancher deficiency) and type 4 (branching enzyme deficiency) produce a proximal myopathy. Type 5 (McArdle's disease) and type 7 (phosphofructokinase deficiency) produce exercise-induced muscle pain and cramp.

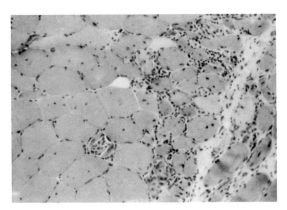

Fig. 21.91 Polymyositis/dermatomyositis complex, showing an inflammatory infiltrate and necrosis and regeneration affecting muscle fibres at the periphery of adjacent fascicles. × 200.

Disorders of lipid metabolism. Long chain fatty acids are the most important substrate for oxidation by the muscle cell during exercise and recovery from exercise. Enzyme defects along the metabolic pathway of lipid lead either to muscle pain and cramp on exercise (*carnitine-palmityl transferase deficiency*) or a progressive proximal myopathy (*carnitine deficiency*). Neutral fat accumulates within the muscle fibres.

Mitochondrial myopathies. This group of disorders is less well defined. The classical pathological feature is the 'ragged red' fibre, due to accumulation of abnormal mitochondria at the periphery of the fibre. The clinical features usually include disorders of eye movement (*chronic progressive ophthalmoplegia*) with or without a limb-girdle myopathy, and variable involvement of the heart, nervous system and other organs.

Myotonic disorders

In myotonia, the muscles are slow to relax after vigorous contraction.

Myotonic dystrophy is a multisystem disorder in which muscular symptoms predominate. The disease is inherited as an autosomal dominant with variable expression. In most cases the main symptom is muscle stiffness with delayed relaxation of grip. Myotonia is also seen in the tongue. Weakness is at first distal in distribution with impaired hand function and foot-drop, but proximal weakness also develops later, notably of the facial muscles, leading to ptosis and a 'transverse' mouth, and of the sternomastoid muscles. Smooth muscle is also involved, with impaired function of the alimentary tract and gallbladder. Defects of cardiac conduction and a cardiomyopathy may also develop. Impaired function of the muscles of respiration leads to hypoventilation and anaesthesia carries a risk of respiratory failure. There is end-organ unresponsiveness to insulin, leading eventually to the development of diabetes mellitus. Progressive ovarian or testicular dysfunction develops. Females often have a poor obstetric history and may give birth to infants with the severe congenital form of the disease. Peripheral neuropathy, posterior subcapsular cataracts and frontal baldness complete the clinical picture.

Muscle biopsy shows a relative selective atrophy of type 1 fibres, marked variation in fibre size and chains of central nuclei.

Myotonic dystrophy is caused by a cell-membrane abnormality and the great variety of manifestations of the disease is probably due to involvement of a wide range of cells throughout the body. Recent evidence shows that the gene defect lies in chromosome 19. Developments in recombinant DNA technology are likely to lead to a greater understanding of this disease.

Myotonia congenita. In this rare condition, muscular hypertrophy is associated with myotonia, which may be localised or generalised.

Periodic paralyses

This group of disorders is characterised by episodes of flaccid weakness during which the patients are either hyper- or hypo-kalaemic. The attacks can last from several hours (hyperkalaemic) to days (hypokalaemic). Weakness may be localised or generalised; in the latter case, progression from proximal to distal muscles is usual. The muscles of respiration and those supplied by the cranial nerves are spared. Rest following a period of prolonged exercise will provoke weakness of the exercised muscles, while mild continued exercise may abort an attack. Areflexia during an attack is usual. Attacks are often provoked by cold and, in the hypokalaemic type, by a carbohydrate meal. Persistent weakness may follow repeated episodes, and myotonia of the eyelids and tongue is seen in the hyperkalaemic type. The hypokalaemic type may be associated with thyrotoxicosis, particularly in patients of Oriental origin.

The basic pathological process is an abnormality of cell membrane of unknown nature which interferes with the control of intracellular sodium and potassium. Muscle biopsy may show vacuoles, derived from the sarcotubular system, in the fibres.

Congenital myopathies

Most cases of congenital myopathy present clinically as the 'floppy infant' syndrome. The infants have very poorly developed musculature and may require ventilator support in the first weeks of life. The prognosis for the child depends on the underlying neuromuscular disease.

Muscle biopsy in the congenital myopathies shows changes of both fibre-type distribution and of muscle structure. These changes are related to the development of the muscle fibre. During normal development, fusion of myoblasts is followed by nuclear margination in which the nuclei move from the entre to the periphery of the fibre. Differentiation of the fibres into types 1 and 2 then occurs with subsequent growth to normal size. If nuclear margination fails, myotubes (p. 21.70) persist (*centronuclear* or *myotubal myopathy*). Defects in differentiation may lead either to a deficiency or a preponderance of type 1 fibres. Both of these abnormalities may be associated with structural changes in the fibre e.g. nemaline rods. These changes in a specific fibre type lead to *congenital fibre type disproportion*.

In general, the disorders which result from early developmental defects lead to progressive weakness and death in 20-30 years. A few adult cases of limb-girdle or facioscapulohumeral syndrome have been shown to be due to similar pathological processes. These later defects are associated with poorly developed musculature in adult life, often accompanied by skeletal deformities, but they are not usually fatal.

Toxic and drug-induced myopathies

Muscle is very susceptible to the direct effects of toxins and some drugs. Most of these compounds act directly on the muscle fibre, causing necrosis. Clinically this leads to a limb-girdle syndrome, sometimes associated with myoglobinuria. The serum creatine kinase is usually increased and provides a sensitive index of muscle involvement. In most cases, removal of the toxin or drug is associated with complete recovery.

Toxins. Many snake bites lead to muscle necrosis. Acute alcoholism may lead to hypokalaemia with extensive fibre necrosis and weakness. In the chronic alcoholic, a progressive necrobiotic myopathy develops which often does not improve with alcohol withdrawal.

Drugs. The commonest drug-induced myopathy is caused by glucocorticoids. Iatrogenic steroid myopathy may be subclinical and has an insidious course. It commonly affects the proximal lower limb muscles, especially the iliopsoas and quadriceps. Its occurrence appears to be related to long duration of treatment and high dosage. The serum creatine kinase level is normal and muscle biopsy shows a severe atrophy of type 2 fibres. Recovery of muscle function is good after stoppping the drug, but recovery is slow.

Other drug reactions include a vacuolar myopathy caused by chloroquine, necrotising myopathy caused by emetine, plasmocid, procainamide and epsilon aminocaproic acid, and a myasthenic-like disorder caused by penicillamine.

Myasthenia gravis (MG)

The classical feature of MG is abnormal fatiguability of skeletal muscles, presenting as weakness on exercising muscles and recovery on resting. It is a disorder of neuromuscular transmission of auto-immune nature (p. 7.26) and may occur at any age, but the peak incidence is in young adults (women more often than men), and it may be associated with organ-specific (notably thyroid) auto-immune disease and also with systemic lupus.

The extrinsic ocular and facial muscles are almost always affected early, causing ptosis and diplopia, and there is commonly difficulty in speaking, chewing and swallowing. Symptoms may remain confined to the eyes (ocular form) but more often generalised muscular weakness develops and respiratory distress may occur, particularly in exacerbations (crises). The disease may progress rapidly, with death in a few months, or slowly over many years, often with fluctuations in severity. The commonest cause of death is aspiration pneumonia due to respiratory muscle weakness.

Antibody to acetylcholine receptors (AChR) of human skeletal muscle can be detected in the serum in approximately 90% of patients with adult-onset generalised MG. The antibody is usually absent in ocular MG and congenital MG (see below) and is only occasionally present in other auto-immune diseases (notably systemic lupus). Some correlation between titre of antibody and severity of MG is seen during the course of the disease in individual patients, but there is no close correlation between anti-

body titre and severity in groups of patients, probably because the antibody is heterogeneous, reacting with various epitopes on AChR. IgG antibody has been demonstrated on the AChR site in muscle biopsies and there seems no doubt that this, probably together with complement activation, is responsible for the neuromuscular block, for the infants of myasthenic mothers frequently present transient features of MG. The immunological injury causes degenerative changes in the post-synaptic membranes (motor end plates), seen by electron microscopy as shrinking of the membrane expansions.

Abnormalities of the thymus have long been recognised in MG. In approximately 90% of cases, there is thymic hyperplasia with formation of B-cell follicles with germinal centres, and in 15% there is also a thymoma of mixed epithelial and lymphocytic type. Thymoma occurs mainly in patients developing MG in middle age. Virtually all patients with a thymoma have a high serum titre of antibody which reacts with the I band of skeletal muscle; its presence is of some value in diagnosing thymoma.

The severity of MG may be reduced temporarily by plasmapheresis. Some of the antibody to AChR is produced in the thymus and long-term improvement may follow thymectomy, particularly in young women without a thymoma; the response is, however, variable, and improvement may be delayed for months. At present, plasmapheresis followed by thymectomy, with or without immunosuppressive therapy, appears to be the most effective treatment available.

A rare congenital form of MG is believed to be due to a genetically-determined defect of AChR; it develops in childhood but may not be noticed for many years. There is also evidence that administration of D-penicillamine, e.g. for rheumatoid arthritis, predisposes to the development of a non-immune form of MG.

Myasthenic (Eaton-Lambert) syndrome. In contrast to myasthenia gravis, this syndrome is associated with muscle weakness which *improves* with repeated exercise. It is usually associated with proximal lower limb weakness and areflexia. It is a well-recognised paraneoplastic manifestation (p. 21.44) of small-cell carcinoma of the bronchus and some other malignancies.

IV: The Eye

Introduction

The pathological changes which occur in the eye and the orbital structures are in many respects similar to those described in other systems of the body. However, owing to the particular anatomical and functional properties of the eye, there are some common ocular disease processes which merit separate consideration. Emphasis is therefore placed on inflammatory, neoplastic and degenerative disorders, corneal disease, glaucoma and degenerative retinopathies, in order to provide suitable examples of pathogenic mechanisms which lead to blindness. The progress of many ocular diseases is followed *in vivo* by a variety of clinical techniques, e.g. slit-lamp microscopy, ophthalmoscopy, angiography and electrophysiological analysis, so that a unique facility exists for clinico-pathological correlation with the changes found in eyes removed surgically or at autopsy.

Applied anatomy

The structure of the eye is shown diagrammatically in Figs. 21.92 and 21.93. Visual acuity depends upon a transparent focusing system (the cornea and lens), transparent media (the aqueous and vitreous) and a normal photoreceptor and neural conducting mechanism. The metabolism of the cornea and lens is maintained by the circulation of the aqueous fluid, which is produced in the ciliary processes and leaves the anterior chamber via the outflow apparatus situated in the inner peripheral cornea adjacent to the root of the iris—the iridocorneal angle. The outflow system is a filter which consists of a series of fenestrated collagenous plates (trabeculae) which are covered by endothelial cells with phagocytic potential. The trabecular network is limited externally by an endothelial monolayer which lines the circumferential outflow canal of Schlemm (drained by episcleral collector channels). The pressure within the eye is normally 15–20 mmHg and depends upon the rate of aqueous production and the resistance in the outflow system. Any marked variation in pressure—*ocular hypotension* or *hypertension*—whether acute or chronic causes an imbalance

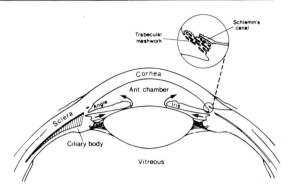

Fig. 21.92 Schematic diagram of the structures of the anterior segment of the eye to show the principal route of aqueous flow.

in vascular perfusion leading to ischaemic damage to the sensitive neural tissues within the eye.

The retina and the pigment epithelium are maintained by blood flow from two separate arterial systems. The inner two-thirds of the thickness of the retinal tissue are supplied by the branches of the central retinal artery while the outer third (the photoreceptor layer) is maintained by the choriocapillaris, which is supplied by the posterior ciliary arteries. Although the optic nerve is supplied by the central retinal artery and the meningeal arteries, the optic disc or papilla is nourished by blood vessels which are derived from the adjacent (peripapillary) choroid. Because of this vascular arrangement, distinctive patterns of ischaemic

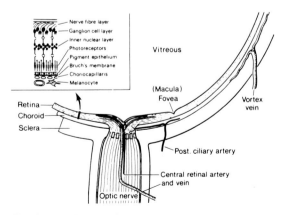

Fig. 21.93 Schematic diagram of the structures of the posterior segment of the eye to show the vascular supply to the choroid, retina and optic disc.

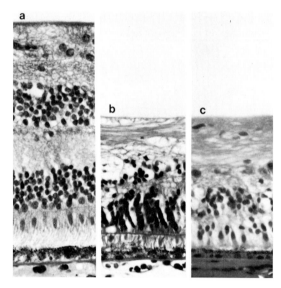

Fig. 21.94 a Normal retina: **b** ischaemic atrophy of the inner retina due to occlusion of the central retinal artery: **c** ischaemic atrophy of the outer retina due to posterior ciliary artery occlusion. × 240.

damage can occur in the visual sensory system according to the anatomical site of the vascular occlusion or impairment (Fig. 21.94).

Infections

Pathogenic micro-organisms can invade the eye from the external surface, the adjacent orbital tissues or via the bloodstream. The cellular response is, in general, similar to that observed in other tissues, but the eye is particularly vulnerable because the lens and vitreous are avascular protein-rich structures ideal for the proliferation of many pathogenic bacteria. An ulcer of the cornea due to pyogenic bacterial infection may measure only a few millimeters in diameter, but it will seriously impair vision, and may necessitate removal of the eye by progressing to perforation, ocular hypotonia and endophthalmitis. While numerous types of micro-organisms can cause eye disease, the following are of particular significance.

Viral infections most commonly involve the cornea and conjunctiva, the adenoviruses and herpes simplex being the most important. The **adenoviruses** (types 3 and 7) cause a conjunctivitis in which there is hyperplasia of lymphoid tissue in the oedematous and hyperaemic conjunctival stroma (*follicular conjunctivitis*). Adenovirus (usually type 8) infection may occur in epidemic form, and can involve the cornea (*epidemic keratoconjunctivitis*). In **herpes simplex** virus infection, *damage to the cornea* is more important than the associated conjunctivitis: the virus infects the epithelium of the cornea, which it destroys in a particular fingerlike or *dendritic* pattern. Herpes keratitis tends to recur, and spread to the corneal stroma, inducing neovascularisation and infiltration by lymphocytes, plasma cells and monocytes from the corneal periphery. The corneal lamellae are disorganised and replaced by fibrovascular tissue which causes corneal opacity. Destruction of the stroma of the cornea is aggravated by the release of collagenases from the damaged corneal epithelial cells and the stromal keratocytes. When scarring impairs vision or when ulceration and secondary bacterial infection threaten to progress to endophthalmitis, it is often necessary to replace the involved cornea by a homotransplant (see p. 7.32).

Trachoma-inclusion conjunctivitis or TRIC infection is caused by chlamydiae (p. 9.34). Infection with *Chlamydia trachomatis* of types A, B and C is common in the tropical zones and causes '**trachoma**', which is responsible for blindness on a massive scale. The chlamydia initially infects the conjunctival epithelium and it can be identified in smears of these cells by the presence of characteristic intracytoplasmic inclusion bodies formed by proliferation of the micro-organism. The conjunctiva is thickened by a dense chronic inflammatory infiltrate containing lymphoid follicles which commonly extends onto and destroys the superficial cornea. The healing stage is associated with extensive corneal and conjunctival scarring and eyelid distortion.

Chlamydia trachomatis of types D–K commonly infects the genital tract (p. 25.2) and causes a milder keratoconjunctivitis in the temperate zones. The lesion is confined to the lower tarsal conjunctiva where there is a low-grade chronic inflammatory infiltration. The inclusion bodies observed in the epithelium in this type of TRIC infection can be detected by direct immunofluorescence or by isolation of the organism in cell culture.

Acute bacterial infection. Primary infections of the conjunctiva and cornea by pyogenic

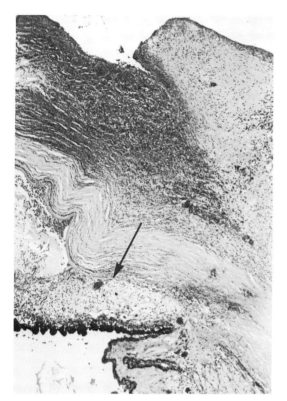

Fig. 21.95 A pyogenic ulcer of the cornea with inflammatory exudation into the anterior chamber and adhesion between the iris and the cornea (*arrow*). × 40.

organisms (e.g. gonococcus, Gram +ve cocci, haemophilus, moraxella and pseudomonas) were previously common and serious causes of corneal ulceration, but are now of minor significance in communities in which topical broad-spectrum antibiotics are readily available. Suppurative corneal ulceration, however, is still important as a secondary complication of pre-existing corneal abnormality, advanced glaucoma, mechanical trauma and viral and chlamydia infection. Application of topical steroids may render the cornea more susceptible to infection.

Histological examination of pyogenic ulceration of the cornea (Fig. 21.95) reveals a massive leucocytic infiltration in the disintegrating corneal stroma. Initially the membrane which forms the posterior corneal surface (*Descemet's membrane*) provides resistance to bacterial spread, but toxin diffusion induces migration of polymorphs into the iris and lower part of the anterior chamber (*hypopyon*) and iridocorneal

adhesion results. Descemet's membrane may prolapse into the corneal deficit to form a barrier. If this barrier breaks down, bacterial penetration is unhindered and abscess formation occurs in the anterior chamber, lens and vitreous.

Chronic bacterial infection. The eye may be affected in systemic microbial infection, e.g. tuberculosis, syphilis and brucellosis, and usually the uveal tract (the iris, ciliary body and choroid) is involved primarily (*uveitis*). A chronic inflammatory process in the choroid (*choroiditis*) can lead to focal destruction of the pigment epithelium and the adjacent retina, which either fuses with the choroid or may be detached by exudation of protein from damaged blood vessels in the choroid and retina. In the iris (*iritis*) and ciliary body (*cyclitis*) the inflammatory process leads to exudation of protein and inflammatory cells into the anterior and posterior chambers and clumps of inflammatory cells adhering to the posterior corneal surface (keratic precipitates) are a classical sign of *iridocyclitis*.

In syphilis, tuberculosis and sarcoidosis, there is widespread destruction of the choroid, ciliary body and iris and the adjacent structures. A similar pattern of tissue destruction is observed in fungal infections. In toxoplasmosis (p. 28.19) and toxocara infection (p. 28.47) the retina is more severely affected.

Uveitis of unknown aetiology

It should be noted that many cases of chronic uveitis are of unknown aetiology, although evidence is accumulating to incriminate a hypersensitivity reaction. The inflammatory infiltration in the uveal tract is predominantly lymphocytic, but the end-result is similar to that described above in the chronic bacterial infections, and ophthalmoscopy reveals punched out areas of depigmentation of the fundus. Involvement of the ciliary body leads to ocular hypotension, which causes choroidal and retinal oedema: the release of toxic substances results in degeneration of the lens, and reactionary fibrosis in the vitreous leads to a traction detachment of the retina. Exudation of proteinaceous material into the subretinal space also contributes to retinal detachment. The end stage of chronic inflammatory disease is a strik-

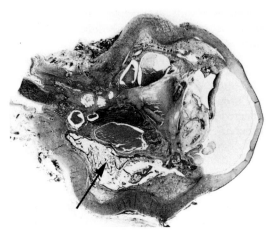

Fig. 21.96   Shrinkage and disorganisation of the eye following inflammation (phthisis bulbi). The retina is detached and the choroid is thickened by oedema and ossification (*arrow*). × 4.

ing shrinkage of the eye with massive subretinal fibrosis and secondary ossification (*phthisis bulbi*) (Fig. 21.96). Conversely, ocular hypertension or secondary glaucoma (p. 21.83) can result from occlusion of the iridocorneal angle by post-inflammatory adhesion between the iris and the cornea (*anterior synechiae*) or by infiltration of the outflow system by inflammatory cells.

Auto-immune disease

Auto-immune reactions occur in the eye in two established disease entities, *lens-induced uveitis* and *sympathetic ophthalmitis*.

(1) **Lens-induced uveitis.** Traumatic breakdown of lens tissue releases lens protein into the anterior chamber or the vitreous and in some circumstances this gives rise to a granulomatous reaction with giant cells due to a complex autohypersensitivity reaction in which both auto-antibodies and delayed hypersensitivity contribute to the destruction of the lens and the adjacent uveal tissue.

(2) **Sympathetic ophthalmitis.** Trauma to one eye which involves damage to or incarceration of either the iris or the ciliary body in the overlying sclera may be followed by a giant-cell granulomatous uveitis in the opposite eye (Fig. 21.97). This secondary inflammatory process may arise months or years after the original

injury and results in extensive damage to the second or 'sympathising' eye.

It is now suspected that release of uveal and retinal antigens from the injured eye stimulates a cell-mediated auto-immune response and that the second eye is the target organ of a delayed hypersensitivity reaction. If the first eye is preserved, it too is damaged by a giant-cell granulomatous reaction in the uveal tissue. Although rare, the threat of occurrence of this complication makes it difficult to decide between surgical repair and immediate removal of the injured eye; the latter procedure abolishes the risk of sympathetic ophthalmitis.

Vascular disease

Retinal ischaemia and haemorrhage. The pattern of ischaemic disease in the ocular tissues can often be related to the anatomy of the blood supply (p. 21.77). Complete occlusion of the central retinal artery by atheroma, thrombus or embolism, results in ischaemic atrophy of the inner two-thirds of the retina, while oc-

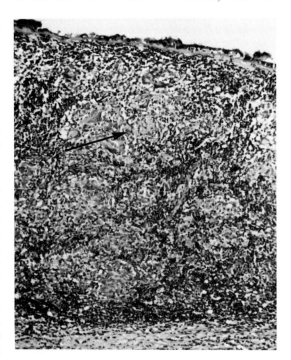

Fig. 21.97   The choroid in sympathetic ophthalmitis; the tissue is infiltrated by a giant-cell granulomatous reaction (*arrow*). × 370.

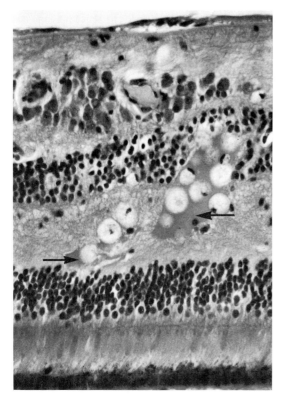

Fig. 21.98 A proteinaceous exudate (*arrow*) in the inner nuclear and the outer plexiform layers; lipid-laden macrophages are prominent. × 300.

clusion of the posterior ciliary arteries causes atrophy of the photoreceptor layer (Fig. 21.94). Important changes occur when there is focal occlusive disease in the retinal blood vessels. The outer plexiform layer is a zone in which there is inadequate resorption of exudate from damaged capillaries. Exudates are seen by ophthalmoscopy as discrete pale yellow areas in the retina and are described as *hard exudates*; resorption by lipid-laden glial macrophages may take several months (Fig. 21.98). The hard exudate is therefore a clinical manifestation of retinal ischaemia. Another feature is the so-called *soft exudate* which is an ill-defined small white area resembling cotton wool in the inner retina. On histological examination, the cotton-wool spot is seen as micro-infarction of the nerve-fibre and ganglion-cell layers of the retina. The damaged segment becomes oedematous and contains the bulbous tips of disrupted axons (*cytoid bodies*) (Fig. 21.99). The bulbous tips result from axoplasmic flow (p. 21.2). Acute focal ischaemia in the retina is

most commonly caused by angiospastic arteriolar disease and is a feature of malignant hypertension. When arteriolar disease is so severe that it leads to haemorrhage, the blood tracks within the nerve fibre layer to produce the flame-shaped haemorrhages seen on ophthalmoscopy. Accumulation of blood in the outer plexiform layer is due to rupture of capillaries and so-called blot haemorrhages are observed.

Haemorrhages are most prominent when venous outflow is impaired by thrombotic occlusion of the central retinal vein. The visual consequences of venous occlusion are less serious than those of arterial occlusion, because dilatation of collateral venous channels within the optic nerve relieves the pressure in the retinal venous system. Retinal oedema often persists and cystic degeneration occurs, particularly in the region of the macula (Fig. 21.100).

One of the important responses to focal retinal ischaemia is vasoproliferation from the blood vessels around the ischaemic area. Although this process is potentially beneficial within the retina, the delicate newly-formed vessels penetrate into the vitreous where they are

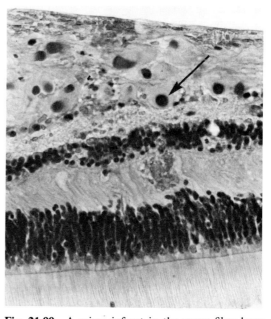

Fig. 21.99 A micro-infarct in the nerve fibre layer of the retina in which the swollen ends of axons (*arrow*) are seen as large darkly-staining round masses surrounded by paler areas. × 300.

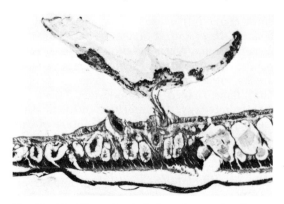

Fig. 21.100   The retina in ischaemic vascular disease due to central retinal vein occlusion. A tree-like growth of blood vessels extends into the vitreous and there is advanced cystic degeneration in the macula. × 40.

a common source of haemorrhage: contraction of fibrovascular scar tissue ensues and may lead to retinal detachment. It has been suggested that the ischaemic retina produces a '*vasoproliferative factor*' which is responsible for the fibrovascular proliferation on the anterior surface of the iris and the inner surface of the trabecular meshwork. Contraction of fibrovascular tissue occludes the iridocorneal angle and causes *secondary (neovascular) angle-closure glaucoma*.

The pathological processes described above are exemplified in **diabetic retinopathy** which is now an important cause of blindness. It is an insidious focal ischaemic arteriolar disease complicated by basement membrane thickening and pericyte degeneration in the capillary walls. The formation of micro-aneurysms in the weakened capillaries is an important feature of diabetes.

Senile macular degeneration. In elderly patients, degeneration of Bruch's membrane and the retinal pigment epithelium in the macular area can result in visual deterioration. This may progress to neovascularisation and subretinal haemorrhage and organisation (senile disciform degeneration of the macula). The pigment epithelium proliferates and contributes to the submacular fibrous mass (Fig. 21.101). The overlying photoreceptors degenerate and loss of central vision is a serious consequence of this disease.

Retinal detachment. Myopia and vascular insufficiency are considered to be important factors in atrophic degenerative disease in the peripheral retina. Vitreous traction causes tears in the atrophic retina; fluid passes from the vitreous into the subretinal space and this leads to progressive retinal detachment and loss of the visual field.

Cataract

The biconvex lens is formed by elongated lens-fibre cells, so named because their cytoplasm extends in the form of two extremely long processes ('fibres') containing transparent crystalline proteins. The cells are enclosed in an elastic membrane, the lens capsule. The malleability of the lens permits rapid fine focusing by tension exerted on the equator by the ciliary muscle via the zonular fibres. The metabolism of the lens is dependent on the composition of the aqueous fluid. As there is a constant production of new lens fibres during life, changes in the composition of the aqueous fluid may result in forma-

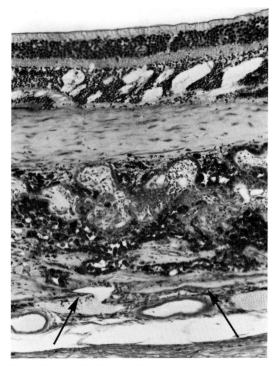

Fig. 21.101   Senile disciform degeneration of the macula, in which there is a sub-macular mass formed by fibrovascular tissue and proliferating pigment epithelium. Bruch's membrane (*arrows*) is penetrated by a vessel from the choroid. × 100.

tion of abnormal, opaque fibres. This may occur in uveitis, keratitis and systemic metabolic disturbances, e.g. in diabetes, hypocalcaemia and steroid overdosage. Such opacification develops in newly-formed fibres i.e. those in the anterior and posterior poles. Trauma to the eye may cause dislocation of the lens or opacification due to tears in the capsule. The most common form of cataract, however, is senile cataract, which is due to degradation of lens proteins in the oldest part, i.e. central nucleus of the lens: this leads to the formation of yellow, and eventually brown, opaque protein. Most cases of cataract can be treated successfully by removal of the opaque lens and insertion of a plastic lens implant.

Glaucoma

Glaucoma is a generic name for a group of diseases in which the intra-ocular pressure increases to a level which impairs the vascular perfusion of the neural tissue and causes blindness. The rise in pressure is usually due to obstruction to the outflow of aqueous, which occurs either as the result of angle closure or as an abnormality within the outflow system.

Closed-angle glaucoma. This may be *primary* or *secondary*. The *primary form* occurs in middle-aged and old people who have a narrow iridocorneal angle and a shallow anterior chamber. In such individuals the iris and lens may come into contact when the iris is in mid-dilatation: this prevents the flow of aqueous through the pupil and pressure builds up behind the iris, which becomes bowed anteriorly and causes further occlusion of the angle. This form of glaucoma is of acute onset, with ocular congestion, corneal oedema and pain.

Narrowness of the iridocorneal angle is attributed to normal variation, and to ageing, which leads to shrinkage of the eye and enlargement of the lens (Fig. 21.102).

Secondary closed-angle glaucoma has many causes, but in enucleated eyes the most common is neovascularisation.

Open-angle glaucoma is an insidious disease of the elderly in which a slowly progressive increase in intra-ocular pressure leads to an ischaemic sectorial destruction of the nerve fibres in the optic disc and this is manifest as a central-field defect which has a characteristic

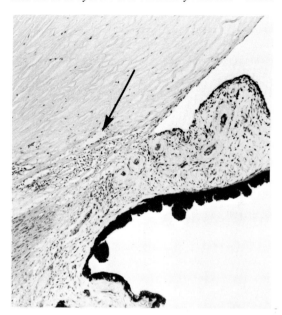

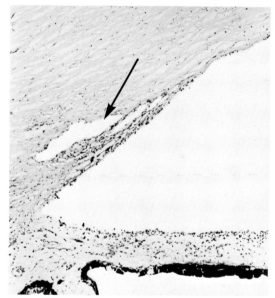

Fig. 21.102 The chamber angle in closed-angle glaucoma (*above*) and open-angle glaucoma (*below*). Note the secondary fusion of trabeculae in closed-angle glaucoma and the preservation of the intertrabecular spaces in open-angle glaucoma. The canal of Schlemm is indicated by arrows. × 75.

arcuate shape. By light microscopy the outflow system in the early stages appears normal (Fig. 21.102), but examination by electron microscopy has shown an accumulation of abnormal collagen within the trabeculae (which narrows

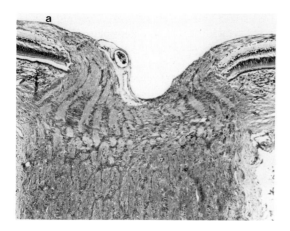

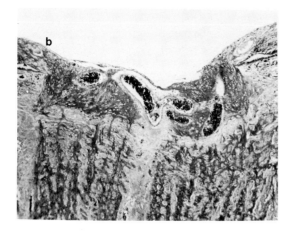

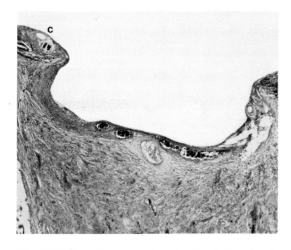

Fig. 21.103   a The normal optic disc: **b** the disc in early glaucoma, showing atrophy of the neural tissue: **c** the disc in advanced glaucoma in which the neural tissue is absent and the lamina cribosa is bowed posteriorly. × 30.

the intertrabecular spaces) and in the extracellular spaces of the outer part of the trabecular meshwork, this increases resistance in the outflow system.

In *secondary open-angle glaucoma*, the outflow system is obstructed mechanically by exogenous material, either particulate or cellular. In acute or chronic inflammatory disease, inflammatory cells accumulate within the intertrabecular spaces, while obstruction by macrophages occurs after haemorrhage or degenerative liquefaction of the lens cortex. The outflow system can also be obstructed by tumour cell infiltration, e.g. by a malignant melanoma of the iris or ciliary body.

The effects of increased intra-ocular pressure

The most serious effects on visual function are due to ischaemic atrophy of the axons in the nerve fibres of the disc and secondary atrophy in the nerve fibre layer of the retina. Excavation or cupping of the disc may become so advanced that it extends into the optic nerve (Fig. 21.103).

The corneal endothelium maintains dehydration of the stroma which is necessary for transparency of the tissue. At high pressure, the cornea becomes oedematous and the epithelium separates (*bullous keratopathy*). At an advanced stage, the uveal tissues become atrophic and fibrosis occurs in ischaemic areas of the iris and choroid; the scleral tissues may stretch to form localised bulges or *staphylomas*.

In infants and children, glaucoma can result from developmental abnormalities in which there is a failure in modelling of the embryonic mesodermal tissues which is found in the chamber angle in the early stages of intra-uterine life. Increasing intra-ocular pressure causes the malleable infantile eye to expand uniformly, and it may become so large that it resembles an ox-eye ('*buphthalmos*').

Tumours

The tumours of the eyelid, conjunctiva and orbital tissues do not differ significantly in morphology and behaviour from those occurring elsewhere. Intra-ocular tumours are rare, but

inal space and causes secondary retinal detachment which is often so extensive that visual loss is out of proportion to the size of the tumour. Microscopically the tumour cells are either spindle-shaped (Fig. 21.104) or round (epithelioid). Epithelioid tumours have a much worse prognosis than mainly spindle-cell tumours, which carry a 60% 15-year-survival rate. Growth within the eye leads to disorganisation and often to secondary glaucoma, while extension usually takes place through intrascleral channels. The choroidal and vortex veins are sometimes invaded with consequent blood spread and distant metastasis, especially in the liver. This tumour is notorious for producing multiple rapidly-enlarging liver metastases as long as 20 (symptom-free) years after enucleation of the affected eye (the big liver and glass-eye syndrome). What happens to the tumour cells in the latent interval is a matter for speculation, but current theories invoke an

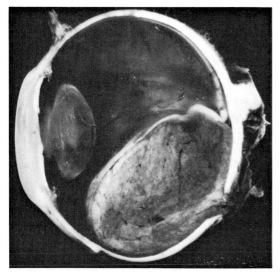

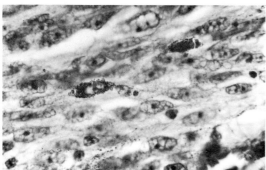

Fig. 21.104 Malignant melanoma of the choroid. *Above*, the gross appearances: the tumour has extended through the sclera. × 2.5. *Below*, microscopy shows this to be an example of the spindle-cell type of tumour. × 525.

are important because of their serious effect on vision and their unusual patterns of behaviour.

Malignant melanoma and **benign naevi** are tumours of adult life and occur particularly in elderly white-skinned individuals. They are derived from the spindle-shaped melanocytes of the uveal tract. **Benign naevi** are common and clinically unimportant, but there is some evidence that occasionally they may undergo malignant transformation. **Malignant melanomas** are unilateral and solitary and are most commonly situated in the posterior choroid. The tumour expands the choroid, penetrates Bruch's membrane and may adopt a characteristic collar-stud shape: alternatively it forms an ovoid mass (Fig. 21.104). Plasma leaks from the tumour, and from the choroid, into the subret-

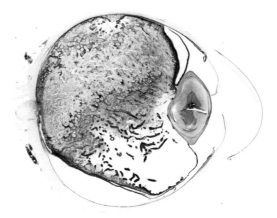

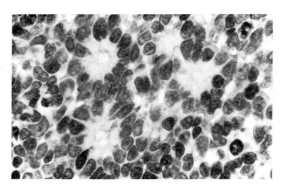

Fig. 21.105 Extensive growth of retinoblastoma within the posterior part of the eye (*above*). × 2·5. The microscopic features include the typical rosettes (*below*). × 525.

immunological suppression of viable metastases.

Retinoblastoma. This is a tumour of infancy, the incidence of which is gradually rising and is now 1 in 20 000 live births in this country. Six per cent of the cases are familial. The genetic basis is complex (p. 13.27), but is of importance in the management of patients. In approximately half the cases, the tumour is bilateral and multifocal within the retina.

On gross examination, the retinoblastoma forms a solid pale-grey, partially calcified and partially necrotic mass within the retina. When the tumour fills the vitreous or detaches the retina, a white mass is seen behind the lens, so that reflected light produces a reflex similar to that in the cat's eye. Blindness in the affected eye causes the child to squint. The tumour is composed of small round or oval cells with scanty cytoplasm and a high rate of mitosis. A tendency to differentiation is seen in the formation of rosettes, which are circular arrangements of the tumour cells (Fig. 21.105). Extra-ocular extension occurs either by spread along the optic nerve into the brain or through the sclera into the orbit. Metastases to visceral organs are a late and unusual event. With early enucleation of the eye or radiotherapy, the survival rate is of the order of 90%.

Glioma of the optic nerve occurs in children and adults. In children, proliferation of glial cells within the optic nerve causes proptosis and papilloedema when the nerve becomes thickened and vascular perfusion in the disc is disturbed. Nevertheless nerve conduction survives and tumour growth declines, so that some authorities consider childhood gliomas to be hamartomatous lesions. By contrast, the adult glioma resembles the glioblastoma multiforme (p. 21.56) in its morphology and behaviour.

References and Further Reading

Central nervous system

Adams, J. H., Corsellis, J. A. N. and Duchen, L. W. (Eds.). (1984). *Greenfield's Neuropathology*, 4th edn., pp. 1126. Edward Arnold, London.

L. J. Rubinstein (1972) *Tumors of the Central Nervous System.* Atlas of Tumor Pathology. Second series, Fascicle 6. pp. 400. Armed Forces Institute of Pathology, Washington.

Russell, D. S. and Rubinstein, L. J. (1977). *Pathology of Tumours of the Nervous System*, 4th edn., pp. 456. Edward Arnold, London.

Treip, C. S. (1978) *A Colour Atlas of Neuropathology.* pp. 208. Wolfe Medical Publications, Ltd., London.

Weller, R. O., Swash, M., McLellan, D. L. and Scholtz, C. L. (1983). *Clinical Neuropathology.* pp. 329. Springer-Verlag, Berlin.

Peripheral nerves and muscles

World Federation of Neurology. Research Group in Neuromuscular Disease (1968). Classification of the neuromuscular disorders. *Journal of Neurological Sciences*, **6**, 165–77.

Mastiglia, F. L. and Walton, J. N. (Eds.). (1982) *Skeletal muscle pathology*, pp. 648. Churchill Livingstone, Edinburgh.

Albuquerque, E. X. and Eldefrawi, A. T. (Eds.). (1983). *Myasthenia gravis*, pp. 512. Chapman and Hall, London.

Chamburg, H. H., Spencer, P. S. and Thomas, P. K. (Eds.). (1983). *Disorders of Peripheral Nerves*, pp. 248. F. A. Davis & Co., Philadelphia.

The eye

Garner, A. and Klintworth, G. (Eds.). (1982). *Pathobiology of Ocular Disease*, pp. 1732. Marcel Dekker, Inc., New York.

22

The Kidneys and Urinary Tract

Fine structure and function

The kidneys are each composed of about one million nephrons, the major functions of which are to remove from the plasma various waste products of metabolism, and to maintain fluid and acid–base balances and normal levels of electrolytes. This is achieved by production of a very large volume of glomerular filtrate, which is subject to selective reabsorption as it passes down the tubules, urine representing what must be discarded for homoeostasis. Although only some 0·5% of the total body weight the kidneys receive 20% of the cardiac output. Nearly all of this passes through the glomeruli, where 22% of the plasma volume (550 ml/min; 800 litres/day) is filtered off, giving a glomerular filtration rate (GFR) of 180 litres per day (120 ml/min). The process of filtration is aided by the unusually high pressure in the **glomerular capillaries** which is due to their unique position between two arterioles. The capillary walls (Fig. 22.1) consist of the vascular endothelium, which is unusual in having cytoplasmic *fenestrations* where the capillary basement membrane is lined only by an extremely thin endothelial membrane. Outside the basement membrane is a layer of visceral *epithelial cells* or *podocytes*, which make contact with the basement membrane by means of cytoplasmic processes—*foot processes* or *pedicels*. In the spaces (slit pores) between the foot processes there is a thin 'slit membrane' with a central bar: this membrane, together with the glomerular capillary basement membrane, is believed to regulate the filtration of macro-molecules and the water flux. Each glomerulus is composed of several lobules, the structure of which is depicted in Fig. 22.2. The capillary loops lie

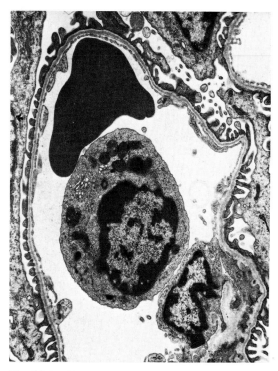

Fig. 22.1 Electron micrograph of glomerular capillary containing a lymphocyte and red cell. Note, from within outwards, the endothelial cytoplasm with fenestrations, the continuous basement membrane, and the foot processes of the epithelium. × 12 000.

at the periphery of the lobules, while the core is made up of mesangial cells and basement membrane-like material. **The mesangial cells** have a number of functions, including a structural supportive role; they also contain actomyosin and may regulate the blood flow through the glomeruli. Thirdly, they have phagocytic properties and, like macrophages, may act

22.1

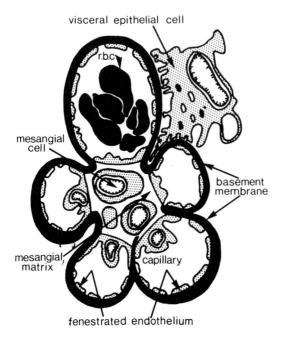

visceral epithelial cell

r.b.c.

mesangial cell

basement membrane

mesangial matrix

capillary

fenestrated endothelium

Fig. 22.2   Diagram of a glomerular lobule in cross section.

which form on the luminal surface of the cells between the bases of the microvilli: there is normally some leakage of plasma proteins into the glomerular filtrate, and this is apparently taken up into these cells by pinocytosis and presumably metabolised by lysosomal enzymes. When, owing to various glomerular lesions, there is increased leakage of protein into the glomerular filtrate, the cells of the proximal tubules come to contain protein-rich droplets—*hyaline droplets* (Fig. 22.26, p. 22.26)—due to increased protein absorption. Finally, the plasma membrane of the basal surface of the cells of the proximal convoluted tubule shows complicated infoldings which also have the effect of increasing the surface area, and are probably important in the passage of reabsorbed fluid into the interstitial tissue, whence it enters the peritubular capillaries.

The cells of the **descending limb of Henle's loop**, and of the thin part of the ascending limb, are relatively simple, and their role in reabsorption is probably largely passive, and dependent

as accessory cells in the immune response by presenting antigen in immunogenic form to lymphocytes.

In its passage along the tubules, all but approximately 1·5 litres of the daily 180 litres of glomerular filtrate, and most of its contained solutes, are reabsorbed. This is a process in which the tubule cells exhibit a high degree of selectivity, and some of the fine structural features of the epithelial cells can be related to their special functions. The epithelial cells of the **proximal convoluted tubule**, whose main metabolic function is sodium resorption, have a prominent brush border, seen by electron microscopy to consist of numerous fine, relatively long microvilli (Fig. 22.3): this feature increases the available cellular absorptive area by a factor of 40, and four fifths of the fluid in the glomerular filtrate, together with most of its contained glucose, amino acids, and much of its sodium, potassium and phosphate are reabsorbed here. Reabsorption of these solutes is an active process, requiring energy and this may account for the large number of mitochondria in the epithelial cells. A third feature of these cells is the presence of pinocytotic vesicles,

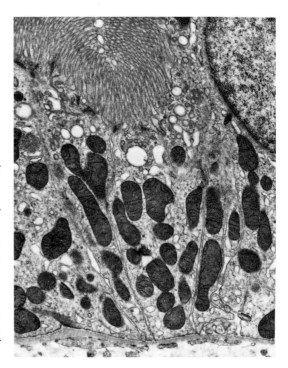

Fig. 22.3   Electron micrograph of parts of two epithelial cells of the proximal convoluted tubule, showing the microvilli (*upper left*) and numerous mitochondria. The basal part of the epithelium rests on a thin basement membrane. × 11 000.

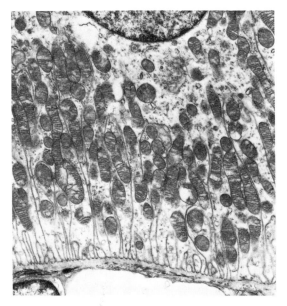

Fig. 22.4 Electron micrograph of the basal part of an epithelial cell of the thick part of Henle's loop. Note large elongated mitochondria situated between the complex infoldings of the basal cytoplasmic membrane. Portion of cell nucleus at top of picture. × 10 000.

on the composition of the tubular and interstitial fluids. By contrast, the cells of the **thick part of the ascending limb** have abundant large mitochondria (Fig. 22.4), and these cells actively remove sodium chloride from the tubular fluid and pass it into the interstitial fluid. This has two effects; firstly, it provides a hypertonic interstitial fluid in the renal medulla, and this allows passive reabsorption of water from the descending and thin ascending parts of Henle's loop; secondly, it renders the tubular fluid hypotonic and facilitates further concentration in the distal convoluted tubule. There is evidence that, like sodium chloride, urea undergoes partial recirculation in this **counter-current system**, thus aiding in passive reabsorption of water. This ingenious concentrating mechanism was suggested by Wirz (1956) (see Black, 1972) and has since become widely accepted. The cells of the thick part of Henle's loop, and of the **distal convoluted tubule**, contain numerous microvesicles, and these may be related to their important functions of deaminating amino acids to produce ammonia, and of providing free hydrogen ion: secretion of NH_4^+ into the lumen by these cells plays an important role in maintaining acid–base balance, and results in an acid urine. Fluid entering the distal convoluted tubule is hypotonic, and isotonicity is restored here by passive reabsorption of water. As the fluid passes through the medulla in the collecting tubules, passive reabsorption of more water is again possible because the concentrations of sodium chloride and urea in the medullary interstitial fluid are high (see above). It is probable that these final adjustments in concentration are mediated largely by *antidiuretic hormone*, which renders the cells of the distal convoluted and collecting tubules more permeable to water. It is also here that aldosterone exerts its effect by stimulating reabsorption of sodium, thus facilitating reabsorption of water.

In addition to these complex tubular functions, there is evidence that some substances are removed from the blood and actively secreted by the tubular epithelium. For example, creatinine and K^+ are reabsorbed in the proximal convoluted tubule, and the amounts appearing in the urine are dependent largely on their secretion, probably by the cells of the thick part of the ascending limb of Henle's loop and of the distal convoluted tubule. Excretion of administered diodone by the kidneys is dependent mainly on tubular secretion, and it may be used to assess tubular function.

In addition to their homoeostatic and excretory roles, the kidneys secrete renin, an enzyme which acts on a substrate in the plasma to produce angiotensin (see p. 10.35). The site of renin secretion is located in the granular cells of the afferent glomerular arterioles, which, together with the macula densa and lacis cells, constitute the **juxtaglomerular apparatus** (Fig. 10.35, p. 10.36). Angiotensin has a direct effect on peripheral vascular resistance, and hence on blood pressure, and also stimulates the secretion of aldosterone by the adrenal cortex. These phenomena, and the fine structure of the juxtaglomerular apparatus, are described on pp. 10.35–8.

Another function of the kidneys is the production of **erythrogenin**, which stimulates the production of red cells (p. 17.4).

Heterogeneity of nephrons. It has long been known that individual nephrons show morphological and circulatory differences—for example, in the length of Henle's loop. Thurau and his colleagues (see Horster and Thurau, 1968) have demonstrated important functional differences between the majority of nephrons and the one-fifth of nephrons originating in glomeruli close to the cortico-medullary junction. By micropuncture of individual tubules, they showed differences in glomerular filtration rates, and differences in responses to low and high sodium loading. These findings may necessitate a reconsideration of various aspects of renal function, both normal and in pathological states, since our present views are based largely on the assumption of a functionally homogeneous population of nephrons.

Pathophysiology of renal disease

Many of the diseases described in this chapter result in disturbances of renal function, and these are considered in more detail later. The four major disturbances which are responsible for most of the clinical features of renal diseases are as follows.

(1) Impairment of blood flow through the kidneys can result in **arterial hypertension (secondary** or **renal hypertension**—p. 14.21): this is encountered commonly in glomerular disease, but can result from extensive renal scarring from various causes, and also from an extra-renal lesion, e.g. narrowing of the main renal artery by an atheromatous patch in the aorta.

(2) **Renal failure ('uraemia')** with accumulation in the body of urea and other nitrogenous waste products and disturbances of water and acid–base balances and of electrolyte levels, can result from *a reduced glomerular filtration rate*, from *tubular injury*, or from a combination of both. *Since lesions which impair renal blood flow reduce the glomerular filtration rate, it is not surprising that renal failure and hypertension are commonly associated.*

(3) There are a number of diseases which injure the glomerular capillaries and render them abnormally permeable to plasma proteins; heavy and prolonged albuminuria results in fall of the level of plasma albumin, and this can set in motion a train of events leading to generalised oedema. *The combination of proteinuria, hypoalbuminaemia and oedema is known as the* **nephrotic syndrome**.

(4) Glomerular injury can result in the escape of red cells which appear in the urine either in small numbers or sufficient to discolour it. *When there is widespread glomerular inflamma-*

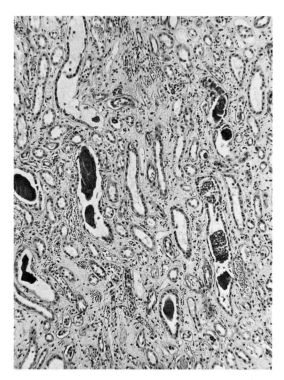

Fig. 22.5   Casts in the distal and collecting tubules. × 90.

tion, as in some forms of glomerulonephritis, such haematuria is accompanied by hypertension and oliguria, a combination known as the **nephritic syndrome**.

Urinary casts. Increased leakage of plasma proteins into the glomerular filtrate results in proteinuria, most of the escaping protein being albumin. This is accompanied by the formation in the distal tubules of solid, cylindrical-shaped bodies, termed casts (Fig. 22.5), *the presence of which in the urine indicates that the proteinuria is attributable to a renal lesion*. When the proteinuria is unaccompanied by escape of cells in the urine, the casts are transparent and are termed *hyaline, colloid* or *protein* casts. Their solid component consists largely of protein— *Tamm-Horsfall protein*—which is secreted normally by the epithelium of the thick part of the ascending limb of Henle's loop and is precipitated to form casts by the presence of plasma albumin in the tubular fluid. When proteinuria is accompanied by escape of inflammatory cells into the tubular fluid or desquamation of tubular epithelial cells, these become incorporated into the casts, giving *cellular casts* when the

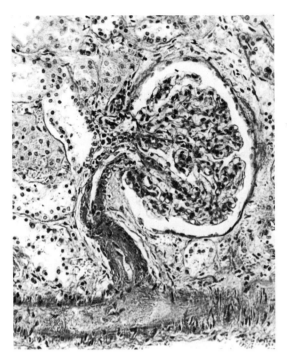

Fig. 22.6 Benign essential hypertension, showing great hyaline thickening of an afferent arteriole. × 180.

cells are largely intact and *granular casts* when the cells are disrupted. Similarly *blood casts* result from incorporation of red cells escaping into the glomerular filtrate or tubule, and *pigmented casts* from incorporation of bilirubin when proteinuria accompanies obstructive jaundice, or from haemoglobin or myoglobin in conditions giving rise to haemolysis or breakdown of skeletal muscle respectively.

Renal changes in hypertension

The arterial changes in hypertension have already been described and their pathogenesis discussed (pp. 14.15–21). The arterial tree of the kidney is usually affected more than other organs and this results in varying degrees of renal damage. In chronic ('benign') hypertension the renal injury is usually slight and there is often minimal functional impairment whereas in malignant (accelerated) hypertension the severe arterial damage commonly gives rise to renal failure.

Chronic ('benign') hypertension. Hypertensive arteriosclerosis of the larger branches of the renal arteries is without any functional effect (p. 14.15); the interlobular arteries may be narrowed in severe arteriosclerosis by the fibro-elastic intimal thickening, but the most significant lesion, **hyaline arteriolosclerosis** (p. 14.17), occurs mainly in the afferent glomerular arterioles which become tortuous, thick-walled and often severely narrowed (Figs. 14.18 and 22.6). These arterial changes tend to cause ischaemia and since the most important lesion is the hyaline arteriolosclerosis of the afferent arterioles, individual nephrons are affected. The capillary tuft of the affected glomerulus shrinks, with wrinkling of its basement membrane. The collapsed capillary tuft later becomes hyalinised and Bowman's capsule becomes filled with collagen, leading to the formation of a solid fibrous ball (Fig. 22.7). The tubule atrophies and is replaced by fibrous tissue often containing some lymphocytes. This piecemeal loss of individual nephrons occurs slowly, so that in the early stages of hypertension the kidney appears normal, but with prominent arteries

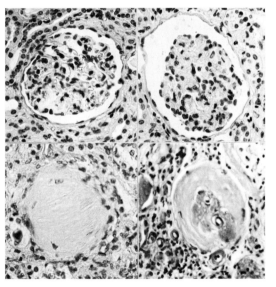

Fig. 22.7 Ischaemic changes in the glomeruli in chronic essential hypertension. The two glomeruli above show partial hyalinisation. The lower left is completely hyalinised and the lower right is collapsed, extensively hyalinised, and encased in fibrous tissue which has formed inside Bowman's capsule. Note its hyalinised afferent arteriole ·(seen below, containing a leucocyte). × 160.

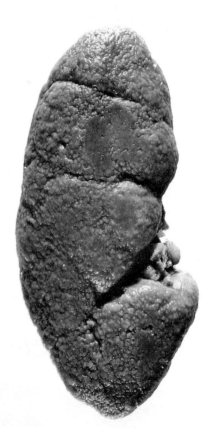

Fig. 22.8   Kidney in longstanding benign essential hypertension, showing slight reduction in size and granularity of the subcapsular surface. × 1.

visible on the cut surface. As more nephrons are lost there is diffuse thinning of the renal cortex and the kidneys become moderately reduced in size. The contraction of the small scars which replace the lost nephrons causes fine depressions on the kidney surface which becomes finely granular in appearance (Figs. 22.8 and 22.9). If enough nephrons are lost there may be hypertrophy of the surviving nephrons which accentuates the roughening of the surface, giving rise to the so-called granular contracted kidney. *The kidneys are seldom very small and while there may be loss of functional reserve, renal function is not significantly impaired.*

Malignant (accelerated) hypertension. This may arise acutely, apparently *de novo*, or may supervene after a variable period of chronic hypertension (p. 14.15), and the appearances in the kidney vary accordingly. In the most acute cases the surface of the kidney is smooth and spotted with tiny petechial haemorrhages. The cut surface may show mottling due to multiple tiny infarcts. The interlobular arteries often show intimal thickening (Fig. 22.10), a form of endarteritis (p. 14.2). Fibrinoid necrosis (p. 11.7) affects mainly the distal portions of the interlobular arteries and the afferent arterioles (Fig. 22.11). The fibrinoid necrosis may extend into the glomerular tuft and often it may have superimposed thrombus (p. 14.18). Other glomeruli show thickening of the capillary walls with reduplication of basement membrane, congestion and capillary dilatation. There is often blood or proteinaceous fluid in Bowman's space and sometimes proliferation of the capsular epithelium may give rise to occasional crescents (p. 22.23). Unlike glomerulonephritis, the minority of the glomeruli are affected and the severe impairment of renal function is due to ischaemia caused by the severe arterial damage and the superimposed thrombosis. The tubules may

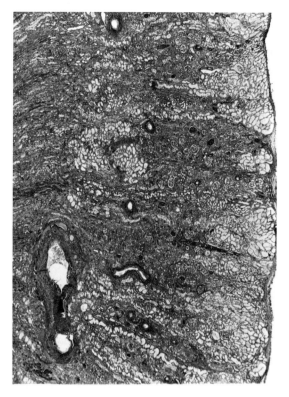

Fig. 22.9   Kidney in benign essential hypertension, showing foci of fine cortical scarring, with enlargement of the tubules in the unaffected cortical areas. Note also the arterial thickening. × 12·5.

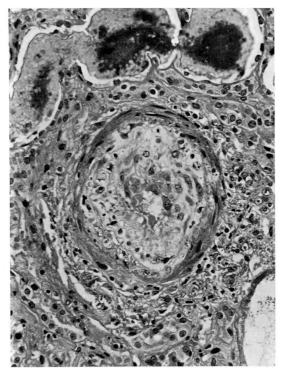

Fig. 22.10 Interlobular artery in malignant hypertension, showing gross intimal fibro-cellular thickening. × 100.

be atrophied or enlarged and usually contain proteinaceous or blood casts.

There is hyperplasia of the renin-secreting cells of the juxtaglomerular apparatus and this morphological change correlates with the very high levels of renin and angiotensin II which invariably occur in malignant hypertension.

In contrast to benign hypertension, renal failure is a common cause of death in untreated malignant hypertension. In treated cases with a more prolonged clinical course chronic renal failure may occur due to ischaemia caused by severe endarteritis of interlobular arteries.

Secondary hypertension. Various grades of hypertension occur in renal diseases and, depending on the height and rate of rise of the pressure, the renal changes of benign and malignant hypertension may be superadded to those of the renal disease which has caused the hypertension.

Other vascular diseases

Renal vessels show the usual features of generalised vascular diseases. **Atheroma** occurs in the main renal arteries and their segmental branches but is much less common than in other arteries of comparable size, and except in patients with diabetes mellitus it is rarely severe enough to interfere with the renal circulation: superadded occlusion by thrombosis is also rare. Disturbances arise more commonly from involvement and narrowing of the origin of one or rarely both renal arteries by aortic atheromatous plaques. This can lead to hypertension (p. 14.21), presumably from ischaemia of one or both kidneys. Compared with essential hypertension, this is a rarity, but it is important to diagnose, for in some cases relief of the stenosis by a bypass operation or removal of the ischaemic kidney has resulted in cure of the hypertension. Renal ischaemia and hypertension may also result from **fibromuscular**

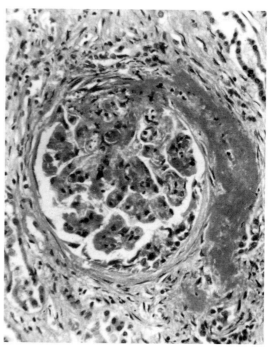

Fig. 22.11 Malignant hypertension. Fibrinoid necrosis of an afferent arteriole and of most of the glomerular tuft. Note also the aggregation of cells in the capsular space (*lower right*) to form a small crescent. × 180.

dysplasia (p. 14.36) of the renal arteries. **Senile arteriosclerosis** in the kidney of elderly normotensive people presents features similar to those of benign essential hypertension and does not seriously impair renal function. The changes of **polyarteritis nodosa** are discussed on p. 22.34.

Finally, the special function of the glomerular capillaries and their unusually high intraluminal pressure render them susceptible to a large group of lesions covered by the terms **glomerulonephritis** and **glomerulosclerosis** (pp. 22.15–41): some of these occur as a feature of systemic diseases, e.g. systemic lupus erythematosus, anaphylactoid purpura and diabetic microangiopathy, while others are attributable to circulating immune complexes although the vascular lesions occur mainly or solely in the glomeruli.

Acute Renal Failure

Renal function is acutely impaired (a) by any condition which causes a severe acute reduction of glomerular filtration, and (b) by acute failure of the renal tubular epithelium.

Acute reduction in glomerular filtration may be classified as (a) *pre-renal*, which is due to the acute circulatory failure of shock; (b) *post-renal*, due to urinary tract obstruction, e.g. blockage of both ureters or acute urethral obstruction by an enlarged prostate, and (c) *renal parenchymal*, usually due to acute glomerulonephritis.

Acute tubular failure is due most often to acute tubular necrosis (see below) in which the tubular epithelium is injured by ischaemia or toxic chemicals. Less common causes of tubular failure include renal cortical necrosis, interstitial nephritis and renal papillary necrosis.

Although it is convenient to classify acute renal failure as above, it will become apparent from the following account that the changes in the kidney are complex and that reduced glomerular filtration is often accompanied by impaired tubular function.

The functional disturbances of acute renal failure are described in the section on the clinico-pathological correlations of acute tubular necrosis (p. 22.10).

'Acute tubular necrosis'

In this condition there is a sudden onset of *anuria* or *severe oliguria* with consequent accumulation of fluid and urinary waste products and disturbances of electrolyte and pH balance. If it is not fatal, this phase is followed by a *diuretic phase* and, in favourable cases, by *recovery* of renal function.

Causal factors

The mechanism of renal failure in acute tubular necrosis is not fully understood, and will be discussed later. At this point it is useful to note the main predisposing factors.

(a) Shock. During an acute state of shock from whatever cause there is a considerable reduction of blood flow through the kidneys and so impaired renal function. In 'acute tubular necrosis', acute renal failure with severe oliguria persists after the state of shock has passed off. This is liable to occur in cases of severe and prolonged shock, for example in association with major injury, prolonged and complicated surgical operations or extensive burns. Severe bacterial infection with endotoxic shock, the trauma of unskilled abortion, retroplacental haemorrhage and postpartum haemorrhage all carry a special risk of acute renal failure. In the bombing of cities in the 1939–45 war, individuals were commonly trapped for some hours under fallen masonry and developed traumatic and ischaemic necrosis of skeletal muscle, particularly in crushed limbs. After rescue, myoglobin and other constituents of muscle from the areas of crush injury diffused into the blood, and myoglobinuria developed. The high incidence of acute tubular necrosis in such cases (**crush syndrome**), and also in the rare condition of acute paroxysmal myoglobinuria, suggests that products of muscle breakdown have a special predisposing effect. Acute haemolysis, as in transfusion of incompatible blood, may also be followed, although much less commonly, by 'acute tubular necrosis'. Operations on the liver and biliary tract are particularly likely to be complicated by 'acute tubular necrosis' (**hepatorenal syndrome**), and although it is likely that shock and disturbance of fluid and electrolytes are at least partly responsible, there may be a special relationship between hepatic trauma and the renal lesion. The prognosis is appreciably worse in cases associated with severe trauma or surgery than in those following incompatible transfusion, complications of pregnancy or chemical poisoning (see below).

(b) Various chemicals are cytotoxic to the tubular epithelium and cause acute renal failure, often together with acute injury to the liver and other organs. At present, the most important examples are the aminoglycoside antibiotics and paracetamol overdosage. Organic mercurial diuretics and various chemicals used in industry, etc., such as Trilene, carbon tetrachloride (used in dry-cleaning), ethylene glycol (antifreeze), phenolic disinfectants and metallic poisons (mercuric chloride and compounds of uranium, arsenic and chromium), can all cause acute tubular necrosis, and various other chemicals have been implicated. In many countries, increasing awareness of the risk has led to the introduction of measures to prevent accidental absorption of most of these chemicals in industry, etc.

Pathological changes

In fatal cases, the kidneys are usually enlarged and the cut surface bulges, due mainly to dilatation of tubules and interstitial oedema. The cortical vessels contain little blood, and the cortex appears pale, with blurring of the normal radial pattern, while the medulla is often dark and congested. Occasionally there are petechial haemorrhages in the cortex.

Microscopically, the glomerular tufts appear normal. Usually there is some granular debris in the capsular space and the parietal cells lining Bowman's capsule may be unduly prominent and cuboidal. The tubular changes are variable and depend on the severity and duration, and on the particular causal agents involved. In many cases, however, the causation is complex, and specific changes cannot readily be attributed to particular causal agents. Also, it is often difficult to identify, in histological sections, which parts of the tubules have been

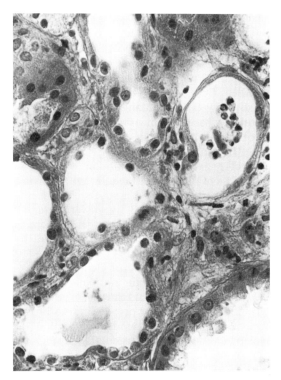

Fig. 22.12 Acute renal failure resulting from post-surgical hypotension. Note the tubular dilatation and flattening of the epithelial cells. Mitotic figures are seen and some cell debris is present in the lumen. × 320.

damaged. At autopsy, the lesion is often obscured by terminal ischaemic changes and post-mortem autolysis.

In cases resulting from shock, etc. (group **(a)** above), both the proximal and distal convoluted tubules are commonly dilated and the epithelial lining is flattened with basophilia of the cytoplasm and mitotic activity (Fig. 22.12). These changes, which are seen as early as three days after the onset, appear to be sequelae to loss of tubular epithelium; the remaining cells become flattened and undergo proliferation, thus restoring epithelial continuity. In the distal convoluted and collecting tubules epithelial proliferation may be pronounced, the cells sometimes forming syncytial masses, particularly around casts (see below). An early change seen by electron microscopy is the loss of the normal brush border from the proximal tubular cells. The time at which these cells regain their brush border correlates well with the return of renal function.

Tubular epithelial necrosis is not conspicuous and in many cases cannot be seen. In a minority there are foci of necrosis, most numerous in the distal convoluted tubule but also occurring in the proximal tubule. This change, which was described by Oliver *et al.* (1951) as **tubulorrhexis**, may be accompanied by disruption of the tubular basement membrane and an inflammatory reaction in the adjacent interstitial tissue. This may progress to scarring and in the event of recovery lead to tubular obstruction and so loss of function of the affected nephrons. The tubulorrhexic lesion and its site in the tubule were demonstrated by Oliver *et al.* by dissection of nephrons. The epithelial necrosis is not conspicuous and is readily obscured by post-mortem autolysis.

From the ascending limb of Henle's loop onwards, the tubules contain proteinaceous and brown granular casts, and in cases associated with haemoglobinuria or myoglobinuria brown pigment casts and rounded granules of pigmented material are particularly prominent.

Distension of the intertubular connective tissue by oedema fluid is conspicuous in some cases, but almost absent in others. The vasa recta of the medulla usually contain groups of nucleated cells which appear to represent erythropoietic foci, a feature which is sometimes seen in the hepatic sinusoids in liver cell necrosis.

The changes described above are seen in acute renal failure resulting from shock, trauma, etc. They occur also in those cases resulting from administration of the nephrotoxic poisons listed above, but in the poisoning cases there is, in addition, more extensive necrosis affecting mainly the proximal convoluted tubule of all or most of the nephrons and resulting from the direct effect of the toxic compounds or their metabolites. This *nephrotoxic change* is often conspicuous but, unlike tubulorrhexis, it does not involve rupture of the tubular basement membrane, and if the patient can be kept alive, e.g. by haemodialysis, it is often repaired by epithelial regeneration without leaving any residual damage or scarring.

Some variation is observed in the nephrotoxic lesions brought about by different chemicals. For example, mercuric chloride tends to affect the whole of the proximal convoluted tubule, and in some instances the necrotic part of the tubule rapidly becomes calcified, resulting in permanent injury. Carbon tetrachloride causes necrosis especially of the terminal part of the proximal tubule, and also perivenular hepatic necrosis. If ethylene glycol is ingested, a small proportion of it is converted into oxalate, crystals of which form in the tubular lumina: in addition to tubular necrosis it may cause death from liver or brain injury or from acute heart failure.

Clinico-pathological correlations. Oliguria lasts from a day or two to about 4 weeks, and is followed by a diuretic phase of much shorter duration. During the **oliguric phase**, renal blood flow and glomerular filtration rate are reduced (see below). Tubular function is also disturbed, so that most of the diminished amount of glomerular filtrate produced is reabsorbed non-selectively across the injured tubular epithelium or denuded basement membrane. Consequently there is oliguria (defined as less than 400 ml urine per day in adults), and the urine comes to resemble in composition a protein-poor filtrate of the plasma. There is thus a progressive rise in urea and other nitrogenous metabolites, and unless fluid and electrolyte intake is carefully regulated, death will result from a combination of uraemia, generalised and pulmonary oedema, and electrolyte disturbances. Acidosis may result from breakdown of endogenous fat and protein, particularly in the crush syndrome or other severe injury. Protein catabolism will aggravate the uraemia and accordingly the most appropriate diet is one which is low in protein and provides sufficient calories to avoid excessive endogenous protein catabolism. One of the most important electrolyte disturbances is retention of potassium, particularly in cases with severe injury and tissue breakdown, and dietary potassium should be carefully controlled. Experience has shown that carefully controlled conservative therapy, including the use of osmotic diuretics such as mannitol, can prolong life in acute renal failure, and where the lesion is reversible, as in acute tubular necrosis, the prognosis has been greatly improved. However, in some cases haemodialysis is necessary. The blood pressure is commonly raised during the oliguric phase.

In the past the oliguric phase was followed by a diuretic phase but this was largely due to fluid overload during the oliguric phase, and with better management this diuretic phase is now short-lived or even inapparent. However, renal concentrating power and homoeostatic mechanisms are only gradually restored, sometimes over many months, and some care is necessary to avoid fluid and electrolyte imbalance. Eventually there is an average of about 80% recovery of previous renal function.

Aetiology and pathogenesis

The pathogenesis of acute renal failure in acute tubular necrosis is complex and by no means fully understood. In the group associated with the various types of shock (p. 10.41) the most obvious possibility is ischaemic injury secondary to impaired renal blood flow. Experimental ischaemic injury, however, results in lesions particularly in the proximal convoluted tubules whereas in those cases attributable to trauma and shock in man the lesion (tubulorrhexis) is focal and usually affects the distal convoluted tubules most severely. Because of this, and because tubulorrhexis may be seen also in cases attributable to nephrotoxic chemicals, it may be that the lesion is produced by some endogenous mechanism which can be set in motion by various causal factors.

Currently four factors are thought to be implicated in the renal failure of acute tubular necrosis: arteriolar vasoconstriction, increased glomerular permeability, tubular obstruction and the backleak of tubular fluid.

Arteriolar vasoconstriction was at one time regarded as the most important factor in the renal failure of acute tubular necrosis and reduction of renal blood flow to less than 50% of normal was demonstrated. Similar reductions in renal blood flow have been found in chronic renal failure without giving rise to oliguria and it was later shown that the reduced flow in acute tubular necrosis was largely confined to the renal cortex. It has been suggested that disruption in the tubular transport of sodium or chloride stimulates renin release and that the renin-angiotensin system mediates the observed vasoconstriction. This mechanism cannot, however, fully explain the facts because angiotensin promotes arteriolar vasoconstriction whilst the cortical ischaemia in acute tubular necrosis is due in part to constriction of the arcuate or interlobular arteries of the kidney.

Increased glomerular permeability is associated with swelling of the glomerular epithelial cells, best seen by scanning electron microscopy, in early post-ischaemic acute renal failure. This process can be mimicked by incubating glomeruli in solutions containing angiotensin, and is a second possible effect of the renin-angiotensin system. There is certainly a correlation between the extent of these glomerular epithelial cell changes and the eventual severity of post-ischaemic acute renal failure in man (Solez *et al.*, 1981).

Tubular obstruction. Micro-dissection studies have shown the presence of long hyaline tubular casts, consisting largely of Tamm-Horsfall protein, which must restrict tubular flow. This is associated with raised intratubular pressure and dilated tubular lumina. The diuretic phase of acute tubular necrosis is associated with a great increase in Tamm-Horsfall protein in the urine and may indicate the flushing out of these casts. Tubular obstruction also leads to afferent arteriolar vasoconstriction which further lowers the filtration pressure gradient. Protein casts and dilated tubules are, however, found in the recovery phase of acute tubular necrosis and hence tubular obstruction cannot be the whole story.

Backleak of tubular fluid can occur through the areas of basement membrane denuded of epithelial cover in acute tubular necrosis, and any rise in intratubular pressure due to obstruction by casts distal to the epithelial loss will increase the amount of fluid leaking back. Tubular obstruction also reduces glomerular filtration, but dextran-clearance studies suggest that this can explain only about 20% of the observed reduction.

It is obvious that the above postulated mechanisms are to some extent inter-dependent, and it is likely that they all contribute to the observed renal failure.

The part played by haemoglobin and myoglobin in acute renal failure is also obscure. In experimental studies, haemoglobin has not been shown to be nephrotoxic in otherwise healthy animals, although it has been shown to cause injury in conditions of dehydration, acidosis and renal ischaemia. Myoglobinuria has been shown to be more prone than haemoglobinuria to be accompanied by acute renal failure, particularly in crush injuries, and it may be that other products of muscle breakdown, in addition to myoglobin, are involved. The more extensive necrosis of the proximal tubules which occurs in cases attributable to various chemicals is more uniform, and is explicable as a direct toxic effect upon the tubular epithelium.

Chronic Renal Failure

Chronic renal failure results when the functions of the kidneys have been so reduced by a chronic disease process that there is retention of nitrogenous waste products normally excreted in the urine, and loss of the capacity of the kidneys to maintain homoeostasis of fluid and electrolytes and acid–base balance in the face of the normal variations of fluid and dietary intake and of physical activity. Changes in hormone production (excess renin and reduced erythropoietin) by the damaged kidneys have also been demonstrated. In most cases hypertension is superadded, and may be of the malignant type, but essential (primary) malignant hypertension may itself cause chronic renal failure. The two commonest causes, however, are chronic pyelonephritis and chronic glomerulonephritis, and there are many others, including polycystic disease of the kidneys, systemic lupus erythematosus, diabetes mellitus, amyloid disease, nephrocalcinosis, gout, irradiation injury and analgesic nephropathy. The pathological changes characteristic of these diseases are described in the appropriate sections: in all of them, severe chronic renal injury may occur, but the resulting chronic renal failure presents biochemical, clinical and morphological changes which are sufficiently similar to warrant a common description.

Biochemical disturbances

Non-protein nitrogen retention. As only a small proportion of functioning renal tissue remains in patients with chronic renal failure, it follows that renal blood flow and total glomerular filtration rate (GFR) are considerably reduced. When GFR falls below normal, the amount of urea removed from the blood falls below the normal level of urea production, and the level in the blood rises. If kidney function remains steady, the blood urea will stabilise at a level at which the normal amount is removed in the glomerular filtrate. To give an example, the normal GFR may be taken as 120 ml per minute and the blood urea level as approximately 30 mg/dl. Since urea is very highly diffusible, the concentration in the glomerular filtrate will also be 30 mg/dl, and the total amount of urea filtered off from the blood will thus be $120/100 \times 30$ mg, i.e. 36 mg per minute. Some reabsorption of urea takes place from the tubule, and the amount excreted is about 25 mg per minute (36 g daily). Consider now the patient with chronic renal failure and sufficient functioning nephrons to provide a GFR of, say, 12 ml per minute. Obviously, this will result in urea retention, which will be reflected in a high blood urea: when the level reaches 300 mg/dl, the 12 ml of filtrate per minute will then contain 36 mg, i.e. the amount normally filtered, and provided that tubular reabsorption is not altered, the normal amount will be excreted. In fact, this is an over-simplification, for urea production varies with dietary protein intake, and there are also variations in the amount reabsorbed from the tubules. In chronic renal failure there is usually distinct polyuria and, as explained below, less reabsorption occurs from the tubules. In spite of these complicating factors, the level of the blood urea gives useful information in chronic renal failure, and is easy to estimate: provided certain precautions are taken, changes in the level reflect changes in renal function. The level of blood creatinine is less influenced by dietary factors and tubular reabsorption and provides a better indication of renal function, but its estimation is less simple.

Urea itself has little or no toxicity, but its retention is an indication of retention of various other non-protein nitrogenous metabolites, some of which are toxic.

Excretion of water. In normal circumstances, the kidneys play the major role in adjusting water loss to suit intake. This is effected by varying the volume of urine from approximately 400 ml to several litres daily. Within these limits, the excretion of urinary solutes is not affected significantly, and the specific gravity of the urine is inversely proportional to the volume, varying between 1·002 and 1·040. In chronic renal failure, the variability of urine volume is commonly lost, and provided sufficient water is taken in, the kidneys excrete daily approximately 2·5 litres of dilute urine of specific gravity approximately 1·010. If water intake is inadequate in this condition, production of dilute urine continues and dehydration results, with consequent fall in blood volume and blood pressure: renal blood flow and GFR are consequently diminished, the volume of urine falls and uraemia increases. If water intake is excessive, the urine volume is little affected, and the patient develops water intoxication and pulmonary oedema. The supervention of heart failure, a common complication of chronic renal failure with hypertension, results in further impairment of renal blood flow and fall in GFR, with consequent oliguria, increase in uraemia, and cardiac oedema (p. 10.32).

The **polyuria** of chronic renal failure is at first sight surprising in view of the small amount of glomerular filtrate produced, but it will be recalled that in the healthy individual, the volume of urine is controlled mainly by the degree of concentration taking place in the tubules, and not by variations in the glomerular filtrate. Obviously, in chronic renal failure the polyuria results from failure of the tubules to effect the normal variations in concentration, and the most likely explanation is that the high concentration of urea in the glomerular filtrate exerts an osmotic diuretic effect similar to that which occurs when a large amount of urea is administered to a normal individual. The effect is not peculiar to urea, and can be induced by giving any substance which diffuses readily into the glomerular filtrate and which is largely unabsorbed in the tubules, e.g. inulin. Normally, 80% of the volume of the glomerular filtrate is reabsorbed in the proximal part of the tubule, but the fluid remaining in the lumen does not exceed isotonicity. In chronic renal failure, the high concentration of urea in the glomerular filtrate results in isotonicity being reached when much less than 80% of the volume has been reabsorbed, and further concentration cannot be achieved in this part of the nephron. In the distal part of the tubule and the collecting tubule, the 'sodium pump' normally results in a high concentration of Na^+ in the adjacent medullary interstitial tissue, and this facilitates

further concentration of the tubular fluid and production of a hypertonic urine. In chronic renal failure (and osmotic diuresis induced in a normal individual) failure to achieve the normal five-fold concentration in the proximal tubule results in a large volume of fluid passing into the distal tubule, and rapid absorption of water here dilutes the Na^+ in the interstitial fluid and so interferes with further urinary concentration.

Electrolyte disturbances. It is a remarkable fact that, in contrast to the blood urea, the plasma concentrations of sodium and potassium are virtually unaltered until the terminal stages of chronic renal failure. In the normal individual, the amounts of Na^+ and K^+ excreted in the urine vary considerably, depending on intake. In chronic renal failure, the range of excretion is limited. Nevertheless, considering that in some cases few functioning nephrons remain, it is apparent that, to maintain homeostasis, considerably more Na^+ and K^+ must be excreted per nephron than normally. This is brought about by the continuous state of osmotic diuresis, referred to above, which pertains in chronic renal failure, diuresis being accompanied by decreased reabsorption of various solutes, including Na^+ and K^+. **Deficiency of Na^+** is a common late effect, for the urinary loss is somewhat inflexible, and deficiency may result from restricted intake of salt or from vomiting and diarrhoea, attacks of which are common in uraemia. Na^+ deficiency in time leads to fall in plasma volume and blood pressure, and to oliguria: nitrogen retention increases and acidosis (see below) supervenes. In some cases of chronic renal failure due to pyelonephritis, sodium loss is severe, and the clinical features may be similar to those of adrenocortical insufficiency (Addison's disease). Correction of Na^+ deficiency in chronic renal failure must be carefully controlled, for administration of too much Na^+ and water can readily induce systemic or pulmonary oedema.

In chronic renal failure, **potassium retention** may arise from excessive intake or as a complication of dehydration and acidosis; in this state, dehydration results in oliguria and reduced K^+ excretion, while acidosis results in exchange of some intracellular K^+ for H^+; both effects raise the level of plasma K^+, and there is a risk of cardiac arrest. **Potassium deficiency** is uncommon in chronic renal failure, but can occur in certain cases of chronic pyelonephritis, where excessive loss of K^+ in the urine can result from secondary aldosteronism attributable, in turn, to excessive Na^+ loss, and producing a picture like Conn's syndrome (p. 26.34).

Another effect of chronic renal failure is **acid-osis**. To conserve acid–base balance, the kidneys must excrete 40–60 mmol of acid (H^+) daily. This is excreted in combination with urinary phosphate and organic acid radicles (e.g. creatinine), and by combination with ammonia as NH_4^+. For homoeostasis, therefore, the glomerular filtrate must provide sufficient dibasic phosphate and other available anions, and the cells of the distal convoluted tubules must produce and secrete an adequate amount of ammonia, which is normally derived by deamination of amino acids. In chronic renal failure, the diminished volume of glomerular filtrate does not contain the normal amount of dibasic phosphate, but tubular reabsorption is also reduced as a result of the continuous osmotic diuresis, and the net amount available for excretion of acid is not very much less than normal until the late stages. Because relatively few functioning nephrons remain, total ammonia production and secretion into the tubules is reduced. There is also some loss of bicarbonate in the urine, whereas normally it is almost completely reabsorbed. As a result of these changes, the patient with chronic renal failure is prone to develop acidosis. In most cases, the **plasma phosphate** level is normal except in the late stages, but if lack of water arises, either from deficient intake or from vomiting or diarrhoea, or if the glomerular filtration rate falls even further as a result of heart failure, phosphate excretion is diminished, the blood level rises and acidosis develops.

The level of **plasma calcium** tends to be slightly low in chronic renal failure, and is further depressed if the level of phosphate rises. In this state, however, acidosis is also likely, and this increases the proportion of plasma calcium in ionic form, with the result that frank tetany does not usually develop, although muscle twitching is common.

Hypertension

This develops in most cases of chronic renal failure, often before there is nitrogen retention, and is sometimes of the malignant type. It may be associated with a decrease in renin response to changes in sodium balance and with an increase in peripheral vascular resistance. The renal changes resulting from hypertension cause further injury to the already damaged kidneys, and progress of renal failure is hastened. Life can be prolonged by antihypertensive drugs and this is now an important aspect of treatment.

Pathological changes

The disease processes most commonly responsible for chronic renal failure are noted on p. 22.12, and their pathological features are described in the appropriate sections. It remains to describe the pathological changes throughout the body which *result from* chronic renal failure, whatever the cause. These changes are neither constant nor specific. **Fibrinous pericarditis**, accompanied by little or no effusion, is common in the late stages, and also **'uraemic pneumonitis'**, consisting of a sero-fibrinous exudate into the alveolar spaces, sometimes fanning out from the hila, and giving a butterfly shadow on x-ray. The changes resemble those of neonatal hyaline membrane disease (p. 16.21), but there is often partial organisation of the exudate. Inflammatory changes occur also in the **gastro-intestinal tract**, including haemorrhagic ulceration and also a pseudomembranous enterocolitis. The cause of these various inflammatory lesions has not been established. **Immunodeficiency**, with a tendency to infections, is known to occur in uraemia, but the fibrinous pericarditis is usually sterile and cannot be explained thus. In some cases, the fibrinoid necrosis of arterioles resulting from malignant hypertension may be responsible for some of the lesions (e.g. Fig. 14.19, p.14.18). The **cardiovascular features of hypertension** are usually obvious in such cases, although cerebral haemorrhage is less common than in essential hypertension. The presence of foci of calcification and of oxalate deposition in the heart and blood vessels may be a prominent feature. Changes have also been described in the pancreas.

Bone changes. Various bone changes may occur, and are termed collectively *renal osteodystrophy* (p. 23.15). They include osteitis fibrosa cystica, osteomalacia, and osteoporosis and in children resemble rickets ('renal rickets'). The variation in calcium and phosphate levels may induce hyperplasia of the parathyroid glands with consequent bone disease (secondary hyperparathyroidism), and raised aluminium levels have been associated with osteomalacia. These bone changes are described in Chapter 23.

Haematological changes in chronic renal failure include a normochromic normocytic anaemia which is due to depressed erythropoiesis and is roughly proportional to the degree of uraemia. There may also be a microangiopathic haemolytic anaemia (p. 17.32) in those patients who develop malignant hypertension, this being one form of the haemolytic-uraemic syndrome (p. 22.45). Patients on long-term haemodialysis may develop foci of macrophages and foreign-body giant cells in lung, liver and the lympho-reticular tissues. This has been attributed to material from the silicone dialysis tubing.

Changes in the nervous system. A variety of mental changes may occur, including disorientation, delirium and psychoses, but there are few obvious pathological changes in the brain. Peripheral neuropathy is sometimes troublesome, particularly in patients on long-term dialysis: it may be greatly improved after renal transplantation. Hypertensive encephalopathy may occur in these cases with malignant hypertension.

Glomerulonephritis

Definition. This term embraces a group of renal diseases in which the lesions are primarily glomerular, other changes in the kidney being the result of the glomerular injury. Lesions due to infection of the kidneys (pyelonephritis) are not included in this group.

Immunological basis

Although no single type of glomerulonephritis is fully understood there is strong evidence that most are due to injury caused by the presence of antigen-antibody complexes in the walls of the glomerular capillaries. Much of this evidence is based on experimental animal work on which there is now a vast literature. (For review see McLuskey 1983.)

Immune complexes may localise within the glomeruli in the following ways. (1) Circulating immune complexes may be filtered out in the glomerular basement membrane. In the acute serum sickness model (p. 7.15) in which a single large injection of a soluble antigen is administered to an animal (e.g. bovine serum albumin to rabbits), antibody appears after a week or so and reacts with antigen still present in the plasma to form immune complexes. If complexes of appropriate size are formed (see below) they are arrested as granular deposits in the walls of blood vessels (Fig. 22.13 and 22.14), especially the glomerular capillaries.

In the chronic serum sickness model, small amounts of antigen are given by repeated (e.g. daily) intravenous injections and there may be extensive glomerular deposition of immune complexes without an acute inflammatory reaction. (2) Antibodies may form to constituents of the glomerular basement membrane. Experimentally, if tissue preparations containing glomerular basement membrane (GBM) of one species (e.g. rat) are injected into animals of other species (e.g. duck or rabbit) then the hetero-antibody which develops is capable of causing acute diffuse glomerulonephritis when injected into animals of the first species. First reported in 1900 by Lindemann, this is usually known as a Masugi type nephritis (*or nephrotoxic serum nephritis*). The antibody becomes bound to the GBM and is seen as a linear deposit by immunofluorescence staining (Fig. 22.15). Various forms of human crescentic glomerulonephritis (e.g. in Goodpasture's syndrome) are known to be associated with auto-antibodies reacting with the GBM.

(3) Until recently, the above two mechanisms were thought to account for immune complex localisation in the kidney, but other mechanisms have now become apparent and may be important. For example, circulating antibodies may react with non-basement membrane glomerular antigens, or with antigens from the plasma which have become trapped within the glomerular basement membrane to form immune complexes in situ.

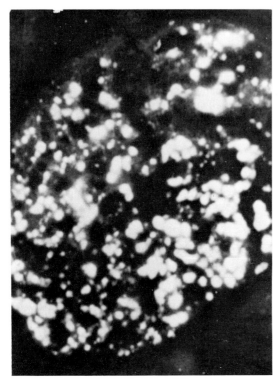

Fig. 22.13 Experimental foreign-protein glomerulo-nephritis. Irregular deposition of immune complexes in the capillary walls, shown by fluorescent antibody to IgG. (Professor R. Lannigan.)

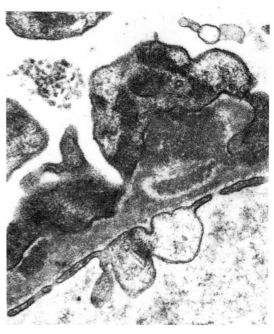

Fig. 22.14 Electron micrograph of segment of glomerular capillary wall in experimental immune complex glomerulonephritis, showing dense nodular deposits in outer part of basement membrane (capillary lumen below; urinary space above). × 25 000.

In some instances non-antibody substances within the glomeruli may activate complement via the alternative pathway and thus cause glomerular damage.

Factors influencing deposition of immune complexes within glomeruli. Why should immune complexes or antigens circulating in the plasma accumulate preferentially in glomeruli?

The kidney receives a relatively large blood supply and the glomeruli are unusual in that their capillaries lie between two arterioles: in consequence, the glomerular capillary pressure is much greater than in other capillary beds. In experimental immune-complex glomerulo-nephritis, reduction of glomerular filtration pressure by partial clamping of one renal artery or one ureter has been shown to reduce the amount of immune-complex deposition in that kidney. In addition, the normal glomerular capillary wall acts as a progressive sieve: very small molecules and ions pass freely through the endothelial layer, basement membrane and

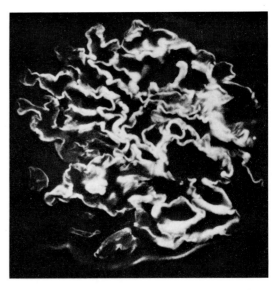

Fig. 22.15 Nephrotoxic-antibody nephritis; linear deposition of nephrotoxic antibody in the glomerular capillary walls, demonstrated by the immuno-fluorescence technique.

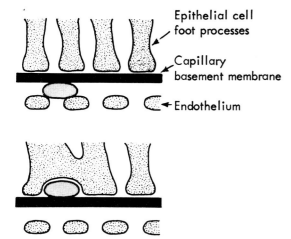

Epithelial cell foot processes

Capillary basement membrane

← Endothelium

Fig. 22.16 The sites of deposition of immune complexes in the glomerular capillary walls. Larger complexes aggregate on the sub-endothelial side of the basement membrane (*above*). Smaller complexes are deposited on the epithelial side of the basement membrane (*below*).

epithelial slit pores to appear in the glomerular filtrate but cells, very large molecular aggregates etc., are kept within the vascular tree by the pore size of the endothelial cells. Between these two extremes, macromolecules and antigen-antibody complexes can penetrate into the glomerular wall (Fig. 22.16) (Germuth and Rodriguez 1973). The depth of such penetration depends not only on molecular size but also on molecular shape: a cigar-shaped molecule may penetrate further through the basement membrane than a globular molecule of the same molecular weight. Molecular charge is also important: the basement membrane and the outer membrane (glycocalyx) of the epithelial cells are negatively charged due to the presence of sialic acid residues and repel negatively charged molecules or immune complexes, preventing them from penetrating the endothelium as readily as positively charged particles of similar size. Some large molecules are able to 'unravel' and penetrate the basement membrane as long fibrous molecules which can then re-assume their former shape after passing through: this phenomenon of 'reptation' may account for the penetration of very large and globular molecules. During conditions of reduced blood flow, the basement membrane, which has a complex layered structure, may allow the passage of larger molecules, because

under such conditions the molecular 'sieve' is less stretched and the pore size is consequently increased.

The mononuclear phagocyte system (p. 4.33) removes foreign material and large protein aggregates from the blood. In normal circumstances it may remove most of the circulating immune complexes. If the system is presented with an excess of such complexes or if it is depressed, e.g. by infections, drugs or neoplasia, then it may be incapable of clearing the blood of circulating immune complexes, some will penetrate into the glomerular capillaries as described above. Other factors include the release of vaso-active agents which increase the permeability of the glomerular (and other) capillaries, and treatment with glucocorticoids which, by contrast, impedes the transfer of macromolecules across the basement membrane. Cognisance of steroid therapy must therefore be taken in any EM assessment of immune complex deposition in the glomeruli.

Immune complex localisation. Depending on their shape and deformability, immune complexes of intermediate or small size may be deposited on either side of the basement membrane, i.e. subendothelially or subepithelially, or within the membrane.

As noted earlier, large immune complexes do not penetrate glomerular capillary endothelium. **Intermediate-sized immune complexes** which penetrate the endothelium are arrested by the basement membrane and so are deposited subendothelially. The mesangial cells exert a clearing effect by phagocytic ingestion of material deposited in this site, and subendothelial deposition is always accompanied by the presence of complexes in the mesangial cells. If the concentration of immune complexes in the plasma is low, and only small amounts reach the subendothelial space, they are removed by the mesangial cells and do not injure the glomerular capillaries. If the amounts deposited are greater, the mesangial clearance system of some of the glomerular lobules may be overwhelmed with consequent development of focal or lobular lesions while very heavy deposition results in diffuse glomerular lesions. **Small immune complexes** are arrested either within the basement membrane or on its outer surface, i.e. subepithelially. In many instances, for reasons given below, immune complexes deposited in this site do not cause acute glomerular injury, but rather a slow and gradual thickening and increase in permeability of the basement membrane.

Mechanisms of glomerular injury by immune complexes. The presence of subendothelial glomerular immune complexes causes damage in at least two ways. Firstly, the complexes activate the complement cascade, with production of the lytic complex which damages the adjacent cells and basement membranes (p. 7.4). Products of complement activation, notably C5a, increase capillary permeability and are chemotactic for neutrophil polymorphs and monocytes which in consequence accumulate in the lesion. These cells phagocytose immune complexes and, in doing so, secrete numerous lysosomal enzymes (p. 4.26), some of which can degrade cell and basement membranes. Secondly there may be local activation of the coagulation cascade, either secondary to complement activation or by cell damage with the release of various enzymes and protein breakdown products. The coagulation system may also be activated locally, with deposition of fibrin in the lumen and walls of the glomerular capillaries, and early administration of anticoagulants in experimental immune-complex nephritis has been shown to prevent some of the glomerular injury. If the injury to the glomerular capillaries is severe, components of the clotting system may escape into Bowman's space where deposition of fibrin promotes the formation of cellular aggregates or crescents (p. 22.23), which further impair glomerular function.

Glomerular manifestations of immune-complex injury. The major histological features of immune-complex glomerular injury can be explained by consideration of the pathogenic mechanism.

1. Hypercellularity is due to an increase in the number of mesangial cells and to arrest and emigration of neutrophil polymorphs and monocytes in response to immune-complex deposition, activation of complement and endothelial injury.

2. Thickening of the glomerular capillary basement membrane as seen by light microscopy (the normal basement membrane can only be appreciated by electron microscopy) has a variety of causes. Large subepithelial, intramembranous or subendothelial deposits of immune complexes, swelling of the damaged epithelial or endothelial cells, or prolongation of long mesangial cell processes between the endothelium and basement membrane (Fig. 22.35) secondary to immune complex deposition can all give rise to a thickened basement membrane. Production of the basement membrane material may also be stimulated by the presence of immune complexes.

3. Crescent formation. The escape of fibrin into Bowman's space stimulates the lining epithelial cells to divide and this, together with an admixture of mononuclear phagocytes, produces a crescent-shaped mass of cells which compresses the glomerular tuft—hence the name of the lesion.

The above changes may affect the whole glomerulus but in some instances where large subendothelial immune complex deposits are involved, the mesangium may be more effective in clearing the complexes from one lobule than from another, resulting in a focal or segmental lesion.

Glomerulonephritis in man

Classification. The widespread practice of renal biopsy is now providing much information about the histological changes of glomerulonephritis and particularly about the early stages, while immunological studies are providing important aetiological clues. However, there is still much to be learned, and classifications of glomerulonephritis must still be regarded as provisional, in the knowledge that modifications will be necessary in the coming years.

In the classification of glomerulonephritis proposed below, we have selected, from the terms in common usage, those which seem to us to indicate best the major glomerular changes. Commonly used alternatives are given in italics.

It must be emphasised that this classification is not intended to be comprehensive. Moreover, some of the types include more than one disease entity. Certain other conditions, e.g. systemic lupus erythematosus, diabetes mellitus and amyloidosis, can give rise to glomerular lesions resulting in clinical syndromes resembling one or other type of glomerulonephritis, and it seems appropriate to discuss them together with or immediately after glomerulonephritis.

CLASSIFICATION OF GLOMERULONEPHRITIS

Acute diffuse proliferative glomerulonephritis
(*Post-streptococcal glomerulonephritis:
post-infective glomerulonephritis*)

Rapidly progressive glomerulonephritis
(*Crescentic glomerulonephritis*)

Diffuse membranous glomerulonephritis
(*Idiopathic membranous glomerulonephritis:
epimembranous nephropathy*)

Mesangiocapillary glomerulonephritis
(*Membranoproliferative glomerulonephritis*)
                                    Type I
                                    Type II

Minimal-change glomerulonephritis
(*Minimal-change nephropathy: lipoid nephrosis:
light-negative glomerulonephritis*)

Focal glomerulonephritis

Chronic glomerulonephritis

Acute diffuse proliferative glomerulonephritis

Clinical features and course. This relatively common type of glomerulonephritis occurs at all ages, although it is more prevalent in children than in adults. It affects males more often than females and usually follows an acute infection with Group A haemolytic streptococci—most often pharyngitis (including scarlet fever), but sometimes infections of the middle ear or skin. In many cases, the disease develops 1–4 weeks after the onset of the streptococcal infection: very often this has settled down and there is a latent period of apparent well-being before glomerulonephritis becomes apparent. Other infections, e.g. with *Staphylococcus aureus* and *Strep. pneumoniae* have occasionally been implicated and acute glomerulonephritis may also complicate falciparum malaria (p. 28.6), toxoplasmosis, schistosomiasis (p. 28.29), and some acute virus infections.

The presenting features include peri-orbital oedema (the eyelids appearing puffy), malaise, fever, and discolouration of the urine due to altered blood in it. The oedema is marked in the morning and may involve the rest of the face and other lax tissues. The blood pressure is usually slightly or moderately raised. The demonstration of haematuria microscopically in otherwise well children following a streptococcal sore throat indicates that renal involvement is often subclinical.

In childhood the disease runs a benign course and some 90% recover completely after an illness lasting a week or two. The mortality, however, increases with age, and exceeds 50% in patients over the age of 65.

Biochemical changes. There is usually a mild or moderate rise in the level of blood urea. The urine is diminished in volume, of high specific gravity, and commonly brownish and turbid ('smoky') from the presence of altered red cells. (*The haematuria, together with oliguria and hypertension, constitute the nephritic syndrome.*) There is moderate proteinuria and, as in all types of glomerulonephritis, the protein is mainly plasma albumin. Quantitative analysis reveals that larger protein molecules, e.g. IgG, are also usually present in appreciable amounts and the proteinuria is thus not a highly selective albuminuria. Microscopy of the urine shows many red cells, moderate or large numbers of neutrophil polymorphs, and hyaline, granular or cellular casts (p. 22.44).

Some patients die in the acute stage from the effects of hypertension, e.g. acute heart failure, or from acute renal failure. In others the glomerular lesions and clinical features persist and get progressively worse, causing death from hypertension and renal failure within two years: these patients are correctly classified as *rapidly progressive glomerulonephritis* (p. 22.22). In a small proportion of patients proteinuria persists long after apparent recovery from the acute attack. Proteinuria for several months is consistent with complete recovery but when it continues for over a year, and particularly when there are also some red cells and leucocytes in the urine, it is very likely that the glomerular injury, although clinically silent, is progressing; such patients are liable to develop *chronic glomerulonephritis*, with hypertension and renal failure, at any time within the next twenty years or so.

Pathological features. In acute diffuse proliferative glomerulonephritis the cortex is pale and distinctly enlarged due to oedema. In fatal cases the cortex is up to twice the normal thickness, pale, and the glomeruli may be just visible with a hand lens as light grey dots projecting from the cut surface.

Microscopically, the appearances are similar in biopsy and autopsy material. The most conspicuous changes are diffuse enlargement and

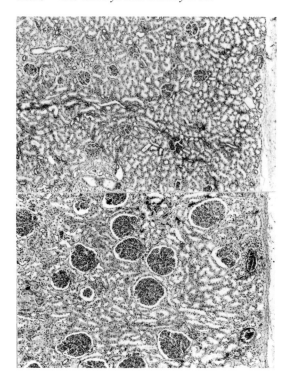

Fig. 22.17 The renal cortex in acute diffuse proliferative glomerulonephritis (*below*) compared with the cortex of a normal kidney (*above*). Note the gross enlargement and hypercellularity of the glomeruli. × 30.

increased cellularity of the glomeruli (Figs. 22.17 and 22.18). The enlargement results in narrowing or obliteration of the capsular space. When a glomerulus happens to have been cut in the appropriate plane, part of the glomerular tuft can often be seen to have herniated into the lumen of the first part of the tubule. The capillary lumina appear narrowed, and the endothelial cells are swollen. Electron microscopy shows the hypercellularity to be due mainly to increase of mesangial and endothelial cells; neutrophil polymorphs and macrophages are also seen but vary greatly in number from case to case.

An additional change in the glomerular tufts is an increase in the number of strands of basement-membrane-like material (mesangial matrix) demonstrable by electron microscopy in the mesangial regions. These strands are normally present between mesangial cells and are made more conspicuous by oedema. In cases which fail to resolve, the material apparently increases considerably and it contributes to the hyaline appearance of the glomeruli in the chronic stage of glomerulonephritis.

Electron microscopy shows localised deposits of granular material, mostly projecting from the outer surface of the basement membrane and giving it a 'lumpy' appearance (Fig. 22.19), while in some cases there are deposits also on the inner surface of the basement membrane.

The epithelial cells do not show widespread fusion of foot processes, although this may occur focally. Some proteinaceous debris, and occasionally red cells, may be seen in the narrowed capsular spaces. In most cases, the epithelium of Bowman's capsule appears normal, but here and there some proliferation may be seen. Epithelial crescents (p. 22.23) are few or absent in typical cases. The changes are represented diagrammatically in Fig. 22.20.

Changes in the rest of the kidney are secondary to the glomerular lesion: there is diffuse oedema, seen as an increase in the loose interstitial tissue between the tubules, and often accompanied by a light scattering of polymorphs or mononuclear cells. The tubules con-

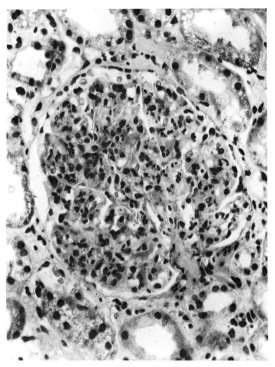

Fig. 22.18 Glomerulus in acute diffuse proliferative glomerulonephritis, showing swelling and increased cellularity of the glomerular tuft. × 200.

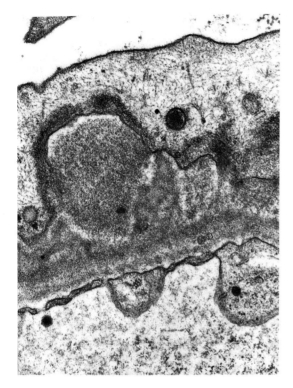

Fig. 22.19 Electron micrograph of part of glomerular capillary wall in acute diffuse glomerulonephritis, showing a large granular sub-epithelial deposit. Note that fusion of the foot processes (lumen below, urinary space above). × 15 000.

tain proteinaceous and cellular casts, including blood casts, and the epithelial cells of the proximal convoluted tubules contain hyaline droplets (p. 22.25). Occasionally there are foci of disruption of tubular epithelial cells, possibly attributable to ischaemia secondary to the glomerular changes. Hypertension is not usually sufficiently severe or prolonged to produce changes in the heart and blood vessels.

With recovery from the disease the glomeruli return to normal, although increased numbers of cells in the mesangial zones of the glomerular lobules may persist for months, and are regarded as a retrospective diagnostic feature.

Clinico-pathological correlation. In acute diffuse glomerulonephritis, light- and electron-microscopy show narrowing of the glomerular capillary lumina attributable to increase in number and size of endothelial and/or mesangial cells and infiltration of polymorphs. Some impairment of blood flow through the kidneys

might be expected, and indeed the renal plasma flow has been shown to be reduced in some cases, but is normal in others. However, the fraction of plasma filtered off by glomeruli (the glomerular filtration fraction) is reduced, and hence *the total glomerular filtration rate (GFR) is also less than normal*. This largely explains the usual rise in the blood urea level, although ischaemic injury of the tubular epithelium may play a part by impairing the functional selectivity of reabsorption.

The factors concerned in the production of oedema and oliguria in acute diffuse glomerulonephritis are not yet fully understood. The point is made several times in this chapter that the *volume* of urine produced, and its *concentration*, are dependent mainly on tubular reabsorption and not on the GFR. Two important factors in tubular reabsorption are, firstly the concentration of solutes remaining in the lumen (i.e. not reabsorbed)—a high concentration of solute, e.g. urea, produces an osmotic diuresis by interfering with reabsorption of water (p. 22.13); secondly, the pituitary anti-

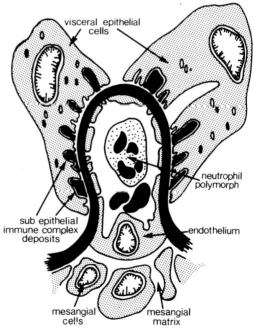

Fig. 22.20 Diagram of a capillary loop in acute diffuse proliferative glomerulonephritis. Note the presence of sub-epithelial immune complex deposits, and an excess of mesangial cells. A neutrophil polymorph is present in the capillary lumen.

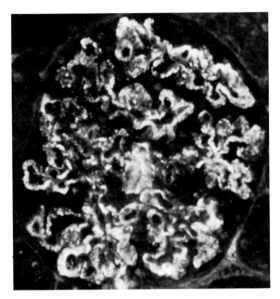

Fig. 22.21   Renal biopsy in acute diffuse glomerulonephritis. Immunofluorescence technique, showing granular and ill-defined deposition of IgG in the glomerular capillary wall. × 350.

diuretic hormone, which increases reabsorption of water. It is not clear what part these and other factors play in the oliguria and oedema of acute diffuse glomerulonephritis: the subject is discussed more fully on p. 10.33. The transient hypertension is presumed to result from decreased renal blood flow.

Unfavourable histological features. Thrombosis and necrosis of individual glomerular capillaries, glomerular haemorrhages, deposition of fibrin and the development of numerous large epithelial crescents are all indications of unusually severe glomerular injury and carry the risk of death in the acute disease. There is no sharp dividing line between such severe cases and rapidly progressive glomerulonephritis (see below).

Following acute diffuse glomerulonephritis, increase in the size and number of mesangial cells may persist for weeks or even months without serious sequelae. Increase in basement-membrane-like material in the mesangial areas is, however, a more serious feature; it is seen together with persistent cellular increase, in those few cases which, after a latent period, develop chronic glomerulonephritis.

Pathogenesis. Immunofluorescence microscopy of renal biopsy material in cases of acute diffuse glomerulonephritis typically reveals granular deposition of immunoglobulin (usually mainly IgG) and components of complement in the glomerular capillary walls (Fig. 22.21). These findings, together with the detection by electron microscopy of dense subepithelial deposits (Fig. 22.19), are strongly suggestive of the deposition of immune complexes, and the diffuse inflammatory glomerular changes also resemble those of experimental acute, serum sickness glomerulonephritis (p. 22.17). As acute glomerulonephritis usually follows a streptococcal infection it is likely that antibodies to streptococcal products, appearing a week or so after the infection, combine with streptococcal antigens still present in the plasma, thus providing immune complexes which would, at first, be formed in the presence of antigen excess. In keeping with this there are usually low levels of serum complement components, consistent with activation of complement by an antigen-antibody reaction, and serum antistreptolysin O (ASO) titres are usually high, indicating previous streptococcal infection. Attempts to demonstrate streptococcal antigen in the glomerular deposits have provided conflicting results: in general, detection of antigen has been reported mostly in biopsy material obtained early in the course of the disease, and it is likely that, later on, the deposited antigen becomes coated, and thus obscured, by an excess of antibody. Still later, immunofluorescence microscopy may reveal complement components alone. The difficulty in demonstrating streptococcal antigen in the glomeruli is not surprising because similar difficulty has been experienced in demonstrating antigen in experimental acute immune-complex glomerulonephritis, in which not only is the antigen known, but powerful antibodies are usually available to facilitate its detection by immunofluorescence microscopy. It is not understood why certain types of Group A streptococci, notably Griffiths types 12, 4, 1, 25 and 49, are nephritogenic, whereas other types and other micro-organisms are not.

Rapidly progressive glomerulonephritis

This usually fatal condition may develop without known predisposing cause, or may follow a streptococcal infection. It can supervene also in patients with the focal glomerulonephritis associated with certain diseases (Table 22.1 and p. 22.33). It can occur at any age, and is commoner in males than females. The clinical features and urinary changes may be indistinguishable at first from those of acute diffuse glomerulonephritis (p. 22.19), but instead of regressing after a week or two, become progressively more severe, and without haemodialysis death usually results from uraemia and hypertension after a period of a few weeks to a year or so. Rarely, proteinuria may be severe enough to give rise to the nephrotic syndrome. In other cases, severe oliguria or even anuria lead to early death.

Rapidly progressive glomerulonephritis is much less common than acute diffuse glomerulonephritis, but because of its severity it makes an important contribution to the number of individuals dying of renal failure.

Pathological changes. The kidneys are normal in size or enlarged due to oedema; on section the cortex is pale, but may show petechial haemorrhages, and the glomeruli stand out conspicuously as grey dots, visible with a lens on the cut surface. In most cases, there is little or no gross scarring and the surface of the kidneys is smooth.

Table 22.1 Rapidly progressive glomerulonephritis

1) Primary
    Idiopathic
    Post-streptococcal
2) Secondary
    Goodpasture's syndrome
    Henoch-Schonlein syndrome
    Polyarteritis nodosa (microscopic form)
    SLE
    Subacute bacterial endocarditis

Microscopy shows the most important changes to be glomerular. As in acute diffuse glomerulonephritis, there is proliferation, probably of both endothelial and mesangial cells, with narrowing of the capillary lumina, and variable polymorph infiltration of the tuft (Fig. 22.22). Although all the glomeruli are affected, some glomerular lobules may be more severely involved than others, and there may be ruptures in the basement membrane, haemorrhages and necrosis and thrombosis of capillaries or lobules.

A surprising feature of the disease is the rap-

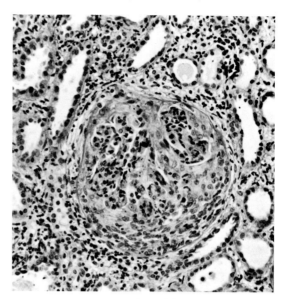

Fig. 22.22 Glomerulus in rapidly progressive glomerulonephritis, showing destruction and fibrosis of parts of the tuft, hypercellularity of the remainder, and formation of a large crescent around the tuft. × 200.

idity with which glomerular scarring may occur: thus in cases with a history of only 2 weeks or so, biopsy may reveal sclerosis of lobules or whole glomeruli, and also fibrous adhesions between the tuft and Bowman's capsule (Fig. 22.23). There is thus a combination of glomerular proliferation, necrosis, thrombosis and scarring, amounting to very severe glomerular injury.

A most characteristic histological feature is proliferation of the parietal epithelium of Bowman's capsule to form **'epithelial crescents'** (Figs. 22.22, 22.23) which occupy the capsular space and surround the tuft. Formation of epithelial crescents occurs in other diseases, for example in subacute bacterial endocarditis, malignant hypertension, and in some cases of acute diffuse glomerulonephritis, but the crescents are neither so numerous nor so large as in rapidly progressive glomerulonephritis, in which they may fill and distend the capsular space of over 80% of the glomeruli. In time, the epithelial crescents are usually replaced by fibrous tissue. Crescents were originally believed to be composed solely of capsular epithelial cells, but there is now evidence from tissue culture that they consist, at least partly, of macrophages, derived from emigrated mono-

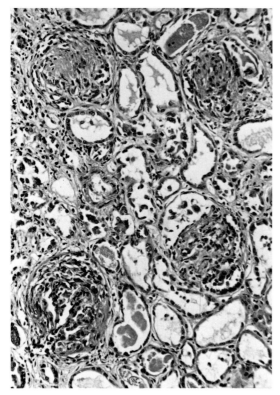

Fig. 22.23 Rapidly progressive glomerulonephritis. The four glomeruli show severe destruction; the lowest one shows crescent formation and the upper two have undergone rapid scarring. The tubules are dilated and there is extensive loss of epithelium. × 110.

cytes (Atkins *et al.*, 1980). Immunofluorescence studies have failed to demonstrate immunoglobulins in crescents, but deposits of fibrin are present and have been shown experimentally to stimulate crescent formation (p. 22.18).

The tubules may be dilated (Fig. 22.23), and usually contain hyaline and cellular casts and red cells and proteinaceous droplets are present in the cells of the proximal convoluted tubules. There may be focal necrosis or irregular tubular atrophy and increase of intertubular connective tissue, presumably due to ischaemia resulting from the glomerular changes.

In some cases hypertension is severe, and the changes of malignant hypertension (p. 22.6) become superadded. There may also be left ventricular hypertrophy and changes associated with uraemia, e.g. fibrinous pericarditis, anaemia and superadded infections.

The glomerular changes result in severely impaired renal blood flow and consequent reduc-

tion in GFR. The clinical and biochemical changes are similar to those in acute diffuse glomerulonephritis, but becoming progressively more severe.

Aetiology. In some cases, rapidly progressive glomerulonephritis follows a streptococcal infection, and these represent the severe end of the spectrum of acute diffuse proliferative glomerulonephritis. They show granular deposition of Ig and complement and sub-epithelial deposits on electron microscopy. In other cases, there is no known preceding infection, and the evidence of immune-complex deposition is sometimes absent. Thirdly, the condition can supervene in a group of systemic conditions which also give rise to the less serious focal glomerulonephritis (p. 22.33). Lastly, the same picture is caused by the development of autoantibody to glomerular basement membrane in Goodpasture's syndrome (p. 22.35).

It is thus apparent that rapidly progressive glomerulonephritis can develop in a number of types of acute glomerulonephritis. Although the prognosis is poor, some cases recover, at least partially, after a period of haemodialysis. The outlook appears to be slightly better in post-streptococcal cases, and treatment by plasma-exchange and a combination of cytotoxic drugs and steroids has given encouraging preliminary results in those cases with Goodpasture's syndrome and in cases with immune complex deposition (Lockwood *et al.*, 1976, 1977).

The nephrotic syndrome

This is described here because it is an important feature of some of the types of glomerulonephritis dealt with below.

The syndrome occurs when prolonged and severe proteinuria results in **hypoalbuminaemia**: this leads to **generalised oedema**, the mechanism of which is described on p. 10.34. The proteinuria is virtually always due to increased glomerular capillary permeability and amounts in adults to the daily loss of 10 g or more of plasma protein. It can be brought about by the glomerular lesions of many different diseases and diagnosis often requires renal biopsy. Conditions other than the renal disease which bring about hypoalbuminaemia, e.g. chronic malnutrition or protein-losing enteropathy, are similarly accompanied by generalised oedema.

Another common feature of the syndrome is

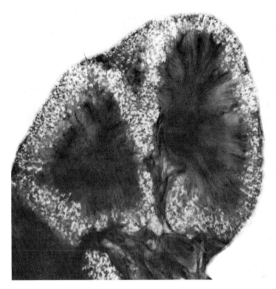

Fig. 22.24 Kidney in nephrotic syndrome, showing abundant cortical deposits of neutral fat and anisotropic lipids. (Photographed using crossed polarising filters.) × 0·8.

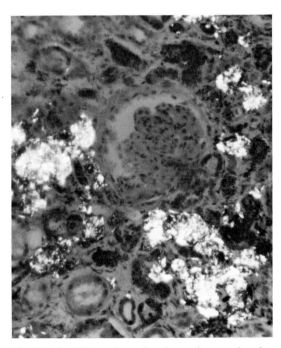

Fig. 22.25 Kidney in nephrotic syndrome, showing abundant anisotropic lipid with some sudanophil neutral fat (dark) in the interstitial tissue and tubules. (Photographed using crossed polarising filters.) × 150.

hyperlipidaemia, increase in levels of lipoproteins of lower density often being considerable. This biochemical change is unexplained and the evidence on its causation is conflicting.

Pathological changes. In addition to generalised oedema, including free fluid in the body cavities, there is a high risk of infections, and before the introduction of sulphonamides and antibiotics a high proportion of patients used to die of pneumonia, peritonitis or meningitis.

The kidneys show striking changes in the nephrotic syndrome. These include generalised enlargement and pallor due to oedema, and frequently a yellow, radial streaking of the cortex due to deposition of lipids (Fig. 22.24). The combination of increased glomerular capillary permeability (responsible for the heavy proteinuria) and hyperlipidaemia results in leakage of relatively large amounts of lipoprotein into the glomerular filtrate: some of this is reabsorbed and deposited in the tubular epithelial cells or in the interstitial tissue of the cortex (Fig. 22.25). There may be accumulation of 'foamy' lipid-laden macrophages and also giant-cell granulomas around crystals of cholesterol. Hyaline droplets due to reabsorption of protein are abundant, along with globules of lipid, in the cytoplasm of the lining cells of the proximal convoluted tubules (Fig. 22.26) and protein casts are present in the distal tubules.

The glomeruli in patients with the nephrotic syndrome show the pathological features of the causal disease. The only feature common to most cases is seen by electron microscopy and consists of fusion of foot processes of the epithelial cells, the cytoplasm of which is closely applied to the outer part of the glomerular basement membrane (Fig. 22.38).

Causes of the nephrotic syndrome are numerous (Table 22.2); they include any condition in which sufficient protein is lost in the urine to cause severe hypoalbuminaemia. In children, minimal-change glomerulonephritis is much the commonest cause, followed by acute diffuse glomerulonephritis and focal glomerulonephritis. In adults, the acute diffuse, membranous and minimal-change types of glomerulonephritis are about equally common, followed by mesangiocapillary glomerulonephritis, renal amyloidosis, diabetes, systemic lupus erythematosus and focal glomerulonephritis.

In some reports, chronic glomerulonephritis

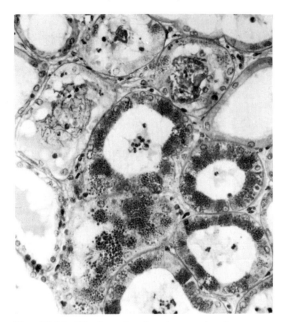

Fig. 22.26 Hyaline droplets in renal tubular epithelium resulting from reabsorption of protein from the filtrate. × 300.

is regarded as a relatively common cause of the nephrotic syndrome. This is probably a matter of nomenclature, for some forms of glomerulonephritis and other renal lesions manifest as the nephrotic syndrome, which may persist for years, and then progress to glomerulosclerosis with reduced renal blood flow and so diminished GFR, leading to renal failure: frequently the proteinuria diminishes as this stage

Table 22.2   Causes of the nephrotic syndrome

1) Intrinsic Renal Disease
    Glomerulonephritis
2) Systematised Disease
    Systemic lupus erythematosus
    Amyloidosis
    Diabetes mellitus
3) Infections
    Syphilis
    Malaria
4) Drugs
    Gold salts
    Penicillamine
5) Malignancy
    Especially lymphoma
6) Miscellaneous
    Sickle cell disease
    Sarcoidosis

develops and the nephrotic syndrome subsides, but in some cases there is a combination of nephrotic syndrome and chronic renal failure.

Diffuse membranous glomerulonephritis

Clinical features. This disease is commoner in males than females, and occurs over a wide age range, although its peak incidence is in middle age. It presents as *the nephrotic syndrome*, i.e. heavy proteinuria, generalised oedema and hyperlipidaemia (see above). The oedema develops gradually, often being first noticed in the face and only partly influenced by gravity. It eventually becomes severe and generalised, with free fluid in the pleural and pericardial cavities. Proteinuria is marked, and as a result the plasma albumin levels falls, usually to below 16 g per litre. The urine often contains small numbers of red cells, and analysis of the protein reveals significant quantities of globulins in addition to the high concentration of albumin: the urine tends to be concentrated and reduced in volume, but can still vary considerably to accommodate fluid intake.

With effective antibiotic therapy for infections (a common and formerly fatal complication of the nephrotic syndrome) the nephrotic stage may pursue an indolent course for many months or years, often ending in chronic renal failure. About 50% of patients are alive 10 years after the onset, and about half of these are in permanent remission. The effects of steroids and cytotoxic drugs on the course of the disease are uncertain; because of the occurrence of spontaneous remissions, their value is difficult to assess.

Pathological changes. The essential change is in the glomeruli, and consists of a diffuse hyaline thickening of the walls of all the glomerular capillaries. In the early stages this is minimal and hard to detect, but it becomes increasingly obvious as the disease progresses (Bariéty *et al.*, 1970; Ehrenreich and Churg, 1968). There is no obvious swelling or proliferation of endothelial or mesangial cells, and no leucocytic infiltration. By light microscopy the capillary walls appear thickened, eosinophilic and hyaline (Fig. 22.27) and silver staining techniques give an appearance of spikiness of the basement membrane (Fig. 22.28). Electron microscopy shows irregular deposition of dense amorphous material in the outer part of the capillary base-

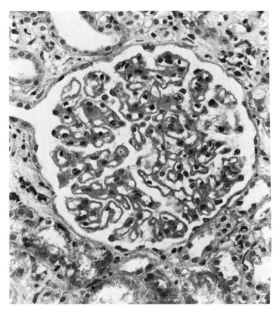

Fig. 22.27 Idiopathic membranous glomerulonephritis. The capillary basement membrane is diffusely and uniformly thickened. × 250.

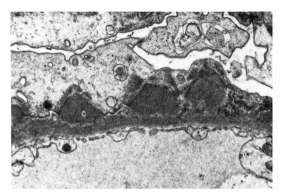

Fig. 22.29 Electron micrograph of segment of glomerular capillary wall in membranous glomerulonephritis (lumen below, urinary space above). The basement membrane is thickened and there are multiple, almost confluent dense deposits on its outer surface. × 16 000.

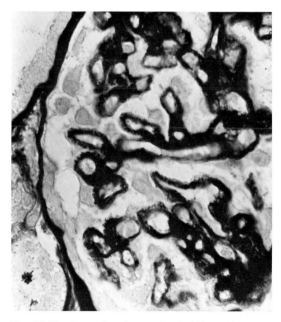

Fig. 22.28 Part of a glomerulus in idiopathic membranous glomerulonephritis, stained by silver impregnation technique and showing the characteristic spiky appearance of the capillary basement membrane. × 475.

ment membrane (Fig. 22.29), and the laying down of new basement membrane between the deposits corresponding to the spikes seen by light microscopy of silver preparations. Eventually the 'spikes' of basement membrane thicken and unite to envelop the deposits and these are gradually replaced by basement membrane, which in consequence, is considerably thickened and irregular (Fig. 22.30). There may also be deposits of dense material between the basement membrane and capillary endothelium, but this is not usually conspicuous and is often absent. At first, the glomerular capillary lumina do not appear to be narrowed, and ischaemic tubular changes are not seen. The other changes seen in the kidneys at this stage are common to the nephrotic syndrome from all causes (p. 22.25).

In the chronic stage of the disease, the thickening of the glomerular capillary walls results in narrowing of the lumina; renal blood flow and GFR are seriously diminished, and uraemia and hypertension develop. Proteinuria diminishes, polyuria often develops, and the oedema tends to subside and may disappear.

Microscopy of the kidneys at this stage shows gross diffuse thickening of glomerular capillary walls, some glomeruli being almost solid eosinophilic hyaline material, while others are less severely affected and still have some patent capillary lumina (Fig. 22.31). Tubular atrophy from ischaemia accompanies the glomerular hyalinisation, and interstitial fibrosis occurs, but lipid deposits, indicative of the preceding

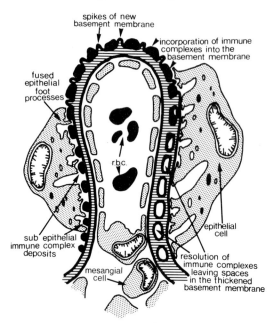

Fig. 22.30 Progression of changes in membranous glomerulonephritis. The sub-epithelial immune complex deposits gradually enlarge and the formation of new basement membrane takes place appearing initially as 'spikes' between the immune complex deposits. The latter are then incorporated into the thickened irregular basement membrane and eventually some complexes may be resolved leaving spaces in the basement membrane.

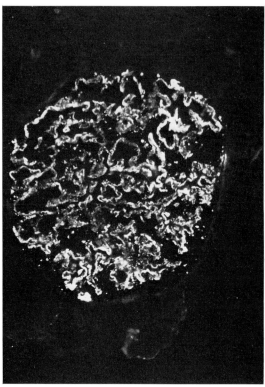

Fig. 22.32 Renal biopsy in membranous glomerulonephritis. Immunofluorescence technique, showing granular deposition of IgG in the glomerular capillary walls. × 250.

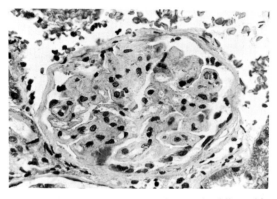

Fig. 22.31 The glomerular change in idiopathic membranous glomerulonephritis which has progressed to the stage of chronic renal failure. The thickening of the basement membrane has resulted in severe narrowing of some glomerular capillaries and obliteration of others.

nephrotic stage, may persist. The kidneys may be slightly shrunken, and may show the super-added changes of hypertension. The pathological features of the chronic stage are compared with those of other forms of chronic glomerulonephritis on p. 22.39.

Aetiology. Examination of renal biopsies by immunofluorescence microscopy shows deposition of immunoglobulin, usually mainly IgG, along the walls of the glomerular capillaries (Fig. 22.32). The deposition is diffuse throughout all the capillaries and at an early stage appears granular. As the disease progresses the deposits increase in size and number and tend to become confluent. Deposition of complement is also usually demonstrable by immunofluorescence: its distribution is the same as that of immunoglobulin but it is deposited in smaller amounts and in some cases is not detectable. The low level of complement deposition may be equated with the absence of inflammatory features (c.f. acute post-infectious glomerulonephritis). These features, together with the dense deposits in the outer part of the basement membrane seen by electron microscopy, and the gradual uniform thickening of the capillary basement membrane, provide a close parallel to experimental immune-complex glomerular injury of the chronic serum sickness type (p. 7.15) and the nephrotic syndrome is a major feature of both conditions. Attempts to demonstrate circulating immune complexes in cases of membranous glomerulonephritis have met with little success and there is some evidence to suggest *in-situ* formation of immune complexes in this type of glomerulonephritis. The nature of the antigen is unknown in most cases, but some cases have associations with infections, e.g. malaria, syphilis and hepatitis B and the corresponding microbial antigens have been demonstrated in the glomerular deposits in such cases. There is an association with malignant tumours and the possibility of a lymphoma or carcinoma should be borne in mind in any middle-aged or old patient presenting with 'idiopathic' membranous glomerulonephritis. Membranous glomerulonephritis may also occur in patients treated with certain drugs, notably penicillamine and gold salts, and also as a feature of systemic lupus erythematosus. In all of these associations, the glomerular deposition of Ig suggests an immune-complex basis, the antigens being assumed to be derived from tumours, drugs, etc., and in those patients with systemic lupus, the deposits have been shown to consist of auto-antigens complexed with auto-antibodies (p. 22.35).

Renal vein thrombosis is now regarded as a complication, rather than the cause, of membranous glomerulonephritis and other conditions associated with the nephrotic syndrome.

Mesangiocapillary (Membranoproliferative) glomerulonephritis

This condition occurs at all ages but particularly in older children. Its presenting features may resemble closely those of acute diffuse proliferative glomerulonephritis, or there may be symptomless proteinuria or development of the nephrotic syndrome.

In general the outlook is poor. The disease continues over a period of years; at some stage the nephrotic syndrome is likely to develop and approximately 50% of patients die within ten

years of chronic renal failure. Some patients do, however, appear to recover. Response to steroids, etc., has so far not been very encouraging, and if renal transplantation is performed the condition tends to recur in the transplant.

Pathological changes. At an early stage the glomeruli show diffuse proliferative change with increase in size and number of mesangial and endothelial cells; the mesangia in particular show increased cellularity and the lobular pattern of the glomeruli is accentuated (Fig. 22.33),

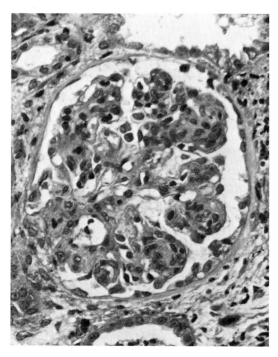

Fig. 22.33 Mesangiocapillary glomerulonephritis. The glomerular lobulation is accentuated, there is increased cellularity, and thickening of capillary walls. × 350.

the disease sometimes being termed lobular glomerulonephritis. The capillary lumina are reduced and there is irregular thickening of their walls. Silver stains show, here and there, a double basement membrane (Fig. 22.34). Two main types are discernible by electron microscopy. In type I, discrete irregular deposits are found on the inner side of the (original) basement membrane, and there is extension of the cytoplasm of mesangial cells between the endothelium and the basement membrane (mesangial interposition). A second layer of basement

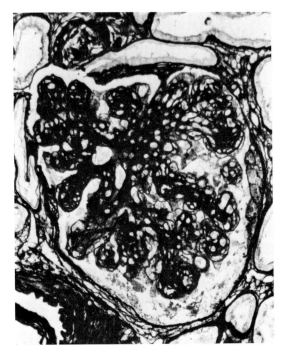

Fig. 22.34 Mesangiocapillary glomerulonephritis. Stained by silver impregnation to show the thickening of the glomerular capillary basement membrane which has a double contour in some peripheral capillary loops. × 350.

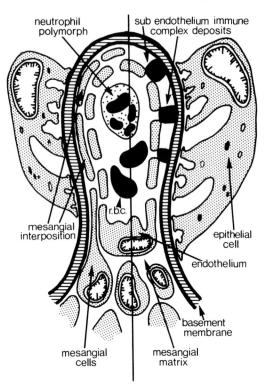

Fig. 22.35 Diagrams of the glomerular capillary loop changes in mesangiocapillary glomerulonephritis.

(a) Type I Mesangiocapillary glomerulonephritis. The diagram depicts the two main features: mesangial interposition and the presence of sub-endothelial immune complexes. For the sake of clarity these have been separated in the diagram. In the actual disease process both features would of course be present at the same time.

membrane is laid down between the endothelium and the mesangial cytoplasmic extension, thus accounting for the double contour seen by some silver stained preparations (Fig. 22.35a). In type II, dense material is deposited within the lamina densa causing a more diffuse thickening of the basement membrane. This has sometimes led to the use of the term **dense deposit disease** (Fig. 22.35b). A type III with both subendothelial and subepithelial deposits has recently been described. The two patterns of deposition are sometimes distinguishable by light microscopy of very thin sections but are seen more readily by electron microscopy. In some cases, particularly of the type II, there is formation of small crescents in the capsule of occasional glomeruli.

As the disease progresses the mesangial cells diminish in number and hyaline material accumulates, while the capillaries become progressively thickened so that glomerulosclerosis and chronic renal failure usually result.

The aetiology of this condition is unknown. In type I, components of complement and immunoglobulin (IgG and/or IgM) are detectable in the capillary walls (Fig. 22.36) and it is likely that the disease is of immune-complex nature. In such cases there is often good evidence of a preceding streptococcal or other acute infection and other associations, e.g. with subacute bacterial endocarditis, sickle cell disease and hepatitis B, have been noted. In type II there is little evidence of immune complex deposition although C3 may be found in the mesangium and around the tubules. In both types, there may be depression of C3 in the plasma and activation of the alternative pathway (p. 7.3) is involved. A factor which activates C3 (*the nephritic factor*) has been detected in the serum in some cases (Davis *et al.*, 1978; West and McAdams, 1978). It appears to be an

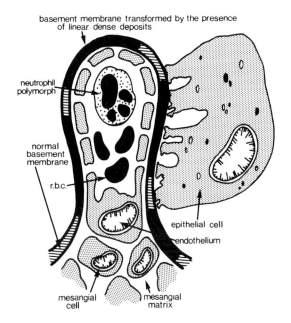

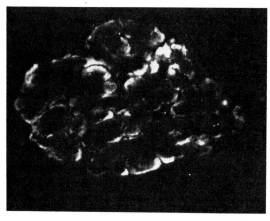

Fig. 22.36 Immunofluorescence staining of two glomeruli in a case of mesangiocapillary glomerulonephritis, showing deposition of IgG at the margins of the lobules. × 200. (Dr H. Moseley.)

Fig. 22.35 (b) Type II Mesangiocapillary glomerulonephritis (Dense Deposit Disease). In this type there is again an excess of mesangial cells and matrix; however the striking feature is the presence of linear dense deposits within the basement membrane.

autoantibody to the C3bBb complex of the alternative pathway.

A familial predisposition is likely in mesangiocapillary glomerulonephritis and in particular there is a syndrome linking partial lipodystrophy and the type II disease.

Minimal-change glomerulonephritis

While this name is not altogether satisfactory, it is preferable to *lipoid nephrosis* because it indicates that the essential lesion is glomerular and that the structural changes are inconspicuous.

General features. The disease has a peak incidence in children between 1 and 4 years old, but occurs in children and adults of all ages. It is by far the commonest cause of the nephrotic syndrome in children. The oedema and proteinuria tend to fluctuate, spontaneous remission and recurrences being common. The blood pressure and tests of renal function are normal. As usual in the nephrotic syndrome (p. 22.24), there is a rise in the level of blood lipids,

including cholesterol, and in the pre-antibiotic era death commonly resulted from superadded infections.

Glucocorticoid therapy has also improved the prognosis, for it cuts short the disease by suppressing the proteinuria. Steroid therapy usually takes 1–2 weeks to show an effect, and the mechanism is quite unknown: there is a risk of relapse on stopping therapy, and at present there is no way of predicting the cases in which this will occur. Relapses may again be treated using steroids or, if necessary, cytotoxic drugs. The prognosis is good (Arneil and Lam, 1967) although a minority of patients eventually develop renal failure with uraemia and hypertension (see below).

The proteinuria is due to increased glomerular capillary permeability, and is usually highly selective, albumin being accompanied by only very small amounts of the plasma proteins of larger molecular size; this contrasts with the less highly selective proteinuria observed in most renal diseases, with or without the nephrotic syndrome. The urine contains lipid-rich protein casts but few or no leucocytes or red cells. A young child with the nephrotic syndrome, normal blood pressure and renal function, absence of microscopic haematuria and selective proteinuria has almost certainly a minimal change glomerulonephritis and it is doubtful whether a renal biopsy is justified in such patients.

Pathological changes. Some patients still die from infection supervening on the nephrotic

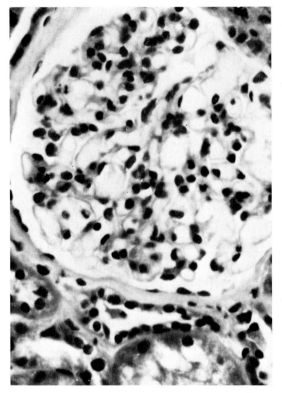

Fig. 22.37 Minimal-change glomerulonephritis. The glomerulus shows no obvious abnormality apart from dilatation of many of the capillaries. × 560.

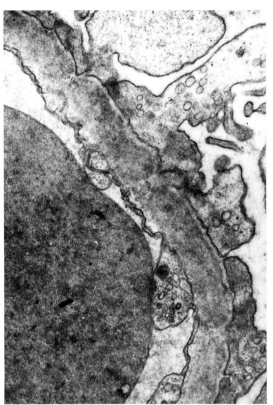

Fig. 22.38 Electron micrograph of glomerular capillary wall in minimal-change glomerulonephritis. The only abnormality is fusion of the foot processes. × 18 000.

syndrome and the kidneys show the usual features of this syndrome (p. 22.25).

Microscopically, the glomeruli look normal apart from an appearance of fixed dilatation of the capillaries; there is no thickening of the capillary walls and no increased cellularity of the glomerular tufts (Fig. 22.37). The most conspicuous glomerular change on electron microscopy is fusion of the foot processes of the epithelial cells, the basement membrane being covered externally by a layer of epithelial cell cytoplasm (Fig. 22.38): the epithelial cells also show an increase in vacuolation and in some cases the basement membrane is slightly thickened with loss of definition of the junction between its inner margin and the cytoplasm of the adjacent endothelial cells.

Aetiology. The nature of this disease remains unknown. Immunofluorescence studies on the glomeruli have been negative for immunoglobulins and complement (surprisingly, some workers have described high levels of circulat-

ing immune complexes in minimal change glomerulonephritis). The disease is occasionally associated with routine prophylactic immunisation and there is evidence that defects in T-cell function may be involved: this is supported by the occasional occurrence of the disease in patients with Hodgkin's disease. In aminonucleoside nephrosis (an experimental animal model with many of the features of minimal change glomerulonephritis), foot-process fusion is associated with loss of polyanion and consequent electrical charge at the interface of the basement membrane and epithelial foot processes: contrary to previous opinion, this antedates the development of proteinuria. As mentioned above (p. 22.17), basement membrane charge is one of the controlling factors in basement membrane permeability.

Focal glomerulosclerosis

At one time thought to be a variant of minimal-change glomerulonephritis, this is now regarded by most workers as a distinct entity. The clinical features are similar to those of minimal-change glomerulonephritis, but proteinuria is less selective and red cells are more commonly present in the urine. Although most of the glomeruli appear normal, those close to the medulla show sclerosis, consisting of deposition of hyaline material with consequent obliteration of capillaries: this change is at first focal but gradually destroys whole glomeruli and extends peripherally to involve more glomeruli. There is associated tubular atrophy. Renal biopsy is only diagnostic if it includes some of the deeper, affected glomeruli. The condition is resistant to steroid therapy although in some cases there may be an initial response. The prognosis is poor, most cases progressing to renal failure although this may take a number of years. The disease tends to recur in renal transplants. Some patients diagnosed from a superficial renal biopsy as minimal-change glomerulonephritis and who eventually develop chronic renal failure are really missed cases of focal glomerulosclerosis.

Congenital nephrotic syndrome. This is a rare familial condition which develops within a few weeks of birth, does not respond to steroids, and has a bad prognosis. The glomeruli may be mostly normal or show various abnormalities and there is usually marked dilatation of the proximal convoluted tubules. Immunological changes have been reported, but the nature of the abnormality is unknown.

Focal glomerulonephritis

This may be defined as a glomerulitis affecting only a proportion of the glomeruli. The lesions usually involve only part of the glomerular tuft, and may therefore be described as **focal** and **segmental**. In many patients the condition is not associated with a known disease, but may accompany mild infections of the upper respiratory tract, probably of viral nature. This 'idiopathic' form usually affects children and young adults, and is characterised clinically by proteinuria and haematuria. The symptoms may subside without residual impairment of renal function, but relapses may occur in association with respiratory infections, sometimes over a period of years (*recurrent haematuria syndrome*) and may eventually lead to chronic renal failure. Focal glomerulonephritis may also accompany a number of other diseases, notably subacute bacterial endocarditis (SBE), systemic lupus erythematosus (SLE), Henoch-Schonlein

purpura, the micro-angiopathic form of polyarteritis nodosa and Goodpasture's syndrome. It must be emphasised that focal glomerulonephritis is not the only renal lesion occurring in these conditions: rapidly progressive glomerulonephritis (p. 22.22) may develop in any of them, and is the usual lesion in Goodpasture's syndrome. Type I mesangiocapillary glomerulonephritis may also occur in SLE, Henoch-Schonlein purpura and SBE.

Pathological changes. The glomerular lesion consists of a cellular proliferation, probably of mesangial cells, affecting the peripheral part of one or more lobules (Fig. 22.39), and in some

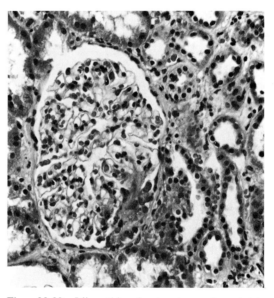

Fig. 22.39 Idiopathic focal glomerulonephritis: early lesion. Note the hypercellularity of the affected part of the tuft on the right. × 200.

cases accompanied by fibrinoid necrosis of capillary loops: within the lesions, individual capillary lumina may be obliterated by eosinophilic thrombus which blends with the necrotic capillary walls. Red cells may be present in the capsular space and in the tubules, and there may also be some proliferation of the epithelial lining of Bowman's capsule, i.e. formation of small crescents (p. 22.23). Lesions may occur in only a small proportion of glomeruli, or may involve the majority. In patients with a long history, old scarred glomerular lesions are usually seen (Fig. 22.40), often adherent to the capsule. Some patients develop the nephrotic

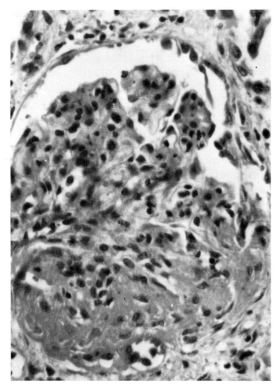

Fig. 22.40 Focal glomerulonephritis: late lesion. The lower part of the tuft is scarred and adherent to the capsule. × 350.

syndrome from heavy proteinuria, and the usual renal changes (p. 22.25) are then seen.

While this account is concerned mainly with focal glomerulonephritis, opportunity is taken below to outline also the additional renal lesions which occur in those diseases of which focal glomerulonephritis is a feature.

Idiopathic focal glomerulonephritis. When it occurs apart from specific diseases, focal glomerulonephritis is usually related to ill-defined respiratory infections, including pharyngitis, 'colds' and 'flu'. In contrast to acute diffuse glomerulonephritis, there is no special relationship with Group A streptococcal infections, and the interval between the respiratory infection and the onset of renal disease is only a day or so. Haematuria is often the presenting feature and is usually of not more than a few days' duration. In most cases, there is only mild proteinuria and the illness subsides with no evidence of residual impairment of renal function. Some patients are subject to recurrences, each associated with a respiratory infection, and

these may occur over many years: there is evidence that chronic renal failure eventually supervenes in a minority of cases. Patients presenting with the nephrotic syndrome have been observed to recover without evidence of residual impaired renal function. The condition is not common: it occurs particularly in children and young adults, more often males than females. Its aetiology is discussed below.

Subacute bacterial endocarditis (SBE). Renal lesions are commonly present in this condition, but in most cases they do not lead to serious impairment of renal function and their practical importance lies mainly in the resulting haematuria, either gross or microscopic, which is of diagnostic value.

As in other organs, infarcts are common in the kidneys in subacute bacterial endocarditis and are usually non-suppurative. Focal glomerulonephritis occurs in about 50% of cases, and tends to develop after some months. Most of the cases have been caused by *Streptoccus viridans* or *Haemophilus influenzae*. Macroscopically, the kidneys are usually of normal size, and show petechial haemorrhages visible on the subcapsular surface and scattered throughout the cortex. Microscopically, a minority of the glomeruli are usually affected, and the focal lesions show capillary thrombosis, fibrinoid necrosis and proliferative changes (Fig. 22.41).

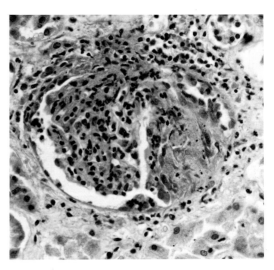

Fig. 22.41 Glomerulus in subacute bacterial endocarditis, showing a large focal necrotic glomerular lesion, with a surrounding inflammatory infiltrate. × 200.

Blood is often seen in the capsular space and tubules, and there may be epithelial crescents. In keeping with an immune-complex-mediated lesion, the serum complement levels are depressed, electron microscopy shows the presence of subendothelial and mesangial deposits and immunofluorescence studies confirm the presence of Ig. Circulating immune complexes have been demonstrated by some workers.

In a minority of patients with subacute bacterial endocarditis, diffuse proliferative glomerulonephritis develops, and may progress to renal failure.

Polyarteritis nodosa. The necrotising arteritis which is the essential lesion of this condition usually involves the larger arteries in the kidneys, with aneurysm formation and/or thrombosis, and renal infarcts are commonly present (Fig. 14.29, p. 14.28). In about one-third of cases, death results from renal failure with hypertension. In the *micro-angiopathic variant* of polyarteritis, the vascular lesions show the same features—fibrinoid necrosis and inflammatory changes—but involve mainly the interlobular arteries (Fig. 14.27, p. 14.27), afferent glomerular arterioles, and also the glomerular capillaries, giving rise to focal glomerulonephritis. As the disease progresses, most of the glomeruli may be involved and renal failure may develop, although hypertension is less common than in the classic form of the disease.

Henoch-Schonlein syndrome (anaphylactoid purpura) occurs mainly in children, and gives rise to a skin rash, joint pains and colic with bloody diarrhoea due to a haemorrhagic exudate into the gut. In some cases there is a focal glomerulonephritis, with haematuria and proteinuria, and this is associated with the mesangial deposition of IgA. Renal failure is either absent or mild and transient, and the kidneys usually recover completely, even after recurrent attacks. Rapidly progressive glomerulonephritis may, however, supervene, particularly in older patients and in some other cases chronic renal failure develops after some years.

Goodpasture's syndrome. In this rare condition, haemorrhage from the alveolar capillaries gives rise to haemoptysis, accompanied by haematuria and proteinuria attributable to focal glomerulonephritis. Pulmonary haemorrhage may become increasingly severe and the renal lesion usually develops into rapidly progressive glomerulonephritis. The glomerular injury is caused by auto-antibody to basement membrane (Fig. 22.42). Although the prognosis is poor, treatment by repeated plasma-exchange and cytotoxic drugs has been reported to give encouraging results (Lockwood *et al.*, 1976).

Systemic lupus erythematosus (SLE). Clinically apparent renal disease occurs in over 50% of patients with this disease, and carries a poor prognosis. The nephrotic syndrome may develop when proteinuria is heavy, and uraemia, with or without hypertension, is an important cause of death. The essential changes are in the glomeruli, which show a great variety of lesions. These include (1) focal glomerulonephritis which is indistinguishable from the proliferative and necrotising lesions described above except that haematoxyphil bodies are sometimes apparent; (2) a focal thickening of the capillary walls with a refractile eosinophilic appearance, known as the wire-loop lesion (Fig. 22.43); (3) hyaline thrombi in individual glomerular capillaries; (4) various combinations of diffuse proliferative and irregular membranous change; (5) diffuse membranous change resembling that seen in idiopathic membranous glomerulonephritis. The duration of these various lesions, and thus the degree of glomerular sclerosis, also vary greatly. Immunofluorescence and electron microscopy provide strong evidence that these glomerular changes represent the spectrum of immune-complex injury as described on pp. 22.17–18. For example, the focal lesion is accompanied by deposition of immunoglobulin and complement in the mesangia and focally in the inner parts of the capillary walls: more extensive deposition of complexes in the inner parts of the capillary walls is seen in the combination of diffuse proliferative and patchy membranous change, while the diffuse granular pattern of deposition, much of it along the outer part of the basement membrane, is seen in the diffuse membranous lesion. Antibody to DNA has been eluted from the kidney tissue in SLE and there is good evidence that DNA is an important, although not the only, antigenic constituent of the pathogenic complexes. Curious tubulo-reticular structures are sometimes seen by electron microscopy in the endothelial cells. Originally thought to be viral, they are now considered to represent a response to injury by various agents, including virus infection. Although re-

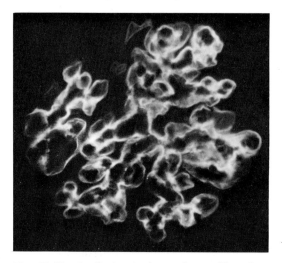

Fig. 22.42 Antibody to glomerular capillary basement membrane in Goodpasture's syndrome, showing the characteristic linear pattern of staining by the immunofluorescence technique.

ported in other conditions, they are seen most often in SLE.

Depending on whether or not the nephrotic syndrome has been present and on the nature and duration of the renal lesions, the kidneys in SLE may be enlarged and pale, of normal size, or small and scarred. The degree of tubular atrophy and interstitial fibrosis will depend upon the nature of the glomerular lesions and there may also be changes resulting from hypertension.

Renal failure is the most important cause of death in SLE and attempts to arrest the glomerular lesions by corticosteroids, cytotoxic drugs and other agents have so far been only partially successful.

Aetiology of focal glomerulonephritis. While focal glomerulonephritis has immunological features, the aetiology is obviously diverse. In some idiopathic cases immunofluorescence microscopy shows heavy deposition of IgA in the mesangium and IgA nephritis ('*Berger's disease*') is now regarded as a distinct entity: the immunological and pathogenic significance of such deposits is obscure although IgA may activate complement by the alternative pathway. In patients with IgA nephritis who progress to renal failure, the disease recurs in renal transplants in 50% of such cases. In other idiopathic cases, IgG and IgM may be found in the mesangium and in a sub-endothelial position in some capillary loops. Although glomerular lesions are focal and segmental by light microscopy, the immunoglobulins have a more widespread distribution by immunofluorescence and electron microscopy. It may be that, for some unknown reason, the focal lesions occur in glomerular lobules in which the mesangial cells fail to clear the subendothelial immune complex deposits (p. 22.17).

The available evidence suggests that the diseases which focal glomerulonephritis accompanies are attributable to abnormal immunological reactions. The evidence is strongest in the case of systemic lupus erythematosus (see above). Henoch-Schonlein syndrome is widely regarded as a hypersensitivity disease, and the antigens which may be concerned include streptococci and certain foods. Lesions resembling those of polyarteritis nodosa occur in serum sickness: fixed immunoglobulins, and in some cases HBsAg, have been observed in the early vascular lesions, although evidence for immune complex deposition in the glomeruli is not convincing.

In subacute bacterial endocarditis the prolonged infection provides a possible basis for

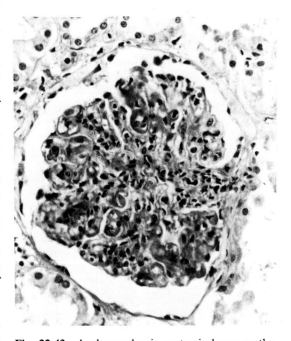

Fig. 22.43 A glomerulus in systemic lupus erythematosus, showing hyaline thickening of some of the capillaries—the 'wire-loop' lesion, and a more diffuse increase in cellularity. × 300.

immunological injury from circulating antigen-antibody complexes (see above), while auto-antibody to capillary basement membrane is demonstrable in Goodpasture's syndrome (*see* Fig. 22.42).

Chronic glomerulonephritis

It is apparent, from the foregoing descriptions of the various types of glomerulonephritis, that an end stage may be reached in which total glomerular function is so reduced that chronic renal failure develops. The time taken to reach this stage, and the rate of progression once it has developed, vary with the type of preceding glomerulonephritis. Hypertension, sometimes of the accelerated (malignant) type, usually develops and aggravates the renal tissue destruction, leading, if untreated, to end-stage renal failure which progresses rapidly to death. In cases where hypertension is absent or less severe, renal failure may progress more slowly, and the end stage may last for several years. Chronic renal failure usually occurs because most of the nephrons have been so severely damaged by the causal disease that they are no longer functional. The remaining functioning glomeruli not only become hypertrophied but also filter off a relatively high proportion of the fluid passing through them. This hyperfunctioning state may itself cause further glomerular injury and consequently further deterioration of renal function.

In over 70% of patients with chronic glomerulonephritis, there is no history to suggest preceding renal disease, and the renal lesions have progressed silently until chronic renal failure develops. In such cases, it is often not possible to decide, even by histological examination of the kidneys, what type of glomerulonephritis has led up to the chronic stage. In other cases, there is a history of previous glomerulonephritis: this may have been an acute attack of post-streptococcal glomerulonephritis years before, or the patient may have had membranous, mesangiocapillary or recurrent focal glomerulonephritis, which has progressed to the stage of chronic renal failure.

Pathological changes and pathogenesis. Both the kidneys are uniformly and equally reduced in size, sometimes only slightly so, but often to about one-third of normal (Fig. 22.44). In those kidneys which are greatly shrunken, the capsule

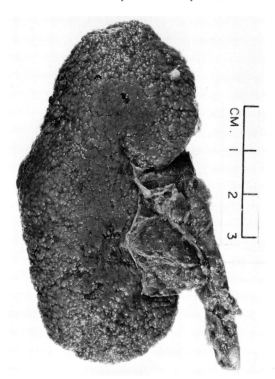

Fig. 22.44 Chronic glomerulonephritis. The kidney is uniformly shrunken, in this case to about half the normal size, and the surface is diffusely granular.

is often firmly adherent and the subcapsular surface uniformly and finely irregular ('*granular contracted kidney*'). There is diffuse thinning of the cortex (Fig. 22.45), which accounts largely for the reduction in kidney size, while the medullary pyramids are also, although less markedly, shrunken. The amount of fatty tissue around the renal pelvis is increased. *In contrast to chronic pyelonephritis, the calyces and renal pelvis are not distorted.*

The renal arteries and their major branches show arteriosclerotic thickening, and in cases complicated by malignant hypertension the cortical mottling and haemorrhages of this condition are superimposed on the changes described above. The other organs and tissues show the changes of chronic renal failure (pp. 22.14–15).

Microscopically, in the small granular kidneys, it is common to find all degrees of hyalinisation of glomeruli. Many are completely hyalinised (Fig. 22.46) and some show partial destruction. A small percentage are normal or nearly so, and may be hypertrophied (Fig.

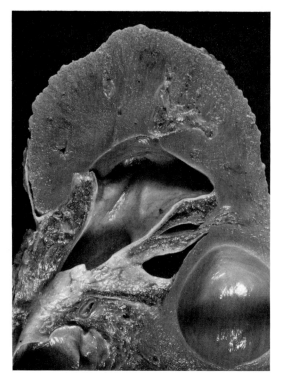

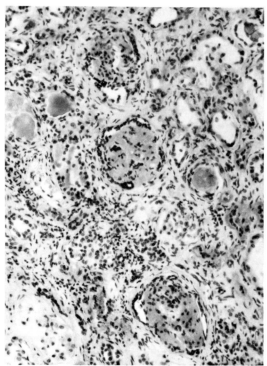

Fig. 22.45 The cut surface of the same kidney shown in Fig. 22.44, showing diffuse cortical thinning. The cyst is incidental. × 2.

Fig. 22.46 Chronic glomerulonephritis, showing hyalinisation of glomeruli; the tubular epithelium is atrophic and there is interstitial fibrosis. × 100.

22.47). In cases in which the kidneys are not greatly shrunken the glomeruli are usually more uniformly damaged: this is seen in the chronic end stages of membranous and mesangio-capillary glomerulonephritis.

The arcuate and interlobular arteries and the afferent arterioles show hypertensive changes which are likely, by causing ischaemia, to have contributed to the glomerular scarring. When malignant hypertension has supervened the consequent changes (Fig. 22.11, p. 22.7) are seen in those glomeruli which have not been destroyed already by the glomerulonephritic process.

The tubules show extensive atrophy, many being completely lost, and there is an increase in the intertubular connective tissue and irregular interstitial aggregation of lymphocytes and usually small numbers of plasma cells. In cases with some near-normal hypertrophied glomeruli, the corresponding tubules are enlarged and conspicuous, and account for the elevations which give the sub-capsular surface its granular appearance. These surviving functioning tub-

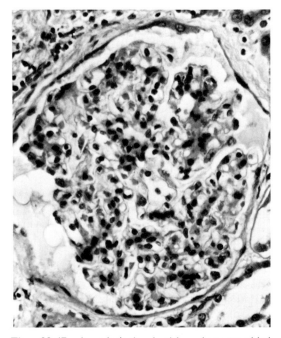

Fig. 22.47 A relatively healthy, hypertrophied glomerulus in chronic glomerulonephritis. × 250.

ules may show hyaline droplets in the epithelial cytoplasm and frequently contain protein casts (p. 22.4), features which relate to the proteinuria. When malignant hypertension has supervened, there may be blood in the capsular spaces and in functioning tubules.

In cases of chronic glomerulonephritis preceded by the nephrotic syndrome, the kidneys may still be enlarged, and lipid deposits may still be visible in the cortex by the naked eye. Although the glomeruli show advanced sclerosis, their appearance may still suggest the type of glomerulonephritis responsible, e.g.

membranous (see Fig. 22.31). All the glomeruli are affected to some extent, and the tubular atrophy is accordingly more uniform, without prominent enlarged tubules; for this reason, the surface of the kidney is often smooth and does not exhibit the granularity usually found in other forms of chronic glomerulonephritis.

Clinical features. Most patients developing chronic glomerulonephritis are between 10 and 50 years old. The clinical features and changes in other organs and tissues are those of *chronic renal failure* and are attributable to *uraemia*, and usually *hypertension* (pp. 22.12-15).

Miscellaneous Renal Diseases

Diabetes mellitus

Renal failure is an important complication of diabetes. It causes death in more than 10% of all diabetics, and in over 50% of those developing diabetes in childhood. The most important contribution to this high mortality is *diabetic glomerulosclerosis*, which can also give rise to the nephrotic syndrome. Hyaline thickening of the afferent glomerular arterioles is also very common in diabetes: it is similar to that already described in hypertensives and old people (p. 14.17), but is more often very severe in diabetics, both with and without hypertension, and affects also the efferent arterioles much more severely than in non-diabetics (Fig. 22.48).

Diabetic glomerulosclerosis. This consists of deposition of eosinophilic hyaline material in the mesangium of the glomerular lobules. The deposits may be discrete rounded nodules, sometimes laminated, situated near the tip of the lobule and therefore appearing peripheral in the glomerulus (Kimmelstiel–Wilson lesion). Such *nodular glomerulosclerosis* affects lobules and glomeruli unequally, and one or more nodules, of various sizes, may be seen in affected glomeruli (Fig. 22.49). The glomerular capillaries are seen around the margin of the nodules, and may long remain unaffected. Aneurysmal dilatation of some glomerular capillaries and also of some arterioles within the kidney is associated with micro-aneurysms elsewhere—in particular within the retina. Diabetic nephro-

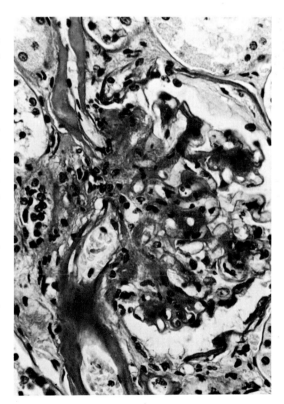

Fig. 22.48 Hyaline change in the afferent and efferent glomerular arterioles in diabetes. Note also the diffuse glomerulosclerosis. × 250.

pathy and retinopathy are almost always associated with one another. Nodular glomerulo-

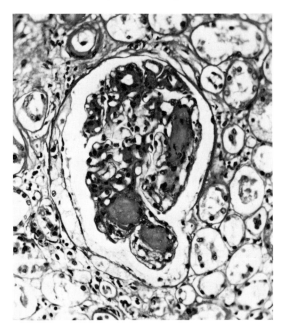

Fig. 22.49 Nodular glomerulosclerosis in diabetes (Kimmelstiel–Wilson lesion). × 205.

sclerosis is usually accompanied by more diffuse deposition of hyaline material in the mesangium of all the glomerular lobules, with associated thickening of the glomerular capillary basement membranes (Fig. 22.48). Electron microscopy confirms this latter change and shows it to affect also capillaries in which the thickening is not sufficiently gross to be detected by light microscopy. This *diffuse glomerulosclerosis* may resemble membranous glomerulonephritis, but shows less uniform basement membrane thickening: it occurs together with the nodular lesion, and may eventually progress to obliteration of most of the capillaries and severe hyalinisation of the glomeruli. Ischaemic changes, including obliteration of the capsular space by collagen and glomerular collapse (Fig. 22.7, p. 22.5) occur, and are presumably related to hyaline thickening of the afferent arterioles. As a result of glomerulosclerosis, secondary atrophy occurs in the tubules, and the kidneys may be reduced in size with thinning of the cortex and a granular surface.

The pathogenesis of diabetic glomerulosclerosis is not understood although it is now generally accepted that the diabetic nodules represent an accumulation of basement-membrane-like material. Whether this represents increased synthesis or decreased removal of basement membrane is not certain. Claims that the nodules formed in relation to beef insulin–insulin antibody complexes have not been substantiated and indeed nodules have been described in diabetic patients untreated with beef insulin. The possibility of auto-antibodies to autologous insulin with immune complex deposition also lacks supporting evidence.

Diabetic glomerulosclerosis has been reported in 25–50% of diabetics at autopsy. In most instances, the nodular and diffuse forms are combined, but in some the diffuse form occurs alone. It is worth while distinguishing between the two forms, for while the nodular lesion is highly characteristic of diabetes, the diffuse lesion is related much more closely to disturbances of renal function. In many cases, diabetic glomerulosclerosis is unsuspected during life, and may be clinically silent. It is commonly associated with proteinuria, and there is usually a progression from asymptomatic proteinuria to the nephrotic syndrome and finally chronic renal failure. As already mentioned, glomerulosclerosis is especially common in early-onset diabetes; its incidence and severity increase with the duration of diabetes. Poor diabetic control increases the chances of the development of renal failure. Hypertension is also common in diabetics and, unless controlled, has an important effect in accelerating the rate of decline of renal function.

Other renal changes in diabetes. Atheroma is very common and often severe in diabetics. In non-diabetics the renal arteries rarely show severe narrowing from atheroma unless they are involved at their origins by aortic atheromatous plaques. In diabetes, however, **severe atheroma** does occur in the main renal arteries and their segmental branches and probably contributes to the high incidence of hypertension.

Other renal changes in diabetes include *papillary necrosis* (p. 22.43) which is a common terminal event, causing or greatly aggravating renal failure. It is well established that poorly controlled diabetics are particularly susceptible to *bacterial infections* (p. 20.64) and a high incidence of urinary tract infections might be expected, particularly as diabetic neuropathy sometimes necessitates catheterisation of the bladder and the glucose in the urine increases

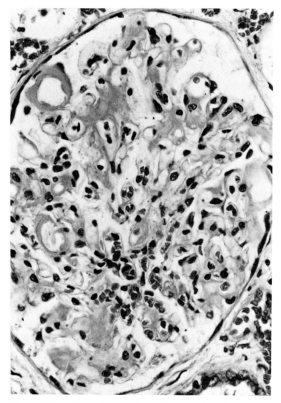

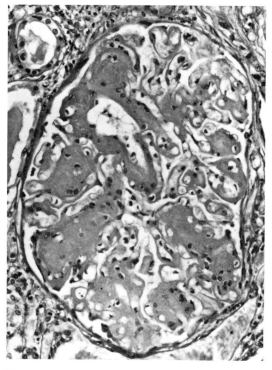

Fig. 22.51 Glomerular amyloidosis, showing thickening and hyaline appearance of capillary walls. × 350.

Fig. 22.50 Deposition of amyloid in the glomerular capillaries at a relatively early stage as compared with Fig. 22.51. × 250.

its nutrient value for many bacteria. Such expectation may have encouraged the widely-held view that there is a high incidence of chronic pyelonephritis among diabetics, but recent epidemiological studies suggest that this is not so. (For discussion see Heptinstall, 1983, p. 1425.)

Amyloid

The kidneys are involved in nearly all cases of amyloidosis secondary to chronic infections, rheumatoid arthritis, etc., and are also commonly affected in primary amyloidosis. The most important site of deposition is around the glomerular capillary basement membrane (Fig. 22.50): this is accompanied by increased permeability, and proteinuria may be sufficiently heavy to cause the nephrotic syndrome. As the deposits increase, capillary narrowing and obliteration ensue, and the glomeruli may be largely replaced by amyloid (Fig. 22.51). Secondary atrophy of the tubules and intersti-

tial fibrosis result from the glomerular lesion, and chronic renal failure gradually supervenes. The kidneys are firm and pale, may be of normal size, enlarged, or shrunken and granular, and the glomeruli are usually visible by naked eye after treating a slice of kidney with Lugol's iodine (Fig. 22.52). In cases with the nephrotic syndrome, the usual accompanying features are seen in the kidneys (p. 22.25).

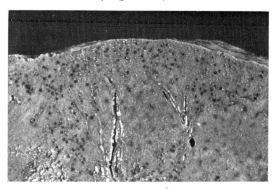

Fig. 22.52 Amyloidosis. A slice of the renal cortex has been treated with Lugol's iodine. The glomeruli contain sufficient amyloid material to be visible as darkly stained spots.

Amyloid is deposited also in the walls of the small blood vessels of the kidneys and upon the tubular basement membranes.

There is a tendency to thrombosis of the intrarenal veins in renal amyloidosis, sometimes extending to the main renal veins, and causing acute renal failure.

Gout

The main features of gout are described on p. 23.52. The excretion of increased amounts of urates by the kidneys may result in crystal formation in the medulla. The crystals are deposited mainly in the collecting tubules where they cause local destruction of the tubular wall and become surrounded by a giant-cell reaction and eventually by fibrous tissue. They are usually at first needle-shaped, but tend to become amorphous. The destructive changes in the collecting tubules result in atrophy of the corresponding nephrons and the kidney may be reduced in size with a granular surface and scarring of the medulla. Urate stones may develop in the renal pelves and may cause renal colic, haematuria and obstruction.

A moderate degree of hypertension is common in gout and is accompanied by the usual renal changes. Polymorphs are often seen in the tubules, but do not necessarily indicate an infection, for it has been shown experimentally that acute inflammation, including polymorph infiltration, can occur around injected urate crystals without superadded infection, and this happens around urate deposits in the acute attack of gout.

In spite of the high frequency and variety of renal changes in gout, renal failure supervenes in only a small proportion of cases.

Renal lesions in pregnancy

There is no doubt that the incidence of renal disease is increased during pregnancy. A factor which contributes to this is the tendency to dilatation of the ureters, attributable to the relaxation of smooth muscle which is a feature of pregnancy, and also to pressure effects of the enlarged uterus. It is probably as a consequence of these effects that urinary tract infection, including pyelonephritis, is a common complication of pregnancy.

Secondly, acute tubular necrosis (p. 22.8), and rarely renal cortical necrosis (p. 22.45), are encountered as complications of pregnancy, particularly in cases of retroplacental haemorrhage, infected abortion and post-partum haemorrhage.

Lastly, pregnancy increases the functional demands on the kidneys, and latent chronic renal disease (e.g. chronic glomerulonephritis) may first become clinically apparent during pregnancy. Essential hypertension may also be aggravated by pregnancy, during which the blood pressure may increase temporarily.

Pre-eclampsia and eclampsia. Albuminuria is a common occurrence in pregnancy, particularly in the last trimester, and may be accompanied by some oedema of the ankles: these disturbances are not of serious significance unless there is also a rise in the blood pressure, when the combination of features is termed **pre-eclampsia** or **pre-eclamptic toxaemia**. This occurs most commonly in primigravida and is usually mild: the changes—oedema, proteinuria and hypertension—do not often increase to alarming degrees, and subside usually within a few days after parturition. But in some cases the features become progressively more severe during late pregnancy, and impaired renal function is reflected in a rise in the level of blood urea. In such cases, hypertensive convulsions may occur, the condition then being termed **eclampsia**. Death may result from uraemia or hypertensive encephalopathy, and considerable judgement is sometimes required to decide whether pregnancy should be allowed to continue to term.

In patients dying from eclampsia, the kidneys are of normal size or slightly enlarged due to oedema: the cortex is pale and the glomeruli may be visible with a hand lens as grey dots projecting from the cut surface. Microscopy (of biopsy or autopsy material) shows diffuse enlargement of all the glomeruli, but without obvious increase in cellularity. The glomerular capillaries characteristically contain very few red cells: their walls appear diffusely thickened, eosinophilic and refractile, and special staining techniques show the thickening to be due to swelling of the endothelial cells. Electron microscopy shows the endothelial cell cytoplasm to be increased in amount and vacuolated: the capillary basement membrane is usually normal, but in severe cases may show some thickening. The epithelial cells may also be enlarged, but do not show fusion of foot processes.

The clinical and histological features of pre-eclampsia indicate impaired renal blood flow with narrowing of the glomerular capillary lumina. There is evidence also of a reduced uterine blood flow in pre-eclampsia, sometimes resulting in placental ischaemia. The causes of the glomerular changes are not known, although intravascular coagulation has been implicated by some investigators.

Hypertension from any cause during pregnancy increases the risks of abortion, premature labour and retroplacental haemorrhage.

Interstitial nephritis

This term is applied to any acute or chronic inflammatory process which particularly affects the interstitium of the kidney, but there is almost invariably some degree of tubular damage. In acute interstitial nephritis, inflammatory oedema is present but paradoxically the cellular infiltrate consists mainly of lymphocytes, plasma cells and macrophages with only a few polymorphs. In chronic interstitial nephritis the main features are interstitial fibrosis and tubular loss and atrophy.

The **aetiology** is diverse; causes of *acute interstitial nephritis* include infection, drug reactions, systemic lupus erythematosus and changes secondary to glomerulonephritis, while an acute rejection reaction is an important cause in transplanted kidneys. Most of these disorders are dealt with elsewhere, but it is interesting to note here that in those cases related to glomerulonephritis and SLE, immune complexes have been found not only in the glomeruli but also in tubular basement membranes, and auto-antibodies to tubular basement membrane have been described in some cases. *Chronic interstitial nephritis* also has various causes, including infection, urinary tract obstruction, ischaemia, x-irradiation and papillary necrosis. One particular form with a marked geographic incidence—*Balkan nephritis*—has been attributed to the toxins of fungi contaminating cereals and pork.

Drugs, chemicals and renal disease

Many drugs are excreted predominantly in the urine and in patients with impaired renal function conventional dosage may result in toxic levels being attained. It is therefore necessary to modify the dosage of many types of drugs in patients with acute or chronic renal failure. A large variety of drugs have now been demonstrated to give rise to renal injury: in some instances this is a direct cytotoxic effect of the drug, in others it represents a hypersensitivity reaction to the drug which may, for example, act as a hapten. Thus the aminoglycoside antibiotics and the cephalosporins can cause *acute tubular necrosis* whilst methicillin, ampicillin, diphenyhydantoins and phenindione have been associated with *acute interstitial nephritis*. Gold salts and penicillamine may give rise to a *membranous glomerulonephritis*. Drug addicts have more than twice the incidence of renal disease in the general population. This may be due in part to the toxic properties of the drugs themselves and partly to the high incidence of infections (p. 15.33) which, occurring in addicts who are often debilitated, with depression of the monoculear phagocyte system, are liable to cause immune complex disease.

Heavy metal poisoning. Industrial awareness of the effects of cadmium fumes in causing emphysema and proteinuria, the introduction of legislation against lead paints and the replacement of mercurial-based diuretics by the thiazides etc., have all resulted in a great reduction in the number of cases of heavy metal poisoning.

The effects of **lead poisoning** have been particularly well documented by Henderson (1958) in Queensland, Australia, where up to 1930 lead paint was used on the wooden verandas of houses. Children playing on the verandas ingested the paint powdered by the strong sunlight and acute lead poisoning was consequently common. Follow-up studies have shown a high incidence of *chronic renal failure* occurring 10–40 years after the acute event. The kidneys are uniformly reduced in size and show gross changes very similar to a chronic glomerulonephritis. Microscopically, however, there is tubular loss and atrophy with severe interstitial fibrosis, while the glomeruli are spared for a long time. Characteristic inclusion bodies are seen in the nuclei of the tubular and other cells.

Analgesic abuse and papillary necrosis. Chronic renal failure is now a well-recognised result of taking large amounts of analgesic drug mixtures, usually containing both aspirin and phenacetin, over a number of years. Other analgesics, such as indomethacin, phenylbutazone and mefenamic acid, have also been implicated. It seems likely that phenacetin, either alone or in combination with another analgesic, is the main pathogenic constituent.

Curiously, the incidence of renal failure from this cause is especially high in Australia, Switzerland and the Scandinavian countries, and is relatively low in other West European countries and in North America. In Australia, the incidence is greater in Queensland with its hot climate than in cooler Victoria and the difference has been attributed to greater fluid loss by sweating in Queensland and so greater concentration of the urine. In most cases 0·5–1 kg of analgesic mixture has been taken annually for some years, either for painful chronic disease such as rheumatoid arthritis or for a vague subjective illness. Most patients are women, often anaemic and with a particular truculent psychoneurotic personality. The first symptoms may be due to recurrent urinary tract infection, or to renal colic due to the passage of sloughed papillae or phosphatic concretions. In many patients, however, the presenting symptoms are due to the hypertension and/or uraemia of chronic renal failure. There may be sterile pyuria and haematuria, although the latter should raise suspicion of a co-existent tumour of the urinary tract (see below).

It is now established that **papillary necrosis** is the primary change in this condition and that this leads to destructive changes in the rest of the kidney. The necrosis affects the distal part of some or all of the papillae and the kidney shows depressed areas on its surface over the necrotic papillae, which appear shrunken: the necrotic distal part may be yellow or white and is demarcated from the living tissue by a red line of congestion. The necrotic tissue appears structureless and may show patchy calcification. One or more papillae may have sloughed off, leaving an irregular ulcerated surface. Atrophy of the overlying cortex ensues so that the gross appearances of the kidney come to resemble those of chronic pyelonephritis with large intervening patches of more normal and sometimes hypertrophied renal tissue. Microscopically, the junction between the dead and living papillary tissue is often indistinct and there may be a zone of partial necrosis. The cortex shows tubular loss and atrophy with a *chronic interstitial nephritis*. Although most commonly seen as a sequel to analgesic abuse,

papillary necrosis may also be found as a complication of urinary tract obstruction or diabetes mellitus.

Pathogenesis. The mechanism of papillary necrosis is not understood. Two basic mechanisms have been postulated—ischaemic and toxic. The appearances are suggestive of infarction and the lesion tends to occur in middle-aged and old people with advanced arterial disease. There is evidence that aspirin-like analgesics induce contraction of the efferent arterioles of juxtamedullary glomeruli, blood from which supplies the medulla. Aspirin-type compounds are also suspected of inhibiting defence mechanisms against oxidising chemicals in the medulla.

The incidence of transitional-cell carcinoma of the urinary tract is increased in patients who abuse analgesics, particularly in those who have papillary necrosis. The peak incidence of tumour formation is some years later than that of papillary necrosis and a carcinogenic effect of the analgesic or its breakdown products has been postulated. Prophylactic removal of the patient's kidneys and ureters should therefore be carried out in those patients treated by renal transplantation for end-stage analgesic nephropathy.

The renal lesion of potassium deficiency

In conditions of potassium depletion and lowering of the plasma potassium level, the kidneys exhibit a striking morphological change consisting of intense hydropic vacuolation of the cells of the proximal tubules (Fig. 22.53), chiefly in the descending straight portion. The lesion is associated with marked loss of concentrating power, but only trivial albuminuria and absence of urea retention.

It occurs most frequently in conditions which cause severe and prolonged diarrhoea, e.g. in ulcerative colitis, or induced by excessive purgation. It occurs also in primary hyperaldosteronism (p. 26.34) and sometimes in Cushing's syndrome or during glucocorticoid therapy. It is a feature of some disorders of the renal tubules including the diuretic stage of acute tubular necrosis and can result from administration of diuretics. Less obvious, acute changes occur during recovery from diabetic coma under insulin therapy, when the plasma potassium falls because insulin promotes the cellular uptake of

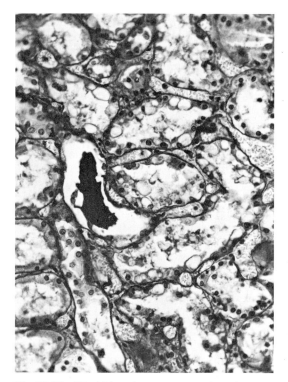

Fig. 22.53 The kidney in severe potassium depletion following prolonged diarrhoea in ulcerative colitis. The cells of the proximal convoluted tubules show gross cytoplasmic vacuolation. × 230.

potassium. Serial biopsies of the kidney have shown the early changes to be completely reversible by restoration of normal potassium levels, and there is no evidence of permanent ill effects.

Renal tubular acidosis

Deficient tubular function is partly responsible for the acidosis which complicates chronic renal failure (p. 22.14). The term 'renal tubular acidosis' is, however, usually restricted to acidosis resulting from a tubular deficiency in the absence of chronic renal failure. It occurs in many conditions and traditionally is divided into two types.

In type I, function of the distal part of the tubule is impaired, with reduced capacity to produce urine of a low pH. This may occur as an inherited tubular defect, or as a result of tubular injury from pyelonephritis, hypercalcaemia, urinary tract obstruction or an autoimmune reaction.

In type II, there is impaired secretion of H^+ by the proximal tubule. This occurs in association with other tubular defects, e.g. aminoaciduria, renal glycosuria, cystinosis, hypophosphataemia.

In both types of tubular acidosis, there is hyperchloraemia, osteomalacia or rickets which is resistant to vitamin D, and a danger of deposition of calcium salts in the renal medulla (nephrocalcinosis) which may cause further renal damage. In type I cases, oral administration of alkali is effective, but in type II this of little value.

Renal changes in disseminated intravascular coagulation (DIC)

A general account of this condition is given on p. 17.68. Many of the predisposing causes, for example shock, systemic lupus erythematosus, malignant hypertension and renal transplant rejection, themselves cause renal lesions, and DIC itself also has serious effects on the kidney. It may, for example, aggravate the renal ischaemic changes of shock, resulting in tubular injury or cortical necrosis (Fig. 22.54). Renal injury in DIC results from obstruction of arterioles and glomerular capillaries by fibrin thrombi (Fig. 22.55). In addition, circulating non-polymerised fibrin and fibrin degradation products pass through the fenestrae of the glomerular capillary endothelium and aggregate subendothelially on the basement membrane and in the mesangia in the same fashion as intermediate-sized immune complexes in focal glomerulonephritis (p. 22.36). There is mesangial hyperplasia and thickening of the basement membrane. Insudation of the walls of interlobular arteries with fibrin may also occur, and stimulate a proliferative endarteritis resembling that of malignant hypertension. The afferent arterioles may also be permeated by fibrin and undergo fibrinoid necrosis, which, as in malignant hypertension, may extend into the glomerular tufts with focal proliferative and necrotic changes. Clinically, the features of renal failure are superimposed on those of the predisposing cause of DIC.

The term **haemolytic-uraemic syndrome** is sometimes used to describe cases of DIC in young children, in whom renal failure, thrombocytopenia and microangiopathic haemolytic anaemia are prominent, usually together with neurological and cardiovascular symptoms.

Rejection of renal transplants

Renal transplantation has not only saved the lives of many thousands of individuals with renal failure but has restored them to good

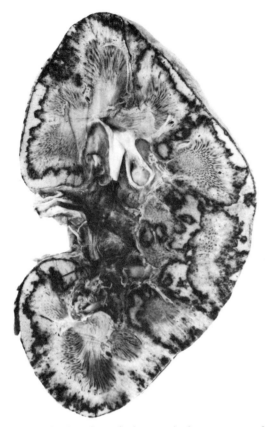

Fig. 22.54 Renal cortical necrosis from a case of eclampsia complicated by retroplacental haemorrhage; the pale necrotic areas with haemorrhagic margins are well shown. × 0·7.

health. The alternative of chronic haemodialysis is much less satisfactory for the patient and is considerably more expensive.

The general immunological aspects of renal transplantation and rejection are discussed on pp. 7.29–31. Problems relating to the transplanted kidney include the technical difficulties involved in the vascular and ureteric anastomoses, acute tubular necrosis which results from the inevitable period of ischaemia when cadaver kidneys are used for transplantation, and immunological rejection of the transplant by the recipient.

Rejection is commonly classified clinically as immediate (hyperacute), acute and chronic.

Immediate rejection, within minutes or hours of renal transplantation, occurs when the kidney donor's ABO blood group is incompatible for the recipient, or when, as a result of pregnancy, blood transfusion or a previous trans-

plant, the recipient has developed cytotoxic HLA antibodies reactive with the donor's cells.

The kidney regains its normal pink colour and starts to produce urine when blood flow is established, but then rapidly becomes soft, cyanotic and anuric. Microscopy shows arrest of polymorphs along the walls of arterioles and venules and in the glomerular and peri-tubular capillaries. Platelets aggregate in the small vessels and thrombosis and haemorrhage occur; unless removed, the kidney becomes necrotic. The process is a type 2 or an Arthus (type 3) hypersensitivity reaction in which circulating antibody reacts with graft antigen. This type of rejection is irreversible and progresses to virtually complete infarction of the kidney, necessitating its removal. Because of improved typing and matching, it is, however, uncommon.

Acute rejection. Many renal transplant recipients have an episode of acute rejection within a few weeks of transplantation. The graft becomes swollen and tender and the patient is pyrexial and oliguric with a raised blood pressure. Microscopically the changes are predominantly cellular or vascular. **Acute cellular rejection** is a cell-mediated or type 4 hypersensitivity reaction (p. 7.18) and the kidney shows interstitial oedema and focal cortical infiltrates of lymphocytes, plasma cells and macrophages. Deposition of immunoglobulin or components of complement cannot be detected by immunofluorescence microscopy. This type of rejection responds to treatment with high dose glucocorticoids, cytotoxic drugs or cyclosporin A,

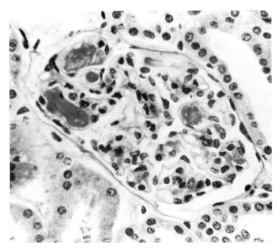

Fig. 22.55 The kidney in DIC. Some of the glomerular capillaries are occluded by fibrin. × 250.

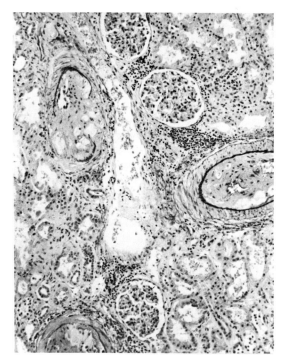

Fig. 22.56 Chronic vascular rejection of a human renal allo-transplant. Note the obliterative intimal changes and disruption of the artery walls. (Professor K. A. Porter.)

and the prognosis is good. **Acute vascular rejection** is a type 2 (cytotoxic antibody) hypersensitivity reaction; lymphocytes etc. are few or absent and immunofluorescence studies show the presence of IgG, IgM and complement components in the walls of blood vessels and of the glomerular capillaries. Platelet thrombi, fibrin and polymorphs are present in the glomerular capillaries and foci of plasmatic vasculosis (p. 11.7) or fibrinoid necrosis are found in the vessel walls. Interstitial haemorrhage may be present and the intima of some vessels is infiltrated by chronic inflammatory cells. If untreated, the process proceeds to cortical necrosis and is associated with micro-angiopathic haemolytic anaemia. Vascular rejection has a poor prognosis and response to steroids is usually only partial.

Chronic rejection may be secondary to an episode of acute vascular rejection when it may start within a few weeks of transplantation, but it also occurs *de novo*, usually after a year or so and presents clinically as a gradual and progressive deterioration in renal function ending

in renal failure. Proteinuria may appear or increase and the blood pressure is raised. Grossly, the kidney is normal in size or enlarged and may appear pale because of ischaemia. Microscopically the changes are vascular and/or glomerular. *The vascular changes* represent a continuation of acute vascular rejection; episodic deposition of platelet- and fibrin-thrombi occurs in the intima of the interlobular and arcuate arteries, which eventually show the circumferential intimal proliferation of endarteritis obliterans, presenting an onion-skin appearance with a marked reduction of the lumen (Fig. 22.56). Lipid-laden macrophages are frequently found in a sub-intimal position. The consequent ischaemia is reflected in hyperplasia of the juxta-glomerular epithelioid cells (p. 10.36) and causes atrophy and loss of tubules and interstitial fibrosis.

The glomerular changes are not specific but mesangial hyperplasia with focal basement membrane thickening is common, giving rise to an appearance resembling mesangiocapillary glomerulonephritis. Various other changes are seen, including focal or segmental glomerular sclerosis and formation of crescents (p. 22.23).

Chronic rejection pursues a relentless but variable downhill course which is resistant to treatment.

Other complications of renal transplantation

Opportunistic infections, notably with cytomegalovirus (p. 13.15), fungi and various bacteria, are a common complication of immunosuppressive therapy in transplant recipients. There is also a significant increase in the incidence of **malignant tumours** in transplant recipients, and particularly of non-Hodgkin lymphomas, which are about fifty times as frequent as in the general population. Another problem is **recurrence of glomerulonephritis** in the donor kidney; this tends to occur particularly after IgA nephropathy, type II mesangiocapillary glomerulonephritis and focal glomerulosclerosis. Glomerulophritis may also develop in the donor kidney in patients transplanted because of pyelonephritis, polycystic kidneys, etc. Occasionally infection, e.g. viral hepatitis, is transmitted from donor to recipient, and rarely cancer, unsuspected in' the donor at the time of transplantation, has grown and spread in the recipient.

Urinary tract infection

Lower urinary tract infection is common and, although debilitating and painful, is usually amenable to appropriate treatment with antibiotics, etc. It may, however, spread to involve the kidneys, infection of which (*pyelonephritis*) is much more serious. The presence of bacteria in the urine (*bacteriuria*) is not necessarily indicative of infection, for normal urine is commonly contaminated by the bacterial flora in the lower urethra and around the urethral meatus. Catheterisation and cystoscopy carry a risk of implanting bacteria of this flora within the bladder despite rigorous aseptic technique and patients who are catheterised repeatedly, or have an indwelling catheter, have a high incidence of cystitis.

As a working rule, *it is generally assumed that detection (by culture) of 10^5 or more bacteria per ml of urine is indicative of a urinary infection.* However, lesser counts may be significant if the patient is voiding large amounts of dilute urine or receiving antibacterial drugs. Conversely, apparently significant bacteriuria is sometimes detected in the absence of clinical symptoms and is known as *asymptomatic or covert bacteriuria*. It is encountered in approximately 1% of healthy schoolgirls, only about one quarter of whom have a history suggestive of a previous urinary tract infection. Tests on younger girls suggest that bacteriuria develops before the age of 3 years. In some of these children asymptomatic bacteriuria is associated with vesicoureteric reflux of urine and in follow-up studies some of these eventually develop chronic pyelonephritis (see below). Symptomless bacteriuria is particularly frequent (about 5%) in pregnant women but fears that it is commonly followed by chronic pyelonephritis appear to be largely unfounded.

Urinary tract infection is much commoner in females than in males at all ages. Defence against such infection (pp. 8.2–3) depends partly on bactericidal properties of the urothelium, due at least in part to coating with IgA antibodies, and partly on normal mechanical function of the tract, including peristaltic action of the ureters and periodic complete emptying of the bladder. The shorter, wider female urethra appears to be a less effective barrier to bacteria than the longer male urethra. The high incidence of urinary tract infections in pregnancy is attributable to impairment of urinary flow, due partly to hormonally-induced relaxation of smooth muscle and partly to pressure of the pregnant uterus on the urinary tract. Other causes of stagnation of urine, with consequent liability to urinary tract infection, include (in both sexes) urethral obstruction by inflammatory scarring or abnormal congenital valve-like mucosal folds, urinary stones, diverticula and tumours of the bladder, congenital malformations such as double ureters, and neurological disorders, e.g. paraplegia or multiple sclerosis, which interfere with emptying of the bladder. In men, prostatic enlargement is the commonest predisposing cause of urinary tract infection.

Urinary tract infection occurring without preceding catheterisation or obstruction is usually due to bacteria normally present in the faeces, in most cases *Escherichia coli*, but sometimes *Klebsiella*, *Proteus* spp. or *Pseudomonas* spp. are responsible. Infection complicating obstruction or instrumentation is commonly of mixed bacterial type. *Esch. coli*, *Proteus* spp. and staphylococci being most often present.

In the early stages of an acute urinary infection, the urine may contain a heavy concentration of bacteria with few cells, but pus cells soon appear; in some instances there may be sufficient haemorrhage from the inflamed mucosa to present clinically as haematuria.

The inflammatory changes in **cystitis** are usually classified as catarrhal, purulent and pseudo-membranous. Pseudo-membranous cystitis is found chiefly in association with chronic obstruction and hypertrophy of the bladder; there is superficial necrosis of the mucosa with fibrinous exudate, especially over the muscular ridges, and the necrotic mucosa is sloughed off in decomposing shreds. The most severe changes are usually observed when there is alkaline decomposition of the urine: haemorrhages into the mucosa are common, and this may become greenish and almost black, while the surface is covered with pus and often a deposit of phosphates. The vesico-uretic valves tend to become incompetent when inflamed and such an infection may ascend the ureters, and cause a pyelitis with similar features. The dilated pelvis may become ulcerated or filled with pus—**pyonephrosis**. Here also, secondary deposit of phosphates may occur. Inevitably, the infection extends to the kidneys and gives rise to **pyelonephritis** (p. 22.51). Often only one renal pelvis is affected in this way, but both may be involved. Most attacks of acute cystitis are 'catarrhal' in nature and of short duration; only rarely does the disease proceed to the more serious forms.

The urinary tract is not infrequently infected from the blood by *Salmonella typhi* in typhoid fever. Usually only a mild catarrhal inflammation is the result, and the condition may be almost a pure bacilluria. The bacilli may persist indefinitely, the patient becoming a 'urinary carrier' (p. 19.45); the establishment of the carrier state is facilitated by almost any anatomical abnormality in the urinary tract. In some cases of coliform infection also, there may be comparatively little inflammatory reaction. Occasionally gonococcal urethritis spreads to the bladder and causes a mild catarrhal cystitis. Coliform bacilli and the gonococcus do not render the urine alkaline, but infection by *Proteus* spp is quickly followed by ammoniacal decomposition owing to splitting of urea.

Malakoplakia. This is an uncommon condition found in some cases of chronic cystitis, and is characterised by the formation of soft rounded pale, yellowish plaques, up to 2 cm across, in the mucosal surface of the bladder. The plaques contrast with the surrounding inflamed mucosa and tend to ulcerate. They consist of cellular granulation tissue containing lymphocytes, plasma cells, and macrophages which have large characteristic granules and hyaline spheres with concentric markings known as Michaelis–Gutmann bodies. These inclusions give a positive PAS-staining reaction: calcium salts may be deposited in them and they also stain positively for iron. Electron microscopy shows them to consist of phagocytic vacuoles containing material probably derived from phagocytosed bacteria. Although uncommon, the condition is important for it may be mistaken clinically for carcinoma.

Tuberculosis. Tuberculous disease of the bladder is, as a rule, the result of direct infection of its mucosa by tubercle bacilli in the urine. It occurs most often in cases of renal tuberculosis, though also in tuberculosis of the genital tract. The bacilli invade the mucosa and give rise to tubercles which then undergo ulcer-

ation. In this way, multiple small ulcers are formed, especially at the base of the bladder, and sometimes the orifices of the ureters are specially involved. The ulcers increase in size and form large areas by confluence. Sometimes there is a considerable amount of caseous thickening of the lining. Secondary invasion by other organisms sometimes occurs, and more acute inflammatory change is superadded.

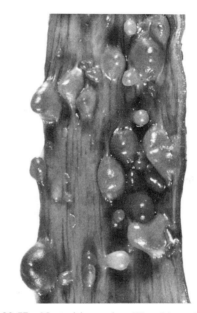

Fig. 22.57 Ureteritis cystica. The thin-walled cysts have formed in sequestered epithelium, but as they enlarged have come to project into the lumen. × 3.

Schistosomiasis (bilharziasis). The bladder is the most frequent site of lesions in this disease, which is caused by *Schistosoma haematobium*. It usually presents clinically as haematuria and in some tropical countries is a common cause of chronic granulomatous cystitis, often with suppurating cystitis due to secondary bacterial infection. It is also a predisposing cause of carcinoma of the bladder. The disease is described on pp. 28.22–9.

Ureteritis cystica. Inflammation of the urinary tract may be followed by formation of multiple small cysts which contain clear fluid and project into the lumen (Fig. 22.57). Apparently foci of epithelium become sequestrated deep to the surface and form these cysts. The change occurs also in the renal pelves and bladder (*pyelitis* and *cystitis cystica*).

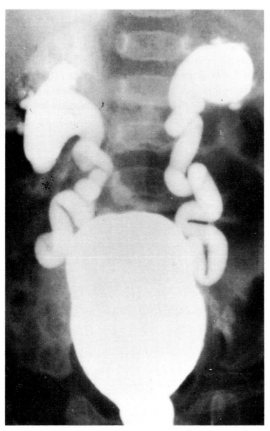

Fig. 22.58 Micturating cystogram on a one-year-old child. Note the reflux of urine up both ureters as far as the renal pelves. On the right side at the upper pole intra-renal reflux is also evident. (X-ray provided by Dr E. Sweet.)

Vesico-ureteric reflux

The importance of this phenomenon, in which reflux of urine occurs from the bladder to the ureters and renal pelves, has been increasingly recognised in recent years (Hodson 1979). Reflux is normally prevented by the oblique course of the ureter through the wall of the bladder, which effects a sphincter-like action during contraction of the bladder. In some individuals, ureteric orifices are displaced laterally with a shorter intramural course and consequently a less efficient valve-like mechanism. Reflux is de-monstrated by micturating cystograms, which show that urine flows back into the ureters and in the most severe cases distends the pelvi-calyceal system of the kidneys and enters the renal parenchyma (Fig. 22.58).

Incidence. The phenomenon has an incidence of less than 1% in young children with a normal urinary tract, but has been shown to be common (40–50%) in those children (nearly all female) who have urinary tract infections. In most cases the reflux is primary in that the urinary tract is otherwise structurally normal, although it may be secondary to various congenital and acquired abnormalities which affect bladder emptying (e.g. bladder neck obstruction, ureteroceles, bladder stones and tumours, benign prostatic hyperplasia, neurological disorders e.g. paraplegia) and so may also occur for the first time in an older age group. In cystitis the valve-like function may also be disturbed. The prognosis in the secondary form obviously depends on its associated condition; the primary form shows a tendency to improve during childhood and may disappear, especially if it is not severe.

In severe reflux, urine may re-enter the renal parenchyma, especially at the upper and lower poles of the kidney where the papillae are compound (fused). In such papillae the mouths of the collecting ducts are held open and refluxing urine flows readily into them. By contrast, the orifices of the collecting ducts of the simple papillae in the mid zone of the kidney have a slit-like opening which collapses on pressure, effectively preventing the entry of refluxing urine. It is of interest that the sites of intra-renal reflux are the sites at which scars are most commonly found in non-obstructive chronic pyelonephritis. Using a very high pressure refluxing system and *sterile* urine some workers have shown it possible to produce renal scars similar to those of chronic pyelonephritis in experimental animals, however in man there is strong evidence that both infection (including asymptomatic bacteriuria) and reflux are necessary to produce such scars and that the kidney is most susceptible to damage in early childhood.

Pyelonephritis

Pyelonephritis is a bacterial-induced inflammation of the renal pelvis, the calyces and renal parenchyma. It can occur in acute and chronic form and affects one or both kidneys, usually in a quite irregular, patchy fashion. Most cases are due to ascending infection of the urinary tract by *Escherichia coli* or, less commonly, other faecal bacteria. Acute pyelonephritis causes death only when bilateral and very extensive. In less severe form, and particularly when recurrent or associated with urinary tract obstruction, it may progress to chronic pyelonephritis, which is an important cause of chronic renal failure. In many instances of chronic pyelonephritis, however, there is no previous history indicative of acute attacks, nor indeed of urinary infection at all. Such cases may be secondary to asymptomatic bacteriuria and vesico-ureteric reflux developing in early childhood (see above). Any structural or functional abnormality of the urinary tract, or lesions which cause chronic or intermittent obstruction, predispose to infection and in these circumstances the infection tends to be severe, to extend to the kidneys causing pyelonephritis, and to be difficult to eradicate.

Causal organisms. Initial acute episodes of urinary tract infection are usually caused by *Escherichia coli* or, less commonly, other faecal bacteria (Enterococcus, Pseudomonas, *Strep. faecalis*, etc.), any of which is often obtained in the urine in pure culture. Patients with recurrent urinary infections, who have usually received previous antibiotic therapy and who may have been subjected to instrumentation of the lower urinary tract, commonly have a mixed infection of these various faecal bacteria.

Pathogenesis

Pyelonephritis may result from bacteria reaching the kidney either by an ascending infection of the urinary tract or by the bloodstream.

Blood-borne infection occurs in acute pyaemia or septicaemia (Figs. 9.8, p. 9.8; 9.9, p. 9.9), and this is seen as a complication of staphylococcal infections, e.g. boils and carbuncles. The bacteria normally present in the distal urethra can also gain entrance to the blood during surgical procedures upon the urethra; in these circumstances, the possibility of blood-borne infection of the kidneys is increased if the lesion which required urethral surgery has also brought about urinary obstruction, e.g. urethral stricture or enlarged prostate (see below).

Ascending urinary tract infection. The commonest site of infection of the urinary tract is the bladder, and it is likely that cystitis is the predisposing factor in most cases of pyelonephritis. As already explained, most attacks of 'spontaneous' cystitis are caused by *Esch. coli*, whereas cystitis following catherisation is commonly a mixed infection. In normal circumstances, the uretero-vesical valves are competent, and, as noted earlier, radiological studies have shown that vesico-ureteric reflux is uncommon, but the competence of the 'valves' is often impaired by cystitis, and reflux of the infected urine then occurs.

When pyelitis has developed, the bacteria may spread into the kidney directly by the lumina of the collecting tubules, or by passing from the submucosa of the inflamed calyces into the interstitial tissue of the renal papillae. Here they proliferate, and an acute inflammatory response occurs, often with abscess formation, eventually involving the adjacent tubular lumina. From here, infection can spread peripherally to the cortex (Fig. 22.59) via both the tubular lumina and the intertubular connective tissue spaces. Thus there develop linear streaks of suppuration with considerable tubular destruction. Since there is haphazard spread of bacteria from variably infected calyces, the renal lesion is not uniform and diffuse, but irregular and patchy.

Significant bacteriuria can reflect inflammation at any level of the urinary tract and exact localisation is often clinically difficult. It is particularly important to determine whether or not bacterial inflammation has involved the renal parenchyma and three factors are often helpful in reaching such a conclusion. The first is the presence of a high titre of serum antibody to the bacterium cultured from the urine. If this is present renal involvement is highly probable. The second is the presence of cellular casts in the urine: pus cells in the urine (*pyuria*) can result from infection anywhere in the urinary tract, but their aggregation into cylindrical

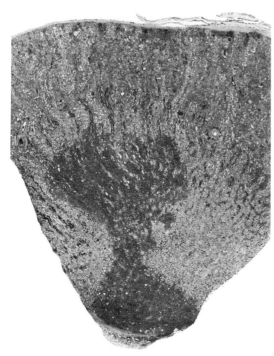

Fig. 22.59   Acute papillitis in pyelonephritis showing severe inflammatory infiltration of the renal papilla extending to the boundary zone. × 5.

casts can only have happened in the renal tubules, thus indicating pyelonephritis. Lastly, if bacteriuria is accompanied by raised serum levels of C-reactive protein then kidney infection is likely.

Predisposing factors

Many of the factors which predispose to pyelonephritis predispose to urinary tract infection in general and have already been discussed. They are listed here for completeness.

i) *Vesico-ureteric reflux.*

ii) *Urinary tract obstruction.* In addition to providing a residual volume of urine (which is an excellent growth medium for bacteria) and predisposing to vesico-ureteric reflux, there is convincing evidence that obstruction *per se* impairs the capacity of the kidneys to resist infection. Chronic urinary obstruction may also cause uraemia and thus lower the resistance to infections in general (p. 22.14).

iii) *Structural abnormalities* of the urinary tract without obstruction also appear to predispose to infection.

iv) In *diabetes mellitus* there is a general susceptibility to infections including cystitis, pyelitis and acute pyelonephritis (p. 20.64).

v) *Age and sex.* At all ages the incidence of pyelonephritis, like urinary tract infections in general, is greater in females than males.

vi) *Pregnancy* (p. 22.42).

vii) *Instrumentation of the urinary tract.*

viii) *Others.* Chronic hypokalaemia, gout and the ingestion of excessive amounts of analgesics (p. 22.43) over a long period can produce renal histopathology similar to that of chronic pyelonephritis. Accordingly these conditions should be kept in mind in the differential diagnosis of chronic pyelonephritis in renal biopsy material.

Incidence

Acute pyelonephritis is a not uncommon disease in young females, including children, and is especially liable to occur during pregnancy. It is less frequent in the male unless there is a pre-existing urinary tract obstruction. The frequency of chronic pyelonephritis is very difficult to assess. In the past it was a somewhat indiscriminate diagnosis and therefore the older scientific literature must be reviewed with caution. Incidences as high as 15% have been reported in general hospital autopsies, but this usually includes cases in which a few cortical scars are present as an incidental finding in otherwise normal kidneys. If the autopsy diagnosis is limited to those cases with severe chronic pyelonephritis, likely to have been of clinical significance, then the incidence is of the order of 1%.

Pathological changes

Acute pyelonephritis

This consists of acute inflammation of the pelvis, calyces and parts of the kidneys, and in severe cases may progress to suppuration. This appears grossly as pale linear streaks of pus bordered by a red rim of congestion, extending radially from the tips of the papillae to the surface of the cortex (Figs. 22.60, 22.61) where adjacent lesions may fuse to produce extensive abscesses. Microscopically, all the features typical of acute inflammation are present in the pelvis, calyces and kidney. Within the kidney

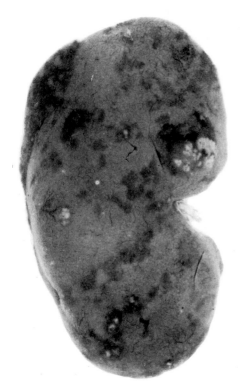

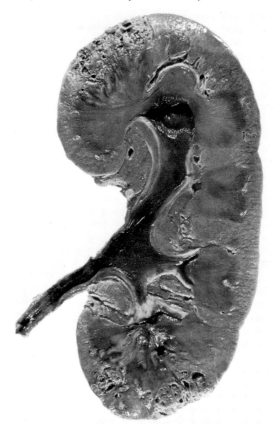

Fig. 22.60 Surface view of child's kidney in acute pyelonephritis, showing small abscesses and areas of haemorrhage. × 1.

Fig. 22.61 Acute pyelonephritis. In this case the lesions are at the upper and lower poles. Note the cortical abscesses and the streaks of suppuration in the medulla. Note also the acutely inflamed pelvis and ureter.

the suppurating lesions cause very extensive but focal tubular destruction. In the cortex there is remarkable sparing of glomeruli and large blood vessels, even when these structures are directly surrounded by intense acute interstitial inflammation. All of these changes tend to be more florid and more extensive if there is obstruction in the lower urinary tract. Obstructed cases often, and very intensely inflamed non-obstructed cases sometimes, develop papillary necrosis (p. 22.44).

Chronic pyelonephritis

The naked-eye appearance of the kidney, calyces, and renal pelvis are of paramount importance in the differentiation of chronic pyelonephritic shrinkage from other types of renal scarring. The pelvic and calyceal walls are usually thickened and their mucosa may be either granular or atrophic: they are always distorted by scarring of the pyramids and the calyces are usually dilated (Fig. 22.62). Pyelography is therefore of great diagnostic value. The degree of dilatation depends on whether or not obstruction or severe reflux is present. The kidney is reduced in size and shows irregular patchy contraction in which the pyelonephritic process has largely destroyed the parenchyma and led to focal scarring and shrinkage. The intervening parenchyma may be normal or may show the changes of hypertension. The cortical surface is depressed over the contracted areas, the cortex and medulla both being consistently narrowed. The cortical surface depressions tend in most instances to be shallower than those produced by ischaemia but they may be very similar, and *the single most important diagnostic feature of the pyelonephritic scar is its close relationship to a deformed calyx.* Microscopically the pelvic and calyceal mucosa may be thickened by granulation tissue and infiltrated by

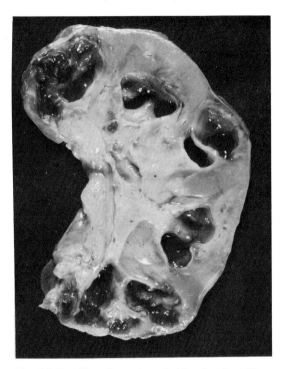

Fig. 22.62 Chronic pyelonephritis, showing dilatation and distortion of the calyces, over some of which the kidney tissue has been largely destroyed and now consists of a thin fibrous layer.

lymphocytes, plasma cells and polymorphs; lymphoid follicles sometimes form and are often responsible for the surface granularity of the mucosa. When the inflammation is florid, the surface epithelium may be lost, the pelves and calyces then being lined by granulation tissue. In cases where the inflammation has subsided, the walls of the pelvis and calyces are atrophic with some scarring.

As explained later, chronic pyelonephritic scarring may vary in extent from involvement of only a small proportion of the renal tissue to extensive renal destruction. When of lesser extent, it is usually an incidental finding at autopsy. The upper and lower poles of the kidney are the areas most frequently affected by scarring (see above).

The scarred areas. There is extensive atrophy and loss of tubules, especially the proximal segments (Fig. 22.63), and this a most important histological feature of chronic pyelonephritis. Tubular atrophy is often accompanied by gross thickening of the tubular basement membranes, and there is an increase in fibrous tissue between the tubules. Commonly partial destruction of tubules results in survival of isolated segments; these become distended with inspissated eosinophilic secretion (presumably produced by the lining epithelium), and the epithelium becomes flattened: these changes occur in groups of adjacent tubules which come to resemble superficially thyroid acini (Fig. 22.64). The interstitial tissue is densely packed with lymphocytes, plasma cells and sometimes neutrophil and eosinophil polymorphs, but in the late stages of the disease the inflammatory cell infiltrate is replaced by dense scar tissue. In such 'burnt out' pyelonephritis, there may be little evidence of active inflammation. The glomeruli in the scarred areas persist for a very long time but eventually a spectrum of glomerular abnormalities appears, the most specific of which is concentric periglomerular fibrosis around a thickened Bowman's capsule (Fig.

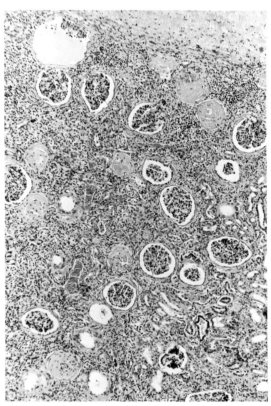

Fig. 22.63 Chronic pyelonephritis. The tubules are greatly atrophied and there is a marked interstitial inflammatory cell infiltrate. Many of the glomeruli still appear normal, but others are completely hyalinised. × 38.

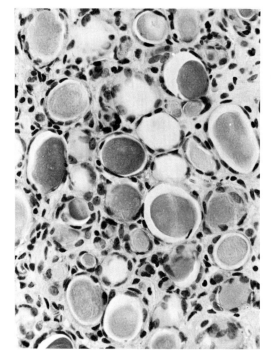

Fig. 22.64 Chronic pyelonephritis. Inspissated colloid-like material in sequestrated portions of renal tubules, presenting an appearance resembling superficially that of thyroid tissue. × 250.

22.65). Other changes are ischaemic and resemble those in essential hypertension: they include gradual hyalinisation of the glomerular tuft and fibrosis within Bowman's capsule (p. 22.5 and Fig. 22.63). Arteriolar and glomerular capillary necrosis occurs only if malignant hypertension has supervened. The arteries show variable degrees of medial and intimal fibrous thickening.

The non-scarred areas. The glomeruli may show compensatory hypertrophy. Other glomerular and vascular changes often develop as a result of arterial hypertension.

Clinical features

Acute pyelonephritis is usually accompanied by acute infection of the lower urinary tract, i.e. cystitis, so that there is frequency of micturition and dysuria. The features of pyelonephritis itself include fever, often with rigors, and pain and tenderness in the lumbar regions. The urine is heavily infected and contains large numbers of polymorphs and often red cells. Microscopy may also reveal cellular casts in which most of the cells are polymorphs; this finding is of particular diagnostic importance, indicating pyelonephritis and not just lower urinary tract infection.

In chronic pyelonephritis there is, in most cases, no preceding history suggestive of urinary tract infection. There may be a long history of vague ill-health with, in children, reduced rate of growth. Commonly, however, the presenting features are attributable to the hypertension or uraemia of chronic renal failure. Depending on whether or not the infection is still active, the urine may contain significant numbers of bacteria (see above), polymorphs and cellular casts. There is usually mild proteinuria, probably secondary to hyperfiltration through the surviving functional glomeruli (p. 22.37). Perhaps because destruction of the tubules precedes that of the glomeruli, the urine tends to be of greater volume and more dilute than in chronic glomerulonephritis. Demonstration by intravenous pyelography of irregular coarse scarring and distortion of the calyces is particularly helpful in the diagnosis of chronic pyelonephritis.

Hypertension in chronic pyelonephritis. Approximately 50% of patients with extensive

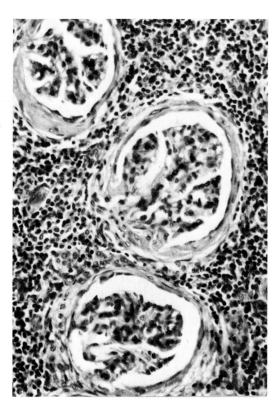

Fig. 22.65 Chronic pyelonephritis. There is periglomerular fibrosis, a heavy chronic inflammatory infiltrate, and almost complete loss of tubules. × 150.

chronic pyelonephritis develop hypertension and in 15 to 20% of these the hypertension is of the malignant type. There has been some controversy over the nature of the relationship between the two conditions, and it has been suggested that the association might result from a predisposition of individuals with essential hypertension to develop pyelonephritis. We do not consider this a likely explanation, for it would not account for the occurrence of hypertension in young patients with chronic pyelonephritis. The obvious explanation is that chronic pyelonephritis, like other conditions giving rise to extensive scarring of the kidneys, commonly leads to hypertension of secondary (renal) type. Admittedly, the mechanism of production of the hypertension of chronic renal disease is not well understood (p. 14.21) but this seems no reason for doubting that it occurs in chronic pyelonephritis.

Tuberculous pyelonephritis

This results from blood spread of tubercle bacilli, e.g. from pulmonary lesions. Like other organs, the kidneys are studded with minute tubercles in acute miliary tuberculosis, but of more importance are the localised renal lesions of tuberculous pyelonephritis which may slowly extend to destroy the kidney(s). Other common sites of blood-borne metastatic tuberculous lesions in the genito-urinary tract are the epididymis in the male and the Fallopian tube in the female, and spread from these sites can give rise to tuberculosis of the bladder. Renal tuberculosis also can spread to involve the ureters, bladder and other pelvic viscera.

   Clinical features. Renal tuberculosis may produce vague illness, with weight loss and fever, or may present with local features such as lumbar pain, dysuria, haematuria or pyuria. *Myco. tuberculosis* can usually be detected in the urine, and pyelography may show distortion of one or more calyces. In most cases, there is neither evidence nor history of tuberculosis elsewhere in the body (although this must, of course, have been present), and even at autopsy active pulmonary tuberculosis is present in only a minority of cases. Renal tuberculosis occurs usually in adult life, and it may be that, as in the lungs, it can remain latent for many years and then flare up: this would account for its occurrence long after any primary lung lesion has healed.

   The incidence of renal tuberculosis in the developed countries has declined along with tuberculosis in general, and it is now uncommon in many of them: its main danger is the involvement of both kidneys to such an extent as to cause renal failure.

   Pathological changes. The initial renal lesion results usually from blood-borne infection, mycobacteria becoming arrested in the cortex, with development of one or more tubercles: these enlarge, caseate and coalesce, while lymphatic and tubular spread leads to tubercles round about, and so the lesion grows as an enlarging patch of caseation. Spread through the adjacent papilla is common, and on reaching the renal pelvis the lesion may soften and discharge its contents, leaving a ragged cavity. Further tubercles develop in the walls of the renal pelvis, caseate and ulcerate; from here infection spreads back into other parts of the kidney, which may then develop multiple caseous lesions (Figs. 22.66, 22,67). The ureter or renal pelvis may become obstructed by tuberculous lesions in their walls, or by plugging with caseous material, and the urine (coming solely from the other kidney) may then be normal. Apart from this, renal pelvic involvement often

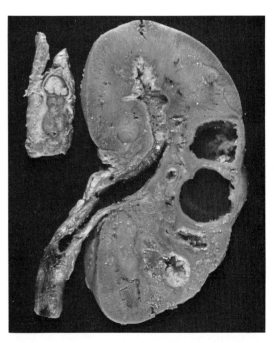

Fig. 22.66   Renal tuberculosis. The kidney contains several caseous lesions, which have discharged into the pelvis. The wall of the uppermost calyx is also caseous and the ureter and seminal vesicle (*inset*) are also involved.

results in haematuria, and the renal lesions tend also to suppurate, giving pyuria.

Xanthogranulomatous pyelonephritis

Xanthogranulomatous pyelonephritis is a distinct form of unilateral pyelonephritis associated with chronic infection (*Proteus* spp in 60% of cases) and obstruction to urinary outflow (often secondary to a staghorn calculus). The patients show a female preponderance and present with fever and loin pain. The kidney is enlarged and on cut section shows dilated calyces lined by yellowish friable tissue which histologically shows the presence of large numbers of foamy lipid-laden macrophages. The latter is presumably secondary to the obstructive element (cf. bronchial obstruction, p. 16.15). The main importance of the condition is its distinction from a clear-cell carcinoma which it may on occasion resemble macroscopically and even microscopically.

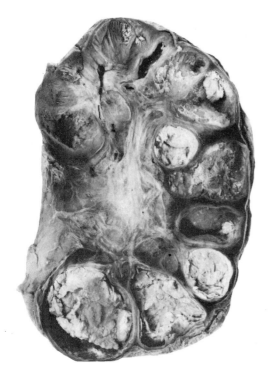

Fig. 22.67 Old tuberculosis of kidney, which has been largely replaced by caseous lesions enclosed by fibrous tissue.

Obstruction of Urinary Tract

Effects of obstruction

Serious mechanical obstruction of the urethra is practically confined to the male sex, and is commonly produced by enlargement of the prostate or stricture of the urethra: occasionally severe phimosis, tumour or calculus are responsible. The chief effect on the bladder is the production of variable degrees of hypertrophy and dilatation. When the outstanding feature is hypertrophy, the muscular part of the wall is thickened and the bands of muscle, which have an interlacing arrangement under the mucosa, enlarge and form prominent ridges or bands with depressions between (Fig. 25.3, p. 25.8). Occasionally one of these depressions may become enlarged and form a projecting diverticulum. When infection occurs, as it often does,

suppuration may occur in such diverticula, and ulceration and even perforation may follow. Urethral obstruction ultimately leads to dilatation of the ureters and renal pelves—bilateral *hydroureter* and *hydronephrosis*.

Hydronephrosis

As noted above, this means a dilatation of the renal pelvis, and may occur on one or both sides. Urethral obstruction is the commonest cause of **bilateral hydronephrosis**. It can result also from pressure of a tumour, or neoplastic infiltration, affecting both ureters, and is a common effect of cancer of the cervix uteri. Occasionally dilatation of the ureters and hydronephrosis are due to congenital abnormality in the posterior urethra, the mucosa of which

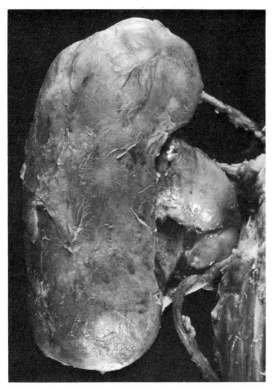

Fig. 22.68 Hydronephrosis with bending of the ureter around an accessory renal artery to the lower pole of the kidney.

forms valve-like folds; renal dwarfism (p. 23.15) may accompany the resulting hydronephrosis. Another cause of bilateral hydroureter and hydronephrosis is neurogenic disturbance of bladder control due to lesions of the spinal cord. In the *megaureter-megacystis syndrome of childhood*, dilatation of the ureters and sometimes of the bladder, progresses despite the lack of any obvious anatomical abnormality. Deficiency of ganglion cells has been postulated by analogy with Hirschsprung's disease of the large intestine, but the evidence is conflicting.

The effects of vesico-ureteric reflux in childhood (p. 22.50) and the effects of hormones in pregnancy in relaxing smooth muscle has already been discussed (p. 22.42). In all these conditions, dilatation of the ureters and pelves is usually moderate. The most striking degree of dilatation is seen, however, in **unilateral hydronephrosis**. This can result from impaction of a calculus, usually at the upper end of the ureter, at the level of the brim of the pelvis, or at the entrance to the bladder. It may be produced

also by a scar, which sometimes follows ulceration due to the passage of a stone, by a tumour of the ureter itself, or pressure of a tumour from outside. In many instances of unilateral hydronephrosis there is a severe narrowing of the ureter, usually just below the pelvi-ureteric junction, but without scarring. The cause of this is unknown; it may represent a congenital structural abnormality or result from some form of neuro-muscular dysfunction. As the renal pelvis dilates the ureter may become kinked at its origin, thus aggravating the obstruction. Kinking of the ureter by an aberrant renal artery to the lower pole of the kidney sometimes appears to be a convincing cause of hydronephrosis (Fig. 22.68), but often the ureter shows the non-scarred stricture described above, and kinking over the artery may occur *after* hydronephrosis has developed. Hydronephrosis is also observed occasionally in congenitally misplaced kidneys.

Structural changes. The effects of obstruction vary greatly. Sometimes a calculus may be firmly impacted, and there may be obvious distension of the pelvis and calyces (Fig. 22.69), or the whole pelvis and calyces may be distended by a branching calculus, though this is more common when infection has been superadded (p. 22.60). In such cases, fibrosis and atrophy of the kidney follow. In other cases, distension is so great that the dilated pelvis may become palpable. As the distension progresses the calyces become flattened, the kidney substance becomes stretched over the dilated pelvis and ultimately may form a mere rind (*intrarenal hydronephrosis*) and the surface of the kidney usually develops a lobulated appearance. Atrophy of the kidney substance may be regular or irregular, so that parts of considerable thickness may be left while the rest is much thinned; the latter result apparently depends on the degree to which the vascular supply is impaired, and the microscopic appearances resemble those resulting from major artery stenosis, i.e. the glomeruli are relatively spared, but the tubules are atrophied. Sometimes the dilatation is mainly in the form of a sac projecting medial to the kidney and there is little effect on the appearance of the kidney itself—*extrarenal hydronephrosis*.

The results of obstruction of a ureter vary greatly. If it is sudden, complete and persistent, production of urine ceases almost immediately and the pelvis does not dilate very much. This

appear, while proteins are added to the fluid by transudation from the wall of the sac. If the obstruction can be relieved before the serious sequelae develop, recovery of function may be considerable, although the dilated calyces and flattened papillae will persist.

Calculi

Urinary calculi are formed by precipitation of urinary constituents, a small amount of organic material also being incorporated. Deposition is favoured by a highly concentrated urine (and is consequently more common in hot climates), and by secretion of excessive amounts of one or other constituents (oxalate, urate, etc.). Calculi develop in the renal pelvis or ureter, or in the bladder, although some of the latter originate in the kidneys, and subsequently enlarge in the bladder.

There are 3 main types of urinary calculus composed respectively of (*a*) a mixture of uric acid and urates—uric acid stones, (*b*) calcium oxalate. Both (*a*) and (*b*) are laid down in acid urines and stones may contain a mixture of both substances: (*c*) complex triple phosphate stones including magnesium, ammonium, carbonate and calcium components (so-called *struvite stones*) which are laid down in alkaline urines and may form an outer laminated deposit upon other stones. They are often associated with urinary infection. Recently 'stones' comprised of pure protein (*matrix stones*) have been described in patients on long-term dialysis. Their pathogenesis is not yet known.

The commonest pure type of stone consists of calcium oxalate whereas only 6% are of uric acid. Most stones consist principally of triple phosphates but contain also some oxalates and urates.

The method of stone formation is complex and ill understood. Urine may be regarded as a supersaturated solution in which a delicate balance is struck between forces favouring solution or precipitation (Fleisch, 1978). Stone formation requires both *nucleation*, a process whereby the stone deposition is initiated, and *aggregation* whereby the stone grows in size. Some urinary constituents can promote the nucleation of others (e.g. urates can nucleate oxalate precipitation) and this provides an ex-

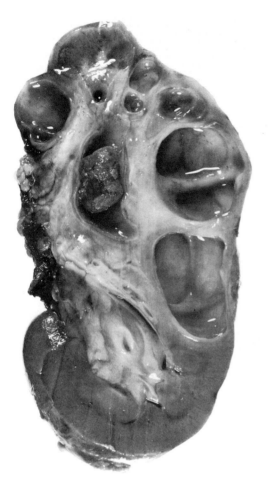

Fig. 22.69 An impacted stone in the renal pelvis, which has caused hydronephrosis and consequent atrophy of the renal tissue. The stone was in such a position that the lower part of the pelvis was not obstructed, and the lower pole of the kidney appears normal.

may result from impaction of a stone. If, however, obstruction develops gradually, or is partial or intermittent, the kidney continues to produce urine and the urinary tract above the obstruction becomes greatly dilated. This may result from pressure of, or infiltration by, a tumour, from movement of a stone, from a stricture, or from kinking of the ureter over a renal artery. When the kidney becomes greatly stretched and thinned, the tubules, and ultimately the glomeruli, become atrophied, and there is a general overgrowth of fibrous tissue. The contents of a dilated pelvis are, of course, at first urine; but, as the condition becomes chronic, the urinary constituents dis-

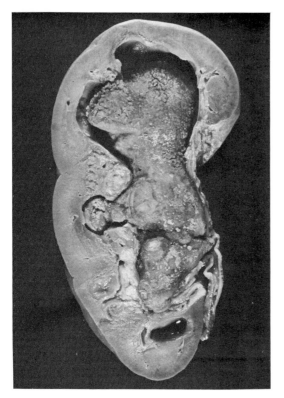

Fig. 22.70   A large 'staghorn' calculus occupying the dilated renal pelvis and calyces.

ever, grow to the size and shape of the dilated pelvis (Fig. 22.70).

A small calculus may pass along the ureter to the bladder, giving rise to renal colic with haematuria. It may be arrested temporarily, usually at the narrow lower end of the ureter. Permanent impaction, usually at the upper or lower ends of the ureter or at the level of the pelvic brim, produces hydronephrosis as already described, and when the obstruction is intermittent the hydronephrosis may be extreme. When the urine is infected with urea-splitting bacteria (e.g. *Proteus* spp.) ammonia is produced and calculi or softer deposits composed of phosphates form in the alkaline urine and are precipitated in the inflamed pelvis. The condition may be accompanied by suppuration (**pyonephrosis**) and ulceration. The large branching 'staghorn' calculi arise in this way and are composed largely of complex hydrated phosphates. A calculus in the renal pelvis, especially when it is movable, may give rise to metaplasia of the lining of the pelvis to stratified squamous epithelium and there is a risk of the development of squamous-cell carcinoma as is illustrated in Fig. 22.71.

Precipitation of sulphonamide drugs may occur in the renal tubules and pelvis unless the

planation for the fact that many urinary stones are mixed in composition. Inhibitors of nucleation and aggregation (e.g. citrates and pyro-phosphates) are also present in the urine and in those patients who are liable to stone formation it may be that the balance is tipped in favour of the promoter. An increase in the urinary excretion of a particular substance is usually an important factor, as for example, in hyperparathyroidism, where the increased excretion of calcium and phosphate in the urine very frequently leads to the formation of urinary calculi. Local factors have long been held to be important and Randall (1940) described stones developing on plaque-like deposits attached to the apices of the pyramids. Such plaques are, however, seen only infrequently, while calcium deposits may be found in the renal papilla of patients who do not have stones.

Renal calculi. Stones in the renal pelvis may be single or multiple. They are sometimes particularly numerous when there is partial obstruction and dilatation. A single calculus may, how-

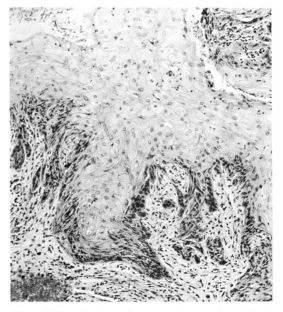

Fig. 22.71   Section through the renal pelvis in nephrolithiasis, showing squamous metaplasia of epithelium and early squamous carcinoma. × 65.

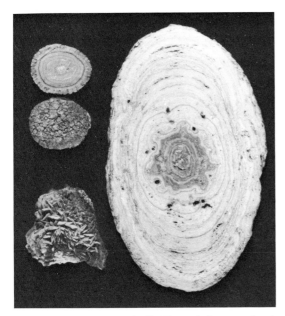

Fig. 22.72 Urinary calculi. *Upper left*, a renal calculus composed of uric acid and calcium oxalate, showing the inner lamellae and rough surface. *Lower left*, a renal calculus composed mainly of calcium oxalate. *Right*, a large bladder stone, which started as a urate stone, probably in the renal pelvis, and subsequently gained layers of phosphates while in the bladder. × 1.

fluid intake is maintained at a high level to promote diuresis. If this is neglected, actual obstruction of tubules, pelves and ureters may result from masses of crystals of the drug or its acetylated form. Acute renal failure from this cause was encountered in the early days of sulphonamide therapy.

Bladder calculi may be single or multiple: they are sometimes numerous and like coarse sand. They are now relatively uncommon in the developed countries. In many cases calculi form first in the renal pelvis, especially uric-acid and oxalate calculi, and pass to the bladder where they increase in size; in other cases they are formed locally. The larger calculi vary greatly in composition and structure, but as a rule there is a nucleus of primary stone surrounded by concentric laminae. The primary stones are composed of urates and uric acid, or are complex triple phosphate stones; very rarely, they consist of cystine or xanthine. The *primary urate stone*, seldom larger than a few millimetres, and often formed first in the renal pelvis, is rounded, hard and brown. The primary oxalate stone is small and very hard with irregular outline, and is often dark brown from altered blood pigment. *Triple phosphate stones* are whitish, often friable, but sometimes hard. They occur in conditions causing hypercalciuria, e.g. hyperparathyroidism, chronic resorptive bone disease, immobilisation in bed, sarcoidosis and the milk-alkali syndrome. In many cases, however, hypercalciuria occurs without known cause. These primary stones may have secondary deposits formed on their surface, and thus *compound or laminated stones* arise. The particular substance secondarily deposited, which need not be in a saturated state in the urine, depends not only on the composition of the urine but also on its pH. Examples of stones are shown in Fig. 22.72. As the composition of the urine varies from time to time, the great variations in the structure of stones can be readily understood. Bladder stones sometimes grow to measure several centimetres, and may weigh over 300 g.

Stones may form without the presence of bacterial infection or inflammation, and lead to mechanical effects—pain and irritation with haematuria, intermittent obstruction, damage to the bladder mucosa with ulceration, etc. When, however, there is secondary bacterial invasion, and ammoniacal decomposition of the urine occurs, then triple phosphates and ammonium urate separate out, often in large amount, and form a further deposit on calculi already formed. Deposits of these substances may occur also in cases of purulent cystitis (p. 22.48) without the previous occurrence of calculi, and form primary inflammatory calculi or irregular deposits.

Tumours of the Kidney and Urinary Tract

Benign renal tumours

The commonest benign tumour **within the kidney** is a small *fibroma* of the medulla derived from the interstitial cells. As it grows it envelops renal tubules, but seldom exceeds 1 cm in diameter and, like most other benign fibrous tissue nodules, its neoplastic nature is doubtful. *Adenomas* are more commonly seen in the end-stage kidneys of patients who are on long-term dialysis or have received a renal transplant. Apart from this they are rare. They usually develop in the cortex, and some have a characteristic appearance with narrow bands of stroma and papilliform ingrowths (Fig. 22.73). They are usually benign, but carcinoma may supervene. In the renal pelvis *villous papillary tumours* are sometimes seen; they correspond to the papillary tumours of the bladder (p. 12.13) and are sometimes associated with them. *Angioma* is another uncommon benign tumour. It may occur in the pyramids or just beneath the lining of the pelvis, and, even when small, may lead to severe haematuria.

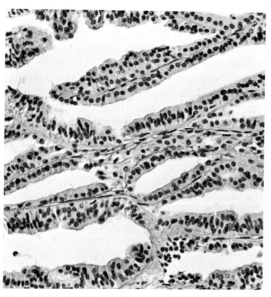

Fig. 22.73 Papillary adenoma of kidney, showing the delicate stroma and the appearances of the epithelium. × 140.

Malignant renal tumours

Malignant tumours are much less common in the kidneys than in several other organs, but two are of importance—*renal carcinoma* and *nephroblastoma.*

Renal carcinoma

Clear-cell carcinoma is the commonest type. It was formerly called *Grawitz tumour* or *hypernephroma.* This last term was based on a superficial resemblance of this type of tumour to adrenal tissue, which led Grawitz to suggest that it arose from adrenocortical tissue misplaced within the kidneys. However, it is now widely accepted that it originates from renal tubular epithelium, and accordingly the term hypernephroma is a misnomer.

Clear-cell carcinoma is often large, and may occasionally form an enormous mass. It may occur in any part of the kidney. On section, there are usually large areas of dull yellowish tissue, interspersed with vascular, haemorrhagic, cystic and necrotic areas, and also broad bands and patches of connective tissue, somewhat mucoid or translucent in appearance (Fig. 22.74). Although the tumour may often appear to be encapsulated, like a benign tumour, it is frankly malignant. It commonly grows into the tributaries of the renal vein and forms thrombus-like masses extending within them, sometimes to the main renal vein and even into the inferior vena cava. Such venous spread is usually followed by metastases, especially in the lungs and bones. Spread also occurs by lymphatics, but often later. Invasion and ulceration of the renal pelvis usually causes haematuria, and in some cases this occurs before distant spread, providing opportunity for complete excision.

Microscopically, most of these tumours are composed of large, uniform cells with abundant clear cytoplasm (Fig. 22.75) rich in glycogen and doubly-refractile lipid. The cells are arranged in places in solid masses, but usually show an acinar arrangement and sometimes papillary processes, or occasionally a papillary

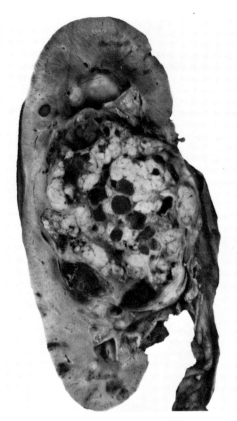

Fig. 22.74 Clear-cell carcinoma of kidney, growing from the central part of the kidney and compressing the renal pelvis. Note the haemorrhagic and gelatinous areas and rounded nodules of whitish tumour.

cystadenocarcinomatous structure (p. 12.20). Some tumours show greater cell pleomorphism and anaplasia, and have a poorer prognosis.

Tumours of purely adenocarcinomatous pattern occasionally occur in the kidney and papillary adenocarcinoma may arise both in the renal substance and in the pelvis, the two types being, however, quite distinct. In some renal carcinomas the cytoplasm of the tumour cells contains large homogeneous acidophilic inclusions. Spindle cell variants of renal carcinoma may also be seen.

Other malignant renal tumours

Nephroblastoma is an embryonic tumour with the features of a rapidly growing sarcoma. It may reach a large size and, though often remaining enclosed within the renal capsule, rapidly invades blood vessels and so produces metastases, chiefly in the lungs. It occurs espe-

cially in the first three years of life, and is known also as 'embryoma', 'mixed tumour' or 'Wilms' tumour' of the kidney. Although rare, it is one of the commonest malignant tumours in childhood and sometimes develops in the fetus and may interfere with delivery.

Microscopically, the tumour is composed of spindle-celled tissue, with formation of acini and tubular structures, and apparent transitions may be seen between the spindle cells and those of epithelial type (Fig. 22.76). There may also be imperfect formation of glomeruli. This tumour is derived from the cells of the kidney rudiment. In some instances it has a more complicated structure, striped muscle fibres being present, and the tumour may have originated from cells of the mesoderm before the differentiation of the myotomes.

Spindle-cell sarcoma is a rare renal tumour and most spindle-cell tumours are, in fact, carcinomas.

Secondary carcinoma in the kidneys is not

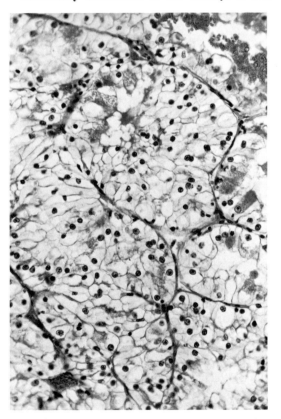

Fig. 22.75 Clear-cell carcinoma of kidney, showing typical empty-looking cells with well-defined walls and delicate stroma. × 205.

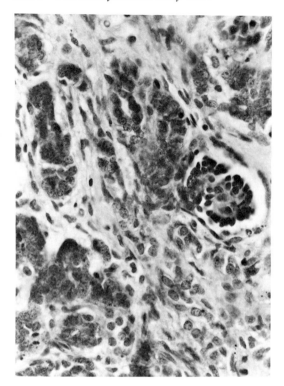

Fig. 22.76 Nephroblastoma, showing spindle-shaped tumour cells and differentiation into imperfect tubules and glomeruli. × 275.

uncommon, although metastases are neither as frequent nor as numerous as might be expected from the large renal blood flow.

Tumours of the urinary tract

Nearly all tumours of the urinary tract arise from the transitional epithelial lining. Chemical carcinogens are of aetiological importance, and as the whole urothelium is exposed to them, it is not surprising that two or more tumours often occur, either simultaneously or sequentially. Because of its relatively large surface area, the bladder is a commoner site of tumours than the ureters or renal pelves, but the trigone appears to be a particularly common site.

It is difficult to adopt the usual classification of benign and malignant for urinary tract tumours, and the following classification takes into consideration the reported experience of the Institute of Urology of the University of London.

Benign papilloma. This is a pedunculated tumour, often less than 1 cm in diameter, which projects into the lumen from a narrow stalk and is composed of fine branching fronds, each of which has a thin central core of vascular connective tissue and a lining which is 3–4 cells thick and resembles very closely the normal transitional epithelium of the urinary tract (Fig. 22.77). The cells are regular, and mitoses are few. Tumours showing this very high degree of differentiation are rare, and are benign.

Well-differentiated transitional cell carcinoma. These tumours may be papillary (Fig. 22.78) or solid, or may contain both types of structure. They comprise the majority of urinary tract tumours.

(*a*) *Papillary.* Tumours of this type have a structure similar to the benign papilloma; they differ, however, in having a thicker epithelial lining composed of more layers of cells. Mitoses

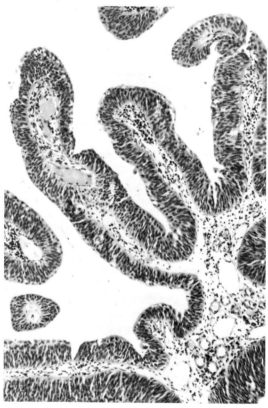

Fig. 22.77 Papilloma of bladder. Part of the tumour, showing the frond-like processes. Where the epithelium has been cut perpendicularly, it is 3–4 cells thick: in other places, oblique section gives a false impression of more cell layers. × 85.

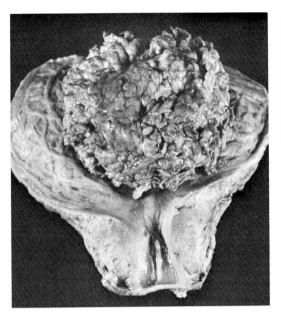

Fig. 22.78 A large papillary carcinoma of the bladder.

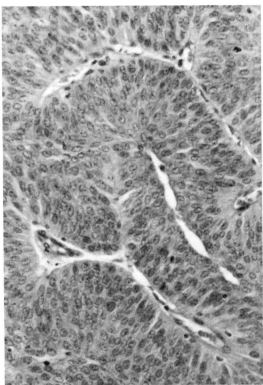

Fig. 22.79 Well-differentiated transitional-cell carcinoma of the urinary bladder. × 350.

are more numerous, and the epithelial cell nuclei show variations in size, but tend to be larger and more deeply staining, giving the impression of crowding of cells. In spite of these appearances, the cells are sufficiently differentiated to be recognisably of transitional type. The base of the epithelium is not as regular as in the benign papilloma and careful search must be made for foci of invasion and extension into lymphatics or venules. Even in the apparent absence of such changes, some of these tumours recur or behave as carcinomas, but the presence of invasion greatly worsens the prognosis.

(b) *Solid.* This has the appearance of a raised plaque attached to the surface by a broad base, and sometimes appearing lobulated or nodular. Microscopy shows solid sheets of epithelial cells with appearances similar to the cells of the papillary tumours (Fig. 22.79), but enclosed by bands of vascular connective tissue. The prognosis is similar to the papillary type, and the detection of invasion is again of great importance.

Some tumours are papillary in their superficial parts, but have a broad base of attachment and deeper solid elements.

Anaplastic carcinoma. This also presents as a plaque raised above the surface, but usually shows central necrosis and thus appears as a sloughing ulcer with raised edges. The epithel-

ium is in solid masses, and may have some resemblance to transitional cells but with obvious cellular atypia and numerous and abnormal mitoses (Fig. 22.80). Foci of poorly-differentiated squamous epithelium are often present. There is frank invasion into the underlying muscle, and lymphatic and venous extensions are often apparent. The prognosis is poor.

Squamous-cell carcinoma also occurs in the urinary tract: in some instances it arises from squamous metaplasia attributable to the presence of calculi and chronic inflammation. In other cases, squamous-cell cancer arises directly from transitional epithelium.

Adenocarcinoma is relatively uncommon. It may arise from transitional epithelium and occurs particularly in congenital extroversion of the bladder, when the epithelium undergoes metaplasia to mucus-secreting type. Another possible origin is from remnants of the urachus around the apex of the bladder.

Clinical features. Both benign and malignant tumours of the urinary tract tend to bleed, and haematuria is the common complaint. In some

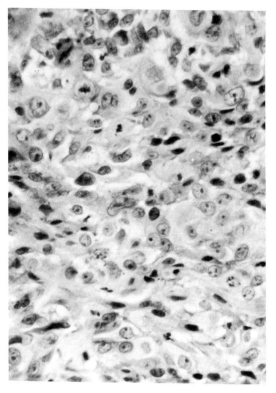

Fig. 22.80 Anaplastic carcinoma of the urinary bladder. × 350.

instances, infection is superadded, and recurrent cystitis is not unusual, particularly with ulcerated malignant tumours. Symptoms may also arise from local invasion or distant metastases.

Aetiology. Bladder tumours, and particularly the transitional cell types, are a well-known industrial hazard in workers in the aniline dye industry, in which 2-naphthylamine has been incriminated (p. 13.19). There is also an increased incidence in workers in the rubber industry, and more recently there is evidence incriminating benzidine and related compounds. The incidence is also increased in cigarette smokers and in people who take high doses of analgesics over a long period (p. 22.44). A high incidence of bladder tumours has been observed in Egypt, and is attributable to chronic schistosomiasis.

Exfoliative cytology. Tumour cells may be found in the urine and exfoliative cytology is a useful screening procedure in high risk groups.

Other tumours. Myxoma and leiomyoma are occasionally encountered, and both leio- and rhabdo-myosarcomas, the last appearing as raised blunt processes.

Congenital Lesions of the Kidneys and Urinary Tract

Congenital cystic kidneys

This occurs in two main forms, one of which does not usually cause illness until middle-age, while the other is usually fatal in infancy.

Adult polycystic disease is the least rare form of congenital cystic renal disease. The kidneys contain large numbers of cysts which enlarge throughout life. Rarely death from renal failure occurs in infancy or childhood, but more than 50% of patients develop symptoms due to hypertension or uraemia in the 3rd or 4th decade; most of the remainder die of unrelated causes.

In adult patients, the kidneys are greatly enlarged and occupied by numerous cysts of various sizes, while little kidney substance may be recognisable between the cysts. Prolonged survival presupposes, of course, the presence of enough functioning renal tissue, but this is gradually compressed by the slowly-enlarging cysts and secondary hypertension or chronic renal failure develops. Each kidney may weigh 1 kg or even more (Fig. 22.81) and be easily palpable. The cysts may be of any size up to 4–6 cm in diameter; they usually contain serous fluid, colourless or brownish, though it may be mucoid, especially in the smaller cysts. Occasionally the cystic change is practically restricted to one kidney. The condition may result from imperfect fusion between the kidney tubules proper and the collecting tubules (which grow up from the extremity of the ureter to meet them) but other embryological explana-

cuboidal or columnar epithelium. Renal enlargement may be sufficient to interfere with birth or, in live-born infants, with respiration. Occasional patients survive longer and develop fatal hypertension in childhood. The condition is associated with multiple hepatic cysts or abnormalities of the small bile ducts in the portal areas.

Medullary sponge kidney shows cystic dilatation of the collecting ducts in the papillae. It is usually bilateral and may affect any or all of the papillae in each kidney. Symptoms usually develop after the age of thirty, and are due to the formation of calculi within the cysts or to superadded pyelonephritis. The cysts are usually less than 5 mm in diameter and their epithelial lining may be single-layered, compound squamous or transitional. The diagnosis may be apparent from intravenous pyelograms. The cause of the condition is unknown and its congenital nature uncertain.

There are now known to be several types of inherited congenital cystic disorders of the kidney, some of which can be detected *in utero* by ultrasonography. It is important to distinguish these from **congenital renal dysplasia**, which is not inherited, and in which abnormal mesenchymal tissues (cartilage, smooth muscle, etc.) develop in the kidneys.

Simple renal cysts are very common and most individuals over the age of 45 have one or more. Occasionally multiple, they show an increasing incidence with age and also in kidneys damaged by pyelonephritis, glomerulonephritis and in end-stage kidneys in patients on chronic dialysis. Such cysts are obviously secondary in nature.

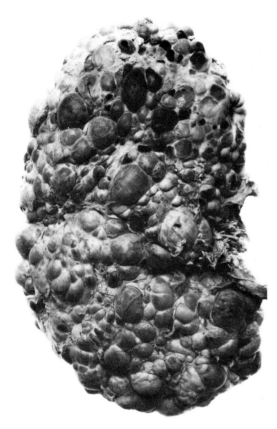

Fig. 22.81 Surface view of congenital cystic kidney, which weighed 1·5 kg.

tions have been proposed. The condition is inherited as an autosomal dominant trait, with a high degree of penetrance and hence the recognition and distinction from infantile polycystic disease (see below) is important in those cases which present in childhood if the appropriate genetic counselling is to be provided. There may be accompanying cystic change in the liver, although not sufficient to disturb hepatic function.

Ten per cent of patients with polycystic kidneys die from subarachnoid haemorrhage. This has been attributed to a high incidence of the congenital abnormality regarded as responsible for berry aneurysms, but there is doubt about this (p. 14.32) and the association may be due simply to the hypertension which commonly develops in polycystic disease.

Infantile polycystic disease is rare and usually causes death shortly after birth. It may be due to an autosomal recessive trait. The kidneys contain multiple elongated radially arranged cysts lined by

Other congenital defects of the kidney

These are numerous and some are comparatively common. Occasionally one kidney, usually the left, is absent—*agenesis*—and there is generally an absence of the ureter also. In such cases, the surviving kidney undergoes compensatory hypertrophy, and its weight may sometimes double; this occurs also in *hypoplasia* of one kidney, which appears usually as an irregular atrophic structure around the upper end of its ureter. If severe, hypoplasia of both kidneys is incompatible with life; minor degrees may cause renal dwarfism. Sometimes the kidneys are fused, most often at the lower pole—'horseshoe kidney': the two ureters pass in front of the connecting bridge. In rarer forms the fusion of the kidneys is more complete and an oval or somewhat irregular kidney results, which varies in position. Occasionally one kidney, more rarely both, lie in front of the sacrum: its ureter is correspondingly short and the arterial blood supply comes from the lower end of the aorta or an adjacent large branch. In these various renal abnormalities the position of the adrenals is usually quite normal. The kidney is originally composed of five lobules and ordinarily their fusion is complete. Sometimes slight grooves on the surface mark the original lobules and the term *fetal lobulation* is applied; the condition is of no importance. The arrangement of the renal arteries is very variable. Ligation of a so-called accessory artery is likely to be followed by infarction of the tissue supplied by it.

The urinary tract

Renal pelves and ureters. The ureter may be double in its upper part or in its whole length; in either case, a partial doubling of the renal pelvis is usually present. When the duplication is complete, the ureter from the upper part of the kidney opens separately into the bladder, or sometimes into the urethra or a seminal vesicle. Such a condition may be present on one or both sides. Narrowing of a ureter without scarring, possibly of a congenital nature (p. 22.58), is a common cause of unilateral hydronephrosis. Such abnormalities appear to favour the occurrence of infection and also its persistence when established.

The bladder. The most important abnormality is a defect of its anterior wall, accompanied by a corresponding median defect of the abdominal wall, the condition being known as *extroversion* of the bladder. The posterior wall of the bladder is thus exposed, and appears as an area of vascular mucous membrane, on which the ureters open. The epithelium of the exposed mucosa undergoes metaplastic alteration, in part into squamous epithelium and in part into a columnar mucus-secreting epithelium resembling that of the large intestine. In the male, the urethra remains open on its dorsal aspect, the condition being known as *epispadias*; in the female there is usually a split clitoris. The symphysis pubis is also usually deficient, though this may occur apart from extroversion of the bladder.

In the posterior **urethra** valve-like folds of the mucosa may cause obstruction with consequent hypertrophy of the bladder and bilateral hydronephrosis. Other abnormalities of the male urethra include *epispadias* (see above), and *hypospadias* in which it opens on the ventral surface of the penis.

References

Arneil, G. C. and Lam, C. N. (1967). Long-term assessment of steroid therapy in childhood nephrosis. *Lancet* ii, 819–21.

Atkins, R. C., Glasgow, E. F., Holdsworth, S. R., Thomson, N. M. and Hancock, W. W. (1980). Tissue culture of isolated glomeruli from patients with glomerulonephritis. *Kidney International* 17, 515.

Bariéty, J., Druet, P., Lagrue, G., Samarcq, P. and Milliez, P. (1970). Les glomérulopathies 'extra-membraneuses' (GEM). Étude morphologique en microscopie optique, électronique et en immunofluorescence. *Pathol. Biol. (Paris)* 18, 5.

Berger, J. and Hinglais, N. (1968). Les depots intercapillaires d'IgA-IgG. *J. Urol. Nephrol. (Paris)* 74, 694.

Boyce, W. H. and Sulkin, N. M. (1966). Biocolloids of urine in health and disease. III. The mucoprotein matrix of urinary calculi. *Journal of Clinical Investigation* 35, 1067–79.

Davis, A. E., et al. (1978) Heterogeneity of nephritic factor and its identification as an immunoglobulin. *Proceedings of the National Academy of Sciences* 74, 3980–83.

Ehrenreich, T. and Churg, J. (1968). Pathology of membranous nephropathy. In S. C. Sommers (Ed.) Pathology Annual 1968. New York. Appleton-Century Crofts, Vol. 3, 145.

Fleisch, H. (1978) Inhibition of promoters of stone formation. *Kidney International* 13, 361.

Germuth, F. R. and Rodriguez, E. (1973). *Immuno pathology of the Renal Glomerulus*, pp. 227. Little Brown, Boston.

Henderson, D. A. (1958). The aetiology of chronic nephritis in Queensland. *Medical Journal of Australia* 1, 377.

Hodson, C. J. (1979). Reflux nephropathy: Scoring the damage. In Hodson and P. Kincaid-Smith (Eds.) Reflux nephropathy. Masson Publishing. New York, p. 29.

Horster, M. and Thurau, K. (1968). Micropuncture studies on the filtration rate of single superficial and juxtamedullary glomeruli in the rat kidney. *Pfluger's Archiv* 301, 162–81.

Lockwood, C. M. *et al.* (1976). Immunosuppression and plasma-exchange in the treatment of Goodpasture's syndrome. *Lancet* i, 711–15.

Lockwood, C. M. et al. (1977) Plasma-exchange and

immunosuppression in the treatment of fulminating immune-complex crescentic nephritis. *Lancet* **i**, 63–7.

McCluskey, R. T. (1983). Immunologic mechanisms in glomerular disease. In Pathology of the Kidney 3rd edn. (Ed. R. H. Heptinstall) pp. 301–387 Little Brown & Co., Boston/Toronto.

Oliver, J., MacDowall, M and Tracy, A. (1951). The pathogenesis of acute renal failure associated with traumatic and toxic injury: Renal ischaemia, nephrotoxic damage and the ischemuric episode. *Journal of Clinical Investigation* **30**, 1307–1440.

Randall, A. (1940). Papillary pathology as a precursor of primary renal calculus. *Journal of Urology* **44**, 580.

Solez, K., Racusen, L. C. and Whelton, A. (1981). Glomerular epithelial cell changes in early post ischaemic acute renal failure in rabbits and man. *American Journal of Pathology* **103**, 163.

West, C. D. and McAdams, A. J. (1978). The chronic glomerulonephritides of childhood: Part II. *Journal of Pediatrics* **93**, 167.

Wirz, H. (1956). Der osmotische Druck in den corticulen Tubuli der Rattenniere. *Helvetia Physiologica et Pharmacologica Acta* **4**, 353–62.

Further Reading

Black, D. A. K. (1972). *Renal Disease*, 3rd edn., pp. 871. Blackwell Scientific, Oxford, London and Melbourne. (A clear account of the pathophysiology and clinical aspects of renal disease.)

Fleisch, H., Robertson, W. G., Smith, L. H. and Vahlensieck, W. (Eds.) (1976). *Urolithiasis Research*, pp. 582. Plenum Press, New York and London. (Reprint of a symposium.)

Heptinstall, R. T. (1983). *Pathology of the Kidney*, 3rd edn., pp. 1695. Little Brown, Boston.

Leaf, A. and Cotran, R. S. (1980). *Renal Pathophysiology*, 2nd edn., pp. 410. Oxford University Press, New York/Oxford.

Meadows, R. (1978). *Renal Histopathology*, 2nd edn., pp. 544. Oxford University Press, Oxford, New York and Melbourne.

Spargo, B., Seymour, A. E. and Ordonez, N. G. (1980). *Renal Biopsy Pathology with Diagnostic and Therapeutic Implications*, pp. 469. John Wiley & Sons, New York, Chichester, Brisbane, Toronto.

Turner, D. R. (1979). Glomerulonephritis. In *Recent Advances in Histopathology*, No. 10, pp. 235–57, Ed. by P. P. Anthony and N. Woolf. Churchill Livingstone, Edinburgh, London and New York.

23

Locomotor System

Diseases of Bone

Normal bone structure

Bone is a specialised form of connective tissue important both for its mechanical properties and in the maintenance of mineral homoeostasis. Certain fundamental concepts of its normal anatomy and physiology are essential to an understanding of its pathology. Normal *bone* consists of cells (osteocytes) lying in small spaces (lacunae) in a matrix formed of collagen fibres, amorphous ground substance and mineral complexes. The mineral consists of calcium and magnesium in combination with phosphate and carbonate, in the complex known as bone apatite. Cell nutrition and respiratory exchange is maintained through this calcified matrix by the fine meshwork of canaliculi that contain extensions of the osteocyte cytoplasm.

Bone formation and resorption. Bone may be formed through the intermediate stage of cartilage (endochondral ossification) or directly from collagen (membranous ossification) but in both these circumstances the production of bone is thought to occur in two stages. Firstly, an uncalcified matrix, *osteoid*, is formed by osteoblasts and secondly, under normal conditions, this is mineralised within 6 to 12 days. The removal of bone (resorption) is generally believed to occur in one stage, mineral and matrix disappearing together. The terms decalcification and demineralisation are therefore to be avoided as they give a false picture of the process in living bone. At sites of bone resorption the bone surface has scalloped edges, *Howship's lacunae*, and these often contain mul-

tinucleated osteoclasts which are probably derived from blood-borne monocytes. Bone is not a static tissue and throughout life the two processes of bone formation and bone resorption continue actively though at a slower rate in adult life than in childhood.

Types of bone. While all bone consists of cells, collagen fibres, ground substance and mineral, different types of bone may be formed depending on the arrangement of fibres and cells. Two main types are found in the human skeleton, woven bone and lamellar bone.

Woven bone consists of fibre bundles running in an irregular, interlacing pattern through a matrix rich in ground substance; the osteocytes are large and closely packed (Fig. 23.1). It is formed whenever bone is rapidly laid down as in the embryonic skeleton, in fracture callus, in Paget's disease and osteitis fibrosa. It is, however, an impermanent structure and, given time, is usually replaced by lamellar bone which is mechanically stronger.

Lamellar bone. The fibre bundles are fine and run in parallel sheets (Fig. 23.2), different sheets having different fibre directions and so giving the whole a stratified appearance. The osteocytes are smaller and less numerous than in woven bone and have more frequent and delicate processes. The histological differences are most clearly demonstrated either by silver stains or by viewing the sections in polarised light. Lamellar bone usually replaces pre-existing cartilage or woven bone in the growing skeleton.

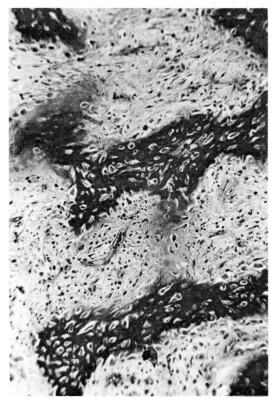

Fig. 23.1 Woven bone, from fracture callus, showing large, closely packed lacunae. × 190.

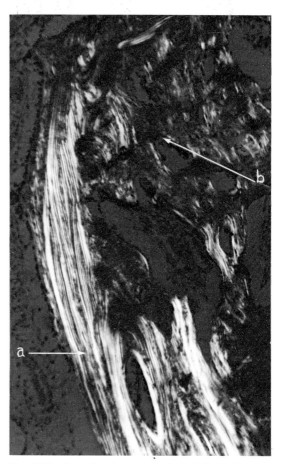

Fig. 23.2 Lamellar bone in polarised light showing the orderly orientation of the bone lamellae (**a**). On the surface are some new-formed trabeculae of woven bone, (**b**) showing lack of lamellar orientation. × 190.

Transplantation of bone (bone grafting)

Bone grafting is a relatively common surgical procedure and the reparative processes are similar to those in the healing of a fracture (p. 5.12). Struts of cortical bone may be used to bridge a gap in a bone or chips of cancellous bone to fill a cavity. Autografts (p. 6.4) are most successfully incorporated for they are the most potent stimulators of host osteogenesis. Though most of the graft osteocytes die, surviving surface osteoblasts (which are most plentiful in cancellous bone) contribute to the formation of the woven bone which anchors the graft to the host bed. Only then do proliferating blood vessels with accompanying osteoprogenitor cells grow into the graft. These cells probably derive from host monocytes, reticular and endothelial cells. Gradually the graft bone and any dead host bone are resorbed by osteoclasts and replaced by new woven bone which is slowly remodelled to form lamellar cancellous or cortical bone. Improvements in microsurgical technique have led to the successful use of vascularised bone transfers for the reconstruction of major bone defects.

The aim of bone banks is to provide stored sterile allografts with low antigenicity, good powers of host bone induction and the ability to be readily remodelled. Antigenicity may be reduced by freezing or freeze drying the graft while union is encouraged by removal of graft marrow allowing easier vascularisation and by implantation at sites of maximum osteogenesis (e.g. within haemopoietic marrow). Xenografts are poorly incorporated and are now seldom used.

Aseptic necrosis of bone

The processes of revascularisation, laying down of new bone and gradual resorption of dead bone involved in the replacement of bone grafts also come into play in the replacement of necrotic bone whether this follows fracture (p. 5.13), hyperbaria (p. 10.22), sickle-cell disease (p. 17.26), Gaucher's disease, the long-term administration of steroids, or is of unknown aetiology. Necrosis involving the medullary cavity is symptomless. However in juxta-articular sites such as the femoral and humeral heads if revascularisation and reossification is incomplete or fails to occur, necrotic trabeculae may eventually collapse with resultant deformity of the joint surface and disabling secondary degenerative changes. A few patients have developed sarcomas at the site of longstanding bone necrosis. Aseptic necrosis is thought to be the cause of a number of eponymous conditions affecting the epiphyses of children (*osteochondritis juvenilis*), the most important of which is Perthes' disease of the femoral head.

Pyogenic Infections of Bone

Acute osteomyelitis

Different terms are applied to inflammation of bone according to the site—periostitis, osteitis proper, and osteomyelitis—but these should not be taken as indicating separate conditions; one may lead to another, and sometimes all three are present together. Although acute osteomyelitis is now rarer in the West, it remains a major problem in developing countries. It is seen most often in childhood though its *relative* incidence is increasing in neonates and adults. The metaphyses adjacent to the more actively growing epiphyses of long tubular bones, i.e. lower end of femur, upper end of tibia, upper end of humerus and lower end of radius, are the sites usually involved, though vertebrae, pubis, clavicle and indeed any bone may be affected.

Aetiology

Bone infection may result from bacterial contamination of a compound fracture, from surgical operation, especially when metal implants are used (p. 23.42), or by spread from an adjacent focus of infection (i.e. to the jaw from an apical tooth abscess). In most cases, however, it arises as a result of haematogenous spread of organisms which probably first settle on the metaphyseal side of the epiphyseal cartilage. Sometimes there is an obvious inflammatory lesion elsewhere such as a boil, paronychia or otitis media, but often a source

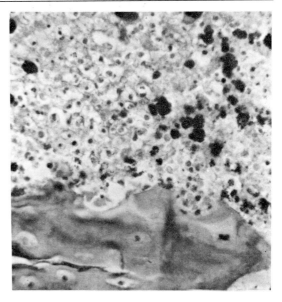

Fig. 23.3 Acute osteomyelitis, showing clumps of darkly stained staphylococci. × 250.

of infection cannot be traced and is probably some slight lesion of the skin or mucous membrane. While suppurative osteomyelitis may be produced by various organisms, by far the commonest cause is *Staphylococcus aureus* which is often penicillin resistant (Fig. 23.3). Streptococci and *Haemophilus influenzae* produce occasional infections especially in infants, while other pyogenic organisms are rarely responsible. A mixed flora is characteristic of osteomyelitis involving the feet of elderly diabetics. An attack of *typhoid fever* may be

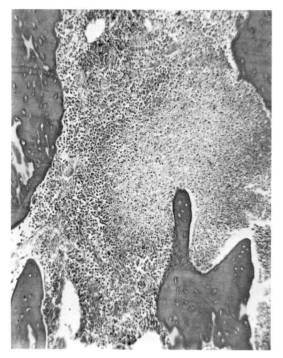

Fig. 23.4 Acute osteomyelitis showing necrosis of bone and marrow and an intense polymorph reaction. ×95.

followed, sometimes many years later, by osteomyelitis, usually in the long bones or spine. Sickle-cell anaemia in children and Gaucher's disease may be associated with osteomyelitis due to *Salmonellae*.

In about two-thirds of patients, organisms may be recovered by blood culture early in the disease but treatment should not be delayed either for the result of the culture or for the appearance of radiological changes, lest fatal septicaemia or irreparable damage to the bone results.

Macroscopic appearances

From the metaphysis the infection may spread widely, so that the medullary cavity becomes largely occupied by pus (Fig. 23.4). In children, as distinct from infants, extension occurs more readily in a transverse direction than onwards into the epiphysis because of the lack of vessels penetrating the epiphyseal plate. The infection, after breaking through the thin metaphyseal cortex, may reach the periosteum which during growth is only loosely attached to the underlying shaft though more firmly anchored at the

epiphyseal plate. A **subperiosteal abscess** thus forms which may spread extensively, bathing a large part or even the whole diaphysis in pus but usually sparing the epiphysis. The abscess may burst through the periosteum and lead to suppuration in the muscles and other soft tissues, and later, if the condition is not treated, may discharge externally. Suppuration leads to increased pressure in the medullary cavity and to thrombosis in blood vessels, which in turn lead to bone necrosis. Suppurative periostitis by itself results in necrosis of only a superficial layer of bone owing to the anastomoses with the endosteal vessels. When there is also medullary suppuration the extent of bone necrosis varies depending on the degree of vascular involvement. If periostitis and osteomyelitis are extensive the affected bone tissue is completely deprived of its blood supply and undergoes necrosis (Fig. 23.5). This is especially the case when, as may happen with a large accumulation of pus under the periosteum, the nutrient artery becomes involved and occluded by thrombus. In extreme cases, death of the whole diaphysis may result, and then the dead bone becomes

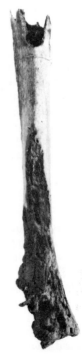

Fig. 23.5 Sequestrum of shaft of tibia from a case of acute suppurative osteomyelitis. Note the partial resorption of the bone at its ends.

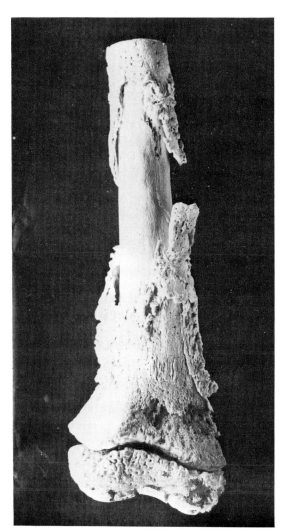

Fig. 23.6 Femur from a case of long-standing suppurative osteomyelitis and periostitis in a child, showing the irregular formation of an involucrum of new bone round the sequestrum.

separated from the epiphysis and forms a large **sequestrum** (Fig. 23.5). Towards its ends, the dead bone may become eroded by granulation tissue, and irregular resorption results; but the part surrounded by pus remains unchanged and smooth-surfaced. Small sequestra may be completely resorbed by osteoclasis. As the infection becomes less acute, new bone is usually produced under the periosteum and this may form an encasing sheath to the dead bone, known as an **involucrum** (Fig. 23.6). This new bone is irregular and is often perforated by openings through which pus may track into the sur-

rounding soft tissues and eventually drain to the skin surface, forming a discharging sinus. The above description applies to the severer forms of the disease which are still commonly seen in tropical countries where delay in treatment and mixed bacterial infections tend to lead to large sequestra and sinus formation. In developed countries, however, good host resistance and the early administration of appropriate antibiotics have reduced the incidence both of large sequestra and of abscesses requiring drainage (Fig. 23.7). Sometimes infection is aborted before any radiological change becomes apparent.

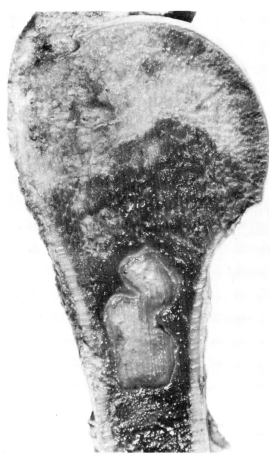

Fig. 23.7 A localised pyogenic bone abscess is seen in the upper end of the humerus of an elderly patient with rheumatoid arthritis treated with steroids. The abscess cavity is surrounded by a rim of granulation tissue. Proximally, the marrow is more diffusely involved.

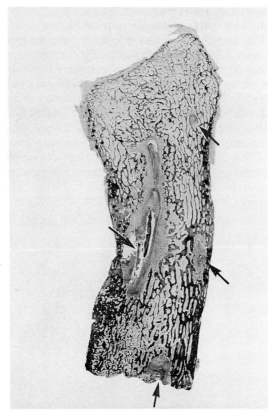

Fig. 23.8 Chronic suppurative osteomyelitis of the fibula following a compound fracture. Several abscesses (*arrows*) are surrounded by fibrosing granulation tissue; the largest contains a small bony sequestrum. There is thickening of the fibula with broad bone trabeculae which gave rise radiologically to increased bone density. (Reproduced by permission from *Applied Surgical Pathology*, Blackwell Scientific Publications).

Complications

Septicaemia or pyaemia. These complications are especially likely to arise in haematogenous osteomyelitis due to staphylococci, where, owing to the production of coagulase by these organisms, the delicate vascular sinusoids in the marrow commonly become thrombosed and suppurative softening of the thrombi allows the organisms to invade the blood. Pyaemia with abscesses in the lungs, kidneys and myocardium and acute ulcerative endocarditis may result even when the osteomyelitis is not extensive or is at an early stage. The causal organisms may be obtained from blood cultures.

Septic arthritis occurs more commonly in the hip and shoulder where the metaphysis is within the joint capsule. Although rare in children it is seen in infants especially when the osteomyelitis involves the femoral neck. *Metastatic blood borne arthritis* involving several joints may complicate infantile streptococcal or pneumococcal osteomyelitis.

Alteration in growth rate. Growth is sometimes retarded, especially in infants, when the germinal cells on the epiphyseal side of the growth plate have been damaged, but occasionally it is accelerated.

Chronic osteomyelitis. Acute osteomyelitis, particularly in adults, may become chronic with recurrent exacerbations of infection, repeated formation of abscesses with discharging sinuses and increasing patchy bone sclerosis (Fig. 23.8). Long continuing osteomyelitis with the discharge of pus may be followed by **amyloid disease** or occasionally by the development of **squamous carcinoma** in the epithelial-lined wall of a sinus.

Neonatal osteomyelitis

Haematogenous osteomyelitis in the newborn presents a rather different picture from the disease in the older child. It may involve one bone only, often the maxilla, or many bones may be affected, so-called *generalised osteomyelitis of the newborn*. It arises sometimes in association with umbilical or other sepsis and is most commonly caused by *Staphylococcus aureus*, often of a penicillin-resistant strain and rarely by *Streptococcus pyogenes* or *Strep. pneumoniae*. In the more severe cases associated with septicaemia there may be accompanying symptoms of pneumonia or gastroenteritis and the infant is desperately ill. The osteomyelitis itself is characterised by the tendency to form a massive involucrum which may be completely resorbed after recovery, by damage to the epiphyseal cartilage causing growth retardation, and by septic arthritis. Involvement of the cartilaginous epiphysis and the joint is due to retrograde spread along the metaphyseal sinusoids which penetrate the epiphysis.

Osteomyelitis in the adult

This condition is relatively rare but may complicate injury or debilitating disease. It tends to involve the diaphysis of the bone rather than the metaphysis or epiphysis. The periosteum in the adult is more fibrous and adheres more firmly to the bone. Accordingly periosteal abscesses are uncommon and large sequestra do not usually form because the cortical blood supply is maintained. However, cortical erosion is common and when much bone is involved pathological fracture may occur. Chronic marrow infection is almost invariable in the adult.

Subacute pyogenic infection

An increasing number of patients now seem to develop a subacute pyogenic infection, often with an insidious onset and relatively little fever or malaise. This may give rise to localised abscess formation of which **Brodie's abscess** is one type (see below). Vertebral osteomyelitis, sometimes due to coliform organisms and associated with urinary or pelvic organ infection, usually has a good prognosis, since bone destruction is soon followed by sclerosis and bony bridging between affected vertebrae.

Brodie's abscess. This is a form of localised, subacute or chronic pyogenic osteomyelitis

which arises insidiously and is usually situated in the metaphysis of a long bone, especially the upper end of the tibia. The central cavity contains pus, which may be sterile, is lined by granulation tissue, and surrounded by reactive bone sclerosis.

Acute periostitis

Acute periostitis may occur as the result of trauma, there being inflammatory oedema with swelling and little accompanying leucocytic infiltration. Apart from this, it is produced by bacterial invasion and is sometimes suppurative. It may result from an external wound or from the spread of bacteria from a skin ulcer, or, in the jaws, from a carious tooth. Haematogenous infection of the periosteum is rare but is a well-known complication of **typhoid fever,** and it may appear months or even years later.

Tuberculosis of Bone

The general background to bone and joint tuberculosis is dealt with here but the morbid anatomical changes in joints are described on p. 23.43. Bone and joint tuberculosis is still a common condition in developing countries especially amongst children. Elsewhere, there has been a continuing fall in respiratory tuberculosis in the last 20 years but this has not been paralleled in bone and joint disease which is responsible for about 3%-5% of new notifications in England and Wales. This represents between three and four hundred new orthopaedic cases each year. With the virtual eradication of bovine infection in advanced countries the human type of bacillus is the chief cause of bone and joint tuberculosis. The infection is thought to arise most often as a result of blood-spread from a tuberculous lesion in lung, urinary tract or lymph nodes though this is identifiable in relatively few patients. Occasionally there is direct spread to bone from an adjacent focus e.g. to ribs from pulmonary infection or to the spine from adjacent lymph nodes. The infection may spread from bone to the contiguous joint and vice versa. In almost all patients the Mantoux reaction is positive. In Britain,

rather less than half the infections are found in the indigenous population, most often in elderly patients who are debilitated through chronic systemic illness such as rheumatoid arthritis, diabetes, alcoholism or in association with corticosteroid administration or drug abuse. Many of these patients have a history of previous tuberculous infection but perhaps because the condition is relatively uncommon there is often considerable delay in diagnosis, in some cases leading to joint destruction and necessitating reconstructive surgery. More than half the notifications of orthopaedic tuberculosis are in patients from the Indian subcontinent, often within 5 years of immigration. Their incidence of infection is 85 times greater than that of the indigenous population. More than half these Asian patients are under 35 years old and teenage boys are most often affected. Although about a quarter of this group has been reported to have additional tuberculous lesions outwith the skeleton, diagnosis appears to be earlier and the outcome more favourable. Occasionally more than one bone or joint is involved. Early diagnosis is important in both groups of patients and persistent monarthritis

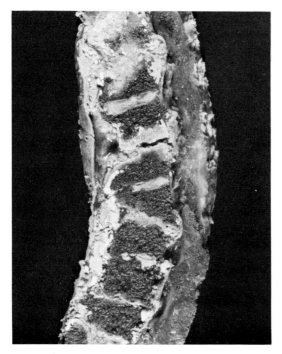

Fig. 23.9   Many thoracic vertebrae are affected by old caseating tuberculosis. Partially calcified caseating material is seen beneath the anterior longitudinal ligament (*on the left*). There is destruction of disc spaces and some vertebral body collapse.

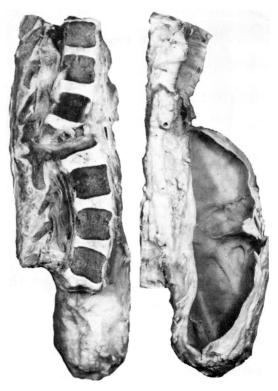

Fig. 23.10   Tuberculosis of spine (Pott's disease). Loss of intervertebral disc and collapse of T.12 and L.1 with paraplegia and formation of psoas abscess.

or bone destruction should lead to biopsy. Culture or histological examination gives the diagnosis in most cases.

Almost half the tuberculous lesions involve the spine and then the knee, hip, ankle and wrist joints in descending order of frequency. Small tubular bones of the hands and feet (see below) are more often affected than the long bones.

Pott's disease of the spine. This is usually a disease of childhood in developing countries, but apart from Asian immigrants it is now seen mostly in adults in Britain. The thoracic, lumbar and cervical vertebrae are affected in that order of frequency. Often more than one vertebra is involved; they are usually adjacent (Figs 23.9, 23.10) but occasionally widely separated. The lesion commonly arises in the vertebral body near the disc. Tubercles develop, followed by extensive caseation or by the formation of granulation tissue leading to bone destruction. The lesion usually progresses more slowly, new bone formation is less and sequestra smaller than in pyogenic osteomyelitis. The

intervertebral disc is involved early. When the infection begins in or spreads to the periosteum, the caseous material is invaded by polymorphonuclear leucocytes and converted into pus. This often extends to form a paravertebral abscess at the front and sides of the vertebra which may spread, especially under the anterior vertebral ligament, to infect other vertebrae (Fig. 23.9). Later the pus sometimes penetrates the sheaths of muscles and tracks along their length (Fig. 23.10). In this way tuberculosis of the lumbar vertebrae may cause a *psoas* or *lumbar 'cold' abscess*, the pus tracking beneath the psoas sheath to point in the inner aspect of the thigh. When the cervical vertebrae are affected, a large collection of pus may form behind the pharynx—*retropharyngeal abscess*. The cold abscess may burst through the skin with the formation of a sinus which tends to become secondarily infected. Such patients are especially liable to develop *amyloid disease*. Bone destruction may result in vertebral collapse anteriorly, and, especially when two adjacent vertebrae are involved, angulation of the spinal column (kyphosis) results (Fig. 23.10).

About a quarter of patients with vertebral tuberculosis develop **paraplegia,** usually as a result of compression of the cord by extradural abscess, granulation tissue, sequestrated bone or disc material. In less than 20% of these patients the infection penetrates the dura to produce an intradural abscess or to involve the cord directly. Occasionally, the tubercle bacilli spread to the spinal subarachnoid space and tuberculous meningitis results. In immigrants, tuberculous paraplegia may occur *without* vertebral disease probably by extension from a blood-borne focus of infection in the meninges.

Healing is by fibrosis and at this stage some new bone formation may be seen. Tubercle bacilli may long remain in caseous material enclosed in fibrous tissue and infection may flare up and cause paraplegia even years after the original infection. Late paraplegia may also result from stretching of the cord over the apex of a severe kyphosis; in the latter case the prognosis is less good.

Tuberculous dactylitis chiefly affects children and may involve a single phalanx or rarely several phalanges of a hand or foot. The infection occurs in the medullary cavity and there is abundant formation of tuberculous granulation tissue which leads to resorption and also expansion of the bone, so that it may be reduced to a shell.

Tuberculous trochanteric bursitis usually arises in young adults. The bursa is replaced by a mass of tuberculous granulation tissue and caseating material which ramifies in the surrounding tissue planes. This is usually associated with tuberculous disease of the trochanter but the hip joint is not involved.

Other Bone Infections

Syphilis of bone

Bone lesions may occur in both congenital and acquired syphilis but are now rare in developed countries.

Congenital syphilis. The commonest form of bone disease in congenital syphilis is **metaphysitis.** The metaphyseal surface of the growth plate is marked by a broad irregular yellowish band which consists of a trellis of unresorbed, patchily calcified cartilage. Bone formation is inhibited and the marrow spaces of the adjacent metaphysis contain fibrous and granulation tissue. In severe cases there may be separation of the epiphysis due to fracture through the delicate cartilage trellis at the metaphysis. **Periostitis,** with the formation of subperiosteal new bone, is sometimes seen. **Saddle nose** results from perforation, destruction and collapse of the nasal septum.

Acquired syphilis. Transient periostitis involving especially the tibia and skull bones occurs occasionally in the secondary stage. The bone changes of tertiary syphilis are also seen in congenital syphilis in older children and adults. These consist of **periostitis** which may be associated with the formation of **gummas.** The bone becomes irregularly thickened and sclerotic (Fig. 23.11) due to the formation of subperiosteal new bone while necrosis and bone resorption may also occur. The tibia, clavicle and skull are most often involved while perforation of the nasal septum occasionally follows a gummatous periostitis.

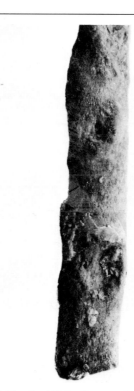

Fig. 23.11 Syphilitic disease of periosteum of tibia, showing nodular thickenings and eroded areas in the bone.

Actinomycosis

Bone involvement usually results from extension of suppuration of the soft tissues. For example, the jaw may be affected by spread from an oral focus or the pelvis from a lesion of the appendix or caecum. The infection is characterised by bone destruction and suppuration with the formation of multiple interconnected abscesses and sometimes fistulae. Large sequestra are rare and there is usually little reactive new bone formation. *Madura disease* may be caused by a variety of actinomycetes or fungi which are soil saprophytes or plant pathogens. It usually affects the foot and results in multiple abscesses with discharging sinuses and extensive bone destruction.

Brucellosis (Undulant fever)

Bone involvement in *Brucella abortus* infections is not common but spondylitis occasionally occurs with back pain due to involvement of the lumbar or thoracic spine. As in tuberculosis, granulomas form and bone is eroded with early involvement of the adjacent intervertebral disc. Rarely small paravertebral abscesses appear. However, in brucellosis, reactive bone formation with the production of vertebral osteophytes occurs earlier: the disease may be self-limiting, healing occurring by bony fusion. Osteomyelitis of long bones is rare (see also pp. 18.4–5).

Effects of Radiation on Bone

For a general description of the effects of radiation see pp. 3.23–9.

Excessive doses of radiation, whether from external sources or following ingestion of a radio-nuclide such as radium, may damage bone and cartilage cells directly as well as by obliterating small blood vessels. Bone may become necrotic and is more likely later to fracture or to become infected. For example, **pathological fracture** of the femoral neck may occur some years after irradiation for pelvic cancer, especially in women. **Osteomyelitis** is particularly likely to follow irradiation of the jaw. In children inclusion of the epiphyseal cartilage plate in the radiation field may damage the cartilage cells causing **retardation of growth** and sometimes premature closure of the epiphysis.

Neoplasia following irradiation

Leukaemia. External radiation of the skeleton tends to affect most severely the haemopoietic cells of the marrow and is a well-established cause of leukaemia (p. 17.54). Leukaemia, however, does not seem a common complication of ingested radium which is incorporated into bone.

Nasal carcinoma. A high incidence of carcinoma of the nose and nasal sinuses has been found up to 50 years after radium ingestion.

Bone sarcoma has occurred in as many as 20% of survivors of those who ingested doses of radium or its salts, but is rare following external radiation. The latent period before development of bone sarcoma is usually from 5–20 years and may be even longer following internal radiation when the tumours may be found anywhere in the skeleton and are sometimes multiple. Post-radiation tumours are usually osteosarcomas, fibrosarcomas or malignant fibrous histiocytomas and are often rapidly fatal from pulmonary metastases.

External radiation of bone carries a relatively small risk of subsequent neoplasia, but due to variation in individual response the 'safe' dosage is uncertain. This small risk is accepted in the treatment of malignancy but, when possible, benign or non-neoplastic lesions, especially in children, are usually treated by other means.

Bone Changes Caused by Vitamin Deficiency or Excess

Vitamin D deficiency (Osteomalacia and rickets)

Definition. Osteomalacia in adults and rickets in infants and children are due to a deficiency in vitamin D which results in an increase in the amount of uncalcified bony matrix (**osteoid**) (Fig. 23.12) and in addition in rickets produces defective mineralisation of the epiphyseal cartilage. These changes may also result from causes other than simple vitamin deficiency. It should be noted that the term osteomalacia is

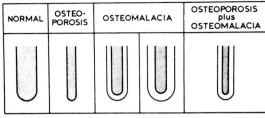

. NORMALLY CALCIFIED BONE   **. UNCALCIFIED BONE (OSTEOID)**

Fig. 23.12 Diagram of bone changes.

applied not only to a disease process but also to the abnormal bone structure.

Sources and functions of vitamin D. 'Vitamin D' includes all the sterols with pronounced anti-rachitic properties. This fat-soluble vitamin exists in two main forms. Vitamin D_2 (calciferol) is produced by irradiation of ergosterol. Vitamin D_3 (cholecalciferol) is present in fish oil and egg yolks, in much smaller amounts in butter and milk and most importantly is synthesised by the action of U.V. light on 7-dehydrocholesterol in the human skin.

The antirachitic effect of sunlight depends on its angle of incidence so that both latitude and season are important, as is the clarity of the atmosphere. While it has been suggested that skin pigmentation may reduce the beneficial effects of U.V. light, diet is another factor prob-ably contributing to the increased incidence of rickets in Asian immigrants. Children brought up in northern cities with their smoky atmo-sphere and few hours of winter sunshine are more dependent on their dietary intake of vitamin D to prevent rickets. The preventive dose is about 400 international units/day for the fair-skinned infant but there is considerable individual variation both in requirements and in sensitivity to toxic effects of hypervitamin-osis. (One international unit has been defined as being equivalent to $0.025\,\mu g$ of pure crystal-line vitamin D). Since naturally occurring sources of vitamin D are scanty, dried milk and cereals for infants and margarine are fortified either by added calciferol or by irradiation. The dietary requirement of the vitamin in adults is uncertain and probably less than 100 inter-national units per day.

The steps in the conversion of vitamin D to its active metabolites are shown in Fig. 23.13. The metabolites are essential for the absorption of calcium from the small bowel, they probably also have a direct effect on bone, promoting resorption and act on the renal tubule to increase phosphate reabsorption. Some recent work suggests that they may also have a direct effect on muscle. The main physiological func-tion of the most active metabolite, $1,25(OH)_2D$

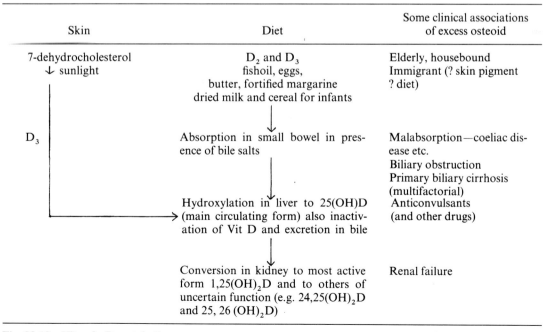

Skin	Diet	Some clinical associations of excess osteoid
7-dehydrocholesterol ↓ sunlight	D_2 and D_3 fishoil, eggs, butter, fortified margarine dried milk and cereal for infants	Elderly, housebound Immigrant (? skin pigment ? diet)
D_3	Absorption in small bowel in pres-ence of bile salts	Malabsorption—coeliac dis-ease etc. Biliary obstruction Primary biliary cirrhosis (multifactorial) Anticonvulsants (and other drugs)
	Hydroxylation in liver to 25(OH)D (main circulating form) also inactiv-ation of Vit D and excretion in bile	
	Conversion in kidney to most active form $1,25(OH)_2D$ and to others of uncertain function (e.g. $24,25(OH)_2D$ and $25, 26\,(OH)_2D$)	Renal failure

Fig. 23.13 Vitamin D metabolism

appears to be under pituitary control and is to increase calcium absorption during the growth spurts of childhood and in pregnancy and lactation. The production of 1,25(OH)$_2$D is stimulated by a low level of plasma calcium (probably in the acute stage via the parathyroid gland) or by a low level of plasma inorganic phosphate: a number of regulatory mechanisms are probably involved.

How vitamin D promotes mineralisation of bone is not clear but whatever the cause, bone laid down in vitamin D deficiency is poorly calcified and the previously-formed calcified trabeculae are covered by osteoid borders of varying thickness. Both osteomalacia and osteoporosis may cause bone weakness clinically and decreased bone density radiologically; it is important to grasp the fundamental difference between them. *In osteomalacia and rickets a normal or even excessive amount of matrix is produced but it is not calcified. In osteoporosis the matrix is diminished in amount but its calcification is normal.* In old people osteoporosis is common and is seen occasionally in association with osteomalacia (Fig. 23.12).

Osteomalacia

Osteomalacia, due to little exposure to sunlight combined with a low dietary intake of vitamin D is now being recognised more often in Britain. Old people, often housebound and living on restricted diets, the coloured immigrant population and food faddists are most often affected. Other causes of vitamin D deficiency and of excess osteoid formation are seen in Fig. 23.13 and discussed on p. 23.15.

Biochemical findings. Although vitamin D deficiency gives rise to failure of calcium absorption, the plasma calcium level is often not lowered. This is probably because the level is controlled by the parathyroids and a tendency to fall is corrected by release of the mineral from resorbed bone and by reduction of calcium excretion.

The most constant abnormality is a low plasma phosphate due partly to vitamin D deficiency and partly to parathyroid overactivity. Increased osteoclastic activity and fibrosis of the marrow is seen in bone biopsies of some osteomalacic patients and in a few the hyperparathyroidism is sufficiently marked for sub-

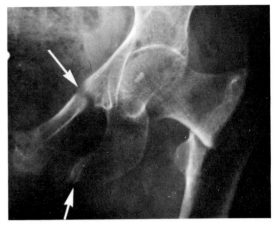

Fig. 23.14 Radiograph of a woman who developed osteomalacia and suffered a pathological fracture of her femur. The radiograph also shows Looser's zones in the pelvic bones (*arrowed*). (Mr John Chalmers, FRCS.)

periosteal erosions to be recognisable radiologically (p. 23.17). Whenever the plasma calcium is low, tetany may occur. The failure of the parathyroids to respond to the hypocalcaemia in these cases may be due to unusually complete coverage of the bone surfaces by osteoid which inhibits osteoclastic resorption.

The serum alkaline phosphatase is often raised, indicating increased osteoblastic activity.

Clinical and radiological features and structural changes. The patient commonly presents with muscular weakness especially noticeable on climbing stairs and with a waddling, penguin gait. Pain is usually vague, aching and poorly localised so that a diagnosis of 'muscular rheumatism' may be suggested. Occasionally a fracture following a mild injury fails to produce radiological evidence of callus formation although uncalcified callus is present in abundance. An incomplete or greenstick fracture in an adult may also suggest the diagnosis. Sometimes **Looser's zones** or pseudo-fractures are seen and when present are almost diagnostic (Fig. 23.14). The radiological picture is of a linear zone of translucency, cutting across at right angles to and usually affecting only one cortex. Looser's zones are painless and are most often found in the pubic rami, ribs, inner scapular borders, neck of humerus and femur, sometimes being bilateral and symmetrical and probably representing bony remodelling at areas of stress. There may be a generalised decrease in bone density, especially noticeable in the peripheral skeleton compared with the spine (c.f. osteoporosis, p. 23.20). In the more severe cases deformity may occur without any fracture, due to the weakening and softening of the bones. The pubic rami may be buckled and pushed forward into a beak (*triradiate pelvis*) with consequent narrowing of the pelvic outlet; the limb bones may be bowed and the spine kyphotic. These severe deformities are seldom seen nowadays except very occasionally in coloured immigrants or in old people who suffered from severe, late-diagnosed rickets or osteomalacia in early life. It must be emphasised that some patients with osteomalacia may show no recognisable radiological abnormality.

Microscopic appearances. Osteoid matrix laid down after the onset of vitamin D deficiency fails to calcify (Fig. 23.15). The osteoid borders covering the previously-formed mineralised bone are recognised most readily in undecalci-

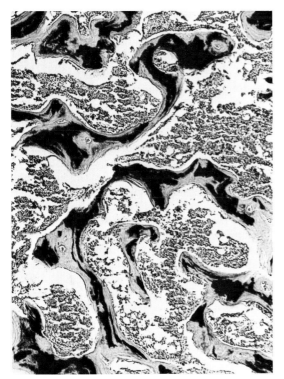

Fig. 23.15 Severe osteomalacia. Undecalcified section stained by von Kossa's method. Only the bone stained black is calcified. There are wide seams of unstained osteoid. No secondary osteitis fibrosa is seen here. × 40.

fied sections stained by von Kossa's method (p. 11.21) in which calcified matrix is stained black and the osteoid remains unstained (Fig. 23.15). Osteomalacia can be diagnosed by bone biopsy preferably of a site containing both cortical and cancellous bone such as the iliac crest. In normal adults less than 25% of the trabecular bone surface is covered by narrow osteoid seams showing fewer than 5 bright lamellae on polarising microscopy. Mineralisation of the osteoid occurs first at its border with bone marked by the **calcification front,** a granular line which stains with toluidin blue and is normally seen along about 60% of the interface between osteoid and bone. In osteomalacia there is an increase in both the extent and the thickness of the osteoid seams and the calcification front is decreased. It is important to realise that when bone turnover is increased as in Paget's disease or osteitis fibrosa the increased trabecular surface covered by osteoid—and usually also by plump osteoblasts—does not indicate osteomalacia unless accompanied by wide seams and loss of the calcification front. The amount of matrix formed in osteomalacia is very variable. It is sometimes markedly increased and the trabeculae are broader than normal probably partly due to an increased amount of formation but also to a decrease in bone resorption. Occasionally, particularly in the elderly, the total amount of matrix is much diminished and the conditions of osteomalacia and osteoporosis exist together (see Fig. 23.12). Mild changes of osteitis fibrosa may be present (p. 23.17) with some marrow fibrosis and osteoclasis of bone not covered by osteoid.

The diagnosis of simple vitamin deficiency osteomalacia may be difficult sometimes on clinical, radiological or biochemical grounds. In any suspected case bone biopsy should be done and undecalcified sections examined. The diagnosis is important because the condition rapidly responds to vitamin D administration.

Rickets

Rickets is the equivalent of osteomalacia in infancy and childhood. In addition to the failure of mineralisation of osteoid matrix as seen in osteomalacia there is failure of mineralisation of the cartilage of the epiphyseal growth plate.

Dietary rickets is chiefly a disease of infancy, being commonest from 6 months to 2 years though 'late' rickets is seen especially in immigrant adolescents, perhaps due to an increased demand for vitamin D during the growth spurt. Rickets is present at birth only in infants born to osteomalacic mothers but it is thought that the infant's supply of vitamin D in the first few months depends largely on transplacental vitamin stored in extrahepatic tissue. Prematurity predisposes to rickets partly due to increased growth rate and partly to defective hydroxylation of vitamin D in the liver.

Biochemical findings. As in osteomalacia, the plasma calcium level is normal or slightly low, but the plasma phosphate is usually below 1 mmol/l (<3 mg/dl) i.e. the normal value (1·3–2·3 mmol/l or 4–7 mg/dl). The plasma alkaline phosphatase is frequently raised.

Clinical and radiological features include muscular hypotonia, skeletal changes, sometimes anaemia and especially in the early stages, tetany.

The ends of the long bones are swollen and this may be particularly noticeable at the wrists. Radiological examination shows wide, irregular, fuzzy, cupped metaphyses, thin bony cortices and the late appearance of epiphyseal centres which are often indistinct. There may be greenstick fractures with deficient callus on x-ray examination, and Looser's zones (pseudofractures) may be seen (see p. 23.12). Deformity results from bending of the soft, poorly mineralised bone and antero-lateral bowing of the femur and tibia is characteristic.

The costochondral junctions tend to be swollen (Fig. 23.16) ('rickety rosary') and 'pigeon chest' due to indrawing of the ribs and protrusion of the sternum is sometimes seen. There may be flattening of the pelvis with constriction of the outlet (of importance during childbirth) and scoliosis may occur. The skull appears square and box-like with bossing of the frontal bones and the closure of the fontanelles is delayed. Dentition may be late.

Microscopic appearances. *In normal bone growth* proliferation of cartilage cells at the epiphyseal plate is followed by mineralisation of the matrix, hypertrophy of the chondrocytes, vascularisation of the lacunae of these hypertrophic cells by metaphyseal vessels, laying down of osteoid on the surface of the mineralised cartilage and finally brisk calcification of the osteoid followed by metaphyseal remodelling. *In rickets* the primary change at the epi-

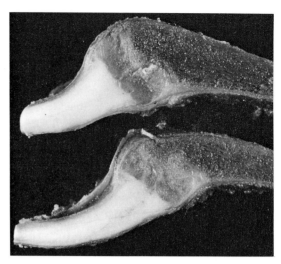

Fig. 23.16 Rickets. Section through two ribs shows marked swelling of the costochondral junctions. The child had a 'rickety rosary' during life.

physeal growth plate is *failure of the normal mineralisation of the cartilage matrix.* As a result the hypertrophic cartilage cells persist for an abnormally long time and as proliferation continues at the usual rate the epiphyseal plate becomes thicker. Patchy calcification leads to some irregular ingrowth of blood vessels but long tongues of cartilage remain projecting far down into the metaphysis (Fig. 23.17). The osteoid matrix which is laid down on the surface of the cartilage is not calcified and, since osteoid is less readily resorbed by osteoclasts, metaphyseal remodelling is also deficient. These microscopic changes account for the gross and radiological appearances of wide, irregular growth plates with flared metaphyses. If the infant has ceased to grow because of other illness or malnutrition, the changes in the epiphyseal plate will not be seen though there will of course be osteomalacic change in the bone as in the adult. Osteoid matrix formed by intramembranous bone deposition also fails to calcify.

Administration of vitamin D leads to resumption of calcification: in the epiphyseal plate this occurs first in the region of those cartilage cells which have most recently become hypertrophic. Since the amount of osteoid laid down is not usually diminished in rickets and its removal is impaired, the bones may become heavier than normal when calcification does occur. Deformities may become less marked

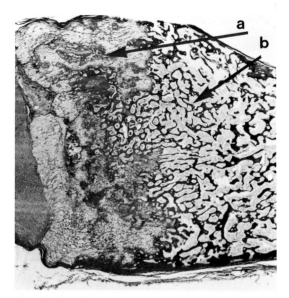

Fig. 23.17 Costochondral junction of rib in rickets. **(a)** The cartilage plate is thickened and irregular. **(b)** The spongy bone is partly uncalcified. × 6·5.

but are not fully corrected so that the child with healed rickets may have permanently bent long bones with bow legs, knock knees or other abnormalities.

Contributory causes of osteomalacia and rickets

It is still uncommon to see dietary rickets or osteomalacia in Britain but failure of mineralisation, alone or associated with other bone abnormalities, may accompany a variety of conditions. The structural changes are as described above but they tend to be less severe and may be modified by other co-existent bone disorders. The more important conditions are as follows (Fig. 23.13).

A. Malabsorption syndromes. Rickets and osteomalacia may occur in coeliac disease and other causes of malabsorption from the gut. They probably result from failure of absorption of vitamin D, though other factors may contribute. There is sometimes an associated osteoporosis.

B. Uraemic osteodystrophy, renal rickets. Bone changes which, in mild degree, are very common, may result from any renal disease which gives rise to prolonged uraemia.

In uraemic osteodystrophy, the bones may show osteitis fibrosa alone or together with rickets (osteomalacia) (p. 23.13), and in any degree of severity. The changes of secondary hyperparathyroidism may be very striking (Fig. 23.20) and associated with a diffuse chief-cell or clear-cell hyperplasia of all the parathyroid glands. **In children,** growth may be stunted, there is often severe osteitis fibrosa, especially in the metaphyses, and bony deformities of the rachitic type develop. **In adults,** there is usually no deformity though bone pain, decreased skeletal radiodensity, subperiosteal erosions and other abnormalities may be present. Occasionally osteosclerosis may be seen especially in the vertebrae, and commonly associated with osteitis fibrosa. When osteitis fibrosa is severe, metastatic calcification may occur in the soft tissues (p. 11.22).

Biochemical changes. The serum phosphate is almost always raised, the serum calcium low or normal and if bone disease is marked the alkaline phosphatase is raised.

Osteomalacia may result from failure of conversion of $25(OH)D$ to $1,25(OH)_2D$ in the damaged kidney while raised parathormone levels may not only follow hypocalcaemia provoked by phosphate retention and poor calcium absorption but be associated with frustrated attempts to increase $1,25(OH)_2D$ synthesis. Improvement may be brought about by massive doses of vitamin D, sometimes as much as 200 times the dose given to cure dietary osteomalacia. Treatment with $1,25(OH)_2D$ or the synthetic analogue $1\alpha OHD$ is easier to control.

C. Dialysis bone disease (dialysis osteodystrophy). Some patients on long-term renal dialysis develop osteomalacia characterised by bone pain, myopathy, a high incidence of pathological fractures and often a failure of response to Vitamin D and its active metabolites. Investigations stimulated by the uneven geographic distribution of these patients have suggested that an important factor is a high level of aluminium in the tapwater used to prepare the dialysate. Since deionised water has been substituted the incidence of bone disease and of progressive fatal dialysis encephalopathy has been reduced.

In some patients similar toxicity may result from the oral ingestion of phosphate-binding aluminium gels. The diagnosis of aluminium-induced osteomalacia may be made by bone biopsy for the metal is demonstrable by histochemical staining or electron-probe analysis within trabeculae at the junction between bone and osteoid. Aluminium toxicity is often associated with hypercalcaemia and should be excluded before assuming that a raised serum calcium in a patient on renal dialysis is due to hyperparathyroidism.

D. Renal tubular osteodystrophy.

(1) *Hypophosphataemic vitamin D resistant rickets.* This condition, which is now known to be inherited by a sex-linked dominant gene, develops in early childhood and is caused by a tubular reabsorption defect of phosphate (and sometimes also glucose) with consequent hypophosphataemia. It may be indistinguishable from dietary rickets, leading to stunting and deformity, though muscle weakness is not seen. It is relieved by phosphate supplements and

vitamin D. It may regress spontaneously but tends to recur in middle age. Renal failure and secondary hyperparathyroidism do not occur. Occasionally non-sex linked hypophosphataemic rickets may present *de novo* in adult life and in some cases is associated with the presence of a mesenchymal tumour whose removal is followed by cure (so-called tumour osteomalacia).

(2) *Fanconi syndrome.* This disease occurs mostly in children, is due to a recessive gene defect resulting in impaired tubular reabsorption of phosphate, glucose, various amino acids and sometimes potassium. There may also be inability to form an acid urine and cystinosis—a metabolic defect of cystine metabolism (Lignac–Fanconi syndrome): patients with these additional defects tend to develop uraemia. Micro-dissection of the kidney has shown a long thin segment at the glomerulotubular junction associated with a short proximal tubule. The bone changes, which are initially rachitic, may later become complicated by osteitis fibrosa, especially in the uraemic cases.

(3) *Distal renal tubular acidosis* is another cause of osteomalacia and rickets. This condition may present at any age and is not usually hereditary: it may follow ureterosigmoid anastomosis. The primary defect is an inability to form an acid urine and the resulting chronic hyperchloraemic acidosis leads to an increased urinary excretion of phosphate and of fixed bases such as calcium and potassium. The patient may present with renal stones, hypokalaemic paralysis or bone disease. Treatment with alkali may prevent renal damage, but otherwise nephrocalcinosis and progressive renal failure result. Secondary hyperparathyroidism may then occur.

E. Anticonvulsant drugs. Long-continued high dosage of several anticonvulsant drugs occasionally leads to osteomalacia, probably by stimulating production of liver iso-enzymes which convert vitamin D to inactive metabolites. Osteomalacia in institutionalised epileptics may also result from lack of sunlight and poor diet.

Hypophosphatasia

In this condition, which clinically closely resembles rickets, there is a low serum alkaline phosphatase and an increase in its substrate, phosphoethanolamine, in the urine. The disease is thought to be inherited as an autosomal recessive, the parents being clinically normal but having either or both of the biochemical abnormalities in lesser degree. The earlier the condition presents the more severe are the symptoms. Infants develop severe bone changes similar to rickets, often most noticeable in the skull vault. Children over six months are stunted with widespread rickets, early loss of deciduous teeth and sometimes premature ossification of cranial sutures

with consequent brain damage. The few patients first diagnosed in adult life present with an increased tendency to fracture. Treatment with vitamin D is ineffective.

Vitamin D excess

Sensitivity to vitamin D varies, but poisoning most often follows very large doses. There is an increase in the blood calcium due partly to increased intestinal absorption and partly to increased bone resorption. Excretion of calcium and phosphorus in the urine rises and renal calculi may form. In addition, there may be widespread metastatic calcification in the kidney, arteries, myocardium and stomach. Hypercalcaemia occasionally develops in infants who are unduly sensitive to the vitamin and have been fed on fortified food.

Vitamin C deficiency (Scurvy)

Scurvy results from vitamin C deficiency and is now a rare disease in developed countries, where it is seen chiefly in elderly people on a restricted diet and in neglected or mentally retarded infants. There is a defect in the synthesis of collagen because ascorbate is a cofactor in the hydroxylation of proline and lysine residues. This defect involves collagen in soft tissue, bone matrix and dentine. Wound and fracture healing are impaired and there is a tendency to haemorrhage because of weakness of the capillary walls.

Bone changes in infants precede the haemorrhagic tendency and are due to failure to lay down bony matrix, associated with the persistence of an unabsorbed calcified cartilage lattice. In contrast to rickets there is no failure of calcification. The cartilage cells of the epiphyseal plate multiply and orientate themselves normally and the intervening matrix becomes calcified, but osteoblasts fail to lay down osteoid and the calcified cartilaginous matrix is only slightly and patchily resorbed (*scorbutic lattice*) so that the epiphyseal plate becomes widened and irregular. Spicules of the calcified cartilage fracture and a very irregular, radiologically dense zone arises at the junction of epiphysis and shaft. The metaphysis itself is weak because of failure of bone deposition, the marrow spaces contain much loose fibrous tissue, and separation of the epiphysis through this site is not uncommon. The pre-existing bony trabeculae in the shaft are thin and delicate (osteoporosis) probably because of continuing normal resorption without bone deposition.

Haemorrhagic tendency. There is a tendency to bleed spontaneously or from trivial injury. The gums are spongy and bleed readily and the teeth may be loosened. There may be haemorrhage into the skin, mucous membranes, joints or subperiosteally.

Subperiosteal haemorrhages cause the severely affected child to lie immobile and to be apprehensive of movement which causes pain. Radiological changes may not appear until subperiosteal new bone is laid down on the surface of the haematoma. Bleeding into the kidney, orbit, brain or adrenals occasionally complicates the picture. The exact cause of fragility of the capillaries in scurvy is not apparent even on electron microscopy.

Failure of healing. In scorbutic patients, skin and flesh wounds and fractures either fail to heal or heal slowly, and old wounds may break down.

Anaemia. Anaemia tends to result from deficiency of iron or folic acid (p. 17.65).

'Battered baby' syndrome (non-accidental injury)

This consists of deliberate and usually repeated injury of a child (generally under the age of 3 years), with soft-tissue and/or bone damage. A history of injury is denied or not offered and the injuries may be mistaken for the lesions of scurvy.

Subperiosteal haemorrhage with subsequent formation of an involucrum of new bone may result from epiphyseal damage in infants. Such lesions at different stages may be seen in several bones. There may also be multiple bruises, fractures of limb bones or more commonly of ribs or clavicle, a ruptured viscus, subdural haematoma or a head injury which is sometimes fatal. The bones are normal radiologically apart from the effects of trauma and there is no haemorrhagic tendency. When clinical and radiological examination are inconclusive, screening blood tests, including the coagulation profile, and measurement of leucocyte ascorbic acid may be helpful. It is important to make the differential diagnosis in order to prevent further assault.

Bone Changes in Endocrine Disorders

Primary hyperparathyroidism

This results usually from an adenoma of one or occasionally two or more of the parathyroid glands (Fig. 26.19, p. 26.30). Less commonly it is caused by hyperplasia of the glands and very rarely it results from parathyroid carcinoma. One or more functioning adenomas may be part of the familial multiple endocrine neoplasia syndrome (p. 26.40). Excess hormone may be produced intermittently. It appears to have a direct action on bone, stimulating resorption. It also inhibits the reabsorption of urinary phosphate and increases calcium absorption from the renal tubule and the gut by its direct action on the tubular epithelium and also indirectly by stimulating the synthesis of $1,25(OH)_2D$ (p. 23.12) in the kidney. The effect of the hormone is to raise the blood calcium from the normal level of 2·5 mmol/l (10 mg/dl) to 3 mmol/l (12 mg/dl) or more. The blood phosphorus falls to 0·7 mmol/l (2 mg/dl) or less and the alkaline phosphatase is increased. A rise in the urinary excretion of calcium follows so that these patients tends to develop *renal calculi* (p. 22.60). Sometimes when the bones are severely affected, *metastatic calcification* of the walls of blood vessels, soft tissues, kidneys and other sites may occur.

Bone changes. Though bone turnover is increased, easily recognisable gross bone changes are infrequent. They tend to occur in the 10% or so with large tumours and high serum levels of parathormone. There is then evidence of increased bone resorption; osteoclasts and Howship's lacunae are prominent on the surface of the trabeculae which become surrounded by delicate, fibrillar fibrous tissue. There may also be 'dissecting resorption' of trabeculae, the central parts being replaced by fibrous tissue (Fig. 23.18). The picture is often one of active bone formation and resorption and the two processes may be seen on opposite sides of the same trabecula. At this stage radiology may demonstrate subperiosteal erosion of the phalanges and of other bones due to patchy replacement of subperiosteal cortical bone by fibrous tissue. As the condition increases in severity the marrow spaces become filled with fibrous tissue— hence the term **osteitis fibrosa**—and the normal structure of bone in both cortex and medulla is replaced by a meshwork of fine, irregular and delicate trabeculae. These often consist chiefly of normally calcified woven bone; narrow

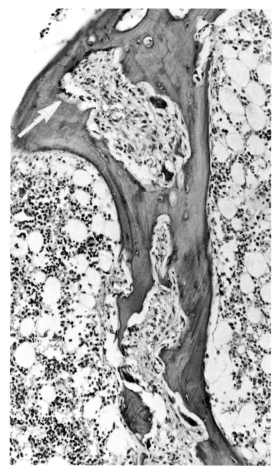

Fig. 23.18 Osteitis fibrosa of hyperparathyroidism. There is osteoclastic resorption of the central part of a bone trabecula with fibrous tissue replacement, so-called dissecting resorption. Some osteoblasts are also seen (*arrow*). × 100.

osteoid borders may be present beneath a row of plump osteoblasts as is sometimes observed in fracture callus and indicate only the rapidity of bone formation rather than a mineralisation defect. Radiology now shows loss of definition between cortex and medullary cavity, the whole bone having a fuzzy, mottled appearance, and because of the loss of normal structure it is more liable to fracture. The loose fibrous tissue is vascular and secondary changes may occur in it as a result of degeneration or haemorrhage. Cystic spaces may form and in areas of haemorrhage the resulting haemosiderin and the large numbers of multinucleated giant cells give rise to the **'brown tumour of hyperparathyroidism'** (Fig. 23.19). The differentiation of

this lesion from giant-cell tumour of bone may be difficult and the possibility of brown tumour should always be considered especially in a site unusual for giant-cell tumour such as jaw, skull or phalanges and above all when the lesions are multiple.

Pyrophosphate arthropathy (p. 23.53) is found in about 15% of patients with hyperparathyroidism.

Effect of removal of the parathyroid tumour. Excision of the parathyroid tumour leads to a fall in the serum calcium level, and within a week bone biopsy may show diminution of osteoclast activity, the bone structure slowly returning to a more normal appearance. Failure of improvement may indicate a second tumour. In some instances tetany has followed immediately after removal of the affected parathyroid, but function of the remaining parathyroid glands, suppressed by the tumour, soon returns to normal.

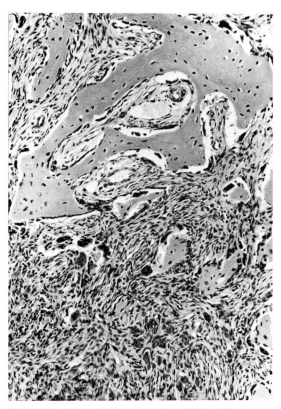

Fig. 23.19 Bone in hyperparathyroidism. Numerous multinucleated giant cells and spindle cells forming a 'brown tumour'. Newly formed bone is seen in the upper part of the photograph. × 120.

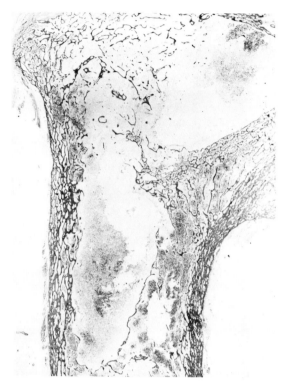

Fig. 23.20 Upper part of femoral shaft from a case of hyperparathyroidism secondary to chronic renal failure. There is osteitis fibrosa and osteoporosis, with severe cancellisation of the cortex. × 1·5.

Secondary hyperparathyroidism. In dietary rickets, osteomalacia, pregnancy, chronic uraemia and some other conditions, there is a tendency to a fall in serum calcium levels and there may be a compensatory increase in parathyroid activity leading to enlargement of the glands. Of these conditions chronic uraemia especially may give rise to bony changes, slight or severe, mimicking those of primary hyperparathyroidism (Fig. 23.20) and in longstanding disease an autonomous adenoma (tertiary hyperparathyroidism) may develop.

Excess of growth hormone

Before puberty (gigantism). There is increased growth of the whole skeleton and growth may continue for longer than normal because of delay in closure of the epiphyseal cartilage plates (retardation of skeletal maturity——see p. 26.7).

After puberty (acromegaly). Bone enlargement occurs and is due partly to subperiosteal proliferation but possibly also to re-establishment of endochondral ossification of the articular cartilage and vertebral end plates. The bones of the hands and feet and the jaw are most strikingly affected (p. 26.6).

Excess of corticosteroids (Cushing's syndrome)

Cushing's syndrome is associated with osteoporosis and has the usual clinical and morbid anatomical features (p. 26.32). Identical skeletal changes are more frequently seen with prolonged cortisone therapy. The porosis is thought to be the result of a reduced rate of bone formation and an increased rate of resorption though osteoclasts are not prominent in histological material. The increased resorption is probably due to secondary hyperparathyroidism induced by a low serum calcium for glucocorticoids inhibit calcium absorption and impair its renal tubular reabsorption.

Thyroid deficiency in infants (cretinism)

Long-standing hypothyroidism in early life results in retardation of both growth and maturation of the skeleton with severe dwarfing. The epiphyses may be irregular, deformed, and radiologically stippled.

Excess of thyroid hormone (thyrotoxicosis)

Prolonged hyperthyroidism may cause osteoporosis. There is an increase of both resorption and bone formation but resorption exceeds formation.

Miscellaneous Bone Conditions

Osteoporosis

In osteoporosis there is a decrease in the amount of bone tissue but the matrix is normally mineralised (Fig. 23.12). It may result from decreased bone formation, increased bone resorption or a combination of both. Osteo- porosis arises in a localised and a diffuse form following various unrelated disorders.

Disuse atrophy (immobilisation osteoporosis, disuse osteoporosis, localised osteoporosis)

Disuse atrophy is found in immobilised or paralysed limbs, e.g. following poliomyelitis or in

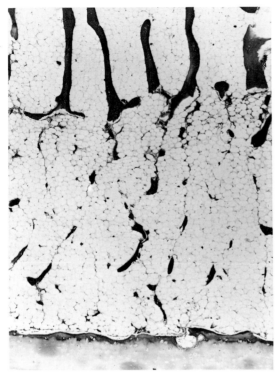

Fig. 23.21 Immobilisation osteoporosis. The articular surface is at the bottom of the picture. The subchondral trabeculae have almost completely disappeared and there is active osteoclasis spreading to involve the normal sized trabeculae above them. × 45.

the old courses of treatment for bone tuberculosis. It may be apparent within weeks and seems to be associated both with loss of muscle action and with loss of weight bearing. It is striking that in even the most severely affected bones cancellous trabeculae remain prominent along lines of stress. The bones become increasingly radiolucent; the trabeculae of spongy bone are scantier and more slender; the cortical bone becomes thinner and more porous due chiefly to opening up of Haversian spaces on the endosteal surface, so-called *cancellisation*. The changes of osteoporosis may be patchy and are usually first recognised radiologically in cancellous bone especially that in the metaphysis and subchondral articular regions, probably because bone turnover is more rapid in these sites. Focal radiological bone changes due to osteoporosis may be mistaken for extension of the local disease responsible for disuse.

An initial increase in resorption is thought to cause the porosis (Fig. 23.21) but later bone deposition and resorption may return to equilibrium. Once muscle activity is resumed there is an increase in bone production and especially in children the bone slowly returns to normal. Occasionally permanent deformity results from *premature epiphyseal fusion* in children. In the initial stage generalised immobilisation may lead to as much as 4% loss of bone mass/month and be complicated by hypercalcaemia and the formation of renal calculi. Similar osteoporosis occurs in astronauts, due to the reduced muscle force applied to bone in the weightless state.

Generalised osteoporosis

Only a small proportion of people with osteoporosis suffer from scurvy, osteogenesis imperfecta or known endocrine abnormalities such as Cushing's syndrome (p. 26.32), thyrotoxicosis or hypogonadism. There is a much larger group of post-menopausal women and elderly men who have generalised bone atrophy causing vertebral collapse and a tendency to fracture. It is known that skeletal mass diminishes in both men and women from the third decade onwards and osteoporosis of the elderly may be regarded as an exaggeration of this age-related bone loss though the cause is uncertain. The increased incidence of osteoporosis after the female menopause and the association of oophorectomy with osteoporosis in younger women suggest that lack of oestrogens plays a part in some cases. In these younger women the bone loss may be prevented by continuing postoperative oestrogen therapy. The possible risk of inducing endometrial cancer, though reduced by the addition of progesterone, prevents the long-term prophylactic use of hormones in all postmenopausal women. Increased effect of parathyroid hormone, longstanding mild negative calcium balance, and relatively slender bones in young adult life are amongst the suggested possible factors. Whatever the cause of osteoporosis of the elderly, and probably many factors contribute to it, bone is lost and not replaced. Search should be made for any treatable hormonal factors, diet should contain adequate amounts of calcium, protein and vitamins D and C and the patient be encouraged to remain as active as possible.

The structural changes of osteoporosis, whether they arise in association with known

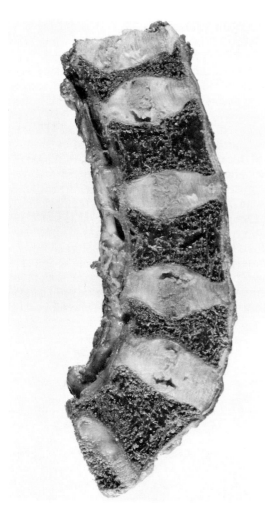

Fig. 23.22 The lumbar spine of this 74-year-old with severe osteoporosis shows bulging of the intervertebral discs and collapse of the vertebral bodies of L1 and L4.

endocrine disorders or with ageing, are essentially the same. Vertebral changes (Fig. 23.22) may be particularly striking with bulging of the intervertebral disc through the weakened end plate (Schmorl's nodes), increased concavity of the vertebrae, collapse with wedging, or less commonly uniform flattening (vertebra plana). These changes cause loss of height, development of a thoracic hump or lumbar lordosis, and the compression fractures are frequently accompanied by pain. There is also a tendency to fracture of long bones from trivial injury, especially at the femoral neck, wrist and upper humerus and for the production of cough fractures in the ribs. The blood calcium, phosphate and alkaline phosphatase levels are usually normal. Bone biopsy may be necessary to exclude osteomalacia, osteitis fibrosa, myelomatosis or carcinomatosis before attributing radiological decreased vertebral density or collapse to osteoporosis.

Paget's disease of bone (Osteitis deformans)

This condition was first described by Sir James Paget in 1877. It was for many years confused with the osteitis fibrosa of hyperparathyroidism. Paget's disease, however, is not a generalised metabolic disorder but a chronic bone dystrophy and the blood biochemistry is usually normal apart from a raised alkaline phosphatase level, indicating increased osteoblastic activity. Urinary hydroxyproline, a measure of collagen breakdown, is increased in parallel with the alkaline phosphatase. The demonstration of paramyxovirus-like particles in the osteoclasts in Paget's disease suggests that there may be an associated slow-virus infection, but infective virus has not been isolated. The condition is commoner in men than women and usually appears after the age of 40.

Sites of occurrence. The lumbar vertebrae and sacrum, skull and pelvis are the most frequently affected bones, though limb bones may also be involved. In about 10% of cases only a single bone, often a vertebra, or even a part of a bone, is involved. The condition may be widespread but is always multifocal and not diffuse (cf. osteitis fibrosa).

Incidence. The condition is almost unknown in Scandinavia and Japan but in Germany and Britain autopsy series show Paget's disease in about 3% of patients over 40 years of age. In only 5% or 10% of these does the disease give rise to symptoms such as bone pain, tenderness, bowing of the lower limbs or increase in skull size.

Macroscopic appearances. In the long bones, the shafts become thickened both subperiosteally and endosteally, so that the bone is enlarged and the medullary cavity is diminished. The femur and the tibia often show forward bowing and the neck of the femur becomes set more nearly at a right angle to the shaft (*coxa vara*). X-rays may reveal cystic spaces and stress

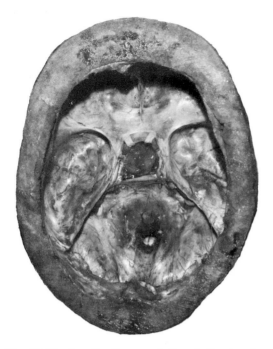

plump osteoblasts without there being any defect in mineralisation. To begin with, bone resorption is most marked and the bone is lighter than normal with a consequent tendency to fracture and bowing deformities. Later resorption decreases and the trabeculae are often thickened with the formation of a *mosaic* or *jigsaw pattern* of irregular cement lines indicating numerous previous phases of resorption and reconstruction (Fig. 23.25). At this stage the bone may be heavier than normal but because of the destruction of the cortical Haversian systems it remains structurally weaker.

Complications. (1) The weakened bones are liable to *fracture*, which in the long bones is often transverse and may be preceded by a stress fracture on the convex surface. There may occasionally be sequelae such as cord compression due rarely to vertebral collapse or more often to bony overgrowth with narrowing

Fig. 23.23 Paget's disease of the skull, showing enormous thickening of the calvarium with loss of distinction of the tables. The sella turcica is much enlarged owing to the fortuitous presence of a chromophobe adenoma of the pituitary.

fractures. The skull enlarges and the calvarium may be three or four times thicker than normal (Fig. 23.23). The distinction between diploë and the tables is gradually lost (Fig. 23.24), and the whole bone becomes fairly uniformly porous and so soft that it may be cut with a knife. (The form of localised rarefaction of the skull known as *osteoporosis circumscripta* is an early stage of Paget's disease.) Similar but less severe changes may be present in the bones of the face. When the vertebrae are involved they tend to collapse anteriorly so that a dorsal kyphus forms and the patient may come to have a crouching stance.

Microscopic appearances. There is simultaneous irregular resorption and regeneration of bone, with fibrosis and greatly increased vascularity of the intertrabecular marrow. In the early stage the picture is often one of intense activity, large osteoclasts and also osteoblasts being abundant, and it may be difficult to distinguish from osteitis fibrosa. Due to the rapidity with which new matrix is laid down some bone is woven rather than lamellar, and osteoid borders may be seen beneath a covering of

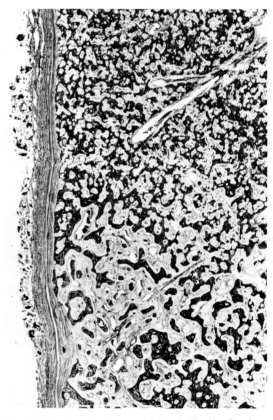

Fig. 23.24 Paget's disease of the skull, showing loss of distinction between the table and the diploë and the variable density of the bone. The marrow is fibrous and highly vascular. × 7·5.

of the vertebral canal. Cranial nerves may be compressed and deafness is a common symptom.

(2) *Osteoarthritis* (p. 23.49) may result from unusual stress on joints caused by the bone deformities.

(3) *High output cardiac failure* may occur when the disease is extensive and there is greatly increased blood flow through the affected bones and the overlying skin.

(4) In Paget's disease there is a thirtyfold increase in the risk of developing *bone sarcoma* in one or more affected bones. The humerus is affected disproportionately often and vertebrae surprisingly seldom. Progressive localised pain should arouse the suspicion of malignant change. The tumours are almost invariably osteolytic and may be osteosarcomas, fibrosarcomas or occasionally chondrosarcomas, often very pleomorphic and with numerous tumour giant cells. The prognosis is very bad because of early pulmonary metastases. Occasionally a giant cell tumour (with a good prognosis) develops especially in the jaw, face or skull.

Fibrous dysplasia

Fibrous dysplasia is a benign fibro-osseous abnormality of bone of unknown aetiology. It is sometimes monostotic, less commonly polyostotic and rarely the polyostotic form is associated with patchy skin pigmentation and precocious sexual development (*Albright's syndrome*). In monostotic cases the lesions are commonly found in a rib (often symptomless), the jaw, femur or tibia, though any bone may be involved. Deformity and exophthalmos may occur when the maxilla or facial bones are affected. In polyostotic cases the femur and tibia are most frequently affected along with various other bones and often the condition is almost but not entirely unilateral. The lesions appear in childhood and new foci may develop even after puberty. When many bones are affected early in life the condition tends to progress with increasing deformity and multiple fractures. Malignant change is very rare.

Macroscopic appearances. The normal bone is sharply demarcated from the whitish, gritty fibrous tissue, often containing cysts and small nodules of cartilage, which expands the bone. The epiphyses of long bones tend to be spared. The typical focus of fibrous dysplasia shows a ground-glass, finely mottled appearance on x-ray and can sometimes be cut with a knife, but lesions in the skull and jaw tend to be more densely bony and indeed often appear radiologically as areas of increased density.

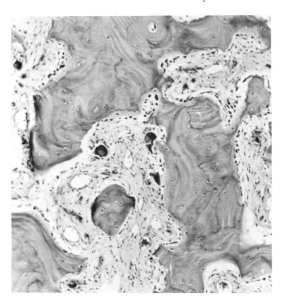

Fig. 23.25 Paget's disease of the femur, showing the typical mosaic structure of the bone, with both active osteoclastic resorption and osteoblastic formation. (Professor J. B. Gibson.) × 90.

Microscopic appearances. There is a loose, small spindle-celled fibrous stroma in which curving and 'lobster-claw' trabeculae of non-lamellar woven bone (Fig. 23.26), apparently devoid of osteoblasts, are scattered. These trabeculae are characteristic and

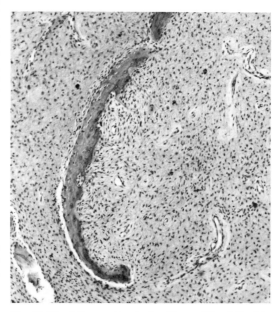

Fig. 23.26 Fibrous dysplasia of bone. The delicately cellular fibrous tissue contains a thin trabecula of woven bone. × 75.

repeated biopsy has shown that they fail to mature to lamellar bone. Groups of osteoclasts and occasional nodules of cartilage may be present.

Eosinophil granuloma

This rare lesion may occur at any age or in any bone but most often presents in childhood or young adult life as one or more lytic lesions involving skull, long bones, vertebra or pelvis. Microscopically the lesions consist of foci of eosinophils and of pale staining Langerhan's cells (probably members of the mononuclear phagocyte system—p. 4.36). There is often a scattering of lymphocytes, plasma cells and neutrophil polymorphs and sometimes Touton-type giant cells. Occasionally there may be difficulty in the differential diagnosis from osteomyelitis or malignant lymphoma. As the lesion ages, foamy lipid-containing macrophages (xanthoma cells) and fibrosis increase with eventual spontaneous healing. Currettage or low doses of radiotherapy are only needed when pain is persistent or pathological fracture seems imminent. In about 10% of patients further bone lesions develop, usually within a few months. The chief concern is whether the bone lesion is the presenting symptom of the Hand-Schüller-Christian syndrome (p. 18.15). However if at the time of diagnosis careful clinical search fails to reveal extraskeletal involvement it is unlikely to develop later.

Digital clubbing and hypertrophic osteoarthropathy

Clubbing of the distal phalanges of the fingers and less commonly the toes is characterised by thickening of the soft tissues with widening of the terminal phalanges; the nails are raised, curved and lose their normal angulation with the cuticle. Clubbing is thought to result from local vascular engorgement and is most often associated with chronic lung disease, bronchial carcinoma or mesothelioma.

Patients with **hypertrophic osteoarthropathy** develop, in addition to finger clubbing, a symmetrical periostitis with subperiosteal new bone formation. This extends proximally from the distal shaft of tibia and fibula and/or forearm bones. There may be a mild arthritis. Hypertrophic osteoarthropathy is almost always a complication of intrathoracic tumour; it may appear early in the course of the disease and disappear after surgical resection of the tumour. Its cause is not known but it may be relieved by vagotomy.

Generalised Developmental Abnormalities of Bone

Osteopetrosis, marble-bone disease (*Albers–Schönberg disease*) is characterised by excessive density of all the bones with obliteration of the marrow cavities and development of leuco-erythroblastic anaemia. It is associated with failure of resorption of the cartilaginous spongiosa and of bone remodelling apparently due to defective osteoclast function. In a few patients matched sibling marrow transplants have been successful in promoting resorption by donor osteoclasts.

Involvement of the skull leads to narrowing of the foramina with deafness and impairment of vision. In spite of their increased density the bones are brittle and fractures occur from slight violence. The disease is transmitted in a severe form as an autosomal recessive character and in a relatively benign form as an autosomal dominant.

Osteogenesis imperfecta (OI) (the brittle bone syndrome) is a hereditary disease of varying severity and some heterogeneity, characterised by osteoporotic bones which are more liable to fracture. The fractures heal readily, occasionally with a mass of hyperplastic callus but immobilisation increases porosis and the liability to further fracture. The defect lies in the formation of type I collagen, often of its $\alpha1$ (I) chain, and a variety of extraskeletal abnormalities including blue sclerae, lax ligaments, thin skin, early onset deafness, thin aortic valves, and brownish teeth due to poorly formed dentine may be found. Paradoxically involvement of extraskeletal tissues is most common in the 80% of patients with mild bone disease inherited as an autosomal dominant (Type I). Although these children have an increased incidence of fracture they do not become severely deformed or dwarfed. In contrast a small number of infants present at birth with many fresh or healing fractures, short limbs (Fig. 23.27) and marked bone deformity (Type II). These are usually sporadic mutations; a few are of recessive inheritance. The most severely affected infants die from intracranial haemorrhage resulting from the poor pro-

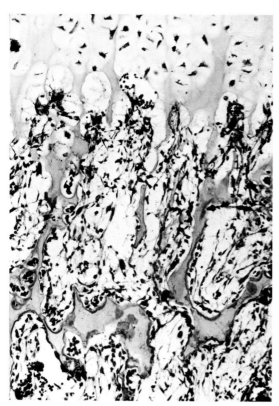

Fig. 23.27 Osteogenesis imperfecta showing numerous osteoblasts but little bone formation at the epiphyseal line. × 115.

tection offered by the almost unossified skull vault or from respiratory failure due to innumerable rib fractures. The few survivors join a heterogeneous group of severely affected infants and children who are of small stature with progressively worsening deformity (Type III). Many have normal sclerae as do a small group of severely affected children with a dominant inheritance (Type IV). It is expected that although this classification is imperfect it will be helpful in genetic counselling.

Pathological appearances. The shafts of the long bones are short and slender with thin cortices and little medullary bone while the epiphyses appear disproportionately broad. Bowing results from multiple fractures. The growth plate is often normal but sometimes disrupted and fragmented by trauma. Vertebrae may be biconcave or wedged due to compression fractures. The more severely affected the patient the higher the proportion of woven bone;

even when bone is very scanty osteoblasts appear plentiful. Lamellar bone is unusually cellular and the crowded osteocytes suggest that osteoblasts are producing less matrix than normal.

Achondroplasia. This remarkable condition, known also as *chondrodystrophia fetalis*, is due to failure of endochondral ossification. It is present at birth and may be diagnosed radiologically *in utero*. The head appears large, the forehead bulging and the root of the nose is indrawn or sunken; the limbs are short and stumpy, sometimes curved, and as there is more growth of the soft tissues than of the bones, the skin of the limbs is in folds. There are vertebral abnormalities with narrowing of the spinal canal in the lumbar region. Obesity is common, and sometimes there is some oedema. The hands are broad with fingers of equal length (trident hands). The characteristic changes depend on the failure of bone formation in cartilage. At the epiphyseal line, the cartilage cells form only short rows, or are irregularly arranged, and there is little or no ossification, hence the failure of growth. The cartilaginous epiphysis is sometimes considerably broadened, and with the small shaft presents a mushroom-like appearance; there may also be areas of softening in the cartilage. The indrawing of the nose results from a shortening of the base of the skull, due to imperfect ossification, sometimes accompanied by premature union of the basisphenoidal and sphenoidal sutures. In fact, all the bones ossified from cartilage are small, whilst intramembranous ossification proceeds normally. There are varying degrees of the condition, and 80% of affected infants are stillborn or die within the first year of life, usually of neurological complications such as hydrocephalus due to undue smallness of the skull base and posterior fossa. The less severely affected child may survive to adult life as a dwarf with short thick limbs, and a tendency to develop neurological problems. Achondroplasia is due to a dominant gene with a very high mutation rate; thus most cases are the result of a mutation in one or other parent, whose chance of producing a second affected child is no greater than that of other normal persons. Achondroplastic dwarfs with a normal spouse produce normal and affected children in equal numbers.

Multiple osteocartilaginous exostoses (*diaphyseal aclasis*) and **multiple enchondromatosis** (*Ollier's disease*) are discussed with benign cartilage tumours (pp. 23.31–32) and a brief account of the **mucopolysaccharidoses** on p. 11.9.

Tumours in Bone

Metastatic tumours in bone

Frequency. Metastatic tumours in bone are commoner than primary bone tumours and probably occur in as many as 70% of cases of disseminated malignant disease. Bone, along with lungs and liver, is the most frequent site of secondary spread. An accurate assessment of frequency depends on meticulous post-mortem study. The true incidence of vertebral metastases for instance is higher than suspected even from sophisticated radiological examinations.

Sites of occurrence. If metastases are present anywhere in the skeleton the vertebral column will almost certainly be affected, especially the thoracic or lumbar regions. Bony secondaries are commonly found in areas where haemopoietic marrow is normally present, i.e. the axial skeleton and the proximal ends of humerus and femur. Skeletal metastases are uncommon below the knee and very uncommon below the elbow. Tumour usually reaches the bone by arterial tumour-cell emboli but it has been suggested that retrograde spread along the vertebral venous plexus may account for the frequent involvement of lumbar vertebrae by tumours of the pelvic organs.

Common primary sites. Tumours which most often give rise to metastases in bone are carcinomas of breast, prostate, lung, kidney, thyroid, melanomas and, in young children, neuroblastomas.

Types of secondary tumours. Bone metastases are commonly *osteolytic* or destructive, and may result in pathological fracture. Thyroid or renal secondaries are highly vascular and may produce marked bone expansion. Resorption of bone trabeculae, especially in metastases from breast cancer, may be stimulated by prostaglandins produced by the carcinoma cells, while in myeloma the cells secrete an osteoclast-activating factor. Hypercalcemia may result from extensive bone destruction or from the production of ectopic parathormone-like peptides by the primary tumour, notably by squamous carcinoma of the bronchus and renal carcinoma.

Sometimes infiltration of the marrow by carcinoma stimulates marked osteogenesis (with a raised alkaline phosphatase). These *osteoplastic*

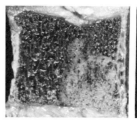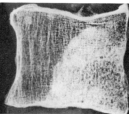

Fig. 23.28   The body of the lumbar vertebra is partially replaced by secondary prostatic carcinoma. The radiograph of a thin slice shows that this has provoked reactive bone sclerosis.

or *osteosclerotic* secondaries arise most commonly in association with prostatic carcinoma (Figs 23.28 and 29) but other cancers, e.g. of breast, lung, stomach and also lymphomas may infrequently give rise to the same picture. Sometimes both osteosclerotic and osteolytic secondaries are present in the same patient.

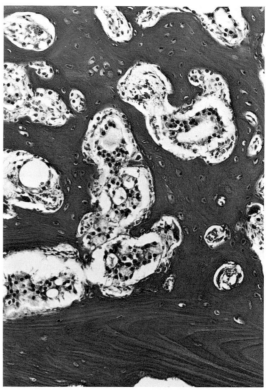

Fig. 23.29   Secondary prostatic carcinoma in bone with reactive new bone formation causing osteosclerosis. × 130.

Extensive osteosclerotic secondaries may cause a progressive anaemia which is often leuco-erythroblastic and associated with splenomegaly due to extramedullary haemopoiesis (p. 17.58).

Occasionally there is widespread diffuse marrow replacement with little bony change.

Solitary metastases. Metastatic tumours in bone sometimes present as solitary lesions and, while this is usually rapidly followed by the appearance of further secondaries, in a very occasional case of renal or thyroid carcinoma, the bony focus may remain the sole metastasis. Only very rarely is surgical resection of both primary and secondary tumour followed by worthwhile remission or by cure.

Primary tumours of bone

The precise diagnosis of bone tumours is sometimes very difficult and it is essential for the clinical and radiological features to be considered along with the naked-eye and microscopic appearances before a final decision is reached. Classification also is not easy, for in some the histogenesis is obscure and in others the very nature of the lesion is uncertain (see Table 23.1).

Classification. *Firstly,* it may be difficult to decide whether one is dealing with a true tumour or a developmental abnormality, e.g. multiple osteocartilaginous exostoses is clearly a hereditary condition and possibly solitary exostosis is a *forme fruste* of this, but, since exostoses, whether single or multiple, may pro-

Table 23.1 Classification of bone tumours

Derivation or type of tumour	Benign	Malignant
Fibrous tissue	Non-ossifying fibroma Desmoplastic fibroma	Fibrosarcoma
Cartilage	Osteocartilaginous exostosis ⟶ Enchondroma ⟶ Benign chondroblastoma Chondromyxoid fibroma	Chondrosarcoma
Bone	Osteoma Osteoid osteoma Benign osteoblastoma	Osteosarcoma (including some Paget's and post-irradiation sarcomas) Parosteal and periosteal osteosarcoma
Unknown	Giant-cell tumour ⟶	Giant-cell tumour Ewing's tumour Malignant fibrous histiocytoma 'Adamantinoma' of long bones
Vascular tissue	Haemangioma Glomus tumour	Haemangioendothelioma Angiosarcoma
Fat cells	Lipoma	Liposarcoma
Haemopoietic	Solitary plasmacytoma ⟶	Myelomatosis Malignant lymphoma
Neural tissue	Schwannoma and neurofibroma ⟶	Neurofibrosarcoma (Malignant schwannoma)
Notochordal tissue		Chordoma

The arrows indicate that these benign lesions may progress to malignancy

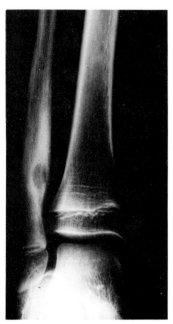

Fig. 23.30 An osteoid osteoma has given rise to an ovoid translucency in the lower end of the fibula. There is a little surrounding reactive bone sclerosis.

gress to malignancy, they are discussed in this section. *Secondly*, in many cases, although the tumour has a distinctive histological appearance, its histogenesis is uncertain; even osteosarcoma is best regarded as a tumour which produces bone or osteoid rather than one which arises from osteoblasts. The number of malignant mesenchymal tissues which may be found in an osteosarcoma points to its origin from a more primitive cell and serves as a reminder that the mesenchymal cell is capable of differentiation in different directions. In spite of these difficulties a classification is worthwhile because when it can be applied to a given tumour it usually helps to indicate its likely behaviour.

In this section certain rare lesions are not discussed but they have been included in the table for the sake of completeness. Lesions of doubtful origin and non-neoplastic lesions simulating bone tumours have been mentioned in relation to the tumours with which they may be confused.

Osteoma

This term is now restricted to rare bony outgrowths of skull bones which sometimes protrude into the orbit or paranasal sinuses. These lesions may be formed of osteoblastic connective tissue and woven bone trabeculae, of extremely dense compact lamellar bone or of a mixture of these components. They are benign but may cause pressure symptoms.

Osteoid osteoma

This is a benign osteoblastic lesion which is usually of less than 1 cm diameter. It occurs chiefly in the long bones of the lower limbs of adolescents or young adults although any bone and age may be affected. The clinical history is of increasingly severe and unusually well-localised pain and tenderness, often relieved by salicylates. Symptoms may be present for some months before the lesion becomes apparent radiologically as a rounded zone of radiolucency (Fig. 23.30). If cortical, there is often massive thickening of the surrounding bone whereas in cancellous bone sclerosis may be minimal. Radio-isotope bone scans which show the osteoid osteoma as a 'hot-spot' are helpful in localisation. Macroscopically, osteoid osteoma is usually a red nodule and microscopic examination shows a very vascular nidus of osteoblastic tissue with formation of many irregular small trabeculae of osteoid or bone undergoing active remodelling (Fig. 23.31). Sometimes the central part of the nidus is more compact. If incompletely removed, symptoms may recur.

Osteosarcoma (osteogenic sarcoma)

Osteosarcoma is a malignant tumour in which osteoid or bone is formed directly by sarcoma cells and is thought to arise from cells of the primitive bone-forming mesenchyme. Apart from myeloma it is the commonest primary malignant bone tumour and occurs more frequently in males than females. About 150 new cases of osteosarcoma are seen every year in the UK.

Age incidence. Osteosarcoma is rare under the age of 5 years and about 75% of patients are between 10 and 25 years old. In more than half of the patients over 40 years old the tumour complicates Paget's disease of bone. Some tumours follow radiation.

Sites of occurrence. Most osteosarcomas arise in the metaphysis of long bones: about half occur around the knee and many others at the upper end of femur and humerus. The tumour

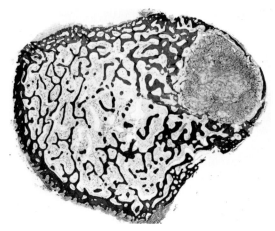

Fig. 23.31 A transverse section of the fibula shows that the small bone trabeculae of the osteoid osteoma have replaced cortical and medullary bone and stimulated slight surrounding reactive sclerosis. × 6.

sometimes occurs in vertebrae, pelvis and skull, especially when associated with Paget's disease but is very uncommon in the small bones of the hands and feet. Multicentric tumours may occur especially in Paget's disease.

Clinical features. Patients often give a fairly short history of increasingly severe pain, worse at night, and this may be followed by swelling, oedema, local heat and dilated subcutaneous veins. Pathological fracture is relatively rare. The serum alkaline phosphatase may be raised. The patient is usually in good general health; if not, the presence of metastases should be suspected.

Radiological and macroscopic appearances. Osteosarcoma commonly arises in the medullary bone in the region of the metaphysis or diaphysis. The epiphyseal cartilage plate may act as a barrier for a while but in about 75% of cases the tumour spreads to the epiphysis. The joint cavity is seldom involved. Osteosarcoma may spread quite rapidly through the bony cortex, without either completely destroying or markedly expanding it, and form a subperiosteal mass (Fig. 23.32) which, in its turn, may burst through the periosteum and infiltrate muscles. When the periosteum is raised spicules of new bone are laid down at right angles to the bone shaft (Fig. 23.33) giving rise radiologically to 'sunray spiculation'. At the junction between raised and normal periosteum, Codman's triangle of reactive bone develops. Neither of these appearances is present in all

cases of osteosarcoma, nor when present are they specific for osteosarcoma; the same appearances may be seen in metastatic carcinoma or even sometimes in infections. Biopsy material should not be taken from an area where reactive bone formation is active as this may increase the difficulty of diagnosis. As well as spread outside the bone, the tumour extends within it, sometimes further than is suspected radiologically, and occasionally separate 'skip' nodules are found proximal or distal to the main tumour. The gross appearances vary according to the amount of tumour osteoid and bone which has been formed. Some tumours contain little bony matrix (*osteolytic*) and these tend to be soft, friable, vascular destructive

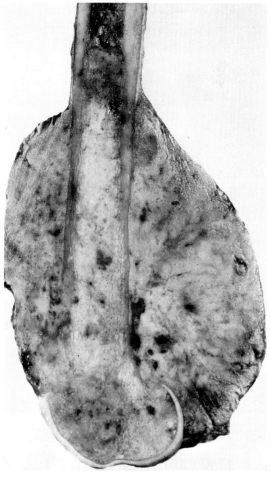

Fig. 23.32 Osteosarcoma of lower end of femur. The medullary tumour has penetrated and partly destroyed the cortex, spreading outwards to form a large subperiosteal mass.

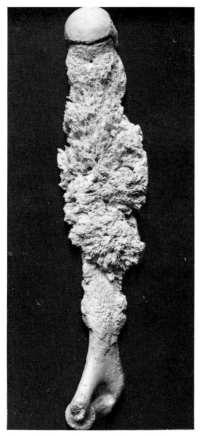

Fig. 23.33 Osteosarcoma of humerus. Macerated specimen to show the characteristic spiculation on the surface of the bone.

lesions with areas of haemorrhage and necrosis. Others may contain much tumour bone (*osteosclerotic*) especially in their central areas: they are dense and of turnip-like consistency in their softer parts. The amount of tumour bone is not related to the age of the tumour nor does it appear to affect the prognosis.

Microscopic appearances. The essential criteria for the diagnosis of osteosarcoma are the presence of frankly sarcomatous malignant cells and the direct formation of tumour osteoid or bone from them. The histological pattern of osteosarcoma is, however, very variable. In addition to tumour bone, some osteosarcomas contain a large amount of cartilage and others much malignant spindle-celled fibrosarcomatous tissue. In the osteolytic type of osteosarcoma the tumour often contains pleomorphic and giant tumour cells with many aberrant mitoses and irregular vascular channels lined by tumour cells (Fig. 23.34). By contrast in the osteosclerotic type, such a mass of tumour bone may be laid down on and between pre-existing trabeculae that malignant cells within the mass of matrix are small and scanty except at the growing edge. Osteosarcomas in Paget's disease are almost invariably of the osteolytic type (Fig. 23.35) and are characterised by their extreme pleomorphism with large numbers of tumour giant cells and numerous osteoclasts.

Metastatic spread. As in most sarcomas spread of the tumour is almost invariably by the blood-stream to the lungs and sometimes to other bones and viscera, lymph node metastases being unusual. Pulmonary metastases occur early and are often believed to have arisen before the patient appears for treatment although at that time they may not be visible radiologically. The five-year survival in osteosarcomas treated by surgery alone is around 30–40%. A rather better prognosis has been reported in young adults and in tumours of the distal skeleton or jaws. Repeated courses of cytotoxic drugs and various forms of immunotherapy are currently being assessed. Osteosarcomas arising

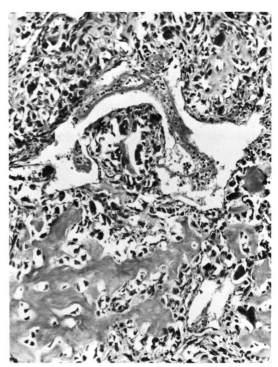

Fig. 23.34 Osteosarcoma. A highly vascular, cellular tumour with osteoid formation well seen in the lower part of the field. × 200.

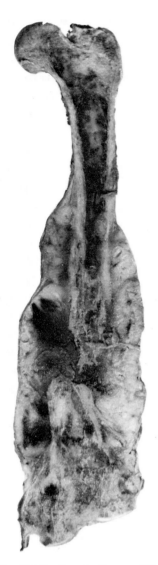

Fig. 23.35 Paget's disease of femur showing a large osteolytic osteosarcoma with pathological fracture.

in Paget's disease have a worse prognosis than those arising *de novo*. In contrast to chondrosarcoma (p. 23.34), local recurrence or seeding of the tumour in the wound is unusual.

Parosteal (juxtacortical) osteosarcoma. This is a rare tumour but worth distinguishing since it has a much better prognosis than medullary osteosarcoma. In most of the reported cases the tumour is metaphyseal and has arisen on the posterior surface of the lower femur or on the upper tibia or humerus. It forms a broad-based swelling arising initially on the surface of the bone and sometimes growing to encircle the shaft, cortical penetration and medullary infiltration being late. Microscopically the tumour usually consists of well-formed bony trabeculae separated by atypical spindle cells; sometimes near the surface the bone is less well formed and there may also be islands of cartilage. The tumour grows slowly and tends to occur in a wider age group than classical osteosarcoma. If the lesion is inadequately dealt with it may recur or become frankly malignant and metastasise, sometimes within two years, sometimes not for twenty years. If it is treated by radical surgery initially the outlook is usually good though this does not apply to the few classical osteosarcomas that present as parosteal tumours.

Periosteal osteosarcomas have a prognosis intermediate between conventional medullary and parosteal tumours. They are relatively small spiculated tumours arising chiefly on the shaft of tibia or femur in young people and contain much cartilage.

Benign cartilage tumours

Osteocartilaginous exostosis (osteochondroma, ecchondroma) is the commonest benign tumour of bone and consists of a bony excrescence. Its outer shell and medulla are continuous with that of the bone from which it arises and it is covered by a proliferating cartilage cap which undergoes endochondral ossification (Fig. 23.36). The lesion may be single or multiple; when multiple the condition is familial and may be associated with some failure of bone remodelling (*hereditary multiple exostoses, diaphyseal aclasis*). Exostoses may arise in any bone formed by endochondral ossification but the metaphyses of long bones, especially the femur, humerus and tibia, are the commonest sites. The lesions are usually first noticed in childhood and adolescence and growth commonly ceases in adult life, the cartilaginous cap sometimes completely disappearing. Malignant change is rare in solitary exostoses but probably about 10% of hospital patients with multiple lesions develop chondrosarcoma, usually in adult life. Exostoses of the axial skeleton or proximal limb bones are much more likely to become malignant than those in the peripheral skeleton (see chondrosarcoma for discussion). So-called *subungual exostosis*, which is often painful, is not an exactly comparable lesion. It arises often following infection or trauma as a result of cartilaginous and osseous metaplasia of the fibrous tissue around the terminal part of the distal phalanx.

Enchondroma is a benign cartilage tumour arising within the medullary cavity, most commonly of the small bones of the hands and feet

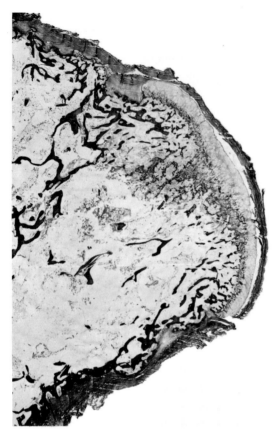

Fig. 23.36 Osteocartilaginous exostosis of humerus consisting of cancellous bone covered by cartilage and perichondrium. Endochondral ossification is occurring. × 8·5.

(Fig. 23.37). The cartilage tumours may be single or multiple and when multiple are thought to arise as a failure of normal endochondral ossification (*multiple enchondromatosis*). In multiple enchondromatosis the hands are almost invariably involved but there may also be lesions in long tubular bones associated with bowing and deformity, especially of the forearm. When the enchondromas are predominantly unilateral the condition is sometimes referred to as *Ollier's disease*. Solitary benign enchondroma may also occur in long tubular bones, particularly the humerus and femur. The tumour arises initially in the metaphysis and may spread into the shaft or occasionally into the bone end if the cartilage plate is closed. Radiologically the lesions are radiolucent, sometimes with spotty calcification and naked-eye examination of an enchondroma shows lobules of bluish-grey cartilage which is often more

gelatinous than normal. Microscopic examination of the benign lesion shows small uniform cells with small and few double nuclei (Fig. 23.38). The lesions of the phalanges and metacarpals, especially in multiple enchondromas, may be unusually cellular without there being any sinister prognostic significance. The common clinical complaints, particularly in the phalangeal lesions, are of swelling or pathological fracture. Malignant transformation in cases of solitary enchondroma is probably rare but about a third of hospital patients with multiple enchondromatosis develop chondrosarcoma. Pain unassociated with fracture, or the onset of enlargement in an enchondroma of the axial skeleton or long tubular bones in an adult should immediately raise the suspicion of malignant change.

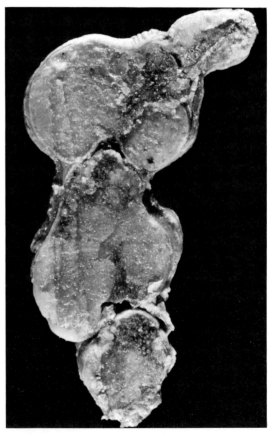

Fig. 23.37 Benign enchondromas of finger. The finger has been amputated just proximal to the metacarpal head. While the joint spaces remain intact each phalanx is replaced by a mass of hyaline cartilage. The cortices have disappeared but periosteum still surrounds the cartilage.

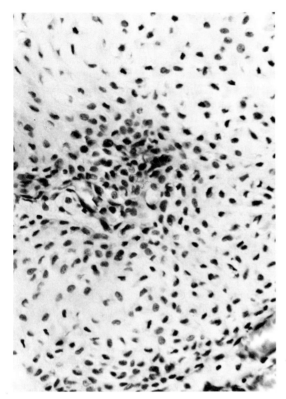

Fig. 23.38 Benign enchondroma from finger in multiple enchondromatosis. The cartilage is highly cellular but the cells are mononuclear and fairly uniform in size. × 250.

Periosteal chondromas usually arise on the metaphyseal surface of tubular bones and cause scalloping of the underlying cortex. Mild degrees of nuclear atypia and binucleate cells do not indicate malignancy.

Chondrosarcoma

Chondrosarcoma is a malignant cartilage tumour and may arise *de novo* or, in about 10% of cases, from a pre-existing benign cartilage tumour. It may be situated within the bone (central) or outwith it (peripheral). The tumour is slightly less common than osteosarcoma and is twice as common in males as in females. In contrast to osteosarcoma, chondrosarcoma is rare under the age of 30 years and most patients are in the 40–70 age group.

Sites of occurrence. About half the lesions arise in the pelvic girdle (Fig. 23.39) and ribs; the proximal femur is another common site. A careful watch should therefore be kept on all cartilage tumours of the axial skeleton, particularly in adults, and increase in size and pain should arouse the suspicion of malignancy. The incidence of malignant change is lower in chondromas of the distal part of the skeleton and is very rare in those of the bones of the hands and feet except for the os calcis and talus.

Macroscopic appearances. *Central tumours.* A central cartilage tumour usually causes slight bone expansion and in slowly growing tumours there is often buttressing of the cortex in response to endosteal erosion. In some cases, the cortex is broken through and the tumour is found growing in the adjacent soft tissue. Sometimes, particularly in large tumours which are especially prone to arise in pelvis and ribs, the exact site of origin becomes difficult to identify and the lobulated tumour is soft, slimy and cystic due to mucoid degeneration of the matrix. Spotty calcification may be present and is sometimes extensive, an aid in the radiological diagnosis of these tumours.

Peripheral tumours may arise *de novo* or from previously existing osteocartilaginous exostoses; the cartilage caps are then much thickened and in the early stages the normally smooth surface may be covered with little

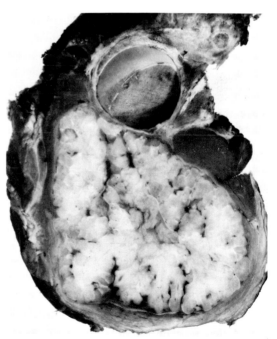

Fig. 23.39 Low-grade chondrosarcoma of pelvis showing the large cartilaginous tumour arising from the ilium.

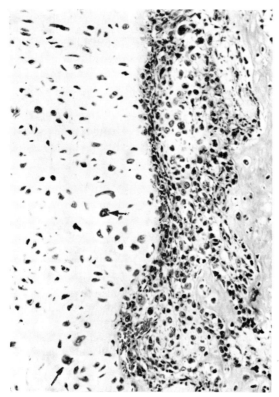

Fig. 23.40   Metastasising chondrosarcoma of ilium. The cartilage cells vary greatly in size and there are several mitoses, two of which are arrowed. × 100.

nodules of proliferating cartilage. Later these tumours may become very large and undergo heavy calcification or myxoid degeneration.

Microscopic appearances. If the cells in a cartilage tumour are pleomorphic and there are abundant multinucleated tumour cells and moderate numbers of mitotic figures, the recognition of malignancy is easy (Fig. 23.40). In slowly growing tumours, however, it may be difficult unless there is an infiltrative growth pattern with sheets of tumour filling the marrow spaces between the preserved meshwork of pre-existing bone trabeculae. The generally accepted criteria of malignancy are the presence, even in only scattered areas, of many chondrocytes with plump nuclei and of moderate numbers of chondrocytes with two or more nuclei (Fig. 23.41). Failure to detect mitoses does not necessarily indicate that the tumour is benign. The best opportunity of assessing the tumour's likely behaviour is in studying material from the growing edge and every scrap of biopsy tissue must be examined micro-

scopically. Biopsies from heavily calcified or degenerate cartilage are useless. Because of variations in histological malignancy in different parts of the same tumour a microscopic diagnosis of chondroma should be viewed with suspicion if clinical and radiological features suggest malignant change. It is particularly important in this tumour that the pathologist should be aware of the *age* of the patient and the *site* of the tumour. Minor changes from normality are much more alarming in cartilage tumours of the axial skeleton, where recurrences may not be resectable, but experience shows they may be largely discounted in growing cartilage tumours in children, in lesions of the small tubular bones and of the soft tissues of the hands and feet, in subperiosteal cartilage tumours and in synovial chondromatosis (p. 23.53).

Implantation. Cartilage cells have low nutritional requirements and this may explain their

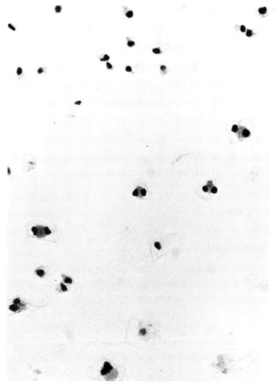

Fig. 23.41   This recurrent low grade chondrosarcoma of pelvis killed the patient by local spread without metastases. The cartilage matrix is well formed and the tumour is not very cellular but there are numerous foci of chondrocytes with plump double nuclei. × 250.

special tendency to implant and grow in soft tissues. This has great practical importance to the surgeon as it means that the site of biopsy must be carefully planned in a suspected case so that the whole of the tissue planes opened up may be excised at the time of definitive treatment. There is a very marked tendency to local recurrence after excision even when the original operation appeared to be clear of the tumour. In order to prevent this in sites where removal of a recurrent tumour would be difficult, such as chest wall or pelvis, a radical operation is often necessary in the first instance.

Course of the disease and prognosis. Chondrosarcoma, in contrast to osteosarcoma, runs a more prolonged course. The patients have often some years' history when they first come to hospital. Excision may be followed by local recurrences which may grow slowly for many years before the patient is finally killed by local involvement of some vital structure. Pulmonary metastases are a less common cause of death. These are tumours which respond most successfully to radical treatment in the first instance where this is surgically feasible. The 15% or so of more malignant, rapidly-growing and metastasising chondrosarcomas may lead to death within a few years but even they may persist for a surprisingly long time. About 10% of low grade chondrosarcomas are associated with, and overrun by, an anaplastic rapidly metastasising sarcoma such as fibrosarcoma, malignant fibrous histiocytoma or osteosarcoma. Chondrosarcoma metastasises by blood spread, frequently to the lungs and has a tendency to direct retrograde spread along veins. Lymph node metastases are rare. In the past the prognosis has been poor, partly as a result of the pathologist's under-diagnosis of the lesion and partly from inadequate initial treatment. However, with adequate surgery more than half the patients should be cured.

Chondromyxoid fibroma of bone

This is a rare benign tumour of bone, important only because of its tendency to be misdiagnosed as chondrosarcoma. It occurs chiefly in the metaphyses of long bones of adolescents and young adults, especially in the lower limb. It usually gives rise to a sharply defined, eccentric, osteolytic defect which bulges the periosteum. The tumour is commonly rather firm and rubbery and on naked-eye examination lacks the gelatinous, slimy features that one

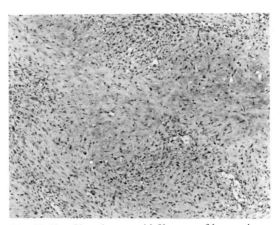

Fig. 23.42 Chondromyxoid fibroma of bone, showing the loose spindle-celled tissue with imperfectly formed cartilage divided into pseudolobules by strands of aggregated cells. × 60.

would expect from the histology. Microscopy shows relatively poorly cellular tissue separated into pseudolobules by curving strands or trabeculae of aggregated cells (Fig. 23.42). The cells of the lobules are spindle-shaped or stellate and lie in a myxomatous vacuolated matrix. The trabecular cells are similar but may show some hyperchromatism, pleomorphism and occasional mitotic figures—features which may lead to misdiagnosis of malignancy. Osteoclasts may also be seen especially at the margins of the pseudolobules. The tumour is benign, and though it may recur, is usually cured by curettage.

Fibrosarcoma

This is a rare malignant tumour which may arise within the medullary cavity (endosteal) or beneath the periosteum (periosteal), usually in adults. **Endosteal fibrosarcoma** affects especially the bones around the knee, though sometimes other sites. In long bones it commonly involves the metaphysis and sometimes the shaft. The tumour in general is osteolytic, and may break through the cortex and into the soft tissues. In parts, however, it tends to infiltrate between pre-existing medullary bone trabeculae without destroying them and sometimes stimulates new bone formation on their surfaces. This gives rise radiologically to a moth-eaten appearance of the bone with irregular areas of translucency and sclerosis. The extent of radiological destruction may thus not indicate the true extent of tumour spread in the medulla. Multiple bones may be involved when the patient is first examined. Microscopically, fibrosarcoma varies from a fasciculated spindle-celled tumour producing much collagen in its more mature parts, to a more cellular tumour with little recognisable fibrous tissue. When present in the same tumour such variations can be misleading. Differentiation histologically from metastatic spindle-celled renal or squamous carcinoma, or from malignant melanoma, may be difficult.

The 5-year survival rate is around 28% though a few patients develop metastases later. In some series prognosis has been linked to the degree of differentiation of the sarcoma.

Malignant fibrous histiocytoma (MFH) of bone

This has been recognised as a soft tissue tumour for many years but only quite recently has it been reported in bone most being formerly diagnosed as pleomorphic fibrosarcomas or osteosarcomas with scanty or dubious tumour bone formation. MFH of bone is rare with a wide age range, and usually presents as an irregular lytic lesion in the metaphysis of a long bone. It may arise in association with long-standing bone necrosis, following irradiation or in Paget's disease. The patient may present with pain, swelling, or a pathological fracture and sometimes there is already a large subperiosteal soft tissue extension.

The histological features are varied. There may be multinucleated tumour giant cells, often with bulky eosinophilic cytoplasm, osteoclast-like giant cells, mononuclear histiocytic tumour cells with folded nuclei (Fig. 23.68), foci of lipid-containing macrophages with Touton-type giant cells, aggregates of chronic inflammatory cells (chiefly lymphocytes) and short fascicles of collagen and fibroblasts radiating from an ill-defined centre producing the so-called cartwheel or storiform pattern. Because of this wide range of features there is a tendency to diagnose any pleomorphic sarcoma as MFH and it is not surprising that there is difficulty in assessing the likely behaviour in an individual case.

Ewing's tumour

In 1921 Ewing described a primary malignant tumour of bone under the name of diffuse endothelioma and since its histogenesis remains uncertain the eponymous title is retained.

Age and sex incidence. Ewing's tumour is rare over the age of 30, and most common between the ages of 5 and 20 years; it is very rare in the first two years of life. Males are slightly more often affected.

Sites of occurrence. The long tubular bones are most frequently involved, e.g. femur, tibia, humerus and fibula but the pelvis and ribs are also affected.

Macroscopic appearances. The tumour appears to originate within the medullary cavity

and in long bones may involve the metaphysis and permeate much of the shaft. It is usually osteolytic and penetration of the cortex with raising of the periosteum and formation of an extraosseous mass may occur early. This subperiosteal elevation may give rise to parallel layers of reactive new bone (onion skin appearance) and less frequently to strands of bone forming at right angles to the cortex (sunray spiculation).

The tumour is usually whitish; some are rather firm while others are very soft, almost puriform.

Microscopic appearances. Ewing's tumour is composed of fairly uniform rounded or polyhedral cells, often with pale nuclei due to the fine dispersion of chromatin. The cell boundaries are indistinct and the cells are arranged in syncytial sheets (Fig. 23.43) without a lobular pattern but divided by broad strands of collagen. Reticulin fibres are scanty and there is often much necrosis. Intracellular glycogen is usually demonstrable by light or electron microscopy. Here and there the cells may be arranged in clusters resembling rosettes but without clearly defined central fibrils. This very inconstant feature is probably the result of degeneration.

Clinical features. Ewing's tumour usually presents with pain and swelling, often of some months' duration. Sometimes fever, anaemia and leucocytosis suggest low-grade osteomyel-

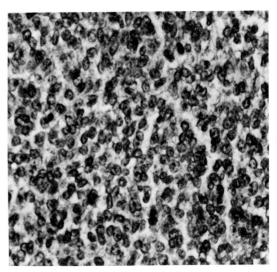

Fig. 23.43 Ewing's tumour of femur showing syncytial structure and uniform cell type. × 450.

itis and the patients with these systemic symptoms have the worst prognosis. The tumour is at first radiosensitive, but frequently recurrence takes place later and secondaries appear especially in other bones and in the lungs. Treatment with cytotoxic drugs following radiotherapy or surgery has led to some improvement in prognosis.

Differential diagnosis. In the absence of clearly distinctive histological features leukaemic deposits, lymphomas, myelomatosis, secondary carcinoma and, in young children, metastatic neuroblastoma must be considered in the differential diagnosis. The increased urinary excretion of catecholamine derivatives in many cases of neuroblastoma and their normal values in patients with Ewing's tumour helps to distinguish between these tumours. Occasionally the true diagnosis becomes apparent only at necropsy.

Malignant lymphoma of bone

Bone is a relatively uncommon site of primary lymphoma.

Age, sex incidence and site. Malignant lymphoma is rare in childhood (cf Ewing's tumour). It is commoner in males, occurs in the metaphysis and in the adjacent shaft of long bones, and may arise also in flat bones and the axial skeleton.

Clinical features. Malignant lymphoma of bone presents with pain and swelling but fever is rare. x-ray often shows a fairly widespread, diffuse, motheaten area of patchy rarefaction. Periosteal new bone formation is not usually conspicuous but there may be patchy reactive bone sclerosis in the medulla. The radiological appearances may suggest a chronic osteomyelitis, and in small biopsies with much necrosis and secondary inflammatory cell infiltrate, considerable difficulty may also arise in making this histological differentiation. The tumour is radiosensitive and the prognosis after radiotherapy is distinctly more favourable than that in Ewing's tumour. About 45% are said to survive for five years and about 30% for ten years. Involvement of regional lymph nodes may occur early or late and may be followed by infiltration in spleen and liver. The lungs tend to be affected only late in the disease. Occasionally leukaemia develops. In every patient with a presumed primary lymphoma of bone, search should be made for involvement of other bones or of lymph nodes since the relatively good prognosis does not apply if the bone lesion is simply the presenting sign of more generalised disease.

Macroscopic appearances. The tumour tends to affect chiefly the metaphyseal region and adjacent shaft, and it is osteolytic so that the bony cortex becomes mottled and rarefied. The tumour penetrates the cortex usually without eliciting any new reactive periosteal bone, and spreads into the adjacent tissues.

Microscopic appearances. Lymphomas of bone were formerly termed 'reticulum-cell sarcomas', but more recent studies suggest that most of them are B-cell tumours of diffuse centroblastic or centroblastic/centrocytic type (p. 18.24). There is sometimes a rich reticulin network, a feature conspicuously absent in Ewing's tumour. Intracellular glycogen is usually absent.

Giant-cell tumour of bone (osteoclastoma)

Giant-cell tumour is an osteolytic, eccentrically placed tumour arising most commonly in the end of a long bone of an adult.

Age. The lesion arises chiefly in the 20–40 age group. The diagnosis should be regarded with suspicion at a site where the epiphyseal cartilage plate is still open as there are several benign lesions in children and adolescents which to some extent simulate giant-cell tumour. Some of these are discussed below.

Site of occurrence. Half of all the tumours occur in the lower end of femur or upper tibia (Fig. 23.44). Another common site is the lower end of radius. Although flat bones may be in-

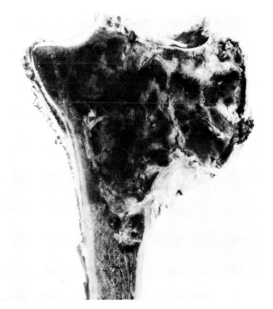

Fig. 23.44 Section of giant-cell tumour of upper end of tibia showing eccentric expansion of the bone end and much haemorrhage within the tumour.

volved, giant-cell tumour is rare in the jaw and in the vertebral column above the sacrum. When the tumour occurs in a long bone it arises almost invariably in the bone end and the metaphysis is involved only later. Accordingly joint symptoms are common.

Macroscopic appearances. Giant-cell tumour is usually located eccentrically and often causes marked expansion of the bone end (Fig. 23.44). It is covered, initially, by a thin shell of subperiosteal bone which may be renewed on the surface as expansion progresses but this may later be breached by the tumour which then extends into the soft tissues. Invasion of the joint through the articular cartilage is uncommon. The tumour is entirely destructive and its cells do not form bone. As a result of its osteolytic propensities patients often present with a pathological fracture. There is none of the subperiosteal sunray bony spiculation seen in an osteosarcoma. The tumour is usually reddish-grey and commonly shows areas of haemorrhage and necrosis. If there has been a fracture or previous treatment by surgery or radiotherapy the picture may be complicated by callus formation, fibrosis and cystic degeneration.

Microscopic appearances. Giant-cell tumour consists of plump spindle or ovoid mononuclear cells abundantly interspersed with giant cells containing many nuclei, sometimes as many as 100 (Fig. 23.45). Fibrous tissue is usually scanty unless the tumour has previously fractured or been treated. Areas of necrosis, haemorrhage, lipid-containing macrophages and cholesterol are sometimes seen. Following surgical treatment there may be recurrence in the soft tissues; neither this nor the presence of tumour in periosteal veins is necessarily of sinister significance.

Prognosis. About half the tumours respond to thorough local removal, more than a third recur and the remaining 10% are liable to become malignant, usually after treatment and recurrence, and to metastasise to the lungs. The tumour may recur as a fibrosarcoma or occasionally as an osteosarcoma. Some help in assessing the prognosis is given by the histology in that tumours which look frankly sarcomatous usually behave badly; however, very rarely, tumours which appear microscopically benign later metastasise.

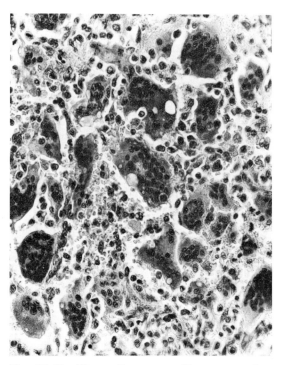

Fig. 23.45 Giant-cell tumour. The mononuclear tumour cells have the same characteristics as the scattered multinucleated cells. × 240.

Lesions likely to be confused with giant-cell tumour

Besides the differentiation of true giant-cell tumour from the benign lesions principally of childhood and adolescence described below, the lesion must be distinguished from the **brown tumour of hyperparathyroidism** (p. 23.18). Since this may not be possible on histological grounds the blood chemistry should be investigated and a radiological search for subperiosteal erosions made, especially if the apparent giant-cell tumour is in the skull or jaw.

Aneurysmal bone cyst. This is probably not a true tumour but has been confused with giant-cell tumour. It is commonest in the long bone *metaphyses* or vertebrae of children or young adults and gives rise to an extremely eccentric osteolytic lesion which may balloon out the periosteum and sometimes involves contiguous bones. Within the thin bony shell the 'cyst' consists of cavernous bloodfilled spaces separated by a brownish spongy meshwork of vascular fibrous trabeculae, the larger of which are reinforced by osteoid or bony strands. Giant cells are smaller and less evenly distributed than in giant-cell tumour (Fig. 23.46). The lesion is benign and is cured by surgery, sometimes even when removal has been incomplete. If untreated it may grow steadily but sometimes heals spontaneously after biopsy. Many

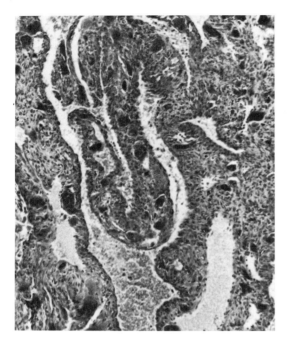

Fig. 23.46 Aneurysmal bone cyst. Vascular spaces lined by fibrous trabeculae with giant cells. × 45.

different tumours may contain areas histologically similar to aneurysmal bone cysts, probably as a result of degenerative change.

Benign chondroblastoma. This rare benign bone tumour of uncertain histogenesis is important because it may be mistaken for a malignant giant-cell tumour or occasionally a chondro- or osteo-sarcoma. Benign chondroblastoma occurs most often in adolescents and is usually located in the epiphysis of long bones, especially around the knee or in the upper humerus. Radiologically there is a well-defined lucent area often with a narrow sclerotic border and sometimes with mottling due to spotty calcification. The tumour may spread across the epiphyseal plate into the metaphysis and rarely into the adjacent joint. Microscopically the lesion consists of fairly uniform small rounded or polygonal cells with a moderate sprinkling of osteoclasts. Plaques of hyaline chondroid or osteoid-like material may be prominent or scanty and in about half the cases a characteristic lace-like web of calcification is deposited around individual cells. The tumour is usually curable by curettage. It may recur but pulmonary metastases are very rare and usually not progressive.

Metaphyseal fibrous defect (non-ossifying fibroma). This is a developmental abnormality which is readily diagnosable radiologically as a small scalloped radiolucent area with a sclerotic edge hugging the metaphyseal cortex in the long bones, particularly the femur, of young children. Such lesions may dis-

appear spontaneously as a result of bone remodelling during growth or enlarge to involve more of the medullary cavity. Macroscopically the tissue is usually orange-yellow and microscopically consists of whorled fibrous tissue with moderate numbers of small giant cells, haemosiderin and in some cases aggregates of lipid-containing macrophages. These lesions, are benign and may heal spontaneously, only requiring curettage when their size makes radiological diagnosis uncertain or pathological fracture likely.

Simple bone cyst. This is a benign non-neoplastic unilocular cystic lesion, probably related to some local disturbance of bone growth and commonly arising in the upper humeral or femoral metaphyses in children and adolescents. As the bone grows, the cyst appears to migrate down the shaft away from the epiphyseal line. It is commoner in males. Attention is frequently drawn to the lesion by pathological fracture and occasionally, following this, the cyst fills in. The appearances are of a smooth-walled cavity containing clear fluid and usually slightly expanding and markedly thinning the cortices. The lining consists of a meagre layer of poorly cellular collagen. When fracture has occurred the fluid may be bloody and the lining transformed to a thick layer of granulation or fibrous tissue with areas of haemorrhage, cholesterol clefts, new bone formation, and osteoclast aggregates which sometimes have given rise to confusion with giant-cell tumour. Rounded balls of fibrin, sometimes calcified, are often conspicuous. The cysts, while perfectly benign, have a strong tendency to recur, particularly if they are near the epiphyseal plate when initially treated.

Chordoma

This tumour arises from notochordal remnants, and usually develops within or in close proximity to the axial skeleton. In post-natal life the notochord persists in the nucleus pulposus of the intervertebral discs. In addition, small remnants are found in the hollow of the sacrum and coccyx and as little gelatinous nodules in the region of the spheno-occipital synchondrosis (*ecchordosis physaliphora*); the latter are, of course, observed merely as incidental findings at necropsy. It is from these ectopic remnants rather than from the discs that most chordomas are thought to originate.

Sites of occurrence. Chordoma usually comes to notice in adult life and most commonly involves the sacrococcygeal region and the spheno-occipital part of the skull base. Cervical, dorsal and lumbar vertebral tumours are much rarer.

Clinical features. Chordomas grow very slowly and commonly cause pressure on adjacent structures. In the sacral region they may become very large and press on the rectum; in the spheno-occipital site the

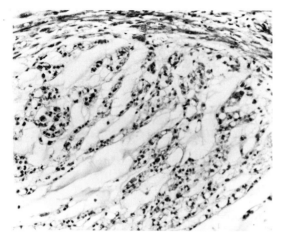

Fig. 23.47 Chordoma from sacrum. Strands of cells, many of them vacuolated, are seen lying in a background of mucinous material. × 140.

symptoms are chiefly due to compression of cranial nerves but pituitary dysfunction may occur. The lat-

ter group are inevitably more quickly fatal. Radiological examination usually shows a lytic bone lesion with a soft tissue shadow and sometimes some patchy calcification. Death usually occurs from local extension of tumour rather than from metastasis.

Macroscopic appearances. The chordoma usually appears well circumscribed in its soft tissue mass but irregularly infiltrates adjacent bone. It is lobulated, greyish, semi-translucent and gelatinous with areas of haemorrhage and softening.

Microscopic appearances. Clusters or cords of cells are surrounded by a sea of mucin (Fig. 23.47). The most characteristic pattern is of cords of syncytial cells radiating towards the margins of the lobules. Some of the rounded or polyhedral cells may appear vacuolated due to intracytoplasmic droplets of mucoid material ('*physaliphorous cells*'). Some spheno-occipital chordomas contain nodules of cartilage. The difficult histological differentiation between chordoma, chondrosarcoma and mucin-secreting carcinoma is best made on a careful assessment of the architecture and on the results of immunohistochemistry.

Diseases of Joints

Normal joint structure

Joints may be categorised as those without a joint cavity, the non-synovial *synarthroses* and those with a joint cavity, the synovial *diarthroses*. In a diarthrosis the bone ends are covered by hyaline articular cartilage and the surfaces lubricated by synovial fluid produced by the synovial membrane which is supported by the fibrous joint capsule.

Articular cartilage. Normal articular cartilage forms a smooth, glistening, slightly elastic covering to the bone ends. It is bluish and translucent in the young, averaging 2–4 mm in thickness; in old age it becomes yellower and more opaque. The matrix consists partly of type II collagen fibres (p. 5.6) which run parallel to the surface in the superficial layer and at right angles to it in the deeper layer. Smaller slender filaments lacking the characteristic banding of collagen surround the chondrocytes. The collagen meshwork entraps a gel of proteoglycans containing chains of chondroitin and keratan sulphate which give cartilage its metachromatic staining.

The chondrocytes lie in lacunae in the matrix and have branching processes which extend into it. Those cells near the surface are flattened and horizontal, the deeper ones are arranged in columns. In the adult a wavy basophilic line marks the junction between the uncalcified cartilage and the small layer of calcified cartilage which interdigitates with the subchondral bone.

Articular cartilage is avascular and the chondrocytes have a low oxygen requirement. Its nourishment is derived from the synovial fluid and probably also, in growing animals, from blood vessels of the subchondral marrow. Exchange between the synovial fluid and cartilage is thought to be promoted by joint movement. Hyaline cartilage has little power of regeneration for repair (p. 5.19).

Synovial membrane forms synovial fluid: it lines tendon sheaths and bursae and covers all the surfaces of joints except articular cartilage and menisci. The synovium may be smooth or folded and may form small villi especially at the joint margins. It is lined by a layer of ellipsoidal cells, one to four cells thick. These intimal cells are not separated by a basement membrane from the underlying tissues which may be areolar, dense fibrous or fatty in different parts of the joint. Two types of intimal cells are distinguished on electron microscopy. It is thought that Type A, the more numerous, are macrophages which produce degradative enzymes while Type B synthesise hyaluronic acid.

The synovial membrane has a rich network of blood vessels, many of which run close to the surface. It is able to regenerate after synovectomy and a lining indistinguishable from synovium may form in adventitious bursae and pseudarthroses (false joints), presumably by metaplasia.

Synovial fluid is a dialysate of blood plasma with the addition of hyaluronic acid which gives the fluid its viscous property. The proportion of hyaluronic acid and hence the viscosity is said to diminish with age. The function of the fluid is twofold: to nourish the articular cartilage and to lubricate the joint surfaces. Under normal circumstances many human joints contain less than 1 ml of synovial fluid. In healthy human joints the fluid contains up to $0.4 \times 10^9/l$ nucleated cells with few polymorphs, about 25% lymphocytes, a few synovial cells and a majority of macrophages, perhaps derived from the synovium.

Albumin and globulin are present in lower concentration in the fluid than in plasma with a preponderance of albumin in the ratio of about 4:1. Glucose levels are normally similar to or slightly less than in the blood.

Infective Arthritis

Acute infective arthritis

In countries where infections with pneumococcus, meningococcus, gonococcus or typhoid bacilli are treated promptly with antibiotics, acute arthritis is now an uncommon complication and, when it does occur, tends to be transient, non-suppurative, and leaves little disability. Many different pyogenic bacteria, including *Streptococcus pyogenes* and *Haemophilus influenzae*, may give rise to **suppurative (septic) arthritis**, but *Staphylococcus aureus* is most often the cause. It is commonest in infants, children and the aged and in seriously ill patients, particularly those receiving immunosuppressant drugs. The knee and hip are most often involved and, especially in infants, more than one joint may be affected.

Path of infection. Acute infective arthritis arises chiefly as a result of haematogenous spread and sometimes a focus of infection such as a staphylococcal boil or a septic throat is identifiable. Infection may spread from adjacent osteitis, especially when the affected metaphysis is within the joint cavity. It is a dreaded complication of reconstructive surgery (p. 23.42) and occasionally follows a penetrating wound or a compound intra-articular fracture.

Clinical features. There are the usual signs of acute inflammation, i.e. local redness, heat, pain, tenderness, oedema, joint effusion and limitation of movement, fever with rigors and often a polymorphonuclear leucocytosis and raised erythrocyte sedimentation rate. Difficulty in diagnosis may arise when, as sometimes happens, a pyogenic infection complicates pre-existing joint disease such as rheumatoid arthritis.

Early non-suppurative stage. The joint effusion contains a large increase of cells, mostly polymorphs. Glucose levels are depressed and, as in most inflammatory arthropathies, protein levels are raised. Synovial fluid and blood cultures should immediately be obtained in a suspected pyogenic arthritis, but are not always positive, and antibiotics should be administered thereafter without delay. The synovium at this stage is intensely red and congested and flecked with yellowish fibrin. Microscopically it shows the features of acute inflammation. If the disease is arrested at this stage the condition resolves with little residual joint damage.

Suppurative stage. If suppuration develops, within a few days extensive cartilage destruction occurs, probably as a result of the increase of proteolytic enzymes from polymorphs and of excess plasmin by bacterial activators. Chondrocytes die and collagen fibres are vulnerable to the effects of trauma. The exposed bone also undergoes necrosis (Fig. 23.48). An acute suppurative arthritis is entirely destructive but once the condition subsides into a subacute or

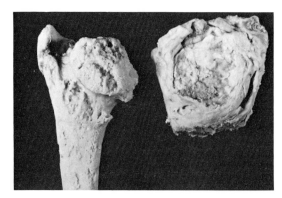

Fig. 23.48 Suppurative arthritis of hip joint. The articular cartilage of both the femoral head and the acetabulum is destroyed and there is erosion of the underlying bone.

chronic stage there is proliferation of granulation tissue within the joint, which is followed by ossification and bony ankylosis. Bony ankylosis occurs more commonly in untreated suppurative arthritis than in tuberculous or rheumatoid disease.

Gonococcal arthritis is uncommon but its incidence is increasing. It is now seen more often in women and homosexual men. The small percentage of patients with gonococcaemia may develop a papular or pustular skin rash accompanied by a migratory polyarthritis which becomes confined to one or two joints. The extensor tendon sheaths of the hands and feet may also be inflamed. Blood cultures are often positive though the synovial fluid is sterile in about half the cases. Specimens from cervix or urethra, rectum and oropharynx should be cultured. The arthritis usually subsides leaving little, if any, disability.

Complications following joint replacement

Infection

Sepsis following joint replacement may be a disastrous complication. Particularly at risk are patients undergoing replacement of a prosthetic joint, the aged, and people with rheumatoid arthritis, diabetes, malnutrition or any condition which impairs the immune response. Meticulous aseptic surgical technique, special attention to haemostasis, shorter operating time and effective air changes in the theatre have reduced the infection rate to less than 2% in hip joint replacements, though it is rather higher in

the knee. Even so, it is still the most commonly seen cause of sepsis in some rheumatology units. About half the infections are with *Staphylococcus aureus* or *epidermidis* but streptococci, pseudomonas and a wide variety of aerobic and anaerobic organisms may be implicated. In about 10% of patients cultures are sterile. Infection may be attributable to bacterial contamination at operation by direct contact or air spread but it may also develop at any time after operation from haematogenous spread of organisms from a focus of infection in urinary tract, gut or other site. Acute or subacute wound infections occurring in the first 3 or 4 weeks postoperatively require to be treated early. With evacuation of any haematoma and aggressive antibiotic therapy the condition may subside.

Infections which develop a year or more after an apparently successful result are often insidious and the course chronic and persistent. In some patients the bacterial flora is mixed, but organisms may be difficult to identify or culture may be sterile. Some bacteria develop a polysaccharide membrane which enables them to form colonies and adhere to smooth surfaces making them less vulnerable to macrophage attack and to penetration by antibiotics. Indeed these infections are often resistant to antibiotic therapy and subside only after removal of the loose prosthesis and its embedding cement along with dead and infected bone and soft tissue.

Reaction to wear products

Joint replacement may be followed eventually by wear of the prosthesis which stimulates a series of changes in the tissues. Necrosis and fibrinous exudation may be striking and result in a mass of soft crumbly material within the joint which raises the surgeon's suspicion of infection. Sometimes the tissues are grey due to small rods of metallic debris contained within sheets of macrophages. These patients may be shown by skin tests to have developed sensitivity to the metal of the prosthesis. If one component of the prosthesis consists of polyethylene, brilliantly refractile shards of this material may be found, the smaller within macrophages and the larger within foreign body giant cells. Both metallic and polyethylene debris stimulate fibrosis. Silicon rubber is most often used for finger-joint prosthesis but also as a buffer between the components of some all-metal joint prostheses. Its wear products are faintly refractile and stimulate a follicular granulomatous reaction within the joint and sometimes also in draining lymph nodes. In many joint replacements acrylic cement, sometimes mixed with barium to assist radiological identification, is used to anchor the prosthetic stem within the medullary cavity. Cement granules dissolve during tissue processing leaving rounded or ovoid spaces surrounded by attenuated giant cells and often containing a few barium granules. Macrophages containing cement have a finely vacuolated, bubbly appearance and may be abundant. Aside from the importance of recognising the source of these foreign materials within the joint, breakdown of cement and excessive wear debris may cause loosening of the prosthesis and pain.

The exact sequence of events is uncertain but perhaps vascular changes result in bone and soft tissue necrosis associated with resorption of bone at its interface with the anchoring cement.

Other joint infections

Tuberculous arthritis

Joint tuberculosis is usually caused by human tubercle bacilli spreading to the synovium directly from an adjacent focus in bone or by the bloodstream from another site (p. 23.7). In the UK, it affects especially debilitated, elderly indigenous patients and immigrants from the Indian subcontinent. The hip or knee is most often involved.

Pathological appearances. There is frequently a moderate joint effusion usually of clear or slightly turbid fluid sometimes containing 'melon-seed bodies' of necrotic synovial fronds and fibrin. Tubercle bacilli can be found in less than 20% of fluids though culture is positive in more. For this reason it is advisable both to culture and to examine histologically a synovial biopsy rather than to rely on synovial fluid examination alone in patients with an undiagnosed monarthritis. Acid-fast bacilli are found in thick (10 µm) Ziehl-Neelsen stained tissue sections in rather more than half the cases and bacteriological culture is positive in about the same proportion.

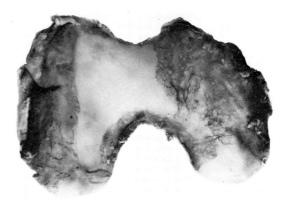

Fig. 23.49 Tuberculous disease of knee-joint. Note the spread of granulation tissue with tubercles over the surface of the cartilage.

The synovial membrane in an affected joint is usually oedematous, congested and hyperplastic and may be studded with tiny yellow foci of caseation. Tuberculous follicles are often readily seen microscopically but occasionally careful search of many sections is required to identify scanty, poorly formed follicles in a background of chronic inflammatory cells. Radiographs at this early stage show soft tissue swelling and some reactive porosis in the adjacent bone. If the condition is promptly and effectively treated, little functional disability results but if diagnosis is delayed, granulation tissue may grow in from the periphery of the joint to cover and replace the articular cartilage (Fig. 23.49). It may also erode the subchondral bone, thus detaching flakes of articular cartilage. The marrow of the exposed bone is likely to be involved with resorption of trabeculae.

When caseous foci form in the capsule and soft tissue, suppurative softening may follow with discharge of pus through the skin and the possibility of secondary infection. During healing fibrous adhesions form across the destroyed joint surfaces and may become ossified if secondary infection supervenes. Joint destruction with discharging sinuses and spontaneous fusion is now virtually confined to countries where the disease is not checked by specific therapy.

Tuberculous tenosynovitis. Tuberculosis may also affect the tendon sheaths, especially of the flexor tendons at the wrist. There is, as in joint tuberculosis, effusion of fluid, the formation of melon-seed bodies and sometimes proliferation of exuberant granulation tissue within the sheath. Extensive caseation with destruction of tendons is rarely seen except in untreated cases.

Syphilitic arthritis

In contrast to tuberculosis, syphilis comparatively seldom gives rise to important joint lesions.

Acquired syphilis. In the *secondary stage* there may be transient arthritis while gummas occasionally arise in the joint capsule in *tertiary* syphilis. Patients with tabes dorsalis sometimes develop neuropathic arthropathy (p. 23.50).

Congenital syphilis. There may be joint pain and swelling in infants and young children with syphilitic epiphysitis. Older children may develop chronic painless effusion, usually of the knees, with some synovial thickening which does not progress to severe joint damage (*Clutton's joints*).

Brucellosis (Undulant fever)

Joint symptoms are the presenting feature in about 25% of cases of undulant fever, the joints being involved in the course of the septicaemia. The arthritis is transient and acute. Sometimes granulomas similar to those of sarcoid or tuberculosis are seen (Fig. 18.1, p. 18.4). Bursae may also be involved.

Arthritis of unknown cause

Rheumatoid arthritis (RA)

Rheumatoid arthritis is one of the connective tissue diseases (p. 23.57), and is characterised by a subacute or chronic non-suppurative arthritis usually affecting several joints. Its course is punctuated by spontaneous remissions.

Age and sex incidence. The disease usually begins between 25 and 55 but may affect both older and younger people. Juvenile rheumatoid arthritis (*Still's disease*) is more often associated with splenomegaly and lymphadenopathy and occasionally pericarditis. Rheumatoid arthritis affects about 3% of the female and 1% of the male population in temperate climates: a small proportion of these patients become severely disabled.

Sites of occurrence. Any synovial joint may be affected but those of the hands and feet are most often involved, the disease often being bilateral and symmetrical. Temporomandibular, crico-arytenoid joints and those of the cervical spine are occasionally involved. Destructive spinal disease may produce instability and neurological complications.

Course of the disease. The onset is often insidious but sometimes acute. The condition may abate after a single attack but more commonly there are repeated relapses and remissions, the joint each time suffering further damage. Involvement of tendons, soft tissue swelling, muscle atrophy, and ligamentous and capsular laxity all contribute to increasing deformity. Sometimes the arthritis progresses to fibrous, occasionally to bony, ankylosis. The tendency is for the rheumatoid disease eventually to burn itself out but even then the joint disability may increase due to further damage from secondary osteoarthritis. During the active phase of polyarthritis, tests for rheumatoid factor are usually positive (p. 23.57).

Clinical and macroscopic appearances. In the early acute stage and during relapse, the joints are acutely inflamed, hot, swollen and tender. There is often fatigue, weight loss and fever; a high ESR, leucocytosis and sometimes a normocytic, normochromic anaemia. The swelling often gives the finger joints a spindle-shaped appearance; it is partly due to synovial effusion which may be turbid but is sterile. There is an increase in cells, sometimes up to $50 \times 10^9/l$ with about 75% polymorphs, and fibrin flakes may be present. The primary changes are in the synovium which is red and congested, oedematous, markedly frondose and often patchily covered by fibrinous exudate (Fig. 23.50). After the early stages it may be heavily pigmented with haemosiderin.

Microscopic appearances. In the florid case there is marked villous hypertrophy of the synovium with synovial cell proliferation, fibrinous and polymorph exudate on the surface, lymphocytes in dense focal aggregates, sometimes with germinal centres, accompanied by a heavy and more diffuse plasma cell infiltrate (Fig. 23.51). These features may persist for an indefinite period after an acute attack; when they are all pronounced, the diagnosis of rheumatoid

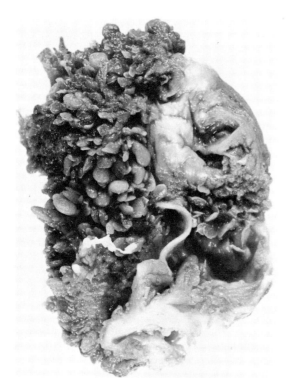

Fig. 23.50 Synovium from a rheumatoid knee joint. The synovial surface is markedly frondose and some of the villi are tipped with white fibrin.

arthritis may be made with fair, though not with absolute certainty. However, the synovium has only a limited range of response to different stimuli and less severe degrees of these changes may be seen in a wide variety of conditions, e.g. following trauma, in joints adjacent to tumours, in psoriatic and various non-specific arthritides and in the late stages of osteoarthritis. Rarely the diagnosis may be confirmed by finding a typical 'rheumatoid nodule' (*see below*) in the subsynovial tissue.

So long as the changes in rheumatoid arthritis are confined to the synovium, the functional disability is reversible, but this is often followed by secondary irreversible changes in other joint structures. Subchondral erosions form at the joint margin and a thin layer of vascular granulation tissue (**pannus**) grows over the joint cartilage, which is eroded and destroyed by enzymes from the cells in the pannus. If the underlying bone is exposed it may be focally replaced by pockets of granulation tissue which may eventually become fibrosed and form adhesions across the joint space: later

ossification sometimes converts this from fibrous to bony ankylosis, especially in the small joints of the carpus and tarsus.

While these changes are going on in the joint, *the bone* at an early stage may become markedly porotic due to hyperaemia and disuse. *The muscles* atrophy and there is wasting and weakness especially of the interossei and sometimes also of the hand flexors. *Tendons* may also become infiltrated by rheumatoid granulation tissue and this leads to pain and disability and sometimes to rupture of the tendon with further deformity. As a result of muscle atrophy and tendon destruction, ligamentous and capsular laxity, the hand in particular becomes greatly deformed with marked ulnar deviation, subluxation and dislocation of joints (Fig. 23.52b).

Changes in other tissues. Subcutaneous lesions known as *rheumatoid nodules* develop over pressure sites in about 20% of patients (p. 23.58). They consist of a central area of fibri-

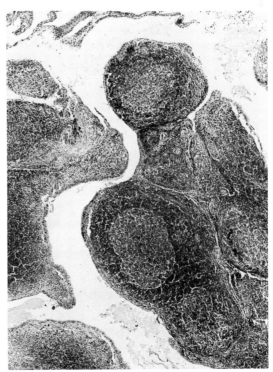

Fig. 23.51 Synovial membrane in chronic rheumatoid arthritis. The synovium shows villous hypertrophy and is extensively infiltrated with lymphocytes, amongst which occur poorly defined germinal centres. Plasma cells also are abundant. × 38.

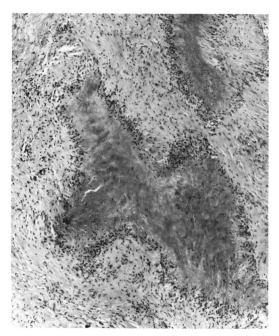

Fig. 23.52a   Rheumatoid nodule from the region of the elbow-joint. × 90.

noid necrosis of collagen surrounded by palisaded histiocytes (Fig. 23.52a). The nodules persist throughout life and are a helpful clinical and histological diagnostic aid. They tend to occur in more severely affected patients and to be associated with a worse prognosis (Fig. 23.52b).

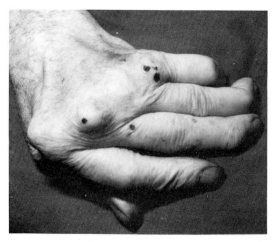

Fig. 23.52b   The hand shows the typical severe deformity of rheumatoid arthritis with marked ulnar deviation of the fingers and muscle wasting. Ulcerated rheumatoid nodules are present over the metacarpophalangeal joints.

Similar nodules are occasionally found at other sites, including the lungs of coalminers with rheumatoid disease (Caplan's syndrome, p. 16.58), the pleura, the heart and pericardium, and the eye.

Rheumatoid vasculitis (p. 14.27) may occur and when severe gives rise to skin ulceration and occasionally gangrene, bowel perforation and myocardial infarction. *Peripheral neuropathy* may also result. *The skin* is often atrophic, thin and papery.

Reactive and hyperplastic changes occur in *lymph nodes* and *spleen* (p. 18.14). The association of RA with marked splenomegaly, leucopenia and diminished resistance to infection is sometimes known as *Felty's syndrome*. About 20% of cases of chronic rheumatoid arthritis coming to necropsy have some evidence of *amyloid disease* affecting the spleen, liver and kidney, although symptoms attributable to amyloid are rare. *Sjøgren's syndrome* (p. 19.9) may accompany rheumatoid disease.

Aetiology. The cause of rheumatoid arthritis is not known. It presents features which suggest that the lesions in the joints and elsewhere are brought about by hypersensitivity reactions. In particular, *rheumatoid factors* are present in the serum of most cases: these consist of IgM or IgG which reacts with antigenic components of the Fc part of IgG, forming immune complexes. Accordingly, rheumatoid arthritis is commonly termed **seropositive arthritis** to distinguish it from a group of **seronegative arthritides**, in which rheumatoid factors are absent.

The aetiology of rheumatoid arthritis is discussed further with the connective tissue diseases on p. 23.58.

Seronegative arthritis

This term is applied to a group of non-infective arthritides in which tests for rheumatoid factor are negative and rheumatoid nodules are absent. The group includes (1) ankylosing spondylitis (2) the arthritides which sometimes complicate psoriasis, ulcerative colitis and Crohn's disease and (3) 'reactive arthritis' which is believed to be a hypersensitivity reaction and may either be associated with infection at a distant site, e.g. in rheumatic fever, bacillary dysentery or Reiter's syndrome or occur as part of a generalised hypersensitivity reaction e.g. in polyarteritis nodosa. There is often considerable clinical overlap between the different conditions. The features of the group, though not all present in each disease, are a tendency to axial skeletal involvement (spondylitis) with radiological evidence of inflammation of the sacroiliac joints, an asymmetrical peripheral arthritis, inflammation of the uveal tract of the eye, an aortitis involving the aortic ring and ulceration of the mouth, intestine or genital tract. There is a tendency to familial aggregation of most of these diseases and for other seronegative conditions to occur within the family. An association has been shown with HLA-B27 especially when there is spinal involvement.

HLA system and seronegative arthritis. The most striking relationship is between HLA-B27 and ankylosing spondylitis (*see below*). The individual with B27 is 300 times more likely to develop the disease than others and 90% of patients with ankylosing spondylitis have HLA-B27. The association between the HLA antigen and the disease has led to the recognition that spondylitis is much commoner than had been suspected, radiological changes affecting perhaps 1–2% of the population and that often, and especially in women, it is a mild, self-limiting condition. Its features appears to be the same in the 10% of patients who are B27 negative. Patients with ankylosing spondylitis may develop peripheral arthritis or attacks of acute anterior uveitis and these have been regarded as complications of the condition. However, both are probably genetically determined since there is a high incidence of B27 amongst patients with uveitis (40%) and with seronegative peripheral arthritis (30%) *without* spondylitis. (About 8% of Europeans have B27 antigen and of these around 75% have no evidence of ankylosing spondylitis.)

Of the groups of patients suffering from psoriasis, Reiter's syndrome ulcerative colitis, Crohn's disease and bowel infections with *Shigellae*, *Salmonellae* or *Yersinia enterocolitica*, those with B27 antigen are more likely to develop arthritis or spondylitis.

Ankylosing spondylitis

This is a polyarthritis which in severe cases may lead to bony ankylosis of the sacroiliac, intervertebral, and costovertebral joints with ossifi-

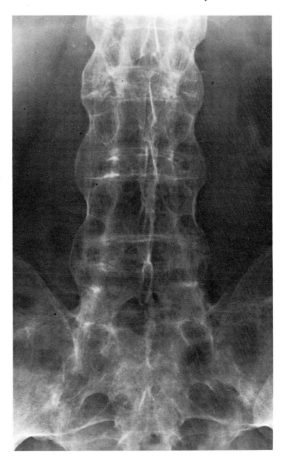

Fig. 23.53a A radiograph shows the typical 'bamboo' spine of late severe ankylosing spondylitis.

cation of spinal ligaments and the borders of intervertebral discs resulting in rigidity of the spine. Sometimes the sternoclavicular and hip joints are similarly involved. The classical form of the disease is much commoner in males than females and usually the onset is in adolescence or early adult life. It is sometimes familial

Course of the disease. There is usually an insidious onset of stiffness in the back with clinical and radiological evidence of inflammation of the sacroiliac joints. The condition is often self-limiting but may progress with exacerbations and remissions until the patient is left with an absolutely rigid back showing the radiological appearances of *bamboo spine* (Fig. 23.53a). When the cervical spine is involved there is danger of atlanto-axial dislocation or vertebral fracture and care must be taken in the handling of the anaesthetised patient. During exacerbations the ESR is commonly raised. The

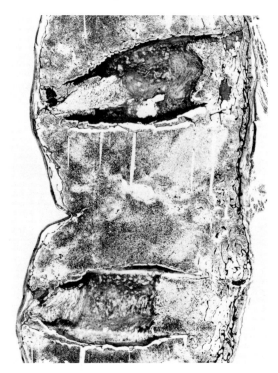

Fig. 23.53b   Bone bridges the lumbar intervertebral discs anteriorly (*on the left*). As a result of endochondral ossification much of the disc has been replaced by bone. There is very severe porosis of the vertebral bodies. (Reproduced by permission from *Applied Surgical Pathology*, Blackwell Scientific Publications.)

hips may be involved transiently, or chronically with final bony ankylosis in the most severely affected patients. Although diminished chest expansion is common, respiratory complications are rare.

Structural changes. The synovial changes resemble those of rheumatoid arthritis. The characteristic extra-articular ossification is thought to result from healing of inflammatory foci at the site of bony attachment of ligaments (enthesis), joint capsule or the outer fibres of the annulus fibrosus. This marginal ankylosis may be followed by endochondral ossification of remaining cartilage (Fig. 23.53b).

Aortic lesions. A few patients with longstanding ankylosing spondylitis may develop aortic valvular incompetence (see p. 15.31).

Leukaemia. Irradiation of the spine in ankylosing spondylitis increases tenfold the chance of the patient developing acute myeloblastic or chronic granulocytic leukaemia.

Psoriatic arthritis

Patients with psoriasis, especially those with involvement of the nails, have a tendency to develop a remittent arthritis which has a predilection for the distal joints of the hands and feet. While the synovium shows much the same nonspecific picture of hyperplasia with lymphocytic and plasma cell infiltrate as in the less florid cases of rheumatoid arthritis, the clinical and radiographic features and the negative test for rheumatoid factor serve to make the distinction. While deformities of the hands and feet may result, the condition is usually less disabling than rheumatoid arthritis. A small number of patients develop spondylitis, of these about 65% are HLA-B27 positive; uveitis may also occur.

Reiter's syndrome

This consists of non-specific urethritis, conjunctivitis and arthritis (p. 25.2) and occurs most frequently in adult males. The knee, ankle, small joints of the hands and feet and sometimes the spine are involved in a transient asymmetric polyarthritis which, unlike gonococcal arthritis, does not respond to penicillin therapy. Tendon sheaths and entheses are commonly affected. While often there is no permanent disability there may be recurrences with a tendency to destructive changes in the feet and sacroiliac joints. The incidence of HLA antigen B27 is high in such cases. The mouth may be involved and skin lesions affect especially the soles and palms. The urethritis is sometimes caused by *Chlamydia trachomatis* which is transmitted sexually (p. 25.2) and isolation of this organism from the joint fluid has been reported, but the syndrome may also follow diarrhoeal diseases including bacillary dysentery, and in most cases the joint fluid is sterile.

Arthritis in rheumatic fever

Rheumatic fever is associated with a sterile transient acute arthritis which is probably a form of hypersensitivity reaction. There is no overlap between rheumatic arthritis and rheumatoid arthritis. The large joints such as knees, ankles and wrists are usually involved and as the inflammation subsides in some joints others become affected. In most patients joint function returns speedily to normal, in a few, there may be some residual stiffness and synovial thickening, especially when the capsule has been involved.

Degenerative Arthropathies

Osteoarthritis

This condition, also termed **osteoarthrosis** or **degenerative arthritis** is the commonest form of chronic joint disease and is characterised clinically by the insidious but progressive onset of joint pain and stiffness. In spite of the name it is not an inflammatory or systemic disease but results from destructive and degenerative changes in the articular cartilage of joints. While any joint may be affected, disease of the hip or knee is most frequent and most disabling.

Osteoarthritis is found chiefly in the elderly. In younger people it is usually seen only when there is an obvious predisposing cause. This 'secondary' osteoarthritis may complicate intra-articular abnormalities such as congenital dislocation of the hip, damage to the cartilage by fracture or loose bodies, or previous inflammation. Extra-articular abnormalities which throw unusual stress on the joint, such as malunion of a fracture, bowing of the legs or scoliosis also predispose to osteoarthritis. The cause of 'primary' osteoarthritis developing in a normal joint is not known, though excessive physical activity or misuse appear to play a part, for some occupations are associated with arthritis in particular joints (e.g. those of ballet dancers' toes).

Structural changes. *Articular cartilage.* The first abnormality recognised by light microscopy is loss of metachromasia in the surface layers. Whether this results from rupture of the superficial collagen network or from depletion of the proteoglycan ground substance following release of enzymes from damaged chondrocytes remains speculative. It is followed by the development of tangential flaking of the surface and this may progress to deeper fissuring or fibrillation. Proliferation of chondrocytes and increased production of ground substance adjacent to the fissures fail to produce healing and loss of the cartilage substance follows so that the subchondral bone may be exposed (Fig. 23.54) seen in radiographs as narrowing of the joint space.

The distinction between age changes and osteoarthritis is difficult. Studies of the hip joint suggest that fibrillation in some sites may be a

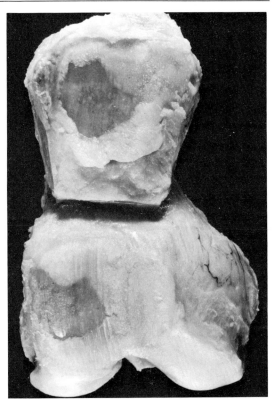

Fig. 23.54 Osteoarthritis of the knee joint has caused complete loss of articular cartilage with exposure of the bone on opposing surfaces of the patella (*above*) and the femur. There is parallel scoring of the joint surfaces.

self-limiting age change while in the load bearing area it is the forerunner of progressive destructive changes.

Bone. While these changes are occurring in the articular cartilage the subchondral bone trabeculae become greatly thickened (Fig. 23.55). When this dense bone is exposed it appears like polished ivory, sometimes grooved in the direction of joint movement (Figs 23.54, 23.58). The superficial osteocytes are usually dead. Fibro-cartilaginous metaplasia tends to occur in any exposed marrow spaces.

Marked bone remodelling results in change in the shape of the joint surface. This is particularly obvious in the flattening and mushrooming of the load-bearing surface of the femoral head in osteoarthritis of the hip joint

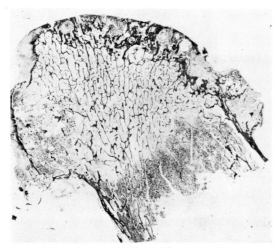

Fig. 23.55 Osteoarthritis of hip joint. The upper surface of the femoral head is flattened and mushroomed and the articular cartilage has largely disappeared. The exposed bone is dense, small osteoarthritic 'cysts' are present and there are peripheral osteophytes.

(Fig. 23.55). Another result is the formation of radiological 'cysts' in the subarticular bone. These are areas where bone has been replaced by loose rather degenerate fibrous tissue sometimes surrounded by new bone trabeculae. Small bony projections (osteophytes) form at the joint margins, giving first an appearance of beading and later of lipping of the joint: they develop as cartilaginous outgrowths which become ossified (Fig. 23.55). The stimulus to cartilage production is not fully understood. The osteophytes cause deformity and limitation of movement. Spontaneous ankylosis does not occur in uncomplicated osteoarthritis.

Synovium. In the early stages the synovium appears normal but when disintegration of the joint surfaces occurs absorption of abraded fragments of cartilage and bone is associated with villous hypertrophy and chronic synovitis followed by subsynovial fibrosis. A chronic inflammatory cell infiltrate may then be seen.

Synovial fluid. Synovial effusion tends to be associated with synovitis, apparently a reaction to debris in the joint. The cell count is slightly raised and only about 15% of cells are polymorphs.

Heberden's nodes. These are small bony elevations on the terminal phalanges of the fingers near the joint line. They may give rise to some deformity and limitation of movement. Some are the result of

osteoarthritis; others result from post-traumatic ossification of para-articular tissues.

Primary generalised osteoarthritis sometimes has a familial incidence, affects multiple joints often in relatively young patients and is almost invariably associated with Heberden's nodes.

Chondromalacia patellae is a condition arising in young people and giving rise to pain, effusion, loss of movement and crepitus of the knee joint. A history of trauma to the patella is often given. Excised patellas show localised softening and degeneration of the articular cartilage, seen first in the deep layers of the medial aspect.

Osteoarthritis of the spine is very common and histological evidence of degenerative changes are present in virtually everyone over the age of 70. Osteophytes may form posteriorly with osteoarthritis of the apophyseal joints and also anteriorly in relation to degenerative changes and narrowing of the intervertebral discs with sclerosis of the bony end plates. The osteophytes may cause symptoms by encroaching on the spinal nerve foramina or, in the cervical region, on the vertebral artery foramen. In the cervical and lumbar regions in particular, intermittent pain and discomfort may be followed eventually by stiffness and limitation of movement.

Spinal osteoarthritis may be distinguished from the changes of *diffuse idiopathic skeletal hyperostosis* (DISH) which chiefly affects elderly males causing aching and stiffness but little limitation of movement. In this latter condition the posterior apophyseal joints are spared, the disc spaces are well preserved and there is calcification and ossification in the antero-lateral aspects of the vertebral column and sometimes in the posterior ligament, especially in the thorax. These vertical osteophytes contrast with the horizontal ones of osteoarthritis. Extraspinal manifestations of DISH may include bony spurs around some peripheral joints and calcification and ossification of ligamentous and tendinous insertions.

Neuropathic arthropathy

Neuropathic arthritis is an accelerated form of degenerative arthritis resulting from the progressive disorganisation of an insensitive joint when subjected to trauma. It is also known as Charcot's joint after his original description in cases of tabes dorsalis and has since been found in many other neurological conditions. The commonest cause nowadays is probably *diabetic neuropathy*, the joints of the feet most often being involved.

The condition results from continued use of an analgesic joint with associated propriocep-

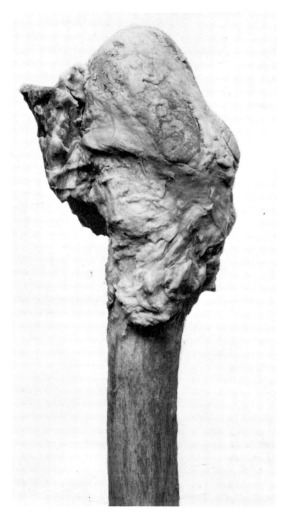

Fig. 23.56 Upper end of femur in neuropathic arthropathy of the hip joint in a patient with tabes. Note the irregular absorption of the head and the mass of new bone below.

tive loss. A cycle of events may occur in, for instance, the knee joint in a case of tabes dorsalis. The ataxia predisposes the joint to minor or major trauma which results in effusion; the swelling and muscular hypotonia increase the instability of the joint and its liability to further damage. Because the joint is painless the patient fails to restrict its use and further injury occurs. The structural changes in this condition are basically those of an extremely severe, and often rapidly progressive, osteoarthritis. The cartilage is destroyed, the bone ends grossly distorted (Fig. 23.56), partly by remodelling and partly by the early formation of very large

osteophytic outgrowths which may fracture and cause further damage. Fracture of the joint surface may also occur and the changes may then be complicated by hyperplastic callus formation. The gross and bizarre radiological changes contrast with the relative lack of pain.

Arthritis associated with gout

Gout is a disease with a hereditary tendency, associated with an incompletely understood disorder of purine metabolism. It results in repeated attacks of acute arthritis which may be followed by chronic degenerative joint changes. Most patients with gout have hyperuricaemia, i.e. a serum urate level of more than 0·42 mmol/l (7 mg/dl) in males; 0·36 mmol/l (6 mg/dl) in females. Hyperuricaemia is much commoner than clinical gout and the higher the serum urate level the greater the likelihood of the patient eventually developing symptoms.

So-called **secondary gout** may arise in the treatment of neoplastic conditions, e.g. leukaemia, with cytotoxic drugs; the hyperuricaemia results from the increased nucleoprotein breakdown. Occasionally secondary gout complicates uraemia, the decreased renal output leading to a raised blood uric acid level.

Age, sex and site. The first attack usually occurs over the age of 40; the disease is much commoner in males, females seldom being affected until after the menopause. In more than half the cases the metatarsophalangeal joint of the great toe is first affected, but the ankle, knee, elbow, wrist and other foot and finger joints may be involved.

The acute attack. In the susceptible subject an acute attack of gout may be precipitated by many factors such as trauma, surgery, overexertion, alcoholic or dietary excess, diuretics and purgation. Some of the drugs given to gouty patients to promote urinary excretion of uric acid may produce an acute attack because they free some of the acid which is bound to plasma proteins and so increase the amount of diffusible uric acid. The acute attack may be related to a rapid rise in serum uric acid rather than to the level reached. Acute gout is sometimes ushered in by pyrexia, leucocytosis and a raised ESR. The onset is sudden, may be nocturnal, and there is excruciating pain in the affected

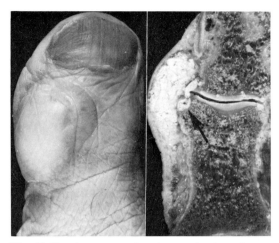

Fig. 23.57 A gouty tophus is seen in the subcutaneous tissue overlying the interphalangeal joint of the great toe. The tophus has produced a little resorption of bone at the joint margin (*arrow*). The articular cartilage is also flecked with white crystalline material.

joint, often the great toe (podagra) or its associated bursa, which shows all the signs of an acute inflammation. Needle-like strongly negative birefringent crystals of monosodium urate may be recognised in the synovial fluid, often within polymorphs (cf. pseudo-gout, see below). The crystal-containing polymorphs release a chemotactic substance which attracts other leucocytes. The ingested crystals damage the membrane-limited phagolysosomes in which they lie, hydrolytic enzymes are released into the cytoplasm and the cell dies, releasing the crystal. Cells in the synovial fluid may increase to $50 \times 10^9/l$ with 70% or more polymorphs. The attack lasts usually for a few days or weeks and is followed by remission, though hyperuricaemia may persist. The cause of the acute attack and of its spontaneous remission is obscure. Even in the first attack crystals, which presumably have accumulated silently, may be seen in the superficial synovium. Shedding of these and perhaps also crystallisation within the synovial fluid may initiate the inflammatory process. Some crystals may be seen in the synovial fluid during remission; their number, size and shape may be important in influencing the severity of the inflammatory reaction.

Chronic gout is associated with the formation of crystalline deposits of sodium urate, often with cholesterol and calcium salts, in relatively avascular collagen, hyaline and fibro-cartilage.

These deposits are known as **tophi** and may be found in the fibrocartilages of the ear, in bursal walls, especially the olecranon and prepatellar bursae, in the Achilles tendon and in the articular cartilage of joints (Fig. 23.57). Tophi are less frequent since drug therapy has become more effective. They may occur at sites of previous acute gouty arthritis or appear insidiously. Tophi are not significantly radio-opaque.

Microscopic examination of alcohol-fixed material from a tophus shows sheaves of urate crystals (Fig. 11.18, p. 11.23) which dissolve in aqueous fixatives. They induce a surrounding very marked foreign-body giant cell and granulomatous reaction.

In joints, urate is deposited in the superficial articular cartilage and appears as opaque white spots like paint. The crystalline deposits may be accompanied by degenerative changes in the articular cartilages. Later, urates may be precipitated in the subchondral and subperiosteal bone giving rise to bone destruction and punched out defects which are radiologically diagnosable. Tophi may occur in relation to synovium or pararticular tissues and sometimes reach great size and destroy cartilage, bone, synovium and capsule, leaving a totally disorganised joint. (Purine metabolism and the aetiology of gout are described on p. 11.23 and the renal changes on p. 22.42).

Pyrophosphate arthropathy

In recent years a condition has been described, chiefly in the middle-aged and elderly of both sexes. It is characterised by episodes of acute or subacute inflammation of one or more large joints, especially the knees. The pain is usually less severe than in acute gout and involvement of the big toe is rare. The differentiation from septic arthritis is important. During the acute stage (**pseudo-gout**) 'rod' and 'tablet' crystals of **calcium pyrophosphate** may be identified in the synovial fluid, mostly within polymorphs. The acute inflammatory response is thought to be precipitated by shedding of crystals into the joint fluid. Calcification may be seen in the menisci of the knee, the articular disc of the distal radio-ulnar joint, the symphysis pubis and also in articular cartilages, ligaments, tendons and joint capsules (**chondrocalcinosis**). While many of these patients with joint calcification have no significant joint disease a number of clinical syndromes have been described. Some patients develop chronic degenerative changes in relatively unusual sites such as shoulder, wrist and carpus. A few progress to severe joint destruction similar to neuropathic arthropathy. About a third of patients have hyperuricaemia and an occasional one has clinical gout but the condition should be distinguished from true gout by the involvement of large joints, the distinctive radiological findings and the characteristic crystals which exhibit a faint positive birefringence in polarised light. Predisposing causes such as hyperparathyroidism, haemochromatosis or diabetes should be sought.

Mixtures of crystals are sometimes found and recently the tiny crystals of *hydroxyapatite* have been recognised by scanning electron microscopy in the joint fluid and synovium of some osteoarthritic joints. It remains uncertain whether the presence of such crystals is the cause or the result of the degenerative changes of osteoarthritis.

Haemophilic arthropathy

Acute haemarthrosis, especially in the knee, is a common finding in haemophilia and the joint may become greatly distended by blood which is gradually resorbed. The synovium becomes hypertrophic and deeply pigmented with haemosiderin. There is a variable amount of inflammatory reaction. After repeated haemarthroses there is often some damage to the articular cartilage partly as the result of ingrowth of hyperplastic synovium and partly from degenerative changes of flaking and fissuring. Degradation of the ground substance may be seen around chondrocytes containing iron.

In addition, organisation of intraosseous haemorrhage may lead to bone resorption and the formation of bone 'cysts', while subperiosteal haematomas may simulate scurvy.

Miscellaneous Joint Conditions

Intra-articular loose bodies

Multiple soft loose bodies are sometimes known as '*rice or melon-seed*' bodies. They are usually formed from fibrin or necrotic synovial tissue and are found in tuberculous and rheumatoid arthritis. Symptoms are those of the accompanying arthritis.

Hard loose bodies may be caused by:

(*1*) *Osteochondritis dissecans*. Here the loose body is derived from part of the articular cartilage and underlying bone which for some reason separates from the surrounding tissue. When completely separated, the cartilaginous part of the body remains viable and may proliferate while the bone dies. Usually one, occasionally several, loose bodies may be present, the medial condyle of the femur being most frequently affected.

(*2*) *Osteoarthritis*. The fracturing of marginal osteophytes is a rare occurrence. It occurs more commonly in the severe osteoarthritis associated with neuroarthropathy.

(*3*) *Fracture of the articular margins*. Occasionally fracture of the articular margins results in one of the fragments of bone entering the joint and acting as a loose body, i.e. in fractures of the lower end of the humerus the medial epicondyle may, in spite of its muscle attachments, form a loose body in the elbow joint.

(*4*) *Synovial chondromatosis or osteochondromatosis*. In this condition multiple nodules of cartilage form by metaplasia in the synovial membrane and may become ossified. Some of the nodules may become detached to lie free in the synovial fluid.

Clinically, hard loose bodies may cause repeated episodes of locking of the joint. Damage to the articular cartilage may result in osteoarthritis (Fig. 23.58).

Pigmented villonodular synovitis (PVNS)

Localised nodular synovitis was formerly called benign giant-cell tumour of tendon sheath or benign synovioma. Women between 30 and 50 are most often affected and the fingers are by far the commonest site (Fig. 23.59). Occasionally similar nodules are found in major joints alone or associated with diffuse PVNS. The lesions consist of firm multilobulated greyish nodules, usually not more than 2 or 3 cm in diameter and sometimes grooved by the underlying tendon. On section there are yellow areas and brownish flecks.

Microscopy shows abundant strands of dense hyaline collagen surrounding groups of histio-

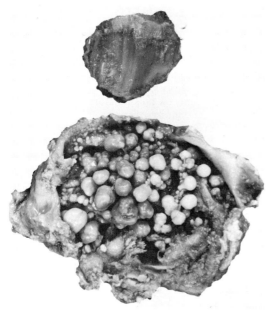

Fig. 23.58 Chondromatosis of synovium of the knee joint. Osteoarthritis of patella.

cytes, often with clumps of foamy xanthoma cells or small foci of haemosiderin, along with a scattering of multinucleated giant cells. Mitoses may be seen and occasionally adjacent

bone is eroded. However the lesion is benign and readily cured by local excision. The 10–20% recurrence rate may be explained by the multinodular growth pattern and by a small amount of diffuse involvement of adjacent tendon sheath or joint synovium.

Diffuse PVNS most often involves the knee or hip joint causing pain, a blood-stained serous effusion and sometimes locking of the joint. The macroscopic appearances are striking. In the early stages the synovium looks like a tangled red-brown beard; matting together of the hyperplastic, pigmented villi later produces a spongy orange and brown pad of great complexity (Fig. 23.60). Microscopically the enlarged villi are covered by hyperplastic synovial cells and contain abundant histiocytes, many filled with lipid or with haemosiderin which is also found in the synovial lining cells and free in the tissue. Multinucleated giant cells and collagen are less prominent than in the localised form. Foci of chronic inflammatory cells are seen especially around the plentiful collagen-collared blood vessels. When the villi become matted together, clefts lined by synovial cells may be confused with the pseudo-epithelial elements of synovial sarcoma.

The condition is difficult to eradicate. It tends

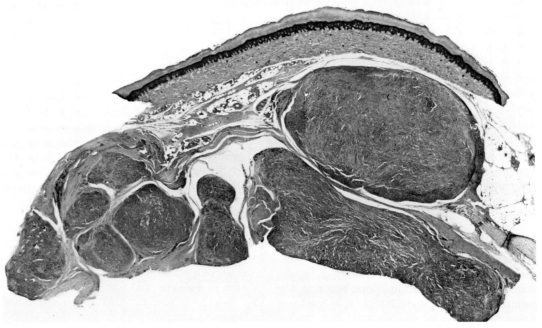

Fig. 23.59 Localised nodular synovitis of tendon sheath. Multiple nodules of pigmented giant-cell tissue are loosely attached to a tendon of the ring finger. × 5·5.

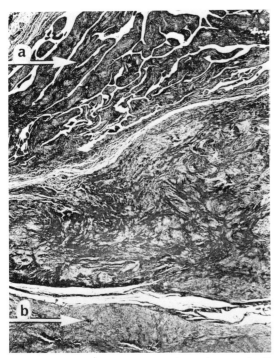

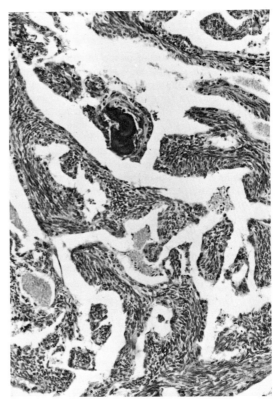

Fig. 23.60 At (**a**) there is diffuse pigmented villonodular synovitis while at (**b**) the villi have become matted together to form a solid mass containing abundant lipid macrophages and haemosiderin. × 10.

Fig. 23.61 Synovial sarcoma showing fibrosarcoma-like spindle cells and clefts lined by cuboidal cells. There is a focus of calcification. This tumour metastasised. × 115.

to recur, may spread to bone, especially when the hip joint is affected, or form a large extra-articular mass in the popliteal fossa or over the femoral neck. Local lymph nodes may be brown from haemosiderin. However this is a benign condition and must be distinguished from synovial sarcoma.

Synovial sarcoma

This rare, highly malignant tumour, also called malignant synovioma, is usually found adjacent to but outside a joint. It occurs most often in the 15–35 age group but has a wide age range. The tumour is most common in the lower limb, around the knee or foot. It is occasionally found in the neck, head and abdominal wall.

Macroscopic appearances. Like many other soft tissue sarcomas, it often has a falsely reassuring appearance of encapsulation due to compression of surrounding tissue. It may be white or pinkish-grey, sometimes with areas of haemorrhage and frequently with spotty calcification which may be sufficient to be seen radiologically.

Microscopic appearances. The tumour consists of fibrosarcomatous and pseudoepithelial elements, either of which may predominate without altering the prognosis. In the fibrosarcomatous tissue there are clefts or gland-like spaces sometimes containing mucinous material and lined by cuboidal or columnar cells (Fig. 23.61). Branching strands of hyaline collagen bearing some resemblance to osteoid are sometimes patchily calcified. Vascular invasion may be seen.

Prognosis. Up to 50% of tumours recur, usually within 2 years of treatment but sometimes much later. Metastases occur in lungs, lymph nodes and other organs. There is a 5-year survival of between 25 and 50% of patients, though some die later of their disease.

Miscellaneous Disorders of the Pararticular Tissues

Ganglion. Ganglia occur in the soft tissue around joints or tendon sheaths, most commonly in the dorsum of the wrist, but also on the palmar aspect and around the knee. They usually develop by myxoid change and cystic softening of the fibrous tissue of the joint capsule or tendon sheath and sometimes have a direct connection with a joint cavity. Rarely they are found within nerve sheaths and may cause symptoms by nerve compression. They consist commonly of a thin, fibrous-walled sac, often rather gelatinous due to the patchy mucoid change, and not lined by synovium. A ganglion contains clear glairy fluid.

Similar lesions occasionally arise in the periosteum, particularly of the tibia and also sometimes within bone, beneath a normal articular surface.

Cyst of semilunar cartilage. The cyst arises in relation to the external semilunar cartilage (lateral meniscus) of the knee and has naked-eye and histological features identical with those of a ganglion. Often it appears to arise in the loose fibrous tissue adjacent to, rather than actually within, the fibrocartilage of the meniscus.

Bursitis. A bursa is a synovial-lined sac and is found chiefly over bony prominences. It may communicate with a joint and is subject to many of the same disorders. Inflammation may arise as a result of repeated trauma as, for instance, in prepatellar bursitis (*housemaid's knee*). The bursa becomes distended with fluid, often with much fibrin, and the synovial lining may show villous hyperplasia or may be replaced by granulation and later by fibrous tissue. Loose melon-seed bodies may form. *Baker's cyst* arises in the popliteal space by herniation of the synovial membrane through the joint capsule. The connection with the articular cavity may be closed by scarring.

Tumoral calcinosis. In this condition radio-opaque calcium phosphate forms small discrete nodules or larger masses around joints, especially the hip, or in soft tissues. It is relatively common in young Africans. The condition is usually initially painless though later there may be pressure on nerves. The overlying skin may ulcerate with discharge of chalky fluid or granular white material. Microscopically the deposits of calcium are often surrounded by macrophages, foreign-body giant cells and dense collagen. Plaques of degenerate collagen may be seen near the deposits. The patients are usually healthy and biochemical changes in the blood are inconstant. The aetiology is uncertain. Suggested causes include traumatic fat necrosis and an abnormality of phosphate metabolism.

Acute calcifying tendonitis. Radiologically detectable calcification within the rotator cuff at the shoulder may be asymptomatic or give rise to attacks of excruciating pain with redness and swelling. The attacks are self-limiting and subside spontaneously. They are precipitated by the rupture of deposits of hydroxyapatite crystals within the tendon often into the subacromial bursa. Sometimes serial x-rays show that the deposit has become smaller.

Polymyalgia rheumatica. This clinical syndrome, which usually affects the elderly, consists of pain, stiffness and tenderness of the muscles of the shoulder and pelvic girdles, with a raised erythrocyte sedimentation rate. There is a mild and often transient non-specific synovitis and about half the patients have evidence of giant-cell arteritis (p. 14.26).

The Connective Tissue Diseases

The concept that the connective tissues of the body comprise a system, subject to its own specific diseases, led Klemperer (1950) to introduce the term *collagen disease*. It soon became apparent that in most types of disease affecting the connective tissues, collagen is neither solely nor primarily involved, and accordingly the term *connective tissue disease* is to be preferred. The diseases most commonly included under this heading are rheumatoid arthritis (RA) and its variants, systemic lupus erythematosus (SLE), rheumatic fever, progressive systemic sclerosis, polyarteritis nodosa and the polymyositis—dermatomyositis complex. The group of diseases is also referred to, somewhat loosely, as the *rheumatic diseases*. It is now apparent that none of these diseases is a primary disorder of connective tissues. Rheumatic fever stands out from the rest in following a specific infection which induces the development of antibodies cross-reactive with the target organ—the heart (p. 15.25). Rheumatoid arthritis, Sjøgren's syndrome, systemic lupus erythematosus, dermatomyositis and progressive systemic sclerosis share the following features. (1) They affect women more often than men. (2) The essential lesion is a vasculitis of small vessels which results in ischaemic and inflammatory lesions in many organs and tissues. (3) They are characterised by a high incidence and wide range of auto-antibodies which react with various components of the nuclei (antinuclear antibodies) or cytoplasm of most types of cell, and by the occurrence of rheumatoid factors which behave as antibodies to IgG. (4) In all, but particularly in SLE and RA, there is evidence that the vasculitis and inflammatory lesions are caused by deposition of autoimmune complexes, i.e. type 3 hypersensitivity reactions. (5) Although these diseases are distinct entities, some patients have a combination of features of two or more of them, e.g. RA and SLE. Because of these common features, it is still appropriate to group the diseases together, and while the term 'connective tissue diseases' does not describe them accurately, it is still widely applied to them.

Polyarteritis nodosa (PAN) is an immune-complex disease which may result from a foreign antigen, e.g. B-hepatitis virus (p. 14.27). Such cases have little in common with the connective tissue diseases, but PAN may occur also as a feature of RA or SLE and is then attributable to auto-immune complexes.

Rheumatoid arthritis (RA)

Because of its high incidence throughout the world, its frequent onset in early adult life and its chronic and disabling effects, RA is one of the most important diseases of mankind. The pathological features of the arthritis and extra-articular lesions are described on pp. 23.44–46, and this account is concerned mainly with the pathogenesis and aetiology.

Pathogenesis. One of the most characteristic features of RA is the development of rheumatoid factors (RFs), and although the mechanisms involved in the destructive inflammatory lesions in the joints and in the formation of rheumatoid nodules have not been fully elucidated, there is strong evidence that activation of complement by antigen-antibody complexes consisting of RF and IgG play a major pathogenic role. RFs consist of immunoglobulins

(IgM and IgG) which behave as auto-antibodies, reacting with antigenic determinants on the Fc of IgG (Fcγ). Although RFs in the plasma react weakly with native IgG to form circulating complexes, they react more avidly with IgG which has been altered by heat, by reacting (as an antibody) with an antigen, or by non-specific binding to the surface of inert material, e.g. latex. In practice, RF is usually detected and assayed by measuring the agglutinating titre of serum for latex beads coated with human IgG (a titre of 1 in 40 or more is usually regarded as a positive result) or by the original Rose-Waaler test which measures the agglutinating titre of serum for sheep red cells sensitised with rabbit IgG antibody (a titre of 1 in 16 or more is regarded as positive). Because RFs differ in their specificity, correlation between these two tests is not complete, but each is positive in approximately 80% of patients with RA, in some patients with various other diseases, and in a small proportion of healthy individuals, very few of whom subsequently develop RA.

Serum RF of IgG class is not readily detected by the above methods because it is not strongly agglutinating, and is assayed more accurately by solid-phase radioimmunoassay (p. 6.12), but in practice this is seldom performed.

The lymph nodes in patients with RA show the features of a humoral immune response (p. 6.37), and immunofluorescence studies in patients with detectable RF (seropositive patients) have shown that RF, mainly of IgM class, is produced by plasma cells in the nodes. Immunofluorescence studies have also shown that some of the plasma cells in the synovium of affected joints produce IgM RF, but many of the synovial plasma cells contain large amounts of IgG which does not behave as RF, i.e. does not bind fluorescein-labelled IgG. However, following treatment of the section of synovium with pepsin, the IgG does bind labelled IgG: the explanation is that IgG RF is self-complexing, possessing both the specific antibody activity of RF and the antigenic Fc components (Fig. 23.62) and treatment with pepsin digests and removes the Fc, leaving Fab capable of binding to the Fc of labelled IgG.

RF-IgG complexes are detectable in the fluid of affected joints, in the walls of small blood vessels, in the interstitial tissue of the affected synovium, and in phagocytes in the synovium

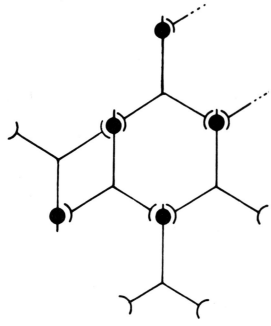

Fig. 23.62 Formation of complexes by IgG rheumatoid factor which acts as both antibody and antigen. The antigen determinant of the Fc is shown as the solid black areas.

and joint fluid. Evidence of complement activation is based on the detection of complement components associated with the complexes, and an observed low level of complement activity, together with the presence of complement activation products, in the joint fluid.

Biopsy of the synovium at a very early stage of RA is not often performed, but the available evidence suggests that the earliest lesion is an acute inflammation accompanied by a vasculitis involving the small blood vessels.

All the features of RA outlined above are consistent with the view that the arthritis is caused by RF-IgG complexes which activate complement and thus induce an exudative inflammation including emigration and activation of polymorphs and monocytes which phagocytose the complexes and, in doing so, release lysosomal enzymes and cationic protein (p. 4.26) injurious to the articular cartilage and synovium. RF in serum has a lower avidity than RF formed in affected synovia, and serum RF in RA patients has been shown to be capable of activating complement, whereas the RF present in the serum of some individuals without RA does not do so: these findings could explain why serum RF is not always associated with disease, and yet a high titre in patients with RA, and particularly the presence of IgG RF, is associated with severe disease.

The extra-articular lesions of RA, notably the lesions of tendons and the nodules which develop subcutaneously and sometimes in various viscera, appear to be caused by RF-IgG complexes in the walls of small blood vessels, but the evidence for this is largely indirect and far from complete.

Various other auto-antibodies are found in some patients with RA, notably antinuclear antibodies, usually in lower titre than in SLE, and antibodies to various cytoplasmic constituents and to collagen. They are, however, of little diagnostic or prognostic significance. An exception is auto-antibody to salivary duct epithelium, which is found in the serum of about 75% of patients with Sjøgren's syndrome (p. 19.9) and in about 25% of RA patients without Sjøgren's syndrome.

While immune-complex disease could explain the major features of RA, there is some evidence that delayed (type 4) hypersensitivity may also play a pathogenic role. Large numbers of lymphocytes are present in affected synovium and joint fluid, and the majority are T (mostly helper) cells. In culture, these lymphocytes produce lymphokines spontaneously and respond poorly to T-cell mitogens, suggesting that they are already activated, perhaps by IgG or an extraneous antigen. These findings might simply mean that T cells are collaborating with B cells in the production of RF, but the presence of lymphokines in the joint fluid suggests that they may also play a role in emigration and activation of phagocytes. A recent review of the pathogenesis of rheumatoid arthritis has been provided by Harris (1984).

Aetiology of RA. As noted above, the local production of RFs in the synovium and pannus of affected joints could account for the arthritis of RA, but it remains to be explained what initiates the production of RF. The answer is not known, but infective agents are likely to be of importance and there is evidence of genetic predisposition. RFs are known to develop in some chronic infections, notably subacute bacterial endocarditis, but usually disappear when the infection is eliminated. Injection of rabbits with autologous IgG antibody complexed with antigen has also been shown to induce production of RF-like immunoglobulins. It therefore seems likely that RF develops as an immune response to the presence of IgG antibody complexed with an antigen. Extensive search has been made for **infective agents** in the synovium and joint fluid in RA patients because it seems most likely that the original antigenic stimulation is provided by an intra-articular infective agent. So far, the results have been disappointing, for although viruses (notably varicella), mycoplasmas and diphtheroids, etc. have been isolated, the results are not consistent, and no particular organism has yet been incriminated. It is, however, possible that infection with various micro-organisms can initiate RF production in genetically predisposed individuals and that, once triggered off, the production of RF in such individuals could be self-perpetuating without the continued persistence of the initiating infection.

The involvement of **genetic factors** is suggested by the high incidence of RA in some families and by the greater degree of concordance for RA in monozygotic than in dizygotic pairs of twins, but it is difficult to distinguish between genetic and environmental factors, e.g. infections. Stronger evidence for genetic predisposition is provided by the high incidence of a particular HLA allo-antigen in patients with RA: for example, in Caucasian patients the incidence of HLA-DR4 (p. 2.13) is much higher than in the general population. Although the significance of such associations is not known, it is possible that the DR antigens on B lymphocytes and monocytes correspond to the Ia antigens in mice and control the immune responses to particular antigenic stimuli (p. 6.25).

Systemic lupus erythematosus (SLE)

This is a chronic disease which is almost ten times commoner in women than in men. It can develop at any age but has a peak incidence in young adults. The disease is characterised by acute and chronic inflammatory lesions, which may occur in almost any organ or tissue, and by the development of various auto-antibodies, most of which are not organ-specific. Many of the lesions appear to be caused by activation of

complement by deposits of auto-immune complexes in the walls of small blood vessels and in various tissues.

The disease may be rapidly fatal, but in most cases it persists for years, usually with periods of remission and acute exacerbations. Improvements in treatment and in the diagnosis of mild cases have increased the 10 year survival rate from about 30% to about 70% over the past 20 years.

Pathological changes. The commoner lesions include polyarthritis, skin rashes, glomerulonephritis, lymphadenopathy, pleurisy and pericarditis. These lesions are inflammatory and may develop acutely and subside, recur, and become chronic. In many cases, the changes are those of acute or chronic inflammation without specific diagnostic features but an acute vasculitis affecting venules and arterioles (p. 14.27) is often seen in the early lesions and is associated with deposition of fibrin and sometimes necrosis in the adjacent tissues. Glomerulonephritis (p. 22.35) develops in about 50% of patients. It is of various types and may give rise to the nephrotic syndrome or to hypertension and/or renal failure: it is the commonest cause of death in SLE. Polyarthritis (80%) is usually mild and, unlike RA, does not result in severe disability. Skin lesions (p. 27.20) occur in about 75% of patients and are commonly induced or aggravated by exposure to sunlight. The typical butterfly rash of the nose and cheeks, which gives the disease its name, occurs in less than 50% of patients. Secondary Raynaud's disease occurs in about 25% of patients: it is due to vasculitis of the small vessels of the extremities and may progress to gangrene and ulceration.

Less common lesions include alopecia, oral ulceration, Libman-Sacks endocarditis (p. 15.37), myositis and myocarditis.

Haematological changes. Anaemia is very common; usually it is mild and normocytic but a haemorrhagic state (see below) may result in iron-deficiency anaemia and occasional patients develop an auto-immune haemolytic anaemia of warm-antibody type (p. 17.29). Leucopenia is also common and auto-immune thrombocytopenia (p. 17.64) is occasionally severe enough to cause purpura. A bleeding tendency may also be associated with the development of antibodies to clotting factors.

Clinical features. The lesions outlined above occur in almost any combination, and a single

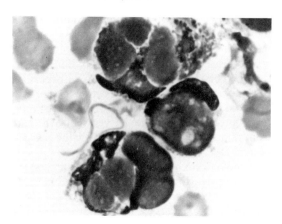

Fig. 23.63 LE cells from a case of SLE. ×600. Three cells are shown with characteristic ingested masses of altered nuclear material. (From a preparation kindly lent by Dr J. M. Robertson.)

feature, e.g. thrombocytopenia, Raynaud's disease or pleurisy, may appear months or even years before the development of other lesions. Neural disorders e.g. confusion, epileptiform fits and psychoses, occur in about 50% of patients. The clinical features are thus wide-ranging and vary greatly from case to case. Some of the lesions are painful, e.g. arthritis and pleurisy, and exacerbations are accompanied by malaise, fever, a raised ESR and loss of weight. Intercurrent infections are common and are aggravated by immunosuppressive therapy.

Immunological features. SLE is perhaps the outstanding example of a non-organ-specific auto-immune disease, a characteristic feature being the large number of auto-antibodies which may develop and which mostly react with components common to many or all types of cell. In the original LE-cell test, whole blood is incubated and stained smears of the leucocytes are examined for LE cells, which consist of homogeneous degraded nuclear material ingested by a neutrophil polymorph (Fig. 23.63). A positive test indicates the presence of antibody to deoxyribonucleoprotein (DNP) which reacts with the nuclei of leucocytes dying during the period of incubation: the antibody-coated nuclear material is degraded by activation of complement which further opsonises it and thus promotes phagocytosis by polymorphs. The LE-cell test has been largely replaced by the more sensitive immunofluorescence technique (p. 6.11) in which sections of suitable fresh tissue, e.g. rat liver, are treated

successively with dilutions of the patient's serum and fluorescein-labelled anti-Ig: anti-DNP is demonstrated by homogeneous staining of the nuclei (Fig. 7.10, p. 7.26) and is found in virtually all cases of SLE, usually in high titre. The test is thus a useful screening procedure; but is not diagnostic of SLE, for it is positive (usually in lower titre) in about 20% of patients with rheumatoid arthritis and other connective tissue diseases, in a number of other miscellaneous conditions, and in a small proportion of healthy individuals.

Antinuclear antibodies to other nuclear constituents are demonstrable by the immunofluorescence test in a proportion of patients with SLE and in some other conditions. They include antibodies to soluble constituents of nuclei (giving a speckled pattern of staining) and antibody to ribonucleic acid (nucleolar staining).

Antibodies to cytoplasmic cellular constituents also occur in SLE and other connective-tissue diseases, but apart from anti-DNP and antibody to 'cardiolipin' which gives a false positive test for syphilis in some patients, the only non-organ specific antibodies of practical importance in SLE are those which react with nuclear DNA. Two such auto-antibodies occur. One reacts only with denatured (single-stranded or ss) DNA and occurs also in other conditions. The second is termed anti-dsDNA because it reacts more avidly with native (double-stranded) DNA (but also with ssDNA): it is detectable by quantitative procedures such as the Farr technique (p. 6.12) or by an immunofluorescence test using slide preparations of the flagellate *Crithidia luciliae*, the kinetoplast of which contains only double-stranded DNA. Anti-dsDNA is detectable in most cases of active SLE and is rarely found in other conditions: serial assay is useful in monitoring disease activity, for exacerbations are preceded by a rise in the serum level and accompanied by a sharp fall.

Pathogenesis of lesions. There is strong evidence that the inflammatory lesions of SLE are caused by activation of complement at sites of deposition of immune complexes in the walls of small blood vessels and in interstitial tissues. The complexes consist of auto-antibodies and their corresponding cellular antigenic constituents (DNA etc.): they are detectable in the serum and circulating complexes may be deposited at local sites, or the antigenic material may be deposited first, followed by union with auto-antibody escaping from the plasma (p. 7.17). Evidence for the pathogenic effects of immune complexes is strongest for the glomerular (p. 22.35) and skin lesions (pp. 27.20–21). In the latter, additional features are involved, for immune complexes can be detected in normal areas of skin in many patients. The induction and aggravation of the skin lesions by ultraviolet light may be due to physical injury to cells with release of auto-antigens, and to the increased vascular permeability of the acute inflammation of sunburn, with exudation of auto-antibodies, immune complexes and complement components.

Once an inflammatory lesion has developed, in the skin or elsewhere, it presumably provides a source of antigens from cell destruction and thus aggravates immune-complex disease and local deposition of antigen. It remains largely unexplained, however, why the sites of lesions vary so greatly from case to case.

A pathogenic role for complement in SLE is supported by the association of hypocomplementaemia with exacerbations of the disease and by the detection of activated complement components associated with the deposits of immune complexes.

Auto-antibodies to platelets and red cells are responsible respectively for the thrombocytopenia and haemolytic anaemia occurring in some patients, and antibodies to leucocytes may contribute to the commonly observed leucopenia. Neuron-specific auto-antibody has been detected by immunofluorescence in some patients with neural disturbances, although deposition of immune complexes in the choroid plexus may also be contributory.

The effectiveness of corticosteroids and other immunosuppressive drugs in many cases is further evidence of the pathogenic role of inappropriate immune responses.

Aetiology. The widely accepted view that many of the lesions of SLE are caused by deposition of auto-immune complexes raises two major questions on its aetiology. First, why are SLE patients unduly prone to develop auto-antibodies? Second, are they unduly susceptible to tissue injury by immune complexes? Neither question has yet been answered satisfactorily.

Genetic factors may be involved in the answers to either or both of the above questions, for although only about 5% of SLE

patients give a family history of the disease, the antinuclear and other auto-antibodies found in SLE have a relatively high incidence in the relatives of patients, and a concordance rate of over 60% for SLE has been reported in pairs of monozygotic twins. Furthermore, tissue typing studies have revealed associations of SLE with various HLA antigens: for example, there is an increased frequency of antigens A1, B5, 7 and 8 and DR2 and 3 in Caucasian patients with SLE and the haplotype A1, B8, DR3 appears to increase the risk of developing SLE by × 5. The nature of these associations is not known: the predisposing HLA antigens may possibly be associated with adjacent Ir genes (p. 2.14) or with defective genes for complement components (see below).

The role of genetic factors has also received indirect support from the regular and spontaneous development of a disease closely resembling SLE in the F1 hybrids of NZB/NZW inbred strains of mice.

The possible causal role of **virus infections** is suggested by the SLE-like disease of NZB/W mice, for these animals are heavily infected with a C-type RNA virus. This does not appear to be the major cause of their disease, but there is evidence that viral antigens and antibodies contribute to the immune complexes and presumably this aggravates the condition, for anti-viral therapy with Ribavirin has been reported to double the lifespan of the mice. In human SLE, particles resembling C-type virus are sometimes observed in renal biopsies, exacerbations of SLE often appear to follow mild viral infections of the respiratory tract, and high serum levels of type II interferon have been reported. In addition to providing immune complexes, virus infections might favour the development of SLE by disturbing the immunity system or by stimulating the development of anti-viral antibodies which act as auto-antibodies, cross reacting with constituents of host cells.

Various **disturbances of the immunity system** have been reported in patients with SLE and also in NZB/W mice: they include defective thymic lymphopoiesis, abnormally high ratio of helper:suppressor T cells in the blood and lymphoid tissues and impaired production of, and unresponsiveness to, interleuken II. Auto-antibodies to T cells have been detected in some patients with SLE and may interfere specially with the function of suppressor T cells, possibly allowing enhanced production of auto-antibodies. There is also evidence suggesting a B-cell abnormality in SLE, but the causes of all these reported disturbances of the immunity system are unknown, nor is it known whether they are of aetiological importance or merely secondary features of the disease.

Defects of complement have been observed in occasional patients with SLE, but recent genetic studies raise the possibility that ineffective ('null') alleles of the genes for individual complement components C4, C2 or B occur in over 80% of SLE patients (see Hughes and Batchelor, 1983): the same defects were observed in over 40% of normal individuals and so, at most, they can only be a contributory causal factor in SLE, possibly by interfering with phagocytosis and destruction of immune complexes. It is, however, of interest that the defects are observed in complement components which are determined by genes in chromosome 6 in close relationship to the HLA loci and that null alleles for particular components are associated with particular HLA antigens. Defects in macrophage function have also been reported in SLE and provide another factor which could interfere with the removal and destruction of immune complexes or antigenic components of dead cells.

In conclusion, many of the lesions of SLE are caused by the presence of immune complexes, and the use of anti-inflammatory and immunosuppressive drugs has greatly improved the prognosis. The undue tendency to develop auto-antibodies and the factors determining the sites of lesions are largely unexplained: multiple disturbances of the immunity system have been observed, but their significance is uncertain. Finally, there appear to be genetic factors which predispose to SLE, but their mechanism is obscure.

Progressive systemic sclerosis. The main features of this rare chronic disease are intimal thickening of small arteries and arterioles, patchy loss of specialised tissue, and replacement fibrosis. In addition to the skin lesion (p. 27.22), the gastro-intestinal tract, heart, skeletal muscles, kidneys and lungs are most often affected. Clinical features include dysphagia from fibrosis and loss of smooth muscle of the oesophagus, disturbances of the gastro-intestinal tract, respiratory insufficiency and repeated infections resulting from progressive pulmonary fibrosis. The interlobular renal arteries are narrowed by severe concentric intimal fibrosis resembling closely that of malignant hypertension: patchy renal ischaemia results, and there may be associated hypertension. Vascular involvement and fibrosis of the dermis bring about ischaemia of the extremities, often with secondary Raynaud's disease. (p. 14.35), and sometimes progressing to ulceration and gangrene. There may also be subcutaneous calcification. Cardiac function may be impaired by myocardial fibrosis, hypertension and lung involvement.

The aetiology of progressive systemic sclerosis is quite unknown. Antinuclear auto-antibodies may be present in the serum, and the condition may be accompanied by rheumatoid arthritis or lesions suggestive of SLE.

The major features of *Sjøgren's syndrome* (p. 19.9), *polyarteritis nodosa* (p. 14.26), *polymyositis* and *dermatomyositis* (p. 21.73) are described in the appropriate systematic chapters.

There is little association between the connective tissue diseases and the organ-specific auto-immune diseases (p. 7.24) except in Sjøgren's syndrome, in which features of both groups are commonly demonstrable.

Tumours and Tumour-like Lesions of Soft Tissues

For practical purposes soft tissues consist of voluntary muscle, fat and fibrous tissue, along with vessels and peripheral nerves supplying them, and their tumours are mesodermal or neuroectodermal in origin. A general survey of these tumours is given in Chapter 12, but it is worth re-emphasising the following points. (1) Although sarcomas may appear well circumscribed on naked-eye examination due to compression of normal tissues at their margin this appearance is misleading. As well as daughter nodules with, at best, a tenuous connection with the main mass, microscopy will show infiltration of tumour along fibrous tissue septa or between muscle fibres, so that surgical 'shelling out' of the tumour inevitably leaves behind these macroscopically invisible tumour extensions and is followed by local recurrence. (2) Sarcomas which arise within a muscle compartment such as the quadriceps femoris remain confined to it until relatively late, when spread to other muscle groups occurs chiefly along vessels or following breaching of the intercompartmental barriers by surgery. The practical implications are that biopsy tracks must be excised at definitive surgery and that removal of the entire muscle compartment often has a good chance of complete local eradication of the tumour. (3) In contrast, a sarcoma which arises outside a muscle compartment, for instance in the groin or antecubital fossa, may extend more widely along neurovascular bundles and involve other tissue planes, making complete excision more difficult. (4) Soft tissue sarcomas most frequently metastasise by the bloodstream to the lungs or, less often, to liver and bone. Though there are exceptions, lymph node metastases are often late and associated with widespread tumour dissemination.

Attempts to evaluate the behaviour and prognosis of a soft tissue tumour depend on a number of factors. An accurate histological diagnosis is essential but it must be admitted that some poorly differentiated tumours cannot be categorised even with the assistance of electron microscopy and immunohistochemistry. However, when a firm diagnosis has been made, say of fibrosarcoma, then it may be useful to attempt to grade this particular tumour in relation to the spectrum of fibrosarcomas, taking into account cellularity, mitotic activity, nuclear pleomorphism and so on. The surgeon considering the grading in conjunction with the equally important clinical staging of the tumour, relating to age, anatomical site, size and evidence of spread, should then be better able to assess the most appropriate type of treatment and the likely behaviour of that particular tumour. Vascular tumours are described on pp. 14.39–43, and tumours of peripheral nerves on pp. 21.64–65.

Benign tumours and tumour-like lesions of fibrous tissue

Although fibromas are found in internal organs such as the kidney they are extremely rare in the soft tissues. Most of the benign fibrous lesions in soft tissues are reactive rather than neoplastic and this probably applies even to the pedunculated skin tags, sometimes described as hard or soft fibromas, which contain a variable

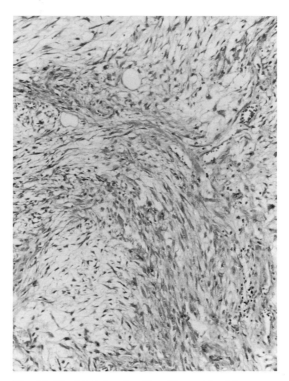

Fig. 23.64 Nodular fasciitis. Plump fibroblasts are loosely arranged and there are pale-staining myxoid foci. A small group of lymphocytes is seen at lower right.

amount of collagen mixed with fat. Localised fibrosis in soft tissue may result from repair following infection, wound healing or the organisation of a haematoma, and is usually not a problem in diagnosis. However, there is a group of benign but very actively proliferating fibroblastic lesions which may be difficult to differentiate from sarcomas, just as early or hyperplastic fracture callus may be difficult to differentiate from osteosarcoma. These lesions (e.g. *nodular fasciitis*, *proliferative myositis*) tend to be rapidly growing but limited in size; they very seldom recur following local excision and never metastasise.

Nodular fasciitis. The usual history is of a rapidly growing tender solitary nodule in the upper limb, especially the forearm of a young adult. Most often the lesion is subcutaneous but sometimes muscle or deeper fascia is involved. Microscopically the nodule consists of a mucopolysaccharide-rich background containing plump fibroblasts arranged in a loose feathery pattern. Myxoid foci and small aggregates of chronic inflammatory cells are seen (Fig. 23.64). Reticulin is plentiful but collagen is scanty. Some

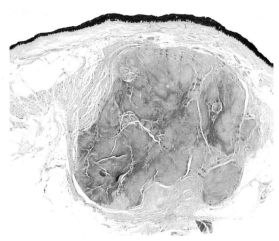

Fig. 23.65 Plantar fibromatosis. Beneath the skin the plantar fascia is greatly expanded by cellular nodules of delicate spindle cells. (Reproduced by permission from *Applied Surgical Pathology*, Blackwell Scientific Publications).

lesions are well circumscribed while others have a sawtoothed edge where capillaries and accompanying fibroblasts extend into surrounding fat. Recurrence after excision is so rare that it calls for review of the diagnosis.

Fibromatosis

This term is applied to a group of conditions whose behaviour and histological features are intermediate between those of a benign fibrous lesion and a fibrosarcoma. Myofibroblasts (p. 5.8) are present in all the lesions.

a) *Keloid.* In some people (Negroes more often than others) excessive amounts of dense hyalinised collagen are formed in the healing of injuries to the skin, resulting in conspicuous firm raised scars. The collagen extends beyond the original site of injury and is associated with large triangular fibroblasts, but growth eventually ceases. Excision is sometimes followed by recurrence.

b) *Palmar fibromatosis (Dupuytren's contracture)* is more common in elderly patients. It begins as a firm nodule in the palm which later extends to form subcutaneous cord-like bands producing flexion contractures usually of the fourth and fifth fingers. In the early stages the lesion may be mistaken microscopically for a fibrosarcoma. The palmar aponeurosis is expanded by highly cellular foci of fibroblasts with little pleomorphism but quite numerous

mitoses. Eventually the tissue becomes almost acellular and tendon-like. *Plantar fibromatosis* is less common, is almost always very cellular, and seldom produces clawing of the toes (Fig. 23.65). Both lesions may be bilateral and are liable to recur following excision of the nodules, probably because there is a field change in the fascia. Fibromatosis may involve the subcutaneous tissue over the knuckles (*knuckle pads*) or the penis (*Peyronies' disease*). More than one of these conditions may occur in the same patient and they are all clearly related.

c) *Musculo-aponeurotic fibromatosis (Extraabdominal desmoid)* is seen characteristically in the thigh, buttock or shoulder. The lesion is white and firm with the consistency and cut surface of a uterine fibroid but it is not encapsulated and infiltrates between muscle fibres, often further than is recognisable by the surgeon's eye (Fig. 23.66). Histologically the diagnosis is most readily made at the margin, where muscle fibres are entrapped: a biopsy from the centre of the lesion usually consists of dense poorly cellular collagen which may be mistaken for scar tissue. The histology is misleadingly bland in view of the aggressive local behaviour of the fibromatosis and the high probability of

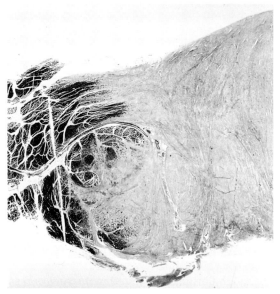

Fig. 23.66 Musculo-aponeurotic fibromatosis. Poorly cellular fibrous tissue has replaced much of the muscle and at its margin is infiltrating amongst the surviving muscle bundles (*left*). (Reproduced by permission from *Applied Surgical Pathology*, Blackwell Scientific Publications).

recurrence. *Abdominal desmoids* are seen characteristically in the rectus abdominis of women during or in the year after pregnancy: their histological picture is the same as the extra-abdominal type but they tend to be smaller, less aggressive and less likely to recur. Neither lesion metastasises.

Myxomas

Myxomas are benign translucent, gelatinous-looking tumours often with cysts containing viscous fluid. They are composed of scanty, delicate, spindle-shaped or stellate fibroblasts separated by ground substance rich in mucopolysaccharide and poor in both collagen and blood vessels. They usually occur as painless lumps within skeletal muscle which may be infiltrated at the tumour margins, but recurrence is rare even after incomplete excision. These benign tumours must be distinguished from myxoid sarcomas of fatty, chondroid or skeletal muscle origin.

Fibrosarcoma

The incidence of fibrosarcoma appears to have dropped in the last few decades partly because of the recognition and reclassification of benign proliferative fibrous lesions such as nodular fasciitis and of locally aggressive, recurrent but non-metastasising fibromatoses. Similarly highly cellular, anaplastic and markedly pleomorphic tumours with numerous tumour giant cells are usually now regarded as malignant fibrous histiocytomas (see below) rather than pleomorphic fibrosarcomas. Electron microscopy and immunohistochemistry have aided in classifying more accurately other spindle-cell sarcomas such as malignant schwannomas (neurofibrosarcomas p. 21.65) and leiomyosarcomas. In consequence, fibrosarcomas are now recognised to be less common than liposarcomas and rhabdomyosarcomas.

Fibrosarcomas may occur at any age but the peak incidence is in the mid-forties. The lower limb is affected most often, and the head and neck least often. The tumours usually involve deep rather than subcutaneous tissue and although they may appear to be well circumscribed rounded masses, satellite nodules are frequently seen. Local recurrence has been reported in about half the patients. Characteristically the tumour consists of interlacing fascicles of spindle cells arranged in a herring bone pattern (Fig. 23.67) and separated by parallel strands of wiry collagen. Unlike liposarcomas and rhabdomyosarcomas, these tumours cannot be sharply divided into subgroups so attempts to grade the tumour histologically are based principally on cellularity, pleomorphism, mitotic activity and the amount of collagen. Richly cellular tumours with little collagen and more than two mitoses/high power field have the worst prognosis, only about a third surviving 5 years, in comparison with 80% survival for the best differentiated fibrosarcomas, some of which may be difficult to separate from fibromatosis.

It is important to be aware that almost 90% of infants with fibrosarcomas have a good prognosis regardless of histological grade.

Malignant fibrous histiocytoma (MFH)

This tumour was first described about 20 years ago but its histogenesis is still controversial. It

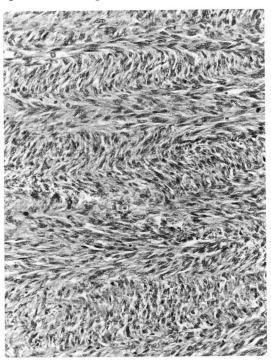

Fig. 23.67 Fibrosarcoma. This cellular tumour has a herring bone pattern due to the interlacing fascicles of spindle cells. Mitoses are plentiful.

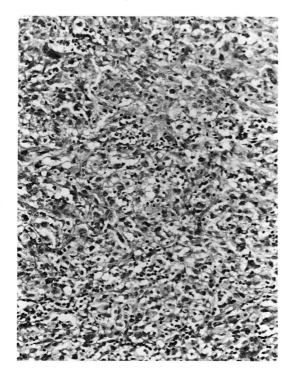

Fig. 23.68 Malignant fibrous histiocytoma, showing pale-staining histiocytes, a scattering of tumour giant cells and some inflammatory cell infiltrate. Elsewhere the tumour was more fibrous and had a storiform pattern.

is thought by some to arise from primitive mesenchymal cells which are capable of differentiating both towards histiocytes with their phagocytic function and to fibroblasts producing collagen. It is the commonest sarcoma of late adult life and is rare before 20. The deep structures of the limbs and the retroperitoneum are most often involved by a multinodular fleshy or myxoid tumour with areas of haemorrhage and necrosis. There are a wide range of histological appearances. Most tumours include areas of plump fibroblastic spindle cells with variable amounts of collagen arranged in short fascicles in a cartwheel (*storiform*) pattern and areas of pleomorphic tumour containing hyperchromatic multinucleate giant cells with bizarre mitoses, plump histiocytes, xanthoma cells and foci of chronic inflammatory cells (Fig. 23.68). Some tumours have nodular foci of osteoclast-like giant cells and others areas of myxoid change. The tumour cells tend to spread along fascial planes and between muscle bundles and almost 50% recur after surgery. About 40%

develop metastases to lung, lymph nodes, liver and bone. Tumours predominantly of a myxoid pattern recur more often but are less likely to metastasise. In general, small superficial tumours on the distal parts of the limbs carry a better prognosis.

Atypical fibroxanthoma is a small, superficial, expanding nodule which occurs in the sun-damaged skin of the head and neck in elderly patients or less often on the extremities of younger patients: it occasionally arises at a site of previous irradiation. It has a similar microscopic appearance to MFH but is benign.

The benign fibrohistiocytic tumour (**dermatofibroma**) and a tumour of limited malignancy, (**dermatofibrosarcoma protuberans**) are described on pp. 27.36–37.

Tumours of adipose tissue

Lipoma

This is the most common benign mesenchymal tumour. Though it may arise anywhere in the body, it is found more often in the neck, back and shoulders of obese middle-aged and elderly women as a soft, symptomless lump which persists unchanged after an initial growth period. Most of these superficial lipomas are removed for cosmetic reasons, while more deeply situated ones in retroperitoneum or mediastinum are symptomless until they are large enough to cause pressure symptoms. The tumour may be recognised radiologically as an ovoid zone of radiolucency surrounded by denser shadows of the compressed adjacent tissues. Lipomas are rounded, well circumscribed, thinly encapsulated masses of yellow adipose tissue which may be very large. They seldom recur following surgery. Multiple tumours may be present and occasionally they are symmetrical. The tumour increases in size by proliferation of fibroblast-like cells which lie around the blood vessels but are hard to see in most cases because they rapidly accumulate fat. Should the patient become emaciated, the fat in the tumour is not utilised—a good example of the failure of tumours to respond to the factors controlling the metabolism of normal tissues.

Other tissues than fat may be present in a lipoma. Large lipomas occasionally contain areas of calcification, bone or cartilage. Myxoid foci are occasionally seen but the lack of lipoblasts and of a network

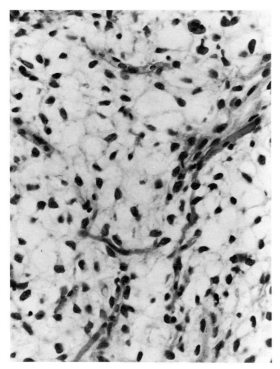

Fig. 23.69 Myxoid liposarcoma. Between the capillary meshwork there is a pale-staining background rich in mucopolysaccharides containing some signet-ring and foamy lipoblasts.

of capillaries should differentiate this from a myxoid liposarcoma (see below). *Fibrolipomas* contain a good deal of mature collagen while the painful *angiolipomas*, usually seen in the forearm of young adults, have a rich capillary network sometimes containing microthrombi. Two related subgroups of lipomas which may be confused histologically with sarcomas are seen especially in the neck and shoulder of elderly men. They are (1) the *spindle-celled lipoma* in which fat and fairly uniform spindle cells with collagen are mixed in varying proportions. When spindle cells are numerous, the lesion may appear alarmingly cellular; sometimes there is a striking vascular pattern. (2) The *pleomorphic lipoma* contains fat and a variable number of bizarre giant cells with peripheral overlapping nuclei ('florets'). Mitoses are scanty in both lesions. Sometimes a mixture of spindle cells and pleomorphic cells is seen in the same tumour. The so-called *intramuscular lipoma* may also give rise to needless anxiety because of the apparent infiltration of skeletal muscle and intermuscular connective tissue by mature lipocytes. These tumours, chiefly of the large muscles of the thigh, shoulder and arm, are found most often in males and complete excision is curative.

Liposarcoma

This is the most common soft-tissue sarcoma in adults; it almost never affects infants and small children. It occurs most often in the thigh, buttock and retroperitoneum and, in contrast to lipoma, usually involves deeper structures, such as the intermuscular fascial planes, rather than the subcutaneous tissues. Liposarcomas vary widely in naked-eye and microscopic appearances and in prognosis.

Well-differentiated liposarcoma is obviously fatty and microscopically simulates a lipoma but contains a scattering of lipoblasts which may contain a single fatty droplet pushing the nucleus to one side, or many small droplets as in the cells of brown fat. Sometimes there may be a scattering of lymphocytes and plasma cells or areas of dense fibrosis.

Myxoid liposarcoma accounts for about half the cases; the tumour appears gelatinous and, on section, thick viscous fluid runs from its surface. Microscopically it is characterised by signet ring or foamy lipoblasts which may be scanty and show little mitotic activity, by a prominent meshwork of capillaries like wire-netting, and by an abundant mucopolysaccharide-rich matrix (Fig. 23.69). Pooling of the mucoid matrix may produce a cribriform pattern similar to a lymphangioma. Neither the well-differentiated nor the myxoid liposarcoma is likely to metastasise but both, and especially the myxoid ones, recur, sometimes repeatedly over many years. The recurrences often have the same histological pattern but sometimes in the myxoid tumours more compact areas of less differentiated rounded cells develop. These **round-cell liposarcomas**, and also the **pleomorphic liposarcomas** (Fig. 23.70), with their large giant cells and high mitotic rate, are more aggressive and liable to metastasise. The five-year survival in limb and retroperitoneal tumours is about 80% in the well-differentiated and myxoid groups and only 20% in the round-cell and pleomorphic groups.

It is important to realise that the presence of lipid within tumour cells does not necessarily imply that the tumour is a liposarcoma, for it may result from degeneration or from the breakdown of infiltrated fat. Conversely, lipid may be extremely scanty in, for instance, a myxoid liposarcoma with few lipoblasts.

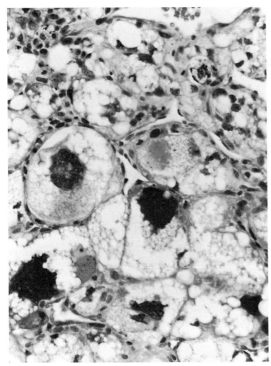

Fig. 23.70 Pleomorphic liposarcoma. Many fatty droplets are present in the cytoplasm of the gigantic lipoblasts with their hyperchromatic nuclei.

Tumours of smooth muscle

Leiomyoma

Benign smooth muscle tumours are found most often in the genito-urinary and gastro-intestinal tracts, especially in the uterus (p. 24.15), less often in the skin and, in contrast to leiomyosarcomas, very infrequently in deeper soft tissues. Cutaneous leiomyomas may arise from the media of superficial veins (angioleiomyoma or vascular leiomyoma, p. 14.40) or from the arrector pili muscles of the skin. The pilar leiomyomas usually form lines or groups of small discrete painful, tender nodules often on the flexor surfaces of the limbs. Solitary examples are found especially in the external genitalia and less often at other sites. These leiomyomas are not encapsulated but merge with the surrounding dermal collagen. They are benign but because of their multiplicity are difficult to treat.

Leiomyomas are composed of fascicles of spindle cells (Fig. 12.45, p. 12.30) which may be identified as myocytes by their longitudinal myofibrils on electron microscopy and sometimes, with special stains, on light microscopy. In cross section, the cytoplasm may appear faintly bubbly while sometimes a single more distinct vacuole indents the nucleus. The nuclei are more blunt ended than those of fibroblasts and occasionally lined up in a palisaded pattern mimicking a schwannoma (p. 21.64). A variable amount of collagen may be mixed with the smooth-muscle bundles.

Leiomyosarcoma

Malignant smooth-muscle tumours are found most often in the retroperitoneum of elderly patients. At the time of diagnosis the tumour is often large and no longer resectable, so that few patients survive, most dying with metastases in the liver and lung. The prognosis is better in leiomyosarcomas of the soft tissues of the limbs, the smaller and more superficial the tumour, the better the outlook. About 10% of the relatively rare and poorly circumscribed dermal tumours and more than a third of the pseudo-encapsulated subcutaneous sarcomas metastasise. The histological differentiation between benign and malignant smooth-muscle tumours may be difficult. Some leiomyomas contain multinucleate and pleomorphic cells so this feature on its own is not a good guide to malignant change. The mitotic rate is more reliable: tumours with 5 mitoses/10 high power fields can be regarded as malignant and those with 1–4 mitoses as potentially so, especially if the tumour is large and shows necrosis and pleomorphism. Occasionally, even apparently benign tumours metastasise.

Tumours of voluntary muscle

Rhabdomyosarcoma is the commonest soft tissue sarcoma of children, adolescents and young adults, but is rare in older patients. It is recognised under light microscopy by the presence of rhabdomyoblasts which vary in their differentiation from rounded or irregular cells with coiled myofibrils (Fig. 23.71a) to spindle and strap-shaped cells. All have eosinophilic cytoplasm, some contain glycogen and the tadpole and strap-shaped cells are most likely to

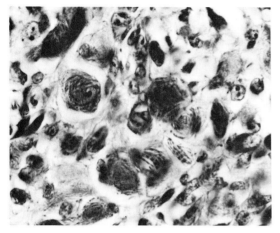

Fig. 23.71a Rhabdomyosarcoma. Large pleomorphic cells in a slightly myxoid background. Coiled myofibrils are best seen in cells below and to the right of centre.

reveal diagnostic cross striations similar to those seen in normal voluntary muscle (Fig. 23.71b). The immunohistochemical demonstration of myosin or myoglobin in the tumour cells or the presence of myofilaments on electron microscopy aid in the diagnosis. Four histological subgroups are recognised.

Embryonal rhabdomyosarcoma occurs chiefly from birth to adolescence, most often involving the head and neck, genito-urinary tract and retroperitoneum. The tumours vary both in their cellularity, often showing poorly cellular myxoid areas, and in the number and differentiation of rhabdomyoblasts. Cross striations are demonstrable in about half the cases. The *botryoid sarcomas* are a variant of em-

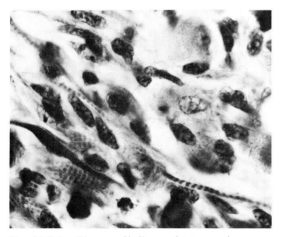

Fig. 23.71b The myofibrils are best seen in cross-striations of the elongated strap cells (bottom right) but these cells are often hard to find.

bryonal sarcoma, so-called because of their distinctive naked-eye appearance of grape-like gelatinous masses. They occur in the submucosa of vagina, bladder, bile duct or nose and project into the lumen.

Alveolar rhabdomyosarcomas chiefly involve skeletal muscle of adolescents and young adults. In this variant, carrot-like or club-shaped tumour cells adhere to the fibrous septae which divide the cells into clumps. Loss of cohesion in the centre of the groups of cells produces the alveolar pattern. Tumour giant cells with peripheral nuclei are common but do not contain cross striations; indeed these are found in only about a quarter of the cases.

Pleomorphic rhabdomyosarcomas are rare and occur chiefly in the skeletal muscles of older people. Cross striations are almost never found, and it is often difficult to separate this group from other pleomorphic sarcomas.

Until recently, rhabdomyosarcomas were almost uniformly fatal, but the prognosis has greatly improved with the combined use of surgical resection, radiotherapy and chemotherapy. The clinical staging of the tumour is the most important factor in estimating survival, but there is some evidence that alveolar tumours are less responsive to treatment.

Benign tumours of voluntary muscle are very rare. They occur occasionally in the head and neck in patients over 40 or under 4 years of age and as polypoid masses in the vagina or vulva in middle-aged women. Their neoplastic nature is doubtful: they may be hamartomas, similar to the cardiac rhabdomyomas seen in children with tuberous sclerosis (epiloia p. 21.48).

Cartilaginous and bony tumours

Benign soft tissue *chondromas* are almost confined to the hands and feet. Most soft tissue chondrosarcomas are deep-seated in the limbs and are of two histological types, a myxoid, prominently lobulated form (*chordoid sarcoma*) with a variable but usually good prognosis (the more myxoid the tumour the better) and so-called *mesenchymal chondrosarcoma* which is highly malignant and metastasising. As the name suggests, the mesenchymal chondrosarcoma consists of two components—sheets of undifferentiated small mesenchymal cells, sometimes with a marked vascular pattern, and lobules of cartilage.

Osteosarcoma arising in soft tissue is rare. Histologically it closely resembles osteosarcoma of bone (p. 23.28). It occurs in an older age group and has a very poor prognosis.

Extraskeletal Ewing's tumour arises chiefly in the paravertebral region and lower limbs and has much

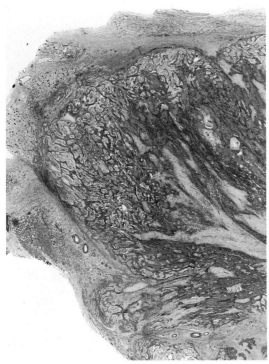

Fig. 23.72 Myositis ossificans. Arcades of woven bone are seen at the periphery of the lesion. Beneath this shell, less well differentiated trabeculae are seen to the right of the picture.

the same age range, histological appearance and prognosis as the bone tumour (p. 23.36).

Myositis ossificans

This condition is entirely benign though in the early stages it may be difficult to distinguish both clinically and histologically from a malignant tumour, hence the alternative term *pseudomalignant osseous tumour of soft tissues*. It occurs mostly in the muscles or subcutaneous tissue of the limbs of young people and in about half the cases there is a history of preceding injury. The patient usually complains of a soft tissue swelling which may increase rapidly. Histologically the central part of the lesion consists of loosely-arranged triangular fibroblasts often with a high mitotic rate and some resemblance to nodular fasciitis (p. 23.64). In places, proliferating cells aggregate into clumps and a distinctively patterned osteoid matrix is laid down which, towards the margin of the lesion, matures to form the more normal picture of woven bone (Fig. 23.72). Eventually arcades of

woven or lamellar bone, sometimes with nodules of cartilage, outline the margin of the lesion which is seen radiologically after 4–6 weeks as a well-defined bony shell. This pattern of peripheral maturation or 'zoning' is helpful in making the diagnosis but the bony shell may be incomplete or even absent, particularly in lesions of the hand. Surrounding or included muscle is sometimes damaged with foci of chronic inflammatory cells and thickened blood vessel walls. If the lesion is close to bone, it stimulates subperiosteal new bone formation which may reinforce the surgeon's suspicion of tumour.

Soft-tissue ossification is found following a variety of soft tissue injuries such as dislocation of the elbow, following tetanus, and after some orthopaedic operations. The ectopic ossification seen in a variety of neurological conditions such as paraplegia and poliomyelitis is usually attributed to forced passive exercise.

Tumours of uncertain histogenesis

Granular cell tumour (Granular cell myoblastoma)

This is a small benign tumour, usually solitary, and found in skin, submucosa or muscle, especially in the tongue. It consists of ribbons or nests of uniform rounded or polygonal cells with small central nuclei and abundant coarsely granular eosinophilic cytoplasm. It is not encapsulated and the clusters of cells extend into the adjacent tissue, sometimes surrounding nerve twigs or growing along muscle fibres. Its histogenesis is uncertain, most favouring a neural origin. This is an important lesion for two reasons: firstly because the overlying squamous epithelium shows pseudoepitheliomatous hyperplasia (Fig. 23.73) and in small superficial biopsies, as obtained for instance from the larynx, this may lead to a mistaken diagnosis of squamous carcinoma if the underlying granular cells are not identified. Secondly, its firm consistency and infiltrating pattern may lead to a mistaken frozen-section diagnosis of breast carcinoma, especially when the tumour cells are scanty and have evoked a marked desmoplastic reaction.

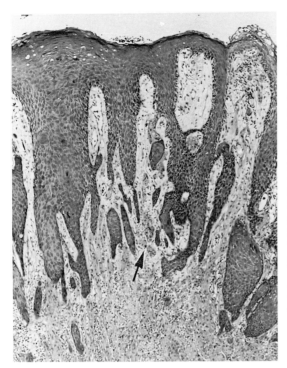

Fig. 23.73 Granular cell myoblastoma of the tongue with marked overlying pseudo-epitheliomatous hyperplasia of the squamous mucosa. Small clumps of granular cells can be made out (*arrow*).

Alveolar soft part sarcoma

The peak incidence of this rare sarcoma is in adolescents and young adults, the leg being most often affected. The favoured site in children is the head and neck and these tumours have a better prognosis in this age group. The patient usually presents with a slowly growing, painless lump, but sometimes with cerebral or pulmonary metastases; only about half the patients survive for 5 years. The histological appearances are of rounded or polygonal cells with abundant eosinophilic granular or vacuolated cytoplasm rich in glycogen. These are grouped into packets and central loss of cell cohesion produces the alveolar pattern (Fig. 23.74). The alveoli are separated by sinusoidal vessels and the frequently observed vascular invasion no doubt accounts for early metastatic spread. This tumour pattern may be mimicked by metastatic renal carcinoma but PAS +ve rod-shaped crystalloid cytoplasmic bodies with a diagnostic ultrastructure are helpful in differentiation.

Epithelioid sarcoma

This sarcoma has been confused clinically and histologically with both granulomatous inflammatory conditions and with carcinoma. The hand, forearm and pretibial regions of adolescents and young adults are most often affected. When the superficial tissues are involved the lesion presents as firm, slowly growing, woody nodules or plaques in the skin, which soon ulcerate. Deeper lesions form indurated, poorly circumscribed multinodular masses around tendons and fascia and symptoms may arise from the involvement of nerves. Microscopically the tumour consists of eosinophilic, epithelial-like and plump spindle cells with scanty mitoses arranged in nodules or festoon-like bands (Fig. 23.75). The nodules are often surrounded by chronic inflammatory cells and show central necrosis, appearances which have been mistaken for a granuloma. Cords of tumour cells may extend between strands of hyalinised collagen mimicking a scirrhous carcinoma. About 75% of these sarcomas recur, sometimes more than once, and 50% metastasise. The course of the disease may be prolonged but involvement of blood vessel walls and regional lymph nodes is ominous. This is one of the sarcomas in which regional lymph node resection may be advisable.

Clear cell sarcoma (Malignant melanoma of soft parts)

This rare, slow-growing, well circumscribed sarcoma may occur at any age but the peak incidence is

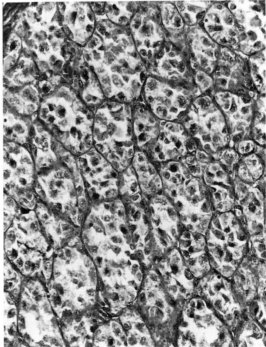

Fig. 23.74 Alveolar soft part sarcoma. Packets of cells are separated by thin-walled, collapsed blood vessels. The cells adhere to the 'alveolar' walls and may contain PAS-positive material in their bulky cytoplasm.

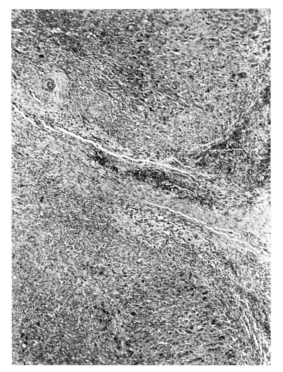

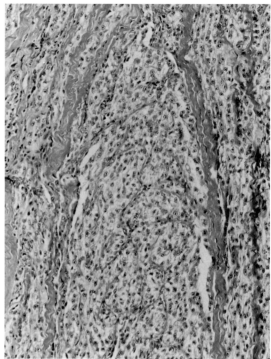

Fig. 23.75 Epithelioid sarcoma. Nodules of epithelial-like cells are rimmed by a chronic inflammatory cell infiltrate (*right*). There is necrosis within the nodules (*left*).

Fig. 23.76 Clear cell sarcoma. Cells with pale-staining cytoplasm and prominent nucleoli are divided into small packets by fibrous septae. Some strands of dense collagen from the invaded tendon can be made out.

between 20 and 40 years and the commonest site is the tendons and deep aponeuroses of the lower limbs. The overlying skin shows no evidence of pigmentation or junctional activity. The rounded or fusiform tumour cells are arranged in compact nests separated by fibrous septa which merge with the adjacent fibrous structures (Fig. 23.76). This packeting of the cells, and their prominent nucleoli, emphasise the histological similarity to melanoma.

About 50% of the lesions contain melanin and in some cases melanosomes in various stages of development have been demonstrated by electron microscopy, features which strongly suggest a neural crest origin. The term 'clear-cell' is perhaps unfortunate for in some cases, and particularly in recurrences, the clear cells are scanty, the cytoplasm being faintly eosinophilic. Recurrence is common, about half the patients die with metastases in the lungs, lymph nodes or bone, and less than a third are cured by the initial excision.

References and Further Reading

Bullough, P. G. (1984) *Atlas of Orthopaedic Pathology*. University Park Press, Baltimore.

Dahlin, D. C. (1978) *Bone Tumors* 3rd edn. pp. 445. Charles C. Thomas, Springfield, Illinois.

Enzinger, F. M. and Weiss, S. W. (1983) *Soft Tissue Tumors*. pp. 840. C. V. Mosby, St Louis.

Harris, E. D. Jr. (1984) Pathogenesis of rheumatoid arthritis. *Clinics in Orthopaedics*, **182**, 14–23.

Hughes, G. R. V. and Batchelor, J. R. (1983) Genetics of systemic lupus erythematosus. *British Medical Journal*, **286**, 416–7.

Smith, Roger (1979) *Biochemical Disorders of the Skeleton*. pp. 293. Butterworths, London.

24

The Female Reproductive Tract and the Breast

The Female Reproductive Tract

The Vulva

The skin of the vulva is part of the body integument and is therefore subject to all the diseases that can afflict the skin elsewhere in the body, such as, for example, psoriasis, pemphigus or lichen planus. Dermatological conditions developing in the vulva tend, however, to be modified by the effects of local heat and moisture, by the easy access afforded to the bacterial flora of the gut and by the changes induced in vulvar skin as a result of its sensitivity to ovarian hormones.

Infections. Many vulvar infections, especially those occurring in debilitated women, are of mixed nature but some are due to streptococci or staphylococci, the latter, and also candida infections occurring with increased frequency in diabetics. The features of the various sexually transmitted diseases which involve the vulva are described for both male and female on pp. 25.1–5.

Atrophy. Thinning of the vulvar epithelium is common; some degree of atrophy occurs as a physiological response to oestrogen withdrawal in all postmenopausal women and is sometimes sufficiently marked to cause narrowing of the introitus.

Vulvar dystrophies. This term is applied to a group of different conditions characterised by disorders of epithelial growth, which occur most commonly in middle-aged women. In *hyperplastic dystrophy* the vulvar skin may show white, red or brown patches which alternate with diffuse areas of corrugation, scaliness or eczematoid change. Histologically, the squamous epithelium shows acanthosis with irregular thickening of the Malphigian layer and long, distorted rete pegs: a variable degree of parakeratosis and hyperkeratosis is often present and there is commonly a chronic inflammatory cell infiltration of the dermis. **Lichen sclerosus et atrophicus** (Fig. 24.1) is characterised by thinning of the epidermis, flattening of the dermo-epidermal junction, hyalinisation of the upper dermis and a non-specific chronic-inflammatory-cell infiltration of the deeper part of the dermis. A *mixed dystrophy* is one in which areas of hyperplastic dystrophy and of lichen sclerosus co-exist in the same vulva.

In most cases of vulvar dystrophy there is no cellular atypia and in these there is no risk of eventual evolution into a squamous cell carcinoma. A proportion of cases, particularly of hyperplastic dystrophy, do however show a significant degree of cellular atypia ('intra-epithelial neoplasia') and these may progress to an invasive squamous-cell carcinoma.

Vulvar intra-epithelial neoplasia. A proportion of vulvar squamous-cell carcinomas arise from atypical squamous epithelium showing varying degrees of cellular atypia: such atypia may be seen in a dystrophic epithelium but also occurs in non-dystrophic vulvar skin. In the atypical epithelia the cells fail to mature, and have an increased nucleo-cytoplasmic ratio and hyperchromatic nuclei: mitotic figures are often seen above the basal layer and are sometimes

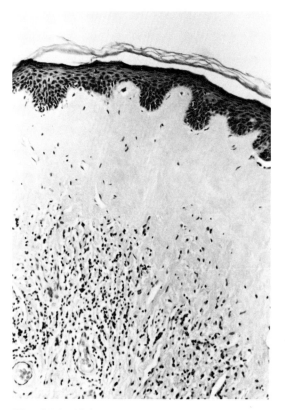

Fig. 24.1 Lichen sclerosus et atrophicus of the vulva. The upper dermis is hyalinised whilst in the deeper part of the dermis there is a non-specific chronic inflammatory cell infiltration. The epidermis is atrophic. × 150.

of abnormal form. Atypia of this type is now recognised to be an intra-epithelial neoplasm (vulvar intra-epithelial neoplasia or VIN). If atypical cells occupy less than the full thickness of the epithelium the condition is classed as VIN I or II whilst if the full thickness of the epithelium is occupied by atypical cells the con-

dition is graded as VIN III and corresponds to carcinoma in situ. Not all cases of VIN III progress to an invasive cancer and a significant proportion spontaneously regress. Progression to an invasive squamous-cell carcinoma is most likely to occur in elderly women or in immunosuppressed young women.

Tumours. A variety of benign skin neoplasms, such as papillomas, fibromas and lipomas, occur in the vulva and this is a site at which benign sweat gland tumours (hidradenomas—p. 22.29) are particularly prone to develop.

Malignant vulvar neoplasms are uncommon and most are *squamous-cell carcinomas*; these tumours usually develop in elderly women and can arise from either an epithelium showing the changes of VIN or an otherwise normal squamous epithelium. The tumour may present as an indurated plaque, an ulcer with hard rolled edges or as a warty mass, most commonly on the labia majora; histologically, it is usually, though not invariably, well differentiated. The tumour spreads first to the inguinal lymph nodes and, because of anastomoses between the lymphatics of the two sides, it is by no means unusual for bilateral inguinal node involvement to occur: later spread is to femoral, iliac and para-aortic nodes. The overall 5-year survival rate for women treated for a vulvar carcinoma is about 70%: the survival rate is 90% for those without lymph node involvement but falls to between 25 and 60% for those with lymph node metastases.

Rare primary malignant neoplasms of the vulva include *adenocarcinoma of Bartholin's gland*, *malignant melanoma* and *basal-cell carcinoma*; metastatic deposits of endometrial adenocarcinoma or choriocarcinoma are also sometimes encountered.

The Vagina

Infection. Vaginal infections are common but many are non-specific in nature and due to lowered vaginal resistance to bacterial invasion, as occurs, for instance, in vaginal epithelial atrophy resulting from oestrogen deficiency. Specific infections, including those transmitted sexually (pp. 25.1–5), may be due to organisms such as *Neisseria gonorrhoeae*, *Mycoplasma*, *herpes virus*, *Chlamydia* or cytomegalovirus, while candida infection, predisposed to by the high glycogen content of the vaginal epithelium, is common; sexually-transmitted infestation with the protozoal parasite *Trichomonas vaginalis* is also very common.

Adenosis. This is characterised by the presence of small glands or cysts in the submucosa of the upper third of the vagina; the epithelium in these may be endocervical, endometrial or tubal in type. This usually asymptomatic congenital abnormality is particularly common in girls whose mothers received synthetic oestrogen therapy during pregnancy and, although innocuous in itself, predisposes to the development of an adenocarcinoma.

Tumors

Squamous-cell carcinoma of the vagina is uncommon; it usually occurs in the upper part of the vagina in elderly women and presents as an indurated patch: the tumour is often poorly differentiated and tends to invade the cervix, paravaginal tissues, rectum and bladder, the 5-year survival rate after treatment being only about 30%.

Adenocarcinoma of the vagina was, until recently, of exceptional rarity, but in the last 15 years a considerable number of clear-cell vaginal adenocarcinomas have occurred in girls aged between 15 and 25, mostly in North America. Common to virtually all of these cases has been pre-existing vaginal adenosis and a history of prenatal exposure to synthetic oestrogens, particularly diethylstilboestrol.

The Cervix

Cervicitis

Cervical infection is common, possibly because the complex deep folds of the endocervical crypts offer a relatively protected haven in which micro-organisms can flourish. The inflammatory response to infection may be either acute or chronic, the histological characteristics of the inflammatory process being exactly the same as those seen in comparable infections elsewhere in the body. Many cervical infections are of a non-specific, and probably mixed bacterial, nature, but specific infection with *N. gonorrhoeae*, *herpes virus*, *Chlamydia*, mycobacteria, *Tr. vaginalis*, *Myco. tuberculosis* and *Treponema pallidum* can occur (pp. 25.1–5).

Cervical ectopy

This term is applied to a red area on the ectocervix which surrounds the external os (Fig. 24.2): this abnormality was previously known as a *cervical erosion* and this term is, indeed, still often used by gynaecologists who tend to regard this as an inflammatory or ulcerative process. An ectopy is, however, usually a physiological change consequent upon an increase in cervical bulk, as occurs at puberty or in pregnancy; this causes an unfolding of the cervix with eversion of the distal endocervix out

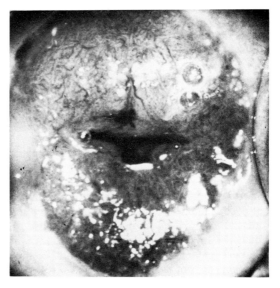

Fig. 24.2 Cervical ectopy as seen through a colposcope. The external os is circumferentially surrounded by thin endocervical epithelium through which the sub-epithelial vessels are clearly visible.

into what is anatomically the ectocervix. The thin endocervical columnar epithelium is relatively transparent and hence the sub-epithelial vessels impart to an ectopy its characteristic redness. The exposure of the delicate endocervical epithelium to the acidity of the vagina results in squamous metaplasia, the squamous cells differentiating from pluripotential basal reserve (stem) cells of the endocervical epithelium. Squamous metaplasia can therefore be seen as a protective mechanism in which the relatively fragile endocervical epithelium is replaced by more robust stratified squamous cells and when this process is complete the ectopy is said to be 'healed'. This area of squamous metaplasia is often known as the '*transformation zone*' and is of considerable importance because most cervical carcinomas appear to originate at this site.

Premalignant disease of the cervix

It is now recognised that a squamous cell carcinoma of the cervix does not usually arise abruptly in · otherwise normal cervical squamous epithelium but evolves over a number of years, probably 10–15, from an epithelium which shows progressively severe degrees of abnormality. The early, or premalignant, stage of cervical carcinoma is characterised by the presence within the squamous epithelium of cells showing a failure of maturation, loss of polarity, excessive and abnormal mitotic activity, an increased nucleo-cytoplasmic ratio and both nuclear and cytoplasmic pleomorphism. Until recently, considerable stress was laid upon both the degree and extent of these intra-epithelial abnormalities. Epithelia in which the cells showed only a minor or moderate degree of abnormality, or in which the abnormal cells did not occupy the full thickness of the epithelium, were considered as *dysplastic* and those in which the full thickness of the epithelium was occupied by abnormal cells were said to show *carcinoma in situ* (Fig. 24.3), a lesion differing from a frank carcinoma only by its confinement within the epithelium and its lack of any stromal invasion. These terms are still widely used but it has become increasingly apparent that the abnormal cells in a dysplastic epithelium are identical in all respects to those in a carcinoma in situ and that the progression from dysplasia to carcinoma in situ occurs as a continuous process, the division between the two types of intra-epithelial abnormality being both subjective and arbitrary. Hence the term '**cervical intra-epithelial neoplasia**' (**CIN**) has been introduced to cover the whole spectrum of premalignant change in cervical epithelium; abnor-

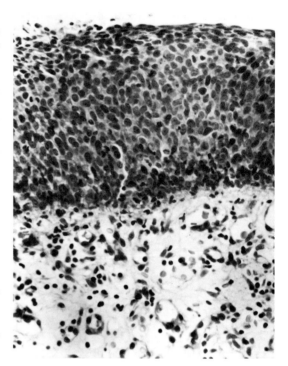

Fig. 24.3   Cervical intra-epithelial neoplasia Grade 3 (carcinoma in situ) of the uterine cervix. The cells in the cervical epithelium show a complete lack of maturation, are pleomorphic and have an increased nucleocytoplasmic ratio. × 275.

malities previously classed as mild or moderate dysplasia are now called CIN I and CIN II respectively and both severe dysplasia and carcinoma in situ are classed together as CIN III. It should not, however, be assumed that all examples of CIN I or II progress to CIN III or that CIN III will invariably proceed to an invasive carinoma. Many cases of CIN, at any stage in the evolution of this abnormality, either remain stationary or regress with probably no more than one-third of cases of CIN III advancing to the invasive stage; indeed, it is almost certain that some, probably many, examples of CIN I and II are not truly neoplastic in nature but represent an atypical cellular response to factors such as viral infection. Currently, however, *there are no available methods for distinguishing a reactive lesion from one which is truly neoplastic or for the recognition of those cases of CIN which will progress to invasive cancer.* Hence all cases of CIN have to be regarded as potentially invasive: fortunately these epithelial lesions, though asymptomatic, are readily detected by cytological examination of cervical smear preparations and their treatment and eradication, by techniques such as cryocautery and laser therapy, are relatively simple. Widespread cytological screening and prompt treatment of intra-epithelial abnormalities appear to have reduced markedly the incidence of invasive cervical carcinoma.

Malignant tumours of the cervix

Ninety-five per cent of malignant cervical tumours are squamous-cell carcinomas and nearly all of the remaining 5% are adenocarcinomas.

Squamous-cell carcinoma

Aetiology and pathogenesis. Epidemiological studies have demonstrated an association between squamous-cell carcinoma of the cervix and early marriage, early pregnancy, a high number of pregnancies, sexual promiscuity, divorce, sexually transmitted diseases, prostitution and low socio-economic status. These findings clearly suggest a correlation with a particular life-style but it is virtually certain that the one common link between these various factors is early onset of sexual activity. It is believed that a carcinogen is transmitted sexually by the male at a time when the epithelium of the cervix is in an unstable state, i.e. when the transformation zone is undergoing squamous metaplasia during late adolescence (see above). The nature of this carcinogenic agent remains uncertain but it is unlikely to be smegma and suspicion has fallen on *Herpes simplex type 2* and certain strains of human *Papillomavirus* (p. 13.14). Certainly the role of sexual transmission is indicated by the fact that barrier methods of contraception are associated with a lower incidence of cervical carcinoma and by the apparent proneness of some men to be 'carcinogenic', their sexual partners having an unusually high risk of developing cervical cancer. Various racial and ethnic factors which were formerly thought to be significant in the aetiology of this neoplasm are now thought to be related principally to the sexual habits of those particular groups.
Macroscopic features. Cervical squamous-cell

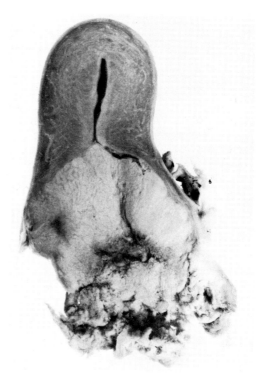

Fig. 24.4   An advanced squamous-cell carcinoma of the uterine cervix.

carcinoma may be predominantly exophytic, *i.e.* it may grow out from the surface as a bulky, friable, papillary or polypoid mass—Fig. 24.4, or endophytic, *i.e.* extending deeply into the cervix, converting it into a hard bulky, nodular mass which eventually ulcerates.
Microscopic features. The tumour tends to infiltrate as irregular sheets of epithelial cells, sometimes with pointed or spiky margins (Fig. 24.5). Formation of epithelial pearls and keratin is unusual but does occur rather more commonly in those neoplasms showing an exophytic mode of growth. A proportion are extremely poorly differentiated.
Spread and prognosis. The tumour invades locally into the uterine body, vagina, parametrial tissues, bladder amd rectum; of particular importance is involvement of the ureters, either by direct invasion of their walls or by compression by extrinsic tumour masses. Lymph-node spread occurs at an early stage to pelvic, inguinal, iliac and aortic nodes but spread by the blood, principally to liver, lungs and bone, does not occur until a late stage. Death is most commonly due to uraemia consequent upon ureteric

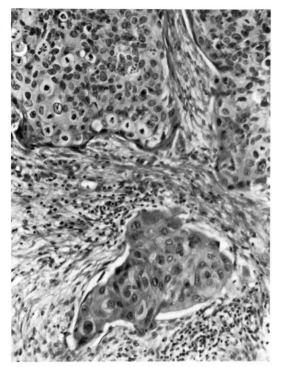

Fig. 24.5 Squamous-cell carcinoma of the cervix uteri, showing infiltrating masses of tumour cells without 'epithelial pearl' formation. Note the numerous mitotic figures. × 165.

obstruction. The 5-year 'cure' rate for patients in whom the tumour is confined to the cervix is, with modern therapy, about 85%, falling to between 50 and 75% for those cases with pelvic invasion at the time of treatment.

Adenocarcinoma

The factors linked aetiologically with cervical squamous cell carcinoma do not apply to cervical adenocarcinoma and indeed the neoplasm is relatively common in nullipara. Some adenocarcinomas of clear-cell type occur in young girls exposed prenatally to diethylstilboestrol.

The tumour grows in the endocervix and is commonly well differentiated: it tends to spread upwards into the myometrium and outwards into the pelvis but the 5-year 'cure' rate is approximately 70%.

The Endometrium

The endometrium is that part of the uterine lining above the level of the internal os and consists of a basal layer, which contains the endometrial stem cells and does not differentiate in response to hormonal stimulation, and a superficial functional layer which is markedly sensitive to ovarian hormones.

Endometrial morphology during the menstrual cycle

An awareness of changing endometrial morphology during the menstrual cycle is basic to an understanding of much of endometrial pathology. The menstrual cycle is divided into three stages; the *pre-ovulatory*, during which the developing Graafian follicle is secreting oestrogens, the *postovulatory*, throughout which the corpus luteum is producing both oestrogens and progesterone, and the *menstrual*. During the pre-ovulatory stage the endometrium regenerates and grows under the influence of oestrogen and is said to be in the proliferative phase (Fig. 24.6); the glands are straight and narrow, the stroma is compact and cellular and mitotic figures are seen in both the glands and stroma. After ovulation, which usually occurs

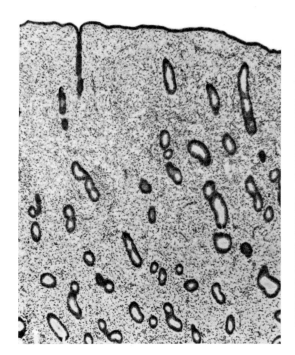

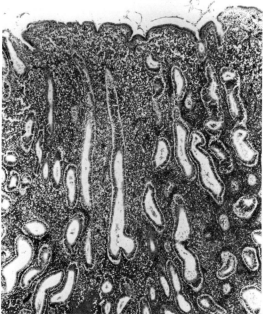

Fig. 24.6 Section of the endometrium on the 10th day of the cycle, showing the appearances of the proliferative phase. The glands are relatively small. × 60.

about the 14th day of the cycle, the endometrium enters the secretory phase, the first morphological evidence of which is the appearance of subnuclear glycogen-containing vacuoles in the glandular epithelial cells (Fig. 24.7); these appear about 36–48 hours after, and are strong presumptive evidence of, ovulation. As the secretory phase progresses the vacuoles disappear, the epithelial nuclei return to a basal position, the glands become increasingly dilated and tortuous and secretions appear in their lumina (Fig. 24.8); because oestrogens increase endometrial intracapillary hydrostatic pressure the stroma becomes markedly oedematous during the mid part of the secretory phase. When the corpus luteum begins to degenerate there is a precipitous fall in oestrogen levels, a rapid regression of the stromal oedema and a sudden decrease in thickness of the endometrium with buckling of the spiral vessels, vascular stasis and ischaemic necrosis of the functional layer. As the oedema regresses the stroma becomes compact and the stromal cells take on a decidua-like appearance. Shortly be-

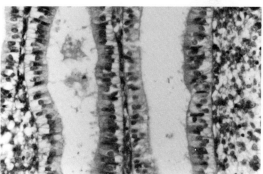

Fig. 24.7   Post-ovulatory endometrium on the 15th day of the cycle. The glands have increased in size and show basal vacuolation. *Above*, × 30; *below*, × 245.

fore breakdown of the endometrium the stroma becomes infiltrated by polymorphonuclear leucocytes and these harbingers of overt necrosis are soon followed by disintegration and haemorrhage, the menstrual phase of the cycle now having been reached. Most of the functional layer is lost during menstruation but the basal layer persists to give rise to the regenerative phase of the next cycle.

The menstrual cycle ensures a recurrent priming of the endometrium for the reception of a fertilised ovum, but menstruation is not an essential biological component of this process.

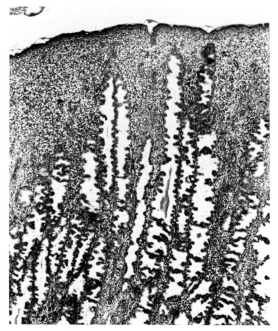

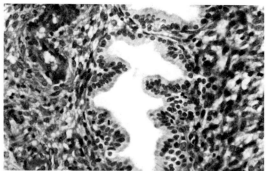

Fig. 24.8 Secretory-stage endothelium on the 25th day of the cycle. The glands contain secretion and are convoluted, presenting a 'saw-tooth' appearance. *Above,* × 30; *below,* × 245.

Endometrial necrosis, and hence resultant menstrual loss, is due solely to the very rapid rate at which oestrogen and progesterone levels fall as the corpus luteum degenerates; in some species oestrogen and progesterone values decline at a much slower rate and endometrial necrosis, and hence menstruation, is avoided, although only at the cost of lengthening the menstrual cycle. Menstruation is therefore the price that women pay for the shortening of their menstrual cycle which allows for a greater number of possible conceptions during their limited years of fertility.

Factors altering endometrial morphology

Pregnancy. The normal cycle will be interrupted if a fertilised ovum implants in the endometrium; when this occurs the corpus luteum persists, the stromal oedema fails to subside completely, the stromal cells become large, plump and polygonal with abundant cytoplasm, the glands enlarge and glandular secretion increases. An unusual endometrial response to placental tissue, whether this be in an intra-uterine or ectopic site, is the **Arias-Stella reaction** in which one or more glands are lined by tall cells with clear cytoplasm and, often, hyperchromatic nuclei; the glandular epithelium shows budding, multi-layering and some degree of pleomorphism and these appearances may be mistaken for an adenocarcinoma. The cells in an Arias-Stella reaction are endometrial glandular cells in a hyperactive secretory state.

Oral contraception. The use of oral steroid contraceptives markedly alters endometrial morphology. The type of pattern seen depends upon the dosage and the type of preparation used, but a very characteristic pattern with the combined type of regime is one of endometrial atrophy in which the glands are small, relatively few, and largely inactive, with a compact stroma showing a variable degree of decidua-like change (Fig. 24.9). Occasionally the stromal cells become spindle-shaped and may appear sufficiently pleomorphic to suggest a sarcoma, but this change is very rare with modern low dosage contraceptives. The endometrium rapidly reverts to normal after stopping oral contraceptives.

Intra-uterine contraceptive devices. The effects on the endometrium vary with the type of device used but focal atrophy and fibrosis are commonly seen; foci of haemorrhage and squamous metaplasia may be present whilst there is frequently a mononuclear cell infiltration of the stroma. Cyclical changes continue in the endometrium but the secretory phase tends to be accelerated.

The menopause. Some slight proliferative activity may occur in the endometrium for a year or two after the menopause but the postmenopausal endometrium undergoes a progressive atrophy and the glands eventually become quite inactive. Stromal fibrosis is not uncommon and this often leads to obstruction of the necks of many of the glands, which tend to become cyst-

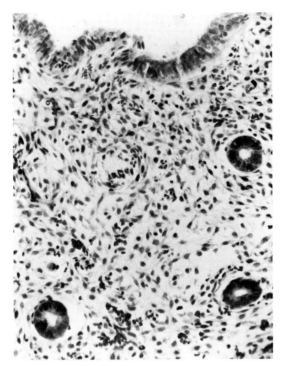

Fig. 24.9 Endometrium from a woman taking a hormonal contraceptive pill. The stroma is abundant while the glands are reduced in number, small and inactive. × 200.

ically dilated; the cystic glands are lined by a thin, inactive epithelium and they thus differ strikingly from those seen in cystic glandular hyperplasia (p. 24.10).

Endometritis

The endometrium is relatively resistant to infection, partly because of the excellent natural drainage which it enjoys, and partly because it is difficult for an infection to become established during reproductive life in a tissue which is regularly shed.

Acute endometritis

An acute inflammation of the endometrium occurs most commonly after an abortion or parturition, especially if fragments of placenta or membranes are retained in the uterus; a variety of organisms, including streptococci, staphylococci, *Esch. coli* and *Pseudomonas*, may be implicated. An acute sterile inflammation can also occur with certain types of intra-uterine contraceptive device and may also complicate irradiation of the uterus.

The inflamed endometrium is reddened and boggy and histologically there is oedema, congestion, a varying degree of ulceration and tissue destruction and a polymorphonuclear leucocytic infiltration. The cellular infiltrate differs from that which occurs as a physiological event during the late stage of the menstrual cycle by being present not only in the stroma but also in the glands where small intraluminal abscesses are commonly seen.

A virulent infection may spread to involve the myometrium and parametrium but complications such as septic pelvic venous thrombosis, pyaemia and septicaemia are nowadays very uncommon in developed countries.

Non-specific chronic endometritis

A chronic inflammation of the endometrium may follow an acute endometritis but is more commonly chronic from the outset. Macroscopically the endometrium may be somewhat thickened but often appears normal. There has been much dispute over the criteria for the histological diagnosis of chronic endometritis, largely because occasional lymphocytes are normally present in the endometrium. Chronic inflammation in this site is, however, characterised by the same features as elsewhere in the body and the diagnosis rests upon the finding of a chronic inflammatory cell infiltration of the stroma; the infiltrate must be of more than trivial degree and although occasionally purely lymphocytic in type there is usually an admixture with, and sometimes a predominance of, plasma cells. Some degree of fibroblastic and vascular proliferation may be present but the inflammatory process is limited to the stroma and does not involve the glands; the normal cyclical changes may continue undisturbed, be accentuated or absent.

Chronic endometritis may follow abortion or childbirth and can occur in association with an intra-uterine contraceptive device, chronic salpingitis or endometrial adenocarcinoma; furthermore, endometrial tuberculosis can masquerade as a non-specific inflammation. Hence, although there do appear to be a very small number of cases of chronic endometritis of apparently idiopathic origin, this diagnosis should not be entertained until all these factors have been eliminated as aetiological possibilities.

Specific endometrial infections

Tuberculosis of the endometrium is nearly always secondary to tuberculous salpingitis and is now uncommon in Western countries. The disease is often accompanied by infertility but this may well be because of the accompanying tubal lesions rather than a result of endometrial damage, for the normal cyclical changes are not usually interrupted by a tuberculous endometritis. Continued menstrual shedding of the endometrium prevents the disease proceeding to the stage of caseation and in premenopausal women the characteristic histological finding is a few small scattered tubercles with little or no central caseation. The tubercles are maximally developed, and so most obvious, in the later stages of the menstrual cycle and diagnostic biopsy in suspected cases should always be undertaken at this time. Occasionally tubercles are absent and the findings are of a non-specific chronic endometritis. The presence of neutrophil polymorphs and eosinophilic debris in the lumen of occasional glands should arouse suspicion. In all suspected cases where tubercle bacilli cannot be detected microscopically, culture and/or guinea pig inoculation should be undertaken.

Endometrial tuberculosis is rare in postmenopausal women but when it does occur there is no obstacle to its progression to caseation. In such cases the endometrium may appear as a thickened whitish-yellow, shaggy lining to the uterine cavity and sometimes the latter is itself filled with caseous material; histologically the endometrium will show confluent caseating tuberculosis.

Schistosomiasis of the endometrium is common in areas where this disease is endemic, e.g. Africa, and can cause infertility. Ova are deposited in the endometrium and usually, but not invariably, elicit a macrophage granulomatous reaction.

Actinomycosis of the endometrium, though rare, is sometimes found in association with an intra-uterine contraceptive device.

Endometrial polyps

The term 'polyp' is a purely descriptive one and does not denote any specific pathological process (p. 12.15); it is, however, usually applied to a focal overgrowth of the endometrium which protrudes into the uterine cavity. Such polyps are common: they may be pedunculated or sessile and are characteristically pink and fleshy with a smooth surface. Histologically a polyp is covered by columnar epithelium and contains endometrial stroma and glands; the latter are commonly either inactive or show patchy irregular cyclical changes but are, in some cases, responsive to oestrogen but not to progesterone and thus show cystic glandular hyperplasia (see below). A pedunculated polyp may undergo torsion, and ulceration of the tip of the polyp may cause bleeding. Malignant change is extremely uncommon.

Endometrial hyperplasia

Two quite separate conditions are included together under the general term endometrial hyperplasia and *a diagnosis of hyperplasia without specification of the type is of no value.*

(a) Cystic glandular hyperplasia

In this condition the uterus is moderately enlarged whilst the endometrial lining is vascular and thickened, often appearing polypoidal. Histologically the endometrium is diffusely involved and the distinction between functional and basal zones is lost. The endometrial glands are straight and cylindrical but of very variable calibre, some being unusually small, but invariably a number are considerably larger than normal (Fig. 24.10). The glands are lined by narrow columnar cells with basophilic cytoplasm; some multilayering may be present but there is no pleomorphism or cellular atypia. The stromal cells are plump and closely packed, giving a hypercellular appearance. As both stroma and glands share in the hyperplastic process the ratio of glands to stroma is approximately normal. Mitotic figures are common in both the stroma and the glands and there may be foci of haemorrhage or necrosis.

Cystic glandular hyperplasia is due to pro-

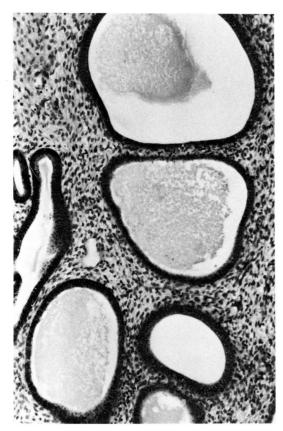

Fig. 24.10 Cystic glandular hyperplasia of the endometrium. The glands, many of which are greatly enlarged, are lined by tall darkly staining cells. × 100.

longed, unopposed oestrogen stimulation of the endometrium, the commonest cause of which is a succession of anovulatory cycles. These occur most frequently in the perimenopausal years but are not uncommon during the menarche and are characterised by the development of a succession of Graafian follicles which mature, fail to release their ova, persist for weeks or months and then degenerate; the consequent fluctuations in plasma oestrogen levels lead to intermittent breaking down of the hyperplastic endometrium and irregular heavy bleeding. Cystic glandular hyperplasia can also be produced by prolonged oestrogen therapy and by oestrogen-secreting ovarian tumours; these should always be considered as possible aetiological factors in postmenopausal women who develop this form of hyperplasia. *Cystic glandular hyperplasia is not associated with an*

increased risk of the eventual development of an adenocarcinoma and does not merit consideration as a premalignant condition.

(b) Atypical endometrial hyperplasia

This may be combined with, or occur independently of, cystic glandular hyperplasia; this form of hyperplasia is, however, invariably focal rather than diffuse and is not simply a late stage of cystic glandular hyperplasia. Atypical hyperplasia is characterised by irregular glandular proliferation without any accompanying stromal proliferation (Fig. 24.11). The glands are increased in number and crowded together, in severe cases being in direct apposition with each other to give a 'back-to-back' appearance: they are irregular in outline and are lined by tall cells with eosinophilic cytoplasm, the epithelium often being multi-layered and forming intraluminal buds. Varying degrees of cellular and nuclear atypia are present and mitotic figures are common and occasionally of abnormal form. In the most extreme cases of atypical

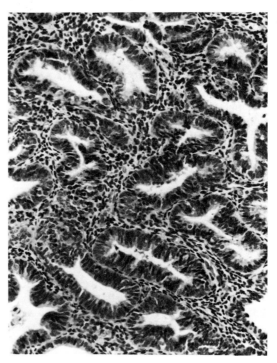

Fig. 24.11 Atypical hyperplasia of the endometrium. Note the crowding of the glands which are of irregular shapes and show evidence of multilayering. × 190.

hyperplasia the distinction from a well-differentiated adenocarcinoma may be almost impossible.

Atypical hyperplasia tends to occur under the same circumstances as does cystic glandular hyperplasia and is most common around the time of the menopause; the focal nature of the abnormality suggests that while cystic glandular hyperplasia is the normal response to prolonged oestrogenic stimulation, atypical hyperplasia represents an abnormal tissue response to this hormonal stimulus. Indeed it is possible that this lesion is a form of intra-endometrial neoplasia rather than a true hyperplasia. Unlike cystic glandular hyperplasia, *atypical hyperplasia is associated with a high risk of progression to an endometrial adenocarcinoma*; the degree of risk is related to the severity of the atypia and in severe cases is in the region of 50%.

Malignant tumours of the endometrium

Adenocarcinoma

The vast majority of malignant tumours of the endometrium are adenocarcinomas: these occur most commonly between the ages of 50 and 60.

Aetiology and pathogenesis. Nulliparous women are particularly prone to develop an endometrial adenocarcinoma: an association between this neoplasm and the triad of obesity, hypertension and diabetes mellitus has also been suggested. There is, indeed, convincing evidence of a link with obesity, but not with hypertension or diabetes

The aetiological role of oestrogens has been much debated but there is now little doubt that such hormones can contribute to the development of endometrial adenocarcinomas, as shown by the frequent occurrence of such neoplasms in women with oestrogenic ovarian tumours and their greatly increased incidence in women receiving long-term oestrogen therapy. Most patients who develop an endometrial adenocarcinoma do so, however, in the absence of such factors and have a normal urinary output of total oestrogens; fractionation of plasma oestrogens has, however, shown that oestrone, which is the most carcinogenic of the natural

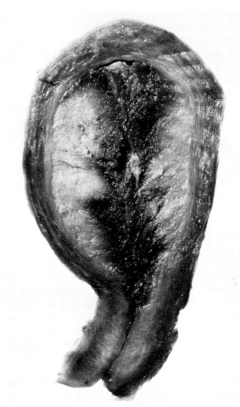

Fig. 24.12 Adenocarcinoma of the endometrium. The tumour has filled and distended the uterine cavity.

oestrogens, forms an unusually high proportion of the total in many of these patients; this is apparently due to an increased capacity for converting androstenedione, of adrenal origin, into oestrone in the body fat (hence the association with obesity).

Although adenocarcinoma may evolve from an atypical hyperplasia, many such tumours arise from an atrophic endometrium.

Macroscopic appearances. The tumour may appear as a localised nodule, plaque or polyp, usually in the upper part of the uterus, but more commonly it presents either as a diffuse nodular or polypoid thickening of the uterine lining (Fig. 24.12), often with superficial ulceration and bleeding, or as a bulky, friable, partially necrotic mass which may fill, or even expand, the uterine cavity.

The uterus may be slightly or moderately enlarged, and the myometrium, although usually focally thinned by invading tumour, is occa-

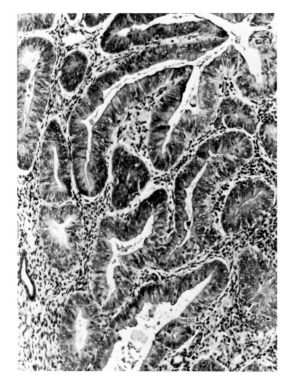

Fig. 24.13 A well-differentiated endometrial adenocarcinoma. × 150.

sionally diffusely thickened by widely infiltrating neoplastic cells.

Microscopic appearances. The neoplasm is commonly a well-differentiated adenocarcinoma (Fig. 24.13) but solid areas, a cribiform pattern and papillary formations are common and sometimes dominant. Foci of intraglandular squamous metaplasia are frequent, and if these are extensive the tumour is sometimes described as an **adenoacanthoma**; definition of the extent of metaplasia necessary for this diagnosis is subjective and arbitrary and there is little justification for regarding an adenoacanthoma as a separate or specific entity. Some endometrial adenocarcinomas are, however, admixed with malignant squamous tissue and such tumours, known as **adeno-squamous carcinomas**, do merit specific identification for they have an unusually poor prognosis. In most endometrial adenocarcinomas, scattered foci of cells with clear cytoplasm are found and occasionally such cells, which are of secretory endometrial type, predominate.

Spread and prognosis. Endometrial adenocarcinoma invades the myometrium at an early stage but, because of the thickness of this muscular barrier, tends to be confined to the uterus until late in the course of the disease. Eventual penetration of the myometrium leads to parametrial infiltration and tumour deposits in the pelvic peritoneum and pouch of Douglas. Extension along the lumen of the tube, a particular feature of growths arising in the cornu of the uterus, can result in implants in the ovaries and broad ligament. Vaginal metastases occur by venous or lymphatic dissemination. Lymphatic spread to the para-aortic nodes occurs at an early stage, but involvement of hypogastric and obturator nodes is a late event. Distant metastases to liver and lung are uncommon and death is usually due to the effects of neoplastic infiltration of the pelvis, including uraemia from ureteric involvement.

The prognosis is related to the degree of differentiation of the tumour and to the clinical stage at the time of diagnosis. The overall 5-year survival rate is in the region of 66%.

Sarcomas of the endometrium

Endometrial sarcomas arise from undifferentiated mesenchymal cells which not only retain their embryonic potential to develop into endometrial stromal and glandular cells but also have a capacity to differentiate into connective tissue cells of a type foreign to the uterus, e.g. cartilage, fat, striated muscle. Sarcomas containing only endometrial-type tissue are known as 'homologous' whilst those in which extra-uterine cell types occur are called 'heterologous'. Further, the neoplastic cells may differentiate along only one cellular pathway to give a 'pure' sarcoma or into a variety of cell types to form a 'mixed' sarcoma.

Thus a sarcoma formed solely of malignant endometrial stromal cells is a *pure homologous sarcoma* whilst a uterine rhabdomyosarcoma is a *pure heterologous sarcoma*. A neoplasm containing both endometrial stromal sarcoma and endometrial adenocarcinoma is a *mixed homologous sarcoma*, and is usually known as a *carcinosarcoma*, while the presence, in such a tumour, of malignant foci of cartilage or striated muscle indicates a *mixed heterologous sarcoma*, commonly known as a *mixed mesenchymal tumour*.

All endometrial sarcomas are rare but the

carcinosarcoma and the mixed mesenchymal tumour are the least uncommon: both usually develop in elderly women and form large polypoid tumour masses which expand the uterine cavity and extend through the endocervical canal to present in the vagina. The prognosis is very poor.

Endometriosis

Endometriosis is a condition in which tissue identical in all respects to the endometrium is found in sites distant from the uterus (Fig. 24.14). The ectopic tissue occurs most commonly in the ovaries, fallopian tubes, pouch of Douglas, uterine ligaments, rectovaginal septum and the bowel; occasionally foci of endometriosis are encountered in laparotomy scars, at the umbilicus or in the skin, while exceptional instances of lesions occurring in lymph nodes, limbs, pleura and lung have been recorded.

The pathogenesis of this disorder is still far from clear but one possible mechanism for its development is the reflux of viable fragments of endometrial tissue through the tubes during menstruation with subsequent implantation on, and growth in, the ovaries and pelvic peritoneum: certainly, endometriosis in scars appears to be due to implantation of endometrial tissue during uterine surgery. A further possibility is that endometriosis arises ectopically as a result of endometrial metaplasia of the peritoneal serosa; this is a feasible hypothesis and it may be that, in fact, such metaplasia is induced by regurgitated fragments of endometrial tissue which, after initiating the process, subsequently die. The occurrence of endometriosis in distant sites cannot, however, be explained except by invoking haematogenous or lymphatic dissemination and it is probable that there is no single pathogenic mechanism which applies to all cases of this condition.

Macroscopically, pelvic endometriosis is seen as small bluish nodules, often with surrounding fibrosis. In the ovaries the lesions are commonly cystic and contain altered blood; these may reach a considerable size, and, because of the dark colour of their contents, are often referred to as 'chocolate cysts'. Ovarian endometriosis is frequently associated with dense adhesions, the ovaries being bound down to the broad ligament or the bowel. Tubal lesions may occur on the serosa or in the wall and, although these often lead to some distortion of the tube, there is virtually never tubal occlusion.

Histologically, the lesions of endometriosis consist of both endometrial glands and stroma. The endometrium is, however, usually functional and hence menstrual type bleeding occurs and often obscures and distorts the original histological appearances; indeed the epithelial component is frequently destroyed and a pres-

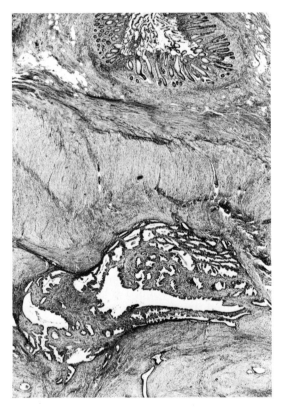

Fig. 24.14 Endometriosis of the appendix and caecum. A focus of endometrial glands and stroma, showing cystic change, is present in the muscular coat of the caecum close to the appendix (*seen at top of picture*). × 12.

umption that the lesion was originally one of endometriosis is then only made possible by the presence of stroma containing many haemosiderin-laden macrophages.

It is the hormonal sensitivity of the endometriotic lesions that is responsible for their role in producing symptoms; recurrent swelling causes pain and repeated bleeding leads to fibrosis. Hence the commonest complaints are of pelvic pain just before and during the menstrual period, deep pain on sexual intercourse and rectal discomfort. Infertility is often noted but the basis for this is obscure; as already remarked, it is not due to tubal occlusion but may result from a disturbance in either tubal motility or ovarian function. The symptoms tend to improve dramatically during gestation in those patients who do become pregnant, and to subside before or at the menopause.

The Myometrium

The myometrium is the thick muscular wall of the uterus and is capable of marked alterations in size, capacity and contractility during pregnancy and labour.

Adenomyosis

This common condition, often misleadingly referred to as '*internal endometriosis*', is characterised by the presence of abnormally sited endometrial tissue within the myometrium, well below the base of the endometrium (Fig. 24.15). The nodules of ectopic tissue may be distributed diffusely, in which case the uterus shows a roughly symmetrical enlargement, or they may be focal, causing a poorly delineated tumour-like asymmetrical thickening of the myometrium. Histologically, foci of adenomyosis are not encapsulated and consist of typical endometrial glands and stroma; the glands are commonly of basal type and hence inactive but cyclical changes and menstrual bleeding sometimes occur. The myometrial lesions can cause dysmenorrhoea and irregular, excessive bleeding with symptoms usually starting during the fourth decade and persisting until the menopause.

Adenomyosis is due to a downgrowth of basal endometrium into the myometrium and continuity of the ectopic tissue with the endometrium can be demonstrated by serial sectioning; the condition is not a form of, and is unrelated to, endometriosis.

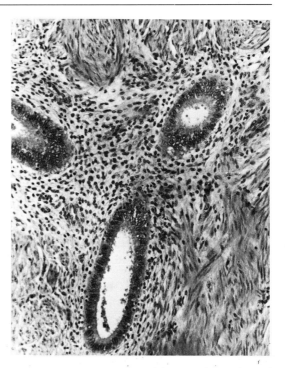

Fig. 24.15 Adenomyosis. A focus of well-formed endometrial glands and stroma lying deep within the myometrium. × 150.

Benign tumours

Leiomyoma. Uterine leiomyomas originate from, and are tumours of, the smooth muscle cells of the myometrium; there is commonly an intermingling with fibrous tissue and these neoplasms are often called 'fibroids'. Myometrial

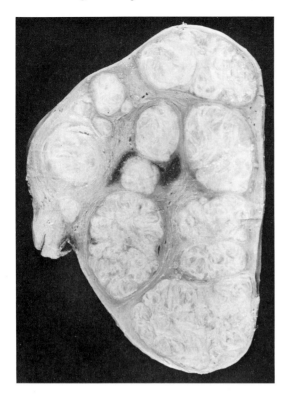

Fig. 24.16 A uterus containing many intramural leiomyomas. The cervix is seen on the left.

leiomyomas are extremely common, being found in at least 20% of women above the age of 35; they are usually multiple (Fig. 24.16) and vary in size from tiny 'seedlings' to huge masses which fill the abdomen. They may be within the wall, i.e. *intramural*, in a *submucosal* site immediately below the endometrium, or lie just beneath the peritoneum to form a *subserosal* tumour. The submucosal leiomyomas bulge into and distort the uterine cavity and the overlying endometrium is stretched and thinned; these neoplasms may become pedunculated and form a polypoid mass within the uterine cavity which can even extend through the cervix into the vagina. The subserosal tumours grow out from the uterine surface, occasionally into the broad ligament, and may also become pedunculated; very rarely such a tumour becomes attached to the omentum or pelvic peritoneum and loses its stalk to become a 'parasitic leiomyoma'.

Leiomyomas have a well-defined, regular outline and a surrounding layer of compressed uterine muscle fibres, giving the appearance of encapsulation; they are firm and their cut surface has a white whorled appearance. Histologically the neoplasms are formed of interlacing bundles of smooth muscle fibres arranged in twists or whorls; some, known as *cellular leiomyomas*, contain densely packed spindle cells with elongated nuclei: rarely the smooth muscle fibres are rounded with central nuclei and clear cytoplasm, tumours containing such cells being variously called *epithelioid leiomyomas, clear cell leiomyomas* or *leiomyoblastomas*. In all except the smallest tumours the appearances are altered to a variable degree by degenerative changes which are due to the neoplasm outgrowing its blood supply and thus fibrosis, hyaline change, calcification, patchy necrosis or fatty change are common. Infarction of a leiomyoma is uncommon but a pedunculated tumour may undergo torsion, whilst a specific form of necrosis, known as *red degeneration*, occurs particularly, but not only, in pregnancy and is characterised by a dull beefy red appearance of the whole tumour; this change may be accompanied by pain and fever and the presence of thrombosed vessels indicates that it is probably due to haemorrhagic infarction of an extensively hyalinised neoplasm. Cells near an area of necrosis may contain large, bizarre hyperchromatic nuclei and form multinucleated giant cells, but this is not an indication of malignant change unless mitotic figures are also present.

Uterine leiomyomas appear to be at least partially under hormonal control, for they occur almost entirely during the reproductive years, enlarge during pregnancy and in women on oral contraceptives, and tend to regress after the menopause; nevertheless attempts to relate them to a hormonal disturbance have been unsuccessful.

Many small leiomyomas are asymptomatic but large tumours can cause pressure effects with pelvic discomfort and frequency of micturition, and complaints of heavy prolonged menstrual bleeding, dysmenorrhoea and reduced fertility are common. Malignant change is rare (see below).

Other benign tumours. Fibromas, lipomas and haemangiomas occur infrequently in the myometrium but **adenomatoid tumours** are less uncommon. They appear as small subserosal nodules, usually in the cornual region, and consist of numerous small channels lined by endothelial-like cells and set in a connective tissue stroma: they are always benign and are probably derived from the serosa, resembling in their fine structure a benign mesothelioma.

Malignant tumours

Leiomyosarcoma. Myometrial leiomyosarcomas are rare and may arise either in a pre-existing leiomyoma or directly from the myometrium. They are less well demarcated in appearance than leiomyomas, often show areas of haemorrhage or necrosis, and are characterised histo-

logically by their cellularity, pleomorphism and mitotic activity, this latter feature being the only one that offers definitive evidence of malignancy. Leiomyosarcomas occur most commonly during the sixth decade and have a poor prognosis.

Endolymphatic stromal myosis. This condition, also known as *stromal endometriosis*, is one in which sheets of benign-appearing endometrial stromal cells permeate the myometrium and infiltrate the myometrial lymphatics. It can recur locally and occasionally metastasises, and is best regarded as an *endometrial stromal sarcoma* of low-grade malignancy.

The Fallopian Tubes

The fallopian tubes play a vital role in sperm and ovum transport and damage to them often results in infertility and sometimes in tubal pregnancy (p. 24.28).

Salpingitis

Classical accounts of acute salpingitis from the pre-antibiotic era described two varieties of this disease: **endosalpingitis,** due usually to a gonococcal infection ascending via the uterine cavity to produce an acute inflammation of the tubal mucosa, and interstitial salpingitis, due commonly to post-abortal puerperal streptococcal infection in which the organisms reach the tube via the uterine lymphatics to establish an acute inflammatory lesion within the wall of the tube.

Acute salpingitis today is virtually always due to an infection which ascends via the uterine cavity and hence takes the form of an endosalpingitis. The disease may occur after abortion, parturition or uterine instrumentation and has a rather high incidence in patients with an intra-uterine contraceptive device; nevertheless most cases occur in the absence of such factors and are commonly due to a mixture of aerobic and anaerobic organisms of enteric type. *Neisseria gonorrhoeae* is now an uncommon cause of acute salpingitis and indeed the ability of this organism to cause an acute tubal inflammation

is doubted by many, who consider that gonococcal salpingitis is usually only transient but inflicts sufficient minor damage to pave the way for the subsequent establishment of secondary, mixed infection. *Mycoplasma, Herpes virus* and *Chlamydia* are now emerging as important causes of acute salpingitis.

In acute salpingitis both tubes are usually involved; they are congested, perhaps slightly swollen, and pus may be seen oozing from the fimbrial ostia, the fimbriae themselves being often swollen, congested and matted. Histologically there is swelling and congestion of the muscosal folds (plicae) which are infiltrated with polymorphonuclear leucocytes; the lumen often contains pus.

Many cases of acute salpingitis resolve but a proportion pass into a chronic stage with polymorphonuclear, lymphocytic and plasma-cell infiltration (Fig. 24.17) and fibrosis; adhesions between the plicae become established and a complex cribiform pattern often results (Fig. 24.18), this being known as **follicular salpingitis**. The chronic inflammatory cell infiltrate may persist but often subsides leaving a legacy of residual scarring and deformity.

An acute salpingitis may also result in a **pyosalpinx** in which the fimbrial ostia become occluded and the tube distended by pus; such a condition may persist but more commonly infection is eliminated and a **hydrosalpinx** results (Fig. 24.19) in which the tube is thin

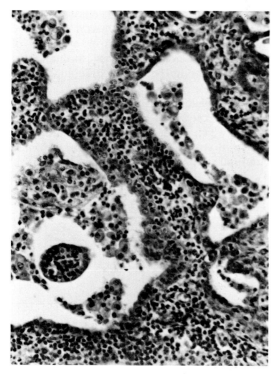

Fig. 24.17 Chronic gonococcal salpingitis. The plicae are fused, thickened and inflitrated with inflammatory cells. Purulent exudate containing polymorphs and macrophages is present in the lumen. × 200.

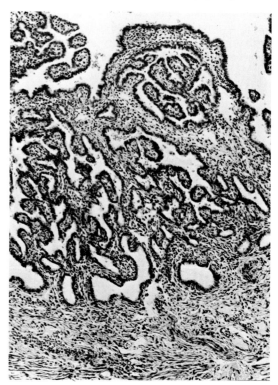

Fig. 24.18 Chronic follicular salpingitis. There is extensive fusion of the plicae, producing blind-ending crypts in the mucosa. × 130.

walled, greatly distended and contains clear watery fluid. The pathogenesis of a hydrosalpinx is not fully understood for the isthmic end of the tube remains patent and there seems no good reason why the fluid should not drain into the uterus.

Tuberculous salpingitis. The fallopian tubes are usually the first part of the female genital tract to be involved in tuberculosis, tubal infection being almost invariably secondary to extra-genital disease and reaching the tube via the blood.

The infected tubes are usually moderately or markedly thickened and the tube deformed and bound down to the ovary by dense adhesions: in the less common exudative form of the disease the tube becomes grossly distended and resembles an ordinary pyosalpinx. Histologic-ally there is a diffuse non-specific chronic in-flammatory cell infiltration of the mucosa and tubercles, usually few in number, are found scattered in the mucosa and submucosa; central

caseation is usually apparent in the tubercles and foci of caseation often become confluent and rupture through the mucosa into the lumen. The mucosa itself is commonly markedly hyperplastic and may sometimes show a degree of atypia, features that can lead to a mistaken diagnosis of carcinoma. The finding of tuber-culous lesions in endometrial curettings usually indicates the presence of tuberculous salpingitis.

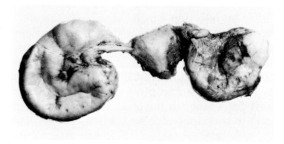

Fig. 24.19 Bilateral hydrosalpinx. Both tubes are extremely dilated and flask-shaped; they are distorted further by adhesions.

Tumours of the tubes

Benign tumours such as fibroma, adenoma, haemangioma and leiomyoma are sometimes encountered but malignant neoplasms are rare.

Adenocarcinoma is bilateral in many cases, is sometimes associated clinically with a characteristic watery vaginal discharge, and has a poor prognosis. *Choriocarcinoma* can develop in the tube as a sequel to a tubal pregnancy.

The Ovaries

Inflammation. Acute inflammation of the ovary occasionally complicates acute salpingitis and this combination may progress to a **tubo-ovarian abscess.** Oophoritis is, however, rare.

Non-neoplastic cysts

Cystic change occurs with some frequency in graafian follicles and corpora lutea. **Corpus luteum cysts** are usually solitary, contain either altered blood or clear amber fluid, are lined by luteinised granulosa and theca cells and, although usually asymptomatic, can rupture and bleed into the peritoneal cavity. **Follicular cysts** are found in the cortex and are small and unilocular. Their smooth lining is formed of flattened granulosa cells which may secrete sufficient oestrogen to inhibit pituitary FSH secretion and lead to anovulatory cycles with consequent endometrial hyperplasia. The cyst fluid is clear and often rich in oestrogens. Multiple follicular cysts occur in a variety of conditions to give the picture of a polycystic ovary; when multiple cysts are associated with thickening of the ovarian capsule, hyperplasia and luteinisation of thecal cells and anovulation, there is often an accompanying clinical triad (expressed either partially or fully) of infertility, obesity and hirsutism which is known as the *Stein-Leventhal syndrome*. The exact pathophysiology of this condition is obscure but it appears that this particular type of polycystic ovary secretes, possibly because of an enzyme defect, an excess of androstenedione.

If the ovaries are subjected to excessive gonadotrophic stimulation, as occurs in patients with a hydatidiform mole and in some women receiving gonadotrophin therapy, cysts, known as **theca-lutein cysts**, may develop in the luteinised granulosa cells of atretic follicles.

Tumours of the ovaries

The many different ovarian tumours are classified on the basis of their cell or tissue of origin, it being believed that these neoplasms arise from undifferentiated cells in mature tissues which retain the same potentiality for differentiation as is possessed by the embryonic cells which are the precursor of that tissue.

A simplified form of the complex classification of ovarian tumours defines five main groups:

   I. Tumours derived from the surface epithelium.
  II. Tumours of sex cord and stromal origin.
 III. Tumours derived from germ cells.

  IV. Miscellaneous tumours.
   V. Metastatic tumours.

I. Tumours derived from the surface epithelium

Approximately 60% of all ovarian tumours, and 90% of those which are malignant, are derived from the surface epithelium: they are collectively known as the **common epithelial tumours**. The ovarian surface epithelium is derived from, and is the mature equivalent of, the coelomic epithelium which in embryonic life overlies the gonadal ridge and from which are derived the müllerian ducts and the tissues to which these give rise, *i.e.* the tubal and endocervical epithelia and the endometrium. Neoplasms arising from indifferent cells in the surface epithelium retain this embryonic potential for müllerian differentiation. In some, the tumour epithelium differentiates along an endocervical pathway, producing the **mucinous neoplasms**; others differentiate into a tubal type of epithelium, forming the **serous group of tumours**, while a third group differentiate along endometrial lines to produce the **endometrioid neoplasms**. Surface epithelial tumours also have a potential for differentiating along Wolffian lines to form uro-epithelium, neoplasms containing such epithelium being eponymously

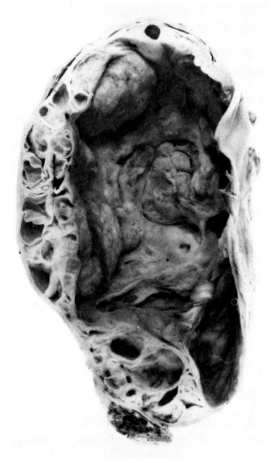

Fig. 24.20   A benign cystic mucinous tumour of the ovary: the multiple locules contained thick mucoid material.

called **Brenner tumours**. The mesonephroid, or clear cell tumours, so called because of a historical misinterpretation of their true nature, are probably a morphological variant of the endometrioid group of neoplasms.

All these epithelial neoplasms can exist in benign and malignant forms and those which are malignant are often grouped together as **ovarian adenocarcinomas**. These are increasing in incidence: they are the commonest fatal tumour of the female reproductive system and form bulky masses which tend to infiltrate locally into the pelvic tissue and seed tumour implants on to the omentum, but they rarely metastasise to distant sites. Patients with ovarian adenocarcinoma have a five-year survival rate of only 30% and little is known of the aetiology of this form of neoplasia; it is thought that recurrent ovulation, which repeatedly inflicts minor trauma on the surface epithelium, and exposure to exogenous ascending material, such as talc or asbestos, may possibly be of aetiological significance.

In addition to the benign and malignant forms, a third category of **tumours of borderline malignancy** or **tumours of low malignant potential** is recognised for epithelial neoplasms. These resemble macroscopically the benign forms but are characterised histologically by changes in their epithelium which suggest malignancy, i.e. multilayering, irregular budding, cellular atypia and mitotic activity, without, however, any evidence of stromal invasion. Most such neoplasms behave in a benign fashion but a few pursue an indolently malignant course.

Benign mucinous tumours (Mucinous cystadenomas) are common and form large cysts with a smooth outer surface; they are usually multilocular and contain clear mucous material (Fig. 24.20). Microscopically the cyst epithelium is formed of tall mucin-secreting columnar cells which in most cases are identical to those lining the endocervix (Fig. 24.21). In a minority, however, the epithelium is of gastro-intestinal type and contains argyrophil and Paneth cells; neoplasms containing this enteric type of epithelium are probably not derived from the surface epithelium and are thought to be teratomas which have developed along only one tissue line. Benign mucinous cysts may attain a huge size and distend the abdomen; torsion may occur, and occasionally the cyst ruptures and

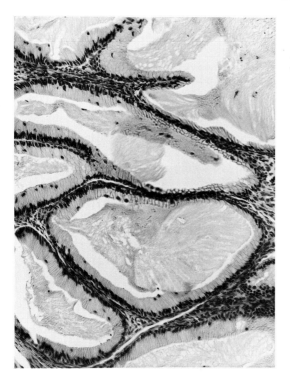

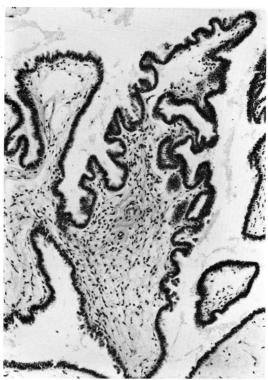

Fig. 24.21 Mucinous cystadenoma of the ovary, showing acini lined by tall columnar epithelium and containing mucous secretion. × 130.

Fig. 24.22 Serous cystadenoma of the ovary, showing papillary processes which are lined by tubal-type epithelium and project into the lumen. × 100.

the contents escape into the peritoneal cavity, where tumour cells may become attached and form seedling growths which continue to secrete mucin (*pseudomyxoma peritonei*). This condition is likely to cause death from matting together and obstruction of the intestine by masses of mucin undergoing organisation.

Malignant mucinous tumours (Mucinous cystadenocarcinomas) are often partially solid, and show the usual features of malignancy.

Benign serous tumours commonly occur as thin-walled unilocular cysts (**serous cystadenomas**) though in some the inner surface shows papillary projections into the lumen. Histologically the epithelium of these cysts is identical to that of the fallopian tube (Fig. 24.22). Serous tumours may also grow as a papillary warty outgrowth on the surface of the ovary (Fig 24.23) and such a neoplasm may give rise to seedling deposits on the omentum and pelvic peritoneum.

Malignant serous tumours are usually cystic (**serous cystadenocarcinomas**) but contain numerous soft papillary ingrowths and are frequently solid in some areas.

Endometrioid tumours are nearly always malignant, benign and borderline forms being very rare. The tumours, usually solid with areas of haemorrhage, are commonly histologically identical with endometrial adenocarcinomas but any type of endometrial neoplasm can occur in the ovary as a form of endometrioid

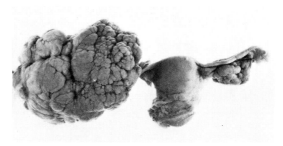

Fig. 24.23 A benign serous surface papillary tumour of the left ovary.

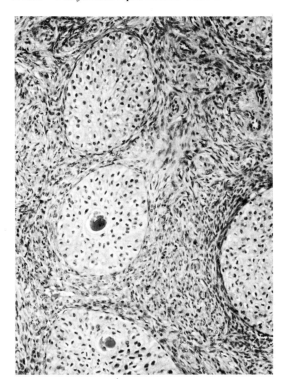

Fig. 24.24   Brenner tumour of the ovary. × 150.

tumour, *e.g. mixed mesenchymal sarcoma*. Although most endometrioid neoplasms originate from the surface epithelium, a minority arise from foci of pre-existing ovarian endometriosis.

Brenner tumours are usually small, solid and benign; microscopically, they consist of rounded islands of transitional-type epithelium embedded in a dense fibrous stroma (Fig. 24.24).

'Mesonephroid tumours' are invariably malignant and show a complex papillary pattern intermingled with sheets of clear cells.

II. Tumours of sex cord and stromal origin

During the early embryonic stages of gonadal development, cords of cells, possibly derived from the surface epithelium and known as sex cords, envelop the germ cells: at this stage the primitive gonad is capable of developing into either an ovary or a testis and the cells derived from the sex cords can differentiate into either the granulosa cells of the graafian follicle or the Sertoli cells of the seminiferous tubules. There is an interaction between the sex cords and the adjacent primitive gonadal stroma, cells from the latter differentiating into either thecal cells or Leydig cells. Tumours derived from tissues of sex-cord or stromal origin retain this bisexual embryonic potentiality and can differentiate into any of these various cell types either singly or in any combination.

Granulosa-cell tumour is the commonest representative of this group of neoplasms. It is usually small, solid, and formed of cells of granulosa type arranged in follicles, trabeculae, islands or sheets; the solid groups of cells often contain tiny cystic spaces filled with eosinophilic fluid and nuclear debris, known as *Call-Exner bodies* (Fig. 24.25). Granulosa-cell tumours frequently secrete oestrogens and can be responsible for signs of precocious puberty in young girls: in older patients the effects of prolonged oestrogenic stimulation of the endo-

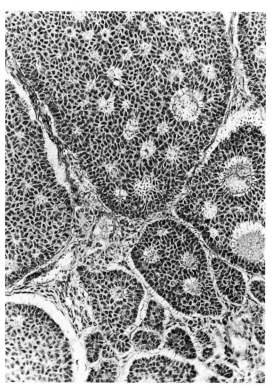

Fig. 24.25   Granulosa-cell tumour of the ovary, showing the characteristic masses of cells forming Call-Exner bodies. × 225.

metrium, *i.e.* hyperplasia and sometimes adeno-carcinoma, lead to complaints of menorrhagia or postmenopausal bleeding. Granulosa-cell tumours are of low-grade malignancy and may recur after many years: the histological features offer no guide to prognosis but the larger the neoplasm the greater is the risk of recurrence.

Many granulosa-cell tumours are pure but some contain an admixture of thecal cells and pure **theca-cell neoplasms** are sometimes encountered: these present as solid, yellowish masses and are formed of plump, lipid-containing, spindle-shaped cells. Theca-cell tumours are often oestrogenic and thus produce symptoms similar to those of granulosa-cell tumours; they are, however, almost invariably benign.

Androblastomas. Neoplasms composed of Sertoli cells, Leydig cells, or any combination of these cells are known collectively as **andro-blastomas**. Pure **Sertoli-cell tumours**, which are formed of well differentiated tubules, and pure **Leydig-cell neoplasms**, formed of sheets of

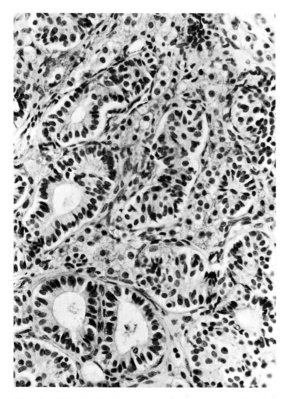

Fig. 24.26 Androblastoma of the ovary showing tubules lined by Sertoli cells and with Leydig cells in the stroma. × 220.

acidophilic Leydig cells and derived either from the stroma or from pre-existing hilar cells, are rare and always benign. **Mixed Sertoli–Leydig-cell tumours** (Fig. 24.26) are slightly more common and show a very wide range of differentiation, most behaving in a benign fashion but a minority pursuing a malignant course; the histological features are of little prognostic value. Pure Sertoli-cell tumours are sometimes oestrogenic but all other types of androblastomas often secrete androgens and produce some degree of virilisation, notably breast atrophy, facial hirsuties, clitoral enlargement, amenor-rhoea, deepening of the voice and temporal recession of head hair.

III. Tumours of germ cell origin

Tumours derived from germ cells may show no evidence of either embryonic or extra-embryonic differentiation: such undifferentiated germ cell neoplasms are known as **dysgermin-omas** and are microscopically identical in all respects to the seminoma of the testis, sharing with this neoplasm also the attributes of early dissemination to the para-aortic lymph nodes and a marked degree of radiosensitivity.

A germ cell tumour may, however, differentiate along extra-embryonic pathways into either placental tissue, resulting in the rare and highly malignant **ovarian choriocarcinoma**, or into yolk sac tissue to produce the equally uncommon malignant **yolk sac carcinoma**: the latter, also known as an **endodermal sinus tumour**, occurs in young girls and, like the yolk-sac tumour of the testis (Fig. 25.15), has a complex histological structure with elements resembling primitive yolk sac, a similarity further accentuated by the ability of these neoplasms to secrete alpha-fetoprotein. These tumours were until recently invariably fatal but many respond well to modern chemotherapy.

Teratoma results from differentiation of a germ cell tumour into embryonic tissues. The embryonic tissues within a teratoma may be fully mature, *i.e.* resemble microscopically those seen in adult tissues, and the neoplasm is then usually benign, or may resemble immature embryonic tissue in which case the tumour tends to behave in a malignant fashion. Most ovarian teratomas are of the mature variety and most

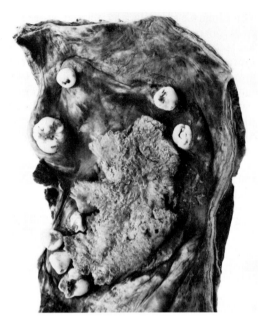

Fig. 24.27a   Part of the wall of a mature cystic teratoma ('dermoid cyst') of the ovary, showing irregular growth of teeth from the inner surface of the cyst wall.

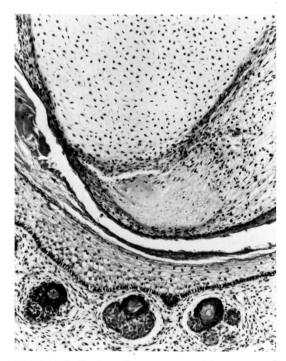

Fig. 24.27b Section of a mature cystic teratoma of the ovary. The cyst cavity is lined by squamous epithelium and shows hair follicles. Note also the nodule of cartilage. × 120.

of these are cystic. The mature cystic teratoma (Fig. 24.27), often misleadingly called a '**dermoid cyst**', accounts for 15–20% of all ovarian neoplasms. It usually takes the form of a large thick-walled cyst containing hairs and pultaceous matter; the cyst is lined by a stratified squamous epithelium and skin adnexae, such as hair follicles, abound; within the wall of the cyst a variety of tissues may be found, amongst which cartilage, bone, teeth, thyroid tissue, gastro-intestinal and respiratory epithelium and neural tissue are the most common. Malignant change supervenes in about 1% of mature cystic teratomas, and usually takes the form of a squamous-cell carcinoma.

Teratomas containing immature tissues are usually solid and occur in children and young adults; although these tumours are malignant, many patients are now being treated successfully by chemotherapy.

Although teratomas classically contain a mixture of tissues, some appear to develop along only one tissue line; thus some, known as struma ovarii, contain only thyroid tissue while others are formed solely of gastro-intestinal epithelium and constitute one form of mucous tumour.

IV. Miscellaneous tumours

Placed in this group are a number of extremely rare tumours of unknown histogenesis, primary malignant lymphomas of the ovary and tumours derived from the non-specialised tissues of the ovary. Amongst the latter group, which includes haemangiomas, lipomas and leiomyomas, is the **fibroma** which merits special attention partly because it is common and partly because this neoplasm can be associated with ascites and hydrothorax (*Meig's syndrome*) which resolve after removal of the ovarian neoplasm.

V. Metastatic tumours

The ovary is a common site for metastatic tumour, especially from the uterus, breast and gastro-intestinal tract. A particular type of metastatic lesion is the ***Krukenberg tumour*** (Fig.

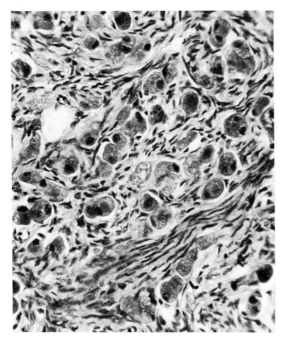

Fig. 24.28 Krukenberg tumour of the ovary, secondary to a primary carcinoma of the stomach. Note the abundant fibroblastic stroma and the large mucin-containing carcinoma cells. × 315.

24.28): this is due to transcoelomic spread of a gastric or colonic adenocarcinoma and is characterised by the presence of mucin-containing 'signet-ring' cells scattered in a fibrous stroma which is extremely cellular and resembles a sarcoma. This florid stromal reaction is seen before the menopause. Metastases in post-menopausal ovaries usually have the same appearances as elsewhere.

Abnormalities Related to Pregnancy

Only a few of the more important aspects of the complex subject of obstetrical pathology will be considered here.

Hydatidiform mole

This is an abnormal conceptus in which an embryo is absent and the placental villi are so distended by fluid that they resemble a bunch of grapes.

Gross appearances. The placental mass is often unduly large and distends the uterine cavity: the villi appear as clusters of tense, translucent, fluid-filled vesicles which commonly measure up to 1 cm and exceptionally as much as 2 cm, in diameter (Fig. 24.29). No trace of an embryo, amniotic sac or umbilical cord is apparent.

Miscroscopically the stroma of the villi is markedly oedematous (Fig. 24.30), often to a degree of complete liquefaction, and no fetal vessels are present. A constant feature is the presence of villous trophoblastic hyperplasia which is variable in degree and involves both the cytotrophoblast and the syncytio-trophoblast; some pleomorphism is often apparent but it has to be borne in mind that the proliferating trophoblast of the normal early placental villi is often moderately pleomorphic.

Epidemiology. Hydatidiform mole occurs most commonly in women aged less than 18 or more than 40; it also shows a striking geographical variation in incidence, being uncommon in Europe and North America, rather more common in Australia and of frequent occurrence in the Far East and parts of Africa, India and Central America. Attempts to explain this regional variation in terms of socio-economic

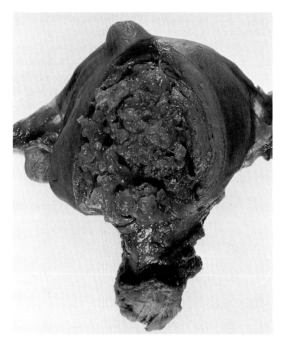

Fig. 24.29 An Opened uterus containing a hydatidiform mole.

status or ethnic group have met with little success. There is also a clear-cut relationship between hydatidiform mole and choriocarcinoma (a highly malignant neoplasm of trophoblast), for about 50% of choriocarcinomas occur in women who have previously had a hydatidiform mole.

Aetiology. In the past, a hydatidiform mole was often thought to be a non-specific consequence of fetal death but it is now realised that it represents an abnormal development of trophoblast. Some light on the cause of this abnormality has been shed by the discovery that 85% of true moles have an XX chromosomal constitution, both X chromosomes being of paternal origin; accordingly, it is postulated that moles arise from the formation and replication of a diploid cell derived from a single sperm that has penetrated a dead or dying ovum. Fifteen per cent of moles have an XY chromosomal constitution, though again both chromosomes are of paternal origin: it is thought that this form of mole is due to the entry of two sperms into an abnormal ovum with subsequent sperm fusion and replication.

Course and prognosis. A mole leads inevitably to abortion, often preceded by unduly rapid

uterine enlargement and haemorrhage. After the uterus has been emptied a woman with a mole has a 5% risk of eventually developing a choriocarcinoma but unfortunately the histological features of any individual mole offer no guide to eventual prognosis, no relationship existing between the degree of trophoblastic hyperplasia and the later occurrence of a choriocarcinoma.

Both hydatidiform moles and choriocarcinoma secrete large amounts of the placental hormone chorionic gonadotrophin (HCG) and patients who have had a mole should be periodically assessed by estimation of their urinary HCG output.

Invasive mole

In most hydatidiform moles the abnormal villi do not invade the myometrium but in 5–10% of moles, the villi not only invade but may even penetrate through the uterine wall; in such cases

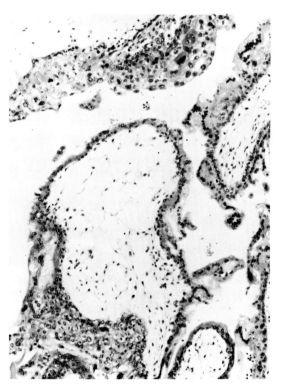

Fig. 24.30 A hydatidiform mole; the placental villi are avascular and markedly oedematous. There is a moderate degree of trophoblastic hyperplasia. × 100. (Dr C.W. Elston).

the myometrial vessels may be breached and emboli of hydatidiform mole transported to distant sites as 'metastases'. Despite this local invasion and distant spread, this form of mole is not malignant; after removal of the mole the 'metastases' will regress spontaneously and there is no increased risk of eventual choriocarcinoma.

Partial mole

This term is applied to placentas in which only a minority of the villi show hydatidiform change, the distended vesicular villi being scattered amidst otherwise normal placental tissue; a partial mole is often accompanied by a fetus, albeit one that is usually grossly abnormal. Histologically the vesicular villi in a partial mole differ from those in a true mole by containing fetal vessels and by the absence of trophoblastic hyperplasia. A partial mole is not simply a variant of a true mole but is invariably associated with, and is an expression of, a chromosomal abnormality in the fetus, most commonly a triploidy but sometimes a trisomy.

Choriocarcinoma

This is a malignant tumour of trophoblast and is formed of both cytotrophoblast and syncytiotrophoblast; it is a unique neoplasm in that, being of purely fetal origin, it is a neoplastic allograft in the mother. The aetiology is unknown but the tumour has a geographic pattern of distribution similar to that of hydatidiform mole, being rare in Western Europe where it occurs no more than once in 40 000 deliveries. The tumour follows a hydatidiform mole in 50% of cases and an unremarkable abortion in a further 25%: the remainder develop, often after a period of months or years, as a sequel to an apparently normal pregnancy, arising presumably from retained fragments of placental tissue.

Because trophoblast has an inherent capacity for invading and eroding blood vessels, the neoplasm is seen within the uterus as a soft, largely haemorrhagic mass (Fig. 24.31). Microscopically, a choriocarcinoma mimics the appearances of an early implanting blastocyst with central cores of mononuclear cytotropho-

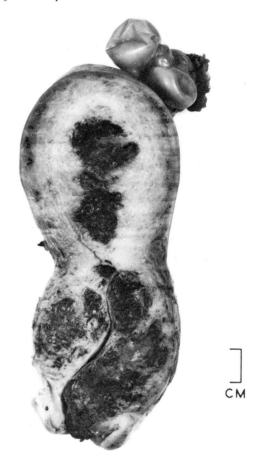

Fig. 24.31   A bisected uterus containing multiple dark haemorrhagic nodules of choricocarcinoma. (Dr C. W. Elston)

blast surrounded by a rim of multinucleated syncytiotrophoblast; the trophoblast shows a variable degree of pleomorphism and mitotic activity but no true villi are present (Fig. 24.32).

Choriocarcinoma invades rapidly and deeply into the uterine wall but penetration is principally by infiltration into venous sinuses rather than by destruction of myometrium. Because of this extensive vascular permeation, blood spread occurs at an early stage, principally to the lungs, liver, brain and vagina; metastasis via the lymphatics is uncommon. Despite this pattern of early spread there have been few neoplasms for which the prognosis has been altered so dramatically by the advent of chemotherapy; *until recently it was always rapidly fatal, but at least 80% of patients are now permanently cured by treatment with cytotoxic drugs.*

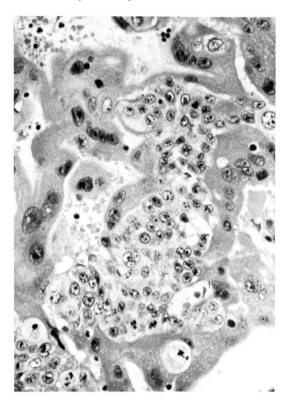

Fig. 24.32 A choriocarcinoma containing both cytotrophoblastic cells and multinucleated clumps of syncytiotrophoblast. × 300. (Dr C.W. Elston).

Ectopic pregnancy

An ectopic pregnancy is one in which a fertilised ovum implants and begins to develop before it reaches its natural site in the uterus. An extra-uterine gestation can develop in the ovary or in the peritoneal cavity but such cases are of extreme rarity and 97% of ectopic pregnancies occur in the fallopian tubes, most commonly in the ampullary portion. Within the tube, the developing placental tissue evokes an inadequate decidual response and not only invades the muscular wall but also erodes the intramural vessels. Erosion of a large vessel may lead to a haematosalpinx and separation of the conceptus from the tubal wall by haemorrhage; furthermore, the invading trophoblast weakens the tubal wall which may rupture, often with considerable intraperitoneal bleeding (Fig. 24.33). Clinically, these complications are usually accompanied by severe pain and other symptoms of an 'acute abdomen' demanding surgical treatment. Following tubal rupture, the conceptus may implant on to the peritoneum and continue to grow as an intra-abdominal pregnancy, but this is distinctly unusual. Despite this range of dramatic complications it is probable that some tubal gestations quietly abort and are resorbed without causing any symptoms.

Many cases of tubal pregnancy are clearly due to tubal obstruction, usually as a consequence of tubal or pelvic infection, while some appear to result from the ovum lodging in a tubal diverticulum. Nevertheless some tubal pregnancies occur in the absence of these lesions and suggested aetiological factors in such cases include increased tubal 'receptivity' because of endometriosis, delayed ovulation with washing back of the fertilised ovum by menstrual reflux, and transmigration of the ovum, *i.e.* an ovum released from the ovary traversing the peritoneal cavity to enter the contralateral tube. The incidence of ectopic pregnancy, particularly ovarian, is increased in women who become pregnant in spite of the presence of a contraceptive intra-uterine device.

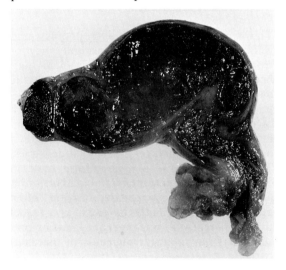

Fig. 24.33 Ectopic (tubal) pregnancy. The fallopian tube is distended with clotted blood and rupture had resulted in intraperitoneal haemorrhage. × 0.7.

Congenital Abnormalities of the Female Genital Tract

During normal female embryogenesis the internal genitalia develop from the two müllerian ducts which fuse distally to form the uterus and upper part of the vagina and remain separate proximally to form the fallopian tubes. The lower part of the vagina develops from the urogenital sinus. The wolffian ducts make no contribution to the female genital tract and undergo atrophy.

The female type of development will occur in neuter embryos and is independent of the presence of functioning ovarian tissue; it is, however, radically altered by the presence of a testis which secretes a substance (not testosterone) that inhibits development of the müllerian ducts and promotes that of the wolffian ducts; this substance has a purely local action and thus a left-sided testis will only influence development of the reproductive tract on the left side of the body. The external genitalia will always develop along female lines unless virilisation is induced during embryonic life by their exposure to testosterone.

Malformations of the female genital tract thus fall into two broad groups, depending on whether the gonads are normal or abnormal.

Malformations in women with normal ovaries

These patients have normal ovaries and external genitalia and usually a normal chromosomal constitution.

(1) Müllerian duct fusion defects. A total failure of müllerian duct fusion will result in a reduplication of the uterus and vagina (uterus didelphys) while lesser degrees of failure can result in a single vagina with double uterus (uterus bicollis bicornis) or a single vagina and cervix with two uterine bodies (uterus unicollis bicornis). The lesser forms of fusion defect are compatible with a normal capacity to become pregnant but are associated with a high incidence of abortion, premature delivery and abnormal labour.

Genetic factors contribute to fusion defects which probably result from a very slight physical separation of the two müllerian ducts at a critical stage of embryogenesis, possibly because of an altered shape of the embryonic pelvis.

(2) Müllerian duct aplasia. Total aplasia is very rare and found only in infants that are also otherwise grossly malformed; unilateral aplasia is slightly more common and results in a hemi-uterus with a single fallopian tube.

(3) Failure of fusion of müllerian ducts with urogenital sinus. A failure of fusion between the two structures that make up the vagina leads to a vaginal atresia; the uterus may be normal but is more commonly hypoplastic or absent (the Rokitansky-Küster-Hauser syndrome).

(4) Persistence of wolffian ducts. Remnants of these ducts are often to be found in the broad ligament and lateral walls of the cervix and vagina and there may give rise to cysts or, very occasionally, neoplasms.

Malformations in women with abnormal gonads

Women of this type, though phenotypically female, often, though not invariably, have an abnormal chromosomal karyotype; if any testosterone-secreting tissue is present the external genitalia will show some degree of virilisation and are often classed as being 'ambiguous'.

Patients with a **pure gonadal dysgenesis** or with **Turner's syndrome** have bilateral streak gonads (a strand of undifferentiated stroma on the back of the broad ligament); both the external and internal genitalia develop along normal female lines but remain infantile throughout life. Many patients with pure gonadal dysgenesis have a normal 46, XY karyotype and at least some cases are inherited as an X-linked recessive trait. Patients with Turner's syndrome have one X and no Y chromosome, the karyotype thus being 45, X; additional features include short stature and often webbing of the neck. Individuals with **mixed gonadal dysgenesis** have a streak gonad on one side and a testis on the other; müllerian development occurs normally on the side with a streak gonad but is inhibited on the other, the external genitalia being ambiguous. **True hermaphrodites**

(p. 25.21) with an ovary on one side and a testis on the other, or bilateral ovo-testes, are very rare and show a variable pattern of genital development.

Some phenotypic females are, in fact, males with a normal karyotype and normally developed internal male genitalia; their external genitalia are, however, female. These patients have bilateral testes which are capable of pro-ducing the factor inhibiting müllerian development; these individuals suffer, however, either from a defect in testosterone biosynthesis, an inability to convert testosterone to dihydrotes-tosterone in target tissues or a complete organ insensitivity to androgen effect, this latter syndrome being known as; **'testicular femin-isation'** (p. 25.22) or, preferably, as **'androgen insensitivity syndrome'**.

The Breast

The female breast is in the unique position of being a gland which is non-functional except during lactation. It is, none the less, subject to hormonal influences, particularly throughout the period of reproductive life, and this prob-ably accounts for most of its pathological changes, which rarely affect the male.

By far the most important disease is *car-cinoma*, which usually presents as a palpable lump. Other lesions are mostly of importance because some of them also produce a lump or lumpiness of the breast, or other symptoms which raise the suspicion of carcinoma, and must therefore be investigated, usually by biopsy. The commonest of these is conveniently termed *cystic mastopathy*. *Fibroadenoma*, a be-nign tumour, is also common, and because of the liability of the breast to injury, *traumatic fat necrosis* is another cause of a hard lump. *Duct ectasia* (dilatation of ducts) and *duct pap-illoma* may each (like carcinoma) cause a dis-charge from the nipple. *Infection of the breast* is rare except during lactation and most *congen-ital abnormalities* are of minor importance.

A basic knowledge of the normal structure of the breast and nomenclature of its various components are essential to an understanding of its more important lesions.

Development and structure

The breast consists of a group of modified sweat glands which develop from 15–25 down-growths of the epidermis. At first solid cords, they develop a lumen and become the major (*segmental*) *ducts*, each of which opens separ-ately at the nipple. Each segmental duct gives rise to the branching duct system of a *segment* of breast tissue. The secretory units are grouped into *lobules*, each of which is supplied with a *lobular ductule*. The lobules of the female breast remain rudimentary until puberty, when a num-ber of smaller *terminal ductules*, ending in solid alveoli, grow from the lobular ductule. The ductule-alveolar units of the lobule become en-sheathed in a loose cellular, mucoid connective tissue. The interlobular and segmental connec-tive tissue is less cellular and more densely collagenous, and during puberty becomes infiltrated with fatty tissue which accounts for most of the enlargement of the female breast at this time.

Apart from a stratified squamous lining close to the nipple, the ducts and ductules are lined by a two-layered epithelium, an inner layer of cuboidal or columnar cells and an outer discon-tinuous layer of smaller, contractile myo-epithelial cells. The epithelium is invested in a continuous basement membrane and the duct system is ensheathed in a layer of loose connective tissue which is rich in lymphatics. There is little or no elastic tissue in the lobules, but an elastic layer surrounds the extralobular ducts.

The ductal epithelium of the mature female breast has some secretory activity, but the secretion is normally reabsorbed. The lobular epithelium undergoes some proliferation and regression during each menstrual cycle and the stroma becomes oedematous during the days preceding menstruation. During pregnancy, proliferation increases and secretory acini de-velop from the terminal ductular alveoli. After the menopause, the breast epithelium atrophies and the lobular connective tissue changes to acellular hyaline collagen: the terminal ductules may virtually disappear, but sometimes become dilated, forming microcysts lined by flattened, attenuated epithelium, a process similar to the atrophic cystic change sometimes seen in the postmenopausal endometrium (p. 24.8). Apart from duct ectasia and duct papilloma, most lesions in the breast are believed to arise from the smaller ducts or within the lobules.

Inflammatory lesions

Acute infections

Acute pyogenic mastitis occurs mainly during lactation and is the result of infection via the ducts or through an abrasion of the nipple. It is most often caused by staphylococci acquired in hospital from the mouth of the suckling infant which has been colonised by the prevalent strain of *Staphylococcus aureus*. Unless effectively treated, staphylococcal mastitis may cause a loculated breast abscess, and extensive destruction and fibrous scarring of the breast may result. Abscess formation may also occur superficial to or deep to the mammary gland. Less commonly acute mastitis is caused by *Streptococcus pyogenes* (Fig. 24.34) and a spreading cellulitis results.

The neonatal infant may frequently show milk secretion caused by transplacental passage of the mother's hormones. This so-called 'witch's milk' is not evidence of inflammation.

Chronic infections

Acute pyogenic mastitis may become chronic if not treated adequately, and infection with pyogenic bacteria may also start insidiously and persist, but these events are rare. Recurrent or chronic low-grade infection of the sub-areolar tissue occurs in some women, with scarring, distortion and sometimes fistula formation.

Tuberculosis of the breast is now rare. It may arise by haematogenous, lymphatic or direct spread, usually from the lungs or pleura. It may remain localised as a single caseating lesion, which sometimes discharges through the skin, or it may spread extensively through the breast. In view of its rarity and the occurrence of other lesions with similar histological appearances, tuberculosis of the breast should not be diagnosed unless *Myco. tuberculosis* has been detected in the lesion.

Non-infective inflammatory lesions

For no good reason, cystic mastopathy (p. 24.33) used to be called chronic mastitis. It is not an inflammatory condition, although inflammation is sometimes seen around a ruptured cyst. Chronic inflammation is a feature of duct ectasia and traumatic fat necrosis.

Failure to establish satisfactory breast feeding is associated with painful congestion and oedema of the breast, which becomes tender and appears clinically to be acutely inflamed. There may also be fever but the condition is not infective and is relieved by effective suckling or removal of milk with a breast pump.

Mammary duct ectasia consists of progressive dilatation of ducts and surrounding chronic inflammatory change. It affects one or more segments of the breast and is rarely palpable, like a 'bag of worms'. The dilated ducts contain inspissated fatty material and their walls are thickened (Fig. 24.35). *Microscopically* the duct epithelium appears thin and the thickened fibrous sheath is usually infiltrated with plasma cells and lymphocytes. Foamy macrophages may be present in the lumen and in the nipple discharge (in contrast to the red cells and tumour cells usually found in the discharge from a duct papilloma). The peri-ductal elastic tissue is usually increased but may show patchy destruction.

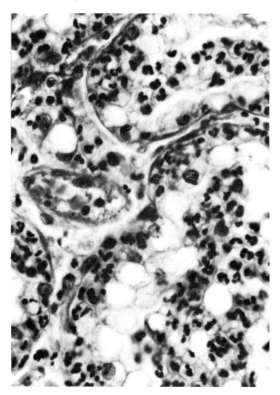

Fig. 24.34 Acute puerperal mastitis showing the secreting mammary acini, heavily infiltrated with polymorphonuclear leucocytes. × 500.

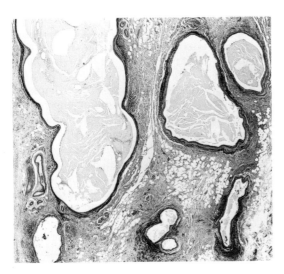

Fig. 24.35 Mammary duct ectasia. The ducts are dilated and filled with fatty material. Their walls show hyperplasia of the elastic tissue. × 13.

Duct ectasia is often symptomless, but there may be a nipple discharge and contraction of periductal fibrous tissue may cause retraction of the nipple and raise the suspicion of carcinoma. Occasionally a dilated duct ruptures into the surrounding stroma, where its lipid contents promote a persistent inflammatory reaction with accumulation of foamy macrophages and giant cells and fibrosis: the microscopic appearances resemble those of traumatic fat necrosis and the lesion may become palpable as a firm lump. Duct ectasia may eventually lead to obliteration of ducts by ingrowth of fibrous tissue.

The aetiology is uncertain: it tends to occur most often in multipara who have not breastfed their babies, but occurs also in nullipara and even in virgins. It has been widely assumed that the inflammatory changes are secondary to the dilatation, but there is some evidence that the inflammation appears first.

The term **plasma-cell mastitis** is sometimes applied to duct ectasia with unusually heavy plasma cell infiltration.

Traumatic fat necrosis. This lesion in the fatty tissue of an obese and pendulous breast is caused by trauma, although in many instances it presents as a hard lump in the breast, often without a history of trauma. The initial necrosis is accompanied by haemorrhage and followed by an acute inflammatory reaction. The necrotic tissue breaks down, sometimes resulting in a central cavity containing oily fluid. The lesion becomes heavily infiltrated by foamy macrophages containing lipid and often haemosiderin, and crystals of lipid may be deposited and stimulate a foreign-body giant-cell reaction (Fig. 24.36). Granulation tissue forms around the lesion and gradually matures into a thick layer of fibrous tissue which, often together with calcification, accounts for the presentation as a firm or hard lump. Macroscopically, the centre of the lesion is usually yellow and may contain cavities filled with oily fluid: this is enclosed in dense white fibrous or calcified tissue. Similar appearances are sometimes seen after minor surgical operations on the breast. The fibrous reaction may result in retraction of the nipple or fixation to the skin, features which increase the clinical resemblance to carcinoma.

Reaction to foreign material. Injection of silicone or paraffin wax to increase the size of the breast is usually without harmful effect,

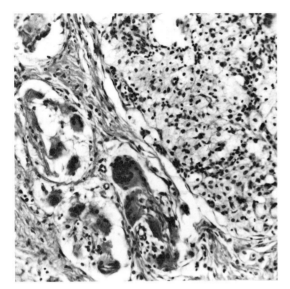

Fig. 24.36 Traumatic fat necrosis of breast, showing lipophages and foreign-body giant cells. × 150.

but can introduce infection, and occasionally induces a granulomatous giant-cell reaction, causing tenderness and nodularity. Microscopically, fragments of the 'inert' material are seen, surrounded by multinucleated giant cells.

Galactocele

This is a cystic swelling of a lactiferous duct which develops during lactation, apparently due to obstruction of the duct. Initially it contains creamy fluid which gradually becomes watery, and it may induce a granulomatous reaction or become infected.

Cystic mastopathy

This term covers a group of changes which very frequently develop in the female breast between puberty and the menopause, and are the commonest cause of a lump or lumpiness of the breast. The changes arise mainly or entirely in the lobular and terminal ducts and include (a) *formation of cysts*, (b) *epitheliosis*, (hyperplasia of ductular epithelium), (c) *adenosis* (enlargement of lobules and formation of new lobules after puberty), and (d) *fibrosis*. Any one of these changes may predominate and they may occur in any combination.

Because of the variety of changes, there is no satisfactory short name for this condition. The old term chronic mastitis is unsuitable: other names include *mammary dysplasia* and *fibrocystic disease* of the breast, but cystic mastopathy seems the least objectionable.

Cyst formation results from localised dilatation of lobular and terminal ductules, and is presumably due to obstruction. Cysts are usually multiple (Fig. 24.37) and mostly less than 1 cm in diameter, although occasional larger ones are not unusual. They are thin-walled and appear blue when seen close to the cut surface of biopsy material. The lining epithelium

often becomes flattened and may be lost in larger cysts. It may also undergo **apocrine metaplasia**, the cells becoming large and columnar with a convex free margin and abundant strongly eosinophilic cytoplasm which near the free margin may contain granules like those in apocrine glandular epithelium. Apocrine metaplasia is of little consequence, even when hyperplastic (Fig. 24.38), for it virtually never becomes carcinomatous. An incomplete layer of myo-epithelium can usually be detected in the walls of the cysts. Like the ductules from which they develop, the cysts are not ensheathed in elastic tissue. Unless haemorrhage has occurred, the cysts contain clear watery or mucous fluid. Occasionally a cyst ruptures and causes an inflammatory reaction in the adjacent stroma, which may be tender or painful. When cyst formation is not accompanied by epitheliosis, the condition is appropriately termed **simple cystic mastopathy**.

Epitheliosis is a term used in the UK to describe hyperplasia of the epithelium of breast ductules. It may take three forms: (a) *solid epitheliosis*, in which the epithelial lining may encroach on or completely fill the lumen with

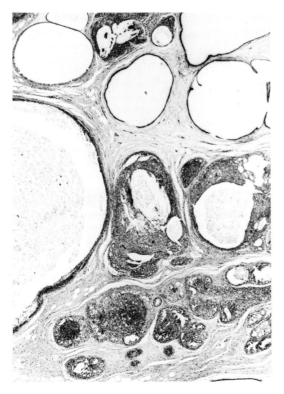

Fig. 24.37 Hyperplastic cystic mastopathy, showing ductular cysts and hyperplasia of epithelium (epitheliosis) in some of the ductules. × 22.

a solid mass of cells (Figs. 24.37, 24.39); (b) *cribriform epitheliosis*, in which the epithelium forms gland-like spaces; (c) *papillary epitheliosis*, in which epithelial processes project into the lumen—they differ from papillomas in usually not having a fibrovascular core (Fig. 24.38).

Cystic mastopathy with epitheliosis is sometimes called **hyperplastic cystic mastopathy** or **cystic hyperplasia**. It is important to distinguish such cases, for the presence of epitheliosis increases the risk of breast carcinoma (see below).

Adenosis. Although lobules develop in the female breast during puberty, they continue to appear and enlarge throughout the period of reproductive life, most markedly during pregnancies, but also in much lesser degree during the secretory stage of each menstrual cycle. This enlargement and increase in number of lobules (Fig. 24.40) is called adenosis. It is a physiological process, but tends to be accentuated in cystic mastopathy.

A pathological process similar to adenosis,

and termed **sclerosing adenosis**, may occur as an isolated phenomenon producing a palpable rubbery greyish discoid mass in the breasts of young women. Commonly it follows incomplete involution after an interrupted pregnancy or lactational failure and involves individual lobules in a patch of breast tissue. Sclerosing adenosis also occurs in microscopic foci in the breasts of women of widely different age groups and may be present along with epithelial proliferative lesions, e.g. papillomas. As in simple adenosis, the changes are always lobular but lack the simple pattern seen in physiological adenosis. Sclerosing adenosis proceeds through a sequence of changes beginning with an early florid, confused picture of proliferation of epithelium and myo-epithelium to form ductular and solid structures which are irregular in size and appear to be invading the stroma (Fig. 24.41a). Mitotic activity may be high at this stage and the lesion may be mistaken for adenocarcinoma. Later, the true epithelial

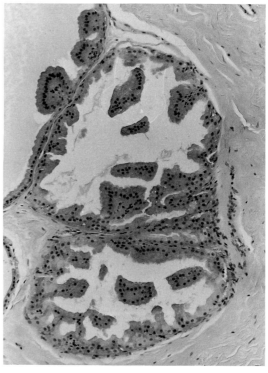

Fig. 24.38 Cystic mastopathy, showing dilatation of ductules and apocrine metaplasia. The epithelium is also hyperplastic, forming projections which differ from the fronds of a papilloma in having no fibrovascular core. × 45.

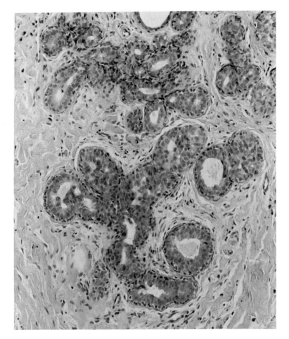

Fig. 24.39 Hyperplastic cystic mastopathy, showing epitheliosis. The ductules are partially or completely filled by hyperplastic epithelium. × 45.

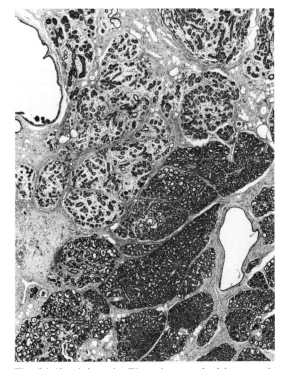

Fig. 24.40 Adenosis. There is a marked increase in the size and number of the lobules. Cystic dilatation of occasional ductules is present. × 22.

elements atrophy and the myo-epithelial cells persist singly and in groups; the stroma becomes more densely collagenous and at this stage the lesion may be mistaken for scirrhous carcinoma. *Sclerosing adenosis does not increase the risk of carcinoma, and its importance lies in the danger of mistaking it for carcinoma, particularly in immediate frozen section diagnosis on biopsy material.* Such errors are best avoided by careful low-power microscopy of the tissue, which reveals that although the epithelial elements give the impression of invading the stroma, they exhibit a *lobular* pattern (Fig. 24.41b). Another misleading feature is the occasional invasion of perineural lymphatics by the epithelial cells, which must not be mistaken for evidence of malignancy. An important feature is the presence of epithelial and myo-epithelial cells in their normal relationship. This two-layered epithellium can usually be seen in some of the ductular elements, at least in the early florid stage of the condition, and helps to distinguish it from invasive carcinoma.

Fibrosis. Increase of fibrous stroma occurs in most cases of cystic mastopathy, but is difficult to assess. In thin women, the normally fibrous breast stroma of young adult life persists with little change even after the menopause, but in obese women there is a progressive replacement of fibrous by fatty tissue, particularly after the menopause. As age advances, the fibrous stroma becomes hyaline and relatively acellular, while the epithelial elements atrophy. It is this collagenisation of pre-existing stroma without obvious fibroblastic proliferation that is responsible for fibrosis of the breast. Occasionally a patch of dense fibrous tissue becomes surrounded by fatty tissue and presents as a palpable hard lump, most often in the upper outer quadrant of the breast.

Patterns of cystic mastopathy. The condition may develop at any time during the period of reproductive life, and the changes persist, and sometimes are first noticed, after the menopause. Whole lobules and groups of lobules are involved, sometimes in one part of one breast, but often in multiple ill-defined areas of one or both breasts. When the changes develop early, they tend to extend and by the age of 30–40 may involve much of the breast tissue. In such extensive cases, the distinction from carcinoma can usually be made readily by clinical examination. The presence of cysts, sclerosing aden-

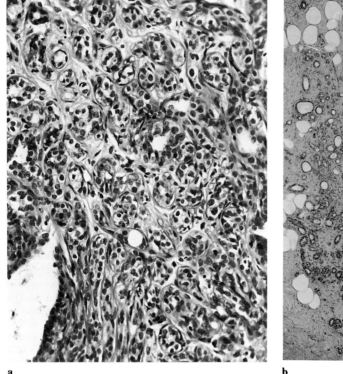
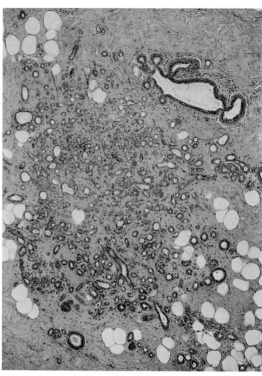

a   b

Fig. 24.41   Sclerosing adenosis of the breast, showing the florid phase (**a**) in which the ductules are greatly increased and atypical, appearing as solid cords of cells invading the stroma. × 200. In (**b**), the changes are much less florid and can be seen to affect a whole lobule. × 20.

osis or fibrosis is often associated with tenderness and pain, particularly before menstruation.

When the condition is localised to one part of one breast, epitheliosis is often a predominant feature, and the condition presents as a patch of induration or discrete swelling which is usually painless and demands surgical excision to exclude carcinoma. Any combination of types of epitheliosis (see above) may be found in such lesions.

Aetiology. It is widely assumed that cystic mastopathy is caused by the influence of hormones on the female breast throughout reproductive life, but this does not explain why the changes are so patchy. An association with menstrual irregularities has been noted, but only in some patients, and there is also a relatively higher incidence in nullipara. Cystic changes in the breast can be produced in animals by administration of oestrogen, but it must be admitted that most patients have no evidence of hormonal imblance.

Relationship to carcinoma. Cystic mastopathy is extremely common and the great majority of patients with it do not develop breast carcinoma. The possibility that its presence increases the risk of carcinoma has long been a matter of controversy. Early histological studies suggested that epitheliosis is an important precursor of carcinoma in situ, but the histological demonstration that one condition progresses to another is notoriously difficult, and most workers now believe that epitheliosis seldom progresses to carcinoma. Follow-up studies in patients with cystic mastopathy have shown that the presence of cysts, apocrine metaplasia, sclerosing adenosis and fibrosis is not associated with a significantly increased risk of carcinoma, but the presence of epitheliosis appears to increase the risk by about 2.5 times.

'Hypertrophy' of the female breast

This must not be confused with the gross mammary adiposity sometimes observed in obese middle-aged women. It usually develops soon after puberty although occasionally it may follow pregnancy. The breasts enlarge progressively and may eventually weigh several kilograms. The condition is usually bilateral but development may be unequal. The term hypertrophy is not really apt since the breast enlargement is due mainly to increase in soft oedematous connective tissue, and sometimes also of adipose tissue. Glandular tissue is not much increased and often appears scanty. The cause of hypertrophy is usually obscure, but rarely it accompanies various hormone-secreting tumours. Treatment by partial excision, with preservation of the nipple and areola, is often successful.

Tumours of the Breast

Benign tumours

Fibroadenoma

This is by far the commonest benign tumour of the breast and arises from within the anatomical unit of the lobule. It is usually regarded as a mixed tumour with both stromal and epithelial neoplastic elements, and occurs chiefly in young women. Sometimes in young girls the fibrous component is inconspicuous and the tumour is then termed a simple *adenoma*. Fibroadenomas are small, well-circumscribed, elastic, round or ovoid masses which may occasionally attain a diameter of up to 7cm. Rarely, they are multiple in one or both breasts. Although encapsulated, they should not be enucleated by the surgeon's finger, for projecting nodules of the tumour may be left behind and give rise to recurrences.

Two forms of fibroadenoma are usually distinguished but many tumours show both types of structure in different areas (Fig. 24.42). In young adults the so-called *pericanalicular type* occurs, in which the epithelial arrangement corresponds roughly to that in the normal breast lobule with an investment of loosely fibrillary connective tissue. The predominantly *intracanalicular* type seen usually in older women shows numerous curved and branching clefts lined by epithelium and produced by the pressure of blunt rounded projections of neoplastic cellular stroma upon ducts and acini. Growth of the lining epithelium merely keeps pace with that of the stroma and the characteristic clefting is produced. When cut across, the surface of an intracanalicular fibroadenoma often appears irregular and granular.

Fibroadenoma is widely believed to develop

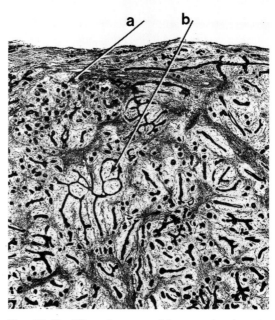

Fig. 24.42 Fibroadenoma of breast, showing the loose periacinar stroma. In places the tumour has a pericanalicular structure (**a**), at other parts an intracanalicular arrangement (**b**). Transitions are seen between the two types. × 16.

within a breast lobule, which it resembles in its loose, cellular stroma and gland-like elements. Multiple small fibroadenomatous areas sometimes occur in association with cystic disease (**fibroadenosis**). Some intracanalicular tumours contain large amounts of smooth muscle and metaplastic bone or cartilage may also develop in the stroma. During pregnancy, a fibroadenoma may enlarge and show secretory activity, and there is some doubt as to whether both elements are truly neoplastic. There is, however, good reason for accepting the stromal cells as neoplastic, for a whole spectrum of tumours of this type occur in the breast, with stromal cells ranging from benign to sarcomatous (see below). The neoplastic nature of the epithelial elements is more doubtful; admittedly carcinoma sometimes develops in a fibroadenoma, but this is very rare, and might simply mean that its epithelium, like that of the normal breast, is not immune to carcinogenic agents. If fibroadenomas are true tumours, the popular belief that they grow by accretion, i.e. by incorporating adjacent breast lobules, is obviously unlikely to be correct.

Giant fibroadenoma: cystosarcoma phylloides. Some intracanalicular fibroadenomas, particularly in women over 40 years old, tend to grow relatively rapidly, often to 10cm or so in diameter (Fig. 24.43); and are commonly known by either of the above names. Occasionally, pressure necrosis of the skin occurs over such a tumour, which ulcerates and resembles clinically a fungating carcinoma. These larger tumours, and occasionally smaller ones, may appear gelatinous and have a more cellular myxomatous or fibroblastic stroma. Indeed, the stroma of this group of tumours shows differences in cellularity, cellular pleomorphism, aberration and mitotic activity ranging from benign (as in the typical fibroadenoma) to frankly sarcomatous, and reflecting their clinical behaviour. Tumours intermediate in this series are cured by adequate excision, remembering that they have finger-like projections (hence the suffix *phalloides*), and that, if these are left behind, successive recurrences are liable to become progressively less benign. Such tumours should not be labelled sarcoma unless the histological appearances of the stromal element are unequivocally malignant. Breast sarcoma is considered further on p. 24.26.

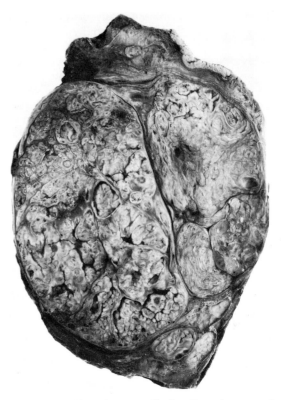

Fig. 24.43   Giant intracanalicular fibroadenoma of the breast. The stroma showed sarcomatous change. × 0·5.

Papillary cystadenoma

This benign tumour is much less common than fibroadenoma. Cysts of varying size are present and within these there is epithelial proliferation. Often these epithelial tumours have a somewhat papilliform pattern but they are composed of adenomatous elements and do not show fibrovascular cores lined by epithelium as in a papilloma. Papillary cystadenoma may become large and, if not removed, may ulcerate through the skin and present as papillary masses on the breast surface. Most are benign but occasionally *cystadenocarcinoma* supervenes. Although this is usually of low-grade malignancy and requires only local excision, occasional cystadenocarcinomas are aggressive and may already have metastasised to lymph nodes at the time of diagnosis. Those in which the infiltrative component is of squamous-cell type appear to be the most dangerous.

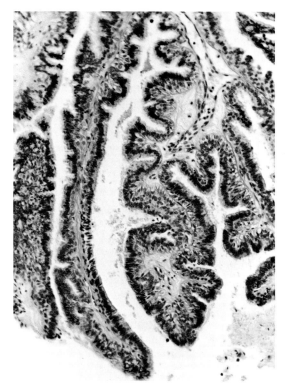

Fig. 24.44 Duct papilloma of breast, showing branching papilliform processes covered by epithelium mainly of columnar type. × 130.

Duct papilloma occurs most often as a rounded pedunculated tumour which forms within and eventually distends a major duct or a lactiferous sinus, in or adjacent to the nipple. A typical papilloma comprises a branching fibrovascular stromal core clothed by a double-layered cuboidal or columnar epithelium (Fig. 24.44), which is sometimes apocrine-like. In time, the epithelium may atrophy and hyalinisation occur. The tumour may be solitary and attain a size of more than 10 mm but sometimes multiple tumours are present throughout the duct system of the breast. The larger tumours are often accompanied by nipple discharge and those in the lactiferous sinus may present with frank bleeding from the nipple. Microscopic examination of such discharges usually shows red blood cells and tumour epithelial cells and often permits distinction from the coloured discharges present in mammary duct ectasia. Sometimes florid papillomas in young women may undergo considerable involution and hyalinisation so that incomplete removal may be followed by apparent cure even when several pregnancies and lactations follow.

Some papillomas of the lactiferous sinuses resemble papillary hidradenoma of the vulva, perhaps reflecting the developmental similarity of the breast to a sweat gland. Another rare lesion of the nipple is the so-called adenoma: double-layering of the epithelium helps to identify it as benign despite stromal distortion.

Papillary forms of epitheliosis occur in hyperplastic cystic disease and it is difficult to draw a clear line between them and papillomatosis; the presence of well-formed fibrovascular stromal cores suggests multiple neoplasms. When such small papillomas are numerous, multiple carcinomas occasionally develop. Carcinomatous change is rare in a solitary papilloma, and only local excision is necessary.

Other benign tumours

These are uncommon but fibroma, myxoma, lipoma, angioma and chondroma are recorded. Granular cell myoblastoma occasionally occurs in the breast and clinically may simulate carcinoma.

Malignant tumours of the breast

Carcinoma

This is among the commonest of human cancers throughout the world (Table 12.3, p. 12.16). Its incidence and mortality rate are particularly high in most of the developed countries, where both have increased slowly for more than 50 years. In this country and in North America it occurs in approximately 6% of women, and the overall 5-year survival is about 50%, although it is much higher in patients without lymph node involvement. It is at least two hundred times more common in women than in men, and while its incidence is highest in old age, it is by no means rare in the third and fourth decades. It usually presents as a palpable lump and for this reason *all lumps in the breast, whatever the age of the patient, must be regarded clinically as possibly malignant until proved otherwise.* Immediate histological examination of frozen sections at the time of operation is of value in enabling the surgeon to decide upon the type of treatment required. Screening procedures involving clinical examination, mammography, xeroradiography and thermography are being applied to the detection of breast cancer at an early stage. Recent reports suggest that two-yearly screening in women over the age of 50 may indeed have some value in increasing survival rates.

Varieties of breast cancer

Carcinoma of the breast arises from the lining epithelium of the duct system. For a variable length of time the tumour cells remain confined within the duct system and may spread extensively before invading the breast stroma. As elsewhere, the distinction between in situ (intraduct) and infiltrating carcinoma is extremely important (p. 12.28). **Carcinoma in situ** takes two main forms which differ in their histological appearances. It was thought originally that one form originated in the ducts and the other in the lobular or terminal ductules, and accordingly they were termed respectively **ductal** and **lobular carcinoma in situ**. Although these names are still in general use, it is now widely believed that the ductal form also usually originates in the lobular ductule. Sooner or later, carcinoma in situ is liable to penetrate the basement membrane at one or more points in the duct system* and invade the stroma to become an **invasive** or **infiltrating carcinoma**, which usually presents as a palpable lump. The tumour is commonly first noticed at this stage. Depending on whether it has arisen from ductal or lobular in-situ carcinoma, infiltrating carcinoma is also classified as **ductal** or **lobular**. The distinction between the two types of in situ carcinoma is important, because the lobular type is more often widespread and is much more prone to give rise to infiltrating carcinomas in both

breasts. The histological distinction between the common forms of ductal and lobular *invasive* carcinoma is, however, less clearly defined.

Ductal carcinoma in situ may spread very extensively within the breast ducts; in some patients it reaches the nipple and the cancer cells may then spread within the epidermis of the nipple and areola: this intra-epithelial spread gives rise to an inflammatory reaction and is known as **Paget's disease of the breast**.

About 90% of infiltrating carcinomas of the breast, whether ductal or lobular, are of **scirrhous** type, with abundant fibrous stroma. Six per cent or so are soft (**encephaloid**) tumours, composed mainly of cancer cells with scanty stroma. The great majority of both types are anaplastic, although some squamous-cell differentiation is not uncommon. The remaining 4% of tumours show various types of differentiation, e.g. to mucoid, adenoid cystic, signet-ring cell or adenocarcinoma.

About 50% of infiltrating carcinomas occur in the upper outer quadrant of the breast, the remainder being distributed equally throughout the rest of the breast. A cancer arising in the axillary tail of the breast may be mistaken clinically for an enlarged lymph node.

Infiltrating carcinoma

Scirrhous carcinoma. As noted above, this is the common form of clinically-apparent breast cancer. It is felt as a hard, almost stony lump, and is usually 1–4cm across at the time of removal. When cut with a knife, it gives a characteristic creaking sensation, rather like cutting an unripe pear, and is seen to be an irregular mass with extensions into the surrounding fibro-fatty tissue (Figs. 24.45, 24.46). The cut surface is firm and pale and often contains yellow foci due to elastosis (see below). *Microscopy* shows the tumour to consist of dense collagenous fibrous tissue among which lie small groups and strands of cancer cells (Fig. 12.28, p. 12.18). Towards the centre, the collagen is particularly dense and often hyaline, and there may be few or no tumour cells, but they are more numerous at the periphery where they are invading the surrounding fibro-fatty tissue. The cancer cells are spherical, often fairly uniform in appearance, with a relatively large round nucleus and few mitoses. Usually there is no obvious structural differentiation, although the

*The term *duct system* is used in this account to include ducts and ductules.

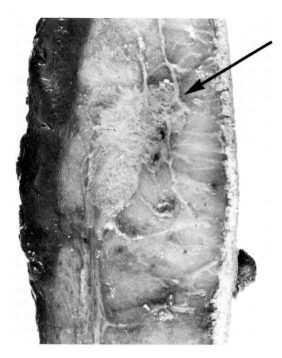

Fig. 24.45 Scirrhous carcinoma of the breast. The skin of the breast, including the nipple, is seen on the right and the pectoral muscles on the left. The cancer is seen on the cut surface (*arrow*) as an irregular paler area, lying in the breast tissue which is mainly fatty.

cells may form occasional irregular gland-like spaces, indicating poorly-differentiated adenocarcinoma.

Ducts and veins incorporated into the tumour often become ensheathed in a thick layer of elastic tissue (*elastosis*), but this is seen also in carcinoma in situ and in some non-neoplastic conditions. The microscopic features outlined above are usually regarded as typical of infiltrating *ductal* carcinoma and are seen in about 90% of scirrhous carcinomas. The remainder show features considered to be characteristic of infiltrating lobular carcinoma: the cancer cells lie in single file between collagen fibres, are arranged in concentric rings about ducts, and sometimes contain mucin, giving a signet-ring appearance (p. 19.30). The significance of these two main patterns is, however, in doubt, for each has been observed to accompany lobular carcinoma in situ, and in some tumours both patterns are observed.

Scirrhous carcinoma does not cause enlargement of the breast. Initially it is a freely mobile

hard lump, but later may become fixed to the deep fascia and/or the skin. Depending on its site, it may cause dimpling of the skin or retraction of the nipple, and if superficial may extend directly to the skin and present as an ulcer with raised edges and a hard base. The spread of breast cancer is described below.

Encephaloid carcinoma is far less common than scirrhous cancer: it forms a well-circumscribed, rounded or multinodular mass, usually of more than 3 cm across on removal, and is characteristically soft (hence encephaloid—brain-like). The cut surface usually shows haemorrhagic and yellow necrotic patches and the tumour may encroach on the skin and form a soft fungating ulcerated mass.

Microscopy shows large masses of tumour cells and scanty stroma (Fig. 12.27, p. 12.18). The individual cells are similar to those of scirrhous cancer, but mitoses are more numerous and a characteristic feature is infiltration of lymphocytes both in the stroma and around the tumour. Some lymphocytes are seen in nearly all encephaloid breast cancers, but when they

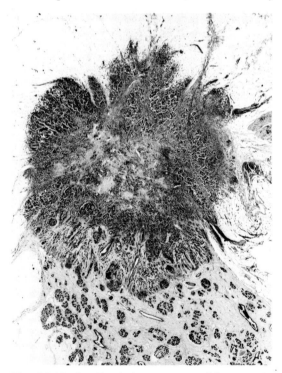

Fig. 24.46 Small scirrhous cancer of breast. The tumour has originated at the periphery of the breast and is invading both the breast tissue and the surrounding fat. Note the claw-like extensions. × 5·5.

are numerous the name **medullary carcinoma** is applied. The prognosis is rather better than for scirrhous cancer, the 10-year survival being approximately 70%. In medullary cancer, it is approximately 90% and the lymphocytes may represent an immune reaction to the tumour. Encephaloid cancers are usually classified as ductal.

Other variants of infiltrating carcinoma are numerous but mostly rare. It is not unusual to observe foci of partial squamous differentiation in an otherwise anaplastic cancer, but pure squamous-cell cancer is very rare. *Mucous (colloid) carcinoma* is usually bulky and, in general, has a better prognosis.

Unusually well-differentiated *adenocarcinoma*, sometimes called *tubular carcinoma*, also has a better prognosis: in some instances the gland-like spaces are so regular and well formed that the appearances may be mistaken for benign adenosis. An important feature is the absence of myo-epithelium. The occurrence of *signet-ring-cell cancer* has been mentioned above.

Spread of infiltrating carcinoma

Unfortunately, at the time of first diagnosis breast cancer is often already widely disseminated. This explains the observation that age-adjusted death rates have remained remarkably stable and that different therapeutic approaches, e.g. radical or local mastectomy, or even simple 'lumpectomy', have little influence on survival.

The axillary lymph nodes are involved at an early stage and in many cases the internal mammary lymph nodes are also affected, particularly by cancers in the medial part of the breast. Later the local skin lymphatics may be permeated, leading to either focal nodularity or more diffuse thickening of the skin known as *cancer-en-cuirasse*. If the skin lymphatics are blocked, lymph drainage is impaired and the skin becomes oedematous and swollen except where it is tacked down by hair-follicles; this produces the characteristic *peau d'orange* appearance of advanced breast cancer. Further lymphatic spread occurs through the connective tissues to the pectoral fascia and muscles and thence to the pleural cavities. In all of these situations microscopy may be required to reveal collections of malignant cells along the lymphatic pathways. Early dissemination may also

occur by the bloodstream: various internal organs and the thoraco-lumbar spine are frequently affected, the latter possibly by retrograde venous spread (p. 12.27). Oöphorectomy, adrenalectomy and hypophysectomy (p. 13.25) have also revealed microscopic metastases in these organs. Metastatic spread to the opposite breast is not uncommon. A second primary carcinoma in the other breast occurs in about 4% of patients and may be identified as such by the presence of intraduct cancer (see below). Lymphatic dissemination of tumour occurs as rapidly in the atrophic scirrhous as in the fast-growing encephaloid carcinoma.

Intraduct carinoma (carcinoma in situ)

As noted on p. 24.40, this is the pre-invasive stage of breast cancer, and is of two main types, ductal and lobular carcinoma in situ, both of which are now believed to arise usually in the lobular or terminal ductules.

Ductal carcinoma in situ at an early stage is seen in the lobular ductule, but has usually extended to the adjacent ducts. At this stage it is symptomless and is discovered accidentally in breast tissue removed for other reasons. In most cases, it invades the stroma and develops into an infiltrating cancer before intraduct spread is extensive, but sometimes it spreads extensively through the duct system before invasion occurs, and the affected major ducts may become palpably thickened. Excision at this pre-invasive stage carries an excellent prognosis. The affected ducts and ductules show a variety of changes: they may be filled with a solid column of cancer cells, the cells may show a cribriform pattern (Fig. 24.47), or they may form an irregularly thickened lining to the duct with trabecular bridges and projections into the lumen (Fig. 24.48). When seen in a ductule or small duct, the appearances may be confused with benign epitheliosis (p. 24.33). The features of malignancy (cell aberration, loss of polarity, mitotic activity, aberrant mitoses, etc.—p. 12.10) are helpful in making the distinction between the two, but it is sometimes very difficult and requires considerable experience. When it involves the medium-sized and larger ducts, ductal carcinoma in situ is recognisable macroscopically: the ducts are distended by solid columns of cancer cells which undergo central necrosis so that lipid-rich yellowish necrotic material

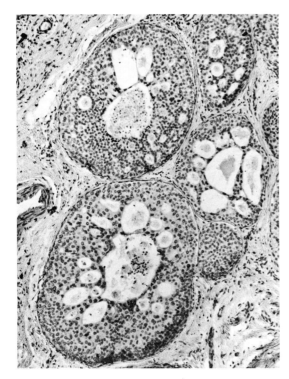

Fig. 24.47   Carcinoma in situ of ductal type. The ductules are filled with carcinoma which in this instance has a cribriform pattern with formation of small duct-like spaces. Note also the larger central spaces containing debris, which have resulted from necrosis. × 100.

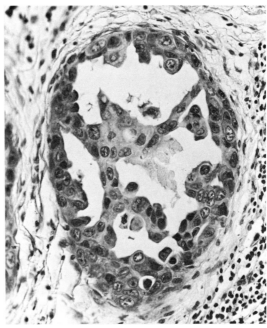

Fig. 24.48   Carcinoma in situ of ductal type, showing the irregularity of the cancer cells and formation of epithelial bridges. × 285.

can be expressed from the cut surface like toothpaste from a tube (**comedo carcinoma**, Fig. 24.51). Calcification of necrotic debris within affected ducts is an important feature in diagnostic mammography. Obliteration of the cancer cells and the duct lumina may result from periductal fibrosis and elastosis, but these changes are always patchy.

When ductal carcinoma in situ extends along major ducts as far as the nipple, groups of cancer cells may enter the deeper layer of the epidermis and spread and proliferate within it over the nipple and areola (Fig. 24.49). The affected skin shows reactive changes in the dermis, with exudation, formation of vascular fibrous tissue and infiltration with lymphocytes and plasma cells. These changes produce a characteristic eczematous condition of the nipple and areola named **Paget's disease of the breast** after Sir James Paget who described it in 1874. The cancer cells are larger than those of the epidermis,

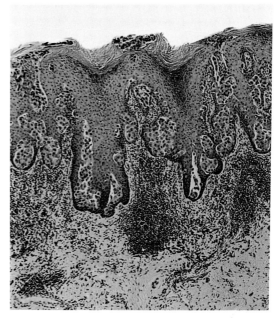

Fig. 24.49   Skin of nipple in Paget's disease, showing scattered groups of carcinoma cells 'Paget cells' in deeper part of epidermis. Note the marked lymphocytic infiltration of the dermis. × 50.

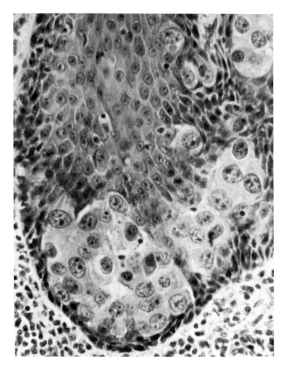

Fig. 24.50 Paget's disease of the breast, showing an epidermal rete ridge containing groups of (large) carcinoma cells. By contrast, the surrounding epidermal cells are smaller and are showing pressure atrophy. × 345.

with pale cytoplasm and a large vesicular, hyperchromatic nucleus and prominent nucleolus (Fig. 24.50). Mitotic figures may be seen and the cells may take up melanin from the adjacent melanocytes. Many of the tumour cells undergo shrinkage necrosis (p. 3.29), with shrivelled cytoplasm and nuclear pyknosis, and in this state are more difficult to recognise. They cause compression atrophy of the surrounding epidermal cells, but never invade the dermis.

Paget's disease is always accompanied by intraduct carcinoma and direct continuity at the nipple can usually be demonstrated (Fig. 24.51). In some patients the intraduct cancer has already invaded the breast stroma; in others it is still contained within the duct system. In either case, mastectomy is essential.

Extramammary Paget's disease of the skin may occur in the vulva, perianal region, axilla, etc., by intra-epithelial spread of carcinoma of the sweat glands in these sites.

Primary intra-epithelial tumours occasionally arise in the epidermis of the nipple. Bowen's disease of the skin and malignant lentigo of the nipple may also produce widespread intra-epithelial growth, but in neither case is there intraduct carcinoma. Squamous carcinoma of the nipple is rare. An even rarer form of benign hyperkeratosis, usually bilateral, may also cause confusion.

Ductal carcinoma in situ may be confined to one part of one breast or may occur in two or more separate foci, presumably because the agents responsible for its development may affect all the breast tissue. Its presence in one breast increases the risk of development of infiltrating cancer in the other, but not sufficiently to warrant removal of a clinically normal breast.

Lobular carcinoma in situ is the less common form of intraductal cancer and is most often found incidentally in breast tissue removed for cystic mastopathy. Cancer cells fill and distend the lobular and terminal ductules of one or more whole lobules (Fig. 24.52). The cells are usually quite small for cancer cells, uniform in appearance and evenly spaced, and mitoses are few, but the nuclear/cytoplasmic ratio is increased: they commonly contain some mucin and sometimes are of signet-ring type (p. 19.30). In distinguishing this lesion from benign aden-

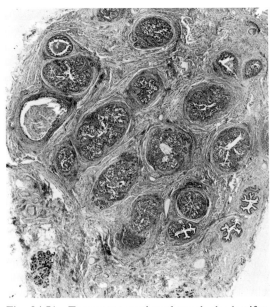

Fig. 24.51 Transverse section through the lactiferous ducts below the nipple in a case of Paget's disease, showing intraduct carcinoma. In some of the ducts the carcinoma shows central necrosis. × 12·5.

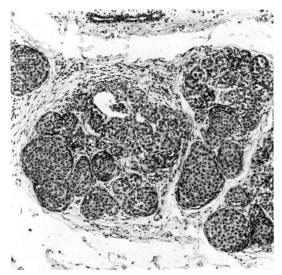

Fig. 24.52 Carcinoma in situ of lobular type. The terminal ductules of the lobule are all filled and distended by carcinoma cells of uniform appearance. × 75.

osis or epitheliosis, *complete filling* and *distension* of all the ductules in one or more lobules is helpful, but a similar change may be seen at an apparently early stage before these two criteria are fulfilled, and is sometimes known as *atypical lobular hyperplasia*.

Lobular carcinoma in situ commonly extends to the medium-sized and sometimes even to the larger ducts by burrowing between the duct epithelium and basement membrane. It does not, however, reach the nipple and is not associated with Paget's disease. It tends to develop towards the menopause, after which the incidence falls, suggesting that it commonly regresses. The change is often multifocal and in 36% of cases is bilateral. Accordingly its presence in a breast biopsy carries a high risk of the subsequent development of infiltrating carcinoma, probably about 25%, both breasts being apparently equally at risk, and removal of a breast with infiltrating lobular cancer is followed by an approximately 30% chance of development of a second infiltrating cancer in the other breast. These risks raise considerable problems in the management of patients with lobular carcinoma, particularly as the prognosis of the infiltrating tumour appears to be rather worse than that of infiltrating ductal carcinoma.

Causal factors in breast cancer

The incidence of breast cancer, like carcinomas in general, increases with age, but the increase occurs earlier than for most cancers, being most rapid between the ages of 30 and 50 years, after which it rises more slowly to a maximum in old age. There is also considerable and unexplained variation in the incidence of breast cancer in different communities, and in general it is much greater in women in the developed countries. The importance of genetic factors is suggested by the high incidence of breast cancer, and by its development relatively early, among groups of related individuals, but the mechanism of such factors is obscure. It has been suggested that lactation reduces the risk of breast cancer, and although this has been disputed it cannot be altogether dismissed, for there is evidence that, in women who feed their babies from one breast only, 80% of cancers developing after the age of 55 years are in the unused breast. However, many of the factors which affect the risk of developing breast cancer within a community appear to be related to the effects of sex hormones on the breast and are discussed below.

Sex hormones. There is good evidence that exposure to the female sex hormones is an important factor in the development of breast cancer. For example, it is rare in men but occurs more often in men treated with oestrogens e.g. for prostatic cancer. In women, the risk is increased by an early menarche, and by a late menopause, and bilateral oöphorectomy below the age of 35 greatly reduces the risk. From these observations and experimental studies it is widely assumed that prolonged exposure of breast epithelium to sex hormones is a major carcinogenic factor. This conclusion is important in relation to the use of hormonal methods of contraception and also in the treatment of breast cancer by altering the patient's hormonal status.

Oral contraceptive pills. In many Western countries, oral contraception has been in widespread use for about 20 years. Most contraceptive pills consist of mixtures of oestrogens and progestogens which, by suppressing the cyclical production of pituitary gonadotrophins, inhibit ovulation and the secretion of sex hormones by the ovaries. The breast is thus subjected to continuous and relatively low levels of sex hormones instead of the normal fluctuating levels. The possibility that this might either reduce or increase the risk of breast cancer was appreciated when the pill was introduced and a number of epidemiological investigations were started to detect these and other possible effects. It may seem surprising that, 20 years later, there is still some doubt about the effects of the pill, but during this period a large number of pills of different composition has been used, some have been withdrawn and others introduced, and women have used oral contraception at various ages and for various periods of time. All these variables have made it difficult to analyse the effects of oral contraception, but above all, the long latent period between exposure to carcinogenic agents and the development of cancer has meant that observations must extend over many years.

In general, epidemiological findings have been reassuring (Kalache *et al.*, 1983). The incidence of carcinoma of the breast has continued to increase since oral contraception was introduced, but the increase has been in women over 45 years old, most of whom have not had prolonged exposure to oral contraception. Recently, however, some workers have reported an increase in breast cancer in relatively young women, more of whom have used prolonged oral contraception: the number of cases reported is small, and other workers have not observed an increase. It is known, however, that nullipara and women who have their first child at a relatively late age have a greater risk of developing breast cancer than those who have their first child while still relatively young. It is therefore possible that the breast epithelium is particularly susceptible to the carcinogenic effect of sex hormones in nullipara and that use of oral contraceptives over a long period before the first pregnancy may increase the risk of cancer. At present, women in this category have not yet entered the age group in which the incidence of breast cancer is high, and more prolonged observation is necessary.

Hormonal dependence of breast cancer

In 1896, Beatson in Glasgow first showed that bilateral oöphorectomy was followed by prolonged remission in some patients with advanced breast cancer and he postulated that such mammary carcinomas required, for their continuing growth, some influence from the ovaries. These observations have been amply confirmed, and it is clear that the growth of some breast cancers is dependent on sex hormones. Bilateral oöphorectomy, and even adrenalectomy and hypophysectomy, have all been undertaken in the treatment of inoperable breast cancer, and more recently the oestrogen antagonist tamoxifen, and aminoglutethimide, which inhibits synthesis of all steroid hormones, have been administered. Such endocrine treatment results in arrest of growth (and sometimes shrinkage) of metastatic breast carcinoma in approximately one third of patients. The period of remission varies greatly, averaging approximately two years, after which growth of the tumour continues in spite of treatment.

Until recently, there was no way of predicting which patients would respond to endocrine therapy, but methods of assay of breast carcinoma tissue for oestrogen receptors have become available and receptors can now be detected in approximately 60% of cancers. There is evidence that carcinomas with demonstrable oestrogen receptors have a better prognosis than those without receptors, and that this is due, at least partly, to the inhibitory effect of endocrine therapy on many receptor-positive tumours. It has also been shown that response to endocrine therapy correlates with the concentration of oestrogen receptors in an extract of the tumour, and that a favourable response is unlikely when oestrogen receptors cannot be detected. The detection of receptors for progesterone has also been shown to be of predictive value, although these are seldom detected in cancers without detectable oestrogen receptors.

Other malignant tumours

Sarcoma. This is much less common than carcinoma. It may arise *de novo* or more commonly supervene in giant intracanalicular fibroadenoma of middle-aged or elderly women, especially after inadequate resection. It is usually well-defined and spindle-celled, myxomatous or pleomorphic. The degree of malignancy is related to cellular aberration and mitotic activity. Some sarcomas show metaplasia with formation of chondroid and osteoid and may resemble an aggressive osteoblastoma, osteosarcoma or giant-cell tumour of bone. In these cases the prognosis is bad and death from pulmonary metastases is the rule. The rare malignant haemangio-endothelioma tends to occur especially in the breast and gives rise to very widespread metastases.

Lymphomas. The breast is an unusual primary site of lymphoma, diffuse centrocytic/centroblastic being least rare. Its distinction from carcinoma at operation is important in order to avoid unnecessary mutilation. Involvement of the breast in disseminated lymphomas and in granulocytic leukaemia is commoner and occasionally provides the first noticeable symptoms. Massive breast involvement is a feature of Burkitt's lymphoma occurring during pregnancy and lactation.

Secondary carcinoma in breast. Spread to the contralateral breast may occur by lymphatic spread from a primary breast cancer. Carcinomas in other organs, e.g. bronchus, may also occasionally metastasise to the breast.

Congenital abnormalities

The absence of one or both of the breasts (*amazia*) is rare; in some instances it has been associated with a corresponding defect of one or both of the ovaries. *Athelia*, or congenital absence of the nipple, is less uncommon and usually bilateral. Hypoplasia of the breasts occurs in association with a similar condition of the ovaries and other parts of the genital system. Additional mammary glands (*polymastia*), may be capable of secretion, although they sometimes lack a nipple. They occur anywhere along the mammary line, but most often below the breasts. *Polythelia* (the occurrence of multiple nipples) is also rare.

The Male Breast

Hypertrophy (gynaecomastia). The male and female breasts are essentially similar until the onset of the secondary sex characters at puberty; in some adolescent males one or both breasts may then enlarge. This is known as **pubertal hypertrophy** and is rarely marked, but may cause pain or discomfort. It is due mainly to increase of stroma and enlargement of ducts, but without lobule formation. The hyperplastic duct epithelium may be surrounded by a zone of oedematous, fibrillary stroma. It tends to regress and operative removal is rarely necessary. Similar changes may occur in old age. Both pubertal and senile hypertrophy are due to changes in levels of sex hormones.

Gynaecomastia occurs in response to high oestrogen levels, for example in chronic liver failure (p. 20.36), in prolonged hormonal therapy for prostatic cancer, and reportedly in workers involved in the manufacture of oestrogens. Less commonly, it is induced by digitalis and some other drugs.

Occasionally hypertrophy results from an underlying endocrine disease such as a feminising tumour of the adrenal cortex. Less often testicular injury is causal. In chromatin-positive *Klinefelter's syndrome* (p. 25.20) the enlarged breasts show lobules comparable with those of the normal female breast. Lobule formation is excessively rare in other forms of enlargement, but is seen occasionally after prolonged administration of oestrogens.

Tumours are rare. Carcinoma may be anaplastic or adenocarcinomatous. Prognosis is often poor because of early spread to lymph nodes and to the chest wall. The possibility that genetic factors are involved or that there is an association with gonadal abnormalities or with exposure to x-irradiation remain unproved. Paget's disease of the male breast is very rare. Metastatic tumour, *e.g.* from a bronchial carcinoma, occasionally occurs and the male breast, like that of the female, may be involved in generalised lymphoid neoplasms and the leukaemias.

References and Further Reading

The female genital tract

Blaustein, A. (Ed.) (1982). *Pathology of the Female Genital Tract*, 2nd edn., pp. 939. Springer-Verlag, New York, etc.

Elston, C.W. (1981). Gestational tumours of trophoblast, pp. 149–61. In *Recent Advances in Histopathology*, No. 11. Ed. P.P. Anthony and R.N.M. MacSween, pp. 287. Churchill Livingstone, Edinburgh, etc.

Fox, H. (Ed.) (1984). *Haines and Taylor's Textbook of Gynaecological Pathology*, 3rd edn. Churchill Livingstone, Edinburgh, etc.

Fox, H. and Buckley, C.H. (1982). *Pathology for Gynaecologists*, pp. 279. Edward Arnold, London.

Fox, H. and Buckley, C.H. Pathology of female infertility (1981) pp. 119–34. In *Recent Advances in Histopathology*, No. 11. Ed. P.P. Anthony and R.N.M. MacSween, pp. 287. Churchill Livingstone, Edinburgh, etc.

Hendrickson, M.R. and Kempson, R.L. (1980). *Surgical Pathology of the Uterine Corpus*, pp. 589. W.B. Saunders, Philadelphia, etc.

Piver, M.S. (1983). *Ovarian Malignancies*, pp. 204. Churchill Livingstone, Edinburgh, etc.

Robertson, W.B. (1981). *The Endometrium,* pp. 201. Butterworths, London and Boston.

The female breast

Azzopardi, J.G. (1979). *Problems in Breast Pathology*, pp. 466. W.B. Saunders Co. Ltd., London, etc.

Kalache, A., McPherson, K., Barltrop, K. and Vessey, M.P. (1983). Oral contraceptives and breast cancer. *British Journal of Hospital Medicine*, **30**, 278–83.

Rosai, J. (1981). Breast. In *Ackerman's Surgical Pathology*, 6th edn. Vol. 2, pp. 1087–1149. C.V. Mosby Co., St. Louis, etc.

25

I Sexually Transmitted Diseases
II Male Reproductive System

I Sexually transmitted (Venereal) diseases (STD)

The intimacy of sexual contact between individuals provides opportunity for transmission of many infections, from the common cold upwards. The risk is obviously greatest when one partner has an infection of the skin or of various mucous membranes, but micro-organisms present in the blood of some individuals, e.g. the virus of B hepatitis, may also be transmitted, probably via minor abrasions sustained in coitus. However, the term STD is widely restricted to infections which are transmitted *mainly* by sexual contact between individuals, and most of them are caused by micro-organisms whose survival apart from the host lesions is very brief. A second common feature of STD is that at some stage they all produce lesions at the site of infection—usually in or about the external genitals and these lesions are highly infective to sexual partners.

Before the introduction of specific antimicrobial drugs, the two most important STD on a global scale were syphilis and gonorrhoea. When penicillin became widely available in the late 1940s, it seemed likely that the incidence of these two diseases would fall, and this did happen initially, but during the past 20 years or so the incidences of these and other STD have risen considerably in many parts of the world, and there is no doubt that the major factors have been (a) the increase in promiscuity of the 'permissive society'; (b) the spread of orogenital and anogenital sexual practices in both heterosexual and homosexual relationships; (c) the great increase in travel and migration, and (d) the widespread use of contraceptive techniques such as the contraceptive 'pill' and intrauterine device which, unlike the condom, do not provide a partial barrier to infection.

Although syphilis and gonorrhoea have both increased, they are no longer the most important of the STD in developed countries, partly because they usually cause symptoms which lead to early diagnosis and curative treatment, and partly because some of the other STD, which are more difficult to diagnose and treat effectively, have increased even more.

The individual lesions of most of the STD are described in the appropriate chapters and the following account simply brings together their main effects on men and women and sometimes on their children.

Syphilis

In pre-penicillin days, this was the most dreaded and important STD and while its incidence has since increased, adequate and early antibiotic therapy eliminates the infection so that in the developed countries the late effects—aortic aneurysm (p. 14.29), gummas, tabes dorsalis and general paralysis of the insane (p. 21.28)—have all but vanished from the autopsy room. A general account of the lesions and stages has been provided on pp. 9.28–30. The primary sore or chancre (Fig. 9.26, p. 9.28) develops early at the site of infection, usually on the external genitals or cervix, occasionally on the lips; the secondary lesions include skin rashes, shallow mucosal ulceration, and condylomata lata. All these lesions are highly infective.

Approximately 25% of primary infections now diagnosed in this country are in homosexual men and the situation is similar in some other countries, e.g. the USA. Largely owing to early treatment and antenatal serological screening, the fetus is now rarely infected and congenital syphilis is rare.

Gonorrhoea

Like syphilis, this is widespread throughout the world. In the male, it affects initially the anterior urethra and its glands, but unless treated effectively progresses to the posterior urethra and vas deferens, where it causes prostatitis, seminal vesiculitis and epididymitis: these latter lesions are more difficult to eliminate and may become chronic. In women, the gonococcus colonises first the glands of the urethra, vagina and endocervix. As in the male, the early infection is easily cured, but it may be virtually symptomless and if allowed to progress it commonly causes salpingitis which is more difficult to treat. Gonococcal lesions are typically pyogenic. The gonococcus has the unusual property of multiplying within polymorphs, which gives a characteristic appearance in smears and aspirates of the lesions (Fig. 8.3, p. 8.11), but the micro-organisms may be scanty and culture may be necessary for diagnosis. The detection of antibody is helpful in diagnosing chronic infection but is not conclusive. Gonococcal virulence and the site of infection are determined partly by variations in the composition of the gonococcal surface pili (p. 8.5). Gonococcal septicaemia (with a skin rash resembling that of meningococcal septicaemia), arthritis, endocarditis and meningitis occur occasionally and are usually due to particularly virulent strains or to a complement deficiency in the host (p. 8.9). Penicillin-resistant strains of gonococci have become widespread and now cause a significant proportion of infections, particularly in the Far East and parts of Africa.

Late effects include posterior urethral stricture in men, an increased risk of tubal pregnancy, and sterility in both sexes.

Subclinical infection is particularly prone to occur in women, and is important in the spread of the disease. Infection of the infant during delivery results in **ophthalmia neonatorum**, a purulent conjunctivitis which, if untreated, can cause blindness.

Chlamydial infections

Chlamydia trachomatis of serotypes D–K causes infection of the genital tract in both sexes and serotypes L1–3 are responsible for lymphogranuloma venereum which involves mainly the lymph nodes draining the genital organs.

Serotypes D–K are the commonest cause of sexually transmitted infective lesions. In men they are the major cause of '**non-specific urethritis**', an acute urethritis which is now much commoner than gonococcal urethritis and in which pathogenic bacteria are not revealed by conventional culture techniques. The urethritis develops a few days after infection and is usually mild, with a thin, slightly turbid discharge most noticeable before the first micturition of the day. Purulent urethritis is more suggestive of gonorrhoea, but the two are often combined, the non-specific urethritis becoming apparent only after eliminating the gonococci by penicillin treatment. Tests for antibodies to *Chlamydia trachomatis* types D–K are useful in excluding infection and high titres are suggestive of active infection. The micro-organisms can be detected microscopically as 'elementary bodies', but the immunofluorescence technique using specific antisera is more reliable, while growth in cell cultures or the chick embryo yolk sac provides the most sensitive method of detection. These techniques have shown that at least 50% of cases of non-specific urethritis in the male are chlamydial and that it is now also a major cause of prostatitis in young men and a common cause of proctitis in homosexual men.

In women, the organism causes mild urethritis, cervicitis and proctitis. The infection can also spread to the tubes and is the major cause of acute salpingitis which, although mild, may persist and cause sterility and tubal pregnancy. In both sexes, acute conjunctivitis may result from auto-infection from the genital region. Maternal infection greatly increases the risk of neonatal death: infection of the infant during birth is the commonest cause of neonatal conjunctivitis and can also cause pharyngitis, otitis media and pneumonia in the neonate.

In both sexes the infection can be asymptomatic and persistent.

Reiter's syndrome consists of acute non-specific urethritis and polyarthritis accompanied in about half the patients by conjunctivitis and sometimes by iritis. It occurs in about 2% of men with non-specific urethritis (both chlamydial and of unknown cause) and is much less common in women with non-specific urethritis. In some instances *Chlamydia trachomatis* has been cultured from the joints. The urethritis and conjunctivitis subside rapidly but the arthritis may persist for some months and relapses of the syndrome occur in about half the patients. As with some other polyarthritides, there is an increased incidence of HLA antigen B27 in those affected (about 90% compared with less than 10% in the general population), indicating the importance of a genetic factor.

Lymphogranuloma venereum (LGV), also called *lymphogranuloma inguinale*, is caused by infection with serotypes L1–3 of *Chlamydia trachomatis*. It occurs particularly in tropical and subtropical countries but is seen occasionally in temperate climates. The disease is almost always acquired by coitus and consists of a small transient primary lesion at the site of infection and gross involvement of the draining lymph nodes.

The primary lesion is a small papule which vesicates and then ruptures to form a shallow ulcer. It occurs on the penis and in women in the vulva, vagina or cervix. Healing occurs in about two weeks. The inguinal nodes become enlarged and painful 2–8 weeks after infection; at first they are discrete but soon become matted together by internodal inflammation and present as a tender, ill-defined lumpy mass which, if untreated, becomes fluctuant and breaks down the overlying skin to form sinuses which discharge pus. In men, the inguinal nodes are involved on one or both sides: in women, the inguinal and/or the pelvic and perirectal nodes are affected, depending on the site of the primary lesion.

Microscopically, the lymph nodes show acute inflammatory change but the enlargement is due mainly to massive aggregation of proliferating macrophages which differentiate into epithelioid cells: the aggregates coalesce and central necrosis followed by heavy infiltration with polymorphs gives the characteristic picture of the stellate abscesses (Fig. 25.1). The surviving lymphoid tissue of affected nodes is heavily infiltrated with plasma cells, but the changes extend to the tissue between the nodes and occasionally there is a generalised lymphadenopathy. These lesions persist for weeks or months and progressive fibrosis and destruction of lymph nodes and lymphatics may lead to elephantiasis of the genital region. In women,

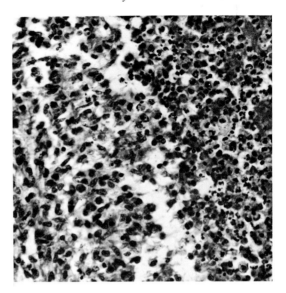

Fig. 25.1 An inguinal lymph node in lymphogranuloma venereum, showing part of the macrophage granuloma (*left*) with central suppuration (*right*). × 320.

scarring in and around the affected perirectal lymph nodes can cause rectal stricture, which is sometimes the first sign of the disease.

Detection of the micro-organism by microscopy of smears of the primary lesion or aspirate of the affected nodes is facilitated by use of the immunofluorescence technique, but growth in cell cultures or the yolk sac is more reliable. The detection of group-specific antibodies is useful diagnostically in communities where the incidence of LGV is low.

Granuloma inguinale (Donovaniasis)

This is a chronic inflammatory condition which causes ulcerating lesions of the external genitals and surrounding skin and in the draining lymph nodes. It is world-wide but uncommon in most of the developed countries. The causal organism, *Donovania granulomatis*, is a small gram-negative bacillus which has exacting cultural requirements and is best grown by yolk-sac culture. The early lesion consists of a subcutaneous nodule which undergoes necrosis and sloughing to form an ulcer. Microscopically it shows aggregates of macrophages containing large numbers of the micro-organism in cytoplasmic vacuoles (*Donovan bodies*), with necrosis, suppuration and formation of granulation tissue. Similar lesions usually develop in the inguinal lymph nodes. The lesions persist for weeks or months and extensive fibrosis of lymph nodes and obstruction of lymphatics may lead to elephantiasis of the external genitals, as in lymphogranuloma venereum.

Genital herpes

Infection with herpes simplex virus (HSV) most commonly causes recurrent lesions of the face, lips and eyes, usually due to HSV type 1, and lesions of the external genitals, usually due to HSV type 2. The incidence of genital herpes has increased very rapidly over the last 20 years: it is spread by sexual contact and only about 50% of those infected develop symptoms or lesions. The primary attack occurs about a week after infection and consists of pain and sometimes fever, arthralgia and headache accompanied by the development of small vesicles: these rupture to form painful, shallow, often confluent ulcers which heal usually within two weeks. In women, the lesions occur on the mucosa of the labia minora and the clitoris, often also on the labia majora and fourchette and sometimes on the cervix, buttocks and thighs. In men the glans penis, frenulum and prepuce are usually involved and in both sexes there may be proctitis, anal and peri-anal lesions. Although the lesions are short-lived, the virus becomes established in the posterior root ganglia where it persists for life and in some patients gives rise to recurrent attacks. These are usually milder than the original attack but can be extremely painful and, by causing dyspareunia, lead to female frigidity and male impotence.

In many people, the infection is symptomless and there are no visible lesions, so that apparently healthy people may transmit the infection to sex partners. The infant of an infected mother may be infected during delivery, and this carries a risk of fatal or severely disabling disseminated HSV infection (p. 23.21).

Diagnosis of an acute attack can usually be made clinically, but syphilis must be excluded. The virus can be detected by electron microscopy of vesicle fluid, by the immunofluorescence technique on smears of suspected lesions, or preferably by inoculation of cell cultures in which the virus has a cytopathic effect (HSV type 1) or produces multinucleate cells (HSV type 2). A fourfold increase in antibody titre is helpful in diagnosing the primary attack and the presence in cervical cytological smears of multinucleate epithelial cells with eosinophilic inclusions is suggestive of infection.

Chancroid

This is largely a disease of tropical regions, but it is now seen in Western countries and the world incidence exceeds that of syphilis. It is caused by sexual transmission of *Haemophilus ducreyi* and presents as one or more papules which become pustular and then break down to form shallow ulcers with ragged undermined margins. Microscopy shows a granulation tissue base with purulent exudate on the surface. The distribution of the genital lesions is the same as in herpes simplex and lymphogranuloma venereum. The ulcers heal slowly with scarring which in the male may cause phimosis or paraphimosis. About half the patients develop painful inguinal lymphadenitis which may suppurate and discharge to form a deep ulcer.

In contrast to the syphilitic chancre, the ulcers are not indurated (hence the alternative name **soft chancre**), but *Haemophilus ducreyi* can sometimes be detected under the prepuce or in vaginal swabs in the absence of lesions and commonly infects syphilitic chancres and other genital ulcers of all kinds: detection of the organism therefore does not exclude other STD. There is no satisfactory serological test.

Other sexually transmitted infections

Among the various micro-organisms which cause vaginitis, two deserve mention because the partners of infected women are often found to be carriers and sexual transmission appears to be the main method of infection. One is the flagellate protozoon *Trichomonas vaginalis* which infects the glands of the urethra and endocervix, causing a mild persistent vaginitis with a green frothy, watery discharge. The living organism can usually be detected microscopically in fresh preparations of the discharge and can be cultured: in men, it is found under the prepuce. The second organism is *Gardenella vaginalis*, a small coccobacillus which is usually associated with *Bacteroides* or other anaerobes and causes a mild vaginitis in which the discharge has an unpleasant fishy odour. Most of the male partners of infected women are urethral carriers. A third common cause of vaginitis, *Candida albicans*, often appears to be non-venereal.

The viral warts, **condylomata acuminata**, are in some instances sexually transmitted and occur on the external genitals: they are caused by a papovavirus.

In conclusion

All the STD described above have increased markedly in incidence in the past two decades and, as noted, most of them can have serious effects on sexual partners and some on the fetus or neonate. Apart from genital herpes, early treatment is usually effective in preventing serious effects and early diagnosis is thus extremely important.

Acquired immune deficiency syndrome (AIDS)

This is apparently a new disease which has appeared in epidemic form since about 1980 among promiscuous homosexual men in the major cities of the USA. It is usually preceded by weight loss, fever and generalised lymphadenopathy lasting for some months (**AIDS-related complex** or **ARC**). AIDS is characterised clinically by multiple and recurrent opportunistic infections, notably by *Cytomegalovirus,* *Pneumocystis carinii*, Epstein-Barr, hepatitis B and herpes simplex viruses, severe candidiasis

and other fungal infections, toxoplasmosis and various mycobacterial infections. About 30% of patients have developed Kaposi's sarcoma (p. 14.41); B-cell lymphomas are also common and some patients develop auto-immune thrombocytopenia. Over 90% of patients die of these complications within two years.

Over 70% of cases in the USA have been in homosexual men, 17% in intravenous drug abusers, presumably from sharing syringes and needles, and 6% in Haitians without known predisposing cause. AIDS has occurred also in patients receiving blood or blood products from high-risk donors, in the female sex partners of drug abusers and bisexual men and in the infants of mothers who are drug abusers. It has not been reported in health workers dealing with AIDS patients. Since 1980, AIDS has appeared in the cities of many countries throughout the world, mostly in homosexual men, and also in Central Africa where the sex ratio is more equal, suggesting transmission by heterosexual contact.

The causal agent of AIDS has been isolated, independently by French and American workers, from ARC and AIDS patients. It is a T-lymphocytotrophic retrovirus which destroys the T-cell population, and although called HTLV-III, resembles visna virus of sheep rather than HTLV-I (p. 13.7). Gallo (1984) has reported positive antibody tests in virtually all AIDS patients and most ARC patients tested, in over 20% of male homosexuals and over 30% of haemophiliacs, whereas normal heterosexual male controls were found to be negative.

II Male Reproductive System

Penis, Urethra and Scrotum

Congenital defects

Hypospadias is the commonest lesion of any importance. The urethra fails to reach the end of the penis, opening usually on its inferior surface or even in the perineum.

Congenital valvular obstruction of the urethra by thin membranous flaps in the prostatic portion is a rare but important cause of urinary obstruction in neonates.

Infections

The most important are the venereal lesions already described, with various sores on the penile skin, and gonococcal and 'non-specific' urethritis, many of the latter being due to *Chlamydia trachomatis*.

Balanoposthitis consists of inflammation of the inner surface of the prepuce (*balanitis*) and adjacent surface of the glans penis (*posthitis*). It is usually caused by various pyogenic bacteria, including occasionally the gonococcus, and is associated with a tight foreskin and lack of personal hygiene. Its prevention is the sole useful short-term benefit of circumcision, though in the long term the risk of cancer of the penis is also reduced.

Urethritis is usually due to gonorrhoea or non-specific sexually transmitted urethritis (p. 25.2). It also complicates cystitis due to *Esch. coli*, etc. and is the usual source of infection of the prostate which, in turn, leads to recurrent urinary tract infection and persistence of gonorrhoea.

Stricture of the urethra is usually a late complication of gonorrhoea, repeated reinfection, inadequate treatment and persistent suppuration in the periurethral glands of the membranous urethra being major factors. It usually occurs in the membranous part of the urethra and causes urinary obstruction with all its complications. Traumatic damage to the urethra by metal catheters, falls astride the perineum or complicating a fracture of the pelvis, also affects the relatively immobile membranous part, and may be followed by stricture.

Tumours of the penis

Papillomas are the least rare **benign tumours** occurring on the penis, usually involving the glans or prepuce. The commonest is the *condyloma acuminatum*, attributable (like the common wart) to a papovavirus. They are reddish papillary growths, sessile or pedunculated, and may become very large. The *giant papilloma* is much less common: it has not been proved to be caused by a virus and shows some cellular aberration and sometimes local invasion. *Condyloma latum*, the flat raised infective lesion of secondary syphilis, may also occur on the glans and prepuce, but is not a true tumour. *Pigmented naevi* may occur on the penis, and the rare *Peyronie's disease* is an example of the fibromatoses (p. 23.64).

Malignant tumours. *Bowen's disease* (p. 27.26) may affect the epidermis of the penis, as also may a rare lesion of uncertain status termed *Queyrat's erythroplasia*, consisting of an irregular hyperkeratotic overgrowth with a heavy inflammatory cellular infiltration of the dermis. Both are regarded as premalignant. *Squamous-cell carcinoma* is also uncommon. It usually develops on the glans or prepuce. As elsewhere, it varies in appearance from an indurated,

ulcerating nodule to a large, cauliflower-like growth. It is uncommon in Europe and North America, but the incidence varies greatly and is relatively high in some parts of Africa. It occurs chiefly in the uncircumcised and is virtually unknown among people practising ritual circumcision within a few days of birth: circumcision around puberty, as practised by Moslems, only partly reduces the incidence. Apart from this factor, the marked geographical and socio-economic variations in incidence probably reflect mainly standards of cleanliness. Inspissated smegma beneath the prepuce, which has been shown to be carcinogenic in mice, may be a causal factor. *Malignant melanoma* may also occur on penile skin and presents the usual features.

Tumours of the scrotum

Most of the many varieties of skin tumour can occur in the scrotal skin, but apart from the quasi-venereal condylomata acuminata (see above) are not common. A particular interest attaches, however, to *occupational squamous carcinoma* at this site, for Pott's description of its occurrence in chimney sweeps in 1775 was the first occupational cancer to be recognised and provided the first hint that a cause for any cancers might be found. The localisation appears to depend on the ability of the rugose skin of the scrotum to retain dirt. Tumours were formerly seen regularly not only in chim-

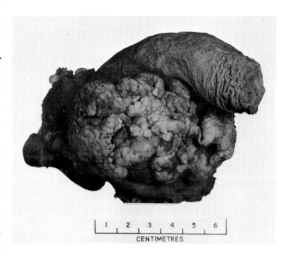

Fig. 25.2 Squamous-cell carcinoma of the scrotum showing ulcerated papillary growth.

ney sweeps (Fig. 12.24, p. 12.17) but also in machine-tool operators, gas-retort workers and men handling arsenic (Fig. 25.2). Precautions to prevent soiling of the scrotal skin with carcinogenic chemicals have greatly reduced the incidence of the condition, but it still occurs.

Prostate, vas deferens and seminal vesicles

Apart from infection, the vas and seminal vesicles are seldom the site of pathological changes. In gonorrhoea and urinary tract infections, the organisms may cause suppuration of the seminal vesicles and spread by way of the vas to involve the epididymis. *Tuberculosis* may extend in either direction along the vas, depending on whether the initial site of infection of the genital tract is by haematogenous involvement of the epididymis, or by extension from the kidney to the urinary bladder and hence to the prostate and vas.

Obstructive lesions of the vas are considered in relation to infertility on p. 25.21.

Prostatitis

Acute prostatitis usually results from spread of organisms from the urethra in gonococcal or chlamydial urethritis or in urethritis complicating cystitis. In the latter, *Esch. coli* and the various other bacteria which commonly infect the urinary tract are responsible. The prostatitis complicating gonorrhoea or cystitis is often suppurative, with formation of multiple abscesses which may coalesce and destroy most of the prostate. Chlamydial prostatitis (p. 25.2) is common but milder.

Chronic prostatitis may result from all of the above infections and also from tuberculosis: the prostate is enlarged and tender but may eventually become extensively fibrosed and shrunken. *Tuberculous prostatitis* shows the usual granulomatous caseating lesions which may involve the whole gland.

Granulomatous prostatitis, with aggregation of epithelioid multinucleate giant cells, is a rare condition of unknown cause: it differs from tuberculous prostatitis in the absence of necrosis and in the usual presence of large numbers of plasma cells. *Allergic prostatitis*, with heavy infiltration with eosinophils, occurs in some patients with asthma.

All these forms of chronic prostatitis occa-sionally cause urethral obstruction and may be mistaken clinically for carcinoma of the prostate.

Benign nodular hyperplasia (BNH) of the prostate

This is also known as simple prostatic enlargement or hypertrophy. It is not neoplastic, but is comparable to such conditions as nodular goitre and cystic hyperplasia of the breast in which there is irregular overgrowth of many areas of an organ with obvious enlargement but a lack of the progressive proliferation to form a discrete mass that marks the true benign tumour. This condition is present in minor and usually asymptomatic form in most elderly men, but in about 5% it is exaggerated and causes urethral obstruction. The central peri-urethral glands of the prostate tend to become hyperplastic and compress those at the periphery.

There is some evidence that these central glands are stimulated by oestrogens, and the peripheral glands by androgens: hence the normal moderate fall in androgen levels in old age, by altering the androgen/oestrogen ratio, might account for the prostatic enlargement. So far from being specially liable, however, eunuchs never develop BNH, though this may relate more to the failure of normal development at puberty than to the hormonal status in later decades. Animal experiments have given inconclusive results.

The mass of tissue that a surgeon removes by a standard 'prostatectomy' consists very largely of the hyperplastic central part of the gland, the remaining peripheral tissue, which is flattened against the capsule, being left behind. The mass so removed varies in size; it is usually between 50 and 100 g but may be much greater. The hyperplasia usually occurs mainly on each side of the urethra (so-called 'lateral lobes') but often there is a localised hyperplasia of the

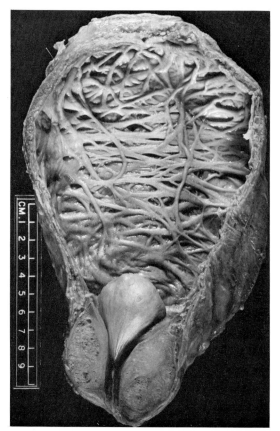

Fig. 25.3 Benign nodular hyperplasia of prostate. The 'middle lobe' is prominent, but the main mass is on each side of the urethra ('lateral lobes'). The compressed peripheral part of the prostate can just be detected as greyer areas in places. Though the urethra is not narrowed, the dilated bladder with prominent muscle bundles provides clear evidence of obstruction. × 0·5.

tissue just behind the urethra to form a rounded lump (the so-called 'middle lobe') which projects into the bladder just behind the urethral orifice (Fig. 25.3). The tissue is usually firm, and its cut surface is white and nodular. It may occasionally show areas of inflammation, abscess formation or infarction.

Effects. Though the urethra in its prostatic segment is greatly distorted, it is not usually much constricted, and the effects on bladder function result from a complex disturbance of the bladder sphincter mechanism by the obtruding prostate rather than simply from obstruction. Accordingly the symptoms of 'prostatism' are more diverse than those of simple obstruction, and the severity of the symptoms is not

closely related to the size of the prostate. There may be acute retention of urine or chronic partial obstruction and sometimes 'overflow incontinence' in which the bladder never empties completely and small volumes of urine are passed at frequent intervals. The pathological consequences are those of obstruction—hypertrophy and dilatation of the bladder, followed in time by dilatation of ureters (hydroureter) and renal pelves (hydronephrosis). If unrelieved, these changes may impair renal function and chronic uraemia may result. *Esch. coli* or mixed bacterial infection of the urinary tract, including pyelonephritis, is often superadded (p. 22.48), and spread of infection to the prostate may precipitate acute retention of urine.

Patchy infarction of the enlarged prostate is common, and this may also result in acute retention.

Microscopically there is usually increase of both the glandular elements and stroma (Fig.

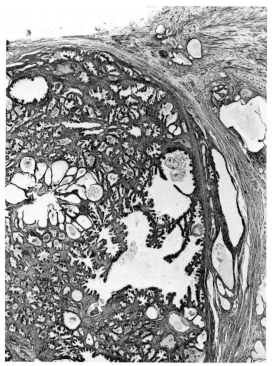

Fig. 25.4 Benign nodular hyperplasia of the prostate. The large adenoma-like nodule that fills most of the field shows predominantly glandular overgrowth, with small cysts. In the actively growing area at top right, glands are hyperplastic but the stroma, with numerous smooth muscle fibres, is much more prominent. × 10.

25.4). The glands are arranged chiefly in acini lined by columnar cells, and there may be small papilliform ingrowths into the lumina (Fig. 25.5). Often some of the acini are dilated and occasionally small cysts are formed: small concentric concretions or *corpora amylacea* are common and deposition of oxalates and phosphates may result in multiple small prostatic stones. The connective tissue stroma usually contains a substantial proportion of smooth muscle fibres. Muscle hyperplasia is most marked in the earlier stages of the process, and muscle may form a very large proportion of smaller lesions. The hyperplastic acini are usually lined by a single epithelial layer, but there may be small foci of more active hyperplasia with the formation of masses of cells, and a cribriform pattern may develop. The relationship between prostatic hyperplasia and carcinoma is considered below.

Carcinoma of the prostate

Even when 'latent' cancer (discussed overleaf)

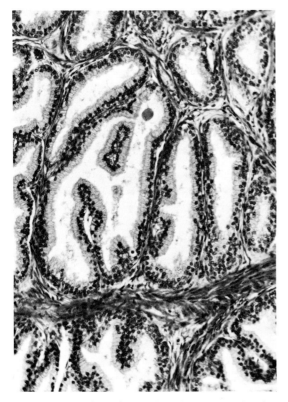

Fig. 25.5 Section of an enlarged prostate, showing hyperplasia of the glandular epithelium. × 130.

is disregarded, this is now one of the commonest cancers of internal organs of males in the developed countries, its mortality rate being exceeded only by carcinomas of the bronchus, stomach and large intestine (Table 12.3, p. 12.16) The age-adjusted incidence and mortality rates have not changed greatly over the past 20 years, and the overall increase is due mainly to the increased number of old men in the population, for this tumour has its principal incidence later in life than most common cancers. Because so many cases are geriatic patients already suffering from other disabilities, the high frequency tends to be disregarded.

The tumour arises anywhere in the prostate, but often in the periphery of the gland (outside the area chiefly affected by BNH) and especially on the posterior surface. The relation to BNH has been much disputed; some carcinomas certainly arise within hyperplastic lesions, but on the whole the evidence suggests that the prior presence of BNH is associated with little if any increase in cancer: neither the presence of BNH itself, nor 'prostatectomy' for BNH as usually practised (leaving behind the chief cancer-bearing area), either reduce or increase the incidence of carcinoma.

Histologically, the carcinoma cells are small and uniform and mitoses are scanty. Most tumours are *adenocarcinomas* of micro-acinar pattern (Fig. 25.6) but often there are areas in which the cells are loosely arranged in columns or more diffusely scattered through the stroma. The cells usually contain some mucin, and prostatic acid phosphatase can usually be demonstrated in them (as in normal prostatic epithelium) by immunohistological techniques: this is sometimes helpful in establishing that metastatic carcinoma has originated in the prostate, in which case there is a good chance that hormonal therapy will be beneficial (see over). A rare variant with larger acini, larger cells and a papillary cystadenocarinomatous pattern, probably arises from periurethral glands.

Mode of spread. The tumour spreads within the gland, and often (but not by any means always) surrounds or invades the prostatic urethra, producing all the effects of urethral obstruction. Because it often arises peripherally, it soon spreads to the surrounding tissues, and has very often metastasised widely and silently before urinary symptoms appear. Spread may be (*a*) *lymphatic*, initially to pre-

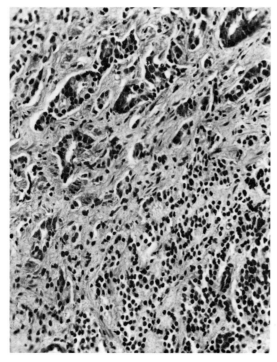

Fig. 25.6   Carcinoma of the prostate. The growth is of scirrhous type, consisting of poorly formed micro-acini (*above*) with transitions to a fine permeation of the tissue by rows of small darkly stained cells (*below*). × 225.

sacral, iliac and para-aortic lymph nodes, but often extending widely, (*b*) *retrograde venous*, to the lumbar and sacral spine, by the mechanism discussed on p. 12.27 or (*c*) by the *bloodstream* causing widespread metastases, with a predilection for the skeleton. Growth of primary tumour and metastases is usually slow. Many patients first present with pain due to bone secondaries; these are usually *osteoplastic*, i.e. they stimulate formation of bone and so appear dense on radiographs. By contrast, most other carcinomatous bone metastases are *osteolytic*.

'Latent' cancer. Microscopic foci of carcinoma are revealed surprisingly often by careful search of BNH prostatectomy specimens, or of prostates obtained at autopsy from men dying of unrelated diseases. The microscopic appearances are indistinguishable from those of clinically overt prostatic carcinoma, groups of closely packed small acini invading surrounding prostatic tissue and sometimes apparently permeating perineural spaces within the prostate.

There is, however, some electron microscopic evidence that these spaces are not lymphatics. The incidence of latent cancers depends largely on the thoroughness of the search: they may be found in 50% of prostates of men in their 50s, and in practically 100% in those over 75 years old. Although morphologically indistinguishable from carcinoma, their frequency is so very much greater than that of clinically overt prostatic cancer that they must either grow extremely slowly or become arrested after initial growth. In fact the incidence of frank cancer in men in whom the lesions are discovered accidentally (in tissue removed because of benign nodular hyperplasia) is little or no more than in the population as a whole (Byar, 1972). On the whole, one must conclude that these lesions are of more interest than practical importance. However, it should be noted that even substantial nodules of frank cancer (too large to call latent) carry a good prognosis if they are removed when the tumour is still confined to the gland: the poor prognosis of prostatic cancer relates chiefly to the large proportion which have spread outside the gland when first diagnosed, and the incidental finding of a latent cancer in a surgically removed prostate is not an indication for anti-cancer therapy or more extensive surgery.

Hormone dependence. At the time of diagnosis, prostatic carcinoma is usually too far advanced for complete surgical removal. Radiotherapy is often of limited value, but approximately 75% of patients are benefitted by therapy which lowers the production of testosterone. The response to orchidectomy is often dramatic, the pain of bone metastases being relieved within hours or days; tumour growth is slowed down or arrested and the tumour masses may shrink. Microscopy shows degenerative changes with cytoplasmic vacuolation and nuclear pyknosis in many of the tumour cells. However, patients who respond usually relapse within a few years, the tumour appearing to escape from the changed hormonal environment.

Orchidectomy is unacceptable to some patients and similar benefit may be obtained from administration of oestrogen which, by suppressing production of pituitary gonadotrophic hormones, inhibits Leydig-cell activity. In elderly men, however, oestrogens tend to aggravate ischaemic heart disease and an alternative treatment at present being investigated is the administration of potent analogues of luteinising-hormone releasing hormone which, after an initial rise of testosterone, results paradoxically in reduced production of luteinising hormone and so a fall in testosterone.

Little attention has been paid to the possibility that androgenic hormones secreted by the adrenal cortex may influence the growth of prostatic carcinoma, but it has recently been suggested that ketoconazole, which suppresses adrenal androgen production, may have a favourable effect (Allen *et al.*, 1983).

Acid phosphatase. Prostatic cancer cells, like normal prostatic epithelium, secrete an acid phosphatase which differs chemically from that produced by other tissues and cells. Conventional chemical assay of the blood level is relatively insensitive and abnormally high levels are detected only when the tumour has spread beyond the prostate. More highly sensitive and specific immunoassay techniques are capable of detecting cancer still confined to the prostate, but unfortunately raised levels occur also in prostatic hyperplasia. Blood levels of prostatic acid phosphatase reflect the response to treatment, e.g. by oestrogen or orchidectomy, relapse being associated with a rise in the level.

Testis and epididymis

It is convenient to consider together these two organs which, along with the tunica vaginalis and lower end of the spermatic cord, make up the testicle (i.e. the contents of the scrotal sac). The epididymis is subject to various infections. Most clinically evident disease of the testis is due to infection, tumour or congenital defect. Many cases of testicular defect are, however, only discovered during the investigation of infertility: the chief causes of which are described on p. 25.18 *et seq.*

Inflammatory lesions

Acute epididymitis is usually a complication of either gonococcal or 'non-specific' urethritis (p. 25.2) or of urinary tract infection; it results in both instances from spread of the infection along the vas, and may be unilateral or bilateral. In most instances, infection is relatively mild and is eliminated without much tissue destruction, but in some cases suppuration develops, followed by stenosis of epididymal tubules and sometimes sterility. The infection does not usually spread to the testis, but when it does, extensive destruction and scarring may result. The bacteria involved in urinary infections are given on pp. 22.48–51.

Tuberculous epididymitis. Tuberculosis of the male genital tract is now uncommon in developed countries. Blood spread to the epididymis from a distant lesion, nearly always in the lungs, results in tuberculous epididymitis with extensive caseation and destruction (Fig. 25.7): if untreated it may involve the scrotal wall and chronic discharging sinuses may develop. Extension to the seminal vesicles, prostate and base of the bladder may occur, and the vas may be focally obliterated. The testis is usually either unaffected or only develops lesions late and usually limited to the tissue immediately adjacent to the epididymis.

Acute orchitis occurs most commonly as a complication of mumps during post-pubertal life. The testis is infected during the viraemic stage, and mumps orchitis develops, usually a few days later than the parotitis, in about 15% of patients. The affected testis becomes acutely tender, swollen and painful due to inflammatory congestion and oedema and rise in pressure within the tunica albuginea. The cellular infiltrate is mainly of lymphocytes and macrophages but occasionally polymorphs predominate. The inflammation subsides in a few days but in about 40% of patients ischaemia due to pressure leads to residual damage, the testis becoming smaller and soft. Fortunately the condition is only occasionally bilateral and sterility rarely results.

Orchitis may occur in other acute viral infections and suppurating orchitis sometimes complicates acute bacterial epididymitis.

Syphilitic orchitis. Apart from the primary sore, the only important site of syphilis in the

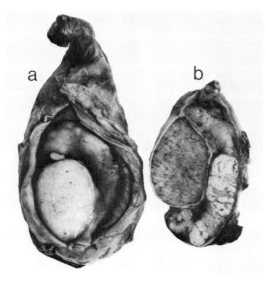

Fig. 25.7 Bilateral epididymal tuberculosis: in **(a)** the irregularly swollen epididymis is seen above the testis; in **(b)** caseation in the other epididymis is shown on section. × 0·7.

male genital tract is the testis, which is involved by tertiary lesions more often than any other tissue except the aorta. The classic gumma causes a hard, painless enlargement of the testis, and on section (Fig. 25.8) is seen as dull yellowish necrotic patches enclosed in greyish translucent granulation tissue or denser fibrous tissue. A diffuse chronic orchitis without gummatous necrosis also occurs, particularly in inadequately treated patients: the testis is largely replaced by granulation tissue infiltrated with lymphocytes and plasma cells, and showing the characteristic periarteritis and endarteritis. The result of both types of lesion is a small fibrosed testis.

Chronic granulomatous orchitis presents clinically as a unilateral painful swelling of the testis, usually in middle-aged men. After a few weeks this subsides leaving an indurated organ with diminished sensitivity to pressure. The lesion is characterised by interstitial inflammatory infiltration of lymphocytes, plasma cells and sometimes eosinophils, and formation of granulation tissue. Destruction of the germinal epithelium is accompanied by infiltration of the tubules with inflammatory cells including many giant cells. Microscopically it bears a superficial resemblance to tuberculosis because the granulomatous reaction centred on the tubules, produces a follicular pattern, but caseation and

tubercle bacilli are absent. The appearances suggest a reaction to spermatozoa or germinal epithelium and an auto-immune pathogenesis has been suggested but with little supporting evidence.

Congenital defects

Apart from germ cell lesions and the intersexes, discussed under infertility (pp. 25.19–22), there are two important and relatively common defects.

(*a*) **Undescended testis** (cryptorchidism). Either one or both testes may be arrested at any point along the track marked by the testicular artery and vein from their origin near the kidneys down through the inguinal canal into the scrotum. Minor degrees with temporary arrest are common, the descent into the scrotum being completed by the age of 4. Descent after that age is unusual. If the testis is otherwise normal there is still some hope of normal function if it can be brought down surgically into

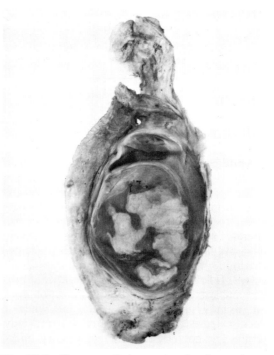

Fig. 25.8 Gumma of the testis, showing a large irregular central pale area of necrosis surrounded by darker granulation tissue. The upper pole of the testis is not yet involved. × 0·8.

the normal cooler environment of the scrotum. In about half the cases, however, there is a marked deficiency of germ cells, and no hope of fertility in that testis. The risk of tumour in the undescended organ (see later) is sufficient to justify removal of any testis that cannot be brought into the scrotum by the age of ten, particularly if there is a functioning testis on the other side. In over half the cases, however, cryptorchidism is bilateral.

(b) Congenital inguinal hernia. In this, the fetal connection between peritoneal sac and tunica vaginalis remains (*persistent processus vaginalis*).

Rare congenital defects include bifid scrotum, absence or duplication of the testis (five have been recorded in one scrotum) and various types of congenital stricture, atresia or absence causing blockage of the outflow pathway via the epididymis and vas.

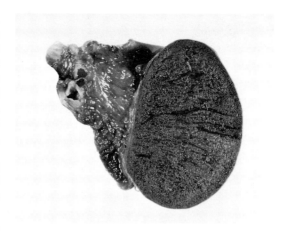

Fig. 25.9 Torsion of testis showing complete haemorrhagic infarction.

may arise from partial persistence of the processus vaginalis. For **varicocele**, see p. 14.38.

Miscellaneous lesions

Hydrocele. This is a collection of clear fluid (usually straw-coloured) within the tunica vaginalis. It can usually be distinguished from testicular enlargement by transillumination. Hydrocele may be part of a general oedema, may result from (and conceal) lesions of the testicle such as inflammation or tumour, and occasionally has no identifiable cause. Pus may also collect within the tunica vaginalis, usually following epididymal infection, and bleeding (*haematocele*) may result from trauma or testicular tumours.

Torsion of the testicle occurs usually during sleep and without obvious cause, and produces a twist of the cord at the inguinal ring. The testicle becomes hard and swollen and extremely painful. Obstruction of the vein results in gross congestion and interstitial haemorrhage and, unless it is corrected within a few hours, infarction is likely to occur (Fig. 25.9).

Cysts are uncommon except in the epididymis. A **spermatocele** is a small cyst containing clear or opalescent, usually colourless fluid in which spermatozoa can be found; it results from obstruction of an epididymal tubule. Other small cysts may arise from embryological remnants. **Serosal cysts** of the spermatic cord

Tumours

About 90% of tumours of the testis arise from the germ cells and most are malignant. They cause well under 1% of all cancer deaths—less than a tenth of that from ovarian tumours, but their importance is enhanced by their peak incidence being in early adult life, during which they are the commonest form of cancer in men and cause one-seventh of all cancer deaths in males in Europe and North America. The spectacular results of early treatment of seminoma, the commonest of the group, and recent equally impressive improvements in the chemotherapy of teratomas, have increased the importance of early diagnosis. The least rare of the germ cell tumours are *seminoma* (40%), *teratoma* (32%), *combined seminoma and teratoma* (14%) and *yolk sac tumour* (2%). Apart from *lymphoma* (7%), other testicular tumours are rare and mostly benign.

Seminoma

This is the commonest malignant tumour of the testis. It is almost unknown before puberty, becomes important in the 20s, has a peak in the 30s and falls sharply in the 50s: this is, of course, in striking contrast to the rise in incidence of most other carcinomas after 50 years of age.

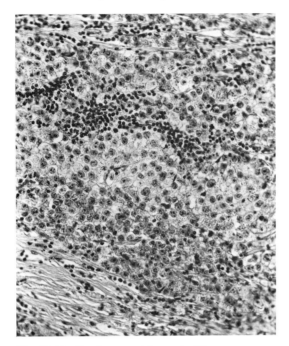

Fig. 25.10 Seminoma of the testis. The tumour consists of large round cells with vesicular nuclei. Note also the lymphocytic infiltration. × 210.

Like all the tumours in this group, it usually presents as a painless enlargement of the testis. *Macroscopically*, it forms a well-defined, firm rounded mass, usually over 7 cm in diameter when removed, replacing all or part of the testicular tissue, but rarely extending through the tunica albuginea or into the epididymis. The cut surface is soft but otherwise resembles that of a potato, being uniformly grey-white, solid and opaque (Fig. 25.11a). Haemorrhage and necrosis are unusual. *Microscopically* (Fig. 25.10) it is composed of large cells bearing a distinct resemblance to spermatogonia, with abundant pale cytoplasm and a large central pale-staining round nucleus: they are arranged in solid masses separated by irregular thin sheets of stroma which is usually infiltrated, sometimes very heavily, with lymphocytes, and often contains sarcoid-like granulomas. Tumour cells can often be seen microscopically in the lymphatics of the spermatic cord, which may be palpably thickened, and metastases occur in the para-iliac and para-aortic lymph nodes, sometimes extending to those in the thorax. Spread may occur also by the blood, metastases usually being first detected in the lungs.

A small percentage of seminomas are more anaplastic, showing greater cell pleomorphism and numerous mitoses, and carry a worse prognosis. In another rare variant, some of the cells resemble spermatocytes.

Seminomas are remarkably radiosensitive and about 95% of patients with spread limited to the para-aortic nodes are cured by orchidectomy and radiotherapy: even those with lung metastases have a relatively good prognosis. Heavy lymphocytic infiltration and granuloma formation are favourable features and may represent an immune reaction to the tumour. Those tumours which cause death usually do so within two years of diagnosis.

The detection of placental alkaline phosphatase in the serum by radio-immunoassay in patients with a seminoma has recently been reported by Jeppsson *et al.* (1983). Raised levels were detected in approximately 40% of patients before treatment and in 75% of those with metastases following orchidectomy. Raised levels are known to be associated with some other types of tumour and their value in diagnosing seminoma and in detection of metastases requires further assessment. Other tumour markers of germ-cell tumours are discussed on pp. 25.16–17.

Teratoma

A general account of these tumours has been given on pp. 12.40–42. In the main, their behaviour in the testis is much like that of seminomas, and treatment with cytotoxic drugs, including particularly cisplatin, has recently achieved remarkable results. It is too early to assess the long-term prognosis, but the two-year 'cure rate' is now similar to that for seminoma. In general, teratomas occur in younger patients, with a few cases in early childhood, the peak in the late 20s, and show a marked drop in the 40s.

In the details of their appearance, however, differences are marked. The cut surface of a teratoma rarely shows the uniform pattern of a seminoma: areas of haemorrhage and necrosis are usually prominent in the more highly malignant tumours (Fig. 25.11b), and cysts are usually seen in the better differentiated examples (Fig. 25.11c). Histologically they fall into several distinct groups, and there is much dispute about their classification and names.

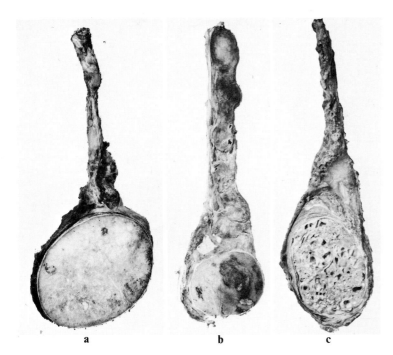

Fig. 25.11 Tumours of the testis. (**a**) Seminoma: typical solid 'potato' appearance. × 0·7. (**b**) Undifferentiated teratoma, mainly solid and haemorrhagic. (**c**) Unusually well-differentiated teratoma with multiple cysts. × 0·5.

Classification

The classification of germ-cell tumours used below is a simplification of the UK Testicular Tumour Panel's recommendations (see Pugh, 1976), which is widely used in this country. The WHO classification (Sobin *et al.*, 1978) is given in parenthesis, but it does not correspond exactly and differs also in regarding embryonal carcinoma as distinct from teratoma, the original definition of which formerly required the presence of multiple tissues. From the clinical viewpoint the name is unimportant, for it influences neither treatment nor prognosis. Of more interest is the origin and relationship of the germ-cell tumours to one another.

(**a**) **Differentiated (Mature) teratoma.** These tumours are made up of a variety of well-differentiated tissues (Fig. 25.12) similar to that occurring in the much commoner benign ovarian teratomas (dermoid cysts—p. 24.23), but unlike the ovarian dermoid cyst they are usually mainly solid and contain multiple small cysts (Fig. 25.11c). If all the tissues are well differentiated the tumour may not metastasise, but small inconspicuous foci of undifferentiated tissue are very often present and may explain why some apparently well-differentiated tumours do metastasise.

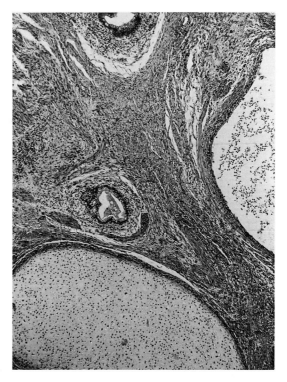

Fig. 25.12 Part of a well-differentiated teratoma of testis, showing a nodule of cartilage, glandular tissue and cystic spaces, lying in a connective tissue stroma containing strands of smooth muscle. × 17

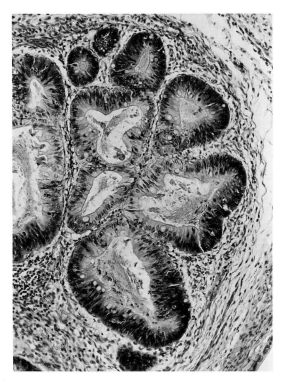

Fig. 25.13 Mucin-secreting glandular tissue in an intermediate teratoma showing dysplasia of the glandular epithelium with crowding of cells and numerous mitoses. × 45

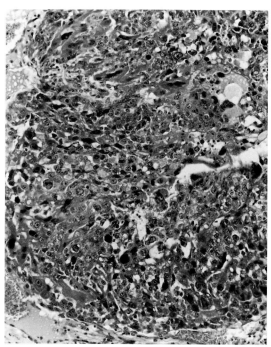

Fig. 25.14 A focus of anaplastic malignant tissue in an intermediate teratoma. The tumour cells show marked variation in size and nuclear hyperchromasia. × 45

(b) Intermediate (Immature) teratoma. These are usually solid tumours and often show patches of necrosis and haemorrhage. They consist of a mixture of tissues of various degrees of differentiation (Fig. 25.13) and areas of malignant tissue which may appear carcinomatous, sarcomatous or anaplastic (Fig. 25.14) and may include trophoblast-like elements and areas resembling yolk-sac tumour (see below).

(c) Undifferentiated teratoma (Embryonal carcinoma) (Fig. 25.11b) consists entirely of malignant tissue resembling the malignant elements of intermediate teratoma.

(d) Teratoma with choriocarcinoma is placed in a separate category because the trophoblastic elements usually metastasise. It is less sensitive to chemotherapy than uterine choriocarcinoma, probably because the latter is of allogeneic (fetal) origin (p. 12.42). Very rarely, a testicular tumour consists entirely of choriocarcinoma and this probably arises by overgrowth of a teratoma by its most malignant element.

Yolk-sac tumour

This occurs up to the age of 4 years and consists of spaces lined by malignant epithelium of varied appearance (Fig. 25.15). A characteristic feature is the presence of alpha-fetoprotein in the cytoplasm, demonstrable by immunohistology. The tumour is moderately malignant.

Combined germ-cell tumours

Fourteen per cent of testicular tumours consist of a combination of seminoma and teratoma, either mixed together or as separate nodules. Various other combinations occur and, in general, the prognosis depends on the most malignant element present. Immunohistological techniques, using antibodies to *human chorionic gonadotrophin* (HCG) and to *alpha-fetoprotein* (AFP) have revealed that extra-embryonic tissues—syncytiotrophoblast (Fig. 25.16) and yolk-sac respectively—occur more frequently in testicular tumours than has been suspected

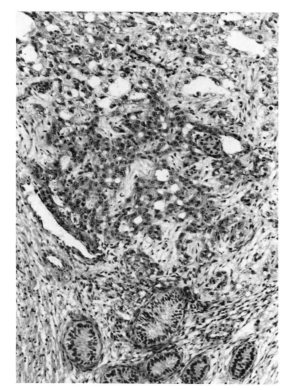

Fig. 25.15 Yolk-sac tumour of the testis of an infant. Surviving non-neoplastic testicular tubules lined by Sertoli cells are seen below. The papillary structure of the tumour (*above*) is not prominent here, but the uniform cell type is well seen. × 11·5.

from conventional microscopy (see Risdon, 1983). For example, about 75% of undifferentiated teratomas contain foci of either or both types of tissue, while 10% of seminomas contain HCG-positive syncytial cells and a smaller proportion contain AFP-positive cells. There is little information on the occurrence of markers for somatic tissues in testicular tumours, but it is becoming increasingly apparent that the stem cells of germ-cell tumours have a wide potential for differentiation and that the features of individual tumours depend on their degree of malignancy and on unknown factors which determine the direction(s) in which they differentiate.

The detection of tumour products in the serum is of value in diagnosis of testicular tumours, in monitoring the response to treatment, and in detecting the development of metastases. This applies to raised serum levels of HCG with choriocarcinomatous tumours and of AFP with yolk-sac tumours and teratomas.

In view of the associations noted above, it is not surprising that the levels of either of these two products are raised in some cases of seminoma.

Causal factors of germ cell tumours

Between 5 and 10% of testicular tumours are associated with cryptorchidism, and while the risk of neoplasia developing in an undescended testis is not great, it is about thirty times that for a normally descended testis. There is also an increased risk in infertile men with small scarred testes (usually of unknown cause). The reason for these associations is unknown, but premalignant change can be seen in a small proportion of atrophic testes, whether undescended or not (Fig. 25.17) and is followed in most instances be the development of seminoma or teratoma within the next few years. Unfortunately the detection of premalignancy would require repeated biopsy. Correct positioning of an undescended testis in early childhood may reduce

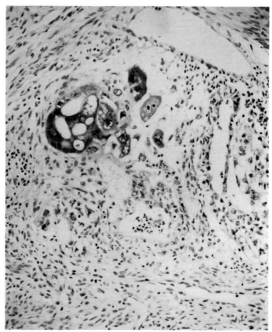

Fig. 25.16 Testicular teratoma stained by the immunoperoxidase technique using antibody to chorionic gonadotrophin. The group of large irregular cells (upper, left of centre) are positively stained and represent trophoblastic differentiation. (By courtesy of Dr R.A. Risdon and the *Journal of Pathology*.)

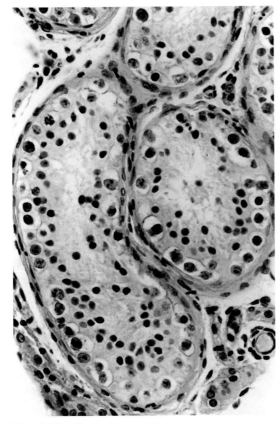

Fig. 25.17 Pre-malignant change in the germinal epithelium in an undescended testis. Note the abnormally large spermatogonia with vacuolated cytoplasm and large hyperchromatic nuclei. (By courtesy of Dr R.A. Risdon and the *Journal of Pathology*.)

the risk of cancer (and of sterility) but the evidence is inconclusive, and where only one testis is undescended there is also an increased risk of tumour in the other.

The incidence of germ-cell tumours in the developed countries has risen steadily over the past 50 years and the age of peak incidence has fallen. No environmental factors have been detected and the increase has been greatest in men in the higher socio-economic classes. It is likely that genetic factors are involved, for the incidence is lower in Negroes and higher in Jews than in Caucasians living in the same country. An association between venereal infections, particularly genital herpes, and germ-cell tumours has also been suggested, but the evidence is inconclusive.

Other tumours of the testicle

Apart from *lymphoma*, these are all uncommon. *Tumours of Sertoli cells* and of *Leydig cells*, fairly common in dogs, are rare in man. They are often hormonally active, the Sertoli-cell tumours usually producing oestrogens. Surprisingly, the Leydig cell tumours produce oestrogens at least as often as androgens. A benign glandular *adenomatoid tumour* is seen occasionally in the epididymis.

Lymphoma accounts for about 7% of testicular tumours. It is usually of diffuse centrocytic/centroblastic type and occurs in elderly men, being the commonest tumour of the testis above the age of 65.

Infertility in the male

At least 10% of married couples are infertile. Though the figures are not very reliable, the responsible partner is generally said to be male or female in roughly equal numbers, with a small group in which both partners have partial defects which combine to prevent conception. This suggests that about 5% of males and of females are infertile. Some cases are psychological, endocrine or drug-induced, but most are due to lesions of the genital tract, chiefly in the testis and Fallopian tubes.

Sperm count. Laboratory examination of a specimen of semen is necessary in most cases of suspected male infertility; it should be delivered to the laboratory within 3 hours. The normal volume is 1 ml or more, averaging 4 ml. The normal sperm count is over 50 million per ml (5×10^9/litre) and is usually well over 100 million per ml. At least 60%, and usually 80%, of the spermatozoa should be motile and of normal morphology. While it is obvious that absence of sperm (*azoospermia*) indicates infertility (provided it is not temporary—see below) it is remarkable that counts below 50 million per ml (*oligospermia*) are associated with greatly reduced fertility. With counts below 10 million fertility is rare and below 1 million it is almost unknown.

Testicular biopsy is often necessary. Practical points are the need for a skin incision large enough to allow inspection of the testis and accurate measurement of its size, a biopsy not too small, and the use of an acid fixative such as Bouin's or Davidson's.

Testicular lesions

Scarring

Gross destruction of testicular tissue by granulomatous orchitis, severe mumps orchitis, gumma or torsion, is, of course, followed by extensive scarring and atrophy and, if the lesion is bilateral, azoospermia. None of these is common however, especially in bilateral form, and the fibrosis found in cases of sterility generally consists of multiple scattered small scars, each involving only a few tubules, in an otherwise normal testis. The cause is usually unknown, but is presumably some mild unrecognised infection in childhood. The production of azoospermia or severe oligospermia by such inconspicuous scarring may seem surprising but it must be remembered that each of the 600 tubules in the testis is nearly a metre long and almost without anastomoses. Within each of the dozen or so sectors, the tubules are very intricately coiled together. With numerous small scars scattered through the testis, the chance of any one tubule having any substantial length free from obstruction is therefore small. The lesion is thus an intratesticular obstruction.

Defective spermatogenesis

The extraordinary activity of the normal spermatogenic epithelium is very readily interfered with, and a fall in sperm count or even azoospermia follows: however, in most such cases depression of spermatogenesis is usually reversible. Possible causes of partial or complete arrest of spermatogenesis are very numerous: the following are the more important.

(*a*) **General causes.** Fever, malnutrition, many poisons, uraemia or indeed almost any severe illness will depress spermatogenesis.

(*b*) **More specific damage** is caused by cadmium, local x-rays and anti-mitotic drugs. In high dosage these cause destruction of the stem cells (the spermatogonia) and so permanent depression of spermatogenesis: in lesser doses, x-rays at least can cause germ cell mutations, though the evidence for this is based largely on animal work.

(*c*) **Temperature.** Spermatogenesis ceases at normal body temperature. Hot baths and tight pants depress spermatogenesis only enough to matter in men with low sperm counts already, but **varicocele** (p. 14.38) can certainly produce azoospermia, and of all causes of impaired spermatogenesis this is the one in which surgical intervention is most likely to cure sterility.

(*d*) **Endocrine disorders.** Development of the testicular tubules in the embryo and spermatogenesis in adult life depend on androgens derived locally from the Leydig cells. These in turn depend on the pituitary. In the adult, LH is the main stimulus to Leydig cell activity. Both Leydig cell androgens and FSH are necessary for tubule activity. Spermatogenesis therefore ceases in most forms of pituitary failure. Most often this is caused by *oestrogen excess*, which suppresses LH and FSH. Oestrogen given in the treatment of prostatic cancer is an obvious example, but *cirrhosis of the liver* provides a more striking one, the rise in endogenous oestrogen seen in many relatively moderate cases of liver damage (p. 20.36) having a very marked effect on the testis. Leydig cells vanish, spermatogenesis ceases (spermatogonia, however, remain, and can resume activity), and there is, in addition, deposition of hyaline material round the tubules between epithelium and basement membrane, which eventually causes irreversible damage.

Germ cell defects

Absence or near-absence of germ cells is usually congenital. The effect is to produce tubular atrophy without loss of Leydig cells, and a rise of pituitary FSH presumably due to the absence of the feed-back hormone *inhibitin* (not yet positively identified) which is apparently produced by active spermatogenic epithelium, and normally suppresses FSH (but not LH). Pituitary activity sometimes produces gynaecomastia. This combination was identified by Klinefelter in 1943. His name, however, is generally used only for the first of the two main forms (below) of germ-cell defect.

(1) Klinefelter's syndrome (of 47XXY type). This, one of the commonest of chromosomal disorders, is the result of the presence of a Y chromosome (which ensures the formation of a testis and masculine development generally) together with a second X, which prevents normal development of the testis. The usual abnormal pattern is thus 47XXY, but variants e.g. mosaics, are not rare and even an apparent normal 46XX karyotype is described. These 'XX males' have parts of the short arm of the Y chromosome transferred to the tip of the short arm of the X, thus transferring male determinants from the Y to the X. A moderate increase in frequency of mental defect is the only important non-genital consequence. A eunuchoid body-build is frequent: FSH levels are high and androgens are usually moderately reduced. There may be gynaecomastia, and carcinoma of the breast is commoner than in normal males. The rare cases with three or four X chromosomes (XXXY, etc.) have a high incidence of congenital defects.

The testis in these cases is very small (5 g or less). The bulk appears to be made up of irregular masses of Leydig cells: among them are occasional tubules lined by Sertoli cells only (similar to those seen in the next group) but most of the recognisable tubules are inconspicuous and hyalinised ('ghost' tubules). In a few cases germ cells persist in an occasional tubule, and localised spermatogenesis occurs. A single well-authenticated case of a fertile man with 47XXY presumably represents an extreme example of this.

Diagnosis in these cases is made easy by the sex chromatin test; this is the only condition of any frequency in which it is positive in males (Figs. 25.18 and 25.19). Using this test, it has been shown that between 1 in 700 and 1 in 1000 male births are 47XXY.

The defect in the testis is not strictly congenital: the testes develop normally until about the time of birth; germ cells then disappear, but tubules remain normal until puberty, when active destruction takes place. The mechanism of this is quite unknown. XXY individuals have been found in all mammals in which such

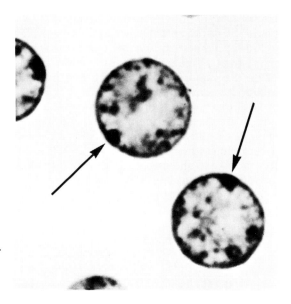

Fig. 25.18 Nuclear sex chromatin, resembling that of normal females, in the Leydig cells of a case of 47XXY Klinefelter's syndrome. Testicular biopsy. × 1500.

chromosomal abnormalities have been sought, and the effects are much the same in all of them.

(2) Germ-cell aplasia (non-chromosomal). (Also called *chromatin-negative Klinefelter's* or the *del Castillo syndrome*.) Here there is absence or near-absence of the germ cells in the testis, of unknown cause but presumed to be congenital. The effects are similar to those of 47XXY, but are (except for the infertility, which is nearly invariable) less pronounced. There is no associated mental defect and a eunuchoid build is less common. The testes are not so small, and the histology is less grossly altered: the tubules

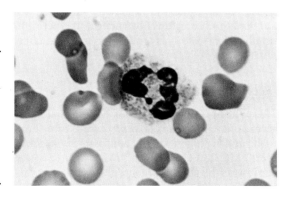

Fig. 25.19 A polymorphonuclear leucocyte showing the typical female sex-chromatin drumstick. × 1000.

are well preserved but reduced in size, and are lined entirely by tall, pale-staining Sertoli cells with no germ cells. Between the tubules there is an apparent excess of Leydig cells. Many cases are partial, with a few fertile tubules, producing oligospermia rather than azoospermia.

Leydig cells in testicular atrophy

In normal men, the Leydig cells have a total volume of about 0·9 ml in each testis, and this quantity remains remarkably constant so long as the normal pituitary stimulus is present. If the tubules in both testes are atrophic, the proportion of the testis occupied by Leydig cells becomes proportionately increased (it may be over 50% in an 47XXY testis) and it is easy to mistake this for hyperplasia (true Leydig cell hyperplasia is very rare in man). When only one testis is atrophic, the Leydig cells appear to be readjusted between the two testes, and little apparent hyperplasia occurs on the affected side.

It is worth remembering that apparent *excess* of Leydig cells in a biopsy in man is nearly always an illusion, produced by tubular atrophy, while *deficiency* is nearly always a sign of pituitary depression.

Non-testicular causes of infertility

These are numerous and sometimes treatable, but account for fewer cases than testicular lesions. They include the following.

(*a*) **Impotence** (i.e. inability to achieve orgasm). This is usually psychological, but may be drug-induced, endocrine (androgen failure, excess of oestrogen or prolactin), neural (spinal cord lesions especially) or vascular. Impotence due to vascular lesions occurs in the Leriche syndrome (p. 14.8). Over half of renal transplant patients have been reported to become impotent after a *second* graft, due to use of both internal iliac arteries to supply the grafts.

(*b*) **Abnormalities which interfere with coitus.** These include penile deformities and extreme obesity.

(*c*) **Obstruction of the outflow pathway.** Part of the vas may be congenitally absent, or it may be interrupted by trauma including operations,

usually for hernia. Sterilisation by bilateral vasectomy must be included here: its occasional failures illustrate the remarkable ability of some tubular structures to re-establish continuity spontaneously after division. Obstruction of the tubules of the **epididymis** may follow any of the epididymal infections described above. Some lesions of the proximal **urethra**, for example stricture or the trauma of prostatectomy, may result in discharge of the semen into the bladder. This is the usual cause of *aspermia* (total absence of ejaculate). In bilateral obstructions of the vas or epididymis or tubular atrophy, the secretions of the seminal vesicles and prostate usually produce an ejaculate even though there is azoospermia.

Surprisingly enough, obstructive lesions have very little effect on the testis itself, no matter how long the duration. The finding of azoospermia with a normal testicular biopsy usually means obstruction, which can sometimes be corrected surgically. Spermatozoa continue to be produced, and collect in the tubules of the epididymis, in time giving rise to 'sperm granulomas' with clumps of sperm heads and macrophages full of brown pigment.

Intersexes

Intersexes are individuals who present some degree of intermingling of the characters of both sexes. Apart from the psychological intersexes, homosexuality and transvestism, with which we are not concerned, the principal varieties are the following.

(*a*) **Chromosomal intersexes.** The commonest varieties are 47XXY Klinefelter's syndrome, considered above, and 45XO Turner's syndrome (p. 24.29). In both of these, and in contrast to the next group, the general anatomy is far less intersexual than the chromosomal picture.

(*b*) **Hermaphroditism.** This term is properly confined to the rare individuals who possess both testis and ovary: there may be an ovary on one side and a testis on the other, or various mixtures of the two. Intermediate forms of sexual development are a natural consequence. Most often the external genitalia are predominantly male at birth and internal genitalia correspond to the gonad nearest to them. Breast development or other signs of feminisation appear at puberty. In most cases the cause is obscure, but some are true *mosaics*—mixtures of XY and XX cells derived from a single zygote. There is strong evidence that this can result from double fertilisation, and can be regarded almost as an extreme case of Siamese twinning, with total fusion at the cellular level. These XX/XY mosaics should not be confused with natural chimeras who consist of XX and XY cells derived from two fertilised ova, or from separate fertilisation of an ovum and its polar body.

(*c*) **Adrenal virilism** (p. 26.35). In this, excessive androgenic hormone synthesis leads to virilisation of the external genitalia in females: the condition is of special importance because, if recognised early, it can often be treated effectively.

(*d*) **Male pseudohermaphroditism.** In this, male external genitalia are imperfectly developed, presumably as a result of temporary failure of testosterone output from the testis *in utero*. In its lesser degree it fades away into such minor conditions as bifid scrotum and hypospadias.

A child of doubtful sex at birth is usually a female with adrenal virilism or a male pseudohermaphrodite: the sex chromatin test distinguishes reliably between them.

(*e*) **Testicular feminisation** is an interesting though rare form of intersex in which there is a genetically determined defect of androgen receptors which renders the target cells insensitive to the male sex hormone. The effect is one of externally complete feminisation, though the patients are XY and possess (undescended) testes. The defect is determined by a gene on the X chromosome, heterozygous females acting as asymptomatic carriers. Offspring of these carriers have equal chances of belonging to any one of the four classes of normal males, normal females, carrier (but otherwise normal) females and affected sterile 46XY phenotypic females.

References and Further Reading

Allen, J.M., Kerle, D.J., Ware, H., Doble, A., Williams, G. and Bloom, S.R. (1983). Combined treatment with ketoconazole and luteinising hormone releasing hormone analogue: a novel approach to resistant progressive prostatic cancer. *British Medical Journal*, **287**, 1766.

Byar, D.P. (1972). Survival of patients with incidentally found microscopic cancer of the prostate: results of a clinical trial of conservative treatment. *Journal of Urology* **108**, 908-13.

Jeppsson, A., Wahren, B., Stigbrand, T., Edsmyr, F. and Andersson, L. (1983). A clinical evaluation of serum placental alkaline phosphatase in seminoma patients. *British Journal of Urology*, **55**, 73-78.

Lennox, B. (1981). The infertile testis. In *Recent Advances in Histopathology, No. 11*, pp. 135-48. Ed. by P. P. Anthony and R. N. M. MacSween. Churchill Livingstone, Edinburgh.

Mostafi, F.K. (1973). Testicular tumours, epidemiologic, etiologic and pathologic features. *Cancer*, **32**, 1186-1201.

Pugh, R.C.B. (Ed.) (1976). Pathology of the Testis, pp. 487. Blackwell Scientific, Oxford and London.

Risdon, R.A. (1983) Germ cell tumours of the testis. *Journal of Pathology*, **141**, 355-61.

Sobin, L.H., Thomas, L.B., Percy, Constance and Henson, D.E. (Eds) (1978). *A Coded Compendium of the International Histological Classification of Tumours*, pp. 116. World Health Organisation, Geneva.

AIDS

Gallo, R.C. *et al.* (1984). Frequent detection and isolation of cytopathic retroviruses (HTLV-III) from patients with AIDS and at risk for AIDS. *Science*, **224**, 500-2.

Sarngadharan, M.G., Popovic, M., Bruch, L. *et al.* (1984). Antibodies reactive with human T-lymphotropic retroviruses (HTLV-III) in the serum of patients with AIDS. *Science*, **224**, 506-8.

Seminars in Oncology (1984). **11**, 1-86. (An informative series of articles on AIDS).

26

The Endocrine System

General features

In considering disturbances of the endocrine system, it is helpful to bear in mind the following important features.

1. *Most hormones have more than one action.* The parathyroid hormone, for example, stimulates the release of calcium from bone and increases calcium absorption from the renal tubules and from the gut.

2. *Most functions under endocrine control are influenced by more than one hormone.* For example, the effects of insulin on sugar metabolism are largely antagonistic to those of growth hormone, thyroid hormone, glucocorticoids and catecholamines: the control of glucose metabolism represents a balance between these various factors.

It follows that the normal endocrine status depends on the balanced functioning of the various endocrine glands.

3. *Negative feedback mechanisms are of major importance in controlling the functions of individual endocrine glands.* In some instances, e.g. the thyroid, control is exerted mainly by the plasma level of the hormone it produces. In other instances, control is mainly dependent on the level of a particular (non-hormonal) compound which the gland regulates, e.g. insulin secretion is controlled largely by the level of the blood sugar and parathyroid secretion by the level of blood Ca^{++}.

4. *The relationships between the nervous system and the endocrine glands are of particular importance.* This is illustrated by the following. (1) The neurohypophysis stores and releases hormones produced in the basal ganglia, while the control of production and release of adenohypophyseal hormones is mediated partly by small polypeptide hormones secreted by nerve cells in the hypothalamus. (2) Many functions are under joint neural and endocrine control, an obvious example being regulation of blood pressure. (3) The autonomic nervous system has a direct influence on the secretory activity of the endocrine glands.

5. *Most of the endocrine glands have a large functional reserve,* and so can function apparently normally when partly destroyed by disease. They also have a high capacity for hyperplasia and can enlarge to meet an increased workload or to overcome defects in their metabolism. For example, individuals who are deficient in iodine (an essential constituent of thyroid hormone) develop thyroid hyperplasia, sometimes visible as enlargement (goitre): by increasing the rate of iodine turnover the hyperplastic gland may be able to maintain relatively normal function.

6. *Lesions in different sites can produce similar clinical features of endocrine disorder.* Thyroid hypofunction, for example, can result directly from chronic inflammatory destruction of the thyroid, usually due to auto-immune thyroiditis; it can result also from any lesion of the pituitary which interferes with the production and secretion of TSH. The secretion of TSH, in turn, may be disturbed by a lesion of the hypothalamus which interferes with the secretion of TSH-releasing hormone. This multiple aetiology applies to other endocrine glands under the control of pituitary trophic hormones, notably the adrenals and gonads.

Immunological techniques in endocrinology

The production of antibodies to various hormones in experimental animals and the rapidly increasing availability of monoclonal antibodies have provided techniques for measuring the concentration of most human hormones in plasma, etc., notably by radio-immunoassay

(RIA) and solid-phase immunoradiometric assay (IRMA). Although problems arise from the presence of breakdown products of hormones which do not correspond in their immunoreactive and hormonal activities, these techniques are a great advance over time-consuming and expensive chemical and biological assay methods and have provided the means for more precise investigation of patients with endocrine disorders. Immunohistological techniques have also contributed greatly to the elucidation of the functions of endocrine cells, particularly in the adenohypophysis (Fig. 26.1).

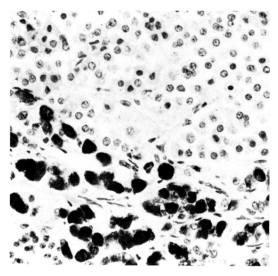

Fig. 26.1 Section of adenohypophysis stained by the immunoperoxidase method, using antibody to growth hormone. The cytoplasm of cells containing growth hormone is stained black. The field includes the edge of a chromophobe adenoma (*above*), the cells of which are devoid of growth hormone (Professor R. B. Goudie.)

Lesions of endocrine glands

Unlike exocrine glands, the endocrines are not connected by a duct system with the lumen of hollow viscera. In consequence, they are liable to become infected only by micro-organisms circulating in the blood. They are also mostly resistant to bacterial infection, an exception being tuberculosis and other chronic blood-borne infections of the adrenals. Viral infections seldom cause serious lesions of the endocrine glands, although the thyroid is sometimes involved in mumps and there is evidence that viral infection of the islets of Langerhans is a contributing cause of type I diabetes mellitus (p. 26.63).

An important group of endocrine disorders results from the **organ-specific auto-immune diseases** which cause destructive inflammation, leading to hypofunction of the thyroid, adrenals and parathyroids, while the common form of hyperthyroidism (Graves' disease) is caused by an auto-antibody which binds to the TSH receptors of thyroid epithelium.

Lastly, all the endocrine glands are subject to **neoplasia**. Most of the tumours are benign adenomas and they are of particular importance because they frequently secrete hormones in uncontrolled fashion. Those arising in the pituitary may, however, compress the surrounding glandular tissue and so cause hypofunction. Carcinomas originating in non-endocrine organs, notably the bronchus, not uncommonly secrete hormones (p. 20.43) and these may produce endocrine disturbances.

This chapter gives an account of the disorders of the major endocrine glands with the exception of the gonads (Chapters 24 and 25) and the endocrine pancreas which, because of its close functional associations with the exocrine pancreas, is considered as a composite organ (pp. 20.55–66).

The Pituitary

The adenohypophysis (anterior lobe)

Despite its importance, the pituitary is a relatively tiny organ which weighs about 500 to 900 mg in the male and often rather more in the female. There is a significant increase in size during pregnancy. The *adenohypophysis* develops from an upgrowth from the roof of the embryonic oral cavity which becomes contiguous with a downgrowth from the developing brain destined to become the *neurohypophysis*. The blood supply to the adenohypophysis is peculiar in that, except for the tissue immediately beneath the capsule, there is no direct arterial supply; blood passes from the capillaries in the hypothalamus into venous portal channels which traverse the stalk and break up into the sinusoids of the adenohypophysis. This arrangement allows hormonal factors secreted by the hypothalamus to influence adenohypophyseal function (see below): it also renders the adenohypophysis liable to ischaemic injury, e.g. during the circulatory collapse of shock, and permits almost complete destruction of the gland by deliberate surgical interruption of the stalk.

The adenohypophysis makes up about 75% of the whole pituitary and produces the following six major hormones of known physiological significance. (1) *Growth hormone* (GH) or *somatotrophin*. (2) *Lactogenic hormone* or *prolactin* (PRL). (3) and (4) The *gonadotrophins—follicle-stimulating hormone* (FSH) and *luteinising hormone* (LH). (5) *Thyroid stimulating hormone* (TSH) or *thyrotrophin*. (6) *Adreno-corticotrophic hormone* (ACTH) or *corticotrophin*.

In addition, the adenohypophysis secretes a number of polypeptides of unknown physiological significance in man.

The hormone-secreting cells

The cells of the adenohypophysis were traditionally classified, on the basis of their morphology and in particular on the presence or absence of basophil or acidophil (eosinophil) cytoplasmic granules, into basophil, acidophil and chromophobe cells. Classification was advanced by Pearse's tri-PAS stain, giving four major cell types. Electron microscopy has demonstrated the presence in many of the cells of secretory granules which differ in size and appearance depending on the hormone(s) stored within them.

Current classification of adenohypophyseal cells is based on immuno-electron microscopy using antibodies to the individual hormones. By this technique, the hormones stored in secretory granules are identified, indicating which hormone is produced by each individual cell. It has been established in this way that FSH and LH are both secreted by the same cell type, while the other four major hormones are secreted by four distinct types of cell.

Somatotrophic cells are roughly spherical, eosinophilic, lie mainly in the lateral wings of the adenohypophysis, and contain numerous secretory granules of 350-500 nm diameter. **Lactotrophic cells** are also eosinophilic and lie mainly in the lateral wings; they contain granules of 275-350 nm. These cells are relatively scanty but are increased in the fetus and in pregnancy due to high levels of circulating oestrogens. **Gonadotrophic cells** are scattered singly throughout the adenohypophysis: they are angular basophilic cells with granules of 275-375 nm and secrete both FSH and LH. **Thyrotrophic cells** lie mostly in the central part of the gland: they are elongated basophilic cells with granules of 50-100 nm. **Corticotrophic cells** are distributed throughout the gland: they are basophilic with granules of 375-550 nm. They synthesise a large molecule which contains also β lipotrophin. **Chromophobe cells,** with pale-staining cytoplasm and few secretory granules, are now thought to be secretory cells which have discharged most of their stored hormone: many of them appear to be lactotrophic cells. The adenohypophysis also contains *stellate cells* which make mutual contact by long processes. Their function is unknown.

Control of adenohypophyseal function

This is highly complex. The major features of the control mechanisms are summarised below and more detail is given in the subsequent accounts of the individual hormones.
1. The role of the hypothalamus. Neurosecretory cells in the hypothalamus produce hormonal factors which pass by the portal venous system (see above) to the adenohypophysis, where they have a stimulatory or inhibitory effect on one or more hormone-secreting cell types. Examples of these factors include growth hormone releasing and inhibiting factors (GHRF and GHIF respectively), thyrotrophin releasing factor (TRF), corticotrophin releasing factor (CRF) and prolactin inhibiting factor (PIF).
2. Control of hypothalamic secretory activity is partly neural and partly humoral. Neural control is exerted by nerves reaching the hypothalamus from other parts of the CNS, and is important in controlling the circadian rhythms of hormone secretion, changes during sleep and rapid responses to stress, etc. Humoral control is by negative feedback mechanisms in which rise in the levels of hormones or metabolites in the plasma inhibits the secretion of stimulatory factors, or promotes secretion of inhibiting factors, in the hypothalamus. This is the classical *long-loop* or *hypothalamic-hypophyseal feedback control*.

3. Direct feedback control. The activity of adenohypophyseal cells is also influenced directly by the levels of hormones and metabolites in the plasma (short-loop feedback control).

4. Mediators of feedback control. As noted above, the short- and long-loop feedback controls are dependent on the levels of hormones and metabolites in the plasma. For those adenohypophyseal hormones which stimulate another endocrine gland (i.e. ACTH, TSH, LH and FSH), the plasma levels of the hormones secreted by the target endocrine glands (cortisol, thyroid hormone and sex hormones respectively) exert feedback control.

Feedback control of secretion of GH (which tends to induce hyperglycaemia) is exerted mainly by the plasma levels of various metabolites, notably glucose.

Thirdly, adenohypophyseal hormones exert some feedback control on their own secretion. For example, a rise in PRL inhibits further PRL secretion: ACTH and GH similarly inhibit their own secretion.

5. In general, the net effect of hypothalamic secretions is stimulatory, but in the case of prolactin, hypothalamic control is largely effected by secretion of inhibitory factors (PIF).

6. The feedback mechanisms are not entirely hormone-specific. For example, thyrotrophin releasing factor (TRF) stimulates secretion of TSH and PRL, and it is capable of either stimulating or inhibiting secretion of GH.

In view of the number of adenohypophyseal hormones and the complexity of their control and interrelationships, it is not surprising that disorders of the pituitary have complex and varied results. Their complexity is further increased by the situation of the organ in the bony sella, for an adenoma of one cell type may secrete excess hormone and yet lead to compression and destruction of the normal pituitary tissue, with consequent deficiency of the other hormones. Moreover, a lesion in or above the sella may produce various effects on the complex functions of both the pituitary and the hypothalamus.

The adenohypophyseal hormones

Growth hormone (GH) is a protein consisting of a single chain of 191 amino acids and constitutes about 10% of the dry weight of the pituitary. It is essential, together with thyroid hormone and insulin, for the normal rate of growth in childhood. This somatotrophic effect has been demonstrated by replacement therapy in hypophysectomised animals and children with hypopituitarism. Deficiency of GH causes dwarfism and obesity: its administration promotes protein synthesis and growth of the bones, organs and soft tissues. GH promotes protein synthesis and reduces the amount of urea excreted. It also accelerates lipolysis in fat depots and provision of energy from fat. It decreases the response of cells to insulin and so tends to raise the blood sugar, although this is not pronounced in man unless GH is administered to hypophysectomised diabetic patients, when it greatly aggravates the diabetes.

GH has been shown, in organ perfusion and tissue culture experiments, to exert the above effects directly. It binds to receptors on various cell types, but the mechanism by which this influences cell metabolism is not known. Part of the effect of GH *in vivo* appears to be mediated indirectly by production of **somatomedins**. These are peptides with amino-acid sequences resembling those of insulin.

Synthesis and release of somatomedins by perfused liver or cultured liver cells is induced by GH together with thyroid hormone and insulin. Somatomedins induce the metabolic changes characteristic of growth and matrix secretion in isolated cartilage, whereas GH is without effect. Somatomedins are also bound by various other tissues. Their effects are not closely parallel to those of GH, for they also exert an insulin-like effect in some tissues.

Immunoassay indicates an average plasma concentration of GH of 2–3 μg/l in adults and about double in children and adolescents, but the level fluctuates considerably throughout the day. Stimulatory factors include exercise, stress and food intake: these effects, together with circadian rhythm, are exerted by the CNS via the hypothalamus. Hypothalamic-pituitary control is mediated by a growth hormone releasing factor, GHRF (which is of unknown composition) and by somatostatin which is inhibitory (GHIF). Feedback inhibition is exerted by a rise of blood sugar and by various other metabolites, and is influenced by some other hormones, including oestrogen.

Chorionic somatomammotrophic hormone, which is produced by the placenta, has structural and biological properties similar to those of GH.

Prolactin (PRL) is a protein in which amino-acid sequences resembling those of GH suggest their derivation from a common ancestral protein. In women, its function is to initiate and maintain lactation in the breast already primed by sex hormones, corticosteroids and insulin. The plasma level in women as measured by immunoassay, is normally below $20\,\mu g/l$; it rises throughout pregnancy, but its action on the breast is inhibited by the rising levels of sex hormones. After delivery, the plasma levels of sex hormones fall rapidly and the high level of PRL initiates lactation. The mammary stimulation of suckling rapidly induces a rise in plasma PRL by neural pathways acting on the hypothalamus, where they inhibit secretion of dopamine which is the major PRL inhibiting factor (PIF). The high levels of plasma PRL induced by suckling both prepare the breast for the next feed and inhibit ovulation, thus explaining the usual temporary state of relative infertility during lactation.

PRL has no known function in men, although the plasma level is only slightly lower than in non-pregnant women.

Gonadotrophic hormones. Maturation and function of the gonads in both males and females is dependent on the two adenohypophyseal gonadotrophic hormones, **follicle-stimulating hormone (FSH)** and **luteinising** or **interstitial cell stimulating hormone (LH)**. FSH is essential for the growth of Graafian follicles and for ovulation, and LH for luteinisation of the follicle following ovulation. Under the influence of these hormones, the Graafian follicle secretes oestrogen, which induces endometrial proliferation, and the corpus luteum secretes progesterone, which inhibits further ovulation and induces endometrial secretory change.

In males, FSH stimulates spermatogenesis and LH stimulates the Leydig cells to secrete testosterone.

Secretion of FSH and LH is regulated by a negative feedback by the sex hormones. This probaby works both directly by influencing secretion of a single releasing hormone (LH/FSH RH) by the hypothalamus. The proportions of FSH and LH secreted depend on the plasma levels of oestrogen and progesterone, and on the stages of the menstrual cycle. They are secreted in pulses and the plasma levels fluctuate rapidly.

These two hormones and also chorionic gonadotrophin are glycoproteins composed of two peptide chains with attached carbohydrate. They all share a common or closely similar α chain and widely different β chains which are responsible for their hormonal activities. It follows that immunoassay, which has replaced bioassay, must be performed with antibodies to the β chains.

The plasma levels increase at puberty: in women they peak at ovulation and increase greatly after the menopause. The levels in men are rather lower than the average levels in women. Some of the effects of these hormones are mediated by activating adenylate cyclase.

Rare cases of infertility in both men and women result from gonadotrophin deficiencies. Excessive production of LH may also give rise to the syndrome of polycystic ovaries and infertility.

Thyrotrophic hormone (TSH) induces proliferation of thyroid follicular cells and synthesis and secretion of thyroid hormone. T_4 and T_3 exert a negative feedback effect in TSH secretion, mainly directly but also via the hypothalamus, which secretes a TSH-releasing factor (TRF). Hypophyseal control is also influenced by various other factors, including dopamine, somatostatin and GH, all of which inhibit secretion of TSH. Plasma TSH is most readily determined by radio-immunoassay: it is undetectable in about 10% of normal subjects, is greatly elevated in patients with untreated primary hypothyroidism, and is suppressed by administration of thyroxine. As explained later, the common form of hyperthyroidism, known as Graves' disease, is due to an abnormal thyroid stimulator, and TSH secretion is suppressed by the high levels of thyroid hormone.

Adrenocorticotrophic hormone (ACTH) is essential for the secretion of glucocorticoid hormones by the adrenal. These steroids operate a negative feedback effect on ACTH secretion, mainly by their direct effect on corticotrophic cells and possibly also via the hypothalamus which secretes an ACTH-releasing factor (CRF). Secretion of CRF is influenced by various neurogenic stimuli and is important in the response to stress, pain, etc. and in the circadian rhythm of ACTH secretion. ACTH binds to receptors on glucocorticoid-producing cells of the adrenal cortex and stimulates them by activating adenylate cyclase. Hypophysectomy or administration of cortisol results in adrenocortical atrophy.

Reliable radio-immunoassay techniques for ACTH have been developed but are not widely available. The plasma level, usually below $50\,ng/litre$ in normal adults, has a circadian rhythm, and the hormone is secreted in short 'pulses'. The level rises in individuals exposed to stress and may exceed 500 ng/litre: high levels are also to be expected, and are observed, in Addison's disease (primary adrenocortical insufficiency) and in patients with 'inappropriate' secretion of ACTH, e.g. by a bronchial carcinoma.

ACTH consists of 39 amino-acid residues of which only the first 20 are necessary for its hormonal effect. It has been synthesised and can be administered repeatedly without development of a refractory state. Its administration causes adrenocortical hyperplasia and increased excretion of glucocorticoid hormones, resulting in gluconeogenesis, atrophy of the thymus and lymph nodes and lymphopenia, etc. (p. 26.31)

ACTH is synthesised as part of a larger prohormone and is released by proteolytic cleavage. The remainder of the molecule, *β lipotrophin*, contains the amino-acid sequences of the endorphins and enkephalin. Endorphins are secreted by the pituitary along with ACTH, but are synthesised also in other parts of the brain and the significance of their production in the pituitary is not clear. ACTH and *β* lipotrophin (*β*-LPH) contain amino-acid sequences which in some fish and amphibians are split off as melanin stimulating hormones (MSH) and control the distribution of melanin in pigment cells. MSH are not, however, secreted in significant amounts as separate hormones in man and the pigmentation of the skin in primary adrenal atrophy (Addison's disease) appears to be due to melanogenic effects of ACTH and *β*-LPH. The latter hormone is lipolytic in animals but appears to have little effect in man.

The secretion of the adrenal mineralo-corticoid hormone most active in controlling sodium and potassium—aldosterone—is not under anterior pituitary control; the factors controlling its release are not fully understood, but one of them is renin, produced by the granular cells of the juxta-glomerular apparatus (p. 10.35).

Adenohypophyseal hyperfunction

Primary hyperfunction of the adenohypophysis is usually due to the development of a hormone-secreting adenoma (rarely a carcinoma). These tumours, which are described on p. 26.10, usually secrete *mainly* one particular hormone, although two or more hormones are produced in excess by some tumours and

various clinical syndromes may result. The most important are acromegaly and gigantism, due to excess of GH, and Cushing's syndrome, caused by excess of ACTH.

Acromegaly and gigantism

These conditions are both due to prolonged and excessive secretion of growth hormone (GH), usually by a pituitary adenoma (Fig. 26.2) but occasionally associated with an increase of GH-secreting cells without a tumour. The adenoma is most commonly of eosinophil-cell type but sometimes chromophobe: electron microscopy shows the characteristic growth hormone secretory granules (p. 26.3), and immunohistology demonstrates the presence of GH in the tumour cells.

In both conditons there is excessive growth of bone and soft tissues and enlargement of most of the internal organs, e.g. liver, kidneys, heart, thyroid and adrenals. Initially, excessive growth hormone secretion is accompanied by normal or occasionally increased secretion of the other adenohypophyseal hormones. The reason for this latter is not fully understood; there may be great muscularity and abnormal strength, sexual precocity in children and increased libido in adults. Glucose tolerance is diminished and in 10% of cases there is frank diabetes mellitus. The blood pressure is often raised and the heart hypertrophied. As the tumour enlarges, however, it compresses and destroys the surrounding adenohypophysis and lack of the hormones other than GH gradually supervenes. Muscle wasting, weakness and asthenia develop and glucose tolerance increases. In some instances the tumour undergoes infarction, cystic change and fibrosis and ceases to secrete excess of GH: the changes in bone and elsewhere then become inactive. At autopsy, it may appear as a thin-walled cyst lined by scanty acidophil cells. The tumour may be locally invasive and may cause other pressure effects (p. 26.10).

Acromegaly means enlargement of the extremities. It results when the GH-secreting tumour develops after fusion of the epiphyses so that the bones cannot elongate but can grow thicker by periosteal ossification. The hands and feet are increased in size, especially in width. The increase is at first mainly in the soft tissues though thickening of bone occurs later.

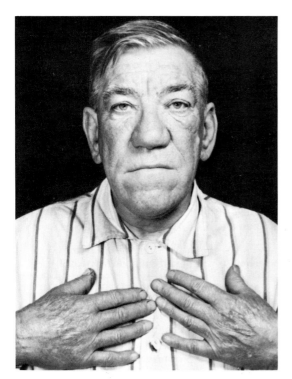

Fig. 26.2 Acromegaly, illustrating the thickening of the nose and enlargement of the lower jaw.

The face is enlarged, especially the nose, which is widened, and the lower jaw is lengthened and its angle widened (Fig. 26.2) so that the teeth project beyond those of the upper jaw. The lips become thickened and there is enlargement of the tongue. The skin is thickened and somewhat warty and the hair is coarse and wiry. In the skeleton generally there is often an increase of bony prominences and there may be roughening of the surface of the bones. Irregular bone growth distorts the joint surfaces and crippling osteoarthritis commonly results. Kyphosis is often present due to irregular vertebral atrophy and hypertrophy. Pain and paraesthesias may result from compression of nerves by bone or soft tissue, e.g. the carpal tunnel syndrome. About 20% of GH-secreting adenomas contain also cells which secrete prolactin; in women, this may result in slight galactorrhoea, as occurs in women with prolactinomas (p. 26.8).

Plasma levels of GH are usually raised, sometimes only slightly, e.g. 5–10 µg/litre, sometimes greatly, e.g. 1 mg/litre. Where the diagnosis is in doubt, it may be confirmed by demonstrating failure to induce the normal fall in plasma GH by oral administration of glucose. Gross acromegaly is rare; lesser degrees are more common and sometimes accompany adenomas of chromophobe type. In either case the condition may become inactive due either to infarction of the tumour or in some cases to development of resistance to GH by the various tissue cells. If mild, such 'fugitive' acromegaly may be difficult to diagnose but enlargement of the sella, demonstrable radiographically, will often confirm the diagnosis. The paranasal sinuses may also be seen to be enlarged as part of the effect of GH on the bones. There is an increased mortality rate in active acromegaly, mostly from heart failure attributable to hypertension, often extensive atheroma, and sometimes to a form of cardiomyopathy with interstitial fibrosis. Bromocriptine, a dopamine agonist, is now used with success in the treatment of acromegalics and sometimes causes shrinkage of the adenoma.

Gigantism is much rarer than acromegaly. It results when excessive GH secretion develops before the epiphyses have fused. A considerable increase in height, sometimes to over 8 feet (2·4 m), may result. Growth is proportionate, so that the bones are both long and thick, the thoracic cage enlarged, etc. Epiphyseal fusion is delayed but occurs eventually. If GH secretion is still excessive, the features of acromegaly then become superadded.

The hormonal changes are as described in acromegaly, and the glucose test described above may be necessary to distinguish between unusually rapid but physiological growth and mild or early gigantism. The stage of adeno-hypophyseal compression and insufficiency usually develops around early adult life and unless treated most patients die from infections or various effects of hypopituitarism. As in acromegaly, there is, in most cases, an eosinophil adenoma, but in 10% a chromophobe adenoma. Small eosinophil adenomas are sometimes found at autopsy with no evidence of previous hyperfunction.

Hyperprolactinaemia. The commonest type of pituitary adenoma is a prolactin-secreting tumour (*prolactinoma*). Such adenomas are often less than 2 mm diameter, but occasionally much larger. There is a suspicion that long-term oestrogen therapy, e.g. in oral contraception, is a predisposing factor. Many adenomas of chromophobe cells have been shown to secrete prolactin (PRL). The larger tumours may cause the local pressure effects of any pituitary tumour (p. 26.10). In some cases, increase in prolactin is symptomless and many of the smaller tumours are found incidentally at autopsy. However, hyperprolactinaemia may cause amenorrhoea and/or sterility in women, and in a minority of cases there is slight or latent galactorrhoea, a drop or two of milky fluid being expressed by pressure. In men, hyperprolactinaemia can cause impotence or reduced libido; these effects are attributable in some cases to inhibition of secretion of LH/TSH releasing hormone in the hypothalamus by high concentrations of PRL, for they are sometimes reversed by bromocriptine, a long-acting dopamine agonist. As noted above, PRL is also produced in excess by some adenomas secreting GH or ACTH.

Hyperprolactinaemia may result also from drugs which interfere with the inhibitory action of hypothalamic dopamine on PRL secretion, e.g. chlorpromazine (which blocks dopamine receptors on prolactogenic cells) and reserpine and methyldopa, both of which deplete the hypothalamus of dopamine.

Adenohypophyseal hypofunction

This may occur from an unknown cause, as a result of lesions arising in the pituitary itself, or from pressure and destruction by adjacent lesions. Pituitary lesions include adenomas, metastatic carcinoma, craniopharyngioma, post-partum ischaemic necrosis, trauma, various infections and macrophage granulomas of unknown nature. Auto-immune destruction occurs rarely in association with the organ-specific auto-immune diseases.

Suprasellar lesions, e.g. craniopharyngioma (p. 21.63) or gliomas, can cause pituitary hypofunction by injury to the hypothalamus, the pituitary stalk, or to the pituitary itself.

The adenohypophysis has large functional reserves and destruction must be extensive to cause deficiencies. In progressive panhypopituitarism, deficiency of growth hormone and gonadotrophins appears first, followed by deficiency of ACTH and of TSH. Occasionally isolated deficiency of any one of the pituitary hormones occurs, the cause being obscure.

The clinical and pathological features of pan-hypopituitarism are described in the syndromes outlined below. Diagnosis may be confirmed by radio-immunoassay of adenohypophyseal hormones in the plasma. *Low plasma corticosteroids with a normal response to ACTH is virtually diagnostic.* If the plasma corticosteroid levels are borderline, other adenohypophyseal hormones may be assayed, preferably under conditions which tend to raise their plasma levels.

The most important examples of pituitary hypofunction are Sheehan's syndrome, pituitary dwarfism and pressure effects of a pituitary adenoma (p. 26.10).

Sheehan's syndrome (Simmond's disease)

This condition is caused by post-partum ischaemic necrosis of the adenohypophysis. It used to be the commonest cause of hypopituitarism but its incidence has fallen greatly with improvements in obstetric care, and where this has happened pituitary adenomas (usually of poorly-secreting type) are now the commonest cause of acquired adenohypophyseal hypofunction (p. 26.10).

Predisposing factors are the enlargement of the pituitary which occurs during pregnancy (p. 26.2), the low-pressure portal vascular supply of the adenohypophysis, and particularly the development of hypotensive shock as a result of difficult labour, often with trauma and excessive haemorrhage.

Clinical features. The first noticeable sign following the causal delivery is failure of lactation, which is due to deficiency of prolactin. Other symptoms develop slowly and in some cases are first noticed a few years after the childbirth presumably responsible for the pituitary deficiency. They include total loss of axillary and pubic hair, amenorrhoea, sterility and loss of libido.

Later, hypersensitivity to cold and other features of hypothyroidism develop, and ACTH deficiency leads to asthenia, hypotension, debility and sometimes fatal collapse. There may be a normochromic anaemia. The fasting blood sugar is usually below normal because the action of insulin is unopposed by growth hormone, corticosteroids and thyroxine, but 'compensatory' fall in insulin secretion usually occurs and averts serious hypoglycaemia. Nevertheless, patients are extremely sensitive to an injection of insulin.

Pigmentation of the skin, as in Addison's disease, does not occur: in fact, the pigment decreases, and the skin has a waxy or alabaster appearance. There is no serious loss of salt and water control, since the secretion of aldosterone is largely independent of the pituitary (p. 26.31). There does seem to be some mineralocorticoid disturbance, however, for *when general metabolism is increased by administration of thyroxine, symptoms of serious adrenal insufficiency, including water and salt loss, may develop.* The neurohypophysis is not usually affected and its function is maintained.

Structural changes. In patients dying soon after the delivery responsible, Sheehan demonstrated extensive necrosis of the adenohypophysis, which he explained by ischaemia resulting from the causal factors noted above. In patients surviving longer, the necrotic tissue is organised and replaced by fibrous tissue.

Other structural changes include atrophy of the thyroid, adrenals, ovaries, uterus and breasts.

Diagnosis may be confirmed by assay of the plasma levels of the pituitary hormones, or the demonstration of adrenal hypofunction and a normal response to ACTH (see above).

Some of the patients originally described by Simmonds exhibited generalised wasting and were probably examples of *anorexia nervosa* which is psychogenic and reversible. The distinction is an important one, as adult patients with panhypopituitarism require life-long treatment with thyroxine, corticosteroids and sex hormones.

Rarely, extensive adenohypophyseal necrosis occurs in sickle-cell disease and in diabetic patients with micro-angiopathy.

Pituitary dwarfism (Lorain–Levi syndrome)

This results from a severe deficiency of growth hormone in childhood. In most cases, there is deficiency of the other adenohypophyseal hormones, but sometimes GH alone is deficient: some of these latter cases are familial.

In approximately one-third of cases, the condition is due to a pituitary adenoma or a craniopharyngioma. Rarely there are multiple adenohypophyseal abnormalities, but more often than not the cause is unexplained.

Impaired general growth is usually noticed after one year of age, sometimes much later: although small, the child is well proportioned (c.f. achondroplasia, p. 23.25) and is not obese. Attacks of hypoglycaemia may occur (c.f. adults with hypopituitarism). The mental state is normal for age and so, being small, the child may seem unusually clever.

If GH alone is deficient, puberty is delayed but eventually occurs normally: the majority, however, also lack gonadotrophins, etc., and do not mature. Human GH is used in treatment, but some children develop resistance to it.

Diagnosis can be confirmed by plasma GH assay before and after provocation by arginine or L-dopa. Conditions which must be distinguished include gonadal dysgenesis (p. 24.29), cretinism (p. 26.18) and also simple neglect of a child, which may be reflected in greatly stunted growth. There is also a condition of dwarfism in which plasma GH is high but somatomedins (p. 26.4) are low.

Adenohypophyseal changes in other diseases

Cushing's syndrome. This is due to excessive secretion of glucocorticoids by the adrenals. In some cases, the cause lies in excessive secretion of ACTH, e.g. by a pituitary tumour or from excessive production of CRF (p. 26.3) in the hypothalamus. Whatever the cause, however, a constant change in the adenohypophysis is enlargement and hyaline change in the cytoplasm of basophilic cells (Crooke's hyaline change). This change (Fig. 26.3) is a consequence of high levels of glucocorticoids, for it is seen also after prolonged therapeutic administration of ACTH or cortisone. The hyaline material does not contain ACTH and electron microscopy has shown it to consist of microtubular material.

Primary hypothyroidism. In untreated patients with this condition, increased functional activity by the TSH-secreting cells is associated with their enlargement, loss of secretory granules, and development of PAS-positive inclusions (Fig. 26.4) seen by electron microscopy to be in cisternae of the endoplasmic reticulum.

There are no characteristic pituitary changes in *primary hyperthyroidism.* In *Addison's*

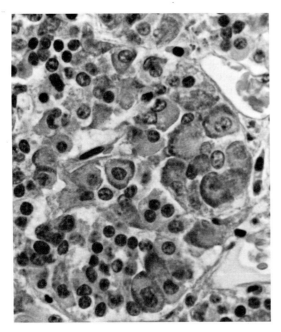

Fig. 26.3 Adenohypophysis in Cushing's syndrome, showing cytoplasmic hyaline change in the basophils. × 500.

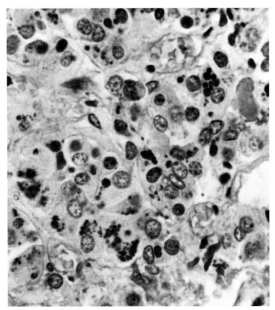

Fig. 26.4 Adenohypophysis in primary myxoedema. The PAS-positive inclusions in the basophil cells show up here as black granules and globules. × 500.

disease, there is an increase in poorly granulated ACTH-secreting cells (p. 26.38).

Pituitary adenomas

Nearly all adenohypophyseal tumours are adenomas, carcinoma being rare. Small adenomas, of 2 mm or so in diameter, are commonly found (if sought) incidentally at autopsy and appear to have caused no clinical effects. Even such small tumours can, however, produce effects by excessive hormonal secretion, and larger tumours can cause both hormonal and pressure effects.

Pituitary adenomas are soft brown tumours, usually sharply defined but with a very thin capsule (Fig. 26.1). Histologically, they consist of cells closely resembling one or other of the normal adenohypophyseal cell types, arranged usually in solid groups with an intervening fine vascular stroma but sometimes forming ill-defined small acinar or papillary structures. Occasional tumours are of more than one cell type, presumably due to variable differentiation of a common tumour stem cell. They are prone to infarction and haemorrhage.

Pressure effects. As it enlarges, a pituitary adenoma may destroy the surrounding glandular tissue by pressure atrophy and erode and enlarge the bony sella. It may rupture the diaphragm, compress and destroy the optic chiasma (Fig. 26.5), causing temporal hemianopia progressing to blindness, and extend into the hypothalamus, causing a variety of symptoms, including disturbances of consciousness, appetite, thermoregulation, and diabetes insipidus. Rarely an adenoma destroys the base of the sella and extends into the nasopharynx, but this is more characteristic of carcinoma.

Hormonal effects. An adenoma sufficiently large to destroy most of the adenohypophysis causes hypopituitarism, the features of which are largely dependent on age and sex. Usually the first effects in adults result from deficiency of gonadotrophins and include loss of libido and sterility, amenorrhoea in women and impotence in men. Deficiency of TSH may be sufficient to cause symptoms of hypothyroidism. Deficiency of ACTH is usually subclinical but the adrenal response to stress may be impaired and the combined deficiency of adrenal glucocorticoids, GH and thyroid hormone greatly increases the patient's sensitivity to insulin.

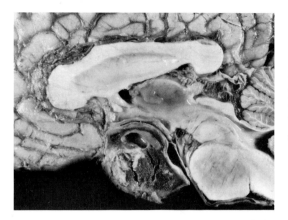

Fig. 26.5 A large chromophobe adenoma of the pituitary which has compressed the optic chiasma. The tumour is haemorrhagic and shows cystic change.

Hypoglycaemic attacks are, however, uncommon in adults. In children, failure to grow and failure of puberty are common features, and hypoglycaemic attacks may occur.

Depending on their cell type, adenomas may produce excess of any of the adenohypophyseal hormones. As such a tumour enlarges, it also produces pressure effects, so that the initial features of hormone excess may be followed by a state of hypopituitarism. *Prolactinomas* are the commonest hormone-secreting adenomas: many are of chromophobe cell type and were formerly regarded as non-secretory but hormone assay has shown that the plasma PRL level is often raised and such tumours contain prolactin in their secretory granules. Other prolactinomas are of eosinophil cell type. The excess of prolactin may suppress release of LH/FSH releasing hormone and cause hypogonadism (an effect which is reversed by administration of bromocriptine): it is important to distinguish this from hypogonadism resulting from the pressure effect of a large tumour. In women, prolactinomas may cause galactorrhoea, although this is usually demonstrable only by manual expression of a few drops of milky fluid. Small prolactinomas are apparently commoner in women than in men and there is a suspicion that their incidence has been increased by oral contraceptives. Less commonly,

chromophobe tumours secrete GH or ACTH. *GH-secreting tumours* are usually of eosinophil-cell type and are responsible for acromegaly and gigantism (see above). As already noted, 20% or so of such tumours also secrete prolactin. *ACTH-secreting tumours* are an important cause of Cushing's syndrome (p. 26.33). The excessive ACTH secretion may also cause skin pigmentation. They are usually small tumours of basophil-cell type and, although neoplastic, their growth and function is often partially inhibited by the high level of plasma cortisol which they induce. Bilateral adrenalectomy may be followed by an increased rate of growth of the tumour and by skin pigmentation. *Thyrotrophic* and *gonadotrophic adenomas* are rare, and in some cases appear to have arisen as a consequence of excessive stimulation of the relevant adenohypophyseal cell type as a consequence of primary hypothyroidism and hypogonadism respectively.

Other tumours and cysts

The commonest **primary tumours** outside the pituitary to cause anterior lobe deficiency by pressure are gliomas and **craniopharyngioma**. The latter is derived from Rathke's pouch, i.e. the craniopharyngeal upgrowth from which the adenohypophysis is developed. It occurs more often above than within the sella and is often cystic (Fig. 21.80, p. 21.63). Cystic tumours or cysts occasionally arise also from the pars intermedia and the cysts may be lined by ciliated epithelium. These are also of Rathke pouch origin and they may cause atrophy of the rest of the gland. Rarely, tumours resembling granular cell tumours (p. 23.71) occur in the neurohypophysis: they are sometimes termed *choristomas* or *pituicytomas*. **Metastases** from carcinoma of the breast or bronchus are not uncommon, and pericapsular deposits occur in some cases of leukaemia. Extra-pituitary tumours in the suprasellar region may involve the nuclei of the hypothalamus and lead to fever, diabetes insipidus, etc. (see below).

The neurohypophysis (posterior lobe)

This is composed of irregular fusiform cells of neural origin, among which are numerous fibres of neurosecretory nerve cells in the supra-optic and paraventricular nuclei of the hypothalamus. Two hormones, *vasopressin* and *oxytocin*, are synthesised by these cells and are transmitted by their modified nerve fibres to the neurohypophysis, where they are stored and released as required. The two hormones are octapeptides and are stored in combination with a common large storage molecule called *neurophysin*.

Antidiuretic hormone (ADH) or vasopressin controls water balance by increasing the permeability of the renal collecting tubules, thus allowing increased re-absorption of water and a more concentrated urine. The name vasopressin is a bad one, for only in very high dosage does it raise the blood pressure. The release of ADH is stimulated by increased osmolarity of the plasma and also by severe hypovolaemia. Conversely, ADH secretion is suppressed by lowered osmolarity of the plasma.

Diabetes insipidus. This is due to deficient secretion of ADH. It is usually caused by a hypothalamic lesion, e.g. head injury, glioma, metastatic cancer or encephalitis. Destruction of the neurohypophysis or high transection of the pituitary stalk do not normally cause diabetes insipidus, as sufficient ADH escapes from the severed neurohypophyseal tract.

The main feature of diabetes insipidus is excretion of a very large volume of dilute urine —often over 10 litres/24 hours. This is accompanied by polydipsia and, if drinking is restricted, the concentration of the urine increases only slightly and severe dehydration results. Onset of the condition is often surprisingly sudden. Apart from inconvenience, the polyuria has little harmful effect unless drinking is prevented. In *psychogenic polyuria*, withholding of fluid results in a concentrated urine without dehydration. Confirmation of the diagnosis of diabetes insipidus is provided by a good response to a dose of ADH.

Oxytocin causes contraction of uterine smooth muscle and expulsion of milk during lactation. It may play a physiological role in uterine contraction during and after pregnancy, and was formerly widely used to initiate labour and to contract the uterus in post-partum haemorrhage, etc.

Women with diabetes insipidus, and therefore presumably deficiency of both ADH and oxytocin, can have a normal labour and lactation, and oxytocin has no known function in males.

The Pineal Body

The function of this minute structure, situated above the posterior part of the third ventricle, is very largely obscure. There is evidence that it secretes hormonal factors, one of which, *melatonin*, is derived from serotonin, and when administered to volunteers induces drowsiness. It is secreted in response to darkness and academics have claimed, somewhat optimistically, that it may explain students' somnolence when the lights are dimmed. Melatonin may also inhibit gonadal maturation and function.

The least rare lesions of the pineal are tumours which occur mainly in childhood. They include gliomas, teratomas and also tumours indistinguishable from seminomas. Effects are produced by pressure on neighbouring structures; thus hydrocephalus, ocular paralyses and deafness from implication of the corpora quadrigemina, also cerebellar effects, giddiness, etc., may result. In young boys, precocious puberty may accompany a pineal tumour of any type. A similar group of changes has been observed with other lesions in the neighbourhood, such as a tumour in the floor of the third ventricle, hydrocephalus, etc. The syndrome is probably not a pineal effect but rather the result of disturbance of nerve tracts possibly related to the pituitary.

The Thyroid Gland

The thyroid gland produces three hormones, **thyroxine**, **tri-iodothyronine** and **calcitonin**. Calcitonin is a polypeptide which lowers the concentration of calcium in the blood. It is secreted by specialised epithelial cells (C cells) which lie between the thyroid acini, and is considered on p. 26.27.

Thyroxine (tetra-iodothyronine, or T_4) and tri-iodothyronine (T_3) are iodinated amino acids which have the effect of increasing heat production in the various tissues by uncoupling oxidative phosphorylation. i.e. increasing oxygen utilisation relative to the rate of formation of high energy phosphate bonds, two processes which are closely linked in the economy of the cell. T_4 is a prohormone and is converted in the various tissues to T_3, the active hormone. T_3 binds to nuclear receptors of cells sensitive to it and influences transcription of DNA and thus the cellular metabolism. T_3 and T_4 are essential for normal physical and mental development and in the metabolism of protein, carbohydrate and fat. Excessive secretion of these thyroid hormones causes the serious disorder known as **hyperthyroidism** while inadequate secretion results in **hypothyroidism** which also has severe pathological consequences. Important physiological mechanisms have evolved to ensure that the amounts of T_3 and T_4 released into the circulation are appropriate to the varying bodily requirements in differing circumstances (e.g. environmental temperature), and, within limits, to compensate for sub-optimal intake of dietary iodine.

Iodine metabolism in the thyroid gland. Iodine ions are concentrated in thyroid cells by a special concentrating or *trapping mechanism* which can be inhibited by perchlorate or thiocyanate ions. Iodide within thyroid epithelium is rapidly *oxidised* by a thyroid peroxidase to an active form which readily enters *organic combination* with the tyrosine present in the glycoprotein, thyroglobulin. This latter is synthesised by thyroid epithelium and stored extracellularly in the colloid within the acini. The organic binding of oxidised iodine results in the formation of mono- and di-iodotyrosine within the thyroglobulin molecule and the synthesis of iodothyronine is accomplished by *coupling* of two appropriate iodotyrosines to give T_3 or T_4.

(The antithyroid drugs thiouracil and carbimazole diminish the organic binding of iodine and the coupling reaction by inhibiting thyroid peroxidase which catalyses both of these reactions.) The hormones, still part of the thyroglobulin molecule, are stored within the colloid until required in the circulation. TSH stimulates pinocytosis of droplets of thyroglobulin by thyroid epithelium. Lysosomes fuse with the pinocytic vesicle and the thyroglobulin is digested, with release of T_4 and T_3, which are transported through the acinar epithelial cells to the vessels within the stroma of the gland. Hormonally inactive iodotyrosines which have not taken part in iodothyronine formation are also released from digested thyroglobulin but these are de-iodinated by a *dehalogenase* enzyme and the released iodide is available for re-oxidation and re-organification.

Due to inborn errors of metabolism one or other of these steps is sometimes defective and this leads to the condition of **dyshormonogenesis**. Thus failure of the iodide-trapping mechanism, defective organification of iodide due to peroxidase deficiency, secretion of abnormal iodoprotein and dehalogenase deficiency each constitutes a different form of dyshormonogenesis and results in a tendency to hypothyroidism.

Control of thyroid secretion. The secretion of thyroid hormone is mainly controlled by TSH. Inadequate plasma levels of T_3 and T_4 cause release of TSH both directly and by release of thyrotrophin releasing hormone (TRH). TSH exerts its effects on thyroid epithelium by activating adenylate cyclase which, by increasing cAMP, stimulates all the processes of thyroid hormone formation and release described above. If prolonged, such stimulation by TSH causes important structural changes in the thyroid: in particular a change of the epithelium from cubical to columnar, proliferation of epithelial cells to form new follicles, and diminution of the volume and concentration of the colloid stored within the acini. These changes may result in **goitre**, i.e. enlargement of the thyroid. When the plasma level of thyroid hormone exceeds the physiological requirements of the body, the production of TRH and TSH are suppressed and the thyroid reverts to its resting

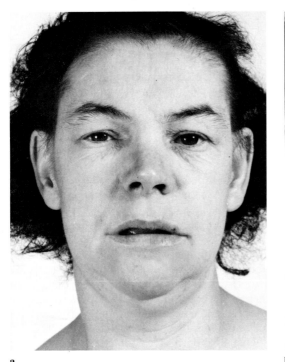 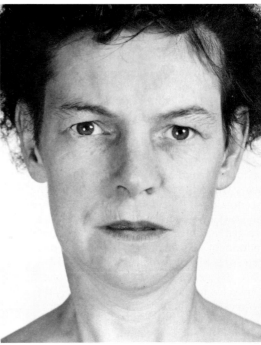

a   b

Fig. 26.6   Myxoedema, (**a**): before treatment, (**b**): after treatment with thyroxine.

state with diminished hormone production, diminished secretion and increased storage of hormone within the eosinophilic colloid which accumulates within the acini.

Hypothyroidism. The effects of subnormal secretion of T_4 and T_3 vary depending upon the severity of thyroid hormone deficiency and the age of onset of the disorder. Infantile hypothyroidism is called **cretinism** and is described on p. 26.18.

In the adult, the syndrome is called **myx-oedema**. In severe cases there is lethargy, slow speech and impaired intellectual function sometimes associated with frank psychosis. The hair, brittle and lustreless, tends to fall out. Hydrophilic mucoprotein ground substance accumulates in the dermal connective tissue causing coarsening of the features (Fig. 26.6) and firm non-pitting oedema of the supraclavicular fossae and dorsum of the hands. Similar mucinous deposits around nerves may impair peripheral nerve function and cause, for example, carpal tunnel syndrome or deafness, while involvement of the tongue and larynx causes a characteristically slurred croaking voice. Despite a poor appetite, the patient gains weight.

The pulse is slow, the basal metabolic rate is lowered, and the patient suffers from constipation, feels cold and is unduly prone to develop hypothermia.

Biochemical abnormalities include a raised serum cholesterol level due to reduced rate of catabolism, but most significant is the low thyroid secretion rate of T_4 and T_3, the concentration of which in the blood can be shown by radio-immunoassay to be abnormally low.

Secretion of TSH is increased, even in patients with early or subclinical thyroid failure, and this is reflected in the appearance in the anterior pituitary of mucoid cells which contain only a few prominent storage granules (vesiculate mucoid cells—Fig. 26.4). There is diminished sexual function and menorrhagia is common due to failure of ovulation and continued endometrial proliferation. All of the above changes, except, of course, the low thyroid hormone secretion rate, are reversed by therapy with T_4 or T_3.

Causes. By far the most common cause of hypothyroidism is primary myxoedema (the atrophic form of auto-immune thyroiditis—see below) but hypothyroidism with goitre is found in Hashimoto's disease, dyshormonogenesis, severe iodine deficiency and as a result of drugs with antithyroid effects. Other causes include extensive surgical resection of the thyroid, therapy with radio-iodine, and hypopituitarism with diminished TSH secretion.

Hyperthyroidism (Thyrotoxicosis) results from excessive secretion of thyroid hormone and causes clinical features which are almost the opposite of those found in hypothyroidism. The patient, though weak, is restless, hyperkinetic and emotionally unstable. The appetite is increased but the patient loses weight. There is increased nitrogen excretion, and sometimes impaired glucose tolerance and glycosuria. The skin is warm and sweating, the pulse rapid and bounding and the cardiac output is increased. Cardiac arrhythmia, particularly atrial fibrillation, may occur, especially in older patients, and cardiac failure may be the presenting feature. Osteoporosis affecting cancellous bone may be present, associated with increased calcium excretion in urine and faeces. Many of the above features are attributable to the raised basal metabolic rate which is, in turn, due to the effects of excessive amounts of thyroid hormone on the tissues. The serum levels of T_3 and less often T_4 are raised and pituitary TSH secretion is inhibited. The common clinical form of hyperthyroidism, Graves' disease, is due to a thyroid-stimulating auto-antibody which reacts with the TSH receptors on the thyroid cell membrane. In such cases there is usually prominence of the eyes (exophthalmos) (Fig. 26.7) apparently caused by a second auto-antibody which reacts with orbital muscle. Less often, autonomous hyperfunctioning thyroid tumour-like nodules lead to thyrotoxicosis, while in very rare cases hyperthyroidism is the result of excessive TSH production in acromegaly.

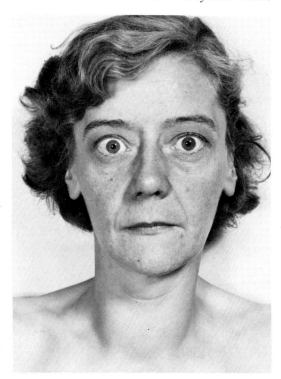

Fig. 26.7 Thyrotoxicosis. Note the prominence of the eyes and the diffuse thyroid enlargement.

Nontoxic (Simple) goitre

Nontoxic goitre is the name given to various non-inflammatory conditions which result in enlargement of the thyroid gland without hyperthyroidism. All forms of nontoxic goitre are probably preceded and for a time accompanied by a phase of impaired thyroid hormone synthesis due to inadequate supply of iodide or to impaired thyroid enzyme activity caused by a genetic defect or exogenous toxic substances. To counteract the diminished secretion of thyroid hormone in these circumstances, more TSH is produced and there is increased activity of the thyroid epithelium, which becomes hyperplastic. These compensatory changes may increase T_4 and T_3 secretion enough to prevent hypothyroidism, but the defect may be so severe that goitrous hypothyroidism results, a condition which some authors would not include under the heading of simple or nontoxic goitre.

Morphologically, the following varieties of nontoxic goitre are recognised; (a) **parenchymatous goitre**, showing hyperplasia of the type illustrated in Fig. 26.8 with little colloid storage; (b) **colloid goitre**, in which there is marked accumulation of colloid (Fig. 26.10). Both types may occur in a *diffuse form* in which the whole gland is involved or in a *nodular form* in which the change occurs in scattered rounded nodules of various sizes.

Epidemiology. Goitre may occur sporadically in any locality. Before the introduction of

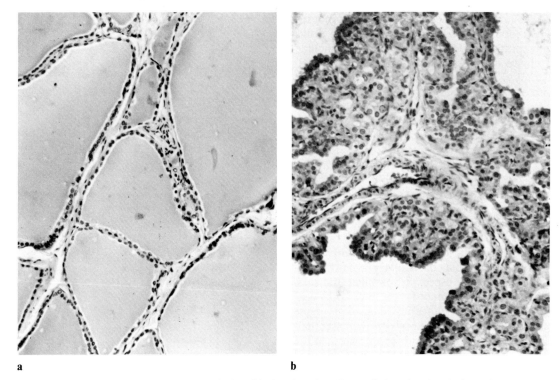

a   b

Fig. 26.8   Normal thyroid tissue (**a**) and thyroid showing the effects of chronic stimulation with TSH (**b**). Note the hypertrophy and hyperplasia of the thyroid epithelium and diminished colloid storage. × 185.

iodised salt, it was unduly common in certain districts (**endemic goitre**), notably in the valleys of Switzerland, the Pyrenees, the Himalayas and in New Zealand; in England in the Derbyshire hills; in parts of Southern Ireland, and in North America in the region of the Great Lakes. Where deficiency of iodine was severe, as in the mountainous regions, e.g. the Alps, the goitre was usually parenchymatous, diffuse at first and becoming nodular later. Thyroid deficiency and cretinism were common, especially where the disease was very prevalent and of severe type. In goitrous districts in Switzerland the average weight of the thyroid at birth was often double the normal and occasionally a congenital parenchymatous goitre was present. In North America, goitre was usually of the colloid type, either diffuse or nodular.

Aetiology. The causation of endemic goitre is not fully understood, but it is known that deficiency of iodine is the chief factor in its production. In remote communities where little food is imported, lack of iodine in the soil and water and in locally produced food is the basic defect. There may be contributory factors which render unavailable any iodine present, such as pollution of water supplies by sulphur-containing organic matter or the presence of much calcium or fluoride. In goitrous disticts, rats, sheep and other animals are also affected. When iodine deficiency is severe, goitre appears in childhood; when it is moderate, goitre is not only less common but also appears later, occurring especially at puberty and during pregnancy and lactation, when there is a drain on the iodine supply. Males are affected less frequently than females. In the early stages especially, treatment by iodine may arrest the thyroid enlargement or cause it to regress. In the region of the Great Lakes and in Switzerland, the administration of small quantities of iodine to school children has resulted in remarkable diminution of the incidence of goitre. In New Zealand and certain other places the results have been less striking, perhaps because of the presence of iodine inhibitors.

Sporadic nontoxic goitre, i.e. that occurring in areas where goitre is not endemic, appears to have three main causes: (1) iodine deficiency due to faulty dietary habits; (2) dyshormonogenesis due to one of a group of inherited defects of thyroid hormone synthesis or secretion (see pp. 26.13, 26.19); (3) the action of chemicals which interfere with thyroid hormone synthesis: excluding antithyroid drugs used in treating thyrotoxicosis, perhaps the most important of these is large doses of iodine given in the form of iodopyrine, or less commonly simply as iodide, as expectorants in asthma or chronic bronchitis. In idiosyncratic subjects this inhibits the iodination of tyrosine; there is a fall in thyroid hormone release, and patients with 'iodide goitre' frequently become hypothyroid. Resorcinol, *para*-aminosalicylic acid and sulphonylureas are other drugs which occasionally cause nontoxic goitre.There is some evidence that certain thyroid auto-antibodies may lead to nontoxic goitre by stimulating growth of thyroid epithelium without causing hyperthyroidism (Drexhage *et al.*, 1980).

Parenchymatous goitre. The initial changes are enlargement of the acinar cells to columnar type and formation of many small colloid-deficient acini. The tissue of the enlarged gland lacks normal thyroid translucency and looks more like pancreas to the naked eye. The changes are at first diffuse, affecting the entire gland, but if the iodine lack persists, foci of excessively active iodine uptake appear, while other parts of the gland become refractory and fail to take up and store iodine; this has been shown by autoradiography of thyroids excised after a dose of radioactive iodine. The hyperactive foci enlarge and compress the adjacent parenchyma so that the gland becomes nodular.

In nodular nontoxic goitre the appearances vary greatly. There may be only one or two nodular masses, or the gland may be studded with them, the parenchyma between becoming atrophied. Following the initially diffuse parenchymatous hyperplasia, the subsequent development of hyperplastic nodules probably depends on the severity of the continuing iodine deficiency, however brought about.

Colloid goitre. In diffuse colloid goitre the whole gland may be affected (Fig. 26.9), or one lobe may be chiefly involved. The affected tissue is tense and firm, and on section presents a translucent brownish appearance due to the accumulation of dense, firm colloid. Indeed, very large acini filled with colloid may be present. Dark red or brown areas due to haemorrhage may be seen, and in places there may be

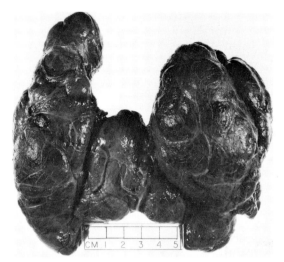

Fig. 26.9 Diffuse colloid goitre, showing general thyroid enlargement.

fibrosis, sometimes with calcification of the stroma. On microscopic examination, the acini are, in general, enlarged and distended with deeply-staining colloid, and the epithelium may be flattened (Fig. 26.10). Cysts may be formed by the confluence of acini. Colloid goitre is much commoner in women than in men, usually appears first at puberty or in pregnancy, and may be dependent on a less severe degree of iodine lack than that associated with paren-

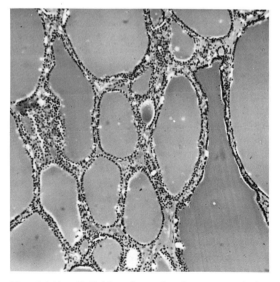

Fig. 26.10 Colloid goitre, showing accumulation of colloid in the acini and flattening of the acinar epithelium. × 40.

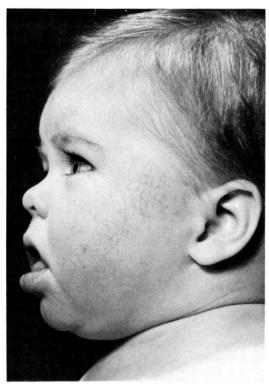 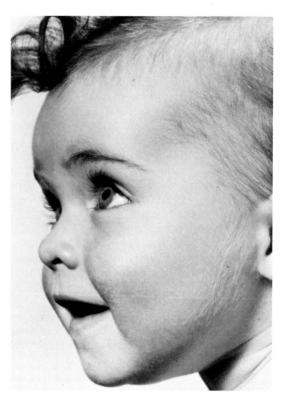

Fig. 26.11   A cretin aged 17 months. *Left*, showing the enlarged, protruding tongue, coarse dry skin and dull expression. *Right*, showing the effects of thyroxine treatment for two months. (Professor J. H. Hutchinson.)

chymatous goitre. This seems to hold generally with regard to the disease in low-lying countries.

Effects. In nontoxic goitre, thyroid function often appears clinically normal, though minor disturbances are not so rare as was once supposed. The enlarged gland may occasionally cause pressure effects on a recurrent laryngeal nerve, the oesophagus or the trachea, and even death by suffocation. Pressure effects are more common when the goitre extends retrosternally. In mountainous regions the thyroid enlargement in children, usually of the nodular type, may be associated with cretinism, the result of severe deficiency of the thyroid hormone. In America, colloid goitre has been associated with some degree of thyrotoxicosis.

Despite much study, it is uncertain whether nontoxic goitre predisposes to the development of carcinoma.

Cretinism

Severe hypothyroidism beginning in infancy is called *cretinism*. Cretins usually seem normal at birth, having received maternal thyroid hormone while *in utero*, but within a few weeks or months it becomes apparent that mental and physical development are retarded. The untreated cretin is a dwarf with severe mental defect, disproportionately short limbs, coarse dry skin, deficient hair and teeth, a large protruding tongue (Fig. 26.11) and pot belly with umbilical hernia. The skeletal changes of cretinism are mentioned on p. 23.19. Routine screening of newborn infants for high blood TSH levels offers hope of detecting and treating congenital hypothyroidism before irreversible intellectual damage develops.

Endemic cretinism occurred almost exclusively in mountainous districts such as Switzerland, where iodine deficiency was severe and endemic goitre common. It is said rarely to appear in a goitrous family until the second or third generation, and cretins of this type are nearly always the offspring of goitrous mothers. Unexplained deaf-mutism is very often present as an additional feature.

The thyroid. In most cases of endemic cretinism a goitre is present, although in some instances the thyroid is atrophic and fibrous. The goitre is nearly always nodular, the parenchyma between the nodules being compressed and atrophic. The appearances are similar to those seen in the nodular goitres of long-standing iodine deficiency.

Sporadic cretinism. This condition, due to congenital absence or hypoplasia of the thyroid tissue, is encountered from time to time in all localities and the causation is unknown. In some cases, no trace of thyroid can be found, although there may be small nodules of atrophied thyroid tissue near the foramen caecum at the root of the tongue. In other cases, the thyroid is small and shrunken, sometimes containing cysts. The thymus is usually atrophic, but the parathyroids are not affected and occupy their usual position.

Dyshormonogenesis. Goitre in sporadic cretinism is very rare, but it occurs as a Mendelian recessive abnormality manifested by congenital absence of some essential enzyme system. In one variety, studied by McGirr and Hutchison in a family of Scottish tinkers, absence of the dehalogenase enzyme, which normally removes iodine from iodotyrosine, allows mono- and di-iodotyrosine to escape from the thyroid into the blood, from which they are excreted in the urine, thus leading to gross iodine deficiency. In another type, iodide accumulates in the gland but thyroid peroxidase deficiency results in failure to oxidise iodide to free iodine, which is therefore not available in the thyroid to combine with tyrosine. Accordingly, iodinated hormone synthesis fails. In some congenital goitrous cretins, deaf-mutism is present, an interesting finding in view of its unexplained frequency in endemic goitrous cretinism.

The thyroid is often greatly enlarged and nodular, and on microscopic examination the epithelial hyperplasia of parenchymous goitre is found.

Less severe genetic defects of thyroid metabolism also occur: in some, the thyroid hyperplasia may largely prevent hypothyroidism.

Auto-immune thyroiditis

In this condition there is infiltration of the thyroid by lymphocytes and plasma cells, associated with abnormalities of the thyroid epithelium and, in many cases, thyroid-specific auto-antibodies in the serum.

Three main variants are encountered: (1) **Hashimoto's disease (lymphadenoid goitre)**— a diffuse and florid lesion causing goitre; (2) **primary myxoedema**, in which the thyroid is shrunken and the epithelium atrophic; (3) **focal thyroiditis** in which patchy lesions occur in an otherwise normal or hyperplastic gland.

Gross appearance. Areas of thyroid affected by auto-immune thyroiditis appear solid and white or peach coloured, lacking the translucent appearance normally presented by colloid stored in the acini. In Hashimoto's disease the gland is firm and there is enlargement, usually symmetrical and of moderate degree; the cut surface has a solid lobulated appearance resembling pancreas on section, and in most cases the capsule is not adherent to surrounding tissues. The shrunken thyroid of primary myxoedema is firm and white while in focal auto-immune thyroiditis ill-defined white patches of about 1 mm in diameter are seen on the cut surface of the gland.

Microscopic appearance (Fig. 26.12). The basic lesion common to all forms is the presence of small acini lined by large cubical epithelial cells with granular cytoplasm and large nuclei which are frequently bizarre in shape. These cells, known variously as Askanazy cells, Hürthle cells, oxyphil cells or oncocytes, owe their eosinophilic (pale pink to bright red) cytoplasmic granularity to the presence of numerous large mitochondria.

The colloid is scanty, usually densely eosinophilic, and may contain macrophages or multinucleated giant cells. Surrounding the abnormal acini, and sometimes invading them, is an infiltrate of plasma cells and/or lymphocytes, accompanied by a variable amount of fibrous tissue.

In *Hashimoto's disease* (Fig. 26.12) the epithelium is all abnormal and is increased in amount. The lymphoid infiltrate is massive and germinal centres may be present. Mitotic figures are very infrequent. The amount of fibrous tissue is variable. Most of the gland in *primary myxoedema* consists of fibrous tissue

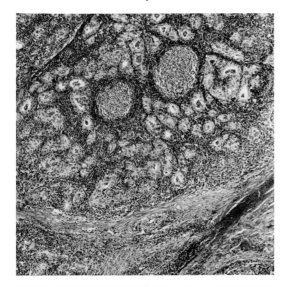

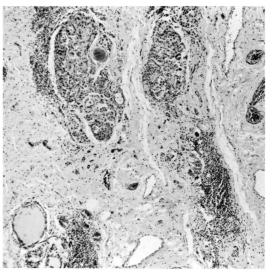

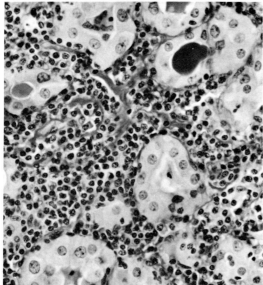

26.13   The thyroid in primary myxoedema. Islands of thyroid tissue, showing the changes of chronic thyroiditis, are embedded in fibrous tissue containing wide vascular channels. × 50.

immune thyroiditis (Fig. 26.14) differs from both these conditions by the persistence of greater or smaller areas of normal or hyperplastic thyroid tissue. The more severe examples, however, approach Hashimoto's disease in extent. It is very common in middle-aged women.

Fig. 26.12   Hashimoto's thyroiditis. *Above*, showing the diffuse lymphoid cell infiltrate, germinal centres, fibrosis and small thyroid acini. × 50. *Below*, showing the lymphocytic and plasma cell infiltrate and change in the epithelium to Askanazy-cell type. × 320.

(Fig. 26.13) containing sparse clusters of small acini lined by Askanazy cells and islets or cysts of epithelium sometimes of squamous type (a feature also seen occasionally in Hashimoto's disease). The lymphocytic and plasma cell infiltration is usually slight and situated mainly around the surviving epithelium. *Focal auto-*

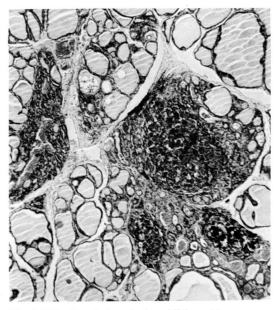

Fig. 26.14   Focal chronic thyroiditis. × 20.

Clinical features. In *Hashimoto's disease* the patient, usually a middle-aged female, has a firm goitre of moderate size. Hypothyroidism is present in about half the cases, and is the rule if partial thyroidectomy is undertaken. The thyroid uptake of iodine is reduced and organification is impaired. An abnormal iodinated thyroprotein, which differs from serum protein-bound T_4 in being insoluble in butanol, is sometimes found in the serum.

Primary myxoedema is characterised by hypothyroidism in the absence of goitre. *Chronic focal thyroiditis* is usually asymptomatic. It is, however, usually present in patients with Graves' disease, and the risk of developing hypothyroidism after partial thyroidectomy is greater if there is extensive focal thyroiditis.

Aetiology. Two auto-antibodies, one against thyroglobulin, the other against a lipoprotein of the membrane of the endoplasmic reticulum of thyroid epithelial cells, are found in high titre in the serum of most patients with Hashimoto's disease. The frequency and titres of such antibodies are lower in primary myxoedema and lower still in focal thyroiditis. There is evidence that most of the autoantibody is formed by the plasma cells which are usually a conspicuous feature of the inflammatory infiltrate of the gland.

Experimental auto-immune thyroiditis can be produced in various animals, including primates, by injecting thyroglobulin in Freund's adjuvant emulsion which enhances immunological responsiveness. The experimental lesions are, however, transitory and their severity, which varies greatly, is related to the genotype, particularly at the histocompatibility loci, of the animal. The lesions parallel the development of cell-mediated immunity to thyroglobulin. Transfer of the disease to normal animals has been accomplished with difficulty using serum or very large numbers of lymphoid cells from affected animals. Mice depleted of T cells by thymectomy and x-irradiation develop persistent auto-immune thyroiditis spontaneously (i.e. without injection of thyroglobulin and adjuvant) and in this model there is a better correlation with thyroglobulin antibody. It has been suggested that loss of suppressor T lymphocytes is important, and this may explain also the enhancement by thymectomy of the spontaneous auto-immune thyroiditis which occurs in an obese strain of chickens. Although

of great interest, these findings have not established the aetiology of human 'auto-immune' thyroiditis: defective function of suppressor T cells may help to explain auto-immunisation but the pathogenic importance of delayed auto-hypersensitivity and/or auto-antibodies is not yet firmly established (see also pp. 7.24–26).

Patients with auto-immune thyroiditis are unduly prone to have, in addition, auto-immune gastritis (p. 19.20) (sometimes accompanied by pernicious anaemia), or auto-immune adrenalitis (idiopathic Addison's disease, p. 26.36). In all these conditions, there is also cell-mediated immunity to mitochondrial antigens, which are not entirely organ-specific and which may account for their co-occurrence in the same individual. The occurrence of all these diseases within certain families suggests that the basic predisposition is inherited. There is a high incidence of HLA antigens B8 and DR3 in patients with primary myxoedema and the other organ-specific auto-immune diseases, but curiously this does not apply to those with Hashimoto's disease, in which the incidence of DR5 is increased.

It remains to be discovered what event triggers the auto-immune process, why the disease occurs mainly in females, what factors determine whether the lesion is focal or diffuse and whether the epithelium becomes atrophic as in primary myxoedema or hyperplastic as in Hashimoto's disease. Nontoxic goitre is unduly frequent in the relatives of patients with auto-immune thyroiditis and, as already mentioned, may be due to auto-antibody which stimulates thyroid growth without causing hyperthyroidism.

Other forms of thyroiditis

Thyroiditis due to causes other than auto-immunity is very rare in Britain. Multiple small abscesses may be found in the thyroid in pyaemia and acute thyroiditis is said sometimes to complicate influenza and typhoid fever.

Giant-cell (de Quervain's) thyroiditis. This variety of subacute thyroiditis begins with the distinctive features of fever and pain in the neck with tenderness. There is a neutrophil leucocytosis and a raised ESR. Elevation of the protein-bound iodine with reduced thyroid iodide uptake is said to be pathognomonic of the disorder. Microscopically, there is polymorphonuclear infiltration followed by lymphocytes and plasma cells; destruction of acini with formation of epithelioid cells and giant cells gives a pseudotuberculous appearance. Israeli workers have recovered a virus having the properties of mumps virus from two cases and have shown the presence of neutralising and complement-fixing antibodies to mumps virus in others. An increased frequency of HLA-BW35 has been observed in giant-cell thyroiditis.

Reidel's thyroiditis. This very rare disease is characterised by enlargement of the thyroid by fibrous tissue of extremely hard consistency; the condition usually affects only one lobe and involves adjacent muscles. Microscopically, the fibrous tissue may be more or less cellular, and in the affected part the acini become atrophic and disappear: fibrous occlusion of thyroid veins is a characteristic feature. Hypothyroidism is unusual. The nature of the disease is unknown; a few cases have been associated with retroperitoneal fibrosis (p. 19.70); other supposed cases may be more properly classified as sclerotic thyroid adenomas or as fibrous variants of Hashimoto's disease.

Hyperthyroidism (Thyrotoxicosis)

Excessive secretion by the thyroid of T_3, and usually also T_4, occurs in three conditions. (1) **Graves' disease**, the most common, is characterised by diffuse thyroid hyperplasia due to the presence of an inappropriaite thyroid-stimulating antibody in the blood. Protrusion of the eyeballs (exophthalmos) and certain other features of the disease cannot be ascribed to the excess of thyroid hormone. (2) **Toxic adenoma** is a relatively uncommon condition in which an autonomous thyroid adenoma produces thyroid hormone in excess of the requirements of the body. (3) **Toxic nodular goitre**, in which excessive hormone is produced in multiple discrete foci within the thyroid, supervenes in older patients who already have a nontoxic nodular goitre. The main features of hyperthyroidism have already been outlined on p. 26.15.

Graves' disease (exophthalmic goitre)

In this disease the **thyroid** shows hyperplasia which is characteristically diffuse, though sometimes one lobe is larger than the other. On section, the parenchyma is less brown and less translucent than normal owing to diminished colloid storage and the gland resembles salivary tissue, being dull greyish-pink in colour and lobulated. However, even in untreated cases, some parts may contain a considerable amount of colloid and the surface may be slightly nodular. The gland is moderately firm and succulent, though if thyroiditis is marked (see below) there may be some fibrosis. The surface veins and arteries may be enlarged but the organ as a whole does not look especially vascular after surgical removal or at autopsy. The appearances may be much modified by treatment.

On microscopic examination, hyperplasia of the epithelium and diminution in the amount of the colloid stored are constant (Fig. 26.15). The epithelial cells of the acini are increased in size and more columnar in type. Numerous small acini are formed, while in the larger ones papilliform ingrowths are often present: both of these factors lead to a great increase in the epithelial surface area. What little colloid remains stains palely and appears watery. These changes reflect increased formation of hormones, which are, however, not stored in thyroglobulin but passed on to the bloodstream. In many cases there is focal auto-immune thyroiditis with lymphocytic infiltration (Fig. 26.14), and sometimes the formation of lymphoid follicles. When such infiltration is widespread, the lesion comes to resemble Hashimoto's disease (p. 26.19), and in such cases hypothyroidism commonly follows partial thyroidectomy.

The alterations described are usually fairly uniform throughout the gland but in places there may be quiescent acini which contain a considerable amount of colloid, especially when, at a later period, the acute symptoms are beginning to subside. The picture may thus be one of hyperplasia and subsequent involution irregularly distributed, even with fibrosis in places.

The administration of iodine tends to reverse the hyperplastic changes in the thyroid; the epithelium becomes more cubical, and colloid accumulates in the acini (Fig. 26.15). These changes after iodine therapy bring about only temporary improvement in the symptoms, and the mode of action of iodine is uncertain. The anti-thyroid drugs derived from thiourea used in the treatment of hyperthyroidism prevent the synthesis of thyroxine and this leads to a strik-

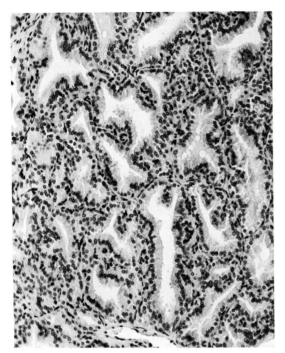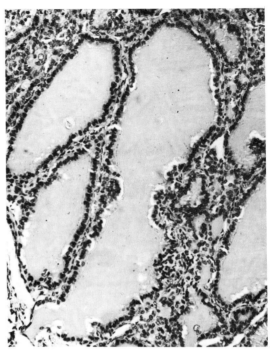

Fig. 26.15 The thyroid in Graves' disease. *Left*, untreated: the epithelial cells are columnar and there is virtually no colloid. *Right*, after treatment with iodine for 10 days. The epithelial cells are cuboidal and some colloid has accumulated. × 125.

ing reduction in the thyrotoxicosis although the epithelial hyperplasia is undiminished or even exaggerated. The histological effects of iodine and of thiouracil on the thyroid are thus antagonistic and when both are administered before thyroidectomy the histological picture in the excised gland is complex.

Other organs. The thymus shows distinct enlargement in three-quarters of the cases, and the thymic lymphoid tissue is increased in amount and contains in its medulla lymphoid follicles with germinal centres. There may also be some enlargement of the lymph nodes. Some observers consider that these lymphoid changes are proportionate to the severity of the disease; they may reflect the auto-immune response of Graves' disease and the usually-associated focal thyroiditis, or they may be due to lowered adrenal cortical function resulting from the accelerated inactivation of cortisol found in thyrotoxicosis. Hypertrophy of the heart occurs in most cases of thyrotoxicosis. There may be neutropenia with relative lymphocytosis. Sometimes, however, there is an absolute lymphocytosis, and this is thought by some to occur in the more severe cases.

Occasionally bilateral patches of myxoedematous thickening appear on the anterior (pretibial) aspects of the lower leg, even while thyrotoxicosis is active. Before partial thyroidectomy was rendered relatively safe by premedication with anti-thyroid drugs, it was recognised that in a few cases spontaneous thyroid involution might culminate in hypothyroidism.

Orbital changes. Exophthalmos in mild cases is attributable to fatty infiltration of the extrinsic muscles of the eye. When proptosis is severe, there is, in addition, increase in amount and oedema of the orbital tissue, and marked lymphocytic infiltration of the extrinsic eye muscles and perivascular connective tissue.

Aetiology. The disease is most common in females, particularly during the reproductive period, and sometimes runs in families, especially in those in which there is an abnormally high incidence of organ-specific auto-immune diseases, e.g. Hashimoto's disease and pernicious anaemia.

It is now apparent, largely from the work of Dr Duncan Adams, that Graves' disease is due to an auto-antibody which reacts with the thyroid epithelial cell surface receptor for TSH (see Adams, 1977). This thyroid-stimulating antibody is detectable in the blood of most untreated patients by an *in vitro* test in which the binding of labelled TSH by human thyroid cell membrane preparations is competitively inhibited by the patient's serum. In some cases, the thyroid-stimulating antibody can cross-react with mouse or guinea-pig thyroid epithelium and causes thyroid stimulation in these animals *in vivo*. In fact this is how the antibody (originally termed *long-acting thyroid stimulator* or *LATS*) was first demonstrated. Thyroid-stimulating antibody has been shown to be quite distinct from TSH.

The auto-immune nature of Graves' disease is supported also by the frequent presence of focal auto-immune thyroiditis and other organ-specific auto-immune diseases (p. 7.24), such as pernicious anaemia. Thyroid-stimulating antibody explains the failure to demonstrate TSH in the serum of patients with Graves' disease, and the failure of administered T_3 to suppress thyroid activity in these patients— findings which indicate that pituitary TSH production in Graves' disease is fully suppressed by the inappropriately high blood levels of thyroid hormone. Further support is obtained from the correlation between the presence of maternal thyroid-stimulating antibody and the occurrence of temporary thyrotoxicosis in the neonate.

Thyroid-stimulating antibody correlates also with pretibial myxoedema. An auto-antibody which reacts specifically with preparations of orbital muscle has recently been demonstrated in the serum of most patients with exophthalmos and may well be responsible for this abnormality (Kendall-Taylor *et al.*, 1984).

Toxic adenoma

Approximately 1% of thyroid adenomas give rise to hyperthyroidism, usually mild and not accompanied by exophthalmos or thyroid-stimulating antibody in the serum.

The tumours are usually single adenomas more than 3 cm in diameter and are composed of small acini resembling those seen in Graves' disease. Towards the centre of the adenoma, stromal oedema and fibrosis may separate the vesicles. Haemorrhage may occur into the

tumour and destroy so much of the epithelium that the hyperthyroidism subsides.

Scanning the neck following administration of radio-iodine shows marked radio-iodine uptake by the tumour, and, because of the autonomous nature of the growth, this cannot be suppressed by T_3. The remainder of the gland does not concentrate iodine since the hormone produced by the tumour results in diminished secretion of TSH by the pituitary.

Toxic nodular goitre

This disorder usually affects patients over 50 years of age who have had nontoxic goitre for many years. The thyrotoxicosis which subsequently develops is usually mild as judged by thyroid iodine uptake studies and hormone levels in the blood. Cardiac arrhythmias and failure may cause the presenting symptoms. Exophthalmos is uncommon.

The macroscopic and histological features are similar to those described in nontoxic nodular goitre (p. 26.15). Autoradiography shows in some cases one or two hyperfunctioning nodules (in effect, and perhaps in fact, toxic adenomas) with complete suppression of radio-iodine uptake by the remainder of the goitre. In other cases, multiple small groups of hyperplastic acini concentrate radioactive iodine though much of the gland is inactive, the appearances suggesting the effect of some extrinsic thyroid stimulator on a gland, part of whose tissue is refractory. Thyroid-stimulating auto-antibody has been reported to be present in low concentration in the plasma in such cases, but this finding is disputed.

Tumours of the thyroid

Thyroid adenoma (Fig. 12.3, p. 12.5) is comparatively common. It has a fibrous capsule, compresses the surrounding gland, and is more often multiple than single. These tumours present varying appearances depending on the extent of degenerative change and the amount of colloid storage. Thus they may be haemorrhagic or cystic and, in the absence of degeneration, they may have the brown honeycomb appearance of colloid goitre on section or be composed of pale, fawn, soft, fleshy tissue.

Microscopically, some are composed of strands and cylinders of epithelium without acinar structure; others consist of very small acini containing little colloid (Fig. 26.16)—such tumours have been called '*fetal adenomas*', but they do not seem to be due to developmental errors. In yet others there may be abundant colloid (Fig. 12.3, p. 12.5. *It is not possible to distinguish between circumscribed hyperplastic changes constituting the nodules in nodular goitres and true adenomatous tumours.* Thyroid adenomas

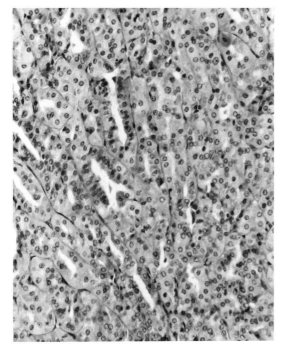

Fig. 26.16 Adenoma of the thyroid of follicular pattern, but with virtually no colloid. × 185.

usually present clinically merely as localised swellings in the gland, but the more cellular ones are sometimes associated with hyperthyroidism. Some adenomas may possibly become malignant in the later years of life. It is often difficult to distinguish clinically and histologically between adenoma and carcinoma in the absence of metastases, but *solitary tumours of the thyroid in children and young adults should be regarded with suspicion.*

Parathyroid adenomas may project into the substance of the thyroid. Simple connective tissue tumours such as fibromas and osteochondromas are rare.

Carcinoma

Carcinoma of thyroid causes about 0·5% of all deaths from cancer in this country. It invades surrounding structures, including the trachea and recurrent laryngeal nerves, and death is commonly due to asphyxia. Its incidence is said to be higher in regions with endemic goitre but this is doubtful. It is known to result in some cases from x-irradiation of the neck in childhood, which was formerly used to treat haemangioma or supposed thymic enlargement. Some of the better differentiated human carcinomas may be TSH-dependent; treatment with thyroxine, which suppresses TSH production, has resulted in regression of established metastases in some cases and is thought to have prevented metastases in others. Also there are records of rapid growth of metastases following total thyroidectomy or the administration of anti-thyroid drugs. A noteworthy feature of well-differentiated thyroid carcinomas, especially in young patients, is the prolonged survival and well-being of the patient despite the presence of metastases.

In well-differentiated tumours, thyroglobulin can usually be demonstrated immunohistologically; this is sometimes helpful in patients presenting with metastatic tumour deposits and a clinically normal thyroid.

Papillary adenocarcinoma is the form most commonly encountered and is sometimes seen in children and young adults, in whom there is often a history of local x-irradiation (see above). The tumour is not well encapsulated, is sometimes only a few millimetres in diameter, and despite its relatively innocuous microscopical appearance it frequently spreads to the cervical lymph nodes, particularly of the side affected (Fig. 26.17). Indeed *all papillary tumours of the thyroid should be regarded as potentially malignant.* Calcified spherules are often present in the stroma and there may be characteristic pale empty-looking 'Orphan Annie' nuclei in the epithelium of these tumours. It was previously erroneously thought that cervical lymph-node metastases of this tumour were 'lateral aberrant thyroid'. Pulmonary and skeletal metastases are rarely found.

Follicular adenocarcinoma. Certain encapsulated tumours, with the gross appearance of adenomas, are carcinomas composed of glandular

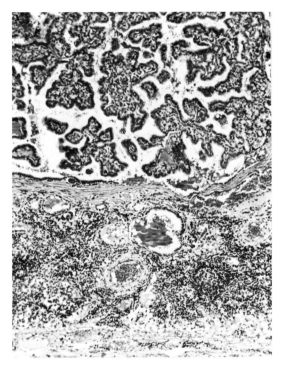

Fig. 26.17 Papillary cystadenocarcinoma of the thyroid in the cervical lymph nodes. × 65.

acini. The best differentiated examples closely resemble normal thyroid but more often there are mitotic figures and aberrant cells; in many cases solid sheets of tumour cells are also present, sometimes of eosinophilic 'Hürthle-cell' type. Malignancy is recognised by invasion of the fibrous capsule and blood vessels, and metastasis is particularly common to bone and lung. Some of these tumours take up ^{131}I, which can be used therapeutically.

Occasionally squamous-cell carcinoma is seen, possibly arising from the thyroglossal duct.

Anaplastic carcinoma. Anaplastic tumours of various types—round-cell, spindle-cell and giant-cell—are relatively common and the majority are probably anaplastic carcinomas rather than sarcomas. They cause respiratory obstruction from rapid enlargement of the gland.

Medullary carcinoma. This tumour consists of solid masses of neoplastic C cells set in a hyaline stroma which in places contains amyloid and is sometimes calcified. Despite its rather anaplastic appearance, the mitotic rate is usually low and survival for many years is com-

mon. Like normal C cells, these tumours secrete calcitonin (p. 27.27). No clinical syndrome of calcitonin excess has been recognised, but medullary carcinoma, being a tumour of apud cells (p. 12.43), is sometimes associated with diarrhoea, carcinoid syndrome or Cushing's syndrome. The blood calcitonin level is usually elevated, especially after pentagastrin or calcium infusion, making diagnosis possible in familial cases before the tumour is palpable.

The tumour may occur alone or as part of the multiple endocrine neoplasia syndrome type 2, in which it is sometimes bilateral (p. 26.41).

Thyroid lymphoma. Tumours of germinal-centre type (p. 18.23) occasionally arise in the lymphoid infiltrate of Hashimoto's disease and tend to metastasise in the lymphoid tissue of the small intestine. Immunohistological demonstration of clonality (p. 2.11) may be required to distinguish between reactive and well-differentiated neoplastic lymphoid follicles. Poorly-differentiated thyroid lymphoma has a better prognosis than anaplastic small-cell carcinoma of the thyroid and the diagnosis depends on the use of immunohistological markers for epithelial and lymphoid cells. Plasmacytoma, which may produce thyroid auto-antibody, is a rare complication of Hashimoto's disease.

Other thyroid disorders

Degenerative changes. Excluding changes in nodular goitre and tumours, degenerative changes in the thyroid are comparatively rare and of little importance. Evidence of damage produced by toxins is found in infections, and there may be actual necrosis of the epithelium. *Amyloid disease*, often accompanied by a remarkable local deposition of adipose tissue, may affect the thyroid either alone or as part of widespread amyloidosis. When well marked, it causes thyroid enlargement (*amyloid goitre*). Amyloid is found in the stroma of medullary carcinoma of the thyroid (see above). Hyaline change, calcification, etc., are often present in the stroma of chronic goitres.

Congenital abnormalities. The isthmus of the thyroid is formed by a downgrowth of a tube of epithelium from the base of the tongue (foramen caecum). The upper portion of this tube above the hyoid bone is lined by squamous epithelium. If this persists and if the buccal end is obstructed, it may give rise to a 'lingual dermoid'. The lower part of the duct below the hyoid bone is lined by columnar ciliated epithelium. **Thyroglossal cysts** may take origin from this part when it does not undergo involution. Such a cyst may rupture on the skin surface, forming a median cervical fistula. Thyroid tissue is sometimes found in the walls of these cysts. Occasionally a mass of thyroid tissue is found in the base of the tongue, the so-called **lingual thyroid**, and the thyroid may then be absent from its normal site. **Congenital absence** and **hypoplasia** of the thyroid are among the causes of sporadic cretinism.

The Parathyroids

The parathyroids are derived from branchial pouch endoderm and usually number four. They are small, yellowish-brown nodules, weighing together about 120 mg, and are difficult to find at autopsy. Usually they are situated in the neck, posterior or postero-lateral to the thyroid but one or more may lie in the upper mediastinum. They consist mainly of *chief* and *water-clear* cells, but with age, increasing numbers of *oxyphil cells* appear, their cytoplasm being rich in eosinophilic granules shown by electron microscopy to be mitochondria. All three cell types are capable of secreting parathyroid hormone and the differences probably relate to their state of functional activity. Oxyphil cells appear to be relatively inactive. During childhood, fat cells appear in the parathyroids and increase up to middle age.

Parathormone (PTH) is a single-chain polypeptide composed of 84 amino-acid residues: hormonal activity resides in the 34 N-terminal residues. The hormone plays a major role, together with vitamin D and calcitonin, in regulating the metabolism of bone and plasma calcium levels. Secretion of PTH is stimulated by a fall in the level of plasma ionic calcium, and the hormone tends to raise the plasma calcium in the following ways. (1) It stimulates osteoclast activity and inhibits formation of bone matrix by osteoblasts, resulting in release of calcium and resorption of bone. (2) It enhances the formation in the kidney of $1,25(OH)_2D$, the most active metabolite of vitamin D (p. 23.12): it thus indirectly increases calcium absorption from the gut and from the renal tubular filtrate. (3) It also has a direct effect on renal tubular epithelium, increasing re-absorption of calcium and inhibiting re-absorption of phosphate.

Secretion of PTH appears to be mediated by adenylate cyclase activation, and a negative feedback control is exerted by vitamin D metabolites. In addition to a low plasma calcium, secretion is stimulated by β-adrenergic agonists, secretin and prostaglandin E_1, while calcium, α-adrenergic agonists and prostaglandin E_2 inhibit PTH secretion.

PTH has been shown to induce its effects by activating adenylate cyclase, thus increasing cellular cAMP. Biological and immunological methods of PTH assay are available, but the results do not correspond closely and the validity of radioimmunoassay depends very much on the particular antibody used.

Calcitonin is produced by the parafollicular (C) cells of the thyroid. Its secretion is stimulated by a rise in plasma calcium. Gastrin, glucagon and β-adrenergic agonists are among the various other agents which enhance secretion of calcitonin.

Calcitonin appears to exert a physiological role by inhibiting the release of calcium and resorption of bone by osteoclasts. It thus inhibits bone resorption by PTH and other agents and lowers the level of plasma calcium. It also enhances renal excretion of phosphate.

Parathyroid hyperfunction

This may be classified into *primary* and *secondary hyperparathyroidism*. In primary hyperparathyroidism, excessive PTH secretion occurs in the absence of any known physiological stimulus and various harmful effects result. Secondary hyperparathyroidism occurs when the glands are exposed to increased stimulation, e.g. when the plasma calcium falls in chronic renal failure.

Primary hyperparathyroidism is usually due to a parathyroid adenoma (p. 26.30) but occasionally to carcinoma or to primary hyperplasia of the chief or water-clear cells affecting all four glands. It may also result from 'inappropriate' production of PTH by non-parathyroid tumours (see below). Primary hyperparathyroidism may occur in as many as 1 in 1000 of the adult population although it is diagnosed much less frequently because the classical presenting features are often absent. It can occur at any age but is commonest in middle age and especially in post-menopausal women.

Presenting features and effects. The presenting features vary considerably depending on whether the symptoms and signs are mainly due to its effects on the kidney or bones or to hypercalcaemia, which may give rise to generalised muscle weakness, tiredness, anorexia, thirst and polyuria. *More than half the patients with primary hyperparathyroidism present with symptoms relating to renal stones*, which are rich in calcium salts and therefore detectable radiologically. Only a small proportion of patients with urolithiasis have hyperparathyroidism, but nevertheless its detection in this group is important. Metastatic deposition of calcium salts may occur in the walls of blood vessels, the lungs and gastric mucosa. Deposition in and around the renal tubules (nephrocalcinosis) is of special importance and may be visible radiologically. It leads to fibrosis, tubular injury and loss of nephrons; it is often complicated by pyelonephritis, and is likely to bring about chronic renal failure. *Symptoms relating to bone changes* (p. 23.17) *are not frequent and overt radiological changes in the bones are recognisable in only about 10–20% of patients, though most have some minor degree of microscopic abnormality.* Obvious bone changes tend to occur in those patients with relatively large and rapidly growing tumours and high levels of calcium and PTH in the plasma. Patients presenting with renal stones tend to have smaller, slower growing tumours and less obvious increases in plasma calcium and PTH.

Associated lesions include duodenal ulceration and chronic pancreatitis. Duodenal ulceration occurs in approximately 15% of patients with hyperparathyroidism and is usually due to the enhancing effect of hypercalcaemia on gastrin. In some instances, however, there is more extensive peptic ulceration due to the association of a parathyroid adenoma or hyperplasia with an islet-cell tumour and pituitary adenoma in the multiple endocrine neoplasia syndrome (MEN) type 1 (p. 26.41).

Hyperparathyroidism may also occur in MEN type 2 (medullary carcinoma of the thyroid or C-cell hyperplasia, sometimes accompanied by phaeochromocytomas) and is usually due to parathyroid hyperplasia and rarely to an adenoma. When exploring the thyroid for a medullary carcinoma, opportunity should be taken to examine the parathyroids.

Diagnosis and sequelae. In suspected cases, repeated plasma calcium assays will usually confirm the diagnosis, but in occasional cases radio-immunoassay of PTH may be necessary. Removal of a functioning parathyroid adenoma is often followed by hypocalcaemia due to suppressed function of the remaining parathyroid glands; this is usually mild and lasts for only a few days. However, in those patients with marked bone changes hypocalcaemia may be severe and more persistent with tetany and psychotic disturbances; this is thought to be due to the avidity of the healing bone for calcium. Treatment with large calcium supplements, vitamin D and restriction of phosphate is necessary. Persistence of hypercalcaemia after removal of a parathyroid adenoma is usually due to the presence of a second, undetected adenoma (approximately 5% of cases) or rarely to metastases from a parathyroid carcinoma. *If possible, all four parathyroids should be identified at operation to exclude the possibility of more than one adenoma.* In some instances no adenoma is present but all four glands are enlarged and hyperplastic. They may, however, differ considerably in size and unless the other glands are inspected an enlarged hyperplastic gland may be mistaken for an adenoma.

Hypercalcaemia is observed in about 10% of patients with a carcinoma. In some instances it is caused by bone metastases and the plasma phosphate is then usually raised. In some cases, however, hypercalcaemia is associated with a fall in plasma phosphate and results from secretion of PTH or prostaglandins by the tumour. Carcinomas of the bronchus (particularly squamous-cell), kidney and ovary, account for most cases of hormonally-mediated hypercalcaemia associated with malignancy. In multiple myeloma there is evidence that hypercalcaemia is caused by an osteoclast-activating factor.

Secondary hyperparathyroidism is compensatory to hypocalcaemia: it occurs, for example, in chronic renal failure and in untreated malabsorption syndromes with osteomalacia. An additional factor in renal insufficiency may be failure of the kidney to convert vitamin D to its active metabolite (pp. 23.11–12).

Occasionally in secondary hyperparathyroidism a parathyroid adenoma may develop, presumably in consequence of the hyperplasia. The hyperparathyroidism is then no longer compensatory: it is sometimes called **tertiary hyperparathyroidism**, and is characterisded by a rising serum calcium level.

Hypoparathyroidism

Deficiency of parathormone secretion results in a fall in plasma ionised calcium and a rise in plasma phosphate. Hypocalcaemia increases the excitability of sensory and motor nerves, with various effects depending on the severity.

Causes. The commonest cause is *accidental removal of the parathyroid glands* during thyroidectomy. The condition sometimes develops following removal of a functioning parathyroid adenoma and it may then be mild and temporary or more severe and prolonged (see above). Thirdly, there is so-called *idiopathic hypoparathyroidism* which, in some instances, is one of the organ-specific auto-immune diseases. *Congenital parathyroid deficiency* may also occur, for example in the DiGeorge syndrome (p. 7.34).

Effects. If severe, hypoparathyroidism results in overt **tetany**. The tone of the skeletal muscles is increased and there may be spasm of the hands and feet in characteristic positions, twitching and jerking movements, and painful cramps of the limb muscles. There may also be generalised convulsions resembling epileptiform fits. These manifestations of motor hypersensitivity are usually accompanied by paraesthesias, often by psychotic disturbances and sometimes even by dementia. In less severe parathormone deficiency, muscle tone may be increased but without obvious twitching, spasms or convulsions. Such latent tetany may be demonstrated by increased responsiveness of neuromuscular junctions to electrical stimuli and by various tests depending upon irritability of the nerves

to mechanical stimuli. The nails tend to be brittle and there is a high incidence of cataract formation.

Idiopathic hypoparathyroidism. This is a rare acquired form of idiopathic hypoparathyroidism; it is commoner in women than men, and in many cases antibody to a cytoplasmic constituent of parathyroid epithelium is demonstrable in the serum by the immunofluorescence technique. The condition is an organ-specific auto-immune disorder (p. 7.25), and is sometimes associated with other disorders of this group, notably primary adrenocortical atrophy, pernicious anaemia, chronic thyroiditis or thyrotoxicosis. Another association is with moniliasis of the fingers and toes. There is no detectable PTH in the plasma and hypocalcaemia with detectable levels of PTH is most likely to be due to pseudohypoparathyroidism, assuming that rickets has been excluded.

Pseudohypoparathyroidism. A familial hereditary disorder, with the clinical and biochemical features of hypoparathyroidism, skeletal defects and metastatic ossification, has been described and given the above title because the abnormalities are not responsive to parathormone, and the parathyroids are actually hyperplastic. The disorder is therefore not due to lack of secretion but to failure to respond to it.

Other causes of tetany

Tetany used to be seen in children with **rickets**, in which there is deficient absorption of calcium from the intestine, although in many cases a compensatory hyperplasia and over-activity of the parathyroids is observed and may prevent tetany. Calcium deficiency may also result from the increased loss during **pregnancy and lactation** and this may lead to tetany. Thirdly, **alkalosis** may lower the level of ionic calcium in the plasma, and tetany is thus seen occasionally in patients with pyloric stenosis and repeated vomiting of acid gastric juice; indeed, even the alkalosis induced by hyperventilation may bring about or aggravate tetany. **Hyperphosphataemia** may also result in hypocalcaemia, e.g. in chronic renal failure.

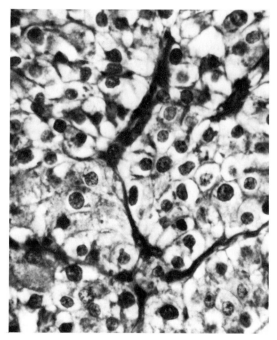

Fig. 26.18 Adenoma of parathyroid from a case of generalised osteitis fibrosa (p. 23.17). Both pale oxyphil and water-clear cells are present. × 500.

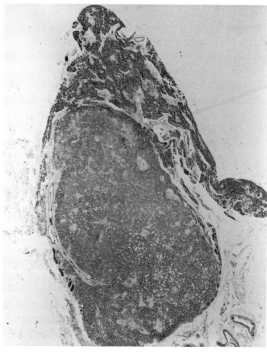

Fig. 26.19 Parathyroid adenoma. The tumour has a thin capsule and is partly enveloped in the tissue of the gland (stained darker) from which it has arisen. × 16.

Parathyroid tumours

The commonest form of tumour is the **adenoma**, and in most cases this has been associated with hyperfunction as described above. It may exceed 5 cm in diameter but is usually much smaller: it is of yellowish-brown colour, occurring most often in the lower glands. Microscopic examination shows that the cells of the tumour are similar to those of the normal gland—chief, water-clear and oxyphil cells in various proportions (Fig. 26.18). In spite of the richness of oxyphil cells in enzymes and mitochondria, pure oxyphil-cell adenomas seldom secrete excess of hormone. The cells are often larger than the normal cells and their nuclei

may be very large in parts of the tumour; this does not indicate any tendency to malignancy. Also a stretched rim of normal parathyroid may be seen at the periphery of the adenoma (Fig. 26.19). These features are not seen in parathyroid hyperplasia. Cells of columnar form may occur and a papillary type of growth may be present in an adenoma, which may project into the substance of the thyroid. As noted earlier, adenomas may occur in two or more parathyroid glands. **Carcinoma** may arise in a parathyroid but is very rare; unless it causes hyperparathyroidism, its histogenesis is usually in doubt.

The Adrenals

The adrenal glands are complex organs, the cortex being mesodermal and the medulla of neural origin. The cortex is the site of synthesis

and secretion of a number of steroid hormones termed **corticosteroids**, which have various important effects on water and electrolyte balance, carbohydrate, protein and fat metabolism, immune responses and inflammatory reactions. The adrenal cortex is essential to life, mainly because of its control of fluid and electrolytes.

The adrenal medulla may be regarded as an effector organ of the sympathetic nervous system, for it secretes the **catecholamines**. By their secretions, both the cortex and medulla play major roles in the response to mental or physical stress, e.g. injury, shock, infections, severe illness and emotional disturbances. Also the medullary hormone adrenaline stimulates release of ACTH by the pituitary, which in turn increases the output of cortisol and related steroid hormones by the adrenal cortex.

The adrenal cortex

Adrenocortical hormones

These are all steroids and fall into three physiological groups, the *mineralocorticoids*, *glucocorticoids* and *cortical sex steroids*.

Mineralocorticoids are so called because they play a major role in the homoeostasis of sodium, potassium and water. The most important one is **aldosterone**, of which, under normal conditions, 150–600 nmol (50–200 µg) is secreted daily into the blood. Aldosterone is synthesised and secreted by the cells of the *zona glomerulosa*, i.e. the peripheral part of the cortex. Its synthesis and release are largely independent of pituitary control, and are stimulated by the renin–angiotensin system (p. 10.35) so that a low sodium concentration in the renal tubule or low renal perfusion pressure, as in hypovolaemia, leads to secretion of aldosterone which increases renal tubular reabsorption of sodium and chloride and so reduces their loss in the urine. The consequent rise in osmolarity of the blood results in secretion of ADH (p. 26.12) so that there is oliguria and fluid retention. Aldosterone also increases the tubular secretion of potassium, thus promoting potassium loss in the urine. Conversely, a rise of plasma (or tubular) sodium or increase in blood volume inhibits secretion of renin and so of aldosterone, with the result that renal loss of salt and water increases. Aldosterone also has a very weak glucocorticoid effect.

Glucocorticoids. These, like aldosterone, are C21 steroids. In man, **cortisol (hydrocortisone)** is the most important, about 50–80 µmol (5–28 mg) being secreted daily; the others of physiological significance are cortisone, corticosterone and 11-dehydrocorticosterone. Synthesis and secretion of glucocorticoids is controlled by ACTH which, in turn, is regulated by a feedback mechanism (p. 26.5).

Glucocorticoids have a number of effects, of which the following are particularly important.
(1) They stimulate production of glucose from protein (*gluconeogenesis*) and antagonise the effect of insulin with consequent rise in blood glucose and deposition of glycogen in the liver, etc.
(2) They inhibit protein synthesis and increase protein catabolism in many tissues, including the muscles and skin.
(3) They enhance the effect of noradrenaline on vascular smooth muscle and thus help to maintain the blood pressure.
(4) When administered in large dosage or secreted in excess, they have the following effects.
(a) *Anti-inflammatory*: this includes limitation of the increased permeability of small vessels and inhibition of emigration, phagocytic and bactericidal activities of polymorphs and monocytes.
(b) *Immunosuppressive*: a cytotoxic effect on lymphocytes with atrophy of the thymus and other lymphoid tissues and lymphopenia. Cell-mediated immunity is affected more than antibody production.
(c) *Inhibition of growth* in childhood by suppressing the secretion of growth hormone and also its effect on tissue cells.
(d) *Cause adiposity* of the face, neck and trunk.
(e) *Cause systemic hypertension.*
(f) *Increase gastric acidity* and predispose to peptic ulceration.
(g) *Inhibit healing* by suppressing formation of granulation and fibrous tissue.
(h) *Cause osteoporosis* by decreasing bone formation and inhibiting absorption of calcium from the gut.
(i) *Cause glucose intolerance* and in some cases overt diabetes.

Glucocorticoids also have a *mineralocorticoid effect*, and while this is much weaker than that of aldosterone, it is important in the treatment of patients with aldosterone deficiency.

Glucocorticoids are synthesised and secreted by cells of the wide intermediate *zona fasciculata* and the narrow inner *zona reticularis* of the adrenal cortex. Their output is largely proportional to the concentration of circulating ACTH. In histological and other investigations on autopsy material from patients dying shortly after acute injury, etc., Symington and others (1955) equated certain changes in the adrenal with active secretion. They observed a correlation with loss of lipid from the cells of the zona fasciculata of the adrenals and with increase in RNA and various enzymes in the zona fasciculata and zona reticularis: these adrenal changes, formerly regarded as indicating functional exhaustion, were considered to reflect *increased* functional activity. As would be expected, destruction of the adenohypophysis is followed by very severe atrophy of the zona fasciculata and reticularis, but persistence of the zona glomerulosa, which continues to secrete aldosterone.

The adrenal sex hormones are ketosteroids: their physiological role is obscure, for the amounts of androgen and oestrogen secreted by the adrenals are insignificant compared with the endocrine activity of the gonads. In pathological conditions, excessive secretion of adrenal ketosteroids can, however, cause premature puberty, virilism in females and very rarely feminisation in males.

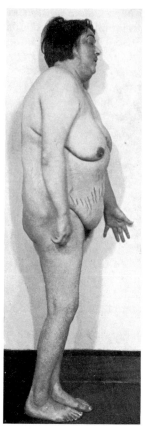

Fig. 26.20   A patient with Cushing's syndrome, subsequently cured by irradiation of the pituitary. Note the characteristic obesity of the face, neck and trunk, dusky cyanosis and facial hair, and striae of the abdominal skin.

Adrenocortical hyperfunction

Three major types of disease result from adrenocortical hyperfunction. The commonest is Cushing's syndrome, which is characterised by excessive production of cortisol. Primary hyperaldosteronism (Conn's syndrome) is rare and so is excessive secretion of adrenal sex steroids except as an additional feature of Cushing's syndrome.

Cushing's syndrome (Chronic hypercortisolism)

Cushing's syndrome results from excessive secretion of cortisol by the adrenal cortex or a cortical tumour. Although its natural occurrence is uncommon, it is important to recognise it as in most cases treatment can relieve an otherwise potentially fatal condition. Closely similar features are observed in patients on prolonged treatment with high doses of glucocorticoids or ACTH.

Clinical features. Cushing's syndrome occurs most often in women over a wide age range but is seen also in men and children. *In all instances, the main features are due to cortisol excess although there is frequently, in addition, excessive androgen secretion resulting in virilism.*

In a severe case, i.e. with grossly excessive cortisol secretion, the features include: (1) *painful adiposity* of the face, neck and trunk which contrasts with the relatively thin limbs (Fig. 26.20); (2) *increased protein breakdown*, with consequent thinning of the skin, generalised osteoporosis and wasting and weakness of the skeletal muscles. The face is highly coloured and the weakened skin becomes stretched along lines of stress, e.g. where fat has accumulated in the abdomen, resulting in purple striae in which the small vessels are visible through the stretched skin. Osteoporosis is particularly important in the spine and may result in collapse of vertebral bodies, with kyphosis, etc. Muscle weakness and wasting are usually prominent features; (3) *systemic hypertension* in most cases; (4) *diminished glucose tolerance*, which is usually only apparent following ingestion of carbohydrate, but in approximately 20% of patients is more severe with a high fasting blood glucose level and glycosuria; (5) an increased tendency to *bacterial infections* and poor healing of wounds, and (6) *arrest of growth in affected children*. Mental confusion and psychoses are also common.

All the above features are explicable on the basis of excessive cortisol secretion. In addition, women with Cushing's syndrome usually show some features of virilism, e.g. masculine distribution of hair, acne, oligomenorrhoea, and sometimes enlargement of the clitoris and deepening of the voice. The changes in the pituitary resulting from hypercortisolism have already been described (p. 26.9).

Unless treated, Cushing's syndrome is likely to result in death from the effects of hypertension, from bacterial infections or from mental depression and suicide.

Diagnosis is based on the observation of abnormally high levels of plasma cortisol in evening specimens of blood (when the level is normally lowest), together with excess of 17-hydroxysteroids (excretory products of cortisol) in 24-hour urine specimens.

Failure of low doses of dexamethasone (a synthetic glucocorticoid) to lower the level of plasma cortisol and failure of plasma cortisol to rise in response to insulin-induced hypoglycaemia provide the basis of further diagnostic tests.

Causation and types. There are three major types of Cushing's syndrome and effective treatment depends on differentiating between them. Firstly, there may be **a cortical adenoma** or **carcinoma** which secretes cortisol in uncontrolled fashion. In such cases, the high cortisol level suppresses ACTH secretion and so the cortisol hypersecretion is wholly resistant to dexamethasone (which suppresses ACTH secretion). About 5% of cases of Cushing's syndrome, including most cases in childhood, are due to a *cortical adenoma*, which is usually 2–6 cm in diameter. Excision is curative. There may be *multiple micro-adenomas* necessitating bilateral

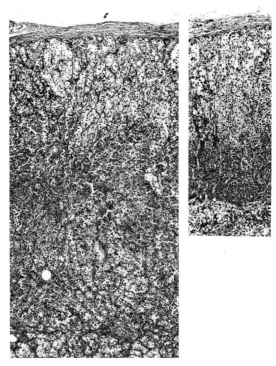

Fig. 26.21 Hyperplasia of the adrenal cortex in Cushing's syndrome (*left*) compared with a normal adrenal (*right*). The zona reticularis is greatly thickened and the cells of the zona fasciculata appear compact. In this instance, the adrenals were appreciably enlarged. × 45.

adrenalectomy. Only 1% of cases are due to adrenal carcinoma.

Secondly, Cushing's syndrome may be due to **excessive secretion of ACTH by the adenohypophysis**. This form of Cushing's syndrome is sometimes confusingly called **Cushing's disease**. In most patients, an adenohypophyseal adenoma of basophil or sometimes chromophobe cell type is responsible. The tumour is usually small and only a minority can be detected by radiography. The plasma ACTH is raised and high doses of dexamethasone, by suppressing ACTH secretion, reduce the output of cortisol. The adrenals show cortical hyperplasia (Fig. 26.21), although they may be depleted of lipid and so not necessarily enlarged. This is the commonest form of Cushing's syndrome in adults and treatment consists of reducing the excessive secretion of ACTH. This can usually be achieved by microdissection of the pituitary adenoma or by irradiation of the pituitary, e.g.

by a cyclotron; it is often possible to relieve the condition by these procedures without inducing hypopituitarism. Results of irradiation are, however, poor when the pituitary is obviously enlarged and it is now believed that in most of the adult cases without a pituitary tumour the primary disturbance is in hypothalamic function. Treatment by adrenalectomy is sometimes followed by hyperpigmentation of the skin.

Thirdly, Cushing's syndrome may result from the **inappropriate secretion of ACTH by a non-pituitary tumour**—the *ectopic ACTH syndrome*. This is most commonly due to small-cell bronchial carcinoma but various other tumours including carcinoids, thymic, pancreatic and even adrenal tumours, may be responsible. The clinical features of this form of Cushing's syndrome are often not conspicuous and wasting and weakness, etc., are likely to be attributed to malignant cachexia. The plasma level of ACTH is high and cortisol secretion is not suppressed by dexamethasone.

Where other methods of treatment are inappropriate, there is the possibility of administering mitotane, a drug which is cytotoxic to adrenal cortical cells.

Iatrogenic Cushing's syndrome. The prolonged administration of high doses of glucocorticoids or ACTH results in the development of Cushing's syndrome and the decision to use such therapy obviously requires careful judgement. Glucocorticoid therapy and certain forms of Cushing's syndrome are followed by a period of adrenocortical insufficiency (p. 26.38).

Hyperaldosteronism

Primary hyperaldosteronism (Conn's syndrome). This was, first described by Conn in 1955: it is due to uncontrolled and excessive secretion of aldosterone, usually by an adrenal adenoma.

Excessive secretion of aldosterone results in retention of sodium, and so of fluid, and, increased excretion of potassium. The sodium and water retention results in *hypertension* which is usually moderate but may be severe and even malignant (accelerated). *Hypokalaemia* is usual but not invariable: if severe it may disturb cardiac rhythm, sometimes causing attacks of syncope, and there may also be attacks of muscular weakness and *hypokalaemic alkalosis* associated with tetany, cramps and

paraesthesias. Hypokalaemia also impairs renal concentrating capacity, resulting in nocturia and polyuria. The plasma sodium concentration is usually raised or in the upper normal range.

Diagnosis of the syndrome in patients with hypertension depends on the demonstration of an increased rate of secretion (or excretion) of aldosterone in spite of a high sodium intake, and a low level of plasma renin during a period of sodium restriction. Both of these criteria are essential as many patients with 'essential' hypertension have a low plasma renin and increased aldosterone secretion occurs commonly as a secondary effect in various conditions (see below). Hypokalaemia can occur from various causes in any type of hypertension. The normal range of plasma aldosterone is 60–440 nmol/l (2–15 μg/dl) and the mean level is 175 nmol/l (6 μg/dl).

Primary aldosteronism is usually due to a single adrenal cortical tumour, most commonly an adenoma (Fig. 12.19, p. 12.14), rarely a carcinoma. In some cases, however, there is no tumour but bilateral hyperplasia of the zona glomerulosa with or without multiple nodules. Excision of the offending tumour is curative. If no tumour is found, removal of one adrenal and part of the other may effect a cure or, if not, facilitate control by drugs, e.g. spironolactone, which inhibit the effects of aldosterone.

Secondary aldosteronism results from increased activity of the renin-angiotensin system (p. 10.37) and is usually a response to hyponatraemia, water depletion, fall in blood volume, impairment of glomerular blood flow or high oestrogen levels, as in pregnancy.

Hypersecretion of adrenocortical sex steroids

The adrenals normally secrete much smaller amounts of sex steroids than the gonads, but clinical sexual disturbances can result from adrenocortical hyperfunction. Least rare is the virilism which is often a feature of *Cushing's syndrome* in women. Secondly, some *adrenal tumours* secrete excess of sex steroids, more commonly androgen than oestrogen, and so may bring about precocious puberty in males and virilism in girls and women. In such cases, there will be an increase in urinary excretion of 17-ketosteroids unaccompanied by hypercortisolism and resistant to suppression by dexamethasone. An ovarian androblastoma has similar effects. Adrenal virilism may result from an adenoma (Fig. 26.22) or a carcinoma. Feminising adrenal tumours are very rare.

Thirdly, adrenal virilism can arise from *deficiency of 21-hydroxylase*, one of a group of enzyme defects described below.

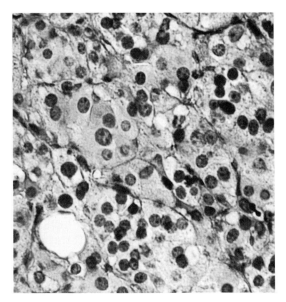

Fig. 26.22 Section of adrenal cortical adenoma associated with virilism. The trabecular structure and variation in the size of cells are common features of adrenal adenomas in general. × 375.

Adrenocortical enzyme defects

There is a group of conditions due to autosomal recessive traits, in each of which there is deficiency of one of the enzymes necessary for steroid hormone biosynthesis.

In one condition, 20-hydroxylase is deficient and steroid synthesis in the adrenals and gonads stops at the cholesterol stage. The adrenals become hyperplastic and greatly enlarged due to accumulation of cholesterol. The external genitalia are of female appearance (in both genetic males and females) and the affected infants usually die.

The least rare member of the group is *deficiency of 21-hydroxylase*, which is necessary for synthesis of both cortisol and aldosterone. This results in increased secretion of ACTH (and, in severe cases, also renin), with consequent adrenocortical hyperplasia. The defect varies in severity in different families. In severe cases, deficiency of glucocorticoids and mineralocorticoids results in features resembling those of Addison's disease. There is, however, an increased secretion of precursor steroids, which do not suppress ACTH secretion. They include the androgen dehydroepiandrosterone (DHEA), which causes masculinisation, so that the female infant is born with partially fused labia and clitoral enlargement and resembles a cryptorchid male with hypospadias ('*female pseudohermaphroditism*'), while precocious puberty occurs in affected males. Less severely affected females may present in childhood with virilism or later because of failure of puberty. In many cases, the defect is not severe, and the adrenal hyperplasia may result in sufficient cortisol and aldosterone production, so that the sex disturbances are the main feature (Fig. 3.12, p. 3.11).

Others in this group of enzyme defects include: (i) a condition similar to 21-hydroxylase deficiency; (ii) deficiency of sex hormones and of cortisol together with excess mineralocorticoid secretion, resulting in sexual infantilism and hypertension; (iii) cortisol deficiency with increased secretion of androgens and mineralocorticoids, resulting in virilism and hypertension.

Early diagnosis of these conditions is very important, for it provides the opportunity to administer the deficient steroid(s), thus restoring the functional balance. In 21-hydroxylase deficiency, for example, cortisol therapy (with extra salt and fluorocortisone if necessary) suppresses ACTH, and so reverses the adrenal hyperplasia and excessive androgen secretion: affected females treated early are sexually normal and fertile.

Primary adrenocortical hypofunction

The function of the adrenal cortex is partly dependent on normal production and secretion of ACTH and gonadotrophic hormones by the adenohypophysis, and, as already explained, pituitary failure results in depression of cortisol production by the adrenals, sex hormones by the gonads, etc. In contrast to such *secondary* failure, primary adrenal hypofunction occurs in spite of normal pituitary function, i.e. the defect lies in the adrenals.

Primary adrenocortical hypofunction can occur as an acute condition in states of severe toxaemia, or it can develop from gradual adrenocortical destruction, usually due to an auto-immune reaction or to tuberculosis.

Acute adrenocortical insufficiency

The fatal effects of bilateral adrenalectomy in experimental animals are due to lack of corticosteroids: death can be delayed by giving salt and prevented by corticosteroids. The same applies to man, in whom bilateral adrenalectomy is performed in the treatment of selected cases of breast cancer, cortical hyperfunction or hypertension.

Acute adrenocortical insufficiency occurs also in some cases of septicaemia, particularly meningococcal, and in severe endotoxic shock: the adrenals become grossly haemorrhagic— *'adrenal apoplexy'* (Fig. 26.23). The cortex, which in fatal cases is largely necrotic, may be visible as a thin yellow layer stretched over the grossly swollen, haemorrhagic medulla. This condition is known also as the **Waterhouse-**

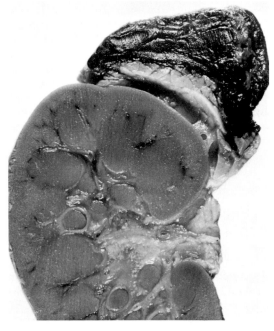

Fig. 26.23 Acute haemorrhagic necrosis of the adrenals in a child who died of meningococcal septicaemia. The adrenal lesion was bilateral.

Friderichsen syndrome and requires immediate and vigorous therapy.

Other toxic infections, e.g. diphtheria, may be associated with marked congestion and small haemorrhages in the adrenals, but these changes are now regarded as consistent with increased cortical activity and do not indicate failure.

The symptoms and biochemical changes of acute adrenocortical insufficiency are due mainly to deficiency of mineralocorticoids and glucocorticoids.

Deficiency of mineralocorticoids results in inadequate function of the distal convoluted tubules: there is failure to re-absorb salt and to secrete potassium, so that *salt deficiency, hyperkalaemia* and *dehydration* (p. 26.31) result. Death is due to a combination of hypovolaemic shock and electrolyte disturbances. Loss of medullary function, which is important in adaptation to hypovolaemia (p. 10.39), is likely to aggravate the condition. These defects can, however, be prevented and reversed by administration of fluid, salt and mineralocorticoid.

Deficiency of glucocorticoids results in failure of gluconeogenesis with consequent *hypoglycaemia* and greatly *increased sensitivity to insulin*. Another effect is *vomiting* which increases the fluid and electrolyte disturbances.

Chronic adrenocortical insufficiency (Addison's disease)

Addison's description, in 1855, of this condition and its relationship to lesions of the adrenals provided the first fundamental contribution to the physiology of the adrenals.

Clinical features. The outstanding features of Addison's disease are weakness and lethargy, loss of appetite and weight, and dizziness due to hypotension. In the absence of these features the diagnosis is unlikely. Libido is usually diminished and the skin pigmented (p. 26.6), particularly the exposed parts, the external genitalia and scars; the pigmentation is increased by skin irritants and in mild cases may be the most noticeable feature. Sometimes, however, it is inconspicuous.

In the absence of high salt intake or steroid therapy, failure of reabsorption of salt in the renal tubules results in *hyponatraemia*, a finding of diagnostic value, and this is accompanied by *chronic dehydration*.

These features result from the combined deficiency of mineralocorticoids and gluco-corticoids, the physiological roles of which are described on p. 26.31. Mineralocorticoid deficiency, as indicated above, results in loss of salt and water, with consequent hypovolaemia, hypotension, weakness and some weight loss. Chronic glucocorticoid deficiency contributes listlessness, mental confusion, hypoglycaemia, increased secretion of ACTH, impaired pressor response to catecholamines and poor reaction to stress. Anorexia, nausea, sometimes vomit-ing, and so weight loss and increased chloride deficiency, are also attributable to lack of glu-cocorticoids.

In addition to these chronic symptoms and signs *there also occur in Addison's disease acute exacerbations or* **crises**, *which are among the gravest emergencies in medical practice, demand-ing energetic investigation and therapy to prevent death.* In these, there occur severe vomiting, which aggravates chloride loss, fall in blood pressure and extreme asthenia with hypoglycae-mia terminating in collapse. Such a crisis may be precipitated by even minor infections, indis-

cretions in diet, or by vomiting or diarrhoea, in fact by anything which depletes still further the blood sodium level. As in acute adrenocortical insufficiency (see above) there is acute salt de-ficiency, dehydration and pre-renal uraemia, and death is liable to result from hypovolaemic shock and electrolyte disturbances.

Pathological changes. The commonest cause of Addison's disease in Europe was formerly destruction of the adrenals by chronic tuber-culosis, which converts both glands into fibro-caseous masses. Where tuberculosis has de-clined, more cases of Addison's disease are now due to atrophy of the adrenal cortex accom-panied by lymphocytic and plasma-cell infiltra-tion (Fig. 26.24). The medulla is relatively un-affected and this shows that loss of the cortex is the main cause of the symptoms of Addison's disease. Antibodies to adrenocortical tissue were first detected in this laboratory (Anderson *et al.* 1957), in the serum of two patients with non-tuberculous Addison's disease, and their presence in over 50% of cases has since been confirmed by various workers. They have been shown to react with lipoprotein of the endo-plasmic reticulum of the cortical cells, and are not found in cases of tuberculous Addison's disease. This finding, and the well-established associations of 'idiopathic' Addison's disease with chronic thyroiditis, thyrotoxicosis, atrophic gastritis and idiopathic hypoparathy-roidism, indicate that it is one of the organ-specific auto-immune diseases (p. 7.24). Less commonly, fungal infections or amyloidosis of the adrenals result in Addison's disease, while rarely destruction of the glands by metastatic tumour is the cause. In all cases the syndrome

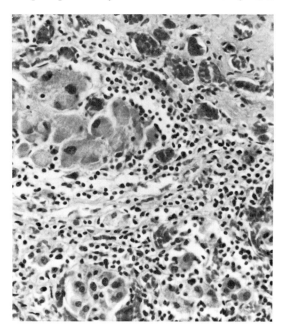

Fig. 26.24 Primary adrenal atrophy (auto-immune adrenalitis) in Addison's disease. Most of the cortical cells have been destroyed and the cortex consists of vascular fibrous tissue. In places there are foci of enlarged cortical cells with associated lymphocytic and plasma cell infiltration. × 320.

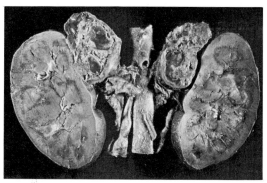

Fig. 26.25 Adrenal glands in tuberculous Addison's disease, showing extensive caseation and enlarge-ment.

of Addison's disease depends upon loss of 90% or more of the cortical tissue.

In tuberculous Addison's disease the adrenals are enlarged, firm and irregular. They are changed into masses of putty-like caseous material, with dense fibrous tissue surrounding it (Fig. 26.25); calcification is frequent and may be detectable radiographically.

In some cases there are no obvious tuberculous lesions in the lungs or lymph nodes.

Apart from the adrenal lesions, the main autopsy finding in Addison's disease is marked wasting of the muscles and adipose tissue. Atrophy of the heart is also striking; it is often more marked than in other wasting diseases, perhaps because of the low blood pressure. The gonads and breasts are also atrophic.

In Addison's disease, the adenohypophyseal basophilic cells which secrete ACTH are sparsely granulated, reflecting increased functional activity. The disturbance of carbohydrate metabolism results in a marked decrease in liver glycogen, the patients are highly sensitive to insulin and attacks of hypoglycaemia are fairly common.

In mild cases of Addison's disease, oral glucocorticoids and a high salt diet may be satisfactory, but in more severe cases the weak mineralocorticoid activity of glucocorticoids is inadequate and mineralocorticoids must also be given.

Diagnosis of Addison's disease is readily confirmed by measuring the plasma level of ACTH and the plasma levels and urinary output of corticosteroids before and during an infusion of ACTH. The distinction between auto-immune and tuberculous adrenalitis in Addison's disease is based on the history and appropriate tests (see above).

Pigmentation and a raised plasma ACTH level readily distinguish primary from secondary adrenal insufficiency.

Adrenocortical hypofunction from 'disuse'

The prolonged high dosage of glucocorticoids now used to treat various conditions results in suppression of ACTH secretion and so atrophy of the fasciculate and reticulate zones of the adrenal cortex. This occurs also in Cushing's syndrome due to an adrenal adenoma. Following removal of the tumour or cessation of prolonged glucocorticoid therapy it may take some months for full restoration of cortical function and reserve, and it may be necessary to administer corticosteroids in gradually diminishing dosage, with increased dosage to cover additional stress imposed by infections, surgical operations, etc.

Secondary adrenocortical insufficiency

This results from pituitary failure with diminished secretion of ACTH and consequently of adrenocortical steroids, particularly glucocorticoids. The condition has been considered on pp. 26.8–9 in relation to hypopituitarism.

Adrenocortical tumours

The commonest cortical tumours are **adenomas**. They occur in the form of comparatively small, rounded, well-defined nodules (Fig. 12.19, p. 12.14), and are usually yellow owing to the large amount of lipid and steroids in the cells; they are sometimes multiple. In the smaller adenomas the cells are arranged in trabeculae and resemble closely those of the zona fasciculata. Particularly in the larger examples, the cells may become large, often contain more than one nucleus (Fig. 26.22) and all transitions to distinctly aberrant forms occur; however these tumours rarely become malignant.

A cortical adenoma may be associated with Cushing's syndrome (p. 26.33) or with precocious puberty in boys and virilism in females. Rarely, an adenoma secretes aldosterone in excess (p. 26.34). It is becoming increasingly apparent that most cortical adenomas synthesise and secrete hormones, although most often in amounts insufficient to give rise to clinical abnormalities. The secretory activity of cortical adenomas may fluctuate considerably, even in those which produce clinical effects, and this may add greatly to the difficulties of diagnosis. **Carcinoma** is sometimes bilateral, although one may be a metastasis. Excessive hormone secretion may persist in spite of much cellular aberration.

The adrenal medulla

Sympathetic nerve endings and chromaffin cells (so named because they reduce chrome salts, producing brown reduction products) secrete catecholamines. Sympathetic nerve endings are the main source of the noradrenaline in the blood, while the adrenal medulla is responsible for intermittent secretion of adrenaline. The blood level of both of these catecholamines is increased almost instantaneously by stressful situations, e.g. by emotion, injury or shock. Part of the stimulus is neural, but histamine, bradykinin and various drugs have a direct stimulating effect. Secretion of adrenaline by the adrenal medulla is in some way dependent on a normal functional cortex, the blood from which is rich in corticosteroids and perfuses the medulla. In turn, adrenaline stimulates secretion of ACTH and so indirectly influences cortical function.

The binding of catecholamines to cell receptors has a profound influence on the function of many types of tissue cell, and its elucidation is not only throwing considerable light on control of cellular function, but has also provided opportunity to develop drugs which activate or block receptors and thus influence cell functions in various ways. Cell receptors for catecholamines have been classified into two major groups, α and β, depending on the relative binding of adrenaline, noradrenaline and related synthetic compounds. This classification has proved useful, but it is clear that neither α nor β receptors form a homogeneous group. Stimulation of at least some β-receptors activates adenylate cyclase activity and so increases the intracellular cyclic AMP (p. 7.4), the effect of which depends on the type of cell stimulated and on the additional effects of various other hormones on it. Stimulation of cholinergic receptors activates guanylate cyclase with consequent increase in intracellular cyclic GMP, which usually produces the opposite effect to a rise in cAMP. The mechanism by which α-receptor stimulation influences cell functions is obscure: in some instances it appears to reduce cellular cAMP.

This profoundly important aspect of cell physiology cannot be considered here in detail, but it must be emphasised that increased secretion of catecholamines in conditions of shock (p.

10.39) is of great importance in maintaining the blood pressure by causing vasoconstriction in the skin and splanchnic circulation: noradrenaline has the greater effect, because it causes vasoconstriction also in skeletal muscles.

In spite of these adaptive effects of adrenal medullary function, the most important effects of adrenal failure are due to deficiency of corticosteroids.

Hypersecretion of catecholamines is observed in patients with a functioning tumour of the adrenal medulla or of chromaffin cells elsewhere, i.e. a *phaeochromocytoma*, the features of which are described below.

Tumours of the medulla

There are three types. Two of them take origin from nerve cells, namely **ganglioneuroma**, a benign tumour containing ganglionic nerve cells and nerve fibres, and **neuroblastoma** or **sympathicoblastoma** composed of embryonic nerve cells or neuroblasts. These tumours are described elsewhere (p. 21.59). Neuroblastoma is much the commoner growth; it occurs particularly in infants and children. It may reach a large size, is composed of soft cellular tissue, and is very haemorrhagic. Secondary growths are often widespread and occur both in other organs and in the bones, the skull often being affected. Similar tumours may arise also from other parts of the sympathetic system. Such tumours may secrete catecholamines other than adrenaline and noradrenaline, especially dopamine, which appears in the urine chiefly as vanillin mandelic acid (VMA) and homovanillic acid (HVA).

Phaeochromocytoma. This third variety of tumour takes origin from the chromaffin cells of the adrenal medulla. It can arise also from chromaffin cells in other sites (see below) and is then sometimes called a *paraganglioma*.

Phaeochromocytoma is a soft, highly vascular tumour, rounded or ovoid and usually less than 5 cm in diameter but sometimes much larger. The cut surface may be solid (Fig. 26.26), grey or pink, but haemorrhages, necrosis and cystic change are common features. It is composed of polyhedral cells, many of which give

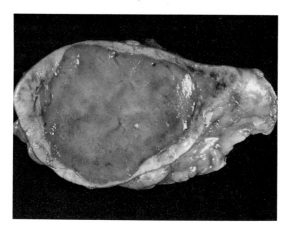

Fig. 26.26 A phaeochromocytoma occupying the adrenal medulla.

the chromaffin reaction, staining a brownish-yellow colour with chrome salts, and rich in glycogen (Fig. 26.27). When placed in formol-saline it imparts a brown colour to the fixative. The cells are arranged in solid groups enclosed in a fine vascular stroma. Cell aberration is common, but the tumour is usually benign.

Clinical features. Phaeochromocytoma occurs mostly between the ages of 25 and 55. The clinical features arise from excessive although usually intermittent secretion of

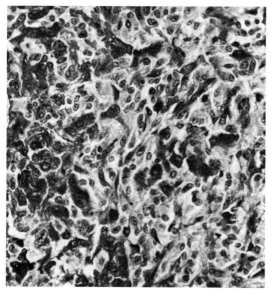

Fig. 26.27 Phaeochromocytoma of the adrenal medulla. The darkly stained elements are cells giving the chromaffin reaction. × 200.

catecholamines. Symptoms include excessive sweating, nervousness, tremors and sometimes psychoses, attacks of blanching or flushing, headache and palpitations; also loss of appetite and weight.

There is hypertension, at first paroxysmal but sometimes becoming continuous; there may also be postural hypotension. The fasting blood sugar is usually raised and the basal metabolic rate increased. Obviously a phaeochromocytoma can mimic various other conditions. In most cases the diagnosis can be confirmed by demonstrating that the daily urinary excretion of VMA is more than doubled. The response to the α-adrenergic blocking agent phentolamine is also of diagnostic value.

The hypertension results in arteriosclerosis, even in young subjects. Occasionally death has occurred from cerebral haemorrhage. Neuro-fibromatosis has been present in 5% of cases. Some families have a high incidence of phaeo-chromocytomas, often bilateral, occurring either alone or as part of the multiple endocrine neoplasia syndrome type 2 (see below). Early surgical removal of the tumour relieves the symptoms. Phaeochromocytomas causing similar hypertension occur in chromaffin tissues outside the adrenal, e.g. in the organ of Zuck-erkandl, but the majority are devoid of excessive hormonal activity. Rarely, phaeochromo-cytomas are malignant and metastasise.

Other adrenal tumours include *lipoma, myelolipoma* and *haemangioma*, all of which are rare. *Melanomas* also occur, as a rule bilaterally. *Carcinomatous metastases* are often present in the adrenals, particularly in bronchial carcinoma, in which both glands may be implicated, the ipsilateral gland being first involved and usually the larger.

Congenital abnormalities

Absence of both adrenals is a rare abnormality, incompatible with life; or one (the right only) may be absent. These abnormalities, and also adrenal hypoplasia, are intimately related to gross defects of the central nervous system, such as micrencephaly or anencephaly.

Accessory adrenals are comparatively common; they are small masses of cortical tissue which can be readily recognised by their brownish-yellow colour. They occur in the surrounding tissues, on the surface or occasionally in the substance of the kidney or liver, and in the region of the ovary or testis, and also at the apex of congenital hernial sacs. Rarely a tumour arises from them.

Multiple endocrine neoplasia (MEN)

This consists of a group of uncommon syndromes caused by hyperplasia or neoplasia of cells which secrete peptide hormones. It occurs in families, having an autosomal dominant pattern of inheritance, but is also seen sporadically. Three types have been described.

MEN type 1 (Wermer's syndrome). The major features include (1) hyperparathyroidism (90%) associated with hyperplasia or one or more adenomas of the parathyroids; (2) functioning pancreatic islet-cell adenoma (80%) which may secrete excess of insulin or gastrin, etc. (3) pituitary adenoma (65%) which may secrete excess of GH, ACTH or PRL, or may be apparently functionless and may cause pressure effects.

MEN type 2a. In this condition, medullary carcinoma of the thyroid is accompanied in 50% of cases by phaeochromocytoma, usually of the adrenal medulla and often bilateral, or arising in other chromaffin tissue. Hyperparathyroidism is a feature of some cases: it is due more often to hyperplasia than to a parathyroid adenoma, and there is evidence that the thyroid and adrenal tumours are preceded by hyperplasia.

MEN type 2b (Sipple's syndrome) resembles type 2a, but parathyroid and adrenal medullary involvement is less common, and neuromas commonly develop in the mucosa of the lips, tongue, eyelids and cornea, causing irregular thickenings. Other features include ganglioneuromas of the intestine and pigmentation of the skin.

These syndromes present in adult life, and their diagnosis usually depends on careful screening of patients with hyperparathyroidism, phaeochromocytoma, medullary carcinoma of the thyroid or pituitary adenoma, for evidence of additional features. Within families, affected individuals have the same types of MEN and usually a similar presentation. The tumours arising in the pancreatic islets, adrenal medulla, etc. are sometimes malignant.

References and Further Reading

Adams, Duncan (1977). Auto-immune disease of the endocrine glands and stomach. In *Immunology in Medicine*, pp. 373–430. Edited by E. J. Holborow and W. G. Reeves. Academic Press, London.

Anderson, J. R., Goudie, R. B., Gray, K. G. and Timbury, G. C. (1957). Auto-antibodies in Addison's disease. *Lancet*, **i**, 1123–4.

Conn, J. W. (1955). Primary aldosteronism. *Journal of Laboratory and Clinical Medicine*, **45**, 661–664.

Drexhage, H. A., Bottazzo, G. F., Doniach, D., Bitensby, L. and Chayen, J. (1980). Evidence for thyroid-growth-stimulating immunoglobulins in some goitrous thyroid diseases. *Lancet*, **ii**, 287–92.

Greenspan, F. S. and Forsham, P. H. (Eds) (1983). *Basic and Clinical Endocrinology*, pp. 646. Lange Medical Publications, Los Altos, California.

Hall, R., Anderson, J., Smart, G. A. and Besser, M. (1980). *Fundamentals of Clinical Endocrinology*, 3rd edn, pp. 788. Pitman Medical, London. (Deals mainly with mechanisms and clinical aspects of endocrine disorders.)

Kendall-Taylor, P., Atkinson, S. and Holcombe, M. (1984). A specific IgG in Graves' ophthalmology and its relation to retro-orbital and thyroid auto-immunity. *British Medical Journal*, **288**, 1183–87.

Sommers, S. C. (1982). The thyroid. In *Endocrine Pathology, General and Surgical*, 2nd edn, pp. 155–203. Ed. by J. M. B. Bloodworth. Williams and Wilkins, Baltimore.

Symington, T., Currie, A. R., Curran, R. C. and Davidson, J. N. (1955). The reaction of the adrenal cortex in conditions of stress. *Ciba Foundation Colloquia in Endocrinology* **8**, 70–84. Churchill, London.

Williams, R. N. (Ed.) (1981). *Textbook of Endocrinology*, 6th edn, pp. 1270. Saunders, Philadelphia, London and Toronto. (An authoritative multi-author text.)

Wills, M. R. and Havard, B. (1983) *Laboratory Investigation of Endocrine Disorders*. pp. 111. Butterworths, London, etc.

27

The Skin

Skin pathology is often regarded as so specialised a subject that it is not suitable for inclusion in a general textbook. But the tissue responses in the diseased skin are basically the same as those that occur in other organs, and it is an ideal organ in which to study the correlation of naked-eye appearances with microscopic changes, especially as the evolution of a lesion may be readily followed by repeated biopsy.

The major functions of the skin include sensory perception, protection against mechanical trauma, UV light and infection (p. 8.2), insulation and temperature control (p. 8.19), conservation of fluid, biosynthesis and excretion and, of course, its aesthetic function. Such functional complexity is reflected in the morphology of the skin which, although at first sight simple, varies considerably depending on site, sex, age, race and environment.

Skin biopsy. In selecting the site for biopsy, it must be appreciated that very early or late lesions often yield less useful information than a fairly early representative lesion. The most satisfactory biopsy is taken by ringing the selected lesion and adjacent normal skin with local anaesthetic and excising an ellipse containing affected and normal skin. The excised specimen should ideally consist of the full thickness of skin down to and including subcutaneous fat. The tissue should not be grasped with forceps but a Gillies hook is helpful to raise and maintain gentle tension on the skin during its removal. Excision should be accomplished with minimum trauma; use of a high-speed punch produces artefacts which often spoil the histology, and many biopsy punches are too small to produce adequate and representative biopsy specimens. Punch biopsies are,

however, of use for immunofluorescence studies. Orientation of the excised skin is essential, and it is helpful to press it gently, under-surface down, on to blotting paper before placing it in fixative (usually 10% neutral buffered formol saline): this prevents distortion during fixation. After 12–24 hours in fixative the tissue is bisected transversely and processed.

Reactive changes in skin disease. The range of responses of the skin to pathogenic agents is limited and many causes can result in similar changes. This is particularly true of inflammatory changes where, for instance, an eczematous reaction, erythema or granulomatous tissue response may be associated with many different aetiologies. *Correlation of the histopathological features with the clinical history and naked-eye appearances of the lesions is nowhere in pathology more important than in the field of skin pathology.* This chapter is intended to cover a representative selection of dermatological conditions, particularly those which have characteristic patterns of tissue reaction.

The microanatomy of the skin. It should be remembered that the microscopic structure of normal skin varies considerably according to body site. This is particularly true in regard to the relative thicknesses of epidermis and dermis and the number and size of adnexal structures. Fig. 27.1 shows in diagrammatic form the main structures that may be identified in a skin section and Fig. 27.2 the different layers of the epidermis.

Terminology in skin pathology

The following terms are in common use to describe pathological changes in the epidermis and require to be defined.

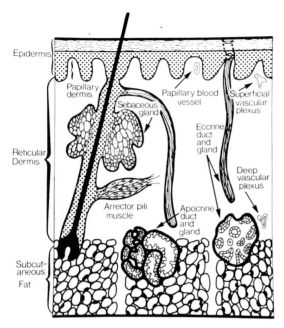

Fig. 27.1   Structures identifiable in section of human skin.

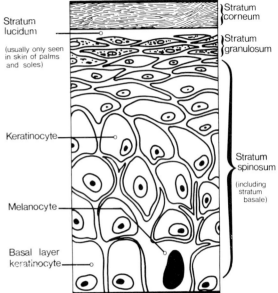

Fig. 27.2   The layers of the epidermis.

Acantholysis. Loss of cohesion between epidermal cells (keratinocytes) with consequent formation of intra-epidermal spaces containing oedema fluid and detached, rounded epithelial cells.

Acanthosis. Thickening of the epidermis, either focally or diffusely, due largely to increase of the stratum malpighii.

Dyskeratosis. Premature, abnormal or individual keratinisation of epidermal cells: the cells lose their prickles and become rounded off, and the nucleus becomes pyknotic. This is seen in some rare benign conditions but more commonly in pre-malignant lesions and carcinoma of the epidermis.

Hyperkeratosis. A thickening of the horny layer, usually accompanied by increase also in the granular layer. As the horny layer normally varies greatly in thickness in different sites, some experience is needed to assess minor degrees of hyperkeratosis.

Parakeratosis. The orderly but abnormal keratinisation of cells so that the keratin layer consists of plump nucleated keratinised cells instead of anuclear squames. It is associated with thinning or loss of the granular layer and is usually seen in diseases of increased cell turnver, whether inflammatory or neoplastic.

Pigmentary incontinence. Loss of melanin pigment from damaged basal epidermal cells and its accumulation, mostly in macrophages, in the upper dermis.

Spongiosis. Intercellular oedema, seen as increased width of the space between epidermal cells and leading, if severe, to formation of vesicles in the epidermis.

Vacuolar degeneration. A degenerative process affecting the basal layer of the epidermis with vacuolization of keratinocytes and pigmentary incontinence (see above). *Hydropic degeneration* and *liquefaction degeneration* are alternative terms used to describe this process.

Hereditary and Congenital Conditions

Genetic factors can produce skin disease in many ways. Common skin disorders such as atopic eczema and psoriasis may have a genetic background: in these disorders the condition has a polygenic (multifactorial) inheritance. Single gene disorders such as Down's syndrome may be associated with skin changes and the largest group of genodermatoses consists of single gene disorders. Recent research has elucidated the pathogenic mechanism producing the cutaneous abnormality in many of these disorders, for example the presence of a steroid sulphatase deficiency in X-linked recessive ichthyosis and various abnormalities of DNA repair in xeroderma pigmentosum. A selection of congenital skin disorders with characteristic pathological features is described below: All of them are uncommon conditions.

Ichthyosis. At least six forms of this condition have been described and it also occurs as a feature of several syndromes. Two forms are important—*ichthyosis vulgaris*, which is determined by an autosomal dominant factor, and a *sex-linked recessive form* confined to males. **The autosomal dominant form,** which is relatively common, develops a few months after birth. Scaly lesions appear on the extensor aspects of the extremities; in unusually severe cases they are large and their appearance has led to the term 'fish scale disease'. The flexures are spared and elsewhere the scales are smaller, like flakes of bran. All grades of severity occur and in some cases the condition accompanies atopic dermatitis. The characteristic feature is hyperkeratosis accompanied by thinning or absence of the granular layer: this is an exception to the general rule that hyperkeratosis is associated with thickening of the granular layer. Treatment is essentially symptomatic but the condition does tend to improve with time.

In the rare **sex-linked recessive form,** the disease starts shortly after birth and may involve most of the skin, including the flexures, but the palms of the hands and soles of the feet are spared. Histologically there is hyperkeratosis, thickening of the granular layer and acanthosis, with occasional mild perivascular infiltration of the dermis with lymphocytes and plasma cells. In very severe forms, the disease may be rapidly fatal, but in other cases it may persist for life.

Congenital bullous ichthyosiform erythroderma. This is a rare autosomal dominant condition where blisters occur in infancy, affecting the limb flexures. This is followed by the development of redness of the skin and verrucous scales. The histological features consist of a peculiar vacuolisation of the upper epidermal layers associated with apparent clumping of keratohyalin. The stratum corneum shows orthohyperkeratosis. This histopathological changes occurring in this condition are sometimes referred to as *epidermolytic hyperkeratosis* and may be seen in some other disorders (Fig. 27.3).

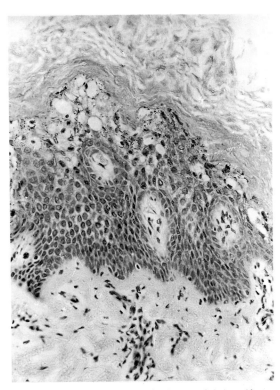

Fig. 27.3 Congenital bullous ichthyosiform erythroderma. Note hyperkeratosis, vacuolisation of upper epidermal cells and irregular clumped keratohyaline granules. × 200.

A non-inherited form of ichthyosis occurs in some patients with a lymphoma or carcinoma. The only histological changes are hyperkeratosis and increase in the granular layer, and such changes occurring alone should raise the suspicion of an internal neoplasm.

Darier's disease (Keratosis follicularis). A familial occurrence of this disease is now widely recognised. Though relatively rare, it is included here because of its characteristic histological features and its confusion with other conditions. The epidermis shows considerable hyperkeratosis and acanthosis, and is thrown into folds. This causes oblique cuts in the preparation of sections and gives rise to the appearance of a core of dermis surrounded by a single layer of epidermal cells, the so-called papillomatosis. Owing to the process of acantholysis, clefts (lacunae) appear in the epidermis and in properly orientated parts of the section these are found just above the basal layer. The two most striking features are, however, the presence of dyskeratotic cells in the epidermis called *corps ronds* and *grains* (Fig. 27.4). *Corps ronds*, which are enlarged keratinocytes, are seen mainly in the upper epidermis in the region of the granular layer. They are easily recognised by their

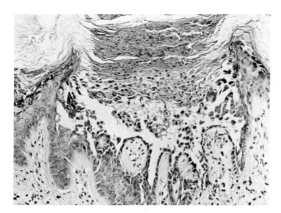

Fig. 27.4 Darier's disease. The corps ronds are seen in the upper layers of the epidermis and the grains underlying the central hyperkeratosis. × 150.

large size (two to three times that of the surrounding keratinocytes) and in haematoxylin and eosin-stained sections by their hyaline-looking eosinophilic cytoplasm (premature keratinisation). Grains are found in the horny layer and differ only in size and shape from the keratinised cells in ordinary parakeratosis. These changes are focal and may involve only very small areas of the epidermis.

This form of benign dyskeratosis must be differentiated from its malignant counterpart which is seen in some types of intra-epithelial neoplasm.

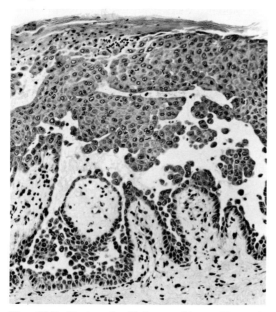

Fig. 27.5 Benign familial pemphigus. Note the acantholysis and papillomatosis. × 175.

Benign familial pemphigus. The essential feature of all forms of pemphigus is acantholysis with consequent formation of bullae, seen as raised fluid-filled blebs. Microscopically, benign familial pemphigus resembles keratosis follicularis (above) in showing acantholysis and papillomatosis (Fig. 27.5). The acantholysis is much more widespread and the epidermis has been aptly likened to a dilapidated brick wall. Dyskeratosis may be seen but is not so severe as in Darier's disease. Areas of grain-like parakeratosis are found overlying the acantholytic epidermis. In cases lacking dyskeratosis, differentiation from pemphigus vulgaris (see below) may be impossible on purely histological grounds.

Urticaria pigmentosa. This is a group of disorders associated with increased numbers of mast cells in the dermis. They include a congenital form and others in which the lesions first appears in adolescence or adult life. It usually presents clinically as widespread pigmented

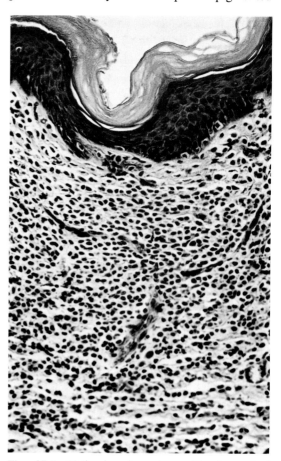

Fig. 27.6 Urticaria pigmentosa. Closely packed mast cells occupy the upper dermis. × 200.

macules which urticate, i.e. develop into pale vesicles with surrounding erythema: occasionally the entire skin surface is involved. The congenital form tends to become gradually milder and may regress completely after puberty.

Histological examination (Fig. 27.6) reveals a normal epidermis apart from an increase in melanin pigmentation of the basal layer. Depending on the severity of the condition part or all of the dermis contains closely packed mast cells. In routine haematoxylin and eosin preparations these are seen as polygonal or hexagonal cells with abundant eosinophilic cytoplasm and well defined dense oval nuclei. Staining by toluidine blue or polychrome methylene blue brings out their typical granular appearance. A few eosinophil leukocytes are also seen. In the urticated phase oedema is evident and may at times be sufficiently severe to cause a subepidermal bulla.

In adults, the intensity of mast cell aggregation varies greatly. In some instances, particularly in the adult form, there may also be aggregation of mast cells in the internal organs, e.g. the spleen, liver and bone marrow, but progression to the fatal systemic mast cell disease is rare.

Adenoma sebaceum. In tuberous sclerosis (p. 21.48), a familial condition of autosomal dominant inheritance, multiple papules are seen on the face, and the name 'adenoma sebaceum' was given to what was mistakenly believed to be late developing 'pilosebaceous naevi'. The lesions are, in fact, angiofibromatous in nature, and there is no abnormality of the pilosebaceous apparatus in this condition.

Virus Diseases

Virus infections of the skin fall into two distinct groups. Firstly, those caused by DNA viruses which integrate into the epidermal cell genome and behave as tumour viruses, producing verrucas (warts). Secondly, those in which the virus replicates within the cell, exerting a cytolytic effect: this occurs in the exanthematous viral infections.

Verrucas (warts) and similar lesions

These common viral lesions of the skin usually affect the hands, feet, knees and face, and are seen particularly in children. They also occur in the genital region. There are several types of viral wart and recent work has shown correlation between clinical and pathological features and the particular subtype of human papilloma virus (HPV). Over twenty human papilloma virus sub-types have now been identified.

Verruca vulgaris and verruca plantaris may be considered together because they are caused by related subtypes of HPV and have closely similar features. They consist of sessile papillary lesions raised above the surface of the skin (except verruca plantaris which occurs on the sole of the foot and, because of pressure, is often flush with the skin surface).

Histologically, the epidermis is thickened and thrown into papillary folds: the rete ridges are elongated and those at the periphery curve inwards giving the lesion in section a cup-shaped appearance. There is hyperkeratosis alternating with parakeratosis.

Studies of G-6-PD iso-enzymes (see p. 2.11) have demonstrated that verrucae arise from a clonal proliferation of epidermal cells and virus particles cannot be detected by electron microscopy in the proliferating cells in the basal part of the lesion. In the older lesions, the nuclei of the more superficial cells are vacuolated (Fig. 27.7) and contain densely basophilic inclusions shown by electron microscopy to consist of aggregates of virions. Both the nucleus and cytoplasm of the more superficial cells contain eosinophilic inclusions which are non-viral in nature.

The histological features of verruca vulgaris and verruca plantaris are very similar, but the latter often shows greater hyperkeratosis.

Growth of these human warts is largely controlled by host resistance: they eventually regress, but fresh crops may develop. They do not become malignant, but may be seen in unusually florid form in immunosuppressed

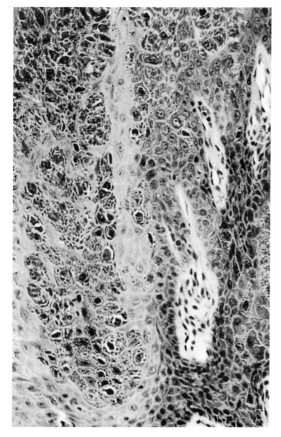

Fig. 27.7 Verruca vulgaris. Margin of a lesion showing the eosinophilic cytoplasmic inclusions and coarse basophilic nuclear inclusions. × 200.

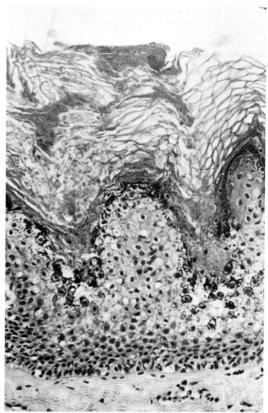

Fig. 27.8 Verruca plana. Vacuolated cells are seen in the upper layers of the acanthotic epidermis. Note the basket weave appearance due to vacuolation of cells of the stratum corneum. × 150.

patients, e.g. following renal transplantation.

Verruca plana occurs most commonly on the hands and face. It presents as a papule with less obvious papillary folding and there is hyperkeratosis but no parakeratosis. The hyperkeratosis has a 'basket-weave' appearance (Fig. 27.8), and there is a corresponding increase in the cells of the granular layer, many of which may be vacuolated. Intranuclear inclusions are not usually seen.

Condyloma acuminatum. The moist regions of the vulva, the penis, and in and around the anus are the sites where condylomata acuminata develop as soft polypoid nodules which can achieve considerable growth into cauliflower-like masses. With irritation and bacterial infection, ulceration may develop, and clinical suspicion of carcinoma may be roused. Histologically, hyperkeratosis is not prominent, but parakeratosis is usually seen with an associated depletion or absence of the granular layer. There is a remarkable degree of acanthosis with fusion and broadening of the rete ridges resulting in marked papillomatosis. However, the cells retain an orderly arrangement and this, together with the appearance of pale cells greatly swollen by intracellular oedema, is helpful in diagnosis. These tumours are caused by a subtype of HPV (p. 13.14) different from that responsible for the common wart, and infection is sexually transmitted. Very rarely they may become malignant.

Molluscum contagiosum is a common contagious lesion caused by a member of the pox-virus group. It occurs mainly in children but also in adults in whom it is commonly transmitted by sexual contact. The lesions are usually multiple, each consisting of a discrete waxy skin-coloured papule, which may grow to about 5 mm in diameter, with a central depression from which a little paste-like material can be expressed. The lesions can occur anywhere on the skin, but are commonly seen on the face and trunk.

Microscopically, a typical lesion consists of a sharply localised overgrowth of epidermis projecting above the surface but mainly downwards into the dermis, which it compresses to form a pseudocapsule (Fig. 27.9). The proliferating basal cells are free of inclusions but the cells just above this level each contain a small intracytoplasmic eosinophilic inclusion known as a molluscum body. As the cells progress towards the surface, this rapidly enlarges and becomes basophilic, forming the Henderson-Paterson body which compresses the cell nucleus into a thin marginal rim (Fig 27.9). Electron microscopy has shown the basophilic bodies to consist of enormous numbers of large virions. In the centre of the lesion the colonised cells break down to form the paste-like material which discharges on to the surface, thus accounting for the central dimple. Without treatment, the lesions may become numerous but eventually they regress.

Exanthematous viral infections

These include a group of conditions in which the predominant effect of the virus is to replicate within and destroy epidermal cells. Examples are *variola* (smallpox) and *vaccinia*, both of which are caused by DNA viruses of the pox-virus group, and *varicella* (chickenpox), *zoster* (shingles) and *herpes simplex*, all of which are caused by *Herpesviruses*. Although these conditions are clinically very different, their individual lesions all show many similarities and may conveniently be considered together. In varicella, variola and primary herpes simplex, the original infection is via the upper respiratory tract or mouth, and in varicella and

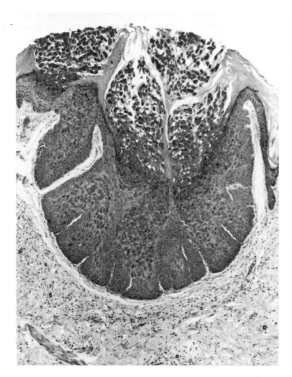
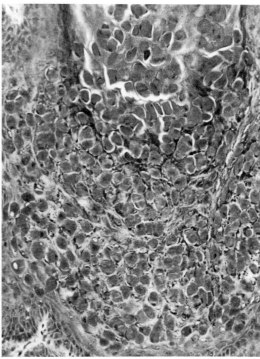

Fig. 27.9 Molluscum contagiosum, showing the whole lesion (*left*, ×70) and the central part (*right*, ×300). The lesion is a sharply localised epithelial proliferation with enlargement and eventual disintegration of the epidermal cells by the Henderson-Paterson bodies.

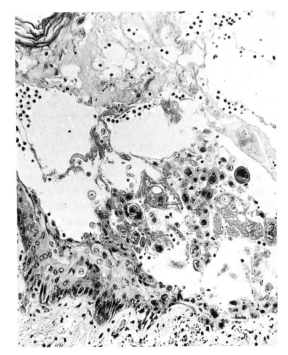

Fig. 27.10 Zoster. Multilocular intra-epidermal bulla, showing large swollen cells (balloon degeneration) and strands of cell walls traversing the bulla (reticular degeneration). × 350.

variola this is followed by a viraemic phase before colonisation of the skin to produce the characteristic lesions. Clinically, the lesions pass through macular, papular, vesicular and sometimes pustular stages. Histologically, in the early stages there may be some increased epidermal proliferation and formation of large cells with a single large or two or three nuclei. However, the major effect is cytotoxic: intracellular oedema results in swelling of the deeper epidermal cells (balloon degeneration) progressing to rupture of the cells to produce a vesicle or bulla (Fig. 27.10). The greatly swollen epidermal cells lining the space become detached and drift into the vesicular fluid. When cell death is rapid, neighbouring cell walls may persist as sheets and strands traversing the vesicle and giving it a multilocular appearance, a feature termed *reticular degeneration*. This is usually pronounced in smallpox, but is seen also in the other conditions.

Variola and vaccinia. The only known cases of variola in the past five years have resulted from laboratory infections. The disease appears to have been eradicated and vaccination is no longer routine practice.

Varicella and herpes zoster are both caused by *Herpesvirus varicellae*. In varicella, which usually occurs in childhood, the lesions are widespread, but tend to occur in successive crops, so that the different stages are seen at the same time. They also differ from those of variola in having a centripetal distribution, being fewer on the extremities than on the trunk and proximal parts of the limbs. They cannot be distinguished with certainty by traditional histological examination from smallpox, although reticular degeneration and pustulation are often less marked and usually they heal without permanent scarring. In immunodeficient or immunosuppressed subjects the lesions may be very numerous and florid and there may be widespread visceral involvement, including a mild virus pneumonia and occasionally mild encephalitis. The virus can persist for years in the posterior root ganglia without causing symptoms, and zoster results (usually in adults) from a recrudescence of this latent infection (Fig. 21.39, p. 21.33). The virus reaches the skin, presumably via the sensory nerves, and produces a crop of lesions which are often preceded and accompanied by severe pain in the area supplied by the individual nerves—most commonly the trunk, face or arm. In immunodeficient individuals, zoster skin lesions may become widespread and there may be visceral involvement.

Herpes simplex is a ubiquitous infection. Most people acquire it asymptomatically in childhood via the oral mucosa: thereafter the virus (*Herpesvirus hominis*) remains latent, but may reactivate (usually during an incidental febrile illness) and produce the typical skin lesions around the lips, etc. Occasionally, more severe lesions occur, usually as part of the original infection, including neonatal generalised herpes, keratoconjunctivitis and an acute necrotising encephalitis (p. 21.33) which is often fatal.

Herpes simplex shares with vaccinia virus the capacity to colonise areas of eczematous skin in children, producing in both cases a condition known as **Kaposi's varicelliform eruption.**

Inflammatory Conditions

Many different conditions, some of known and others of unknown aetiology, are arbitrarily grouped under the heading of inflammatory diseases. This is not so irrational as it may seem because those varied diseases show different degrees and facets of the changes of inflammation.

Dermatitis

Much confusion has been caused by the rather indiscriminate use of the terms *dermatitis* and *eczema* to describe similar conditions. It is now widely accepted that the two terms are synonymous, and in this text dermatitis will be used. The term covers the inflammatory response of the skin to a wide variety of pathogenic agents ranging from contact with external primary irritants to a hypersensitivity reaction to various antigens, both exogenous and endogenous.

External primary irritants such as strong acids or alkalis produce an acute inflammatory response similar to that seen in other tissues and the dermatitis subsides once the irritant has been removed.

The hypersensitivity group is complex and imperfectly understood. Many chemicals which cause dermatitis following contact with the skin are haptenic (p. 6.2) and require to combine with an epidermal protein to become immunogenic. The hypersensitivity, which is of delayed type (p. 7.23) is termed contact dermatitis and may resolve on preventing contact with the hapten, but in some cases becomes self-perpetuating.

Dermatitis caused by drugs and other haptenic or antigenic material after absorption by mouth or some other route may be of atopic type (p. 7.22) or the result of immune-complex deposition (p. 7.23).

Various other clinically recognised disorders are of unknown cause, e.g. pompholyx, seborrhoeic dermatitis, lichen simplex chronicus (formerly neurodermatitis) and exfoliative dermatitis.

In all these conditions, various degrees of itching, erythema, exudation and scaling characterise the clinical picture. Whatever the cause, the basic microscopic picture is similar, and it is convenient to speak of the *dermatitis reaction* which, like any inflammatory process, may be acute, subacute or chronic. The pathologist can only report on the type of dermatitis reaction and can rarely suggest the aetiology without having recourse to the clinical history and findings.

Acute dermatitis. The earliest change is spongiosis (intercellular oedema) which separates the keratinocytes; this is followed by infiltration of the epidermis by polymorphs, macrophages and lymphocytes. Focal degeneration and lysis of keratinocytes occurs, with consequent formation of vesicles which may enlarge into bullae (Fig. 27.11). Depending on the stage at which biopsy is performed, the vesicles may

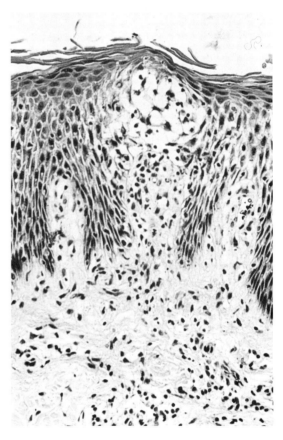

Fig. 27.11 Acute dermatitis, showing an intraepidermal vesicle containing leucocytes and degenerate epithelial cells. × 200.

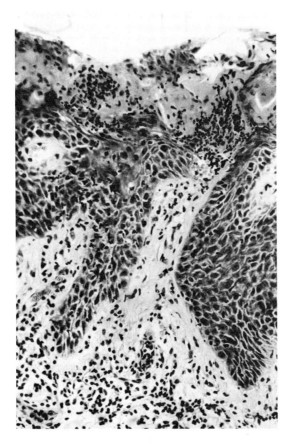

Fig. 27.12 Subacute dermatitis. Note the tip of the dermal papilla in contact with the serous exudate and debris on the surface. × 300.

contain cell debris, fibrin, neutrophil polymorphs and lymphocytes. Disordered keratin formation may result in focal parakeratosis which, together with dried inflammatory exudate and cell debris, forms loose or firmly adherent surface crusts. Depending on the severity of the reaction, the dermis may be hyperaemic and oedematous with perivascular aggregation of eosinophil and neutrophil polymorphs and lymphocytes.

As with other vesicular or bullous lesions, an early typical lesion should be selected for biopsy. The histological picture is similar in the acute phase of any clinical form of dermatitis including, for example, the lesion of **pityriasis rosea,** a common condition with typical clinical appearances.

Subacute dermatitis. As the acute stage subsides the lesions become less vesicular and although spongiosis and vesiculation may persist, they are usually less obvious. The epidermis becomes acanthotic with deepening and then fusion of the rete ridges. There is also parakeratosis with formation of surface crusts which include a mixture of fibrin, degenerating leucocytes and bacteria. Occasionally a vesicle may rupture on to the surface, leaving a naked dermal papilla covered by fibrin and debris (Fig. 27.12) and forming the so-called *dermatitis pit.* There is less oedema and vascular congestion in the dermis, but it is more heavily infiltrated with inflammatory cells, mainly lymphocytes and macrophages with only an occasional neutrophil leucocyte. **Nummular dermatitis** is the classical example of this stage of dermatitis although it occurs also as a phase of others, particularly atopic dermatitis. Stasis dermatitis, associated with impaired venous return from the lower limbs, may show the same changes with, in addition, scattered deposits of haemosiderin in the dermis.

Chronic dermatitis. An outstanding feature of this stage is marked acanthosis with elongation of the rete ridges. Hyperkeratosis with areas of parakeratosis are evident and there is a corresponding patchy thickening of the granular layer. Small foci of spongiosis may be seen but no vesicles (Fig. 27.13). The upper dermis is infiltrated with moderate numbers of lymphocytes, macrophages, fibroblasts and occasional eosinophil leucocytes. The walls of the small blood vessels often show hyaline thickening with reduction of their lumina, and there may be scarring of the dermis. These changes correspond to the clinical picture of thickened, leathery skin referred to as 'lichenified', seen in many types of chronic dermatitis. The most characteristic clinical condition is, however, **lichen simplex chronicus.**

The prognosis of dermatitis is variable. Acute and subacute phases can be quickly controlled by the use of appropriate topical treatment and, in the case of contact and irritant dermatitis, by removing the patient from the source. Chronic dermatitis, particularly of the hands and feet, is often extremely resistant to treatment and may persist for life, varying in intensity but never regressing completely.

There are several conditions which, although not classified clinically within the dermatitis group, show histopathological features which may be indistinguishable from those of derma-

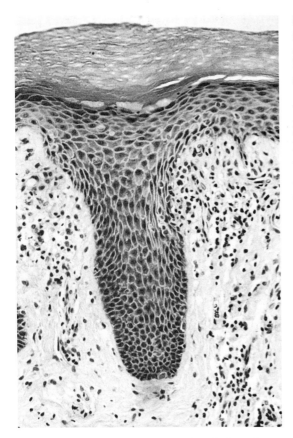

Fig. 27.13 Chronic dermatitis. There is hyperkeratosis, elongation of the rete ridges and a perivascular inflammatory infiltrate in the upper dermis. × 300.

titis. These include *chronic superficial dermatitis* (the benign form of so-called *parapsoriasis*), some *annular erythemas* and certain *psoriasiform reactions* where the appearances may be difficult to distinguish from chronic dermatitis. Generalised exfoliative dermatitis (generalised erythroderma) shows some of the features of sub-acute or chronic dermatitis but there is normally a fairly heavy perivascular lymphocytic infiltrate in addition to the epidermal features. This condition may be the result of several different aetiologies including psoriasis, dermatitis, a drug reaction and occasionally a malignant lymphoproliferative disease.

Acne vulgaris

This is very common in adolescents of both sexes. It begins about puberty, varies greatly in severity and duration and eventually subsides, although sometimes not until the mid-twenties. Acne affects mainly the face, chest and upper back but may extend to the deltoid regions and down to the buttocks.

The earliest structural change is blockage of the opening of the pilosebaceous follicle by a mass of keratin: this is seen as a **comedo** (blackhead) which is dark because of melanin deposition. Secretion of sebum continues in the blocked follicle until the sebaceous gland undergoes pressure atrophy. Meanwhile the follicle may become grossly dilated with keratinous debris and sebum (*cystic acne*). More commonly blockage is followed by suppuration, the pus discharging on to the surface (*pustular acne*). The skin commensal *Propionibacterium acnes* appears to thrive in the blocked follicle: it splits neutral fats of sebum into free fatty acids which are intensely irritating. Sometimes the wall of the distended follicle is disrupted and the contents escape into the dermis where they induce a macrophage granulomatous reaction with foreign-body giant cells. Granulation tissue is formed and permanent scarring results which occasionally progresses to keloid formation.

Extensive investigation has failed to elucidate the basis of acne: the influence of androgens on sebum production may be important, and the tissue reaction is probably aggravated by the fatty acids produced by bacterial enzymic activity of sebum. The use of long-term low-dose oral tetracycline therapy has done much to alleviate acne and reduce the tissue reaction and scarring.

The bullous diseases

These comprise pemphigus, pemphigoid and dermatitis herpetiformis.

It is possible to separate the pemphigus group from the others by histological examination but only if an early representative biopsy is taken. Secondary infection and degenerative changes rapidly alter the histological features. Ideally a small lesion should be taken within 12 hours of its appearance. Pemphigoid and dermatitis herpetiformis show histologically a sub-epidermal blister formation in contradistinction to the pemphigus group of disorders where the blister forms within the epidermis.

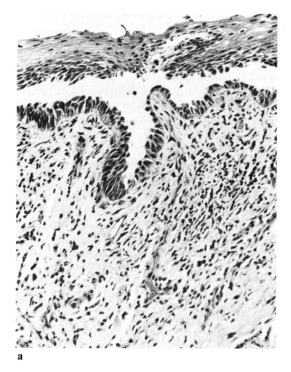

a

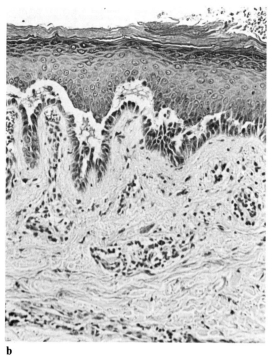

b

Fig. 27.14   Pemphigus vulgaris. **(a)** Acantholytic bulla in buccal mucous membrane. × 150. **(b)** Intraepidermal bulla containing acantholytic cells, best seen just above the basal layer of the epidermis. × 150.

Pemphigus

Three major types of pemphigus are recognised: *pemphigus vulgaris*, *pemphigus vegetans* and *pemphigus foliaceus*. In the latter two types bullae may not be detectable clinically although histological examination will reveal the characteristic changes at the edge of the lesion. Pemphigus is a serious disorder and the vulgaris and vegetans types, if untreated, may cause death. Systemic corticosteroids and immunosuppressant drugs have greatly improved the prognosis. Pemphigus foliaceus is more benign and can often be satisfactorily controlled by one of the more potent topical corticosteroid preparations.

The bulla of pemphigus is intra-epidermal and arises as a result of acantholysis of epidermal cells which produces a horizontal plane of cleavage in the epidermis. The diagnosis of pemphigus can sometimes be made by microscopical examination of scrapings from a blister floor. This is called a Tzanck smear and the finding of rounded acantholytic epidermal cells confirms the clinical diagnosis.

Pemphigus vulgaris is an uncommon disease of the middle-aged. It is characterised by the development of rather flaccid bullae of the skin: they appear in crops, soon rupture and leave a raw surface which does not granulate.

In this condition (Fig. 27.14), the cleavage takes place above the basal layer, this layer remaining intact due to its attachment to the dermis by cytoplasmic processes. The bulla contains serum and somewhat condensed, rounded-off keratinocytes. A few polymorphonuclear leucocytes and eosinophils may also be present within the bulla. The underlying dermis shows slight oedema and a sparse infiltrate of polymorphs and eosinophils.

Pemphigus vegetans. In pemphigus vegetans the early lesion is identical with that of pemphigus vulgaris. As the disease progresses, however, the epithelium proliferates and the characteristic acantholysis is not seen. There is marked acanthosis of a verrucose type and intra-epidermal 'microabscesses' composed almost entirely of eosinophil leucocytes (Fig. 27.15). The inflammatory infiltrate in the upper dermis includes many eosinophil leucocytes and is much more pronounced than in pemphigus vulgaris.

Pemphigus foliaceus. In pemphigus foliaceus

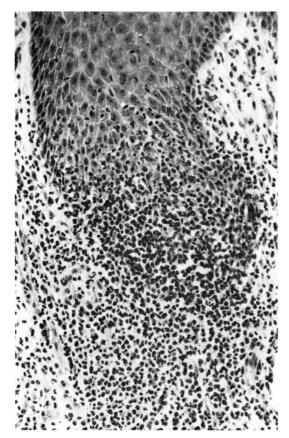

Fig. 27.15 Pemphigus vegetans. An early intraepidermal abscess composed of eosinophil leucocytes at the tip of an elongated rete ridge. × 300.

the acantholysis occurs high in the epidermis, usually just below the stratum corneum (Fig. 27.16), and if the biopsy is not carefully taken or the tissue is roughly handled the superficial layer may be lost, making the diagnosis difficult. Careful examination of the surface, however, will reveal acantholytic cells.

Mucosal lesions of pemphigus. While all forms of pemphigus are usually regarded as skin diseases, many cases begin as 'ulcers' of the mouth or genitalia. These may precede the skin lesions by as long as two years. The histological changes in mucous membranes are similar to those in the skin, viz. acantholytic bullae (Fig. 27.14a). However, because of the moist conditions within the mouth or on the vulva, maceration occurs rapidly and the roof of the bulla is quickly lost, making histological diagnosis extremely difficult. The demonstration that patients in the active stages of pemphigus have

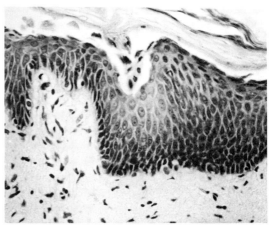

Fig. 27.16 Pemphigus foliaceus. Subcorneal bulla containing occasional acantholytic cells and some leucocytes. × 200.

serum antibodies to an intercellular antigen of squamous epithelium, demonstrable by indirect immunofluorescence staining, has contributed greatly to the accurate diagnosis of the condition. Fig. 27.20 and p. 27.15.)

Dermatitis herpetiformis. This chronic condition usually appears after the age of 30. It presents as grouped crops of extremely itchy urticarial papules and vesicles, most commonly on the shoulders, lips, nose, external genitalia and over the sacrum. The early lesion is a subepidermal vesicle (Fig. 27.17) which rapidly enlarges into a bulla. There is no acantholysis. Difficulty may arise if an older lesion is biopsied as the epithelium regenerates rapidly and grows along the floor of the bulla which thus appears intra-epidermal. The subepidermal bulla is filled with serous exudate and contains leucocytes, the majority of which are neutrophil polymorphs. The underlying dermis is oedematous and there is a considerable leucocytic infiltration. A useful diagnostic feature is the presence of papillary tip microabscesses—oedematous dermal papillae packed with eosinophil polymorphs—at the margins of the bullae (Fig. 27.18). Their detection may require examination of multiple sections. In late lesions significant numbers of eosinophils may also be present in the dermal papillae.

In the majority of patients there is also a gluten-sensitive enteropathy with jejunal villous atrophy. Symptomatic relief of dermatitis herpetiformis can often be obtained by administra-

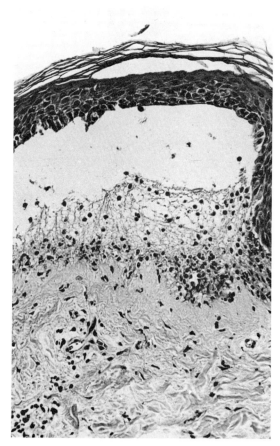

Fig. 27.17 Dermatitis herpetiformis. Subepidermal bulla containing fibrin and leucocytes. × 200.

tion of the drug dapsone. The enteropathy may respond to a gluten-free diet.

Pemphigoid

This consists of a bullous disease which may affect mainly the skin (*bullous pemphigoid*) or the mucous membranes (*benign mucosal* or *cicatricial pemphigoid*). The early lesion, as in dermatitis herpetiformis, consists of a subepidermal bulla which contains relatively few inflammatory cells, including some eosinophils, and which soon becomes intra-epithelial as a result of extension of epidermal cells over the base. There is usually little dermal involvement until later, when neutrophil and eosinophil polymorphs aggregate both in the bullae and in the adjacent dermal papillae.

Bullous pemphigoid presents as an itchy ery-

thema with development of large tense bullae, particularly on the flexural aspects of the limbs. After a few days the blisters burst and healing usually occurs. The condition, which is seen mostly in the elderly, is recurrent but often subsides after some months or years. It responds to systemic corticosteroid therapy. Its distinction from dermatitis herpetiformis is helped by antibody studies (see below).

Benign mucosal pemphigoid affects the mucous membrane of the mouth, the genitalia and the cornea and conjuctiva. The lesions resemble those of bullous pemphigoid and there may be some skin lesions. Scarring of the cornea and conjunctiva may seriously affect vision.

Epidermolysis bullosa. This group of blistering disorders is usually inherited as a genetic disease and there are autosomal dominant and recessive forms of the disorder. Clinically all

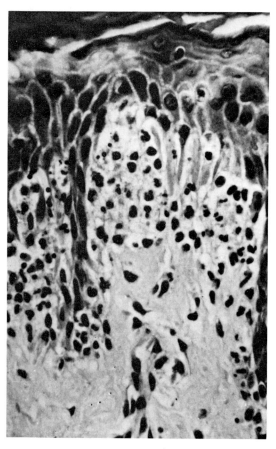

Fig. 27.18 Dermatitis herpetiformis. 'Eosinophil abscess' in an oedematous dermal papilla at the margin of a bulla. × 350.

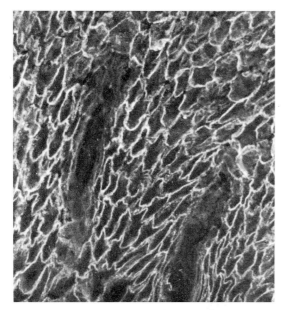

Fig. 27.19 Pemphigus vulgaris. Intercellular immunofluorescence staining in squamous epithelium. Indirect immunofluorescence technique. × 300.

patients develop blisters and some forms of epidermolysis bullosa result in severe scarring. The histopathological appearances in many types of the condition are essentially those of subepidermal blistering with relatively little inflammation in the underlying dermis. Precise diagnostic classification however, normally requires ultrastructural and other studies.

Immunofluorescence tests in the bullous diseases

In recent years, application of immunofluorescence (IF) tests (p. 6.11) has contributed greatly to the differential diagnosis of the bullous diseases. In the *indirect IF test*, a suitable fresh tissue substrate, such as rabbit or preferably (in our experience) baboon oesophagus, is treated successively with the patient's serum and fluorescein-labelled anti-immunoglobulin. In the *direct IF test*, unfixed cryostat sections of the patient's skin are treated with fluorescent-labelled anti-immunoglobulins and antibodies to complement components.

In the *pemphigus group*, circulating antibody (of IgG class) to a constituent of the intercellular substance of squamous epithelium is demonstrable, during active phases of the disease, by the indirect IF test (Fig. 27.19). The titre

reflects the severity of the disease and may be used to monitor therapy. The direct IF test shows antibody and complement bound to the intercellular substance.

In *dermatitis herpetiformis* the direct IF test shows small granular deposits of IgA on the basement membrane in the prevesicular lesion and the adjacent skin. Antibody is not detectable in the serum.

In *bullous pemphigoid*, specific circulating antibodies may be demonstrated by direct and indirect IF testing. They bind to the basement membrane zone of stratified epithelium as homogeneous linear deposits principally of IgG (Fig. 27.20), and they also fix complement. In *benign mucosal pemphigoid*, fixed immunoglobulin, usually IgG, rarely IgM, together with complement, or sometimes IgA, is demonstrable on the basement membrane in many cases, while in some patients antibody reacting with basement membrane is detectable in the serum. Neither in bullous pemphigoid nor in benign mucosal pemphigoid can the titre of circulating antibody be used as an indicator of the severity of the disease or as a monitor of therapy, since such antibodies may be demonstrated in many cases long after clinical resolution has occurred.

In *erythema multiforme* the IF findings are

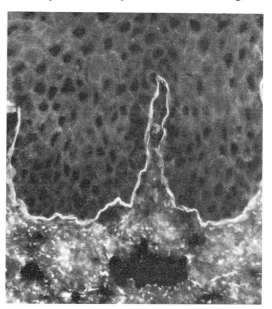

Fig. 27.20 Bullous pemphigoid. Homogeneous linear immunofluorescence of basement membrane. Direct immunofluorescence technique. × 300.

inconstant and not diagnostic. Occasionally deposits of IgG and/or C3 are detectable in the walls of the small dermal vessels.

Immunofluorescence studies in lupus erythematosus are described on p. 27.21.

Erythema multiforme

This is an acute disorder seen at all ages and is sometimes recurrent. As the name suggests, there is a variety of clinical and histological appearances; in some the cause may be known, e.g. drugs or infections, while in others it is obscure. Typically the eruption involves the face, hands, and forearms. It may appear as a number of 'target lesions', each consisting of a circular erythematous area of skin with a pale centre. The lesions vary greatly in severity and size: there may be macules, papules, blisters or pustules and haemorrhagic necrotic areas. A severe, sometimes fatal, form is the *Stevens–Johnson syndrome* in which extensive erosive lesions occur on the skin and mucous membranes.

Histologically, in the classical type of erythema multiforme, a diagnostic picture of an area of coagulative necrosis of the epidermis is seen, and this area may be raised above the underlying dermis by bulla formation (Fig. 27.21). The dermis shows oedema and there may be haemorrhage, with an acute necrotising capillaritis or vasculitis. More commonly there is a scattered perivascular cellular infiltrate consisting of varying numbers of neutrophils, eosinophils, lymphocytes and histiocytes. A frankly bullous form occurs without necrosis of the overlying epidermis, and differentiation from other causes of subepidermal bullae may not be possible histologically.

In the severe forms of erythema multiforme, including the Stevens–Johnson syndrome, early and intensive systemic corticosteroid therapy may be life-saving.

Toxic epidermal necrolysis

This term is used to describe a clinical disorder where the epidermis becomes necrotic and peels off in sheets, the appearances resembling a scald or burn. It is now clear that this clinical picture embraces two pathological entities. One of these occurs in childhood and is sometimes referred to as the staphylococcal scalded skin

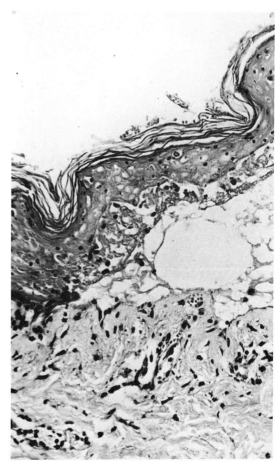

Fig. 27.21 Erythema multiforme. Subepidermal bulla roofed by necrotic epidermis. Regenerating epidermis can be seen at the left of the picture. × 200.

syndrome. This is a condition caused by staphylococcal toxin and the histopathology shows a high-level split in the epidermis, often subcorneal in location. The second form of toxic epidermal necrolysis occurs in adults and may be associated with a drug reaction. In this group the blister formation is usually found in the region of the dermo-epidermal junction and this condition may be related to erythema multiforme.

Scaling disorders

Psoriasis. This common, extremely chronic disorder is estimated to affect about 2% of the population. It usually appears first between the

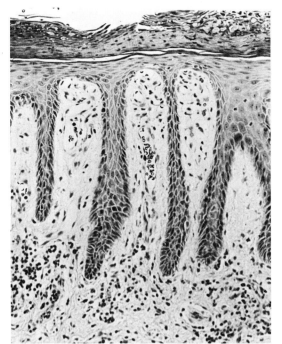

Fig. 27.22 Psoriasis. The surface is covered by a parakeratotic scale containing numerous polymorphonuclear leucocytes. The rete ridges are elongated and the suprapapillary epidermis is thinned × 150.

ages of 15 and 30 years. The lesions are slightly raised, sharply demarcated, red or pink, round or oval plaques with a fine scaly surface, varying in diameter from millimetres to centimetres. They may occur anywhere on the skin, but are commonest on the knees, elbows and over the sacrum. About 25% of patients show a peculiar pitting of the finger and toe nails and about 5% develop a chronic polyarthritis with absence of rheumatoid factor.

Characteristically there is parakeratosis with marked thinning of the epidermis over the dermal papillae which are oedematous and broadened at their tips. The rete ridges are greatly elongated and club-shaped (Fig. 27.22). There is usually a light chronic inflammatory cellular infiltration of the dermis. A characteristic feature of the early lesion is migration of neutrophil polymorphs into the epidermis, where they accumulate in and beneath the parakeratotic horny layers to form scattered '*Munro micro-abscesses*'.

The above histopathological description corresponds to established plaque psoriasis and it

must be remembered that the histopathological features of the condition may vary with the stage of the disease. *Guttate psoriasis*, which consists of small scaly patches of psoriasis often affecting the trunk and particularly common in young people, shows a histopathology sometimes indistinguishable from subacute dermatitis. The most important condition to consider in the differential diagnosis of the pathology of psoriasis is a form of dermatitis known as *seborrhoeic dermatitis*. The presence of spongiosis in this disorder is a useful clue.

Lichen Planus is a relatively uncommon disease which often has a sudden onset and tends to persist: it affects both skin and mucous membranes. The skin lesions are intensely itchy: they consist of violaceous papules with a shiny surface and the chronic lesions show various degrees of hyperpigmentation. Characteristic

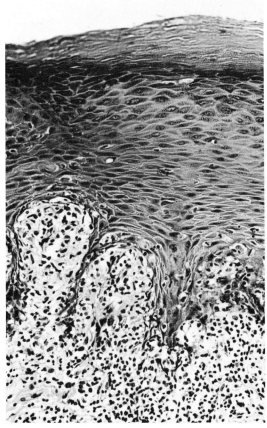

Fig. 27.23 Lichen planus. Note the hypertrophy of the granular layer and the saw-tooth appearance of the rete ridges. × 200.

sites for the eruption are the wrists, trunk, external genitalia, legs and buccal mucosa. Delicate networks of white lines (Wickham's striae) may be seen on the surface of the lesions.

The papule of lichen planus has characteristic microscopic features (Fig. 27.23). There is marked hyperkeratosis with focal increase in the granular layer. The epidermis is acanthotic and the rete ridges assume a pointed outline, giving a saw-tooth appearance. There is often some swelling and disintegration (liquefaction degeneration) of the basal layer of the epidermis, and colloid bodies, probably derived from effete basal cells, may be seen in the lower epidermis and also in the upper dermis, which is heavily infiltrated with lymphocytes and occasional macrophages. The upper border of this infiltrate is in contact with the epidermis and may actually invade the basal layers, causing the dermo-epidermal junction to be indistinct. Lesions in the mucosa present a similar appearance although the hypertrophied granular layer is not so obvious. (Normally there is no granular layer in some areas of mucous membranes).

The histopathological differential diagnosis of lichen planus includes lichenoid drug eruptions, lupus erythematosus and lichenoid solar keratosis.

Vascular Disorders

Vascular changes of some sort commonly occur in most inflammatory disorders of the skin. However, in some disorders the vascular changes seem to be the major histopathological feature. In the various causes of erythema the microscopic features are those of dilatation of superficial blood vessels with a surrounding cuff of chronic inflammatory cells, predominantly lymphocytes. In chronic urticaria again there may be some dilatation of blood vessels and dermal oedema with increased numbers of cells around blood vessels. In urticaria, however, the infiltrate is more polymorphous with neutrophils, eosinophils and mast cells present in addition to lymphocytes.

The term vasculitis is the subject of much confusion both at a clinical and pathological level and there is no completely satisfactory classification system. Many classifications are based on the size of blood vessels involved in the process (see p. 14.22) and the type of associated inflammation. Some evidence of structural damage to blood vessel walls is usually necessary before one can use the term vasculitis. In the following sections the problem of so-called cutaneous angiitis will be discussed briefly in addition to the group of conditions which include erythema nodosum and nodular vasculitis.

Erythema nodosum, nodular vasculitis and erythema induratum (Bazin's disease)

These three conditions are all characterised by nodular lesions of the subcutaneous fatty tissue of the lower extremities. While there are differences in aetiology and clinical course they cannot be clearly distinguished histologically and the appearances vary with the age of the lesion. They all produce tender subcutaneous nodules or thickenings of the legs, sometimes with reddening of the overlying skin. The lesions consist of areas of inflammation and fat necrosis with subsequent repair. In the early stages there is an infiltrate of polymorphonuclear leucocytes and lymphocytes in the subcutaneous fat. Inflammatory infiltration of the walls of small veins, which may be the basic lesion, is seen and in the more severe cases endothelial proliferation and thrombosis may occur (Fig. 27.24). As the nutrition of the fat is impaired, foci of epithelioid cells and giant cells appear in response to liberated fat. In severe cases necrosis resembling caseation may be seen. These changes gradually subside and at a later stage the process of healing with fibrosis is observed.

It will be appreciated that the extent of the histological changes will be dependent on the severity or acuteness of the condition. In ery-

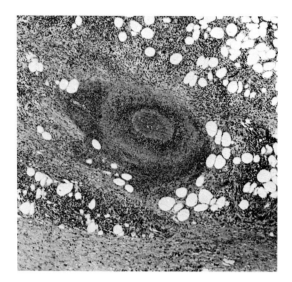

Fig. 27.24 Erythema nodosum. Thrombophlebitis of subcutaneous vein with surrounding inflammatory reaction in adipose tissue. × 30.

thema induratum the fat necrosis may be so extensive that the lesion ulcerates, discharging caseous material on the surface.

Cutaneous angiitis—anaphylactoid (Henoch–Schönlein) purpura; necrotising or allergic vasculitis

Until recently it was customary to consider such disorders as anaphylactoid purpura and allergic vasculitis, etc., as separate entities. It is, however, now generally accepted that these are all variations on a single theme based on the deposition of immune complexes and complement in or around the vessel walls and the consequent Arthus-type inflammatory reaction. The majority of the small dermal vessels involved in this process are venous channels and it therefore seems appropriate to use the term angiitis rather than the previously used term of arteritis.

These conditions must be distinguished from the small haemorrhagic areas of bleeding into the skin (purpura) seen in association with increased venous pressure (stasis) or in deficiency states such as scurvy. In such cases histological examination will show merely extravasation of red cells into the dermis with perhaps some swelling of the capillary endothelium. Later the red cells disintegrate and collections of

haemosiderin-laden macrophages indicate the site of previous haemorrhage.

In true angiitis there are conspicuous changes both in the vessel wall and in the tissues surrounding the vessels. The cutaneous lesions of angiitis tend to occur in dependent parts of the body where there is some slowing of the venous return. The lower limbs are particularly affected where, in addition to a certain amount of slowing of the venous return due to the site, there is further slowing of the blood flow due to cooling which increases the viscosity. The combination of slowing of the circulation and increased viscosity is thought to favour the deposition of immune complexes which initiate the pathological changes. In the early stage activation of complement by deposited immune complexes attracts neutrophil leucocytes in and around the walls of the small cutaneous vessels. Many of these neutrophils disintegrate, releasing proteolytic enzymes which further damage the vessel wall. At this stage the endothelium is swollen and there is dense perivascular poly-

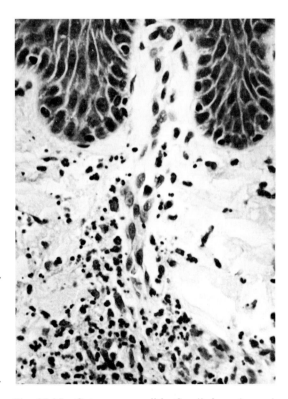

Fig. 27.25 Cutaneous angiitis. Small dermal vessel showing polymorphonuclear infiltration in and around the wall. × 350.

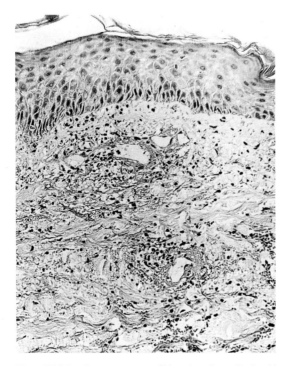

Fig. 27.26 Cutaneous angiitis showing fibrinoid necrosis of dermal vessels. There is haemorrhage under the epidermis and a marked perivascular inflammatory infiltrate. × 200.

morphonuclear leucocytic infiltration which invades the vessel wall. Much nuclear dust is seen from the disintegrating polymorphs and at this stage the term *leucocytoclastic angiitis* is often used (Fig. 27.25). The damage to the vessel wall allows red cells to escape into the tissue (purpura) and deposition of various amounts of fibrin. The vessel wall finally undergoes necrosis and becomes surrounded by a mixture of fibrin and polymorphonuclear leucocytes (Fig. 27.26)—*necrotising angiitis*. Despite the extensive involvement of these small cutaneous vessels, ulceration of the overlying epidermis occurs only rarely (*purpura necrotica*). This immune complex angiitis may be seen following acute bacterial infections, adverse reactions to drugs, as a manifestation of systemic lupus erythematosus and as a cutaneous manifestation of visceral malignancy.

Connective Tissue Diseases

Lupus erythematosus

Two basic types of this condition are recognised: (1) chronic discoid lupus erythematosus (CDLE), which is confined to the skin and is benign, and (2) systemic lupus erythematosus (SLE), in which visceral vascular lesions predominate (see p. 23.59) and which may be fatal, usually from renal involvement (p. 22.35). It may run its entire course without cutaneous manifestations. Intermediate forms between these extremes are encountered and transition from one type to another occurs, but is rare. In the systemic form of the disorder the cutaneous lesions are sometimes identical to those seen in chronic discoid lupus erythematosus.

Histologically, it is not usually possible to distinguish unequivocally between the two forms of lupus erythematosus, for many features are common to both. There is hyperkeratosis with plugging of follicular orifices (Fig. 27.27), liquefaction degeneration of the basal layer and epidermal thinning (Figs. 27.28, 27.29). In the dermis there is lymphocytic infiltration, particularly around the dermal appendages, focal oedema and occasionally haemorrhages: colloid bodies may be present in the upper dermis. A diagnosis of lupus erythematosus should not be made in the absence of liquefaction degeneration which, together with various degrees of the other features described, may provide a picture suggestive of the diagnosis. Similar findings may, however, be seen in lichen planus, and the clinical history and findings must be taken into account in interpreting a biopsy. Immunofluorescence tests are helpful in diagnosis and distinguishing between the two types of lupus erythematosus. In both condi-

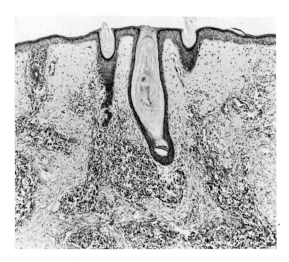

Fig. 27.27 Chronic discoid lupus erythematosus. Flattening of rete ridges, follicular plugging and focal lymphocytic infiltration of the dermis are seen. ×40.

tions, direct IF tests (p. 6.11) reveal in most cases granular deposition of immunoglobulin (usually IgG and IgM) and complement components in the vicinity of the basement

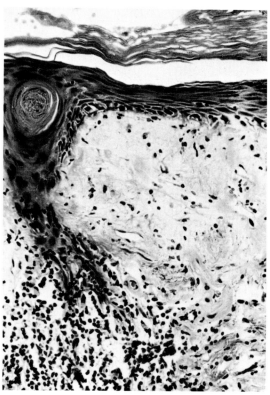

Fig. 27.29 Systemic lupus erythematosus. Liquefaction degeneration of the basal layer with oedema and fibrinoid change in the collagen of the upper dermis. ×200.

membrane of *affected* skin. In most cases of SLE a positive result is observed also in areas of clinically *normal* skin from *exposed* areas, whereas such areas are negative in CDLE.

In SLE antinuclear antibodies, usually in high titre, are almost always demonstrable by immunofluorescence. Rheumatoid factor is also sometimes present in SLE, 'standard' serological tests for syphilis (p. 9.31) often give (false) positive reactions, and occasionally auto-antibodies to red cells or platelets develop. Indeed, SLE is notable for the high incidence and variety of auto-antibodies (p. 7.26). In CDLE, the incidence of autoantibodies is much lower.

Morphoea (scleroderma) and systemic sclerosis

Much confusion has been caused by the use of the term scleroderma to describe two different diseases, *morphoea* and *progressive systemic sclerosis*. **Progressive systemic sclerosis** (p. 23.62) is a generalised condition, involving the skin

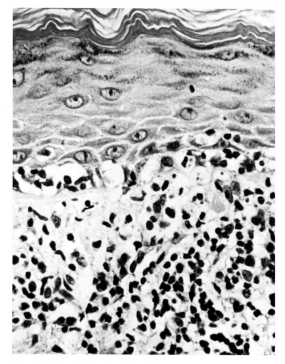

Fig. 27.28 Chronic discoid lupus erythematosus. Liquefaction degeneration of the basal layer of the epidermis. ×300.

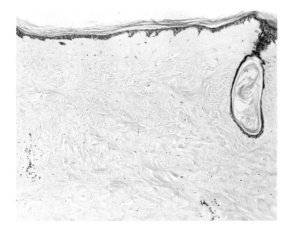

Fig. 27.30 Morphoea. Note the flattening of the rete ridges and the increase in thickness of the dermal collagen. Dermal appendages are absent. × 40.

Lichen sclerosus et atrophicus. This is a disease of unknown cause, affecting primarily the dermal connective tissue, and is conveniently described here. It is seen in the vulva as white patches which clinically may simulate malignancy, but it also occurs elsewhere in the skin in both sexes. Histological examination shows a characteristic picture of hyperkeratosis over a thinned epidermis which shows liquefaction degeneration of the basal layer. In typical cases, a split is seen at the epidermal–dermal interface, and the upper dermis has a pale hyaline appearance (Fig. 24.1, p. 24.2) with virtual absence of elastic fibres. A linear band of lymphocytes and histiocytes is present at the upper margin of the reticular dermis.

and other organs. Scleroderma should be used only as an alternative name for morphoea, which consists of areas of hardening of the skin and does not affect the viscera. Both are chronic diseases, developing most often in the 3rd–5th decades, and affect both sexes.

Morphoea (scleroderma) consists of localised patches or larger areas of thickening and hardening of the skin. In the early stages, an erythematous halo is seen at the margin of the lesion. Microscopy shows thickening of the dermal collagen extending into the subcutaneous tissue, together with a light chronic inflammatory cellular infiltrate. The lesions spread for a variable period and then regress with depigmentation and thinning of the epidermis and loss of rete ridges, sweat glands and hair follicles and their surrounding fatty tissue (Fig. 27.30). The dermal collagen fibres appear swollen and coarse elastic fibres can be seen lying parallel with the surface.

Progressive systemic sclerosis. The histological picture seen in this condition may be similar to that of localised scleroderma or morphoea. However, occasionally the only pathological features present may be some atrophy of the skin and its appendages but with the maintenance of the normal overall architecture (Fig. 27.31) so that the appearances are those of 'the skin in miniature'.

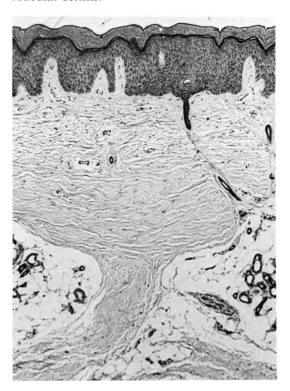

Fig. 27.31 Progressive systemic sclerosis. The microanatomy of the skin is maintained but the sweat glands and subcutaneous fat are much nearer the surface. Although from different regions of the skin, this figure and Fig. 27.30 are taken at the same magnification, illustrating the difference between systemic sclerosis and morphoea. × 40.

Granulomatous Diseases of the Skin

The tissue response of granulomatous inflammation is seen in many varied skin disorders and most commonly represents a host response to an exogenous microbial organism or some other foreign material. Evaluation of cutaneous granulomatous inflammation usually requires a search for specific organisms with special stains although it must be remembered that in many infectious conditions the causal organisms are hard to find. Some of the conditions which may produce granulomatous disease in the skin have been discussed in previous chapters. These include tuberculosis, leprosy, sarcoidosis, syphilis and deep fungal infections. Among the non-microbial materials that may excite a granulomatous foreign body response are keratin and hair, paraffin and greases, plant materials such as thorns, minerals including beryllium, zirconium and asbestos, tattoo pigment, calcium and bone.

Three granulomatous skin lesions, lupus vulgaris, granuloma annulare and necrobiosis lipoidica, require a brief description.

Lupus vulgaris. Tuberculosis of the skin is rare nowadays, but occasional examples of lupus vulgaris are still seen. It presents as one or more reddish-brown patches, usually on the skin of the face, in which small yellow-brown macules ('apple-jelly nodules') may be discerned by viewing the lesion through a glass slide pressed onto the skin. The nodules consist of well-defined tubercles with little or no caseation. The lesion lies in the dermis and often extends up to the epidermis through which it may eventually ulcerate. The condition progresses slowly and results in scarring with atrophy of the skin and disfigurement. Tubercle bacilli are rarely detectable in suitably stained histological sections.

Granuloma annulare and necrobiosis lipoidica. These two conditions form what are known as *palisading granulomas*. Granuloma annulare is seen mainly in children and young adults, as varying numbers of non-itchy, raised annular papules, often on the fingers and the backs of the hands. It may also affect the subcutaneous tissue and is then closely similar to rheumatoid

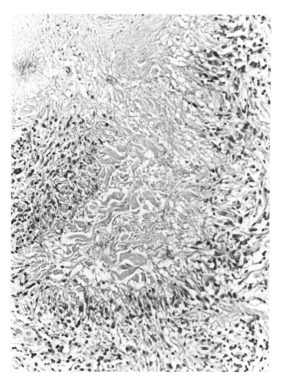

Fig. 27.32 Granuloma annulare. The lesion consists of a central acellular area of necrosis which is surrounded by a palisade of macrophages and, more peripherally, a mixture of chronic inflammatory cells. × 150.

nodules (p. 23.46). Necrobiosis lipoidica has been associated traditionally with diabetes, but may also occur in non-diabetics. The lesions appear most often in the legs, as reddish patches which slowly spread and have a yellow centre. Scarring occurs and ulceration is occasionally seen.

In both conditions a central area of collagen degeneration is surrounded by an infiltrate of macrophages (Fig. 27.32). Multinucleated giant cells may be present and differentiation of the two conditions may depend on clinico-pathological correlation. However, the granuloma formation in necrobiosis lipoidica tends to be more 'untidy' and extends more deeply than the pallisading granuloma seen in granuloma annulare.

Tumours of the Skin

The skin is a large and complex organ in which the epidermal cells are labile and thus continuously dividing. They are also directly exposed to many carcinogenic agents in the environment and it is therefore not surprising that epithelial tumours are numerous. The skin is the site, above all others, where many malignant tumours which would otherwise prove fatal can be treated effectively by early detection and excision.

Skin tumours can be classified readily according to cell type. Epithelial tumours may arise from the epidermis, sweat glands or hair follicles: dermal tumours may arise from the fibrous, vascular, nervous or lymphoreticular elements and a third group arises from melanocytes. Some of the most important tumours, such as squamous carcinoma, have been dealt with already in Chapter 12 as local representatives of more general types, but many other tumours are peculiar to the skin.

Epidermal tumours

Embryological studies have revealed that the keratinocytes of the skin undergo specific differentiation at an early stage in development; three distinct cell lines are produced and form the surface epidermis, the pilo-sebaceous complexes and the sweat apparatus. This probably explains the differing biological behaviour of tumours arising from the epidermis and its appendages.

Two sharply distinct types of tumour arise from the surface epidermis, the *squamous group* and the so-called *basal-cell group* which includes basal-cell papilloma (verruca senilis) and basal-cell carcinoma (rodent ulcer). Tumours of the sweat glands form a heterogeneous group and are discussed later.

Basal-cell papilloma (verruca senilis) is a common benign warty growth seen most often on the trunk of older people. It appear as a soft, raised, flattened, sessile, brown patch, usually with a rough surface, Microscopically it consists chiefly of basal-like cells, with relatively little differentiation into keratinised cells unless irritated: keratin is however formed, often in fairly large amounts, characteristically in spherical masses (horn cysts) within the epithelium and sometimes reaching the surface (Fig. 27.33). Melanocytes are usually present among the basal-like cells and melanin is often abundant, accounting for the pigmentation which may cause clinical confusion with malignant melanoma. Mitoses are usually absent, growth

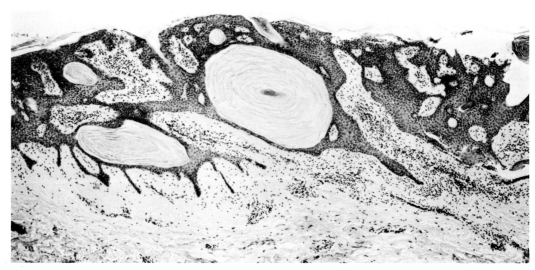

Fig. 27.33 Basal-cell papilloma. A flat papillary tumour composed of basal-like epidermal cells. Note the several 'pearls' of keratin formation within the epithelium. × 50.

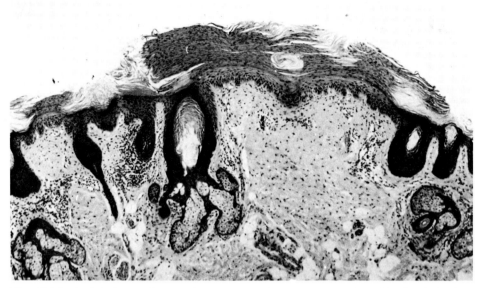

Fig. 27.34 Actinic keratosis, showing a patch of epithelial atrophy with dysplasia, hyperkeratosis and parakeratosis. × 25.

is slow and malignancy so rare that cases can mostly be explained as coincidences or mistaken diagnoses. The name **seborrhoeic keratosis,** sometimes applied to these tumours, indicates their common occurrence on so-called seborrhoeic sites (forehead, chest and back).

'Squamous' group

The cells of these tumours form neoplastic stratified squamous epithelium. Cancer originates in stem cells in the basal layer (p. 12.4) and the tumour cells show various degrees of differentiation towards squames. In the benign tumours, the undifferentiated basal layer is only one cell thick, and the differentiated cells and the keratin more conspicuous than in normal skin, but with increasing malignancy the undifferentiated cells become more numerous and keratin formation diminishes, though in skin tumours it hardly ever disappears altogether.

Squamous papilloma is the benign member of this group. Most are viral in origin, and seen usually on the hands of children **(juvenile warts),** on the soles of the feet of those who use communal changing-rooms **(plantar warts),** and about the genitalia of those exposed to venereal infection **(condylomata acuminata).** If one excludes viral tumours, and the keratoses dealt with in the next section, the squamous papillomas (Fig. 12.15, p. 12.12) are probably very rare. Malignant change in a skin papilloma is extremely rare, though occasionally genital tumours show an exuberant growth hard to distinguish from malignancy.

Squamous keratosis. This is the best name for the premalignant lesions of this group. When the aetiology is known, such terms as *actinic* or *arsenical keratoses* are commonly used, and in old people they may be called *senile keratoses,* but the lesions are indentical. They are typically dry, rough-surfaced thickenings, arising usually in an area of skin which shows, by its thinness (Fig. 27.34), inelasticity and irregular pigmentation, the effects of prolonged exposure to sunlight or other carcinogens: the face and the back of the hands are the usual sites.

Histologically one sees all stages from the slightest thickening and irregularity of the epidermis to large lesions with gross irregular hyperplasia of the epithelium, a massive overlying layer of keratin, and greatly enlarged rete ridges, the cells of which appear to be on the brink of invasion. The hallmark of these lesions is the presence of alternating columns of hyperkeratosis and parakeratosis. Nuclear pleomorphism, frequency of mitoses and disordered, irregular cellular differentiation usually increase in parallel with the above changes. Sometimes, severe cytological changes occur in the presence of relatively minor general hyperplasia, and the term **carcinoma in situ** of

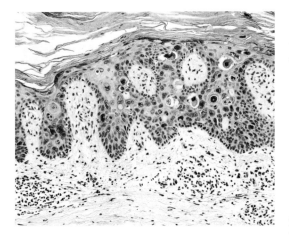

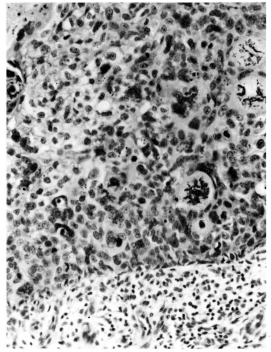

Fig. 27.35 Bowen's disease of the skin. *Above,* showing the large, abnormal cells in the epidermis. × 60. *Below,* showing more cellular detail, including enlarged and clumped nuclei and aberrant mitoses. × 160.

the skin might reasonably include this condition.

Squamous keratosis, from whatever cause, is the most important precursor of invasive squamous-cell carcinoma of the epidermis.

Bowen's disease. Although this is an epidermal hyperplasia which may progress to squamous-cell carcinoma, it is very different from squamous keratosis. It may arise anywhere in the skin, but nearly always in non-exposed areas. While squamous keratosis blends into surrounding skin, which is itself abnormal, Bowen's disease is sharply circumscribed from normal skin, forming rounded, reddish patches which enlarge slowly over a period of years. The epidermis in the affected area shows marked hyperplasia, with deep but fairly regular rete ridges and usually not much keratin: cellular de-differentiation is prominent, and large cells with multiple large clumped nuclei are a characteristic feature (Fig. 27.35). The importance of recognising Bowen's disease, which is another form of carcinoma in situ, is twofold. First, it may look like (and is often treated for years as) a patch of psoriasis or other chronic skin disease. Secondly, defective and irregular differentiation of the epidermis, which in a squamous keratosis showing carcinoma in situ would mean imminent invasion, in Bowen's disease is compatible with many years of continued limitation to the surface—even though ultimate invasion may occur.

Squamous-cell carcinoma. The description of squamous-cell carcinoma in Chapter 12, and the discussion on its aetiology in Chapter 13, make it unnecessary to say much of this important skin tumour. The great majority are better differentiated than the average mucosal squamous carcinoma: this, combined with accessibility, makes for a relatively good prognosis. Dissemination, when it does occur, is by the same routes of local, lymph and blood spread as with other carcinomas. It may arise anywhere on the body surface, but in most countries the face, the pinna of the ears and the backs of the hands are the commonest sites. The muco-cutaneous junctions are also important sites, but the tumours mostly arise on the mucosal side of the junction: thus, most lip tumours arise from the red margin, most anal tumours within the canal, and most penile tumours from the glans. In the vulva, however, most squamous carcinomas arise in the true skin of the labia majora, the modified skin of the labia minora being a less common site.

The tumours of the exposed surfaces presumably arise chiefly from the effect of ultra-violet light in sunlight. Industrial exposure usually produces tumours of the hands and forearms, but with carcinogens which penetrate the clothes, such as the lighter mineral oils and dusts like soot (Fig. 12.24, p. 12.17) and powdered arsenic, the scrotum becomes an important site probably because its rugose surface traps dirt. The relation of circumcision to cancer is a particularly interesting one (p. 25.6). The majority of penile cancers are associated with an intact foreskin and a low standard of personal hygiene.

There is a small but clinically important group of squamous carcinomas which arise in areas of old scars caused by burns, at the edges of long-standing ulcers (the so-called *Marjolin's ulcer*) and in sinuses, presumably as a result of hyperplasia following prolonged attempts at healing.

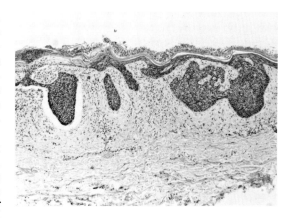

Fig. 27.36 Basal-cell carcinoma, showing the apparently multicentric origin from the base of the epidermis. × 32.

Basal-cell carcinoma (rodent ulcer)

The typical basal-cell carcinoma begins as a slow-growing, flattened nodule of the skin of the face. The centre breaks down, forming a shallow ulcer, but the periphery of the nodule persists to form a smooth, slightly raised margin to the ulcer which, as the tumour grows, illustrates well the characteristic raised, 'rolled' edge of ulcerated malignant tumours. If not successfully treated, the ulcer spreads slowly, and ultimately erodes deeper and destroys the underlying structures of the face. Death results, if at all (for nowadays treatment is rarely so unsuccessful), from destruction of mouth and nose, or from invasion of the cranial cavity, most often via the orbit.

Neither lymph spread nor blood spread is seen except as the greatest of rarities. This is the only common malignant tumour other than those within the cranial cavity (where conditions are exceptional) which shows this extreme disinclination to metastasise, a finding that remains entirely unexplained.

Histologically, the tumour begins with groups of small dark basal-like cells, apparently sprouting from the undersurface of intact epidermis (Fig. 27.36). These cell groups enlarge and grow down into the dermis, forming clumps with an outer layer of columnar cells which resemble the basal layer of the epidermis. Instead, however, of the keratinocytes which one would expect to see arising from this basal layer, the centre of each clump is occupied by a solid mass of darkly-staining spheroidal cells (Fig. 27.37). The term basal-cell carcinoma in-

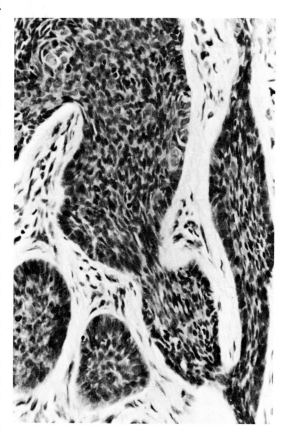

Fig. 27.37 Basal-cell carcinoma. The dermis is invaded by clumps of small, darkly-staining tumour cells resembling basal epidermal cells. The peripheral cells in places present a palisaded appearance. × 250.

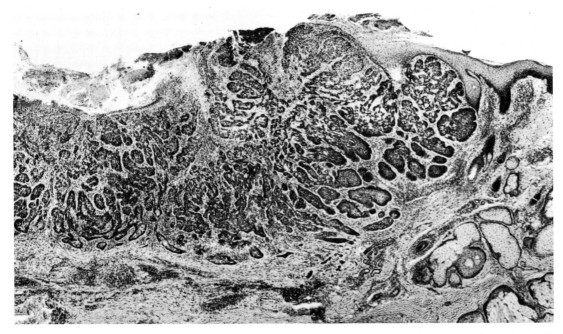

Fig. 27.38   Basal-cell carcinoma, showing the flat, shallow ulceration. Note the extension laterally which accounts for the 'rolled' border. × 33.

dicates the similarity of the tumour cells to the basal-cell layer of the surface epithelium, but should not be taken to imply that they originate from the basal layer of the surface epidermis.

Continued proliferation of the cell masses beneath the epidermis gives rise to a nodule: breakdown of the overlying epidermis and central part of the tumour results in ulceration and infection (Fig. 27.38). The characteristic rolled border is due to lateral invasion of the tumour under the intact epidermis.

The detailed histology of these tumours varies considerably, but the well-defined single peripheral columnar layer ('palisading'—one of several different uses of this word in pathology), and the predominance of 'basal' cells, are constant. The cell masses may be large and uniform, or narrow and ribbon-like. Small patches of squamous differentiation or even keratinisation may cause confusion with squamous carcinoma if one is not aware of their frequency in basal-cell carcinomas. Small cystic spaces form at times, some genuine, some the result of stromal degeneration. Inclusion of a few melanocytes from the original epidermis is common, and occasionally the tumour is sufficiently heavily pigmented to cause clinical confusion with

melanoma. Little attention should be paid to the number of mitoses, which can be surprisingly numerous for such slowly-growing tumours. One variety meriting special mention is the sclerotic type, in which the stromal reaction to the tumour is unusually marked and small thin strands of epithelium are buried in dense fibrous tissue: this results in the edge being ill-defined and may lead to inadequate excision with consequent 'recurrence'.

Sites. Though they can be found anywhere on the skin (except the palms and soles) most basal-cell carcinomas occur in a relatively restricted area of the face, in front of the ears, above the mouth and below the supra-orbital ridges. In this area, sunlight produces far more basal-cell carcinomas than squamous carcinomas (in some parts of Australia it is the exception for a fair-skinned man to reach the age of 75 without having had at least one basal-cell carcinoma on the face). In other sites the reverse holds, and a radiation-induced basal-cell carcinoma of the trunk, for instance, or one arising in the margin of a varicose ulcer of the skin, is much less often seen than the corresponding squamous carcinoma.

Tumours of sweat glands (hidradenomas)

These form a distinct group of varied and often bizarre histological appearances but characteristically they exhibit a two-layered epithelium and show evidence of mucin secretion. Arising from the **eccrine sweat glands** are three main types: (1) from the intra-epidermal portion of the sweat duct, the *eccrine poroma*; (2) from the intradermal portion of the sweat duct, (*a*) the *nodular* and (*b*) the *tubular hidradenoma*. The nodular type (Fig. 27.39a) consists of solid masses and cords of cells forming occasional duct-like structures containing mucin. The tubular type (Fig. 27.39b) consists of branching duct-like structures lined by a double layer of epithelium and containing mucin embedded in a prominent fibrous stroma; (3) arising from the secretory coils, the *eccrine spiradenoma*. Most eccrine sweat gland tumours are benign although nodular hidradenomas may exhibit local invasion and recurrence after removal. True metastasising sweat gland tumours (hidradenocarcinomas) are rare. The **apocrine sweat glands** may also give rise to tumours, the commonest being the benign *hidradenoma papilliferum* of the vulva and the *cylindroma* or turban tumour of the scalp.

Tumours of pilo-sebaceous follicles

These are even less common than sweat gland tumours. True sebaceous adenomas are very rare. An uncommon tumour which probably arises in the hair matrix is the so-called '*benign calcifying epithelioma*' of Malherbe (pilomatricoma). This forms a slowly growing encapsulated rounded mass lying under the skin, arising anywhere on the body surface and at any age but most commonly in the first two decades. Calcification occurs in over 70% and may be extensive and spectacular, sometimes with ossification. The tumour epithelial cells are small, darkly-staining and regular and form disproportionately large masses of keratin in which ghosts of the cells that have formed it can often be seen. Rupture of the capsule may be followed by a foreign-body giant-cell reaction, which appears to predispose to the calcification, although direct calcification of ghost-cell areas of keratin in the intact tumour may also occur.

Keratoacanthoma (molluscum sebaceum). This tumour-like but self-healing lesion is much commoner than any of the true hair follicle tumours. It occurs predominantly on the face of adults. A nodule in the skin appears and grows rapidly for about eight weeks, producing a rounded, slightly umbilicated mass of 10–20mm diameter (Fig. 27.40). It stops growing, the central dimple enlarges and becomes dry and scaly, the central plug is discharged and the lesion heals: the whole process usually takes about six months.

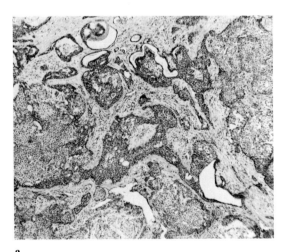

a

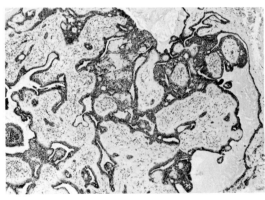

b

Fig. 27.39 Hidradenomas of intradermal sweat duct origin. **(a).** Nodular hidradenoma, consisting of solid masses of pale-staining cells with occasional duct-like structures (which contain PAS-positive material). **(b).** Tubular hidradenoma, showing the typical branching duct-like structures lined by two-layered epithelium and embedded in a hyaline stroma. × 30.

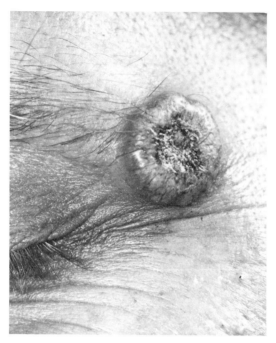

Fig. 27.40   Keratoacanthoma. Clinical photograph of an eight-week-old lesion near the eye. A firm rounded nodule with epidermis stretched over the edge, and a central crater where the keratin core is exposed. × 1·5.

Histologically, the resemblance to squamous carcinoma is very close during the active phase, so much so that it was only after 1950 that it won general recognition as a distinct lesion which did not require to be treated as a carcinoma. The appearances which mimic invasion are, however, considered by some to result from rapid irregular overgrowth of a group of hair follicles (Fig. 27.41). During the stationary phase, the epithelium so formed is progressively keratinised, and the resulting mass of keratin is finally discharged. Recognition of this lesion is obviously of great importance in treatment. An important diagnostic feature is the superficial nature of the lesion, well seen in Fig. 27.41: the apparently invasive deep surface lies at or above the level of the skin appendages. In the later stages, polymorphs migrate into the epithelial masses, a feature not usual in squamous carcinoma. It is important to examine histologically the edge of the lesion, which shows abrupt transition from normal to the hyperplastic epithelium. These features are of value in distinguishing the lesion from squamous car-

cinoma, although this is not always possible even when the clinical history is taken into account.

Self-healing squamous-cell carcinoma of the skin. This is a rare familial disorder which begins usually in early adult life and is characterised by the appearance at intervals of tumours of the skin, mostly, but not exclusively, of the exposed parts, which are indistinguishable histologically from squamous-cell carcinomas. After some months of activity, each lesion in succession undergoes involution by keratinisation of the infiltrating columns of cells and discharge of the dead cells leaving shallow depressed pits. It is quite unrelated to keratoacanthoma.

Melanocytic tumours

The following account attempts to give a clear if somewhat oversimplified explanation of a complex series of phenomena, interpretation of which is still controversial.

Early in fetal life specialised cells migrate from the neural crest and settle in the skin, the uveal tract of the eye and the leptomeninges, in which sites they are known as melanocytes.

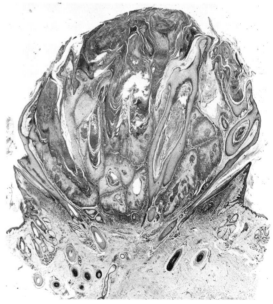

Fig. 27.41   Keratoacanthoma. A lesion about the same age as Fig. 27.40. Note the resemblance to squamous-cell carcinoma. × 12.

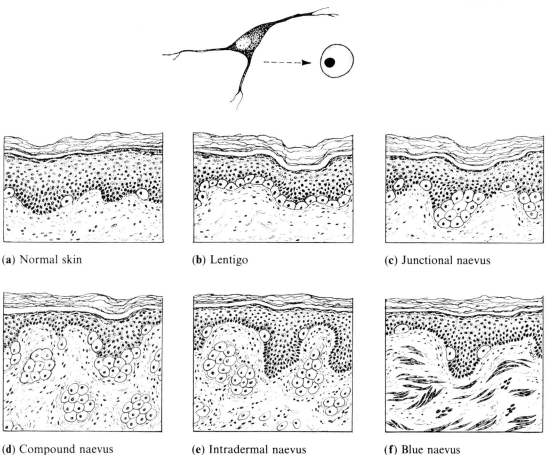

(a) Normal skin   **(b)** Lentigo   **(c)** Junctional naevus

(d) Compound naevus   **(e)** Intradermal naevus   **(f)** Blue naevus

Fig. 27.42 Diagram of the origin and evolution of pigmented naevi. At the top of the diagram the dendritic melanocyte, the cell of origin, is seen. Stained by the DOPA reaction, this has a triangular body with long branching processes (dendrites). In fixed tissue sections this cell appears rounded with clear cytoplasm. The distribution of melanocytes in normal skin is seen in **(a)**. Replacement of the basal layer of the epidermis by melanocytes is the **lentigo (b)**. Focal proliferation of melanocytes is the **junctional pigmented naevus (c)**, and this proliferation at the dermo-epidermal junction is called **junctional change.** Some of these nodules descend into the dermis to become adult naevus cells and the combination of junctional change and intradermal naevus cells is the **compound pigmented naevus (d)**. Junctional activity ceases and masses of mature naevus cells lie in the dermis, the **intradermal naevus (e)**. Occasionally melanocytes en route from the neural crest may be arrested in the dermis where they form the **Mongolian spot or blue naevus (f)**.

Melanocytic tumours arise from these cells. Those melanocytes which migrate to the skin come to lie among the basal cells of the epidermis in the ratio of 1:10 to 1:5, depending on the anatomical site. The number of melanocytes per unit area of skin is constant irrespective of race or skin coloration.

Occasionally some melanocytes fail to reach the epidermis, developing within the dermis to form a Mongolian spot or a more compact mass termed a blue naevus (p. 27.36).

During infancy, the balance between the normal ratio of melanocytes to basal epidermal cells breaks down at a few or many sites: the melanocytes multiply too rapidly and become too numerous to be accommodated in their normal position. The lesions resulting from this proliferation of melanocytes are known as pigmented naevi. While precise details of the evolution of these lesions is not known, the probable course is shown in diagrammatic form in Fig. 27.42.

Initially the proliferating melanocytes replace the basal layer of the epidermis over a given area and at this stage the lesion is known as a *lentigo* (Fig. 27.42b). (This should not be confused with an ephilis or freckle, in which there is an increase in melanin pigmentation of the basal layer without an increase in the numbers of melanocytes). The next stage is more focal proliferation of the melanocytes and the formation of small nodules within the epidermis which bulge downwards into the dermis: this lesion is known as the *junctional naevus* (Fig. 27.42c). Eventually the basement membrane is disrupted and some of the nodules or packets of melanocytes pass down into the dermis. At this stage, where there is a combination of junctional activity and nests of melanocytes in the dermis, the lesion is known as a *compound pigmented naevus* (Fig. 27.42d). The melanocytes which reach the dermis soon lose their melanin-synthesising enzymes, become smaller and lose the power to proliferate and are known as *naevus cells*. At or around puberty, in the majority of instances junctional activity ceases, the naevus cells in the dermis undergo further maturation and a certain amount of fibrosis occurs. At this stage the lesion is known as an *intradermal naevus* and may remain as such for life. (Fig. 27.42e).

While the above account is thought to represent the normal evolution of these lesions it should be emphasised that *maturation may be arrested at any of the stages described*. In addition, *similar stages of melanocytic proliferation may occur in adult life*, either after exposure to ultraviolet light or from as yet imperfectly understood hormonal changes.

The principal types of pigmented naevus are described below. They are extremely common lesions: few people have none at all and some have many: the mean number per person is said to be 18.

Lentigo. Clinically this presents as a flat blemish on any part of the skin surface, varying in colour from pale brown to deep black. *It is not possible to distinguish these lesions clinically with any certainty from junctional naevi.* Histologically one sees stretches of the basal layer of the epidermis replaced by melanocytes, which appear in fixed tissue sections as rounded cells with abundant clear cytoplasm. Many of the melanocytes contain varying amounts of fine granular brown melanin pigment. In the under-

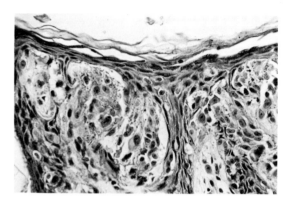

Fig. 27.43 Junctional pigmented naevus. Note the groups of melanocytes lying in the deeper part of the epidermis. × 200.

lying dermis, macrophages containing coarser granules of darker melanin pigment are usually seen.

In older persons, on sun-exposed skin, a variant of the lentigo, the *lentigo maligna*, may be encountered (p. 27.34).

Junctional pigmented naevus. As already stated, the clinical appearance of the junctional naevus is virtually indistinguishable from the lentigo. In older lesions, examined with a lens in a good light, small areas of darker speckled pigmentation, corresponding to the nests of junctional activity, can be detected.

Histologically the junctional naevus is composed of rounded aggregates (or packets) of melanocytes which, while occurring at any level of the epidermis, tend to be in the lower layers and to bulge down into the underlying dermis, giving the undersurface of the epidermis an irregular configuration (Fig. 27.43). It is this proliferation of melanocytes at the dermoepidermal junction which gives the junctional naevus its name.

Compound pigmented naevus. This is the commonest type of pigmented naevus in late childhood. Clinically such lesions are usually raised above the surface: they may be papillomatous in appearance and vary in colour from pale brown to black. In some instances the hair follicles are increased in number and abnormally large, and various numbers of coarse dark hairs can be seen growing from the surface of the lesion. Rarely such hairy pigmented naevi may cover an extensive area of the skin surface (giant hairy naevus). Such cases may also be associated with diffuse meningeal melanomato-

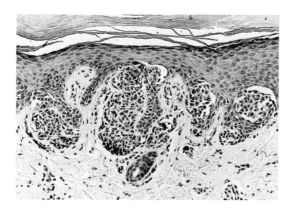

Fig. 27.44 Compound pigmented naevus. Some groups of proliferated melanocytes lie in the deeper part of the epidermis. Other groups have become separated from the epidermis and lie in the superficial dermis. × 100.

sis and can undergo malignant transformation in childhood (see below).

Histologically compound naevi show junctional activity in the overlying epidermis. In the dermis are loose aggregates of rounded inactive-looking cells, some of which contain granules of melanin pigment. The deeper these cells lie in the dermis, the smaller they tend to be (Fig. 27.44). The cells are often called naevus cells but in order to avoid confusion with other naevi (e.g. angiomas) they should always be referred to as pigmented naevus cells. In the connective tissue of the dermis between the nests of pigmented naevus cells are found varying numbers of macrophages containing coarser granules of melanin pigment. The gross colour of pigmented naevi depends largely on the numbers and content of these macrophages.

'Dysplastic naevus'. This term has been applied by Elder et al. (1980) to certain atypical naevi that seem to have an increased risk of progression to malignant melanoma. Clinically, these lesions tend to be multiple, flat and relatively large with irregular borders and variable pigmentation. Histological characteristics include melanocytic proliferation at the epidermodermal junction with some cytological atypia and other changes in dermal blood vessels and connective tissue. The disorder may be familial and the terms '*B-K mole syndrome*' and the '*familial atypical multiple mole melanoma (FAMMM) syndrome*' are sometimes used to describe this inherited form of the condition.

Juvenile melanoma. (Spitz naevus). This variant of the benign compound pigmented naevus is important because it may sometimes be mistaken histologically for a malignant melanoma, especially if the age of the patient is not known. It is commonest in children although no age group is exempt. Junctional proliferation of melanocytes is present but sometimes relatively sparse. At the epidermodermal junction and in the papillary dermis the naevus cells are often bizarre and atypical with large, sometimes multiple nuclei and with large amounts of eosinophilic cytoplasm. In the deeper dermal portions of the lesion there is a tendency for the tumour cells to become smaller and more regular, resembling the intradermal naevus cells of a compound naevus. The overall low power architecture of a juvenile melanoma tends to be symmetrical and this is a helpful feature in distinguishing it from invasive malignant melanoma. Melanin pigment is rarely prominent in typical juvenile melanoma. Other histological features which are of importance for diagnosis are pseudo-epitheliomatous hyperplasia and the presence of numerous large dilated vascular channels (Fig. 27.45). It is this latter feature which accounts for the reddish colour of these lesions to the naked eye.

Intradermal pigmented naevus. The vast majority of pigmented naevi in adults are of the intradermal type. Clinically these are similar in appearance to compound pigmented naevi, being sometimes raised and warty (Fig. 27.46), sometimes flat. Histologically there is no junctional activity in the epidermis although there may be an increase in the number of normal-

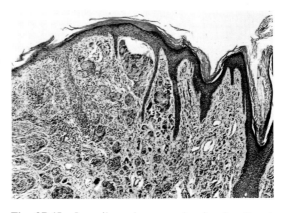

Fig. 27.45 Juvenile melanoma, showing junctional activity and extensive dermal infiltration. Note also the pseudo-epitheliomatous hyperplasia and dilated vascular channels. × 30.

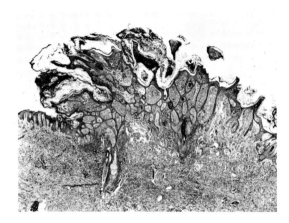

Fig. 27.46   Intradermal pigmented naevus of warty type. The dermal papillae are filled with naevus cells which extend widely in the underlying dermis. × 14.

looking melanocytes. The dermis is occupied by cells similar to those seen in the dermal component of the compound naevus (Fig. 27.47). In older lesions, particularly in the deeper parts,

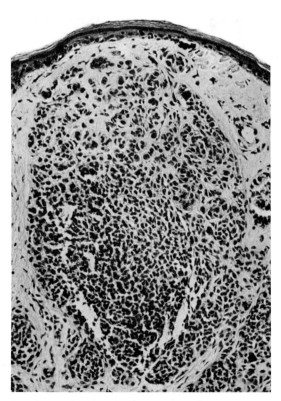

Fig. 27.47   Section through an intradermal naevus, showing collections of so-called 'naevus cells' underneath the epidermis. × 220.

there is often considerable fibrosis and some of the nests of pigmented naevus cells merge imperceptibly into bundles of elongated cells which bear a close resemblance to neurilemmal cells or sensory nerve endings, both of which, like melanocytes, are of neural crest origin. Such appearances are of no practical significance.

Relationship of pigmented naevi to malignant melanoma

Malignant melanoma is exceedingly rare before puberty. The main exception to this is in the case of the giant hairy pigmented naevus, a significant number of cases of which have been reported where death resulted either from metastases from the skin or from diffuse meningeal melanomatosis.

After puberty any pigmented naevus with junctional activity has the potential to undergo malignant change, but the proportion of lesions which undergo such change must be extremely small as malignant melanoma is not a common tumour.

Histological assessment of a junctional naevus from an adult is often difficult, and multiple sections of a suspicious lesion should be examined. Features of the proliferating melanocytes which should raise the suspicion of malignancy include a high mitotic rate, a cell size appreciably larger than the adjacent keratinocytes and the presence of melanin pigment and aberrant melanocytes in the superficial part of the epidermis.

Prophylactic excision of all pigmented lesions in adults is clearly impractical and the clinical features which warrant complete excision and examination are given on p. 27.36.

Malignant melanoma

This tumour, which arises from melanocytes, spreads locally and also by the lymphatics and blood to produce metastases. It arises in four main forms, described below.

Lentigo maligna or **Hutchinson's melanotic freckle** is a slowly growing, flat lesion of varying shades of brown, arising on the sun-exposed skin of the elderly. While this is essentially malignant melanoma *in situ*, it may be present for up to 20 years with different areas simultaneously developing and regressing. Over a

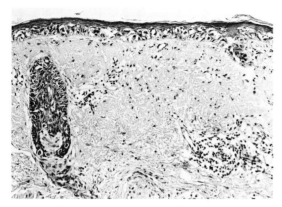

Fig. 27.48 Lentigo maligna. Melanocytes of variable appearance form a continuous deep layer in the epithelium and are seen also in the pilosebaceous unit. The dermis shows pronounced solar elastosis. ×30.

period of observation the lesion may thus appear to move within the skin. Eventually invasive malignant melanoma may develop. Histologically the basal layer of the epidermis is replaced by dysplastic, pleomorphic melanocytes which have a high nuclear-cytoplasmic ratio, and which may aggregate to give collections of spindle-celled junctional activity (Fig. 27.48). While there is little tendency to extend through the epidermis to the surface, the dysplastic melanocytes do extend into the skin appendages. Solar elastosis (degeneration and matting of the dermal elastic tissue) is usually present. The areas of regression show various degrees of epidermal atrophy, upper dermal telangiectasia, fibroblastic reaction and melanin lying free or within macrophages. Invasive malignant melanoma arising on the basis of a lentigo maligna has a relatively good prognosis.

Superficial spreading melanoma. This is a slightly raised, variably coloured lesion which can occur anywhere on the skin. The colour varies from brown in actively melanogenic areas to blue, white or red in regressed and regressing areas. The area of visible abnormality is usually smaller than in lentigo maligna. Invasive malignant melanoma generally develops from superficial spreading melanoma *in situ* in 5 to 7 years. Histologically there is a population of dysplastic and pleomorphic melanocytes at the epidermal-dermal junction (Fig. 27.49): these cells spread through the epidermis rather like the carcinoma cells in Paget's disease (p. 24.43). The invasive tumour which

results shows a variable histology but the cells often resemble epithelial cells. Diagnosis rests not on the invasive component but on the presence of abnormal melanocytes in the adjacent epidermis. Prognosis is worse than that for invasive melanoma arising in lentigo maligna, but somewhat better than that of nodular malignant melanoma.

Acral lentiginous and **mucosal melanomas.** These variants have recently been described as arising on the soles and palms and on mucosal surfaces respectively. They are characterised by melanocytic abnormality of the adjacent epidermis or mucosa which is similar to that of lentigo maligna except that actinic damage is not seen and the epithelium does not show atrophic changes. The prognosis is worse than that of superficial spreading melanoma.

Nodular melanoma. The above three types of malignant melanoma are characterised by a clinically detectable phase of melanoma *in situ* ('horizontal growth phase') from which an invasive melanoma ('vertical growth phase') develops. In nodular malignant melanoma there is neither clinical nor histological evidence of a horizontal growth phase. The invasive tumour apparently arises by transformation from a morphologically and numerically normal melanocyte population. The histology shows an epithelioid or spindle cell malignant melanoma (Fig. 27.50) with junctional activity confined to that area of epidermis immediately overlying the tumour. This variant carries the worst prognosis.

Other types of melanoma include the rare tumours which develop in congenital (bathing trunk) naevi and blue naevi. In some cases the patient presents with metastases and the primary tumour cannot be found.

The prognosis for patients with primary malignant melanoma is related to the depth of invasion of the tumour in the dermis, which may be assessed by comparison with the skin appendages (Clark, 1969) or by measuring the thickest part of the tumour (Breslow, 1970). The outlook is best when invasion is confined to the superficial dermis and worst when it has extended into the subcutaneous fat. Other morphological features which correlate with prognosis include the histogenetic types of melanoma (see above), the extent of ulceration, mitotic rate and local invasion of lymphatics.

Metastases occur commonly in the lymph

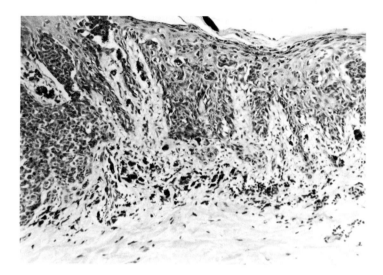

Fig. 27.49 Superficial spreading melanoma, showing proliferated dysplastic cells at the dermo-epidermal junction and in groups within the epidermis. On the left, invasion of the dermis has occurred. The black cells in the dermis are macrophages laden with melanin. × 80.

nodes and also by blood spread, particularly to the liver, brain, lungs, bowel and bone marrow. Widespread metastases may also appear in the skin, where they differ from the primary tumour in the absence of junctional activity and of an inflammatory flare. Metastases from deeply pigmented primary melanoma sometimes produce little or no pigment.

Clinical features suggesting that a pigmented naevus or melanoma *in situ* has undergone aggressive change include alteration in colour, spreading of pigment to the adjacent skin, itching, bleeding, ulceration, increase in size and the development of satellite lesions. Such changes in character of a pigmented lesion in an adult warrant its excision and examination. Any new pigmented lesion developing after the age of 20 years should be regarded with suspicion and excised for histological assessment. Diagnostic biopsy is only justified where total excision requires a very extensive or disabling resection.

Blue naevus

In these lesions there are accumulations of deeply pigmented cells in the dermis (Fig. 27.42f). These are melanocytes in the sense that they produce melanin: they correspond to no normal human cell but have some homology with the frog melanophores. The lesions are blue in colour as a result of an optical effect due to their depth beneath the surface. Occasionally elements of blue naevi and ordinary pigmented naevi occur together in one tumour (the **'combined naevus'**), producing a very confusing histological picture. Malignancy in blue naevi is very rare. Other conditions where dermal melanocytes occur include the common mongolian blue spot which represents a bluish discolouration of the skin, particularly the sacral area, present at birth and which tends to resolve in time, and the naevi of Ota (around the eye) and Ito (in the scapulo-humoral region).

Dermal tumours

With a few exceptions, these are less common and less important than the epithelial tumours. They are, however, too numerous in variety for any systematic treatment here and what follows consists only of notes on some of the more interesting kinds. Reference should be made elsewhere for fibromas (pp. 12.31; 23.63), lipomas (pp. 12.3; 23.66) and angiomas (p. 14.39) and their variants, which include several important skin tumours. Neurofibromas and schwannomas will be found on p. 21.64, and lymphoid tumours of the skin are discussed on p. 27.38.

Histiocytoma (Dermatofibroma)

This common lesion is usually found on the limbs and the clinical appearances are those of a smooth firm cutaneous papule. The histological appearances are rather variable but the main feature is the accumulation in the mid-

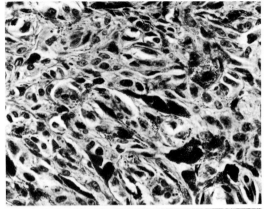

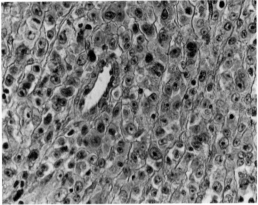

Fig. 27.50 Examples of nodular melanoma, illustrating the wide range of morphology. *Above*, a large spindle-celled tumour with abundant melanin production. *Below*, a tumour of epithelioid appearance with no obvious melanin production in this field. × 250.

dermis of a localized collection of macrophages and fibroblasts (Fig. 27.51). Blood vessels may occasionally be prominent in these lesions and when this is so haemosiderin pigment is also widely distributed throughout the lesion, particularly in macrophages. The term sclerosing haemangioma is sometimes given to the variety of dermatofibroma that shows fibrosis in association with vessel proliferation. Lipid-laden macrophages and multinucleated giant cells are also commonly seen in certain examples of dermatofibroma.

Dermatofibrosarcoma protuberans

Fibrosarcoma of the skin is represented by this lesion, which arises usually *de novo* from the skin of the trunk. It has the histology of any low-grade fibrosarcoma, and when small a characteristic hour-glass shape, with a base in the dermis and two nodules, one superficial pressing the epidermis outwards (hence 'protuberans') and one larger invading the deeper tissues. It is slow growing and rarely metastasises but recurs persistently after any but the most ruthless excision.

Lymphomas

The skin may be involved in all forms of malignant lymphoma although mycosis fungoides is the commonest single type of lymphoma that presents with skin lesions. Hodgkin's disease presenting in the skin without evidence of Hodgkin's disease elsewhere is extremely rare although this diagnosis is often mistakenly made on skin biopsy. Leukaemic deposits may be found in the skin and occasionally non-specific general dermatological symptoms such as erythema, pruritus and ichthyosis may be a sign of underlying malignant lymphoproliferative disease.

Mycosis fungoides. Mycosis fungoides is a T-cell lymphoma which primarily involves the skin but after many years disseminates to lymph nodes and other organs in a high proportion of those patients who do not die from other diseases. The characteristic histological changes may be preceded for many years by pruritic eruptions with non-specific histological

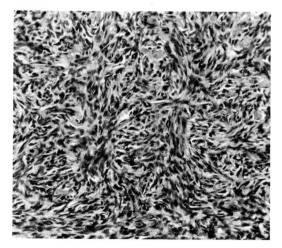

Fig. 27.51 Histiocytoma, showing the characteristic whorled pattern. × 154.

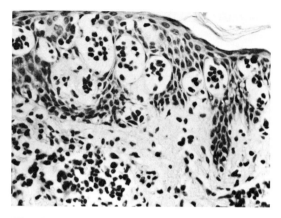

Fig. 27.52 Mycosis fungoides. Several Pautrier 'microabscesses' are seen in the epidermis. In the upper dermis there is a pleomorphic cellular infiltrate. × 265.

appearances in which only an occasional atypical cell raises the suspicion of its true nature. Serial biopsies may be necessary before the histological diagnosis can be made despite strong clinical suspicion of mycosis fungoides.

During the second and third stages of the disease, i.e. the stages of induration of the skin and the development of nodules of tumour respectively, skin biopsy usually shows characteristic changes. These consist of infiltration of the upper dermis by atypical lymphoid cells which usually vary considerably in size, shape, staining characteristics, nuclear appearances and mitotic activity. The lesions may contain also variable numbers of lymphocytes, plasma cells, plasmacytoid cells, free red blood cells, macrophages and occasional neutrophil polymorphs. There is a tendency for these mononuclear cells to infiltrate the epidermis and accumulate within epidermolytic spaces. In such situations they are known as 'Pautrier microabscesses' (Fig. 27.52), (a misnomer because they do not contain pus). While not invariably present, their presence is of considerable help in differentiating longstanding dermatitis from mycosis fungoides, and should always be sought by examination of multiple sections.

B-cell lymphoma. Skin involvement in B-cell lymphoma is less common than mycosis fungoides. Clinically the lesions tend to resemble one another and rarely show epidermal involvement. Multiple purplish dermal nodules are the most common presenting feature. The histopathological appearances consist of a dense, relatively monomorphic dermal infiltrate, sometimes also involving subcutaneous tissue. The epidermis is usually not involved and there is often a small band of papillary dermis that is free of infiltrate (the so-called grenz zone). The histopathological differentiation of B-cell cutaneous lymphomas from other non-malignant conditions can at times be difficult (see pseudolymphomas *below*).

Pseudolymphomas. There are many different dermatological diseases that show the histological features of a heavy dermal lymphocytic infiltrate with some degree of cytological atypia and may thus be confused with true malignant lymphoma. The most common of these conditions include the various lymphocytic infiltrates such as that of Jessner, lymphocytoma cutis and its variants, lymphomatoid papulosis and various inflammatory disorders such as syphilis, actinic reticuloid and insect bite reactions. The differentiation of these disorders from true lymphoma may on occasions be extremely difficult. Some features which favour a diagnosis of lymphoma are a very dense infiltrate, marked cytological atypia, mitotic figures, necrosis of dermal connective tissue and blood vessels, a monomorphic infiltrate without a mixture of other cell types and an infiltrate that extends to the subcutaneous fat. *Clinical details are of paramount importance in accurate histopathological assessment of lymphocytic infiltrates in the skin.*

References and Further Reading

General skin pathology

Ackerman, A.B. (1978). *Histologic Diagnosis of Inflammatory Skin Diseases*, pp. 863. Lea and Febiger, Philadelphia.

Lever, W.F. and Schaumburg-Lever, Gundula (1983). *Histopathology of the Skin*. 6th edn., pp. 848, Lippincott, Philadelphia.

Mackie, R.M. (1984). *Milne's Dermatopathology*, Revised 2nd edn., pp. 368. Edward Arnold, London.

Montgomery, H. (1967). *Dermatopathology* (2 vols.) Hoeber Medical Division, Harper and Row.

Pinkus, H. and Mehregan, A.H. (1981). *A guide to Dermatohistopathology*, 3rd edn., pp. 591, Appleton-Century Crofts, New York.

Clinical aspects of skin diseases

Fitzpatrick, T.B., Eisen, A.Z., Wolff, K., Freedberg, I.M. and Austen, K.F. (1979). *Dermatology in General Medicine*, 2nd edn., pp. 1884, McGraw-Hill, New York.

Rook, A., Wilkinson, D.S. and Ebling, F.J.G. (1979). *Textbook of Dermatology*, (2 vols.) Blackwell Scientific, Oxford.

Cutaneous malignant melanoma

Ackerman, A.B. (1981). *Pathology of Malignant Melanoma*, pp. 393, Masson, New York.

Breslow, A. (1970). Thickness, cross-sectional areas and depth of invasion in the prognosis of cutaneous melanoma. *Annals of Surgery* **172,** 902–8.

Clark, W.H. Jr., From, L., Bernadino, E.A. and Mihm, M.C. Jr. (1969). The histogenesis and biological behaviour of primary human malignant melanomas of the skin. *Cancer Research* **29,** 705–27.

Elder, D.E., Goldman, L.I., Goldman, S.C., Greene, M.H. and Clark, W.H. (1980). Dysplastic naevus syndrome: a phenotypic association of sporadic cutaneous melanoma. *Cancer* **46,** 1787.

McGovern, V.J. (1983). *Melanoma: Histological Diagnosis and Prognosis*, pp. 197, Raven Press, New York.

Soft tissue tumours

Enzinger, F.M. and Weiss, S.W. (1983). *Soft Tissue Tumors*, pp. 840, Mosby, St. Louis.

Cutaneous lymphomas

Burg, G. and Braun-Falco, O. (1983). *Cutaneous Lymphomas, Pseydolymphomas, and Related Disorders*, pp. 542, Springer, Berlin.

Lennert, K. (1978). *Malignant Lymphomas other than Hodgkin's Disease*, pp. 833, Springer, Berlin.

28

Diseases Caused by Parasitic Protozoa and Metazoa

Introduction

Parasitic diseases result from infection by protozoa, helminths (worms) and some arthropods. They have an immense influence on the lives of man and all lower vertebrates, producing a great variety of illnesses with effects ranging from the rapidly fatal through the chronically morbid to the incidental and asymptomatic. About 30 000 species of protozoa and a similiar number of helminths are known, most of them free-living, the minority parasitic. Of these, only 20 or so genera of protozoa and about 100 species of worms afflict man. Yet the genus *Plasmodium* alone—the cause of the malarias—is a major, sometimes *the* major public health problem in 70 countries with one-third of the world's population at risk from infection. In Africa alone, it is estimated that malaria kills directly or indirectly one million children each year. Similarly, the two species of hookworm may be found in one-quarter of all people on earth and are a significant cause of chronic anaemia and consequent debility and loss of work output.

Parasitic diseases are not synonymous with tropical diseases. Although parasitic infections (sometimes called *infestations*) are more common in warm climates, 'tropical diseases' are also the natural results of poverty, overcrowding, malnutrition, lack of clean water and of adequate disposal of excreta. The interactions of these factors with the prevailing parasites constitute medicine in the tropics. In developed countries, many parasites are endemic at a low level, e.g. amoebae and hydatid cysts, and several at a high level, such as threadworms, *Toxoplasma* and scabetic mites. New diseases have emerged, for example the acquired immune deficiency syndrome (AIDS, p. 25.5) with its fre-

quent opportunistic infections by ubiquitous but normally non-pathogenic parasites such as *Pneumocystis* and *Cryptosporidium*. Also nearly one billion passengers travel by air each year around the world; visitors to endemic zones can bring back their newly-acquired parasites to developed countries before the incubation periods are over and present clinically at home. These considerations emphasise the significance of parasitic illnesses in all nations and the necessity of recognising them.

This chapter gives a synoptic account of the pathological changes induced by the major parasites, along with brief clinical descriptions. Life cycles, usually considered an unnecessary burden on the memory, are kept to the minimum needed for understanding the disease processes. the importance of immunopathology is emphasised and the outlines of diagnostic tests are stated. For further details of the life cycles of parasites and accounts of their intermediate hosts—whose epidemiology frequently determines the geographical prevalences of the diseases—the student is referred to standard texts on parasitology and medical entomology (p. 28.48).

Some **general features of parasitology** are worth introducing at this point:—

1. The intensity of infection, i.e. the number of parasites present in a host, determines whether an infection is asymptomatic, mild or debilitating. A few hookworms or schistosomes are of minimal clinical consequence; hundreds may be fatal.

2. In the absence of effective host resistance, protozoa can replicate within the host and may build up fatal intensities e.g. in cerebral malaria and African trypanosomiasis. At the other extreme, as with *Entamoeba histolytica*, the host may pass cysts chronically and suffer no ill

effects. By contrast, most helminths do not multiply in the host, but increase in number by repeated infections. In endemic zones, recurrent infections tend to produce episodes of acute illness, with slow accumulation in the host, culminating in severe chronic disease in the small proportion of sufferers with the highest infection intensities.

3. Resistance to parasites is a vast and complex subject. Man is resistant to some protozoa which nevertheless can cause 'opportunistic' infection (p. 8.1): an example is *Pneumocystis carinii*, a cause of severe, sometimes fatal pneumonia in subjects with depressed immunity. Other protozoa multiply readily in man and cause disease in most or all of those infected, but they stimulate an immune response with consequently increasing resistance. Such acquired immunity helps to explain the varying features of infection by a parasite in different age groups in endemic zones and also the different patterns of disease seen in non-immune visitors as compared with inhabitants who have been exposed to infection all their lives and have acquired a degree of protective immunity. Thus, unprotected visitors to malarial zones acquiring *Plasmodium falciparum* infection may die of cerebral malaria, but this is hardly ever seen in local inhabitants. In the latter, acute malaria is mainly seen in childhood and during pregnancy (p. 28.5).

4. The mechanisms by which parasites cause disease in the host vary enormously. In the schistosomiases, the damage is wrought by a hypersensitivity reaction to the eggs laid by the worms. At the other end of the scale, the lesions of the amoebiases are due almost entirely to tissue necrosis caused directly by the amoebae; the host's contribution is a mild inflammatory reaction.

5. In the highly endemic zones—the tropics and subtropics—multiple parasitism is the rule. The interactive effects are still unclear, but a typical African peasant may harbour hookworms, schistosomes, ascarid worms and a filarial worm, in addition to a chronic low level of malarial parasitaemia.

6. The pathophysiology of parasitic infections is complicated by the close interdependence, in susceptible populations, of infection, nutrition and immunity. This is particularly important in those parts of the world where malnutrition is common. Infections such as malaria and hookworms reduce nutrition by causing chronic ill health; malnutrition increases the severity of many protozoal, bacterial and viral illnesses; and heavy parasite loads impair nonspecific and immune cellular defence mechanisms. Yet, as an illustration of our lack of full understanding of the complexities involved in these relationships, there is the paradoxical observation that severe oedematous malnutrition in children (kwashiorkor) appears to protect them against the cerebral form of malaria.

7. Finally, a few parasites are known to be associated aetiologically with cancer: *Schistosoma haematobium* with bladder cancer, opisthorchiasis with cholangiocarcinoma and malaria with Burkitt's lymphoma. In none of these is the parasite known to produce any carcinogenic agent; rather, they appear to act as promoters or by causing immunosuppression.

Diseases Caused by Protozoa

Protozoa are small unicellular eukaryotic cells which range in size from 1 to 150 μm, although most parasitic species are at the smaller end of the scale. They have short generation times, high reproductive rates and variable means of evading the host immune response, so that protozoal infections are generally more persistent than most bacterial infections. Their life cycles vary from the simple and direct (i.e. no intermediate host), as with amoebae, to the complex and indirect as exemplified by the leishmanias, with their elongated flagellate forms in the sandfly alternating with the smaller rounded, non-flagellate forms in the cells of man.

The major human protozoal diseases are malaria, the leishmaniases, the trypanosomiases and amoebiasis. In developed countries, the commonest is toxoplasmosis.

Malaria

This ancient disease is still the scourge of the tropics and subtropics. Africa, the Middle East, Asia and China, and Central and South America are all endemic zones, with tens of millions of cases annually. Non-endemic countries see malaria frequently as an imported but uninvited guest in travellers. Temperate areas in the USA and Europe have been cleared but elsewhere attempts to obliterate the disease have been hindered by lack of finance, wars and political upheavals, acquisition of resistance to insecticides by the mosquito and to drugs by the parasite. Consequently, in most endemic areas the aim is now suppression rather than elimination.

Four species of *Plasmodium* affect man: *P. falciparum*, *P. vivax*, *P. malariae* and *P. ovale*, of which *P. falciparum* is the most important. Malaria is a complex multisystem disease. Its main features include attacks of fever and shaking chills, acute and chronic anaemia, hepatosplenomegaly, acute and chronic renal disease, increased susceptibility to malnutrition and to other infections, low birth weight infants, shock syndromes, and death in a proportion of cases.

Life cycle (Fig. 28.1). Females of *Anopheles* species of mosquito are the vectors of malaria. They bite man to obtain a blood meal necessary for the development of their own progeny.

When man is bitten by an infected mosquito, *sporozoites* (10 μm long) are injected. These rapidly leave the circulation and enter hepatocytes, where asexual multiplication occurs and the progeny, called *merozoites* (1 μm diam.) are released into the circulation when the infected liver cells rupture (Fig. 28.2). This exo-erythrocytic schizogony (literally: multiplication outside the blood) takes from 5 to 15 days, depending on the *Plasmodium* species, and determines the incubation period of malaria.

The merozoites enter red cells and become *trophozoites*; at first, they have a ring form (Fig. 28.3), but then enlarge to fill the cell. Further asexual division occurs, forming a *schizont* composed of many merozoites (Fig. 28.4). The developing parasite feeds on the haemoglobin and brown breakdown pigment called haemozoin is seen in the red cells. The erythrocytes rupture, releasing the merozoites which then in-

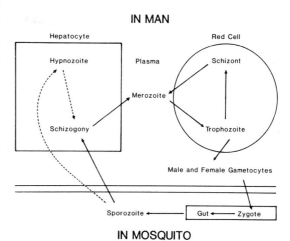

Fig. 28.1 Life cycle of malaria parasites. The hypnozoite pathway (interrupted line) applies only to *P. vivax* and *P. ovale*.

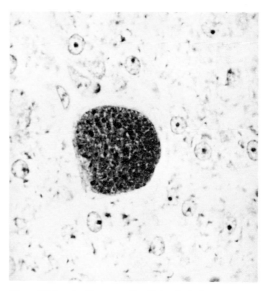

Fig. 28.2 A liver cell distended by numerous merozoites in the early stage of malarial infection. × 1000.

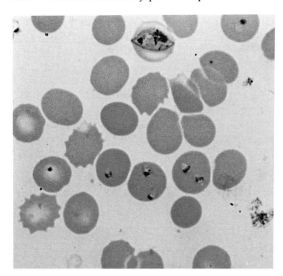

Fig. 28.3 Blood smear showing ring forms of *Plasmodium falciparum* in red cells. Some cells contain two parasites. The large crescentic form also present is a gametocyte. × 1000.

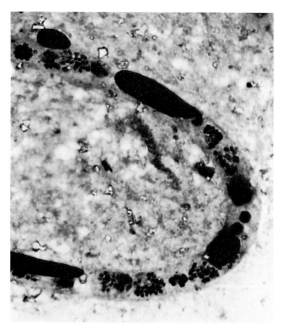

Fig. 28.4 Plasmodium falciparum schizonts inside a cerebral capillary in a fatal case of cerebral malaria. The numerous merozoites which fill the red cell schizonts are seen as tiny black dots. The large nuclei belong to endothelial cells. × 1250.

vade other red cells. This erythrocytic cycle is characteristically synchronous; it takes 48 hours in *P. vivax*, *P. ovale* and *P. falciparum* and 72 hours in *P. malariae* infections and this determines the periodicity of the clinical paroxysms of fever and chills in acute malaria.

Some merozoites do not develop asexually but differentiate into male and female *gametocytes*. The mosquito takes these up in a blood meal from an infected individual; they fuse in the mosquito gut to form a zygote which multiplies to produce thousands of sporozoites. These enter the mosquito's salivary gland and are injected into man at night over the next two weeks or so.

In *P. vivax* and *P. ovale* infections, the relapses (see below) are now known to be the result of persistent liver parasites called *hypnozoites* (literally: sleeping animals) which develop directly from the sporozoites. They lie dormant as 4 μm bodies in hepatocytes, emerging months or years later to release merozoites into the blood.

Malaria may also be contracted from infected blood by blood transfusion and by syringes shared among intravenous drug abusers. Transplacental infection is uncommon; it presents as anaemia and splenomegaly in early infancy. The morphology of the various parasite forms in the erythrocytic cycle are characteristic for each species and serve to differentiate them diagnostically. As will be described, *P. falciparum* infections are potentially fatal, while the others are not. This is due to several factors: 1. *P. falciparum* produces more merozoites from the schizogony cycles in the liver and red cells than the other species, and so causes higher levels of parasitaemia. 2. Red cells harbouring *P. falciparum* have 'knobs' on the cell memmembrane which make them adherent to endothelium. They are sequestered in the capillaries of the viscera where they impede blood flow and cause ischaemic damage. Another consequence of such sequestration is that schizonts of *P. falciparum* are not seen in peripheral blood except in severe cases. 3. There is a possibility that *P. falciparum* parasites make a toxin which acts systemically.

Clinical features. Malaria presents with sudden onset of fever, headache, myalgia and a haemolytic anaemia. In the first attack, the bouts occur at regular intervals, coinciding with the release of merozoites from burst red cells:

every two days with *P. vivax* ('benign tertian' malaria), *P. ovale* ('ovale tertian' and *P. falci-parum* ('malignant tertian'), and every three days with *P. malariae* ('quartan malaria'). Elimination of parasites in the blood is curative for *P. falciparum* and *P. malariae*, but *P. vivax* and *P. ovale* malarias may relapse months or years later in the absence of intervening re-infection (see above). In endemic zones with constant re-infections, an acquired humoral immunity is built up in survivors. Passive immunity from maternal antibodies lasts about six months from birth, then waves of severe infection ensue but become less severe after a decade or so. Thereafter, attacks of acute malaria occur most often in pregnant women because the maternal sinuses of the placenta provide a particularly favourable site for intra-erythrocytic schizogony.

Pathological changes

The anaemia of malaria is multifactorial, and in endemic zones is commonly complicated by iron and folate deficiency. The most important factor is destruction of parasitised red cells, producing the general features of a haemolytic anaemia (pp. 17.19–22): haemolysis occurs both intravascularly and by extravascular destruction in the spleen, but *splenectomy makes malaria worse by impairing parasite clearance.* Blood films show a variable parasitaemia, usually affecting 2% or less of the red cells except in falciparum infections when, in spite of sequestration of infected cells up to 30% parasitaemias may be seen in non-immunes; levels over 25% are commonly fatal. The anaemia is normochromic; there may be a reticulocytosis, and a leucopenia with relative monocytosis is common. Dyserythropoiesis (p. 17.34) is uncommon. A variably positive Coombs' test does not correlate with the haemoglobin level, and immune haemolysis of parasitised and non-parasitised cells by bound antibody or immune complexes (which appear in the blood in malaria) is therefore apparently of minor importance. A probable exception to this is in *blackwater fever*, an acute intravascular haemolysis during falciparum malaria in non-immunes following quinine therapy: the effects are those of massive haemolysis, notably prostration, fever, acute anaemia, shock and

acute renal failure. The renal tubules are filled with debris and haemoglobin products, and show acute tubular necrosis which is not a toxic effect or due to blockage, but a result of the state of shock (p. 22.8).

The lymphoreticular system. Malaria causes hyperplasia of the lymphoreticular system and the prevalence of malaria in a community may be gauged by the proportion of children with palpable spleens. In the acute attack, lymph nodes, spleen and liver enlarge and become dark browny-grey as does the bone marrow. The sinusoids are congested with parasitised red cells and haemozoin pigment is plentiful in

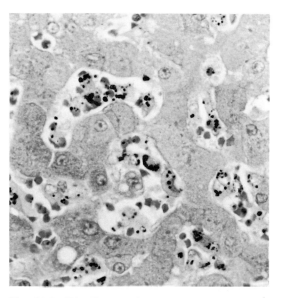

Fig. 28.5 The liver in falciparum malaria: parasitised red cells are just visible and there are plentiful dark granules of haemozoin within the Kupffer cells. × 1000.

splenic macrophages and Kupffer cells (Fig. 28.5). Sinus histiocytosis is seen in the lymph nodes and spleen. Following clearance of parasites from the blood, the pigment in the liver is carried in macrophages from the sinusoids to the portal tracts. The haemopoietic marrow is hyperplastic and contains abundant haemozoin pigment.

Tropical splenomegaly syndrome (TSS). Some adults in areas endemic for falciparum malaria develop massive splenomegaly without obvious cause, i.e. not due to schistosomiasis, cirrhosis or portal vein thrombosis. The spleno-megaly is likely to be related aetiologically to malaria because (1) it is restricted to endemic zones; (2) patients with TSS have higher mean levels of antimalarial antibodies in the serum than controls, and also a very high serum IgM level; (3) it is rare in people with sickle-cell trait, who are partially protected against malaria, and (4) the splenomegaly regresses with long-term antimalarial treatment. The main clinical effects of TSS are those of hypersplenism and

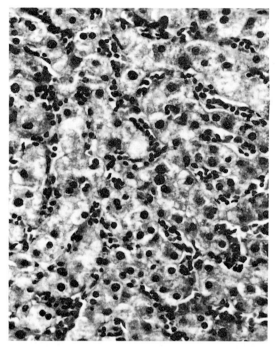

Fig. 28.6 The liver in tropical splenomegaly syndrome: the sinusoids contain numerous mature lymphocytes—hepatic sinusoidal lymphocytosis. × 400.

a dragging pain in the left flank. Parasitaemia is very scanty or absent.The spleen may weigh 3 kg or more and on section is firm and dark red. Histologically there is hyperplasia of both the red and white pulp, but minimal or no pigment. The most characteristic histological change is hepatic sinusoidal lymphocytosis (Fig. 28.6). The syndrome is probably an idiosyncratic immunological response to malaria and is better termed **hyper-reactive malarial splenomegaly.**

The kidney. The renal tubules are damaged during blackwater fever and in the shock state of algid falciparum malaria (see below). Circu-

lating immune complexes are commonly present in malaria, and two types of immune-complex glomerulonephritis occur. The first is a clinically mild and reversible acute proliferative glomerulonephritis seen in some non-immune patients with acute *P. falciparum* infection. The second, '*quartan malaria nephrotic syndrome*', occurs in a small percentage of children with chronic *P. malariae* infection. Biopsy shows focal or diffuse membranous glomerulonephritis and, later on, sclerosis of glomeruli. Deposits of *P. malariae* antigen, immunoglobulin and complement can sometimes be detected in the glomerular capillary walls. The condition has a poor prognosis; it does not respond to antimalarials, and progresses to chronic renal failure.

The malarias of *P. vivax*, *P. ovale* and *P. malariae* cause much chronic ill health but, apart from the quartan malaria nephrotic syndrome, are seldom fatal. *P. falciparum* infection has a fatality rate that is highest in children in endemic areas and in non-immune visitors who are not taking effective antimalarial prophylaxis: its more serious effects include severe acute anaemia, blackwater fever, pulmonary oedema, algid malaria, hyperpyrexia and cerebral malaria.

Overwhelming infection with parasitaemias around $10^{12}/l$ of blood is responsible for hyperpyrexia and anaemia and for the *algid malaria shock syndrome* with peripheral vascular collapse: disseminated intravascular coagulation also occurs but is not common. Severe pulmonary oedema may be seen after treatment has commenced and is due to both shock and over-enthusiastic intravenous infusions in patients with impaired renal function.

Cerebral malaria is the major cause of death in falciparum malaria in non-immunes. Clinically, there is clouding of consciousness, fits, and sometimes focal neurological signs. Intensive therapy saves some patients, and residual neurological deficits are uncommon. In fatal cases the brain is swollen due to congestion and oedema, often with petechial haemorrhages in the subcortical white matter (Fig. 28.7). Gross haemozoin pigmentation is not a feature and nor is infarction unless the patient has been maintained on a ventilator after brain death. Microscopy shows microvascular congestion and large numbers of parasitised red cells sticking to the vascular endothelium. Changes sometimes present include pericapillary demyelination, pericapillary ring haemorrhages (Fig. 28.8) and focal perivascular glial proliferation—the Durck granuloma, which is a response to focal ischaemic necrosis and may be accompanied by disruption of vascular endothelium and plugging of small vessels with agglomerated red cells and fibrin. These advanced lesions probably represent irreversible brain damage and are seen only if the patient lives for some days after the onset of clinical cerebral malaria. The pathogenesis of the condition is not yet certain. The sticky red cells block the capillaries, and there is also kinin activation in severe malaria which will render the small vessels leaky and cause intracapillary haemoconcentration and red cell sludging. Immunological reactions have also been postulated to play a role. The demyelination and ring haemorrhages appear to be related to vascular disruption; a similar picture is seen in systemic fat embolism.

The malarias are diagnosed by finding the parasite in the blood. Serodiagnosis is still

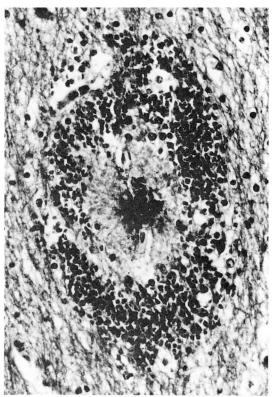

Fig. 28.8 A ring haemorrhage in cerebral malaria. The central vessel is plugged with fibrin and the immediate surrounding white matter is necrotic. Peripheral to that is a ring of red cells (stained black). × 400.

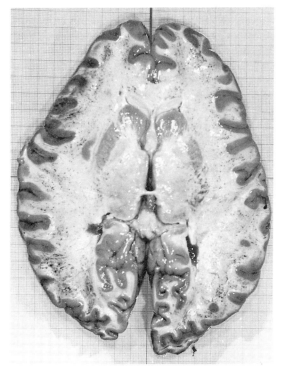

Fig. 28.7 The brain in cerebral malaria. Petechial haemorrhages are widespread throughout the white matter.

being developed but is aimed more at epidemiology than at individuals. A light parasitaemia is most readily detected by examining thick films (Fig. 28.9), but the thin film is usually needed to recognise the infecting species.

Burkitt's lymphoma (p. 18.26) is limited geographically to highly endemic malaria zones, where it forms the commonest malignancy in childhood. In these zones, most or all children are infected with both the Epstein-Barr virus and malaria parasites, and in a small proportion of these the T cell immunosuppression associated with malaria apparently allows the oncogenic potential of EBV in B cells to be expressed as a B cell lymphoblastic lymphoma.

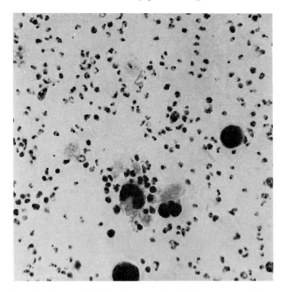

Fig. 28.9 Thick film of blood in falciparum malaria, showing trophozoites of varying sizes and some leucocytes. × 1000.

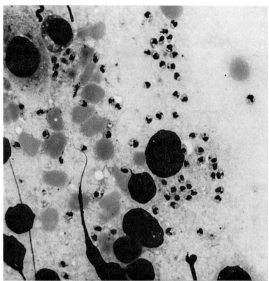

Fig. 28.10 Numerous Leishman-Donovan bodies in a splenic aspirate from a case of visceral leishmaniasis. The comma-shaped bodies next to the nuclei are the kinetoplasts. × 1000.

The leishmaniases

These diseases are caused by flagellate protozoa of the genus *Leishmania*. With few exceptions they are zoonoses, i.e. infections primarily of animals with man as an incidental victim. Transmission is by the bite of sandflies. Some 400 000 new cases occur worldwide *per annum*, and these include visitors to endemic zones. Three broad clinicopathological groups of diseases result (Table 28.1). The taxonomy of the leishmanias is complex, and enzyme analysis of the parasites is used to distinguish the various species producing similar lesions.

The leishmanias are intracellular parasites, and cell-mediated immunity is therefore involved in resistance and in their elimination. After an infective bite, injected leishmanias are taken up by macrophages, transform into non-flagellate *amastigotes* (literally: no whip) and multiply by binary fission. The amastigotes of all species are morphologically similar: they are round or ovoid bodies of 1·5–3 μm diameter with a thin cell membrane, a dense nucleus and a rod-shaped kinetoplast in the cytoplasm. They are also known as Leishman-Donovan (L-D) bodies (Fig. 28.10).

Cutaneous leishmaniasis is generally a localised self-healing condition. At the site of a bite, a papule develops and breaks down to form a

Table 28.1 The types and geographical distribution of leishmaniasis

Disease	Parasite	Distribution
1. Cutaneous leishmaniasis ('oriental sore')	*L. tropica* *L. major*	Africa, Asia, Middle East.
	L. mexicana	South and Central America.
2. Mucocutaneous leishmaniasis ('espundia')	*L. brasiliensis*	South and Central America.
3. Visceral leishmaniasis ('kala-azar')	*L. donovani* *L. infantum*	Asia, Africa, S. America. Southern Europe.

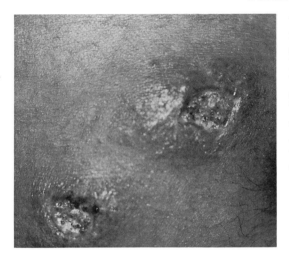

Fig. 28.11 Two lesions of cutaneous leishmaniasis near the umbilicus. The erythematous papules have broken down to form crateriform ulcers. (Slide kindly supplied by Dr D. Evans, London School of Hygiene and Tropical Medicine.)

crateriform ulcer (Fig. 28.11). Secondary bacterial infection often supervenes, but healing takes place over weeks or months, leaving a scar. Microscopically, the early lesion consists of aggregated dermal macrophages filled with amastigotes (Fig. 28.12); later there is an intense infiltration of lymphocytes and plasma cells followed by necrosis and gradual elimina-

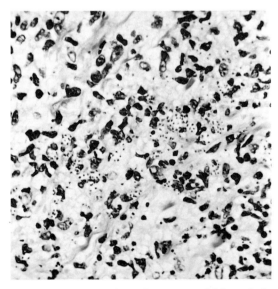

Fig. 28.12 Early lesion of cutaneous leishmaniasis. Amastigotes are seen as abundant small dark bodies within dermal macrophages. × 250.

tion of the parasites. Giant-cell granulomas and fibrosis herald the healing process. There is subsequent immunity to re-infection by homologous *Leishmania* species. L-D bodies can usually be detected microscopically in an aspirate or biopsy of the lesion, or if necessary by culture. Occasionally the host response in cutaneous leishmaniasis is inadequate and large areas of the skin become and remain filled with heavily parasitised macrophages. This condition of **diffuse cutaneous leishmaniasis** is analogous to lepromatous leprosy (p. 9.23) and indeed there is evidence of a similar immunopathological spectrum of host-parasite relationships in both conditions.

Mucocutaneous leishmaniasis. *L. brasiliensis* infection starts like ordinary cutaneous leishmaniasis, with lesions on the head, leg or trunk. These heal, but months or years later lesions may reappear at mucocutaneous junctions, commonly in the nose and the upper lip. These secondary lesions do not heal, but progress destructively, eroding skin, mucosa and cartilage and often causing gross disfigurement. Secondary bacterial infection complicates the picture. There is necrosis and a mixed inflammatory infiltrate including macrophage granulomas, in which the parasites are scanty or undetectable. The pathogenesis is ill-understood but hypersensitivity reactions associated with a strong but ineffective host immune response, are probably involved.

Visceral leishmaniasis The term *kala-azar* is Hindi for 'black fever', so named because fair-skinned patients become hyperpigmented. The disease is the result of anergic failure to react to the intracellular parasites, which disseminate throughout the lymphoreticular system and haemopoietic marrow from the skin lesion that follows a bite. Consequently, there is hepatosplenomegaly, lymphadenopathy, cachexia, fever and pancytopenia. The incubation period is about two months, and without treatment the classical *L. donovani* disease is usually fatal either from chronic debility or from intercurrent bacterial infection such as pneumonia. In the form of the disease caused by *L. infantum*, subclinical illness and recovery from infection are common.

The pancytopenia results from hypersplenism and marrow replacement by parasitised macrophages. The susceptibility to secondary infection is multifactorial; leucopenia, T-cell suppression, and deficient antigen handling by parasitised macrophages all contribute. There is also a polyclonal B-cell proliferation in the tissues, producing a characteristic high level of IgG and IgM in the serum, only part of which is anti-leishmanial antibody.

The liver in visceral leishmaniasis is large and pale; the spleen is massively enlarged, commonly weighing 3 kg or more, and on section is firm and red. The red marrow is hyperplastic. Histologically, amastigotes are abundant in the macrophages of the liver, spleen, marrow,

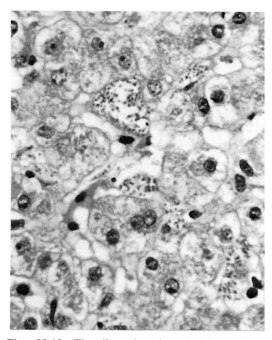

Fig. 28.13 The liver in visceral leishmaniasis. Hypertrophied Kupffer cells are filled with small L-D bodies. × 400.

lymph nodes and lamina propria of the gut, but necrosis is rare. Liver sinusoids are distended by hypertrophied parasitised Kupffer cells (Fig. 28.13); sinus histiocytosis and paracortical cell depletion are seen in the lymph nodes, and there is gross hyperplasia of the splenic red pulp. Plasma cells are also increased in these organs. The nearest analogy to this disease is *Mycobacterium avium-intracellulare* infection in immunosuppressed patients, where all the macrophages of the lymphoreticular system become filled with acid-fast bacilli, yet without necrosis or formation of tubercles.

Visceral leishmaniasis is diagnosed by finding L-D bodies in smears from spleen or marrow aspirates (Fig. 28.10).

The trypanosomiases

Insect-transmitted flagellate of the genus *Trypanosoma* cause two entirely distinct diseases in man—the African trypanosomiases (sleeping sickness) and South American trypanosomiasis (Chagas' disease). The trypanosomes in the blood (*trypomastigotes*) in both diseases are undulating elongated slender cells, 15–30 μm long, with a nucleus and a posterior kinetoplast with a flagellum arising from it (Fig. 28.14). In fresh

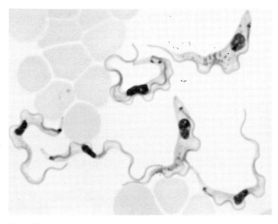

Fig. 28.14 *Trypanosoma cruzi* in a blood smear. The flagellum is seen arising from the kinetoplast body. × 1200.

preparations they wriggle rapidly and continuously and can be detected at low magnification by the disturbance they create among the adjacent red cells. In African trypanosomiasis the parasite remains extracellular in location, but in Chagas' disease it enters tissue cells and assumes a small *amastigote form* (like a *Leishmania*) and transforms back to the trypomastigote form during subsequent episodes of parasitaemia.

African trypanosomiases

About 45 million people in West, Central and East Africa are at risk from sleeping sickness, which is fatal without treatment. Related trypanosomes are an even more important cause of disease in cattle so that much of the African savannah is uninhabitable by livestock. The human disease may occur in epidemics and depopulate large areas. Two forms of the disease are seen: that caused by *Trypanosoma brucei gambiense* in West and Central Africa is restricted to man, whilst that caused by *Trypanosoma brucei rhodesiense* in Central and East Africa has a reservoir in game animals, and is the more fulminant form. All trypanosomiases in Africa are transmitted by tsetse flies. Transplacental transmission is very uncommon.

The parasites multiply by binary fission at the site of the tsetse fly bite. The ensuing oedema and inflammation result in a trypanosomal chancre. Invasion of the blood follows and various grades of parasitaemia persist until terminated by death or treatment. The trypanosomes may divide in the blood to peak numbers exceeding $1.5 \times 10^9/l$.

Clinical features and course. Clinically, there is fever, anaemia, mild splenomegaly, lymphadenopathy, a puffy face and skin rashes. Sooner or later after blood invasion has occurred, the trypanosomes enter the central nervous system. Headache, behavioural changes, neurological signs and altered sleep rhythm gradually lead to semi-coma. Death follows from inanition and secondary infection, within months in the florid East African form and within months to years in *T.b. gambiense* infection. In *T.b. rhodesiense* infection, there are heavier parasitaemias, often cardiac involvement and in some cases an immune-complex glomerulonephritis or disseminated intravascular coagulation.

Immunological factors. The parasitaemia of both forms of African trypanosomiasis is periodic. Antibodies are produced to trypanosomal antigens and opsonise the parasites, which are cleared from the blood by phagocytes in the liver, spleen, etc. However, a few parasites with different surface antigenic determinants survive and they multiply to produce a new wave of parasitaemia. Further antibody production follows, but the same phenomenon occurs, and the results are repeated episodes of parasitaemia at roughly weekly intervals and increasingly high levels of IgM in the blood. This phenomenon of **antigenic variation** by the parasite and subsequent multiplication of new

clones of parasites non-reactive with the 'old' antibodies thus allows the trypanosome to evade the host immune response. A B-cell mitogen may also be produced by the parasite since only a fraction of the IgM is anti-trypanosomal antibody. There is a general depression of immune responses which contributes to the development of intercurrent infection. One cause of the anaemia in trypanosomiasis is immune adherence of antibodies and immune complexes to erythrocytes, which may undergo 'bystander lysis' (p. 7.4) in the spleen.

Pathological changes. The spleen and lymph nodes show sinus histiocytosis and plasma cell proliferation, with depletion of the T-cell zones. A chronic valvulitis and myocarditis with involvement of the cardiac conducting system is seen in some East African cases.

When the central nervous system is involved, the CSF protein and IgM levels rise and lymphocytes, morular cells (see below) and also trypanosomes are found in it.

The neural lesion is a **meningo-encephalitis.** Grossly, the meninges are congested and on section there is patchy oedema and congestion of the white matter. In acute cases, there is narrowing of the ventricles due to brain swelling, but in longstanding *T.b. gambiense* infections there may be some cerebral atrophy and secondary hydrocephalus.

Microscopy shows the features of a chronic meningitis and focal encephalitis, particularly in the brainstem. Lymphocytes and plasma cells infiltrate the meninges and the perivascular spaces to produce perivascular cuffing. There is neuronal degeneration and reactive gliosis, and near vessels the characteristic morular cells of Mott are to be seen (Fig. 28.15). These are plasma cells containing large refractile vesicles stuffed with IgM. (*Russell bodies*)

The cause of neuronal injury in trypanosomal encephalitis is one of the mysteries of tropical pathology, and trypanosomes are rarely, if ever, seen in the brain tissues. The lymphoid cells are of B-cell type, and abundant antibody is present, yet the features of type 3 (immune-complex) hypersensitivity, such as vasculitis or polymorph infiltration, are not seen, and the absence of T cells militates against a delayed hypersensitivity reaction. Neither antibodies to neuronal elements nor trypanosomal toxins have been demonstrated convincingly.

Diagnosis of African trypanosomiasis de-

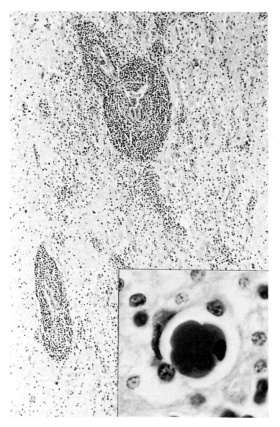

Fig. 28.15 Pons in a case of *Trypanosoma rhodesiense* infection. There is encephalitis with marked perivascular cuffing by lymphocytes. × 100. Inset: a morular cell of Mott—a plasma cell distended by large Russell bodies containing IgM. × 1000.

pends on finding the parasites in the blood, lymph node aspirate or CSF. In late *T.b. gambiense* infection, blood trypanosomes may be exceedingly scanty, and haemoconcentration techniques may be needed. A raised CSF IgM concentration is almost pathognomonic of cerebral trypanosomiasis.

South American trypanosomiasis (*Chagas' disease*)

At least 10 million people in South and Central America are infected with *Trypanosoma cruzi*, the causal agent of Chagas' disease, though not all show clinical disease. The clinical syndromes are firstly *acute Chagas' disease*, with a mortality of 5-10%, followed by a latent asymptomatic period of 10-20 years, after which *chronic Chagas' disease* becomes manifest

in about 30% of infected people; it frequently presents with congestive cardiac failure, and this is the commonest single cause of admission to adult medical wards in many South American hospitals.

Initial infection is usually acquired in childhood when an infective reduviid bug takes a blood meal and deposits flagellate forms of *T. cruzi* in its faeces on the skin. The victim rubs the parasites into the skin when scratching the bite. Transmission may also occur transplacentally or by transfusion of infected blood. The parasites enter dermal macrophages, in which they transform into amastigote forms and multiply. The local inflammation and oedema produce a trypanosomal chancre or chagoma. If the parasite enters near the eye, the resulting eyelid oedema and conjunctivitis are known as Romana's sign. After about two weeks, the amastigotes transform back into trypomastigotes and spread by the blood to infect many types of cell, including myocardium, glial cells of the central nervous system, cells of the myenteric plexus in the gut and cells of the lymphoreticular system.

The main clinical features of the **acute systemic disease** are due to myocarditis, encephalitis and lymphadenopathy. The heart is dilated, the muscle soft and focally haemorrhagic, and microscopy shows clusters of amastigotes in the myocardial cells (Fig. 28.16): rupture of these cells induces a lymphocytic, plasma cell and macrophage reaction with phagocytosis of the parasites.

Antibodies to *T. cruzi* persist in the **latent phase,** and although chemotherapy may abolish the transient phases of parasitaemia, the tissue amastigotes persist.

Chronic Chagas' disease has two main aspects: cardiac failure and the megasyndromes. There is cardiomegaly, heart block, arrhythmias, increasing congestive failure and embolic phenomena from mural thrombosis in the left ventricle. The megasyndromes are caused by gross dilatation of the alimentary canal, principally the oesophagus and colon, with the symptoms of stasis.

The **heart** may weigh up to 1000 g. All the chambers are dilated and there is often an apical aneurysm. Histologically, there is chronic inflammation, fibrosis of the myocardium and scattered hypertrophied muscle fibres, but at this stage parasitised myofibres are few and are

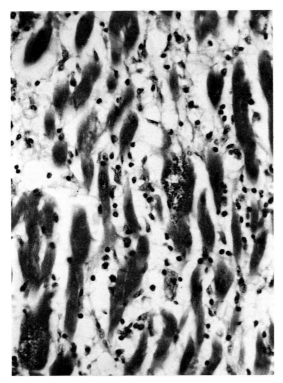

Fig. 28.16 Acute chagasic myocarditis. The myocardium is oedematous and inflamed, and clusters of tiny black dots (amastigotes of *Trypanosoma cruzi*) are seen in two myocytes. × 400.

found in less than 50% of cases. Inflammation and fibrosis also affect the conducting system with reduction of nodal ganglion cells. The dilated alimentary tract shows thinning of the wall with variable mural inflammation and scarring. Myenteric plexus ganglion cells are greatly reduced in number.

These chronic lesions are probably caused by delayed hypersensitivity reactions to parasitised muscle and neurones, and possibly also by cytotoxic antibody. During the acute phase of the disease, trypanosomal antigens are released from disrupted infected cells. These antigens bind to other cells and render them susceptible to later attack by the host's anti-*T. cruzi* response. It is possible that, in the majority of those infected, low levels of cell-mediated immunity result in a balanced state in which both host and parasite survive.

Chagas' disease is diagnosed by finding the parasite in the blood or by specific serology. In the latent or chronic phases, parasitaemia is often very low and sometimes the diagnosis can be confirmed only by allowing an uninfected reduviid bug to feed on the patient and examining it later for vector stages of the parasite.

The amoebiases

Two types of amoebae are pathogenic for man, the most important being the intestinal amoeba *Entamoeba histolytica*. Many other intestinal amoebae are described, such as *Entamoeba coli* and *Iodamoeba buetschlii*, but these are harmless commensals and are important only because they may be mistaken for *E. histolytica* or *vice versa*. The second type of pathogenic amoeba is free-living and the most important is *Naegleria fowleri*, which causes a meningo-encephalitis.

Entamoeba histolytica

Infection with this parasite can cause **amoebic dysentery** and **amoebic 'abscesses'** in the liver and other viscera. Some 10% of the world's population carry *E. histolytica* in their bowel. The proportion is highest in the cities of the tropics and subtropics, but no country is free of infection. Man acquires amoebae by ingesting food or water contaminated by cysts derived from human faeces, there being no animal reservoir. The cysts are hardy and resist drying: following ingestion, they excyst in the small intestine and release four motile trophozoites, which are 20–30 µm in diameter and have a single nucleus (Fig. 28.20). They are anaerobic, feed on gut bacteria and multiply by binary fission. Most people who are infected are asymptomatic healthy carriers; the amoebae reside in the lumen of the proximal colon and do not damage the mucosa but encyst to form quadrinucleate cysts that are excreted in the faeces.

It is now evident that the occurrence of invasive, symptomatic disease, to which the term amoebiasis should be properly restricted, depends on both parasite and host factors. By enzyme chromatographic studies, many different strains (or zymodemes) of *E. histolytica* have now been identified, only a few of which have caused invasive disease in man. The other strains, though morphologically identical, appear to be non-pathogenic. The luminal enterobacteria are also probably involved in the expression of pathogenicity by some synergistic action with the amoebae. There is clinical evidence for acquired resistance to re-infection by *E. histolytica* after recovery from invasive disease. Conversely, certain immunosuppressive states such as pregnancy and steroid therapy predispose to invasive disease, but the mechanisms of natural resistance are unknown.

Pathogenic amoebae lyse cells and tissues; direct contact between amoeba and target cell is necessary and it appears that the target cell membrane is made leaky so that cytoplasmic ions escape and the cell dies. The host inflammatory reaction is variable and induced by cell injury rather than directly by the amoebae. Healing of the lesions is usually accompanied by minimal scarring, and, in contrast to many other parasitic infections, no recognisable hypersensitivity reactions contribute to the pathology of amoebiasis.

Intestinal amoebiasis. Invasion usually occurs in the caecum and sigmoid colon, rarely in the ileum and appendix. There is early superficial necrosis of the mucosa with adjacent oedema (Fig. 28.17) and the amoebae then invade the submucosa (Fig. 28.18) where they tend to spread laterally. This undermines the mucosa and produces the characteristic flask-shaped ulcer (Fig. 28.19). The ulcers may stay discrete or become confluent with sloughing of large areas of mucosa. Secondary bacterial infection contributes to the abundant mucus secretion.

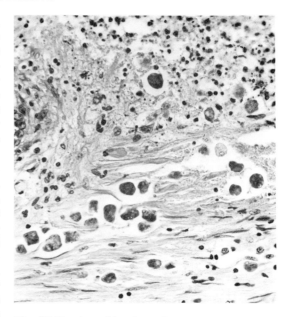

Fig. 28.18 Amoebic ulcer of the colon. The upper part of the field consists of necrotic mucosa and exudate. Below this, the amoebae are seen digesting the submucosa, but with remarkably little cellular reaction. × 200.

The stools are foul-smelling, loose, mucoid and tinged with blood.

The early invasive lesion may heal spontaneously or progress to pan-colonic ulceration and dilatation and sometimes perforation, with consequent peritonitis, which has a high mor-

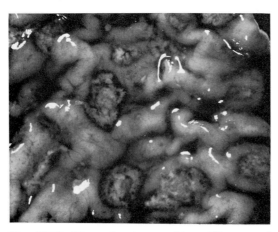

Fig. 28.17 The colon in amoebic colitis; several discrete small ulcers are present and the adjacent mucosa is oedematous.

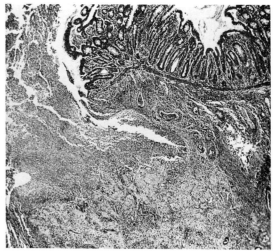

Fig. 28.19 Undermining ulceration in intestinal amoebiasis. The necrosis is extending laterally under the muscularis mucosae. × 32.

tality and is more likely to occur in patients misdiagnosed as ulcerative colitis and treated with glucocorticoids.

Histologically, the mucosal cells degenerate and the amoebae are often best seen in the adjacent mucous exudate. They appear rounded in form, or amoeboid with pseudopodia, and when invasive they contain phagocytosed red cells (Fig. 28.20). The lesions are infiltrated by plasma cells, macrophages and lymphocytes and sometimes polymorphs due to secondary infection. As the trophozoites invade deeper, they are concentrated at the advancing edge of the lesion, and the overlying mucosa shows ischaemic necrosis.

Proctosigmoidoscopy often shows scattered foci of ulceration surrounded by oedematous mucosa, appearances which differ from those of ulcerative colitis and Crohn's disease and may suggest the correct diagnosis. Confirmation of the active disease can usually be made by identifying the motile amoebae in a fresh specimen of stool: healthy carriers and patients with chronic indolent disease excrete only cysts. The amoebae can also usually be detected by biopsy of an ulcer. The indirect immunofluorescence test for antibody to *E. histolytica* is usually positive in amoebiasis and negative in healthy carriers. **Amoeboma** or *amoebic pseudotumour*

of the colon is an uncommon complication of intestinal amoebiasis. After invasion of the submucosa, the infection may remain localised and form a large mass of granulation and fibrous tissue, which may obstruct the lumen. The differential diagnosis is with carcinoma of the colon.

Extra-intestinal lesions may affect the skin, liver and some other internal organs.

Amoebiasis of the skin is an uncommon complication of colorectal disease. It usually results from direct spread to the anus or vulval area or to the skin around a colostomy site. Penile amoebiasis is the result of anogenital intercourse with an infected person. All the skin lesions ulcerate with a foul slough. There is marked epidermal hyperplasia at the edges, which may easily be mistaken histologically for squamous-cell carcinoma, but numerous amoebae can usually be seen at the ulcer margin.

Hepatic amoebiasis arises as a complication of or sequel to colonic invasion. Trophozoites are carried in the portal venous system to the liver where they multiply and produce small zones of necrosis of liver cells: these enlarge and become confluent, producing one or more cavities (**tropical or amoebic 'abscesses'**), which may grow to more than 10 cm in diameter and are usually in the right lobe. Clinically, they present as fever, polymorphonuclear leucocytosis, hepatomegaly and right hypochondrial pain. Jaundice is uncommon.

Grossly, an abscess has a shaggy pale peripheral necrotic rim and central thick reddish-

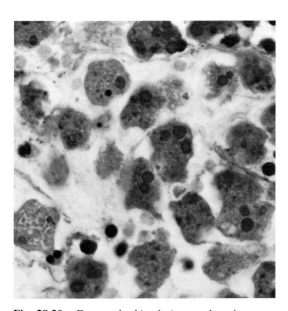

Fig. 28.20 *Entamoeba histolytica* trophozoites near a colonic ulcer. In addition to the nucleus, they also contain phagocytosed red cells (stained dark). × 100.

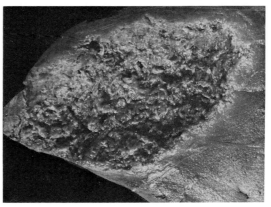

Fig. 28.21 Amoebic liver 'abscess' in the periphery of the right lobe of the liver. The shaggy necrotic lining is enclosed in a thin layer of fibrous tissue.

brown fluid (often likened to anchovy sauce) composed of necrotic liver-cell debris, fibrin and blood (Fig. 28.21). Histologically, trophozoites may be numerous or scanty in the wall of the cavity. Surrounding the zone of necrotic cells, the liver is oedematous and chronically inflamed (Fig. 28.22); polymorphs are not present in or around the cavity, which is therefore not really an abscess.

Without treatment, hepatic amoebiasis is usually fatal, although occasionally the amoebae are eliminated spontaneously. Clinical diagnosis is supported by a characteristic pattern on ultrasonography and a high titre of antibody to *E. histolytica*. Concurrent intestinal amoebiasis is found in less than 50% of cases, and the stool may be negative even for cysts. Aspiration is generally reserved for very large 'abscesses' and those about to rupture, as indicated by a local friction rub. Modern chemotherapy is very effective for this condition.

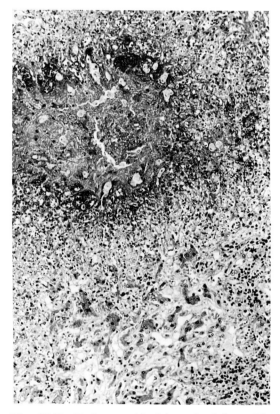

Fig. 28.22 Early amoebic 'abscess' of liver. The liver is inflamed and oedematous, and there is a central zone of necrosis. The amoebae are seen as pale bodies toward the periphery of the necrosis. × 125.

Complications include rupture and spread beyond the liver. Rupture into the pleural, peritoneal or pericardial cavities has a considerable mortality. From the pleural cavity, the infection can spread to the **lungs** with the formation of a pulmonary 'abscess' and a bronchopleural fistula; necrotic material may then be coughed up. Haematogenous dissemination to **other organs**, including the **brain**, occasionally results in amoebic 'abscesses' similar to those in the liver.

Naegleria fowleri

Primary amoebic meningo-encephalitis. *Naegleria fowleri* is a cosmopolitan amoeba, living in warm waters such as natural hot springs. It can parasitise man when he swims in infected water; the amoebae pass into the nasal passages and through the cribriform plate, entering the central nervous system along the olfactory neuroepithelium (*Herpes simplex virus* follows a similar route to cause encephalitis). These amoebae damage host cells in the same way as *E. histolytica* (see above). Children are usually affected and there is no evidence of a predisposing immunodeficiency. The clinical course of the meningo-encephalitis is rapid and fatal unless treated aggressively from an early stage. The cerebrospinal fluid has a raised protein level and contains red cells and polymorphs and motile amoebae 10–20 μm in diameter. The brain is swollen with a purulent meningitis and the olfactory bulbs are destroyed. On section, foci of haemorrhagic necrosis are seen in the grey matter. Histologically, there is a mixed inflammatory cellular infiltrate in the meninges; the amoebae are seen in the perivascular spaces from where they infiltrate into the nervous tissue (Fig. 28.23).

Giardiasis

Infection with *Giardia lamblia* is world-wide. It is acquired by ingesting cysts contaminating food or water. The life cycle is similar to that of *Entamoeba histolytica* except that it colonises the small bowel and infections are not so chronic.

After ingestion, the cysts break open in the duodenum, releasing trophozoites which then

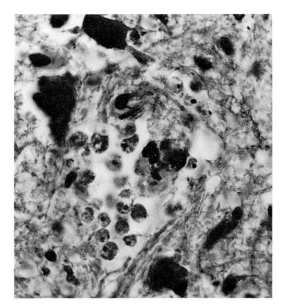

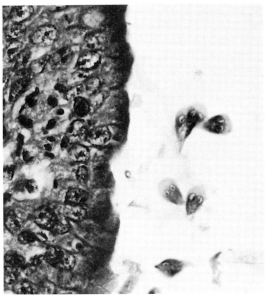

Fig. 28.23 Several trophozoites of *Naegleria fowleri* in the Virchow-Robin space around a vessel in the pons. ×800. (Section kindly supplied by Dr D. Warhurst, London School of Hygiene and Tropical Medicine.)

Fig. 28.24 The binucleate trophozoites of *Giardia lamblia* adjacent to jejunal epithelium. ×1000.

multiply by binary fission so that, within a few days, millions of parasites cover the surface of the villi of the small intestine. The trophozoites are pear-shaped, 15 μm long, and adhere to the enterocytes by their sucker discs. They do not invade the mucosa. Usually giardiasis is a self-limiting condition, although the immunological means of eliminating the parasite are not well understood. About 70% of infections are asymptomatic; the minority cause a diarrhoea lasting some weeks. Fewer than 10% of patients suffer chronic diarrhoea with malabsorption.

How the giardias induce diarrhoea is still uncertain. The condition tends to be severe in patients with deficient IgA production. The histology of the symptomatic cases shows jejunal villi varying in architecture from normal to subtotal atrophy (p. 19.51), and malabsorption is usually associated with this change. Trophozoites are seen near the surface of the mucosa (Fig. 28.24). Plasma cells are plentiful in the lamina propria and increased intra-epithelial lymphocytes are usual, but the microvilli are less atrophic than is usual in coeliac disease. In patients with defective IgA production, plasma cells are scanty but submucosal nodular lymphoid hyperplasia may be present. Pathophys-

iological mechanisms proposed for giardiasis include the physical covering up of the villi by the parasites, direct damage to the enterocytes, luminal substrate competition, bacterial synergism and immunopathological reactions involving antibody.

Giardiasis is diagnosed by finding cysts in the faeces or trophozoites in jejunal aspirate and biopsy material. The indirect immunofluorescence test for circulating antibodies to *Giardia* in positive in 90% of patients with chronic infection and malabsorption.

Toxoplasmosis

Toxoplasmosis is a very common world-wide infection caused by the protozoon *Toxoplasma gondii*. From serological studies in many populations, it is evident that about 20% of people have acquired the infection by the age of 20 years, and up to 50% by the age of 70. The infection is usually asymptomatic, but a small minority develop one of the following clinical syndromes: (1). acute acquired toxoplasmosis, (2). congenital toxoplasmosis. (3). ocular toxoplasmosis, and (4). toxoplasmosis in the immunocompromised host.

Life cycle. The definitive host for *T. gondii* is the cat, in whose intestinal epithelium there is a sexual reproductive cycle via schizogony and gametogony to produce oocysts. A wide variety of other mammals (including man) may act as intermediate host, and in these, two forms of the parasite exist: proliferating trophozoites (or *tachyzoites*) and *bradyzoites* in tissue cysts. The trophozoite is a crescentic cell about $6 \times 2 \mu m$ without a kinetoplast. It is an intracellular parasite which proliferates by binary fission, causing disruption and death of the host cell. In the early phase of infection, it avoids destruction by phagocyte lysosomes. The tissue cysts are found in many host cells and contain a few to thousands of bradyzoites (Fig. 28.25), which are smaller than the tachyzoites.

Man acquires toxoplasmosis by ingesting either oocysts from cat faeces or tissue cysts in the undercooked meat of other intermediate hosts, such as sheep, cow and pig. The cysts rupture in the intestine, releasing parasites which rapidly penetrate the intestinal cells and enter macrophages. These intracellular tachyzoites are then disseminated via lymphatics and the bloodstream throughout the body and enter many host-cell types, particularly those of heart muscle and the central nervous system. Inside these cells the tachyzoites replicate and cause necrosis. In time, the host mounts a combined humoral and cell-mediated immune response to the parasite. The latter is the more important in inhibiting the spread and multiplication of the tachyzoites. Finally, in the uncomplicated case, the parasites persist as bradyzoites in tissue cysts—*the latent infection phase.* The cysts remain in various parts of the body for many years and possibly for the duration of the host's life.

Clinico-pathological features

Acute acquired toxoplasmosis. This presents clinically as malaise and fever; if severe, there may be myocarditis and encephalitis. Moderate splenomegaly is usual and in the later stage there may be lymph-node enlargement. The disease thus mimics infectious mononucleosis or lymphoma. It may last from weeks to a few months but nearly always there is complete recovery. In the affected tissues, multiplication of the tachyzoites is associated with necrosis and focal inflammation. The lymphadenopathy, which usually involves the posterior cervical nodes, has characteristic though not pathognomonic histological features. The architecture of the node is retained and there is follicular hyperplasia and sinus histiocytosis. The most suggestive diagnostic feature is focal aggregation of epithelioid macrophages in the paracortex and within the follicles themselves (Fig. 28.26). Although the nodes are involved in the acute phase of infection, parasites are rarely seen in them.

Congenital toxoplasmosis. About 30% of women who acquire toxoplasmosis in pregnancy (usually asymptomatically) transmit the infection to the fetus via the placenta. A woman who already has toxoplasma antibodies cannot transmit infection. If the infection occurs in the first trimester, the result may be abortion or severe congenital morbidity: the risk of severe fetal disability decreases progressively the later the infection and most fetuses infected during mid or late pregnancy are born free of disease.

The classic tetrad of congenital toxoplasmosis is hydrocephalus or micrencephaly, chorioretinitis and cerebral calcification. Widespread intracerebral dissemination of tachyzoites

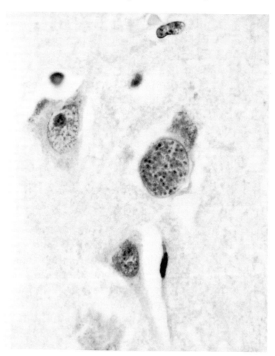

Fig. 28.25 *Toxoplasma* tissue cyst: numerous bradyzoites are seen as small dots inside a cyst in a cerebral neuron. $\times 1000$.

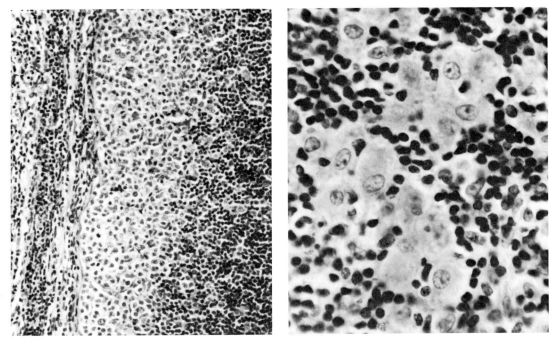

Fig. 28.26 Lymph node in toxoplasmosis. *Left*, a lymphoid sinus filled with cells of uncertain origin. ×175. *Right*, showing the large macrophages which are scattered singly and in small groups throughout the node. ×475.

results in much cerebral necrosis and inflammation. This damage is caused partly by the destructive effect of tachyzoites, but hypersensitivity reactions are probably also involved. The ensuing tissue swelling and vascular thrombosis produce hydrocephalus (Fig. 28.27). Peri ventricular dystrophic calcification is characteristic. Milder sequelae of congenital infection can take months or years to appear and include chorioretinitis and squints, deafness, mental retardation and epilepsy.

Ocular toxoplasmosis. Infection of the uveal tract of the eye is usually secondary to congenital rather than acquired infection. The retina and choroid in the posterior part of the eye are mainly involved, and the condition presents with blurred vision and pain. After the acute necrosis and inflammation have died down, the tissue cysts persist and the infection may become active again at any time.

Toxoplasmosis in the immunocompromised host. People who have previously acquired *T. gondii*, with or without manifestations of disease, may suffer a devastating relapse if their immune defences, particularly cell-mediated immunity, are impaired. The tissue cysts rupture

and release the bradyzoites. These enter adjacent cells, become active tachyzoites and cause

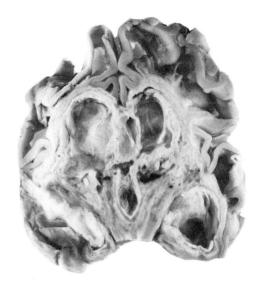

Fig. 28.27 Congenital toxoplasmosis. Coronal section of the brain of a 2-month-old infant. There is extensive cystic and gelatinous degeneration of the cerebral hemispheres and hydrocephalus.

necrosis. The organs most commonly damaged are the brain and the heart; if untreated, the encephalitis may be fatal.

The diagnosis of toxoplasmosis is made either by finding parasites in the tissues, or by serology. Infected tissue may also be injected into mice which are examined for toxoplasmas six weeks later. Serological tests include the Sabin-Feldman dye test which utilises live tachyzoites, and a variety of immunofluorescence tests and complement-fixation tests using soluble antigens. A rising titre of IgM antibody indicates recent infection.

Cryptosporidiosis

Cryptosporidiosis was long assumed to affect only animals, but is now recognised increasingly as a cause of diarrhoea in man. It affects particularly patients with the acquired immunodeficiency syndrome (AIDS, p. 25.5).

Cryptosporidium is a common parasite of cattle, sheep and domestic animals. It has a life cycle similar to that of *Toxoplasma* in the cat intestine (but does not produce tissue cysts and is not invasive). Frequently-exposed healthy people such as vets may ingest oocysts and develop a mild self-limiting diarrhoeal illness as the parasite damages the enterocytes of the gut. However, in patients with defective cell-mediated immunity, the infection is more severe and chronic, affecting both large and small bowel: there is profuse, cholera-like diarrhoea which is often fatal.

Biopsy shows regeneration of mucosal crypts and inflamed lamina propria. The trophozoites of *Cryptosporidium* are seen as 2–3 μm haematoxyphilic dots on the glycocalyx of the mucosal cells (Fig. 28.28). Diagnosis may also be made by finding oocysts in a faecal smear.

Pneumocystis pneumonia

Chagas originally described the organism *Pneumocystis carinii*, believing it to be a developmental stage of a trypanosome. Its life cycle is not yet precisely determined, and while probably a protozoon, it may be a fungus. However, it is ubiquitous and inhaled by everyone, yet

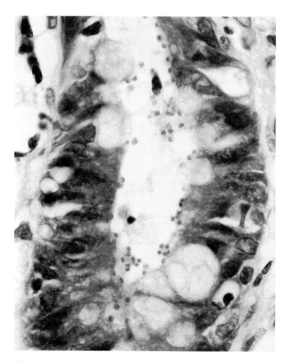

Fig. 28.28 *Cryptosporidium* colitis. The small round parasites are seen on the surface of the epithelium of the intestinal crypts. × 1000.

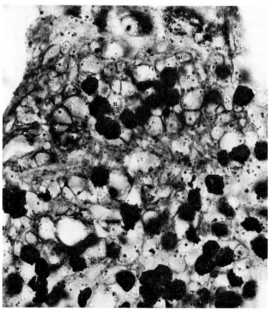

Fig. 28.29 *Pneumocystis carinii* in lung alveolus. The cysts have polygonal shapes and some stain very darkly. Trophozoites are seen as tiny black dots inside the cysts (Grocott silver impregnation). × 1250.

causes disease—an interstitial plasma cell pneumonia—only in neonates and immunosuppressed people.

As a pathogen, it multiplies in the alveolar spaces of the lungs. Clinically there is dyspnoea, unproductive cough and cyanosis. In transplant patients the symptoms develop about six weeks after the start of immunosuppressive therapy. The chest x-ray has a characteristic uniform reticulonodular pattern of bilateral shadowing. The disease may resolve spontaneously or after treatment. In fatal cases, the lungs are consolidated and appear dry and grey. Histologically there is a chronic inflammatory infiltrate in the interstitium with many plasma cells except in patients with a B-cell deficiency. The alveoli and terminal bronchioles contain foamy material in which there are ovoid and crescentic 'cysts' of about $5\,\mu m$ diameter, within and around which there are numerous tiny trophozoites (Fig. 28.29). Minimal cellular reaction is seen within the alveoli in acute cases. The foamy material is phagocytosed in those who recover.

The diagnosis is made by finding cysts in bronchial washings or in a lung biopsy.

Diseases caused by helminths

Helminths (worms) comprise two main phyla, the platyhelminths (flatworms) and the nematodes (roundworms). Flatworms are divided into cestodes (tapeworms) and trematodes (flukes). The size range of parasitic worms is enormous; at one end of the scale are some nematode larvae 0·1 mm long, and at the other are some tapeworms which can reach 10 m in length.

Man may be infected by adult tapeworms in the gut lumen or by larval stages in many viscera; one tapeworm (*Taenia solium*) can have both effects. The trematode flukes reside in blood vessels, bile ducts, lungs or the gut. The more numerous species of nematodes are even more diverse, between them parasitising virtually every tissue.

Broadly speaking, helminth-induced disease relates to the intensity of infection. A plot of the numbers of parasites per host against numbers of people infected by that parasite usually follows a Poisson distribution: most people have relatively few worms and suffer mildly or not at all, whilst a minority with a heavy infection have considerable morbidity and mortality. With only a few of the helminthiases is a single worm able to induce significant disease: examples of this are an *Ascaris* worm obstructing the bile duct, and a hydatid cyst blocking the flow of CSF in the brain.

In some infections, the sheer number of worms and their products appears sufficient to account for disease (e.g. the hookworms and ascarid infections). In others, such as some filariases, the more severe disease states may be associated paradoxically with a reduced parasite load but a high degree of hypersensitivity to worm antigens. In schistosomiasis, to take an intermediate example, the severity of disease depends on both the intensity of infection and the host immune reaction.

Immunity to helminth infections is variable and reflects both the intensity of exposure and individual resistance. Even in the most heavily endemic areas where, for example, 95% of the population may have ascarid intestinal worms, a few people with presumably similar exposure to infection do not acquire, or do not keep, the worms. This probably represents a high innate or rapidly acquired immune resistance. Among those with demonstrable parasites, there is a spectrum of clinical, parasitological, pathological and immunological phenomena which indicate not only a wide range of resulting infection intensities but also a very complex set of host-parasite relationships. Their crucial interaction is well exemplified by *Strongyloides stercoralis* infection, where immunocompetent people may have a few worms in the gut for years with no ill effects, and yet can suffer an overwhelming disseminated infection if their cell-mediated immune defences become defective. This implies that, for this parasite at least, the immunity system is constantly operating in the bowel to contain the infection, even though it cannot eliminate it.

Eosinophil leucocytosis is a common feature of nearly all helminth infections (in contrast to its absence in protozoal diseases). The cause is generally assumed to be immunological, with eosinophil chemotactic factors produced by type 1 (immediate) and type 4 (delayed) hypersensitivity reactions, both of which are common in worm infections. The function of the eosinophil is obscure, although there is evidence that in one disease, schistosomiasis, it is associated with resistance to infection.

Diagnosis. The finding of a raised eosinophil count often starts a search for faecal and urinary ova, or larvae in the blood. The relevance of any positive parasitological findings to a patient's problems should always be considered carefully. For example, a middle-aged expatriate working in Africa who presents with blood in the stool, has a mild eosinophilia and is excreting ova of *Schistosoma mansoni*, may still have a carcinoma of the caecum as the cause of his symptoms.

As with all parasitic infections, diagnosis of helminthic diseases should be made by finding the worm. Serological techniques may eventually prove easier, more reliable and perhaps cheaper, but current methods of worm antibody detection are plagued by cross-reactions between species (particularly with the nematodes) and by a lack of distinction between previous and new, active infections. The specificity, sensitivity and availablity of such tests will undoubtedly increase in the future.

Trematode infections

Trematode worms (also known as flukes) cause chronic infections in many tissues of man, including the bowel lumen, the blood vessels, the lungs and the bile ducts. Apart from the species causing schistosomiasis, they are hermaphrodite, and they all utilise specific freshwater snails as intermediate hosts (see Fig. 28.30). By far the most important trematodes are the blood vessel flukes—the schistosomes—which cause cystitis, intestinal ulceration, hepatic fibrosis, portal hypertension and splenomegaly. These parasites, and the two liver flukes (*Fasciola* and *Opisthorcis*), which live in the bile ducts, will be described in this section.

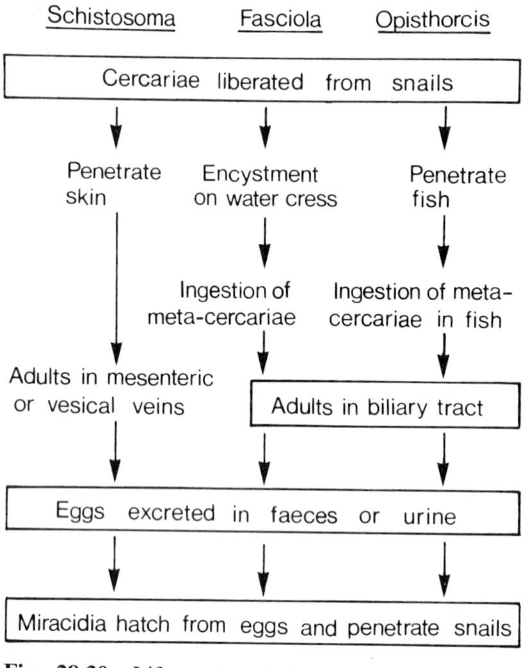

Adult trematodes do not multiply in the human host. The presence of the few worms in the majority of those infected is tolerated with little inconvenience; overt clinical disease follows when the number of parasites is large or when the adults and/or eggs are in an ectopic site in the body.

Fig. 28.30 Life cycle of the parasitic trematode worms.

Schistosomiasis (Bilharzia)

The three main *Schistosoma* species, *S. haematobium*, *S. mansoni* and *S. japonicum*, between them infect 10% of the world's population. The resulting disease, schistosomiasis, is the most important parasitic disease after malaria, and its global incidence is increasing. *S. haematobium* causes urinary schistosomiasis; *S. mansoni* and *S. japonicum* both cause hepatosplenic and intestinal schistosomiasis. Table 28.2 gives further geographical, pathological and parasitological details. *S. japonicum* infection is a zoonosis; the other two species affect only man.

Table 28.2 Summary of the major features of the schistosomiases

Schistosome	Distribution	Habitat of adult worms	Features of ova	Pathology of chronic phase
S. mansoni	Africa, South America, the Caribbean	Mesenteric and portal veins	Lateral spine	1. Hepatic fibrosis, portal hypertension, splenomegaly. 2. Intestinal erosions and polyps. 3. Pulmonary hypertension and right ventricular failure.
S. japonicum	China, South East Asia, the Philippines	Mesenteric and portal veins	Rudimentary lateral spine	As for *S. mansoni*
S. haematobium	Africa, the Middle East	Perivesical and rectal veins	Terminal spine	1. Chronic cystitis, hydronephrosis, bladder carcinoma. 2. Rectal lesions. 3. Pulmonary hypertension and right ventricular failure.

The simplistic equation: 'Man + Snails + Water = Schistosomiasis' is valid because of the high reproductive potential of the life cycle. The peak age of infection is in the first two decades of life, and in many areas the prevalence at this age approaches 100%. Thereafter the prevalence and intensity of infection decline, but in those with moderate to heavy infections, schistosomiasis causes chronic morbidity, with a mortality estimated at 2–10%. It is a predominantly rural disease, a scourge of peasant farmers, and is acquired through contact with water. Children in particular, with their high infection levels, indiscrimate habits of excretion, and predeliction for playing in water, are very important in propagating the disease.

Life cycle (Fig. 28.30). Schistosome eggs in urine or faeces hatch in fresh water and the emerging larva (*miracidium*) penetrates a snail of the appropriate species. After further development in the snail, vast numbers of *cercariae* are released into the water. These are elongated, actively motile larvae, of 360 × 60 μm with a forked tail (Fig. 28.31) and head glands that secrete cytolytic substances. They can penetrate human epidermis in less than 5 minutes, during which the tail is lost, and the larva is then termed a *schistosomulum*. After a few days in the dermis, it enters a venule and is arrested in the lung, where it grows. It then migrates via the systemic circulation to the liver and enters portal veins where final maturation takes place. Thereafter, the adult schistosomes migrate by the bloodstream to their definitive locations: *S. mansoni* and *S. japonicum* to the mesenteric and portal veins and *S. haematobium* to the perivesical venous plexus and rectal veins. Attached to

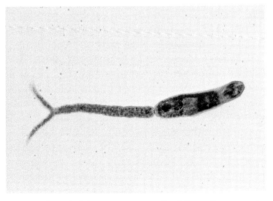

Fig. 28.31 Schistosome cercaria. Note the constriction where the head detaches from the forked tail on skin penetration. × 220.

the endothelium of the veins by their suckers, male and female worms pair up and live in connubial bliss, the female lying in the gynaecophoric canal of the male (Fig. 28.32). They feed on red cells and excrete a dark haemozoin pigment very similar to that produced by malarial parasites. A month after skin penetration, *S. mansoni* and *S. japonicum* worms start laying eggs; this commences after about 8 weeks with *S. haematobium*.

The adult males are about 10 mm long and the females are about 15 mm, depending on the species. Each worm pair of *S. japonicum* lays about 3000 eggs daily, and *S. haematobium* and

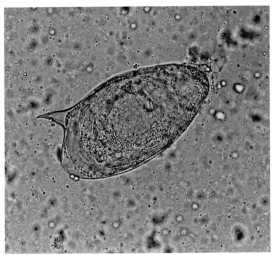

Fig. 28.33 Egg of *S. mansoni* with characteristic lateral spine containing the granular-appearing miracidium. × 400.

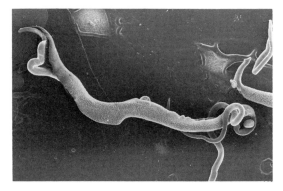

Fig. 28.32 Scanning electron micrograph of a pair of *S. japonicum* worms. The female is longer, thinner and smooth, and lies in the gynaecophoric canal of the male, whose surface appears speckled. × 15.

S. mansoni about 300. Schistosome worms can live for over 20 years, although the mean lifespan is usually 3–5 years. Infection usually increases steadily as new larvae are acquired. Data on *S. mansoni* infections in Brazil indicate that those people with 10 or fewer pairs of worms in the body have little significant clinical disease. Individuals with severe liver fibrosis (*see below*) have 150 to 300 worm pairs. The highest number of worm pairs recorded at autopsy is 1608 in a case of schistosomal colitis. The presence of adult worms in the veins induces no direct host reaction, for during their maturation the schistosomula become non-antigenic by acquiring a coat of host molecules, especially A,B,H and Lewis blood group glycolipids, and this acts as a protective disguise.

The eggs are characteristic in shape and size for each species: those of *S. mansoni* (Fig. 28.33) and *S. haematobium* are about 140 × 60 μm and those of *S. japonicum* are 85 × 60 μm.

The position of the spine on the eggshell is a distinguishing feature (see Table 28.2). The larval miracidium inside the egg is viable for about 3 weeks. After this it degenerates if the egg has not hatched in water. A proportion (roughly half) of the eggs are excreted in the faeces or urine, the rest being retained. *It is the host reaction to the eggs that causes the significant pathology in schistosomiasis.*

Clinical and pathological changes

The various phases of infection have their distinct clinico-pathological features. The host develops an immune response to the antigenic secretion of the head glands of miracidia and to surface antigens of the miracidia and ova. Penetration of the skin by cercariae causes a transient local inflammatory reaction. In many cases this is clinically evident as a rash—'swimmers' itch' or *cercarial dermatitis*. It is probably a hypersensitivity reaction and may account for the modest resistance to re-infection that develops in schistosomiasis. Atopic (type 1), delayed (type 4) hypersensitivity and IgG antibody-dependent eosinophil reactions are thought to be involved. Before or shortly after the onset of egg-laying by the worms, there may be a **constitutional reaction** to a heavy synchronous infection, particularly if this is the first exposure. Fever, cough, diarrhoea, urticaria, hepatosplenomegaly, and a marked eosinophil leucocytosis characterise this phase, known as the *Katayama syndrome*, which may last for days or weeks. The types of hypersensitivity involved are unclear: it has some features of a type 3 (immune-complex) reaction but other types of reaction, kinin activation and even endotoxic shock, may also be involved.

However, neither cercarial dermatitis nor the Katayama syndrome constitute the major problems in schistosomiasis. The reaction to the eggs is the important feature. Wherever the eggs are found, in the liver, bowel or bladder, or in other sites such as the skin, the venule they are in is disrupted and a cellular reaction occurs around the egg. This involves polymorphs initially, then macrophages, lymphocytes and eosinophils, and the evolution of an **epithelioid-cell granuloma** (Fig. 28.34) with giant cells and sometimes central necrosis. Plasma cells accumulate around the granuloma. Like granulomas due to other agents, schistosomal granulomas heal with fibrosis. The eggshell and

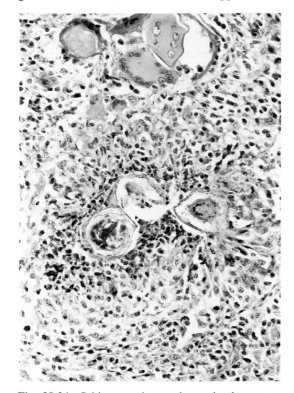

Fig. 28.34 Schistosomal granuloma; in the centre, three eggs are seen inside an epithelioid-cell granuloma with eosinophils and plasma cells. At the top, part of an older granuloma is seen with giant cells phagocytosing fragments of eggshell. × 235.

miracidium are phagocytosed, although many eggs resist full degradation and remain as calcified shells. The characteristic fibrosis and scarring of organs in schistosomiasis are the result of coalescence of fibrosis around thousands or millions of eggs. The cause of the florid reaction to schistosome eggs is immunological, a classic example of a type 4 (delayed) hypersensitivity.

Of course, many eggs leave the body by penetrating the mucosal surfaces of the bowel or bladder without becoming trapped in a granuloma. The mechanism by which they do this is another obscure aspect of schistosomiasis. Although it has been suspected that the miracidium inside the egg secretes a cytotoxic enzyme to aid its migration out of the body, there is no good experimental evidence for this. Alternatively, it is possible that the host cell reaction in some way mediates excretion of eggs. Excretion of eggs is accompanied by inflammation of the mucosae with the focal erosions at the sites of escape of eggs: this causes the **acute cystitis, colitis and ileitis** seen in schistosomiasis.

S. mansoni and *S. japonicum* infections

These parasites affect predominantly the bowel and liver. Roughly half the eggs laid in the portal and mesenteric veins are carried to the liver, the rest remaining in the bowel wall or passing into the lumen.

The liver. The eggs lodge in the portal venules and induce the inflammatory reaction with granulomas. Over months and years, the granulomas heal with fibrosis, and gradually the portal tracts become linked by fibrous tissue. In heavy infections, e.g. with over 100 worm pairs, there is often massive fibrosis around major portal tracts. This scarring may be up to 2 cm across and is known as **Symmers' pipestem fibrosis**—the pictorial analogy is with the white stems of clay pipes being thrust into the liver substance (Fig. 28.35). Such fibrosis is not a true cirrhosis because the lobular architecture is maintained beyond the portal fibrosis. The reaction to the schistosome eggs also induces biliary proliferation, but not obstruction. Blood vessels also proliferate with the formation of shunts between hepatic arterioles and portal venules.

The effects of schistosomal liver disease depend on the intensity of infection. If this is

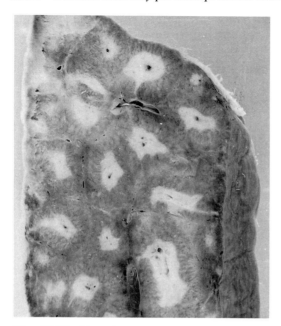

Fig. 28.35 Liver in heavy *S. mansoni* infection showing Symmers' pipestem fibrosis. (Picture kindly supplied by the Wellcome Museum of Medical Science.)

light, there is little clinical upset, but when pipestem fibrosis is marked there are several secondary phenomena. The most important is **portal hypertension**, due to the fibrosis and the intrahepatic arterio-venous shunting. Oesophageal varices and haemorrhage, ascites and splenomegaly with hypersplenism (p. 17.32) follow (although the splenomegaly is in part a consequence of reactive lymphoid hyperplasia). Because the lobular architecture is preserved, liver function is unaffected by schistosomiasis, and the liver can deal with the metabolites of an absorbed blood meal from oesophageal haemorrhage, repeated episodes of which are characteristic of hepatosplenic schistosomiasis: hepatic encephalopathy does not follow unless the liver is severely damaged by ensuing hypovolaemic shock. *Because schistosomiasis is such a prevalent disease, it is the commonest single cause of portal hypertension in the world.* Just as schistosomiasis does not cause cirrhosis, nor does it predispose to hepatocellular carcinoma. *S. haematobium* does not significantly affect the liver.

Macroscopically, the liver is usually enlarged and nodular; on cut section, fine fibrosis or the massive Symmers' fibrosis is evident. Histolog-

ically, schistosome eggs are seen in epithelioid cell granulomas in the portal tracts with a diffuse eosinophilia. Dark brown haemozoin pigment granules are found in portal macrophages and Kupffer cells. In the areas of fibrosis, hyalinising granulomas and some eggshell remnants are seen.

The spleen is enlarged up to 1·5 kg. It is firm and dark, and histologically there is lymphoid hyperplasia, pigment deposition and an occasional egg.

The intestine. All three schistosome species affect the bowel. *S. mansoni* and *S. japonicum* eggs affect the whole bowel from duodenum to rectum; *S. haematobium* eggs are usually confined to the appendix and large bowel. The acute inflammatory lesions around eggs in the gut wall and passing through the mucosa (Fig. 28.36) cause bleeding and diarrhoea: grossly they appear as small raised granular foci with haemorrhagic points. *Schistosomal polyps*, consisting of masses of eggs in the submucosa and inflamed hyperplastic mucosa may develop in the large bowel (Fig. 28.37). They are usually due to a pair of worms blocking a draining venule and pouring eggs continuously into it. The polyps can obstruct the lumen and can form the apex of an intussusception. Elsewhere,

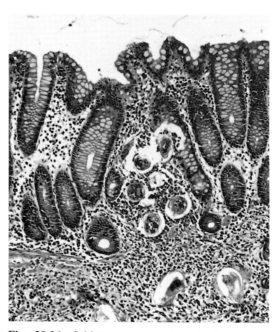

Fig. 28.36 Schistosome eggs in colonic mucosa. One has broken into a gland. Note the marked inflammatory cell infiltrate. × 125.

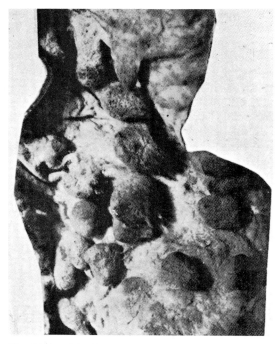

Fig. 28.37 Multiple schistosomal polyps protruding from colonic mucosa. (Picture kindly supplied by the Wellcome Museum of Medical Science.)

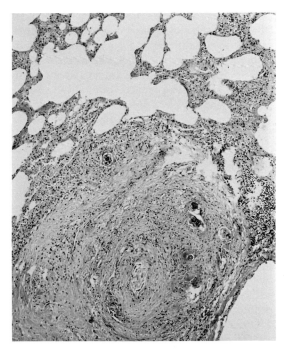

Fig. 28.38 Schistosomal pulmonary hypertension. Small pulmonary artery with eggs and fibrosis. × 80.

there may be focal fibrosis of the bowel. In the serosa and mesentery, nodules composed of eggs, granulomas and fibrosis are occasionally found—so-called '*bilharziomas*'. Despite the widespread intestinal disease, schistosomiasis does not cause malabsorption. Nor does it predispose to colorectal carcinoma. Specimens of acute appendicitis in endemic areas often contain schistosome eggs in the submucosa, but there is no aetiological relationship between the two diseases.

When porto-systemic venous anastomoses are established in schistosomal portal hypertension, eggs can pass from the abdominal veins to the lungs. This also occurs in *S. haematobium* infections, because the pelvic veins drain into the inferior vena cava. The eggs impact in the pulmonary arterioles and induce a granulomatous reaction with arteritis and fibrosis (Fig. 28.38). If the infection is heavy, arterial plexiform lesions associated with pulmonary hypertension are formed throughout the lungs, and right ventricular failure develops in a small proportion of cases.

S. haematobium infection

The urinary bladder. Eggs laid by worms in the veins of the bladder induce a heavy inflammatory reaction in the mucosa and underlying connective tissue. Eggs passing through the mucosa cause focal erosion of the epithelium. The clinical effects are a painful cystitis and haematuria (characteristically at the end of micturition), which can lead to chronic iron deficiency. Historically, Egypt, where *S.haematobium* is highly prevalent, was known as the 'land of menstruating males'.

Cystoscopically, the mucosa appears granular. The inflammation causes a reactive hyperplasia of the urothelium, and in a very heavy infection gross polyps (Fig. 28.39) result from the hyperplasia and the underlying masses of inflammatory tissue around eggs (Fig. 28.40). Thus in the acute stage the mucosa appears hyperaemic, and thickened. Histologically, eggs are seen in the venules, in and under the mucosa, surrounded by a heavy diffuse eosinophil infiltrate and granulomas. The hyperplastic epithelium is often metaplastic, with glandular or squamous appearance. Adult worms are commonly seen in veins in the outer part of the bladder wall.

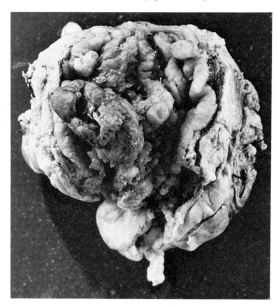

Fig. 28.39 Large polyps in the urinary bladder in severe *S. haematobium* infection.

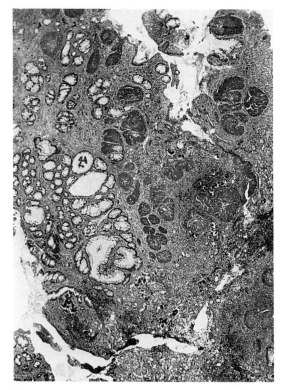

Fig. 28.40 Schistosomiasis of the urinary bladder, showing glandular metaplasia of the surface epithelium, chronic inflammation and fibrosis. × 80.

As the infection becomes chronic, there are several additional features. Retained eggs tend to calcify and remain in the bladder wall: eventually they are so numerous that a plain x-ray of the pelvis will show the viscus as a thick calcified ring. The muscular coat and sub-mucosa become rigid as a result of the granuloma-induced scarring, and this may affect bladder contraction, so that emptying is incomplete. Secondary bacterial cystitis with coliforms and *Salmonellae* follows in a proportion of cases. Microscopically, vast numbers of calcified eggs are seen embedded in a fibrous stroma, beneath an attenuated epithelium often of stratified squamous type.

The ureters are commonly affected by *S. haematobium*, and the pathology is similar to that in the bladder. Inflammation and fibrosis at the lower end of the ureter cause obstruction, and hydronephrosis develops in up to a quarter of infected children in some parts of Africa. However, treatment by anti-schistosomal drugs results in relief of the **obstructive uropathy** in most early cases.

Carcinoma of the bladder. *Heavy S. haematobium infection predisposes to bladder cancer, which accounts for about one-quarter of deaths from this infection and has a peak incidence between 40 and 60 years.* Unlike the usual bladder cancer, the schistosomiasis-associated tumour is usually a well-differentiated squamous cell carcinoma. It grows from the posterior or lateral wall and projects into the bladder lumen, forming a keratinising mass, but also invades through the wall and later metastasises. Its aetiology is obscure: neither the worms nor the eggs have been shown to produce any carcinogenic agent. Currently, the best explanation is as follows: (1) chronic urinary schistosomiasis causes squamous metaplasia of the urothelium and predisposes to Gram −ve bacterial cystitis; (2) the bacteria (e.g. *Esch. coli*) produce nitrosamines by breakdown of dietary nitrites and nitrates excreted in the urine; (3) the carcinogenic nitrosamines act on the squamous epithelium as initiating agents, and (4) the persistent inflammation and epithelial irritation induced by the schistosomal infection act as promoting factors.

Other organs. Worms in the pelvis can lay eggs in other organs of the genito-urinary tract. Thus schistosomal granulomas are commonly found in the epididymis, testis, prostate and seminal vesicles. In women, the ovaries, fallopian tubes and cervix are affected; in the cervix, the inflammation and epithelial proliferation may be so marked as to simulate carcinoma. Schistosomiasis has, however, no aetiological relationship to cervical carcinoma although that tumour is particularly common in developing countries. In both sexes, itchy nodules in the groin areas can result from ectopic egg deposition in the dermis.

The **intestinal** and **pulmonary lesions** in *S. haematobium* infections have been described on pp. 28.26–27.

Other lesions in schistosomiasis

Schistosome worms do not always follow the classical migration pathways, and adults may end up anywhere in the body. If they pair and lay eggs, typical granulomatous inflammation results. Thus schistosomal lesions in lymph nodes, skin and pancreas are not uncommon. The most severe 'ectopic' schistosomal lesions are found in the *central nervous system. S. japonicum* worms can inhabit the veins inside the skull, and *S. mansoni* and *S. haematobium* worms can live within vertebral veins. In the neural tissue, the eggs and inflammation produce space occupying lesions, resulting in focal neurological signs and sometimes paraplegia. Obviously, diagnosis can be made only by biopsy of a lesion.

As noted above, hydronephrosis often results from schistosomal urinary obstruction; less frequently, schistosomal granulomas form in the kidney. Circulating immune complexes are present in schistosomiasis, and an immune complex glomerulonephritis of mesangiocapillary type (p. 22.29) has been described in *S. mansoni* infections (but not with other species). This lesion is, however, much less common than obstructive uropathy resulting from *S. haematobium* infection.

Diagnosis

Schistosomiasis is diagnosed by finding the eggs. All three species excrete eggs in the faeces, and they may be seen microscopically in faecal suspensions. Alternatively, a biopsy of rectal mucosa can be pressed between two slides and examined for eggs. Histological examination of rectal and liver biopsies is overall a less sensitive method, but biopsy is necessary to diagnose the grosser lesions such as bilharziomas. Similarly, in urinary schistosomiasis, examination of urine sediment for eggs is straightforward; cystoscopy and biopsy is used for complex lesions. The schistosome species is identified by the shape of the egg and the position of the spine (p. 28.23).

Serology for schistosomiasis, using egg antigens and the enzyme-linked immunosorbent assay technique, is very sensitive. However, most of the available tests do not discriminate old from new infections, and they are used mainly for epidemiological purposes.

Fascioliasis

Sheep and cattle are the main definitive hosts of *Fasciola hepatica*; sheep liver-rot is a veterinary problem in most sheep-raising areas of the world. Man is only occasionally infected.

The metacercariae are ingested with contaminated water-cress (see trematode life cycle, Fig. 28.30) and excyst in the duodenum, releasing larvae which penetrate the gut wall and migrate in the peritoneal cavity. They then burrow

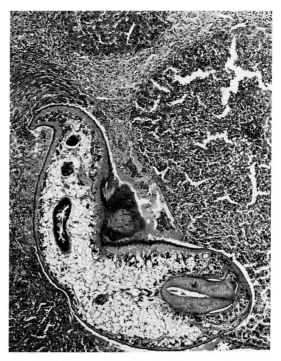

Fig. 28.41 Young *Fasciola hepatica* worm burrowing through the liver. × 80.

directly into the liver parenchyma, leaving a trail of necrosis and inflammation (Fig. 28.41). In the acute phase, the patient has a tender enlarged liver, fever, and eosinophil leucocytosis. Rarely, a subcapsular haematoma develops and ruptures, causing intra-abdominal haemorrhage. The worms gain access to the bile ducts where they mature into leaf-like adults (about 30 × 10 mm) and remain attached to the biliary mucosa, laying their eggs in the bile.

The adult worms induce hyperplasia of the biliary epithelium, periductal inflammation and some fibrosis. Most patients have only a few worms; the hepatic symptoms subside and there is spontaneous recovery after a year or so. Heavier infections may cause obstructive jaundice. During their migration, worms may get lost and appear in the subcutaneous tissues of the abdomen as itchy nodules. Unlike opisthorciasis, fascioliasis does not predispose to the development of cholangiocarcinoma.

The diagnosis of fascioliasis can be difficult because eggs are usually scanty in the faeces: serology is helpful when they cannot be found.

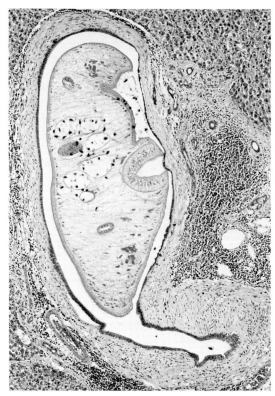

Fig. 28.42 *Opisthorcis* adult attached to the biliary epithelium by its sucker. There is marked periductal fibrosis. Several small dark ova are seen in the coiled uterus of the worm. × 65.

Opisthorciasis

The most important of the three *Opisthorcis* species affecting man is *O. sinensis* (formerly *Clonorchis sinensis*). Up to 75% of people in the focal endemic zones in the Far East may be infected but, as with most helminthiases, only those with heavy infections—in this case, hundreds to thousands of worms in the liver—suffer symptoms and permanent organ damage.

The metacercariae ingested during consumption of raw fish excyst in the duodenum and pass through the ampulla of Vater into the biliary system. The adults do not invade but attach to the biliary tract epithelium, mainly in the intrahepatic bile ducts but also in the common bile and cystic ducts and the gallbladder. They are flat in shape, measure about 16 × 4 mm and feed on the epithelium (Fig. 28.42). Reactive hyperplasia of the biliary epithelium, periductal inflammation and fibrosis follow. The worms live for up to 20 years, each releasing a thousand or so eggs daily into the bile. Only occasionally are eggs deposited in breaches of the epithelium, where they provoke a granulomatous reaction.

Unlike fascioliasis, necrosis does not occur during invasion of the liver, and disease symptoms come late. Serious effects result from worms obstructing bile ducts with consequent secondary infection and suppurative cholangitis, bile retention cysts, biliary stones (often containing a dead worm), and cholecystitis if worms or stones obstruct the cystic duct. Biliary cirrhosis and pancreatitis are rare complications. Damage to the bile duct can also lead to a chronic carrier state with *Salmonella* sp., an effect similar to that seen in urinary schistosomiasis. In milder symptomatic infections there is tender hepatomegaly. A low grade eosinophil leucocytosis is common.

Intrahepatic cholangiocarcinoma is relatively common in patients with a heavy *Opisthorcis* infection. The worms probably act as promoters by their irritatant action on the biliary epithelium.

Opisthorciasis is diagnosed by finding the eggs in the faeces.

Cestode diseases

Adult cestodes or tapeworms are flat, ribbon-shaped, segmented worms of sometimes vast length which reside in the intestinal lumen of a definitive host. Their life cycle requires an intermediate host, in which the larvae often take the form of cysts in the tissues. Man can be infected with both adult and larval stages although it is the larval forms which are most harmful. The important human cestode infections are the *taeniases, cysticercosis, hydatid disease* and *diphyllobothriasis*. All cestodes have a common life cycle (Fig. 28.43): the adult in the

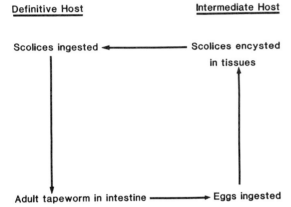

Definitive Host   **Intermediate Host**

Scolices ingested ◄————————— Scolices encysted
                                        in tissues

Adult tapeworm in intestine ————► Eggs ingested

Fig. 28.43 Life cycle of *Taenia* and *Echinococcus* tapeworms.

intestine sheds into the faeces gravid segments containing numerous eggs. The eggs contaminate the soil, are ingested by an intermediate host, and hatch into *oncospheres* or larvae, which invade through the intestinal mucosa and disseminate to various viscera; in the infections to be considered here, this spread is haematogenous and the larvae develop into cysts that contain one or more tiny rounded bodies termed *scolices*, which are the heads of future adult worms. When tissues containing the cysts are eaten by carnivores, including man, a scolex attaches to the gut mucosa by means of suckers or hooks and grows into a chain of segments (*proglottids*). Self- or cross-fertilisation of segments occurs and the distal gravid segments are shed.

Taeniases

Man is the only definitive host for *Taenia solium* (the pork tapeworm) and *Taenia saginata* (the beef tapeworm). The worms are cosmopolitan and about 100 million people are infected. Like all cestodiases, their epidemiology depends less on climate than on the distribution of the intermediate hosts. The worms are acquired by eating undercooked or raw measly (i.e. cyst-containing) meat from domestic pigs (*T. solium*) and bovines (*T. saginata*).

The final length of an adult *T. solium* is about 6 metres, whilst *T. saginata* can reach 8 metres. They consist of hundreds of 1 cm square, flat segments (Fig. 28.44), and their lifespan is up to 25 years. Usually only one worm is present in the intestine and it generally has little effect on the host. Symptoms of mild dyspepsia and fullness are common but there is no malabsorption or weight loss. Psychological upset on seeing moving segments in the faeces or occasionally the unpleasant sensation of a segment wriggling through the anus are more relevant consequences. In the early phase of infection, there may be a mild eosinophil leucocytosis.

These infections are diagnosed by finding

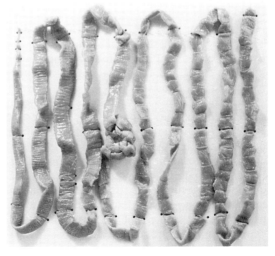

Fig. 28.44 An adult *Taenia* tapeworm. The head (scolex) is the small section at the top left. The mature gravid square segments are evident in the distal half. (St Thomas's Hospital Medical School Pathology Museum.)

either segments or eggs in the faeces; although the eggs of the two species are identical, their segments may be differentiated by the pattern of the uterus. Parasitologically and clinically, the significant difference is that while eggs of *T. saginata* cannot develop further in man, those of *T. solium* can do so, resulting in cysticercosis (see below).

Diphyllobothriasis

Diphyllobothrium latum is a relatively uncommon intestinal parasite of temperate zones. A larva is eaten in infected fresh-water fish, and grows into the longest of all helminths, measuring up to 10 metres. Like the *Taenias*, usually only one tapeworm develops and it lives for about 20 years attached to the ileal mucosa.

Pathologically, the only serious effect of infection arises from the worm's consumption of dietary vitamin B_{12} in competition with the host (p. 17.38). In Finland, 10% of people with diphyllobothriasis have some degree of megaloblastic erythropoiesis, but only 2% are actually anaemic as a result. In other parts of the world, diphyllobothriasis is asymptomatic.

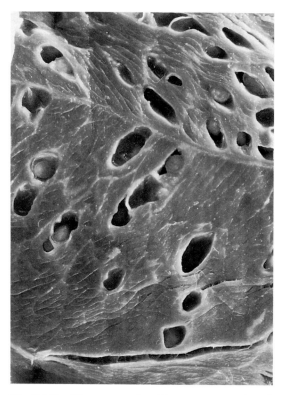

Fig. 28.45 Human muscle with numerous cysticerci. In many of them, the scolex can be seen as a solid ball within the bladder-like cyst. (St Thomas's Hospital Medical School Pathology Museum). ×2.

Cysticercosis

The relationship between man and *Taenia solium* is most unusual in that man can be host to both the adult and the larval form; the latter results in cysticercosis.

The larvae form 5 × 10 mm cysts which act as space-occupying lesions in many viscera and cause particular damage if located in the brain or eye. Less than 25% of people with cysticercosis also harbour an adult *T. solium* in the bowel, the majority of cyst infections being acquired by ingesting eggs from the environment rather than by regurgitating back into the stomach a gravid segment of the host's own tapeworm. The cysts grow slowly and the incubation period may be several years.

The disease is common in many tropical and subtropical regions where, like tuberculosis, it is a far more frequent cause of cerebral lesions than primary brain tumours. A patient may have hundreds of cysts distributed in skeletal

muscle (Fig. 28.45), subcutis, heart, the central nervous system and the eye. The cyst is a fluid-filled bladder containing one scolex (Fig. 28.46). While it is alive, it elicits little or no inflammatory reaction. After some years, it dies and stimulates the formation of florid granulation tissue with foreign-body giant cells but little tissue eosinophilia. Finally, the degenerate shrunken cyst becomes calcified and enclosed in a fibrous capsule.

Cysts are most frequent in **skeletal muscle** where they are usually asymptomatic and often discovered by chance when an x-ray reveals calcified nodules in the **soft tissues**. They may present as soft nodules under the skin. In the **brain**, the cysts act as space-occupying lesions in the meninges, parenchyma and ventricles. Because the nervous tissue is soft, the cysts may grow to 2 cm in diameter: focal neurological signs and epilepsy are frequent, and hydrocephalus can result from a blockage of the third ventricle or aqueduct by a cyst. As the cysts

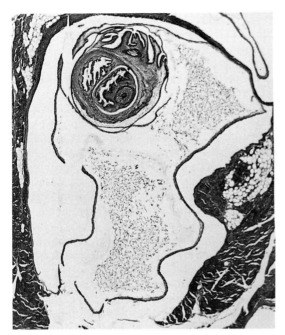

Fig. 28.46 Cysticercus in muscle. Inside the cyst is the scolex, which is inverted. The central targetoid structure is a sucker. × 20.

die, the host reaction can aggravate the clinical effects, and may cause symptoms in previously silent infections. The mortality from neurocysticercosis may exceed 10%. In the **eye**, cysts are found in the retina, vitreous or anterior chamber; optic shadows and blindness may follow, with secondary reactions such as conjunctivitis, uveitis, retinitis and finally optic atrophy.

Diagnosis of cysticercosis may be difficult. Biopsy of a subcutaneous lump will give a ready answer, but confirmation of neurocysticercosis is not always possible. Computerised axial tomography shows up most cysts, and can monitor their disappearance with medical therapy. Serological diagnostic techniques are improving, but cases with only central nervous system involvement may be seronegative.

Hydatid disease (Echinococcosis)

Hydatid disease, caused by the larvae of *Echinococcus granulosus*, is the most serious tapeworm infection in man. One or more large cysts in the viscera behave as chronic space-occupying lesions. Medical therapy is so far poor, and surgery is difficult with the risk of dissemination of cyst material: this is a 'metastasising' parasite.

Life cycle. The adult tapeworms are 5-9 mm long and live in the small bowel of dogs. Eggs eaten by sheep and cattle, which are the main intermediate hosts, develop into hydatid cysts in their viscera. Offal containing cysts is consumed by the dogs. Man acquires cysts by eating eggs from dog coats and faeces. Man is probably not always a dead end for the parasite, since some African tribes in endemic areas lay out the bodies of their dead to be eaten by canine carnivores. Hydatid disease is prevalent in sheep-raising countries in all latitudes: early this century, up to a third of the population of Iceland had cysts, and in Southern Australia half the dogs are infected with adult *E. granulosus*. The disease is a major problem in the Middle East, North and sub-Saharan Africa, and South America.

Pathological changes. When eggs are ingested by man, the oncospheres hatch out, pass through the duodenal mucosa, and then by the portal vein to the liver, where cysts may develop or the embryos may disseminate by the bloodstream to other organs. The cyst grows slowly, reaching 1-5 cm in diameter by 6 months, and a final size of 5 to over 20 cm. Whatever the tissue, a hydatid cyst has a similar structure (Fig. 28.47). There is a surrounding host fibrous capsule enclosing the cyst wall, which is 1 mm thick, white, acellular, soft, chitinous and laminated. Inside is a thin cellular lining, the germinal membrane, from which develop the scolices. Smaller cysts (daughter cysts or brood capsules) develop from the germinal membrane inside the main cyst and these also generate scolices (Fig. 28.48). Thus fertile cysts contain myriads of scolices, which are visible as grains of 'hydatid sand' in the otherwise clear or slightly yellowish cyst fluid. The fibrous capsule and parasite cyst wall may rupture, spilling fragments of germinal membrane which can form new hydatid cysts nearby. Scolices cannot, of course, develop further in man.

An infected person may have one or several hydatid cysts: 50% of them are in the **liver**, usually in the right lobe, where they produce hepatomegaly and occasionally obstruct the portal vein and bile duct. Cysts in the **lung** are rather less common, causing pressure collapse

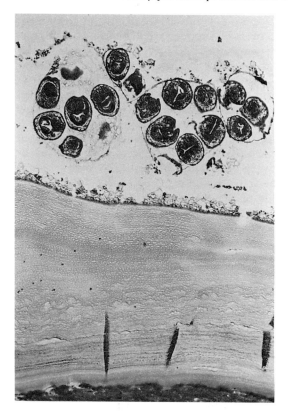

Fig. 28.47 The lining of a hydatid cyst. From the bottom upwards are the host fibrous capsule (stained dark), the pale laminated cyst wall, the thin cellular germinal membrane and, lying in the cyst cavity, three brood capsules containing rounded scolices. ×95.

of the affected lobe, haemoptysis and pleural effusion. Any other organ of the body can be involved, notably the **spleen** (hydatids are the commonest form of splenic cyst) and the **breast**. In the **peritoneal cavity**, where the host reaction is slight, multiple cysts expand to produce great abdominal swelling. **Bone** hydatids occur in about 2% of cases and are very difficult to remove: in the vertebrae, they produce relentless spinal cord compression and vertebral collapse. Similarly, cysts in the **brain** cause focal signs and obstruct the flow of CSF with resulting hydrocephalus (Fig. 28.49). In addition to causing pain, cysts in the **kidneys** are an uncommon cause of renal failure. *In areas of the world where hydatid disease is highly prevalent, all tumours in any organ should be suspected of being hydatids until proved otherwise.*

In addition to the pathological effects of organ compression, allergic reactions occur if a cyst ruptures spontaneously or through trauma or surgery. The spillage of hydatid antigen results in a type 1 (anaphylactic) reaction with

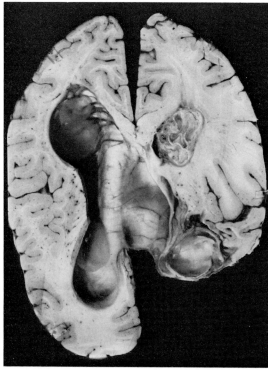

Fig. 28.49 Hydatid cysts in the brain. Several cysts are seen in the lateral ventricle and have caused hydrocephalus. On the right is a collapsed cyst with convoluted internal cyst walls.

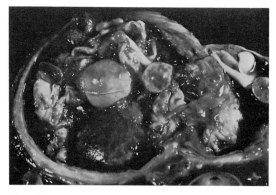

Fig. 28.48 Hydatid cyst of liver. Several daughter cysts, some collapsed, are lying in the main cyst. Note the fibrous capsule around the cyst.

dyspnoea, cyanosis and circulatory collapse; in suspected cases of a cyst in the liver, needle biopsy should not be attempted for this reason. The treatment of a hydatid cyst is problematic. Surgery is still the choice for accessible cysts causing clinically-important compression, but care is needed not to spill any of the contents. To prevent metastasis of fertile germinal membrane, hepatic cysts are instilled with formaldehyde after exposure, before proceeding with their removal. Recurrent peritoneal cysts are a common complication of inadequate surgery on the liver. Lung cysts are easier to remove intact, using positive pressure ventilation.

Overall, the mortality of diagnosed hydatid disease is about 10%. Although there is evidence of an immune host response to hydatid antigens, there is no effective resistance to infection.

Diagnosis. Serology is reasonably specific, and the old Casoni skin test, which had too much cross reactivity, is no longer performed. In some cases there is an eosinophil leucocytosis. Radiology and ultrasound examination are useful to locate hydatid cysts, which are readily recognisable histologically. Occasionally a lung hydatid ruptures into a bronchus, and hooklets from dead scolices may be seen microscopically in the sputum.

Nematode infections

Nematodes are cylindrical smooth worms which grow to adult size by several moults. They are dioecious, i.e. of separate sexes, and they tend to be long-lived. With the exception of *Strongyloides stercoralis*, their life cycles include an obligatory phase outside the human host. Some of the species require also an intermediate host.

The most important nematode infections are the intestinal worms and the filariases. Also considered in this section are trichinosis, guinea-worm infection, and the larva migrans syndromes.

Intestinal nematodes

Intestinal nematodes are ubiquitous, and even if man avoids infection by those adapted to him alone, he may be parasitised by the larvae of roundworms living in the gut of lower animals (see *larva migrans*, p. 28.47).

The most important intestinal nematodes are *Enterobius vermicularis*, *Trichuris trichiura*, the two hookworms (*Necator americanus* and *Ancylostoma duodenale*), *Ascaris lumbricoides* and *Strongyloides stercoralis*. Their life cycles are of varying complexity (see Fig. 28.50) and they are acquired either by ingesting ova or by active penetration of the skin by larvae living in the soil. None of them has an intermediate host,

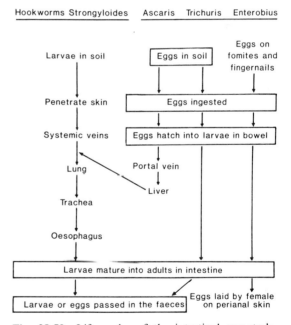

Fig. 28.50 Life cycles of the intestinal nematode worms.

but one of them, *Strongyloides stercoralis*, is unique in that it can maintain its cycle entirely within the human body. The other species have a finite lifespan and the infections die out unless new worms are acquired. Further details of these parasites are given in Table 28.3.

Table 28.3   Features and effects of the common intestinal nematodes of man

Parasite	Adult female: length in mm	Location	Lifespan	Clinical effects
Enterobius	10–12	Colon, appendix	4 weeks	Pruritus ani; rarely intra-abdominal abscesses.
Trichuris	30–50	Colon	1–2 years	Diarrhoea, rectal prolapse.
Hookworms	10–12	Jejunum	5 years	Blood loss, iron-deficiency anaemia, pneumonitis, dermatitis.
Strongyloides	2	Ileum	Unknown (persists by autoinfection)	Diarrhoea, malabsorption, pneumonitis, dermatitis: hyperinfection, visceral dissemination.
Ascaris	200–400	Ileum	1–2 years	Bowel and bile duct obstruction, pneumonitis.

Enterobiasis (Oxyuriasis)

This condition is world-wide and possibly the commonest human infection after the common cold. It is caused by *Enterobius vermicularis*, and has many synonyms including *oxyuriasis*, *pinworm* and *threadworm* infection. The highest prevalence is in children.

The worms are acquired by ingesting eggs, either one's own or from the environment (Fig. 28.50). The larvae in the eggs hatch in the ileum and the mature worms move to the appendix (Fig. 28.51) and large intestine where the males and females mate. The gravid females migrate out of the anus at night and each lays about 10 000 eggs on the peri-anal skin and then dies. The eggs are dispersed on bed clothes, personal clothes, the floor and the walls, and some are picked up under the fingernails to autoinfect the subject later on. This cycle of infection lasts 4 to 6 weeks; the ubiquity of the eggs accounts for the ease of re-infection.

The clinical phenomena are primarily itching of the peri-anal skin (*pruritus ani*) and, in women, the vulval skin. This is a reaction to the worm proteins and the eggs. The adult worms in the bowel lumen have no significant local effect; as initiators of acute appendicitis they are probably unimportant.

An uncommon complication of enterobiasis is seen if a gravid female worm migrates up the female genital tract, by which route a worm can reach the peritoneal cavity. When it dies it provokes an intense eosinophil and granulomatous reaction with central necrosis and abscess formation. Thus endometritis, salpingitis, serosal nodules and liver abscesses can occur. The abscesses are bacteriologically sterile and the contents are greenish-white. In the liver, they can masquerade as metastatic tumour deposits in patients undergoing laparotomy for bowel cancer.

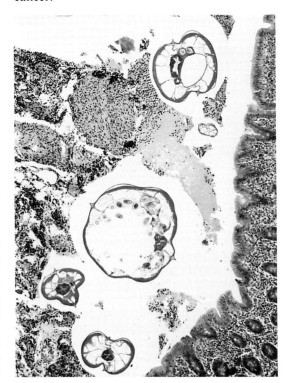

Fig. 28.51   Lumen of the appendix, showing cross-sections of *Enterobius vermicularis* adults. The paired lateral spines on the outer cuticle of the worms are characteristic. × 80.

Adult worms may be seen in the stools or around the anus at night. Examination of faeces for ova is unrewarding, and the easiest method of diagnosing enterobiasis is by applying clear sticky tape to the anal skin of the subject after sleeping. The eggs adhere to the tape and can be identified by examining it microscopically.

Trichuriasis (Whipworm infection)

Trichuris trichiura is also widespread and about 500 million people are affected throughout the world. Like ascariasis, trichuriasis is particularly common where human faeces are used as fertiliser ('night soil'). Eggs are ingested with soil or vegetables and hatch in the ileum. The mature adults are about 50 mm long and live in the colon and rectum with their thin anterior end attached to the mucosa and the long, wider,

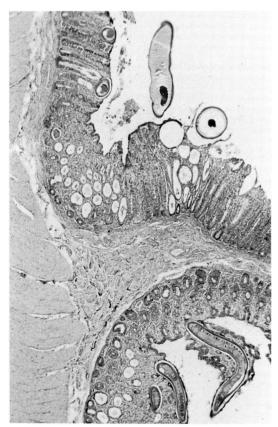

Fig. 28.52 Colonic mucosa, showing several *Trichuris* worms. The narrower anterior ends are buried in the mucosa whilst the broader posterior ends lie in the lumen. × 28.

coiled posterior part (the 'whip') hanging in the lumen (Fig. 28.52). The female lays about 5000 eggs per day into the faeces.

Mild infections are symptomless. Heavy infections with hundreds of worms are associated with diarrhoea, and occasionally rectal prolapse in children. The mucosal damage from the physical attachment can also lead to significant blood loss and iron-deficiency anaemia if more than 1000 worms are present. Eosinophil leucocytosis is common in the early stages of infection. Diagnosis is made by finding eggs in the faeces or by seeing the worms on sigmoidoscopy.

Hookworm infection (Ancylostomiasis)

Hookworm infection of the bowel is one of the most important human afflictions. At least 700 million people are infected and a proportion suffer debilitating chronic anaemia as a consequence. The two species of human hookworm, *Necator americanus* and *Ancylostoma duodenale*, have similar morphology and life cycles (Fig. 28.50). They are both found in the tropics and subtropics and *A. duodenale* also extends into temperate regions.*

Life cycle. The parasite has an obligate phase in the soil, where eggs deposited in faeces hatch into larvae. The larvae actively penetrate human skin, usually bare feet, and are carried in the venous blood to the lungs. Whilst developing, larvae break into the alveoli, crawl up the airways to the pharynx, and are swallowed. The mature adults reside in the jejunum, attached to the villi. *N. americanus* females lay about 5000 eggs per day, and *A. duodenale* up to 20 000 eggs per day.

Clinical and pathological features depend on the intensity of infection and on previous exposure. Repeated infection sensitises the host so that penetrating larvae cause an intensely itchy dermatitis—'*ground itch*'. This inflammation may be a manifestation of resistance, because partial immunity does develop to the infection. During the phase of migration through the lungs, a heavy infection can induce an eosinophil leucocytosis and a pneumonitis, although this is not as severe as Loeffler's pneumonitis seen in ascariasis.

*In 1909 the forerunner of the Rockefeller Foundation was instituted for the sole purpose of eliminating hookworm infection from the USA and Puerto Rico.

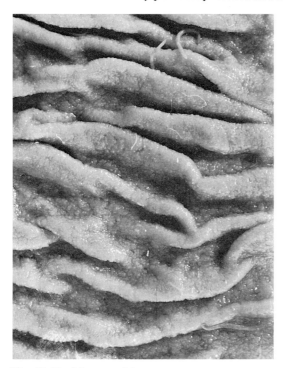

Fig. 28.53 Mucosa of ileum with three hookworms attached (two towards the top, one near the bottom of the picture). (St Thomas's Hospital Medical School Pathology Museum.)

The most important clinical effects arise from the attachment of the worms to the jejunal mucosa (Fig. 28.53). The worm is 10 mm long: it attaches to the mucosa by grasping a villus in its mouth, wriggles continuously and sucks blood from the villus. It also secretes an anti-coagulant, and even when a hookworm detaches and moves to another part of the mucosa, bleeding continues for a while. Each *N. americanus* worm causes loss of 0·03 ml of blood daily, and *A. duodenale* loss of 0·1 ml per day. An individual may harbour up to 2000 worms, but even a few hundred cause **chronic iron-deficiency anaemia**, which is often aggravated by a diet low in iron. The worms live for about 5 years and are a very important cause of debility from anaemia. Infection is diagnosed by finding the eggs (identical in the two species) in the faeces.

Strongyloidiasis

Infection with *Strongyloides stercoralis* is endemic in the tropics and subtropics with an estimated 100–200 million cases. An unusual feature affecting the life cycle of this worm is the ability of its eggs to hatch and invade without being excreted by the host. By this means, the parasite can persist for decades after a person has left an area of infection. Recent surveys of British ex-servicemen who were prisoners of war in Burma between 1941 and 1945 have shown that up to 20% of them still carry *Strongyloides stercoralis* in their bowel.

The life cycle of *S. stercoralis* (Fig. 28.50) is similar to that of the hookworms. However, the adult females are smaller (2 mm long), lie buried in the ileal mucosa and produce eggs parthenogenetically, i.e. a male worm is unnecessary, and has rarely been demonstrated in man. The eggs hatch in the lumen of the intestine, and most of the larvae are passed with the faeces. Some larvae mature into infective forms by the time they reach the anus and can penetrate the peri-anal skin directly, pass via the lungs to the bowel and maintain the infection even in the absence of fresh invasion from parasites in the soil. This *auto-infective cycle* is, however, usually prevented, by protective immune mechanisms in the bowel (p. 6.37), from producing a heavy infection except in subjects with defective cell-mediated immunity, in whom massive auto- infection occurs. Not only do larvae penetrate the skin to re-cycle and increase the parasite load, but they can also invade the bowel mucosa and disseminate via the blood stream and lymph throughout the body—*the 'hyperinfection syndrome'*.

As with the hookworms, the phase of larval invasion by *Strongyloides* can produce skin eruptions and pneumonitis. The ileal mucosa is inflamed and the villi focally blunted. In moderate infections, the patient may have some diarrhoea and mild malabsorption, and eosinophil leucocytosis is usual.

The hyperinfection syndrome of strongyloidiasis is life-threatening. The typical cases are people with chronic *S. stercoralis* infection (usually asymptomatic) who are treated by immunosuppressive drugs, e.g. following organ transplantation, or who are grossly malnourished or develop a neoplasm, e.g. a lymphoma, which depresses immunity. There is severe diarrhoea, malabsorption, hepatomegaly and prostration. In addition to the effects of widespread visceral spread of larvae, *Escherichia coli* septicaemia is common, the bacilli entering the

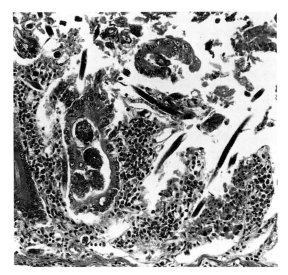

Fig. 28.54 Ileal mucosa in *Strongyloides* hyperinfection. Inside the crypt on the left are four cross-sections of the adult female worm. Above and to the right, several thinner elongated larvae are seen. × 200

blood through breaches in the bowel mucosa. The entire gut is dilated, oedematous and haemorrhagic. Microscopically, the mucosa is grossly inflamed and distorted by innumerable adult worms and larvae (Fig. 28.54). Larvae are seen also in the liver, lungs, brain and meninges, and are surrounded by an inflammatory reaction with eosinophils. The syndrome is fatal unless treated, and it is a diagnosis to be considered in immunocompromised patients with unexplained multi-organ damage.

Strongyloidiasis is diagnosed by detecting larvae in the faeces. In the hyperinfection syndrome, larvae can be found in large numbers in a gastric aspirate and sputum, as well as in the stools.

Ascariasis

Ascaris lumbricoides is by far the largest intestinal nematode, measuring 20–40 cm in length and 5–6 mm in diameter. Much of the pathology of acariasis is due to worms obstructing viscera.

The condition is world-wide and about 800 million people are infected. The reproductive efforts of *Ascaris* are remarkable, each female laying about 200 000 eggs per day into the faeces. Consequently, infection is prevalent where hygienic standards are low, especially if human faeces are used as an agricultural fertiliser.

The life cycle is complicated (Fig. 28.50) because the larvae hatching from ingested eggs have to pass through the lungs during their maturation. They invade the ileal mucosa, travel by the portal vein to the liver and then in the systemic venous blood to the lungs, where they moult twice and enter the alveoli: after this, their passage is as for the hookworms (p. 28.37).

Clinical and pathological features. Light infections are symptomless. The overt clinical and pathological effects of ascariasis occur in two phases. During **the larval migration phase**, a heavy synchronous infection (from ingesting a hundred or more eggs) results in a transient hepatitis and pneumonitis as a reaction to the migrating larvae. The pulmonary symptoms include cough, dyspnoea, fever and sometimes haemoptysis. Chest x-ray shows widespread dense pulmonary infiltrates and there is an eosinophil leucocytosis. This condition, known as

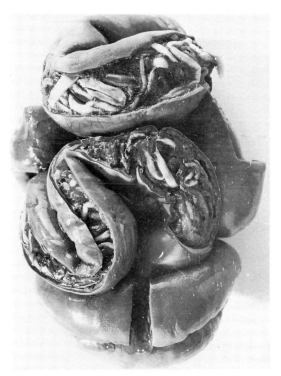

Fig. 28.55 *Ascaris lumbricoides* causing small bowel obstruction. A long bolus of worms fills the lumen. (St Thomas's Hospital Medical School Pathology Museum.)

Loeffler's syndrome, comes on 5 days after ingesting the eggs and lasts about 10 days. The lungs are focally consolidated and microscopy shows interstitial pneumonia and eosinophils and fibrin in the alveoli around the small *Ascaris* larvae. The pneumonitis is more severe than that seen in hookworm infection because a heavy synchronous infection is commoner in ascariasis and also because the larvae moult in the lungs, releasing more antigenic material.

Once the worms have matured in the ileum, the **adult worm phase** of the disease ensues. Generally fifty or more worms are needed to produce symptoms although ascariasis is one of the few helminth diseases where a single worm, by blocking at a critical site, can cause morbidity and even death. Tangled masses of worms can produce intermittent or complete intestinal obstruction, commonly at the ileo-caecal valve (Fig. 28.55). They may also form the centre of a volvulus, and rarely, by obstructing the lumen of the appendix, may cause acute appendicitis. Serious complications arise if an ascarid enters and blocks the bile duct; biliary colic and sometimes ascending cholangitis and liver abscesses may follow. Should the adult female ascend into the liver and deposit eggs there, a granulomatous abscess may form around the degenerating worm and eggs. Blocking of the pancreatic duct is a known but unusual cause of pancreatitis. Rarely, the worms also perforate the intestine, with resulting peritonitis. The wanderlust of *Ascaris* is dramatically shown when adults occasionally appear from the nose, mouth, urethra or vagina. In addition to their physical effects, these large worms can compromise the nutrition of the host; it is estimated that a child with 26 ascarids loses one-tenth of the total dietary protein intake to the worms.

There is some evidence of a partial acquired immunity to *Ascaris* in older people. The worms live for 1 to 2 years, and transmission is often seasonal. The infection is diagnosed by finding the eggs in the faeces. In Loeffler's syndrome, larvae may also be seen in the sputum.

Filariasis

This group of diseases is caused by several genera of tissue-dwelling, long thin filarial worms. All are transmitted by biting insects, the adult worms live as paired couples in man, and the females produce embryos called *microfilariae*. These are worm-like motile larvae, ranging in length from 150–300 μm (Fig. 28.56). In onchocerciasis, the microfilariae wander in the dermis and ocular tissues, but in the lymphatic filariases and in loiasis, they live in the blood. When a suitable insect bites an infected person, the microfilariae are ingested and develop into larval forms infective for man. Morphologically, the adults and microfilariae are characteristic for each species of filaria. Some of the major features of the filariases are shown in Table 28.4.

Lymphatic filariasis

The clinical, parasitological and pathological features of infection with *W. bancrofti* and *B. malayi* are similar and are considered together.

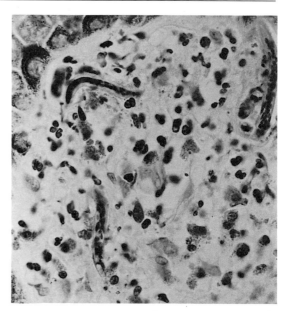

Fig. 28.56 Microfilariae of *Onchocerca volvulus* in the upper dermis after treatment with diethylcarbamazine (see text); they are degenerating and are surrounded by eosinophils. × 750.

Table 28.4   Types and features of filariasis

	Female parasite (size in mm)	Intermediate host	Numbers affected ($\times 10^6$)	Geographical distribution	Effects
Lymphatic filariasis	*Wuchereria bancrofti* (100×0.25) *Brugia malayi* (100×0.25)	*Culex* mosquito *Mansonia* mosquito	400	Sub-Saharan Africa, India, S.E. Asia, Pacific islands, Central and S. America S.E. Asia (*Brugia*)	Lymphadenitis, elephantiasis Tropical pulmonary eosinophilia
Onchocerciasis	*Onchocerca volvulus* (500×0.3)	*Simulium* blackfly	40	Sub-Saharan Africa, Central America	Subcutaneous nodules, dermatitis, blindness
Loiasis	*Loa loa* (70×0.5)	*Chrysops* fly	20	West and Central Africa	Migratory subcutaneous swellings

Life cycle. The larvae are injected into the skin by a mosquito and migrate by lymphatics to the draining lymph nodes. During the next year, they develop into adults and reside in the afferent lymphatics and the cortical sinuses of the nodes. The females release microfilariae into the lymph from where they pass into the blood. Microfilariae do not circulate in the blood constantly, but stay in the lung capillaries during the day and emerge into the peripheral circulation at night. This nocturnal periodicity is thought to depend on the oxygen tension of the blood during sleep and corresponds with the nocturnal biting habits of the vector mosquitoes. In the endemic zones, filarial worms are acquired progressively from infancy onwards, with peak prevalence in early adulthood. The adult worms live for 10 to 18 years and there is some degree of concomitant immunity against infection. In many places, infection rates are 50% or more but, as with most helminth infections, the majority of those infected (i.e. those with detectable microfilaraemia) remain free of symptoms.

Pathological changes

The adult worms are located predominantly in the lymph nodes of the groin and axilla. The essential clinico-pathological features arise from the host reaction to the adult worms, particularly degenerating ones. No toxic factor is secreted by these worms and, with the exception of the syndrome of tropical pulmonary eosinophilia (see below), the microfilariae do not cause lesions.

Living worms in the lymphatics cause a perilymphatic inflammation and fibrosis, but do not occlude the channels. However, their physical presence has a dilating effect with subsequent lymphatic incompetence and lymphoedema. Degenerating worms elicit a predominantly cell-mediated immune response with a granulomatous reaction, eosinophilia and fibrosis (Fig. 28.57) and this blocks the afferent lymphatics. Eventually the dead worms calcify.

In the early years of infection, there may be recurrent episodes of **acute filariasis** with fever, lymphadenitis and retrograde lymphangitis. The pathogenesis is not clear, but there is thought to be a transient Arthus-type reaction to worm antigens or secondary bacterial infection in the dependent limb. After many years, signs of overt **chronic filariasis** develop in a small proportion of those infected. The permanent lymphatic dilatation and obstruction caused by the adult worms results in transudation of protein-rich lymph into the dependent tissues. The regions commonly affected are the legs and arms, the scrotum, and sometimes the breasts and vulva. The lymphoedema induces a chronic inflammatory and fibroblastic reaction in the dermis and subcutis, with ensuing hardening and gross enlargement of the soft tissues—**elephantiasis** (Fig. 28.58). Histologically there is dilatation of dermal lymphatics and the epidermis is often so hyperplastic that

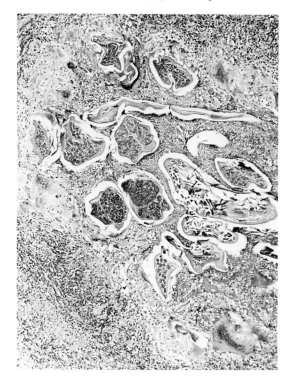

Fig. 28.57 Adult *Wuchereria bancrofti* in a lymph node. Fragments of the coiled worm with a giant-cell granulomatous reaction. × 70.

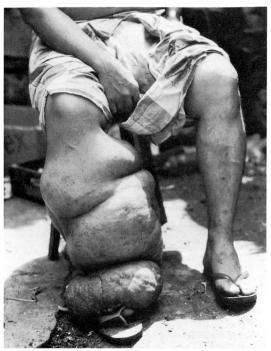

Fig. 28.58 Gross elephantiasis of the right leg due to *Brugia malayi* infection. (Photograph kindly supplied by Dr R. Muller, Commonwealth Institute of Parasitology.)

the skin of the foot takes on a verrucose appearance—'*mossy foot*'. Secondary bacterial infection of the limb contributes some of the damage in elephantiasis of the leg. At this late stage, chemotherapy for filariasis does not reverse the elephantiasis. Within the scrotum, lymph may accumulate in a hydrocoele in which microfilariae are sometimes found. If intra-abdominal lymph nodes are infected and obstructed, the lymph can leak back into the peritoneum and produce ascites, and also from the bladder wall into its lumen, resulting in chyluria.

Tropical pulmonary eosinophilia. A small percentage of people with either *W. bancrofti* or *B. malayi* infections suffer from nocturnal attacks of fever, asthma and eosinophil leucocytosis. They have very high serum levels of IgE (some of which is anti-filarial antibody) but microfilariae are not found in the blood. Chest x-ray reveals widespread pulmonary infiltrates, and lung biopsy shows microfilariae surrounded by a granulomatous reaction. It appears that these individuals develop a type 1 (atopic) hypersen-

sitivity reaction to microfilarial antigens, and that this syndrome is a form of 'occult filariasis' in which microfilariae are effectively cleared from the blood by the host immune reaction. A parallel hypersensitivity probably underlies the production of elephantiasis and the other sequelae of chronic lymphatic filariasis: the affected victims react more strongly than usual to degenerating adult worms, and thus incur more lymphatic damage.

Diagnosis. The microfilariae are found in the blood (by nocturnal sampling) only in the early stages of lymphatic filariasis, and it may be difficult to distinguish the chronic disease from other environmental causes of lymphoedema such as silicone lymphadenopathy. The diagnostic value of serology is limited by the wide antigenic overlap with many other nematodes, and also by the disappearance of antibodies in chronic infection; although of little use in endemic areas, serology is of diagnostic value in transient visitors to endemic areas. Eosinophil leucocytosis is characteristic only in the early stages of filariasis.

Onchocerciasis

Onchocerciasis is a chronic disease caused by *Onchocerca volvulus* (Table 28.4). Infection begins in infancy and in many endemic zones everyone is affected by the age of 20. It is a rural disease and the vectors breed by swift streams and rivers; as with schistosomiasis, dams and hydroelectric schemes provide new breeding sites for the vector. Depending on the local prevalence and intensity of infection, up to one-third of people in some villages may be partially sighted or blind because of onchocerciasis, which is also known as *river blindness*. Consequently, many fertile valleys in tropical Africa are abandoned by the population to avoid the disease.

Life cycle. The larvae transmitted by an infected *Simulium* fly migrate via lymphatics to subcutaneous sites over bony prominences, particularly over the iliac crests, ribs, shoulders and cranium. There they mature into pairing adults, the males and females lying coiled around each other. Often they induce a fibrous

reaction and become palpable nodules, or *onchocercomas* (Fig. 28.59). During a lifespan of some 10–15 years, female worms liberate hundreds of thousands of microfilariae, which can live up to 30 months. They do not enter the blood, but wander through the adjacent dermis where only a small proportion will be taken up by a biting vector.

Pathological changes

The presence of the adults in non-critical body sites is of no great direct significance, the microfilariae being responsible for the more serious effects. This is in contrast to lymphatic filariasis where the adults cause the major effects. Microfilariae of *O. volvulus* do not secrete any known toxin, and apart from fibrosis they induce no reaction until they degenerate and cease to be motile, when they elicit an eosinophil, mast-cell and histiocytic reaction. Degeneration may occur through natural ageing or from the administration of microfilaricidal drugs.

The intensity of the lesions caused by the presence of microfilariae in the dermis depends on the intensity of infection and on the strength of the host reaction. Skin testing with onchocercal antigens has shown that those with the strongest delayed hypersensitivity reaction have the most active dermatitis with the least number of microfilariae in the skin. Conversely, those with many microfilariae may have little reaction. This is reminiscent of lymphatic filariasis where those reacting more strongly to worm antigens have the more severe disease. The reaction around degenerating microfilariae depends also on antibody-dependent eosinophil cytotoxicity: IgG antibody binds to the microfilarial surface and mediates degranulation of eosinophils, with injury to the microfilariae. A similar phenomenon occurs in the skin in schistosomiasis, when schistosomula are damaged by antibody-dependent eosinophil cytotoxicity.

Skin lesions. Clinically, the majority of people with untreated onchocerciasis have relatively mild dermatitis. There is pruritus, and in the early stages a rash of small discrete papules. As a result of chronic microfilaria-induced inflammation and scratching, the skin eventually becomes hyperplastic and lichenified. Finally it loses its elasticity, becomes atrophic, focally depigmented and hangs in folds.

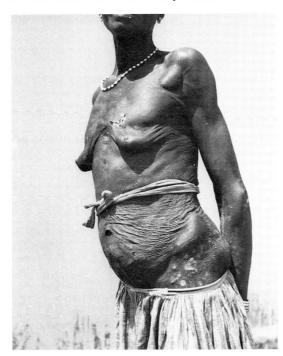

Fig. 28.59 Chronic onchocerciasis. Subcutaneous nodules containing adult worms (onchocercomas) are visible on the shoulder and the iliac crest. Also present are the depigmented areas (above the skirt) and hanging folds of skin from chronic dermatitis.

Histologically, variable numbers of microfilariae are seen in the upper dermis (Fig. 28.56). There is an inflammatory reaction with infiltration of eosinophils, lymphocytes, plasma cells and macrophages, both perivascularly and focally around microfilariae. The coiled adults in onchocercal nodules (Fig. 28.60) are surrounded by a variable chronic inflammatory cell infiltrate and eosinophil reaction with much fibrosis. When they degenerate, they are phagocytosed by giant cells.

Eye lesions. Although the skin lesions are distressing to the patient, the ocular damage in onchocerciasis is more disabling. Eye lesions are a consequence of heavy and chronic infection with a high density of microfilariae in the dermis of the peri-ocular skin. Microfilariae reach the anterior parts of the eye via the ciliary vessels and the bulbar conjunctiva; they may reach the posterior parts—the retina and the vitreous—via the optic nerve.

The clinico-pathological sequelae in the eye are as follows: (1) punctate keratitis, seen as transient fluffy white spots on the cornea, results from an oedematous inflammatory reaction to degenerating microfilariae. (2) sclerosing keratitis, which is a wave of granulation tissue coming in from the limbus and permanently scarring the cornea. This is a significant cause of blindness. (3) microfilariae may also float free in the fluid of the anterior chamber, cause iritis and the formation of anterior synechiae with secondary glaucoma. (4) in the posterior chamber, foci of microfilaria-induced retinitis and depigmentation occur. Damage to the optic nerve may cause optic atrophy.

Lymph nodes. The groin and axillary nodes usually show perifollicular fibrosis. In those people with very severe, ulcerating dermatitis, the nodes may have marked follicular hyperplasia and be enlarged. Lymphoedema and elephantiasis are rarely found in this disease.

It is an important feature of onchocerciasis that the main form of current treatment is with diethylcarbamazine, a microfilaricidal drug that has little or no effect on the adult filariae: it does not kill microfilariae *in vitro*, but induces an acute inflammatory response to them, probably by unmasking antigens on their surface. As a result, there is fever, and inflammation develops wherever microfilariae are present in the body, with an acute aggravation of symptoms and signs of the disease. This is known as the *Mazzotti reaction*, and is distinctive enough to be used as a diagnostic test for onchocerciasis. In the presence of a heavy infection, however, such rapid induction of a widespread reaction may be dangerous.

Diagnosis is made by demonstrating microfilariae in skin snips; small fragments of skin are snipped off with a razor blade, immersed in saline, and examined later for emerging microfilariae. This also provides a guide to intensity of infection. Blood eosinophilia is usually marked in onchocerciasis except in advanced and burnt-out cases.

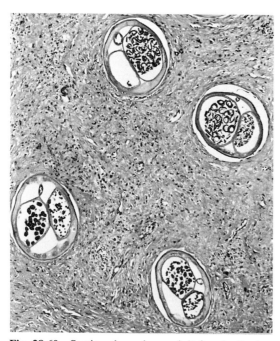

Fig. 28.60 Section through an adult female *Onchocerca volvulus* in the subcutaneous tissues. Several cross-sections of the coiled worm are seen, with the uterus containing many microfilariae. × 75.

Loiasis (Eye worm infection)

Infection with the filarial worm *Loa loa* (Table 28.4) is characterised by fleeting areas of subcutaneous oedema although many infections are asymptomatic.

Life cycle. The *Chrysops* fly ingests the microfilariae from an infected host and injects infective larvae when it takes a blood meal. The worms mature and mate in the subcutaneous tissues and the females deposit microfilariae which enter the capillaries and circulate in the blood. The female adults live for 4–17 years.

Effects. Neither adults nor microfilariae elicit any significant direct injury. The adults move continuously in the superficial tissues, and induce local allergic erythematous and oedematous swellings ('Calabar swellings') which last a few days. These may occur anywhere on the body but are found particularly around the orbit and in the extremities: they are hot, itchy, and may be painful, so that joint movement is impaired. The worm may also cross the eye in the subconjunctival tissues—moving at about 1 cm per minute—where it causes allergic irritation. A rate but serious phenomenon is men-ingoencephalitis. *Loa loa* is the most frequent filarial invader of the central nervous system, and microfilarie may be found in the CSF.

Histologically, granulomatous reactions are seen around degenerating adults in the skin, and a similar reaction to microfilariae presumably underlies the meningoencephalitis. As with onchocerciasis, treatment of loiasis with diethylcarbamazine may temporarily aggravate the disease as the worms and microfilariae degenerate.

Loiasis characteristically induces a marked eosinophilia of $20 \times 10^9/l$ or more. The diagnosis is made by seeing the migrating worm in the eye, and by finding the microfilariae in the blood, where they appear during the day (like their vector fly).

Other nematode infections

Dracunculiasis (Dracontiasis)

Infection with the 'Guinea-worm', *Dracunculus medinensis*, is a classic example of a rural, water-borne, seasonal disease arising from the contamination of water used for drinking and washing. Its effects are a blistering and cellulitis of the limbs which, by making movement painful, reduces the productive activity of farmers, often during the harvesting period.

Over 50 million people are affected throughout Africa, the Middle East and India, with local prevalence rates of over 50%. The infection occurs where people immerse their limbs in wells or cisterns used also for drinking water and colonised by small crustacean *Cyclops*. When infected individuals immerse their limbs, *Dracunculus* larvae escape into the water (see below) and are ingested by *Cyclops*, in which they develop into a form infective for man in about two weeks. When infected *Cyclops* are swallowed in the water, they are digested and larvae are released into the gut. They burrow through the gut wall, and migrate through the abdomen to the subcutaneous tissues where they mature and mate; the males then die and are absorbed. The gravid females exhibit geotropism and migrate to the extremeties, in most cases to the lower limbs. The female is now a cylindrical white worm of about 60 cm × 1.5 mm

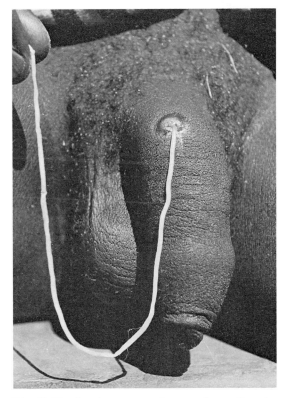

Fig. 28.61 A guinea-worm, *Dracunculus medinensis*, being withdrawn from a blister on the shaft of the penis. (Picture kindly supplied by Dr R. Muller, Commonwealth Institute of Parasitology.)

with some 3 million larvae in its uterus. The worm's head glands secrete irritant (and antigenic) substances which induce a blister in the overlying skin. This is itchy and painful. The blister bursts, and on contact with water, the female extrudes larvae, gradually emerging further out of the skin, until without intervention, it is completely expelled by four weeks (Fig. 28.61). Not all gravid worms emerge onto the skin; some degenerate in the deep tissues and calcify, and may be detected by x-ray.

The complete life cycle from ingestion of larvae in *Cyclops* to expulsion of larvae from the body takes a year, and coincides with the annual dry season when water levels are low and hence densities of *Cyclops* and of expelled larvae in the water are high.

There is no protective immunity to guinea-worm and repeated infections occur. The clinical features are (1) awareness of a moving subcutaneous worm, (2) allergic phenomena such as urticaria, fever, nausea, diarrhoea and vomiting just before the blister formation, and (3) the local skin reactions to the female worm. If the worm bursts in the tissues during larval expulsion, there is a severe reaction due to the worm antigens and larvae, with cellulitis, myositis and abscess formation. Secondary bacterial infection often supervenes, and acute arthritis can result if the lesion is near a joint. The skin lesions are also a focus for infection with tetanus spores. During infection, blood eosinophilia is usual.

The diagnosis of guinea-worm infection is usually obvious. The time-honoured treatment is to accelerate the emergence of the adult female by daily immersion of the site of exit and gradually winding the worm out onto a stick. Antibiotics may also be required.

Trichinosis (Trichinellosis)

Trichinella spiralis is a parasitic nematode worm with many hosts, including the pig, boar and rat. The parasite is acquired by eating the flesh of an infected animal and is thus found only in carnivores. Man is infected by eating undercooked pork, usually in sausages, and is a dead-end for the parasite, because, although a suitable host, his flesh is now seldom eaten.

Larvae are released from cysts in ingested muscle and mature into adult worms in the ileum. About a week later the fecund females release numerous larvae which invade the mucosa and spread by the blood. (The adult worms are later expelled from the gut by an immune reaction.) Larvae in the blood invade many tissues. Those entering skeletal muscle fibres become encysted and remain alive, while in other organs they are destroyed by a granulomatous and eosinophil reaction.

The human disease often occurs in epidemics originating from a single source of infected meat. The clinical effects depend on the intensity of infection: 90% of infections are light, but symptoms usually develop when there are more than 10 larvae per gram of skeletal muscle: they include the classical picture of diffuse myalgia, facial oedema and fever, with an eosinophil leucocytosis. Very heavy infections (up to 5000 larvae per gram of tongue muscle have been observed) result in a myocarditis, pneumonitis and encephalitis, and are sometimes fatal. In one autopsy, James Paget noted more 'creatures (worms) than the whole population of the earth'.

During the invasive stage, biopsy shows a marked myositis, but the infected muscle cell becomes a 'nurse cell' in which the larva ($100 \times 6\,\mu m$) lies coiled up in a hyaline cyst wall (Fig. 28.62) and remains alive for some years before it eventually dies and becomes calcified.

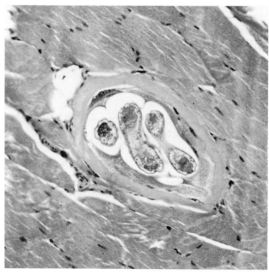

Fig. 28.62 Larva of *Trichinella spiralis* within a skeletal muscle cell ('nurse cell'). A hyaline layer has formed round the coiled parasite. × 200.

Definitive diagnosis is made by muscle biopsy although serology may be helpful.

Larva migrans

Many helminths whose definitive hosts are lower animals can nevertheless infect man. Their larvae enter the body (see below) and wander locally or systemically, but are unable to mature to adult forms in the wrong host and soon die, causing inflammatory lesions in their wake. Two types of disease result, *cutaneous* and *visceral larva migrans*.

Cutaneous larva migrans. The commonest cause is infection with dog hookworm larvae, which penetrate the skin and move in the deep dermis in a serpiginous fashion at a rate of a few centimetres a day, provoking an itchy erythematous raised reaction—*creeping eruption*. Another parasite group causing cutaneous larva migrans is the bird schistosomes; their cercariae can penetrate human skin and induce an itchy cercarial dermatitis. Outbreaks of this condition have occurred in the UK from swimming in snail-infested gravel pits.

Visceral larva migrans is caused by ingestion of eggs of several species of zoophilic worms, the commonest being the *Toxocarae*. Adult *Toxocara canis* ascarid worms live in the intestine of dogs in all parts of the world and their eggs are deposited in the faeces. Children acquire visceral larva migrans by ingesting eggs in contaminated soil or food. The larvae are released from the eggs in the gut, penetrate the gut wall, and disseminate by the blood to many organs.

The clinicopathological features depend on the location of the larvae. Pulmonary infection causes cough and dyspnoea, while liver and CNS involvement result respectively in hepatomegaly and focal neurological signs with fits. Fever is common and a marked eosinophil

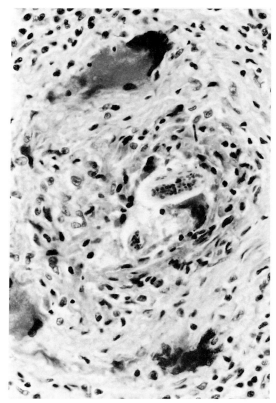

Fig. 28.63 Larva of *Toxocara canis* in a giant-cell granuloma. The fragments of the larva are recognisable by their multiple small nuclei. The lesion was in the pons of a 2-year-old child. × 230. (Section kindly supplied by Dr C. Scholtz, London Hospital Medical College.)

leucocytosis (over 20×10^9/l) is usual. In the tissues, small larvae measuring about $400 \times 20\,\mu$m are surrounded by a giant-cell granulomatous reaction with aggregation of eosinophils (Fig. 28.63). The most important manifestation of toxocariasis is involvement of the eye, resulting in a granulomatous endophthalmitis which clinically may resemble a retinoblastoma and lead to unnecessary removal of the eye.

Further Reading

Binford, C. H. and Connor, D. H. (Eds) (1976). *Pathology of Tropical and Extraordinary Diseases*, Vols. 1 & 2. Armed Forces Institute of Pathology, Washington, D.C.

Katz, M., Despommier, D. D. and Gwadz, R. W. (1982). *Parasitic Diseases*. Springer-Verlag, New York.

Muller, R. (1975). *Worms and Disease*. Heinemann, London.

Index